Bray's
clinical laboratory
methods

Bray's
Clinical laboratory
methods

Revised by

JOHN D. BAUER, M.D.

Director, Laboratories, DePaul Hospital; Director, Laboratories, Faith Hospital;
Director, Northland Clinical Laboratory; Assistant Professor of Pathology,
Washington University School of Medicine, St. Louis, Missouri

PHILIP G. ACKERMANN, Ph.D.

Biochemist, DePaul Hospital; Consulting Biochemist to Faith Hospital and
Homer G. Phillips Hospital; Research Associate, Reproductive Biology
Research Foundation, St. Louis, Missouri

GELSON TORO, Ph.D.

Research Associate, Reproductive Biology Research Foundation;
Director of Biochemistry, Missouri Clinical and Biochemical Laboratory,
St. Louis, Missouri

With 174 illustrations and 16 color plates

Seventh edition

The C. V. Mosby Company

Saint Louis   1968

Preface

This new edition is drawn from lectures to residents in clinical pathology and to medical technology students. All chapters have been extensively revised, enlarged, and brought up to date by the inclusion of much new material. The references have also been updated and most old ones omitted. Chapters such as "Methods in Microbiology" and "Clinical Chemistry" have been rewritten, and glossaries have been added to two of the chapters. Despite these changes, the handy size of the book has been maintained by eliminating outdated material and methods.

A section on quality control has been added which includes suggested control procedures for clinical chemistry, hematology, blood banking, parasitology, and tissue examination.

In the chapter on clinical chemistry the introductory section has been expanded with discussions of the principles and techniques involved not only in colorimetry and spectrophotometry but also fluorometry, electrophoresis, chromatography (paper, thin-layer, gas-liquid), and automation. New or additional methods have been introduced for glucose, urea nitrogen, iron, iron-binding capacity, and bilirubin, including a discussion of the problems involved in the preparation of calibration curves for this latter substance.

The methods for enzymes have been collected in one section, which has been greatly enlarged and expanded. Alternate procedures are given for the more important enzymes such as the phosphatases, transaminases, and lactic dehydrogenase. Methods have been added for the determination of aldolase, alpha-hydroxybutyrate dehydrogenase, ceruloplasmin, creatine phosphokinase, and ornithine carbamyl transferase, along with a brief discussion of many of the enzymes involved in inborn errors of metabolism.

The material dealing with tests for thyroid function has been enlarged to cover new developments, and a section on basal metabolic rate was included for completeness.

The expanded chapter on methods in hematology includes methods for hemoglobin electrophoresis, glucose-6-phosphate dehydrogenase deficiency, immunoelectrophoresis, and antibody identification. Several black and white as well as color photomicrographs have been added. Mention is made of the Kleihauer method for hemoglobin F, classification of immunoglobulins, and lymphocyte culture and its role in tissue transplants.

"Examination of Biologic Fluids" includes the investigation of joint fluid, the RA cell, and Gm groups and the rheumatoid factor. Amniotic fluid analysis is included in this chapter as well as in the discussion of erythroblastosis fetalis.

The chapter on microbiology includes newer methods for the diagnosis of tuberculosis and recent enzymatic and fluorescent methods for the investigation of bacteria. Newer media for the diagnosis of *Neisseria, Mima,* and *Herellea* are included as well as a short discussion of the L forms of bacteria and *Mycoplasma pneumoniae.* Several differential diagnostic tables have been added as well as a short section on the diagnosis of viral diseases.

We wish to express our appreciation to T. J. Cooper, M.D., for his critical review of many of the chemical methods and to Sam Frankel, Ph.D., for his many helpful suggestions in regard to the enzyme determinations.

Edith Rich, Ph.D., freely gave her time and experience to review the chapters on microbiology and mycology.

In an already crowded schedule, A. S. Wiener, M.D., found time to review the chapter on blood groups and made many helpful suggestions and corrections.

The responsibility for errors and omissions rests with the authors.

The cooperation of members of the Department of Pathology at DePaul Hospital is gratefully acknowledged. Toshio Nishi, M.D., willingly accepted additional workloads to make this revision possible.

The majority of the photomicrographs added in this edition were skillfully produced by K. Cramer Lewis of the Department of Medical Illustration, Washington University School of Medicine, St. Louis, Missouri. Miss Marilyn J. Harris produced the line drawings and diagrams. The source of other photomicrographs used is gratefully acknowledged in the legends.

John D. Bauer, M.D.
Philip G. Ackermann, Ph.D.
Gelson Toro, Ph.D.

Contents

1 Laboratory rules and quality control, 1

2 Urinalysis, 11

3 Examination of semen and pregnancy tests, 87

4 Methods in hematology, 95

5 Blood groups, blood typing, and crossmatching, 232

6 Clinical chemistry, 283

7 Gastric, duodenal, and pancreatic juice analysis, 443

8 Stool analysis, 452

9 Methods in parasitology, 459

10 Examination of biologic fluids (serous fluids, cerebrospinal fluid, synovial fluid, amniotic fluid, sputum, pus), 507

11 Methods in microbiology, with reference to methods in virology, 526

12 Methods in mycology, 629

13 Water and milk examinations, 652

14 Serology, 655

15 Toxicology—poisons and drugs, 684

16 Methods of tissue examination, 705

Appendix, 722

Color plates

1 Crystalline and amorphous sediment in acid urine, 52

2 High-power field showing crystalline and amorphous sediment in alkaline urine, 52

3 Hormone test for diagnosis of early pregnancy, 91

4 Blood cells, 126

5 Red blood cell series, 132

6 Red blood cell pathology, 156

7 White blood cell pathology, 189

8 *Entamoeba histolytica*, 467

9 Ova of intestinal parasites, 471

10 Malarial parasites, 497

11 Gonococci in a cervical smear showing well-preserved pus cells and the characteristic clear spaces around the organisms, 557

12 *Haemophilus ducreyi* from a chancroid, 584

13 Donovan bodies of granuloma inguinale, 584

14 Tubercle bacilli in sputum, 594

15 *Torula* in spinal fluid, 639

16 *Histoplasma capsulatum* in bone marrow smear, 641

Chapter 1

Laboratory rules and quality control

LABORATORY RULES

All requests for laboratory examinations should be made in writing and contain the patient's full name, his hospital number, the type of specimen furnished, the clinical diagnosis, and the specific examination desired.

Upon entering the patient's room the technologist should identify herself and state the reason for her presence (blood test, etc.). Prior to any procedure she must identify the patient by checking his name band or name plate. Do not identify the patient by bed number or by asking his name.

Keep good records. The record should contain not only the patient's identification, the test, and its result but also the procedure used. For example, in biochemistry, specify the dilution used and the spectrophotometer reading; in bacteriology, include the various media used and their reactions.

Each laboratory must have an accession book that lists all incoming specimens, their final disposition, and the results of the tests. An adequate filing system must allow easy access to records.

QUALITY CONTROL[1]

Every phase of laboratory work requires a quality control program to guarantee reproducibility and accuracy of laboratory results.

As shown by several laboratory surveys,[2, 3] there is a need for uniform, reliable laboratory methodology and for careful standardization of methods, with repeated checks on the standards themselves. Quality control programs instituted by public health departments, The College of American Pathologists, and The American Society of Clinical Pathologists represent concentrated efforts toward persistently precise, accurate, and reproducible laboratory results. Well-organized, but expensive quality control programs are commercially available for almost every field of laboratory activity.

Continued education

Since laboratory medicine changes rapidly, the staff must be kept well informed by refresher courses, workshops, educational films, and seminars. An active program of interdepartmental postgraduate education is a valuable asset. Each laboratory section should be provided with an up-to-date procedure book and policy manual. The latter must be available to all other departments of the hospital. A program to invite senior nurses of hospital divisions to spend a day or two in the laboratory pays rich dividends in understanding and cooperation.

Motivation

The practice of laboratory medicine is a profession motivated primarily by service to the patient. Inadequate training or knowledge must not be tolerated since very often the patient's treatment depends on the results of laboratory tests.

1

Automation and computers[4-6]

The coming years will see far-reaching changes in the anatomic and clinical laboratory. This area, which generates such a multitude of clinical data, is particularly amenable to the use of digital computers. In a few years almost 75% of all laboratory tests will be processed by automated equipment. Automated laboratory results can be fed directly into a computer programmed to detect errors and "outside" laboratory results. The laboratory information is then filed on tape and merged with the patient's previous laboratory and clinical data. All this information can then be sent to the nurses' stations on the hospital floors, to the business office, and back to the laboratory.

QUALITY CONTROL IN BLOOD BANKING

A blood bank control kit, together with a self-check unit,* assures the laboratory that its equipment, reagents, and techniques are functioning properly. The control kit includes group A_1, A_2, B, O, Rh-positive, O, Rh-negative, O, and D^u-positive test cells and Coombs control cells coated with antibodies. These cells can be used for reverse (serum) grouping of donor or recipient blood, or they may be used for identification and control of blood grouping sera, for titration of saline-reacting isoagglutinins in serum, and for titration of immune anti-A and anti-B antibodies. Group A_2 cells can be used to control absorbed anti-A blood grouping serum (anti-A_1) and to identify anti-A_2 antibodies in serum. Group O, Rh-positive cells, which contain a number of Rh factors, can be used for screening for Rh antibodies and for titration of these antibodies. The positive Coombs control cells may be used to check the adequacy of antigamma globulin (Coombs) sera. Group O, Rh-negative cells, homozygous for c and e, are more sensitive to and reactive with anti-c and anti-e antibodies. Group O, D^u-positive cells may be used to check the D^u technique.

The self-check unit consists of unknown cells and unknown sera for laboratory study that may present some problems in group identification or crossmatching.

*Hyland Laboratories, Los Angeles, Calif.

The self-check unit is followed by an explanatory letter containing test results and a discussion. The Commission of Continuing Education of the American Society of Clinical Pathologists has a similar check sample for immunohematology which includes samples and the presentation of the problem, followed later by a critique.

Various check samples from the American Society of Clinical Pathologists may be used as quality control for many phases of clinical pathology.

QUALITY CONTROL IN CLINICAL CHEMISTRY[7-9]

Sources of error: In addition to errors in the actual reading of the colorimeter there are other errors attributable to the use of the colorimeter that result from a fluctuating light source, stray light, imperfectly matched cuvettes, and nonlinearity of the response of the photocell and the milliammeter. There are also many other sources of error in chemical determinations. These include errors in pipetting due to dirty pipettes or improper technique, incorrect or fluctuating temperature of a water bath, and errors in preparation of reagents and standards. Careful attention to all details of a given procedure will decrease the magnitude of errors but will never eliminate them completely.

In discussing errors involved in a given determination the terms "precision" and "accuracy" are used. The terms are not synonymous. The results of repeated analyses on the same samples duplicating each other indicate **precision.** If the results of repeated analyses are all very close to each other, the method is high in precision. The results of an analysis or of the average of a series of analyses approaching the true or correct value refers to **accuracy.** Precision can be readily estimated by methods that will be mentioned later. The determination of accuracy is not always simple since the **true value** of the concentration of a substance in a biologic system may not be known. Usually the accuracy of a method is judged by analyzing for the constituent by a number of different methods involving different types of chemical reactions and often using as reference those methods that are too long and complicated for routine use. The problem is not always simple, as illustrated by the fact that although relatively precise blood sugar methods have been in use for nearly 40 yr. there is still some discussion as to the "true" level of glucose in the blood.

Precision and accuracy: In the laboratory one can check the accuracy of a method by comparing results obtained on samples of known concentrations that have been analyzed previously by more competent workers or by the use of commercially available control sera, which are usually obtained in a lyophilized form and are quite stable under refrigeration. But the serum must be used within a short period after reconstitution. Even here, errors are possible. Care must be taken to add exactly the right amount of pure water and to make certain that the material is completely solubilized. Usually the control sera are quite reliable, but it should not always be assumed that they are absolutely correct. In cases of unexplainable discrepancies it is often advisable to try another sample from a different lot of the serum or even that of a different manufacturer.

In the laboratory there is generally more interest in the precision of a method or how well repeated analyses are reproduced on the same sample. The accuracy of a method is often difficult to determine. The clinician may be more concerned with the precision of the result. If, for example, the blood sugar level is reported on one specimen as 100 mg.% and a second specimen taken at a later date is 110 mg.%, does this represent a true change in the glucose level or is the difference within the limits of laboratory error and can significance be attached to the difference in reported levels? Obviously the more precise the method, the more meaningful are small differences.

The determination of the precision of a method and of the significance of differences between determinations is carried out by determining the **mean** and **standard deviation.** This is a mathematic computation of the different values obtained in a test series and the difference from the average value.

Calculation of standard deviation: The standard deviation (S.D.) is calculated after performing a number of determinations on the same sample under the same conditions and recording the results. From these results one obtains the mean or average value by adding all the results and dividing by the total number of determinations (at least 15). The difference of each value from the mean is obtained. Each of these differences is squared and all are added. This total is divided by the number of determinations minus 1 and the square root of this value is taken as 1 S.D. This is expressed mathematically as

$$\text{S.D.} = \sqrt{\frac{\Sigma\ (\bar{x} - xi)^2}{N - 1}}$$

where Σ is the symbol used for summation, $\bar{x}$ is used to denote an average, xi denotes the separate determinations, and N is the number of determinations (Table 1-1).

Table 1-1. Calculation of standard deviation using daily PBI values

No. of determinations	Results ($\mu g\%$)	Difference from mean value	Difference from mean value squared
1	5.8	0.0	0.00
2	5.9	0.1	0.01
3	5.9	0.1	0.01
4	5.8	0.0	0.00
5	5.7	0.1	0.01
6	5.9	0.1	0.01
7	5.7	0.1	0.01
8	5.6	0.2	0.04
9	5.8	0.0	0.00
10	5.7	0.1	0.01
11	5.7	0.1	0.01
12	5.9	0.1	0.01
13	6.0	0.2	0.04
14	5.7	0.1	0.01
15	5.9	0.1	0.01
	87.0		0.18

$$\text{Average} = \frac{87.0}{15} = 5.8\ \mu g\%$$

$$\text{S.D.} = \sqrt{\frac{0.18}{14}} = \sqrt{0.0128}$$

$$1\ \text{S.D.} = \pm 0.11\ \mu g\%$$

$$2\ \text{S.D.} = \pm 0.22\ \mu g\%$$

$$3\ \text{S.D.} = \pm 0.33\ \mu g\%$$

At the start of a quality control program the control limits may be set at ±3 S.D. from the average. In Table 1-1 ±3 S.D. is ±0.33 μg%, or a range of 5.5-6.1 μg%.

After the control program is well established the limits should be narrowed to ±2 S.D. In Table 1-1 this is ±0.22 μg%, or a range of 5.6-6.0 μg%.

Standard deviation is a measure of the **spread of values**; the greater the standard deviation, the greater the differences between individual determinations and the less precise the method. It may only be used at the concentration level at which it was determined. The standard deviation is sometimes expressed as a percent of the average $\left(\dfrac{\text{S.D.}}{\overline{x}} \times 100 \right)$. This is known as the **coefficient of variation**. This coefficient of variation may be applied to results at any level of concentration.

When the standard deviation of a reasonable number of measurements (at least 15) is determined, subsequent determinations will show that approximately 68% of all values will fall within ±1 S.D. from the average. Approximately 95% of all values will fall within ±2 S.D., and 99.7% of all values will fall within ±3 S.D.

One major criterion of a good clinical laboratory is that the day-to-day determinations of a given constituent have a satisfactory degree of precision. This can best be done by analyzing one or more samples of known concentrations each day and comparing the results. These samples should be similar in constitution to the regular laboratory specimens and should have a definite unvarying concentration. These criteria are best met by a number of commercially available quality controlled lyophilized sera. Sometimes pooled serum obtained from excess serum from laboratory specimens can be used. However, this serum may be less stable, even when divided into small quantities and kept frozen. Only the quantity required for a day's work is thawed at one time. The absolute amount of all of the constituents present in this sample is more difficult to establish.

In setting up a quality control program the control sera are analyzed each day along with regular specimens for the desired constituents. A record is kept of the values obtained and they are usually plotted on a quality control chart. After obtaining an average value and a standard deviation from a number of measurements one should find that only about 5% of the subsequent measurements should fall more than 2 S.D. from the average. A typical quality control chart is shown in Fig. 1-1.

Ordinarily the points are more or less distributed at random about the average. Points more than 2 S.D. from the average are considered a danger signal indicating that the procedure and calculations should be checked. Since 1 point in 20 will in theory fall by chance outside the limit

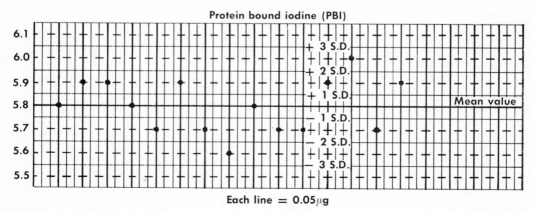

Protein bound iodine (PBI)

Each line = 0.05μg

Fig. 1-1. Quality control chart.

of 2 S.D., 1 point just outside the limit is no cause for concern. If the points fall outside the limits for 2 or 3 days, something is wrong in the procedure. The possible sources of error can often be spotted earlier.

The previously mentioned methods will still not determine whether the technique is precise enough for ordinary purposes. One could compare the standard deviations for a given procedure with those of other laboratories, but such data are not always available. Another approach has been suggested. If, for example, the limits of normal values for fasting blood sugar are taken as 90-120 mg.% and for serum sodium as 131-143 mEq./L. (the actual normals may vary with the method, but those mentioned will serve for illustrative purposes), then the normal range for glucose is 105 ± 15 mg.%, while the normal range for sodium is 137 ± 6 mEq./L. It seems reasonable that the precision of these methods should not be more than a fraction of the normal range. The narrower the normal range, the more precise the method must be to allow distinction between normal and abnormal subjects.

One proposed criterion is that allowable limits of variation (± 2 S.D.) should not exceed $\pm\frac{1}{4}$ the difference between the limits of the normal range, or in terms of percentage:

$$\frac{\text{Upper limit of normal range} - \text{Lower limit}}{\text{Average of normal range} \times 4} \times 100$$

It is suggested that the limits should in no case exceed $\pm 10\%$. For most commonly measured blood constituents this leads to ranges of 2.2% for sodium and chloride; 5% for calcium; 8% for glucose, NPN, total protein, inorganic phosphate, and potassium; and 10% for many other constituents. Preferably the coefficient of variation should be kept within these limits. If a given method leads to much greater values, the method should be studied very carefully for sources of error. It may be necessary to change the method.

QUALITY CONTROL IN COAGULATION

All clotting procedures must be standardized to a high degree, including apparently unimportant details such as frequency and degree of tilting of a test tube to observe clotting. Normal controls must be run with each test and both test and control should be performed in duplicate.

Equipment

Water bath: The thermostatic control must maintain a constant temperature of $37°$ C. A thermometer should be kept in the water bath and checked frequently. The water bath must be wide enough to accommodate an adequate number of test tubes, e.g., for the thromboplastin generation test, and should allow free visualization of the tubes by indirect light. The fish tank type of water bath with flat glass surfaces is preferred.

Method for visualization of clotting: An electric clot timer is suggested. Another method which, with experience, is reproducible is 60-degree tilting of the test tube at regular intervals in the water bath until the clot forms. This method is somewhat difficult if clot formation is poor, e.g., in hypofibrinogenemia. Excessive agitation must be prevented. A diffuse light source is important. The platinum wire method is reproducible and can often be mastered quickly.

Centrifugation: As the number of platelets in plasma depends on the speed and size of the centrifuge, centrifugation should be carefully standardized. For many purposes a refrigerated centrifuge is advisable, or a small centrifuge can be placed in a refrigerator.

Glassware: Glassware must be scrupulously clean and should not be scratched. Disposable plastic tubes are ideal for clotting procedures. Accurate, slow-emptying pipettes are important since the average amount handled varies from 0.1-0.3 ml. Test tubes should be uniform in size because variation in size alone may alter the result of coagulation tests, e.g., the disintegration of a blood clot in the fibrinolysin test.

Reagents: Blood must be carefully obtained without contamination by tissue thromboplastin and without stasis. The proportion of anticoagulant to blood must be accurate. The specimen should not be exposed to $37°$ C. for longer than 5 min. It can be kept in the refrigerator as long as 2 hr. Immediate return of a blood specimen to the laboratory is imperative. Best results are obtained if the blood is drawn in the laboratory. If this is not possible, double-walled jars with ice-water jackets or 37° C. water jackets are taken to the patient's room.

Siliconization: To preserve the number and function of platelets, contact with a rough glass surface must be prevented by a nonwettable surface such as provided by siliconization. Smooth plastic surfaces or paraffinized areas closely duplicate the effectiveness of siliconized material.

Technique

Details such as temperature, pH, timing, etc. must be carefully standardized. The standard deviation of various tests should be determined after repeating the same test at least 15 times. (See discussion of quality control in clinical chemistry.)

QUALITY CONTROL IN HEMATOLOGY[10]

The sources of error in hematology can be classified as follows:
1. Errors related to methods of sampling. Capillary blood obtained from an inadequate puncture wound may lead to counts that are higher than those obtained from venous blood.
2. Errors in preservation of the specimen. Improper mixing, inadequate or excessive amounts of anticoagulant, and incorrect type of anticoagulant as well as a leaking stopper may lead to inaccurate counts and hematologic tests.
3. Technical errors related to the instruments.[11] Inaccurate or dirty pipettes, inadequately standardized automatic pipettes, unmatched or dirty cuvettes, and poor standards may all add up to inaccurate laboratory work.

Many of the errors related to a specific test such as white count, red count, hematocrit, etc. are included in the discussion of the various tests.

Methods for detection of errors

Controls are available for hemoglobin determination, hematocrit, white blood cell count, and red blood cell count.

Celltrol* is a control for red blood cell counts and hematocrit determinations. It is available in normal and below normal range values. It serves as a control of technique as well as of equipment. A similar product, Leukotrol,* is a suspension of stabilized white blood cells available in normal and above normal range values of white cell counts. Both products can be used as controls for manual and electronic counts.

The results of daily analysis of hematology controls are plotted on a graph to show daily variations and to indicate any possible trend toward inaccurate results. All control tests are done in duplicate and the standard deviation of duplicate tests should be calculated daily. (See discussion of quality control in clinical chemistry.)

The mean corpuscular hemoglobin of normal blood can also be used as a control. The mean and the standard deviation can be recorded daily.

Acuglobin† is a hemoglobin standard consisting of a solution of cyanmethemoglobin and is useful for daily standardization of hemoglobin determinations. It is suggested that the standard be diluted 50% with Aculute diluent† to include low hemoglobin values in the control setup.

Estimation of total white cell count from stained blood smear:

No./high-power field (hpf)	Estimated total count
2-4	4000-7000
4-6	7000-10,000
6-10	10,000-13,000
10-20	13,000-18,000

Fragile leukemic cells may disintegrate in the Coulter counter; therefore the total white count should be estimated from the slide as a check on the Coulter counter result.

Estimation of platelets: A peripheral blood smear may be used to judge the platelet count:

Less than 1 platelet/oil-immersion field— decreased number of platelets
Several platelets with occasional clumps— adequate supply of platelets

---

*Chas. Pfizer & Co., Inc., New York, N. Y.
†Ortho Pharmaceutical Corp., Raritan, N. J.

More than 25 platelets/hpf—increased number of platelets

If one counts the number of platelets in 10 oil-immersion fields and multiplies the total figure by 2000, the result closely approximates the platelet count as obtained by the Reese-Ecker method.

The standard deviation of various tests should be determined and result of normal, high, and low controls plotted daily on graph paper. (See discussion of quality control in clinical chemistry.)

QUALITY CONTROL IN MICROBIOLOGY

Most of the points described in detail in this section apply, with some variation, to all phases of laboratory work.

Safety rules: Quality control begins with a properly designed bacteriology laboratory equipped with a safety hood that pulls air from the laboratory to the outside. A number of safety rules should be enforced at all times when working with bacteria, such as careful technique, working over a gauze pad soaked with 5% phenol solution, the use of safety pipetting devices, and periodic washing of all equipment with 5% phenol solution. An alcohol-sand flask should be available for cleaning inoculating loops prior to flaming. All bacteriologic waste material must be autoclaved prior to leaving the department. Contaminated swabs or dressings must be wrapped before disposal.

Quality control procedure must be observed in the handling of every specimen, from collection and transportation to the laboratory, handling by the technologists, plating, choice of media, recording of findings, and incorporation of the findings into the patient's record.

Collection: A representative, adequate specimen must be obtained from a suitable source or area under conditions that prevent contamination. It must be collected in sterile, labeled, covered containers that allow ready access to the material.

Transportation: Transport media are not needed if the culture can be done at the bedside or in the outpatient department and if the material can be sent immediately to the laboratory for pro-

cessing. When specimens are collected in areas removed from the laboratory, **holding media** should be employed. They provide a moist environment with a low nutrient content and low oxidation-reduction potential. They maintain the status quo of the culture material so that sensitive bacteria such as *Neisseria gonorrhoeae* and *Shigella* do not suffer. Dacron-tipped swabs sealed in foil-lined envelopes are satisfactory for throat cultures. Control studies using known organisms must be employed to check continued adequacy of the holding media.

Handling by the technologist: The technologist must be adequately trained and have the opportunity for further training (seminars, journals, meetings, etc.). A detailed laboratory manual should be available to point out step by step the proper preparation of smears, the technique of staining, and the best methods of inoculating various media and of obtaining (picking) an isolated colony. The gram stain can be checked by applying matchhead-sized dots of known grampositive or gram-negative bacteria to the slide. Reference cultures of known bacteria must also be employed to check the adequacy of every new batch of media. The technologist should be familiar with characteristics of pathogenic bacteria and with chemical and physical factors that govern the response of media to bacteria. Mimeographed forms that list the various procedures used for identification of bacteria and that allow space for recording the results of these procedures are suggested to help in the proper identification of bacteria. Known CO_2-sensitive and anaerobic bacteria can be used to control the adequacy of the CO_2 jar and of anaerobic procedures. For the latter, methylene blue is superior because, if the culture does not grow, the fault may be in the stock culture and not in the anaerobiosis. The media used, the biochemical reactions employed, and the sensitivity disks applied must all be checked with known bacteria of known characteristics and sensitivities.

Stock cultures: Most of the steps just outlined employ reference cultures (Table 1-2). Such cultures are commercially

Table 1-2. Recommended strains of stock cultures*

Genus	NCTC	ATCC
Acinetobacter anitratus	7844	15308
Aeromonas liquefaciens	7810	9071
Alcaligenes faecalis	655	
Bacillus subtilis	3610	6051
Clostridium sporogenes	533	10000
Clostridium welchii	6719	9856
Enterobacter aerogenes	10006	13048
Enterobacter cloacae	10005	13047
Escherichia coli	9001	11775
Klebsiella aerogenes	418	15380
Mycobacterium phlei	8151	
Mycobacterium smegmatis	8159	
Nocardia brasiliensis	10300	
Nocardia caviae	1934	
Proteus morganii	10041	
Proteus vulgaris	4175	13315
Pseudomonas aeruginosa	7244	7700
Salmonella typhi	786	
Salmonella typhimurium	74	13311
Shigella dysenteriae I	4837	13313
Shigella sonnei	8220	
Staphylococcus aureus	8532	12600
Staphylococcus epidermidis	4276	
Streptococcus agalactiae	8181	13813
Streptococcus dysgalactiae	4669	
Streptococcus faecalis	8213	
Streptococcus hominis	8618	7073
Streptococcus pneumoniae	7465	10015
Streptococcus sanguis	7863	10556

*From Cowan and Steel: Manual for the identification of medical bacteria, London, 1965, Cambridge University Press.

available.* Pure cultures obtained daily in the laboratory can be carried on stock culture media for prolonged periods when stored in the refrigerator. Periodic transfer of these cultures can be arranged as shown in Table 1-3. Freeze-drying equipment allows lyophilization of young cultures suspended in sterile serum. Standardized lyophilized preparations of bacteria such as DriBac† are commercially available.

Serology: Serologic tests employed in bacteriology are only meaningful if they are accompanied by a negative and a positive control. Titrated sera from the first specimen should be frozen and retitrated with the second specimen.

Recording and reporting of laboratory results: An accession book should show the date (and time if necessary) when the culture was received and should identify the patient (name and hospital number) and the material as well as the

*American Type Culture Collection (ATCC), Rockville, Md.; National Collection of Type Cultures (NCTC), Central Public Health Laboratory, London, England.

†Warner-Chilcott Laboratories Division, Warner-Lambert Pharmaceutical Co., Morris Plains, N. J.

Table 1-3. Conditions for maintenance of test organisms*

Genus	Medium	Incubation Temp. (°C.)	Incubation Time (hr.)	Storage (°C.)	Interval between subculture (mo.)
Acinetobacter	Nutrient agar	37	18	5-25	3
Aeromonas	Nutrient agar	37	18	5-25	3
Alcaligenes	Nutrient agar	37	18	5-25	3
Bacillus	Nutrient agar	30	48	5-25	12
Clostridium	Cooked meat	37	48	5-25	12
Enterobacter	Nutrient agar	37	18	5-25	6
Escherichia	Nutrient agar	37	18	5-25	6
Klebsiella	Nutrient agar	37	18	5-25	3
Mycobacterium	Dorset egg	37	48-72	15-25	6
Nocardia	Dorset egg	37	48-72	15-25	3
Proteus	Nutrient egg	37	18	5-25	3
Pseudomonas	Peptone water agar	30	18	5-25	3
Salmonella	Dorsett egg	37	18	5-25	12
Shigella	Nutrient agar	37	18	5-25	6
Staphylococcus	Nutrient agar	37	18	5-25	3
Streptococcus	Cooked meat or	37	18	5-25	3
	blood broth	37	8	5	1

*From Cowan, and Steel: Manual for the identification of medical bacteria, London, 1965, Cambridge University Press.

physician. After completion of identification of the bacteria the date of completion of the test and the final diagnosis are entered in the accession book. If identification requires a prolonged period of time, the reporting system must be organized in such a way that the physician is certain to receive the results of the completed work. Many bacteriologic results only reach the record room and not the physician. An interim report should assure the physician that the laboratory is still working on a case that requires several weeks.

QUALITY CONTROL IN PARASITOLOGY

As in all other phases of clinical pathology, adequately trained personnel with knowledge and experience are necessary for the correct identification of parasites.

Specimens

Stool specimens are unsuitable if they contain barium, oil, iron, or bismuth. They should not be contaminated with urine, toilet paper, or water. Specimens should be brought immediately to the laboratory.

Procedures

Approved routine procedures arranged in sequence of suggested performance should be available in the procedure book. No single test is satisfactory for all specimens. Each specimen should be examined at least three times.

Errors in diagnosis may occur if details of even the "simplest" method such as the preparation of wet mounts are not adhered to.

It is necessary to preserve positive specimens and to collect slides so that they are available for teaching and training. Prepared slides are commercially available.* The United States Public Health Service Communicable Disease Center has available for loan many excellent teaching films. A variety of animals harbor representatives of various intestinal parasites and can be used to

supply living specimens. The following are sources of parasites[12]:

Roundworms (pinworms): Pinworms similar to human pinworms are found in the hindgut of the cockroach. Puppies may supply hookworm and whipworm eggs. Adult pig *Ascaris* is indistinguishable from that of man. Stools from monkeys or chimpanzees contain motile *Strongyloides* larvae.

Tapeworms: Laboratory mice may harbor the dwarf tapeworm. Eggs of cat and dog *Taenia* are indistinguishable from human *Taenia*. Adult worms may also be obtained.

Trematodes: Freshwater snails harbor a variety of larval trematodes. When placed in tap water they may liberate cercaria.

Protozoa: Monkey and chimpanzee feces often contain *Balantidium coli, Endamoeba histolytica, Endamoeba coli, Iodamoeba* species, *Trichomonas hominis,* and ciliates. Guinea pig feces contain *Balantidium coli, Giardia, Trichomonas,* and *Endamoeba.* Laboratory mice supply *Giardia, Trichomonas, Amoeba,* and other flagellates.

The motility of amebas can be demonstrated at room temperature using *Endamoeba terrapinae,** which grows readily in culture.

QUALITY CONTROL IN THE TISSUE LABORATORY

As in all other sections of the laboratory, the techniques employed in the tissue section should be standardized and follow methods recorded in a procedure manual.

Facilities and equipment must be adequate to take care of the work load and must be kept in perfect working condition. Routinely used reagents in the various "staining rows" and of the mechanical tissue processor are changed regularly according to a schedule posted in the laboratory on which the technician enters the date the reagents were changed. Merely replenishing them is not enough. All special and biochemical

---

*General Biological Supply House, Inc., Chicago, Ill.; Tropical Biologicals, San Juan, Puerto Rico.

*May be obtained from General Biological Supply House, Inc., Chicago, Ill.

staining procedures include a known control cut from blocks stored for this purpose. A negative bacteriologic or biochemical stain is of no value unless it is accompanied by a suitable control slide.

The technician should be familiar with the characteristics of "a good slide" and with the various steps to remedy any defects. Slides and smears should be spot-checked during the staining procedure as soon as the first slides are completed to prevent repetition of the same defect in an entire day's work.

Color standards[13]: The key to good staining and thus to correct interpretation of a slide is the color given by various dyes. As it is difficult to accurately describe shades of a color which should result from a correct staining procedure, a color standard has been suggested. Such a standard can be provided by a stamp collector's color guide in booklet or card form which contains hundreds of color shades. The color obtained by a stain can be checked against the ideal color selected from the guide.

REFERENCES

1. Quality, quality control and automation for the clinical laboratory, St. Louis, 1963, The Catholic Hospital Association of the United States and Canada.
2. Editorial: Southern Med. J. **59**:1118, 1966.
3. Flokstra, J. H., Varley, A. B., and Hagans, J. A.: Amer. J. Med. Sci. **251**:646, 1966.
4. Pratt, A. W., and Thomas, L. B.: In Sommers, S., editor: Pathology annual, New York, 1966, Appleton-Century-Crofts, vol. 1.
5. Juergens, J. D., and Roseyear, J. W.: Proc. Staff Meet. Mayo Clin. **39**:818, 1964.
6. Seligson, D.: Mod. Hosp. **106**:109, 1966.
7. Henry, R. J., and Dryer, D. L.: In Seligson, D. editor: Standard methods of clinical chemistry, New York, 1963, Academic Press, Inc., vol. 4, p. 205.
8. Mainland, D.: Elementary medical statistics, Philadelphia, 1952, W. B. Saunders Co.
9. Commission of Continuing Education: Manual for workshop on statistical methods in the clinical laboratory, Chicago, 1965, American Society of Clinical Pathologists.
10. Dorsey, D. B.: Amer. J. Clin. Path. **40**: 457, 1963.
11. Clinical laboratory instrumentation repair and maintenance, an institute for the medical technologist, St. Louis, 1962, The Catholic Hospital Association of the United States and Canada.
12. Crowson, S. H., and Wideman, F. D., editors: Guidebook for instruction in medical technology, Pilot edition, Alabama project, 1963, N.C.C.M.T.
13. Lhotka, J. F.: Stain Techn. **41**:65, 1966.

Chapter 2

Urinalysis*

URINE SPECIMENS

Most specimens of urine examined are random samples. Special problems require special methods for collection; e.g., specimens obtained in the investigation of orthostatic albuminuria, alimentary glycosuria, level of urobilinogen, renal function, glucose tolerance, etc.

Since some urinary characteristics and components are not stable and since urine is an excellent culture medium, all specimens should be collected in clean containers and examined within 30 min. If the latter is not possible, the specimens should be stored in the refrigerator. Sediments are unstable even at refrigerator temperature if the urine is alkaline.

COLLECTION

Twenty-four-hour specimen: Empty bladder at the beginning of the period (e.g., 8 A.M.) and discard urine. Save all urine voided during the next 24 hr. At the end of the period (e.g., 8 A.M. the next day) empty bladder and add this to the specimen. Keep urine in refrigerator in a wide-mouth collection bottle large enough to hold about 2000 ml. A variety of tests require special preservatives.

Preservatives for special tests:
Addis count: 0.5 ml. 40% formalin
Vanillyl mandelic acid (VMA): 10 ml. concentrated hydrochloric acid
Catecholamines: 1 ml. concentrated sulfuric acid
Aldosterone: 10 ml. chloroform
Steroids: 1-2 ml. toluol

*Refer to Kark et al.,[1] Kushner,[2] and Berman[3] for a general review of this subject.

The **creatinine level** of the specimen is a good check on the adequacy of the 24 hr. collection since it averages 1.6 gm./24 hr.

The total 24 hr. specimen must be carefully measured or the volume can be calculated on the basis of weight and specific gravity.[4]

Night specimen: Collection of this specimen should begin at least 3 hr. after the evening meal. Supper at 5 P.M. Empty bladder at 8 P.M. and discard urine. Save all urine voided during night and empty bladder at 8 A.M. (before patient has breakfast or begins work) and add this to the specimen.

Day specimen: Empty bladder at 8 A.M. (before patient has breakfast or begins work) and discard urine. Save all urine voided during the day; empty bladder at 8 P.M. (at least 3 hr. after the last meal) and add this urine to the specimen.

First morning specimen: It is the specimen of choice because it is concentrated. It is collected in a clean container and covered with a tight-fitting lid. Random specimens are less satisfactory because their dilution and therefore the concentration of their solutes may vary considerably. On the other hand, postprandial specimens are more likely to contain protein and glucose.

Afternoon specimen: Urobilinogen is best evaluated in a specimen obtained between 2 and 4 P.M.

Clean-voided midstream specimen: The external genitalia are washed with soap and water and rinsed with sterile water and a 1% aqueous merthiolate solution.* Female patients are asked to kneel over a bedpan or stand astride the toilet bowl while the labia are held apart by a gloved assistant. Men must keep the foreskin retracted. The initial portion of the urine stream is allowed to escape while the midstream portion is collected into a sterile wide-mouth container with a fitted sterile lid. This specimen is suitable for culture and should be plated within 2 hr. or refrigerated. (See Chapter 11.)

Collection of urine from newborn babies and infants: This collection presents special problems that are often difficult to solve as evidenced by the many, occasionally drastic, methods suggested.

1. Tube method: a plastic tube and plastic funnel are strapped to the genitalia. The tube may be replaced by a rubber finger or a plastic bag with an adhesive ring.†
2. Midstream-catch method: With love and patience this method suggested for adults can be used on children.
3. Gauze-pad method: A method similar to the one described for the collection of sweat in fibrocystic disease can be utilized. A gauze pad is used to collect the urine and is then centrifuged in a centrifuge tube containing a golf tee. The tee will hold the gauze at a distance from the bottom of the centrifuge tube and will allow clear urine to collect in the lowermost portion of the tube.
4. Catheterization: Not recommended.
5. Suprapubic aspiration: This method is suggested for critical quantitative bacteriology.

PRESERVATION

If a chemical preservative is added, state on the label the one used.

Preservation of the urine will prevent:
1. Conversion of urea to ammonium carbonate (alkaline fermentation) by urea-splitting organisms
2. Destruction of glucose by yeasts or bacteria
3. False positive albumin tests due to the presence of bacterial protein

4. Degeneration or destruction of organized sediment—pus, blood, and casts

Methods

Refrigeration: Keep all specimens cold whether or not a preservative has been added. Refrigeration prevents the growth of bacteria and helps to preserve casts, red and white blood cells, epithelial cells, and an acid pH.[5]

Chemical preservation:

Toluol (toluene): Add enough to form a thin layer over the surface. The toluol may be skimmed off or the urine pipetted from beneath it. It does not interfere with tests.

Phenol or tricresol: Add 1 drop/oz. urine. This is an excellent preservative and is often used in specimens forwarded to distant laboratories.

Thymol: Add a small crystal (about 5 mm. diam.) for 3 or 4 oz. of urine. An excess in solution may give a false positive albumin test and may interfere with the test for bile.

Formalin (40%): Add 1 drop/oz. urine. This preserves the urinary sediment especially well, but formalin prevents the Obermayer test for indican, reduces alkaline copper solutions (Fehling and Clinitest) used in the tests for sugar, and may in large quantity give a precipitate with urea that interferes with the microscopic examination.

Formaldehyde tablets:* Preservative tablets issued by life insurance companies liberate formaldehyde from methenamine. One tablet is used for 2 oz. of urine. It slightly increases the specific gravity.

Chloroform: Add a few drops at a time until some of them remain on the bottom after mixing gently. It reduces alkaline copper solutions (Fehling) and is not a very good preservative.

Special preservatives: Certain tests require special preservatives (see p. 11).

TESTS FOR PRESENCE OF URINE

Any considerable amount of **urea** is considered a positive test for urine. Most

*Eli Lilly & Co., Indianapolis, Ind.
†Aloe Scientific Division, Brunswick Corp., St. Louis, Mo.

*R. P. Cargille Laboratories, Inc., New York, N. Y.

body fluids contain small amounts of urea, and some urines from patients with hydronephrosis may contain little or no urea.

Tests for urea:

1. Evaporate nearly to dryness a few drops of the fluid on a glass slide, add a drop of pure white nitric acid (or saturated solution of oxalic acid), and cover with cover glass. Crystals of urea nitrate (or oxalate) can be recognized with the microscope if urea is present.

2. Remove any albumin present by making acid with dilute acetic acid, boiling, and filtering. In a Doremus-Hinds ureometer add a small amount (usually 1 ml.) of the fluid to a fresh hypobromite solution prepared by mixing equal parts of sodium hydroxide solution (40%) and potassium bromide solution (Br 1, KBr 1, H_2O 8). Nitrogen indicates presence of urea. A rough estimate of the amount can be determined in this way since the instrument indicates the grams of urea in the amount of fluid used.

3. To about 2 ml. of the specimen in a test tube add a drop of phenol red indicator and adjust to a faintly acid reaction (yellow). Add 2 drops buffer solution (for urea) and 2 drops urease solution. Incubate (water bath) at 37° C. or hold in closed hand for 10-15 min. A red color indicates the presence of urea.

Test for creatinine: An appreciable amount of creatinine is indicative of the presence of urine.

Conclusion: The presence of urea, creatinine, and chloride in amounts usually found in urine not contaminated by protein is highly suggestive of urine.

PHYSICAL EXAMINATION OF URINE

AMOUNT

Normally the amount varies with the substance to be excreted (food and fluid intake, stage of digestion, and state of metabolism) and with the loss of fluid in perspiration and in expired air due to temperature and exercise as well as with the condition of the circulation and of the kidneys. The amount is in proportion to the weight, but men secrete relatively more than women, and children more than men. Adults secrete about 1 ml./kg./hr. and children about 4 ml. Normal for adults is usually 1200-1500 ml. in 24 hr. The first day or two after birth the amount varies from 20-50 ml.; 5-10 days after birth from 150-250 ml.; and in infants, from 200-400 ml. After about 10 yr. of age the amount is that of adults. The ratio of the night to the day specimen is usually 1:2, 3, or 4 in adults. In children the ratio is variable and not reliable. This ratio is reversed (nocturia) in renal impairment and is an early sign of such impairment.

Increase: The amount is increased above the normal (**polyuria,** usually over 2500 ml.) by excessive fluid intake, by chilling of the skin, by intake of diuretics, during absorption of exudates, during absorption of fluids in edema, in many nervous diseases, with hypophyseal tumors, in hydronephrosis, in tuberculosis of the kidney, in compensating chronic nephritis, in diabetes insipidus, and in diabetes mellitus. In diabetes mellitus, polyuria is due to the presence of large amounts of glucose to be excreted so that the specific gravity is still high. In diabetes insipidus the specific gravity is very low. Polyuria should be distinguished from frequency, which occurs in cystitis, pyelitis, and hypertrophy of the prostate, and means "a frequent desire to empty the bladder."

Decrease: The amount is decreased below normal (oliguria, usually under 750 ml.) by decrease of fluid intake, by fluid loss (hemorrhage, vomiting, diarrhea, fever, etc.), during the formation of exudates or in edema, by impaired circulation (decompensated heart disease), and in acute nephritis.

Anuria or total suppression of urine formation occurs in collapse, in some cases of acute nephritis, and in complete obstruction to the urinary outflow. With obstruction on one side only, the other kidney may also not function (reflex anuria). In the lower nephron syndrome[6,7] that occurs in burns, in transfusion reaction, in the crush syndrome, in traumatic shock, and in thyroid and liver disease and following many types of operations, there is oliguria that progresses to anuria and results in renal azotemia and uremia. Anuria should be distinguished from retention or inability to void, which may be due to obstruction of the urethra by clotted blood, stricture, or prostatic hypertrophy.

RESIDUAL URINE

The urine obtained by catheter immediately after the patient has emptied the bladder voluntarily is known as residual urine. Normally there is no residual urine.

ODOR

The normal odor of urine may be modified by the presence of acetone, which imparts a fruity odor, or by bacterial decomposition, which produces an ammoniacal odor. In 1954, Menkes and associates[8] described maple syrup urine disease, a syndrome occurring in infancy and characterized by cerebral dysfunction and maple syruplike odor of urine. An offensive odor may be due to bacterial action in the presence of pus.

COLOR

Normally urine is some shade of yellow because of a mixture of pigments such as uroerythrin, urochrome, porphyrins, etc. The color will vary with the specific gravity; if the urine is diluted, it will be straw colored and almost deep orange if concentrated.

Variations in color:

Yellow. Normal pigments in abnormal amounts.

Very pale yellow or greenish yellow or practically colorless. Severe iron deficiency, chronic kidney disease, and diabetes mellitus and insipidus. The kidney is unable to produce pigments.

1. Chlorosis. Due to faulty iron metabolism and decreased hemoglobin.
2. Chronic nephritis. Due to polyuria and impaired kidney function.
3. Diabetes mellitus and diabetes insipidus. Due to polyuria.

Orange. Urine is usually concentrated in fever, in inadequate water intake, and in excessive water loss through sweat.

1. Abnormal pigments.
   (a) Bilirubin. Gmelin test and modification; iodine test.

(b) Medicines. Rhubarb, senna, and santonin in acid urines. Acriflavine, which suggests bile but does not give bile tests. Santonin imparts a yellow color to acid urine and a pink color to alkaline urine.
(c) Foods. Carrots (carotin). Soluble in petroleum ether; bile is not.

Green. Often due to blue pigment mixed with yellow urine.

1. Normal pigments in abnormal amounts.
   (a) Increased indican when oxidized upon standing. Obermayer test.
2. Abnormal pigments.
   (a) Bile when oxidized upon standing. Bichloride test.
   (b) Methylene blue. Sometimes used as urinary antiseptic or in "kidney pills." Evans blue. (See discussion of indican.)
   (c) Chromogenic bacteria such as *Pseudomonas aeruginosa*. Culture.
   (d) Riboflavin.

Red

1. Normal pigments in abnormal amounts.
   (a) Uroerythrin. Soluble in amyl alcohol. Absorption bands at 525-540 mμ and at 490-500 mμ.
2. Abnormal pigments and porphyrins.
   (a) Blood pigments.
      (1) Hemoglobin (hemoglobinuria). Benzidine test. Often dark red, resembling Coca Cola.
      (2) Myoglobin. Benzidine test. Spectroscopic test.
      (3) Red blood cells (hematuria). Microscopic test.
      (4) Porphyrins (porphyrinuria). These do not give the benzidine test. Often wine colored or dark purplish red. The urine may be normally colored on voiding, but darkens on standing.
   (b) Chromogenic bacteria such as *Serratia marcescens*. Culture.
   (c) Medicines.
      (1) Pyramidon and antipyrin. No indicator reaction. A large amount of sodium hydroxide destroys the red color.
      (2) Mercurochrome. Fluorescent. Stains epithelial cells, pus cells, and casts pink. Precipitates with acid unless acetone is present and may be filtered out.
      (3) Mercury oxycyanide. Does not fluoresce. Acts like methyl red indicator. Is not precipitated by acids and shows no spectroscopic bands.
      (4) Phenolsulfonphthalein, phenolphthalein, chrysarobin, senna, rhubarb, cascara, and santonin in alkaline specimens. These act as indicators and are yellow in acid urines.
      (5) Pyridium. Foam is yellowish. If much drug is present, dilute acid

gives no change, and sodium hydroxide produces a white cloud. If dilute, there is a slight indicator reaction. Does not interfere with benzidine test, but does with test for urobilinogen. Does not fluoresce. The absorption band is similar to that of urobilin. May be precipitated out if made acid with dilute hydrochloric acid, then concentrated (not over 35° C.), and placed on ice.

   (d) Food. Beets may give a red color (complex pigments, anthocyanins) that has an indicator reaction like methyl red.

Black
1. Normal pigments in abnormal amounts.
     (a) Marked increase of indican. Blue-black, often with metallic scum. Obermayer test. Color is soluble in chloroform.
2. Abnormal pigments.
     (a) Melanin. Ferric chloride test.
     (b) Phenol derivatives. Ferric chloric added to distillate gives amethyst color.
     (c) Alkapton bodies. Blackens upon adding alkali. Color not soluble in chloroform.
     (d) Old blood. Benzidine test.
     (e) Argyrol. Dark purplish red. Digest with nitric acid and hydrogen peroxide, dilute, and add hydrochloric acid. Silver chloride will precipitate. Or treat with ferric chloride. The color disappears.
     (f) Porphobilin. Product of porphobilinogen.

Milky
1. Normal substances.
     (a) Phosphates. Clears upon addition of acetic acid.
     (b) Urates. Clears upon warming.
2. Abnormal substances.
     (a) Chyle. Fat microscopically. Examine for microfilaria.
     (b) Pus. Microscopic.
     (c) Prostatic secretion. Microscopic.
     (d) Protein-phosphate compounds. Colloidal.
     (e) Bacteria.

TRANSPARENCY AND TURBIDITY

Normally fresh urine is clear except when earthy phosphates are precipitated from alkaline specimens.

Clouding may be due to the following:

1. Amorphous **phosphates** or **carbonates**. These dissolve upon addition of dilute acetic acid; the former without and the latter with gas.
2. Amorphous urates. These dissolve upon warming.
3. Calcium oxalates. There is no change on heating, but clearing is produced by the addition of dilute hydrochloric acid.
4. Pus, blood, and epithelial cells. These are found upon microscopic examination. In alkaline urine, pus is usually mucoid, while it is crumbly in acid urine. About 200 white blood cells/mm.^{2} or about 500 red blood cells/mm.^{2} produce turbidity.
5. Bacteria. These are seen microscopically. They are not removed by filtering through paper unless some inert substance such as kaolin or sawdust is first added, and this is not always satisfactory.
6. Fat. This gives a milky appearance. It is seen microscopically and may be removed by ether. Chyluria may be parasitic (filaria, *Echinococcus*) or nonparasitic in origin (thoracic duct obstruction, trauma, tumor, or infection of the lymphatics).
7. Colloidal particles. The cause for these is not known. The urine cannot be cleared by filtering or centrifuging. The particles are not visible in microscopic examination and are not removed by ether. The particles might be agglomerated by electrolytes or by colloidal particles of opposite electric charge such as mercuric chloride or sulfosalicylic acid. Many urines may be cleared by adding lead acetate and filtering; this will remove many coloring substances, but the method is not suitable for clearing urines for the albumin tests.

Except for microscopic examination, clouding due to causes 1, 2, and 3 may be removed by filtering through paper or by centrifuging.

HYDROGEN ION CONCENTRATION OF URINE (pH)

NORMAL VALUES: Normally the pH varies from about 4.8-7.5, with an average of about 6.6. At body temperature it is about 0.2 lower than at room temperature. The night urine has a low pH because of the respiratory acidosis that develops during sleep. In the morning and after meals the pH rises (alkaline tides).

The pH of a pooled specimen is therefore often in the range of pH 6.0.

On standing, urine becomes alkaline due to liberation of ammonia by urea-splitting bacteria. The pH must therefore be measured in fresh urine.

Kidney in acid-base metabolism[9]

The pH of urine depends largely on the acid-base composition of the blood. Normal metabolism produces an excess of acids (H ions) consisting mainly of mineral acids such as sulfuric and phosphoric acids which are excreted by the kidneys (**fixed acidity**). Carbonic acid produced by metabolism of carbohydrates is eliminated by the lungs (**volatile acidity**). In pathologic conditions nonmetabolized organic acids such as beta-hydroxybutyric acid (diabetes) or lactic, citric, and pyruvic acids significantly add to the acidity of the urine. Because of the very adequate buffering systems of human urine (NaH_2PO_4, creatinine, beta-hydroxybutyric acid, etc.) the kidney can excrete up to 480 mEq. acid/day. Most titrable acidity is present as acid phosphate (NaH_2PO_4) which forms part of a reversible reaction.

$$H^+ + Na_2HPO_4 = NaH_2PO_4 + Na^+$$

In **acidosis** most phosphate is excreted as NaH_2PO_4 and in **alkalosis** as Na_2HPO_4. Normally the largest number of H ions is excreted as NH_4 (**ammonium**) which is synthetized in the kidney and excreted in amounts depending on the systemic acid-base balance. Microelectrodes have recently been used to measure partial O_2 and CO_2 pressures in the urine of the renal pelvis and of the urinary bladder. The P_{CO_2} varies greatly in acidosis and alkalosis. In **respiratory acidosis** (CO_2 retention) and in **metabolic acidosis** (diabetic ketosis, starvation, uremia) the urine is usually acid, whereas in **respiratory alkalosis** (hyperventilation) and **metabolic alkalosis** (vomiting, administration of alkalies) the urine is usually alkaline. In metabolic acidosis there is an increased titratable acidity (total excretion of acid) of the freshly voided urine, whereas in metabolic alkalosis the titratable acidity is decreased. There are exceptions to this rule, such as renal failure

(inability to form ammonia) and renal tubular diseases (e.g., Fanconi and Milkman's syndromes), in which weakly alkaline urine (pH 6.5) may be excreted in the presence of systemic acidosis.

Potassium deficiency and hyperaldosteronism produce alkaline urine.

The urinary pH is important in the treatment of certain conditions; e.g., it should be kept alkaline during treatment with sulfonamides and for the prevention of formation of uric acid and calcium oxalate stones. It is kept acid to prevent bacteriuria and the formation of "alkaline stones" such as calcium carbonate or calcium phosphate stones.

METHODS OF MEASURING pH:

Nitrazine test paper*: It may be used for approximate values. Apply a drop of the urine to the test paper with a glass rod, and in 1-2 min. compare with the color chart, the colors of which vary by steps of 0.5 from pH 4.5 (yellow) to pH 7.5 (blue). Do not dilute urine. If urine is alkaline, test for ammonia with litmus paper. Heat urine gently and allow the vapor to come in contact with litmus paper held in the mouth of the test tube. The paper will turn blue and on drying will turn red again (volatile alkalinity).

Litmus paper: It is not sensitive enough.

Labstix*: Indicators are methyl red and bromthymol blue.

SPECIFIC GRAVITY AND REFRACTIVE INDEX

Specific gravity is a measure of the concentration of solutes in the urine and thus of the concentrating and diluting power of the kidney, a very complicated function involving osmosis, countercurrent, ultrafiltration, excretion, and secretion mechanisms.

The specific gravity of the glomerular filtrate is 1.010; therefore a fixed urinary specific gravity of 1.010 indicates poor tubular resorption. On the other hand, a high specific gravity may indicate dehydration or presence of abnormal solutes.

NORMAL VALUES:

Adults:

    Random specimen, 1.001-1.035

    24 hr. specimen, 1.015-1.018

---

*E. R. Squibb & Sons Division, Olin Mathieson Chemical Corp., New York, N. Y.

Newborn babies:
Random specimen, 1.002-1.004
Middle age and over:
Progressive decreases of specific gravity

METHODS:

Urinometer: Mix urine well and allow to come to room temperature. Float the instrument in the specimen, giving it a slight twist to see that it is completely free. Read the bottom meniscus and correct figures for temperature, protein, and sugar. Most urinometers are calibrated at 20° C. A difference of 3° C. gives a correction of 0.001, to be added if above and subtracted if below the proper **temperature.** If amount is small, dilute with 1 or 2 parts water and multiply last two figures of reading by 2 or 3.

For each **1% albumin** the specific gravity is increased 0.003. For each **1% glucose** it is increased 0.004. **Preservative tablets** also increase the specific gravity.

As the specific gravity determination of urine may suggest renal disease or rule it out, it is important to check the accuracy of the urinometer. A couple of matched instruments to cover the entire range from 0-40 may be preferable to a single **urinometer.**

Urinometer controls:

Distilled water at 15.5° C.	Specific gravity 1.000
0.85% saline solution at 15.5° C.	Specific gravity 1.006
5% saline solution at 15.5° C.	Specific gravity 1.035

An error of ±0.003 renders a urinometer reading unsatisfactory.

Falling drop method: Dogramaci[10] described a method for the determination of the specific gravity of a very small amount of urine. The method employs graded series of oily solutions made up by mixing kerosene and bromobenzene in varying proportions ranging in specific gravity from 1.000-1.060. A drop of urine is added to each bottle and is observed to determine whether it rises or sinks in the test solution. The method is similar to the copper sulfate method for blood specific gravity.

Speegrav*: This instrument, which is temperature-compensated, determines the specific gravity photoelectrically, thereby eliminating inaccuracies of the hydrometer readings.

Refractometer* (TS meter, total solids meter): This instrument, which is temperature-compensated, is calibrated in terms of specific gravity for urine and requires only 1 large drop of the sample, thereby eliminating most "quantity not sufficient" amounts. The total urinary solids can be determined by converting the specific gravity reading to total solids by the use of a conversion table.

Total solids: The specific gravity may be used to determine roughly the total solids of the urine. The last two figures of the specific gravity of the 24 hr. specimen multiplied by 2.33 (Häser's coefficient) give the gm./L. For the average man of 150 lb., the total solids are about 60 gm./24 hr.

A more accurate way of measuring the total solids is the determination of the osmolarity of urine, calculated from the freezing point or by using the refractometer method.

OSMOLALITY AND FREEZING POINT DETERMINATION

OSMOLALITY: The determination of the osmolality of urine is helpful in the clinical management of water and electrolyte disturbances. When a solute is added to a solvent, the freezing point of the solvent is lowered and the osmotic pressure is raised proportional to the molal concentration of the particles. Osmolality is the number of osmoles of a solute per kilogram of solvent (water) and it is directly related to the depression of the freezing point of an aqueous solution below that of water. Solutions of widely varying osmolalities have the same specific gravity; therefore changes in urinary osmolality may not be reflected in the specific gravity.

FREEZING POINT DETERMINATION: The freezing point determination is essentially a measure of the **salt concentration** of the urine and is not materially influenced by large molecular substances such as proteins. The higher the water content,

---

*Biological Research, Inc., Bridgeton, Mo.

*American Optical Co., Buffalo, N. Y.

the closer the freezing point will be to zero.

METHOD:

Osmometer[11, 12]: An osmometer is an instrument that determines the concentration of free particles in a solution, the osmolality, by means of measuring the freezing point. The osmolality is proportional to the freezing point. The lower the freezing point, the higher the osmotic pressure. The instrument is calibrated in milliosmoles and requires about a 2 ml. sample.

Normal 24 hr. excretion:
Males: 767-1628 mOsm./24 hr.
Females: 433-1146 mOsm./24 hr.

It remains to be seen whether the determination of the osmolality is superior to the determination of the specific gravity or to the measurement of the total solids by refractometer in the clinical evaluation of kidney function or of acid-base balance.

CHEMICAL EXAMINATION OF URINE

PROTEIN

Heller ring test: Into a clean dry test tube pour 2 or 3 ml. pure white nitric acid. Filter urine through paper, allowing urine to trickle gently down the opposite dry side of glass to form a layer over the acid. Observe for a grayish ring at the line of contact. Do not report a negative reaction until the test has stood for 3 min. For observing the slightest possible trace of albumin, hold the finger behind the line of contact, facing a window with the eyes on the level of the contact ring. A grayish ring indicates albumin or some interfering substance, e.g., mucus, urea, uric acid, nitrates, bile acids, proteoses, Uroselectan, and resins.

The specific gravity of the nitric acid should be 1.42. If the acid develops a yellow tinge (nitrous acid), aerate it.

Grade as follows:

Protein: trace; can just be seen from above. A finger moved can be seen.
Protein 1+ (about 0.1%): ring is quite dense but not opaque from above. A finger moved under the glass can be seen from above.
Protein 2+ (if just opaque, 0.2-0.3%): with this amount the ring is opaque when viewed from above, and the clinical quantitative

method should be done on a 24 hr. specimen.
Protein 3+: if ring is very dense, over 0.5%.

Heat and acetic acid test: Filter urine and fill test tube two-thirds full. Heat upper fingerbreadth (2 cm.) and observe for clouding. Clouding may be due to phosphates, albumin, or some interfering substance. Add 2 or 3 drops of dilute acetic acid and observe again. Clouding due to phosphates will disappear. Repeat the heating and the adding of acid twice in order to make sure that the specimen is sufficiently acid, observing each time. A persistent cloudiness indicates albumin or some interfering substance.

For detecting the slightest trace of albumin, slant the tube with the upper end toward the window over a dark background and compare the upper boiled portion with the lower portion. Allowing the tube to stand a few minutes will bring out the reaction more plainly. But grade promptly, as correlation is lost after standing.

Grade as follows:

Protein 1+: diffuse cloud
Protein 2+: granular cloud
Protein 3+: distinct flocculi
Protein 4+: large flocculi, dense, sometimes solid

Modification of heat and acetic acid test: When the specific gravity of a specimen is low, mucin and nucleoprotein may interfere with the usual heat and acetic acid test. Many insurance companies require the following modification which eliminates the mucin and nucleoprotein.

To the filtered urine add one-fifth its volume of saturated sodium chloride solution and about 5 drops glacial acetic acid. Heat the upper fingerbreadth (2 cm.) to boiling. The salt holds nucleoprotein in solution, and the acid dissolves the mucin so that any clouding may be considered to indicate the presence of albumin or globulin.

Kingsbury-Clark method (sulfosalicylic acid test): If urine is alkaline, acidify with acetic acid, filter, and divide into two portions. To one portion add 3 parts 3% aqueous sulfosalicylic acid to 1 part urine. A cloud forms if protein is present. Compare with the other portion of filtered urine. If a cloud forms, heat to boiling. Albumin and globulin do not clear on boiling; Bence Jones protein disappears upon boiling and reappears upon cooling. Cloudiness due to urates will disappear when warmed moderately. Sulfosalicylic acid also precipitates mucus, proteoses, and x-ray contrast media.

The density of the precipitate can be compared with commercial Kingsbury-Clark standards,* allowing some measure of quantitation.

Method of reporting:

7.5 mg./100 ml.	Negative
Up to 20 mg./100 ml.	Trace
Up to 30 mg./100 ml.	+
Up to 50 mg./100 ml.	++
Up to 75 mg./100 ml.	+++

Priodax and Telepaque, trade names for iodoalphionic acid and iodopanoic acid, respectively, give albumin-like reactions with sulfosalicylic acid and with nitric acid but not with heat and acetic acid. This pseudoalbuminuria may last for 2 or 3 days.[13]

Hypaque sodium, trade name for sodium 3,5-diacetamido-2,4,6-tri-iodobenzoate, likewise produces pseudoalbuminuria, and because of its high iodine content (59.87%) it gives a black color with the Benedict test for sugar.

Carinamide gives interfering reactions in albumin tests. With the Heller test the reaction is the same as with resins—soluble in ether, alcohol, and alkali. With the heat and acetic acid test a precipitate occurs at room temperature (as it does in the presence of nucleoproteins) and disappears upon warming (as in the presence of urates). It is soluble in ether, alcohol, and alkali. With sulfosalicylic acid the reaction is similar to that with heat and acetic acid. (See discussion of Albutest.)

Colorimetric tablets and strips (Albu-Stix and Albutest†): This protein test is based on the phenomenon of a "protein error of indicators" which is based on the principle that at a fixed pH certain indicators will have one color in the presence

of protein and another color in the absence of protein. The pH is 3, and the indicator is tetrabromphenol blue. These tests are simple, rapid, accurate, sensitive, specific, and capable of being used with turbid urine. If a tablet is used, place tablet on clean surface and put 1 drop urine on tablet. After urine drop has been absorbed, add 2 drops water and allow penetration before reading. Compare color on top of tablet with color scale. If a strip is used, dip yellow end in urine and compare color of dipped end with the color scale. These methods also give negative results after the administration of tolbutamide (Orinase), penicillin (massive doses), and sulfisoxazole (Gantrisin), drugs which frequently lead to false positive results when turbidity, heat, and acid methods are used.

Esbach quantitative method: Dilute filtered urine to a specific gravity of 1.006-1.008. For example, if the specific gravity is 1.012-1.016, dilute with an equal amount of water and multiply the result by 2. Acidify with dilute acetic acid if necessary. Fill an Esbach tube to the mark "U" with the urine and add Esbach reagent to the mark "R." Mix gently by inverting the tube 12 times. Stopper and leave in upright position for 24 hr. The height of the precipitate gives the amount of albumin in gm./L. when no dilution is necessary. Correct for dilution and report in percent and in gm. protein/24 hr. output.

The amount of precipitate is not exactly proportional to the amount of protein present, and therefore the Esbach tube is graduated empirically.

Esbach reagent:
1. Picric acid, 1 gm.
2. Citric acid, 2 gm.
3. Distilled water up to 100 ml.

The Kingsbury-Clark method can also be used quantitatively.

Significance: Normally no protein is demonstrated in urine by the usual tests. Pathologically, protein may be present because of mixture with exudates from the urinary tract or from extraneous sources (menstrual flow and hemorrhage). This is known as **false** or **accidental albuminuria.** About 80,000-100,000 pus cells/ml. (80-100/mm.[3]) will give 0.1% albumin.

---

*Aloe Scientific Division, Brunswick Corp., St. Louis, Mo.

†Ames Co., Inc., Elkhart, Ind.

Howard[14] found that about 24,000 red blood cells in 14 ml. urine or 0.01 ml. prostatic secretion or 0.04 ml. fluid from the seminal vesicles in 15 ml. urine gave a positive test for protein.

True proteinuria is the result of filtration of plasma proteins through the hypothetical pores of the glomerular membrane. The proteins of relatively low molecular weight and small size pass through first, e.g., hemoglobin, molecular weight 68,000; albumin, molecular weight 70,000; and then globulin, molecular weight 165,000. Fibrinogen, the molecule of which is much larger, escapes only in severe renal disease. If albumin is excreted in large amounts, the serum albumin-globulin ratio will be altered. Urine proteins are similar to plasma proteins and can be demonstrated by **paper electrophoresis.** (See discussion of Bence Jones protein and serum electrophoresis.) Clinically the terms **albuminuria and proteinuria** are used synonymously.

Functional albuminuria is temporary following sufficient strain (severe muscular exercise, emotional stress, etc.) and is not accompanied by renal lesions. Albuminuria of newborn infants (first few days of life), albuminuria of normal pregnancy (about half of the cases), intermittent or cyclic albuminuria (orthostatic and hypostatic), and albuminuria of adolescence are examples of true albuminuria without definite renal lesions. Albuminuria with only temporary renal lesions (cloudy, swelling, and ischemia or hyperemia) is found in febrile reactions, after trauma, in severe anemias, in preeclampsia and eclampsia, and after ingestion of toxic substances (about one fourth of the cases of ether anesthesia). Albuminuria with definite renal lesions is found in acute and chronic nephritis, tuberculosis of the kidney, neoplasms of the kidney, nephrosis, infections of the kidney, severe poisoning (metals), and polycystic kidney.

Removing protein from urine: To remove protein from the urine when it interferes with other tests, make the urine acid with dilute acetic acid and boil. Cool, make up to the original volume, and filter.

Bence Jones protein[15]

Bence Jones protein occurs with or without other proteins. It is found in 40% of the cases of multiple myeloma and in some cases of tumor metastasis to bone, chronic leukemia (lymphocytic), and amyloidosis. It may be present alone or, more often, with albumin. During electrophoresis it migrates sometimes with the alpha globulin, sometimes with the beta globulin, and sometimes between the two as its composition varies.

If the Heller ring test with concentrated nitric acid or the sulfosalicylic acid test is negative for protein, Bence Jones protein is absent, and no further procedure is indicated. If either test is positive, make a ring test with concentrated hydrochloric acid (Bradshaw test). If this test is negative, no further procedure is indicated; if it is positive, proceed with the following test.

Toluene sulfonic acid (TSA) test[16]:
Principle: TSA reagent precipitates Bence Jones protein but does not precipitate albumin. It unmasks globulin only if present in high concentrations.

Technique: To 2 ml. urine add 1 ml. reagent (12% in acetic acid) by allowing it to slowly (15-30 sec.) run down the side of the test tube (10 × 75 mm.). Flick the tube with finger to mix.

Interpretation: Any precipitate occurring within 5 min. is a positive test for Bence Jones protein. It is excluded by a negative test. If the test is positive, proceed with the heat precipitation test.

Heat precipitation test:
Principle: Bence Jones protein precipitates at 60° C. It disappears at 100° C. and reappears on cooling to 85°-60° C.

Technique: Dilute the specimen with normal (protein-free) urine, make acid (pH 5, Nitrazine paper) with 25% acetic acid, and let stand 5 min. If a precipitate forms, nucleoproteins are present. Filter through Whatman paper No. 42 or No. 44. Insert a thermometer into the filtrate and heat slowly (in water bath) to boiling. If Bence Jones protein is present, clouding will begin at 40° C., and precipitation will be complete at 60° C. The precipitate will disappear upon boiling a few minutes. Upon cooling the precipitate reappears and begins to disappear again below 40° C.

To separate Bence Jones protein when albumin is present, filter at boiling temperature. Albumin will be filtered out. Test the filtrate for Bence Jones protein.

Differential extraction of uroproteins and Bence Jones protein: If there is massive proteinuria, the previously mentioned methods fail. Naumann[17] described a differential extraction method of uroglobulins and Bence Jones protein to solve the difficulties encountered in the diagnosis of Bence Jones proteinuria in the presence of advanced renal proteinuria.

Paper electrophoresis of urine: This can be used to demonstrate Bence Jones protein.

Concentration of urine protein for electrophoresis by dialysis: If the concentration of protein is greater than 1%, no dialysis is necessary. Otherwise filter 10-100 ml. urine of 24 hr. specimen into No. 26 cellophane dialysis tubing.* Dialyze 12-24 hr. against 1000 ml. phosphate buffer (pH 6.0) in a cold room or refrigerator. The buffer is made up as follows:

> Na_2HPO_4, anhydrous, 12.78 gm.
> $NaH_2PO_4 \cdot H_2O$, 86.95 gm.
> Distilled water to make 9 L.

Dissolve 200-300 gm. polyvinyl pyrrolidone (PVP) in 1000 ml. buffer. Several hours will be required. Place the urine tube in a rotating dialyzer installed in a refrigerator. It will take from 24-48 hr. for the urinary proteins to become adequately concentrated. Centrifuge the concentrated protein in a hematocrit tube and apply clear supernatent (6-12 λ) to electrophoresis paper or gel.[18, 19]

Other methods: The method using collodion bags and glass suction apparatus† for concentration of proteins is somewhat easier and faster than the previously described procedure.

In the Beckman microzone electrophoresis system, 40% carbowax dialyzing solution is used.

---

*Visking Corp., Chicago, Ill.
†Carl Schleicher & Schnell Co., Keene, N. H.

Aminoaciduria

The renal threshold for amino acids is high so that only small amounts of amino acids are normally found in urine. Paper chromatography (two-dimensional technique) can be used to identify the various amino acids. The amino acids that normally occur in larger quantities are glycine, taurine, histidine, glutamine, and cystine. The other amino acids, e.g., tryptophan, tyrosine, serine, and alanine, occur in much smaller amounts.

TESTS FOR AMINO ACIDS: The total excretion of amino acids can be evaluated by measuring the total free alpha amino nitrogen in urine and determining its ratio to total nitrogen or creatinine.

Specific amino acids can be determined by paper, column, and thin-layer chromatography as well as by thin-layer electrophoresis.

Qualitative identification by paper chromatography[20]:

Principle: The method is based upon the different speeds with which compounds travel in two phases—a solid phase and a liquid phase. The liquid or mobile phase is usually an organic solvent saturated with water, whereas the stationary (solid) phase is water saturated with organic liquid and held stationary within the paper.

Most amino acids can be separated by two-dimensional chromatography. Separation can usually be obtained with solvents partially miscible with water. The filter paper serves as an inert support holding the stationary aqueous phase. As the solvent flows through a section of the paper containing the unknown substances, a partition of the substance occurs between the mobile organic phase and the stationary phase.

Reagents:
Solvents:
1. Phenol. Dissolve 100 ml. metal-free water in 400 ml. liquid phenol* by gentle warming. The solvent may be stored in a dark bottle in a refrigerator where separation into two layers will occur. Before the solvent

---

*Mallinckrodt Gilt Label.

is used, the bottle is shaken, and the desired quantity of emulsion is removed and gently warmed to form a solution. A beaker containing 100 mg. NaCN in 4-6 ml. water is placed in the cabinet. The liberated HCN retards the decomposition of phenol. A beaker containing 0.3% NH_3 may also be placed in the bottom of the cabinet.

2. Lutidine-ethanol. A mixture of 55 ml. 2,6-lutidine, 25 ml. ethanol, 20 ml. water, and 2 ml. diethylamine is prepared. This mixture is completely miscible. (Room must be adequately ventilated.)

Stain: 0.25% ninhydrin in acetone (ninhydrin sprays may be obtained commercially).[20]

Technique: See discussion of urinary sugar chromatography.

Thin-layer chromatography: This system of chromatography uses glass instead of paper as the inert support. This method is more sensitive than paper chromatography; dilutions of 10^{-9} can be detected. It is much quicker; 30-40 min. are usually sufficient for sharp separation. Quantities as small as 0.02 μg can be separated.

Hydrated silica is used most frequently as slurry spread in a thin layer (250μ thick) on a glass plate. The plate is spotted with the unknown solution and then placed upright in a closed chamber, with the spotted edge immersed in the solvent at the bottom of the chamber. The solvent rises through the silica layer by capillary attraction and separates the different components of the applied material. The plate is then dried and the spot components are visualized by various staining methods.

Thin-layer electrophoresis: This method also utilizes slurries applied in a thin layer to glass plates, which are then sprayed with buffer and connected to trays filled with buffer by means of wicks. The samples are applied to one end of the plate and separation is achieved in an electric field. The separated sample components are detected by spraying with dyes.

Test for amino acid nitrogen[21, 22]:

Principle: Most amino acids react with ninhydrin to form a blue color when heated at a pH of over 3. The reaction is almost exclusively with the alpha nitrogen. Not all amino acids will give the color and the different amino acids give slightly different amounts of color on a molar basis, but the method is satisfactory for most clinical purposes. Some other nitrogen compounds also give a color with the reagent. In the method given the use of a nonaqueous solvent greatly reduces the interference of urea, and ammonia is eliminated from urine by a preliminary treatment.

Reagents:

1. Carbonate buffer. Dissolve 14.3 gm. anhydrous sodium carbonate and 2.66 gm. sodium bicarbonate in water and dilute to 1 L.

2. EDTA buffer. Dissolve 50 gm. disodium EDTA (ethylenediaminetetraacetic acid) in about 900 ml. water, then add 18.7 ml. glacial acetic acid and 10 ml. 1N sodium hydroxide. Dilute to 1 L. Check the pH and adjust to 3.7 if necessary.

3. Ninhydrin reagent. Dissolve 200 mg. ninhydrin in 100 ml. ethylene glycol. The material may dissolve rather slowly. This solution is stable for a few weeks in the refrigerator.

4. Sulfuric acid and sodium tungstate solutions for the preparation of a Folin-Wu filtrate (q.v.).

5. Amino acid nitrogen stock standard. Dissolve 0.286 gm. glycine, 0.525 gm. glutamic acid, and 1 gm. sodium benzoate in about 400 ml. water. Add 4 ml. concentrated hydrochloric acid and dilute to 500 ml. This solution is quite stable.

6. Working standard. Dilute 5 ml. stock standard and 0.5 ml. 1N sodium hydroxide to 100 ml. This solution contains 1 mg. amino acid nitrogen/100 ml. The pH of the diluted standard should be approximately neutral. Check the pH before diluting and add a few drops of acid or base to bring it in the range of pH 6-8.

Procedure for urine: Check the pH of the urine. If it is not neutral, roughly titrate 5 ml. urine with acid or base (approximately 1N is usually satisfactory) to a pH of 7 (paper) and add this amount of acid or base to 5 ml. urine used in making the dilution. Dilute the urine quantitatively with water. For 24 hr. urine volumes over 2 L., dilute 5 ml. to 25; for volumes between 1 and 2 L., dilute 5 ml. to 50; and for lower urine volumes, dilute 5 ml. to 100. Pipette 2 ml. diluted urine to a 25 ml. Erlenmeyer flask. Add 0.5 ml. carbonate buffer and mix well. In the lower end of a one-hole rubber stopper that will fit the flask insert a rolled-up square of filter paper until it projects about 15 mm. from the bottom of the stopper. Moisten the paper with a few drops of 1:10 sulfuric acid and insert stopper into flask, taking care that the filter paper does not touch the sides of the flask. Allow to stand at room temperature for 2-3 hr., then remove stopper and discard paper. Add to the flask 2 ml. EDTA buffer and mix well. Also mix together 2 ml. diluted standard, 0.5 ml. carbonate buffer, and 2 ml. EDTA buffer and prepare a blank by repeating the procedure using water instead of standard. In test tubes place 0.5 ml. of the mixtures from the sample, standard, and blank. Add to each tube 6 ml. ninhydrin reagent and mix well. Heat tubes in boiling water bath for 20 min., then cool. Read standard and samples against blank at 570 mμ.

Calculations: Since the diluted standard containing 1 mg.% amino acid nitrogen and the diluted urine are treated similarly:

$$\frac{OD\ sample}{OD\ standard} \times 1 \times Dilution\ of\ urine =$$

Mg.% amino nitrogen in urine

$$Mg.\% \times \frac{Total\ volume\ in\ ml.}{100} =$$

Total mg. amino nitrogen excreted

Significance: Amino acids are increased in liver impairment, gout, pneumonia, diabetes, leukemia, extensive tissue necrosis, and inborn errors of amino acid metabolism (tyrosinuria, phenylketonuria, cystinuria, alkaptonuria, and melanuria).

Other conditions leading to aminoaciduria include progressive muscular atrophy, hyperthyroidism (liver damage), cortisone therapy, and renal defects due to poisoning with oxalic acid, phosphorus, etc. The previously mentioned congenital diseases must be recalled—Wilson's disease, galactosemia, Fanconi syndrome, cystinuria, and Hartnup disease.

DENT'S CLASSIFICATION OF AMINOACIDURIA (MODIFIED AFTER HOLT):
Renal aminoaciduria—due to defective tubular reabsorption of certain amino acids; leads to increased renal excretion
1. Generalized:
   Fanconi syndrome
   Cystinosis
   Galactosemia
   Wilson's disease
   Rickets
2. Specific:
   Cystinuria
   Glycinuria

Overflow aminoaciduria—increased plasma amino acid concentration; accounts for hyperexcretion of urinary amino acids
1. Generalized:
   Liver disease
   Premature and newborn infants
   Megaloblastic anemias
   Lead poisoning
   Muscular dystrophies
   Wilson's disease
   Leukemia
2. Specific:
   Maple syrup urine disease
   H disease
   Phenylketonuria

Abnormal excretion of products derived from amino acids
   Alkaptonuria
   Oxalosis
   Tyrosinosis
   Pyridoxine deficiency
   Folic acid deficiency

RENAL AMINOACIDURIA:

FANCONI SYNDROME: Aminoaciduria occurs as part of a multiple renal defect that leads to glycosuria, stunted growth, and hypophosphatemic rickets. Other features are proteinuria, polyuria, inability to form acid urine, and loss of potassium.

CYSTINURIA: Cystinuria represents a congenital defect in the reabsorption of cystine, lysine, ornithine, and arginine. The demonstration of cystine and other amino acids in the urine helps to distinguish this disease from cystinosis, a generalized disease involving cystine. The main clinical feature of cystinuria is recurrent cystine calculus formation. Lewis described the cyanide nitroprusside test for cystine.

Cyanide nitroprusside test for cystine: To 5 ml. urine add 2 ml. 5% sodium cyanide solution; mix and allow to stand for 10 min. Add 5% sodium nitroprusside drop by drop and shake. If the test is positive, a red color will result.[23]

WILSON'S DISEASE: In Wilson's disease the copper deposition in the kidneys may lead to aminoaciduria. The primary defect is of the ceruloplasmin, the plasma copper-binding protein.

GALACTOSEMIA: Galactosemia may be accompanied by aminoaciduria.

OVERFLOW AMINOACIDURIA:

MAPLE SYRUP URINE DISEASE[24, 25]**:** This is a congenital defect in which the odor of the urine resembles that of maple syrup. Valine, leucine, and isoleucine are increased in the urine.

H DISEASE: This is a congenital aminoaciduria accompanied by a pellagra-like rash and neurologic changes (cerebellar ataxia). It has also been referred to as Hartnup disease and Hart's syndrome.

PHENYLKETONURIA[26] **(PHENYLPYRUVIC OLIGOPHRENIA):** This is a laboratory finding in a hereditary form of mental deficiency. Phenylpyruvic acid appears in the urine. Normally phenylalanine is metabolized in the liver to tyrosine. Absence of phenylalanine hydroxylase in the liver leads to accumulation of phenylalanine in the plasma and to increased excretion of phenylpyruvic acid in the urine. The disease is inherited through a single autosomal recessive gene so that both parents of a patient must have the genic defect. The patients are mentally retarded and have epileptic seizures. **Phenylpyruvic acid** appears in the urine after phenylalanine has become elevated in the plasma. Normal phenylalanine plasma level is 1.65 mg./100 ml. and phenylpyruvic acid appears in the urine at phenylalanine plasma levels of 8-11 mg./100 ml. Since milk contains phenylalanine, an affected infant will show a rise in the phenylalanine plasma level 1 or 2 days after the first few feedings, usually just about the time the infant is ready to leave the hospital. The **urine phenylpyruvic acid level** or **phenylalanine level** will not be elevated until the infant is 1-6 wk. old.

Ferric chloride test: To about 5 ml. urine add a few drops of dilute sulfuric acid and a few drops of ferric chloride solution. A dark green color that disappears after a few minutes is positive for phenylpyruvic acid or some interfering substance.

If the color is obtained, remove creatinine with Lloyd reagent (a specially prepared silicious earth) and repeat the test.

Interfering substances are chlorpromazine, aspirin, and acetoacetic acid. The test may not be positive in infants until after 2 or 3 wk. of age. The urine may be dried on **absorbent paper (filter paper)**, and the test can be made even after several months. The mother is instructed to put pieces of filter paper into the diaper, and a small portion of the filter paper can be either used for the chemical test or attached to the chromatography paper.

Paper chromatography: See p. 21.

Phenistix: A reagent strip, Phenistix,* allows routine screening of all infants. Large amounts of urates and phosphates do not interfere with the strip test but do influence the older ferric chloride method.

Though not related to the problem of phenylketonuria, it should be mentioned that Phenistix may be used to test the urine of patients receiving antituberculous therapy for para-aminosalicylic acid (PAS) and its metabolites.

Phenylalanine bioassay (Guthrie test): Performance of this test during the first week of life of the infant is compulsory in many states. In an affected infant it may be positive 24 hr. after the first milk feeding.

Principle: Germination of spores of *Bacillus subtilis* is markedly enhanced by the presence of phenylalanine in a medium containing an inhibitor to spore germination. One drop of blood taken from the infant's heel is collected on a special filter paper disk, which is then placed on the streaked medium. The area of bacterial growth around the specimen disk is compared with areas of growth around control disks containing known amounts of phenylalanine. Elevated phenylalanine plasma levels may be found before urine levels are increased. Ames* prepares a kit (Pheniplates) to screen 325 newborn infants.

*Ames Co., Inc., Elkart, Ind.

Quantitative fluorometric phenylalanine determination in blood: This is the method of choice as both the Guthrie method and Phenistix may produce false positive results.[27]

Principle: The test is based on the fact that the fluorescence of the phenylalanine-ninhydrin-copper complex is greatly enhanced when formed in the presence of a peptide such as leucyl-alanine. Since the test is often performed on infants, the directions are given for use of only a small amount of serum. With microtechniques even smaller amounts can be used.[28]

Reagents:

1. Succinate buffer, 0.6M, pH 5.88. Dissolve 16.21 gm. sodium succinate ($Na_2C_4H_4O_4 \cdot 6H_2O$) in water containing 8 ml. 1N hydrochloric acid and dilute almost to 100 ml. Mix well and check the pH. Adjust if necessary and dilute to 100 ml. Store in refrigerator.
2. Ninhydrin, 0.03M. Dissolve 0.534 gm. ninhydrin in water to make 100 mm. Store in refrigerator.
3. Leucyl-alanine, 0.005M. Dissolve 0.100 gm. of the peptide in 100 ml. water. This solution is not stable. It may be divided into small aliquots and kept frozen until needed. If the test is run only occasionally, it may be more convenient to use either sterile ampules containing 1 mg./ml. of peptide* or preweighed vials containing 2 mg. of the peptide† to be dissolved just before use.
4. Fluorescence reagent: On the day of use mix together 5 vol. solution 1 (succinate buffer), 2 vol. solution 2 (ninhydrin), and 1 vol. solution 3 (peptide).
5. Copper diluent. Prepare daily by mixing together 3 vol. of solution containing 2.66 gm. anhydrous sodium carbonate and 113 mg. Rochelle salt in 1 L., and 2 vol. solution containing 200 mg. crystalline copper sulfate/L.
6. Trichloroacetic acid, 0.6M. Dissolve 9.8 gm. trichloroacetic acid in water and dilute to 100 ml.
7. Phenylalanine standards. Dissolve 5, 10, and 20 mg. phenylalanine in 100 ml. solution containing 7.5% bovine albumin. Also prepare a blank solution containing only the bovine albumin. Divide the standards and blank in small aliquots in test tubes, stopper securely, and keep frozen, thawing as needed. The standards are made up in bovine albumin so that when the standards are treated like the serum samples the final pH will be the same in all.

Procedure: Add 0.1 ml. serum or heparinized plasma to 0.1 ml. trichloroacetic acid in a small test tube. Mix well and allow to stand for 10 min. Treat 0.1 ml. aliquots of the blank and standards similarly. After they stand for a while, centrifuge strongly. To 0.5 ml. supernatant add 0.80 ml. mixed reagent and incubate at 60° C. for 2 hr. Cool by immersion in tap water, then add 5 ml. copper diluent. Mix and determine the fluorescence within 1 hr. Use filters with an activating wavelength of 365 mμ and a secondary filter at 515 mμ. Either read standards and samples against blank or read all tubes against water and subtract blank reading from that of standards and samples.

Calculation:

$$\frac{\text{Sample reading}}{\text{Standard reading}} \times \text{Conc. of standard} =$$

$$\text{Conc. of sample}$$

The readings are corrected for the blank and the standard reading closest to the sample reading is used. The three standards used are equivalent to 5, 10, and 20 mg.% phenylalanine.

Normal values and interpretation: By this method the normal range for adults is 0.9-2.2 mg.%; for newborn infants, 1.6-2.6 mg.%. Newborn infants with low birth weights have a slightly higher range, 3.7-4.7 mg.%. In contrast, phenylketonuric children have levels of 16-46 mg.%. Heterozygous parents of phenylketonuric children have slightly higher values than the normal adult population, with a range of 1.4-2.5 mg.%.

---

*Mann Laboratories, New York, N. Y.
†Sigma Chemical Co., St. Louis, Mo.

Phenylalanine tolerance test[29]: This test is useful for the diagnosis of heterozygotes. A dose of 200 mg./kg. of L-phenylalanine is divided into two portions; one-half is given initially and the other half is given 30 min. later. A discriminant score of 3.51 ± 0.374 is normal, while heterozygotes have a score of 2.32 ± 0.374.

ALKAPTONURIA (ALKAPTON BODIES): This is a rare congenital (single recessive gene) metabolic disease in which the enzyme homogentisic acid oxidase is absent. The error in the metabolism of phenylalanine and tyrosine leads to the accumulation and excretion of homogentisic acid which cannot be metabolized. The patient is clinically well until the later years of life when black pigments are deposited in the bones and joints (ochronosis). Urine may appear normal upon voiding but turns reddish brown or black upon standing or upon becoming alkaline. The reaction begins at the surface. Alkapton bodies reduce copper but not bismuth. They do not ferment. Similar reactions are given by hydroquinone.

Tests:
1. Add excess of 10% sodium hydroxide and shake. The urine will quickly turn black.
2. Add 10% ferric chloride drop by drop. A bluish green color will develop and then fade.
3. Benedict qualitative test will produce a yellow precipitate.

TYROSINURIA[30]: This is a rare congenital defect in which p-hydroxyphenylpyruvic acid appears in the urine and gives a positive Millon reaction.

Millon test: With the aid of heat, 1 ml. Hg is dissolved in 2 ml. concentrated nitric acid and then diluted with 2 parts water, allowed to stand for several hours, and then filtered. This reagent is added to urine in equal parts, and the mixture is heated to the boiling point. A red precipitate appears if tyrosine or p-hydroxyphenylpyruvic acid is present.

HOMOCYSTINURIA[31]: This is due to a congenital (recessive gene) defect in the metabolism of methionine, leading to excessive amounts of homocystine in the urine. Clinically the disease is character-

ized by mental retardation associated with ocular, vascular, and skeletal changes. Cystinuria and homocystinuria can be distinguished by high-voltage paper electrophoresis.

Other inherited enzymatic defects that have been described are as follows: argininosuccinic aciduria, hyperglycinemia, histidinemia, and hyperprolinemia.

SUGAR REDUCING SUBSTANCES

Glycosuria results from diabetes and other endocrine disturbances, intravenous glucose infusion, ingestion of large amounts of sugar, renal tubular disorders, brain lesions, and stress. About 70% of normal pregnant women show an intermittent temporary glycosuria that appears to be of no clinical significance.[32]

If a sensitive quantitative method such as the glucose oxidase method is used, measurable amounts of glucose are found in all urine specimens of normal individuals; 91% have from 1-15 mg./100 ml. glucose, with a mean of 7 mg./100 ml. The Clinitest method does not "pick up" 7 mg./100 ml. but will record 15 mg./100 ml.

Tests for identification of sugar reducing substances

To test for the presence or absence of sugar reducing substances in the urine follow the procedure indicated (Fig. 2-1).
1. Benedict reagent heated at 100° C. (boiling) for 5 min. will be reduced (positive reaction) by glucose, fructose, lactose, galactose, and pentose. No reaction (negative reaction, blue color remains) indicates the absence of sugar or any other reducing substance. Clinitest tablets* can also be used.
2. Specific enzyme test for glucose.
3. Benedict reagent heated at 55° C. for 10 min. will be reduced by fructose and pentose (and glucose over 4%). Pentose can be tested for with orcin test and paper chromatography on the original sample. Fermentation with bakers' yeast removes

---

*Ames Co., Inc., Elkhart, Ind.

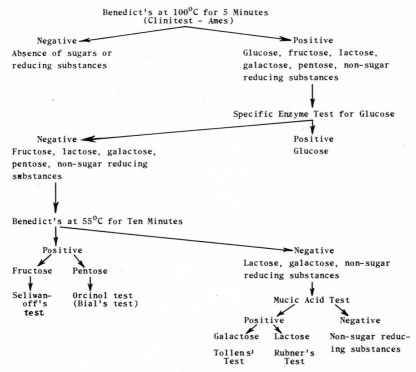

Fig. 2-1. Differentiation of urinary reducing substances.

glucose and fructose. Fructose can be confirmed by the Selivanoff test or paper chromatography on the original sample.

4. If step 3 is negative, do mucic acid test. Lactose and galactose will produce mucic acid; nonsugar reducing substances will not. Galactose (pentose and glucuronic acid) will give a positive Tollen test (phloroglucinol-hydrochloric acid reaction). Lactose will give a positive Rubner test.

Other tests that can be utilized in the identification of sugars are polariscopy and phenylhydrazine crystal formation.

GLUCOSE, FRUCTOSE, LACTOSE, GALACTOSE, AND PENTOSE:

Benedict qualitative test:

Principle: The reagent consists of copper sulfate, sodium citrate, and sodium carbonate. Substances containing free keto or aldehyde groups reduce the soluble cupric salt to insoluble yellow to red cuprous oxide.

Technique: Place 5 ml. Benedict qualitative reagent in a test tube, add 5 drops (or 0.25 ml.) urine, mix, and place in boiling water bath 5 min. or boil over flame 1-2 min. A green, yellow, or red color with a yellow or red precipitate is positive. A clear or cloudy blue color with a grayish precipitate is negative. Allow to cool at room temperature before discarding as negative.

The test may be positive with as little as 0.02% glucose or other reducing substances.

Reagent:

1. Copper sulfate, CP, crystals, 17.3 gm.
2. Sodium or potassium citrate, CP, 173 gm.
3. Sodium carbonate, crystals (or 100 gm. anhydrous salt), 200 gm.
4. Distilled water to make 1000 ml.

Dissolve citrate and carbonate by heating in about 700 ml. water. Dissolve the copper sulfate in about 100 ml. water and pour into the other fluid. Cool and make up to 1 L.

Rough estimate of amount of sugar in urine from qualitative test: This is help-

Table 2-1

Benedict	Glucose (%)	Reaction
Red	3	4+
Reddish yellow	2	4+
Greenish yellow	1	3+
Yellowish green	0.7	2+
Green	0.3-0.5	1+
Bluish green	0.2-0.25	Trace
Greenish blue	0.1	Trace
Blue (gray precipitate, if any)	None	0

ful in following diabetic patients. Read the tests promptly without setting aside to cool. Consult Table 2-1.

Clinitest tablets: They form a standardized self-heating method for quantitative determination of urine sugar by a copper reduction method. A color chart provides a rough estimate of the amount of sugar present.

Phenylhydrazine reaction (osazone test): To a small test tube add 1 vol. 10% phenylhydrazine hydrochloride and 2 vol. 10% sodium acetate. Add 4 vol. urine to the reagent, mix, and heat in boiling water bath for 45 min. Remove and let stand for at least 1 hr. Microscopic crystals are formed by glucose, galactose, fructose, lactose, and maltose. These crystals have characteristic melting points and differ in shape and size.

Paper chromatography in the identification of sugar in urine[33-35]: Since chromatography is of importance in the identification of soluble substances (sugars, amino acids, porphyrins, steroids, etc.), this method is described in some detail.

Principle: Separation and identification is dependent on the different solubility of each sugar (or any other solute) in water, which is absorbed by the filter paper and thus considered to be the stationary phase, and in an organic solvent, which is immiscible but saturated with water and thus considered to be the mobile phase. The filter paper acts as an inert support for the stationary phase. The solvent is shaken and mixed with water. Then it is allowed to separate so that two layers are produced—a water-rich layer

used as the stationary phase and a water-poor layer used as the mobile phase. The mobile phase is allowed to flow past the urine spot, carrying with it the sugar and displacing it from its original position. The sugar (or any unknown solute) is identified by its R_f value, which is one of its specific physical constants. Since the R_f value of identical substances under identical conditions is the same, known control sugars should be run with the unknown specimen. The R_f value of a soluble substance is the ratio of the distance moved by the solute from its application (loading) point to the movement of the solvent past the application point of the unknown.

$$R_f = \frac{\text{Movement of solute}}{\text{Movement of solvent}}$$

Reagents:
Solvents (choice of two):
1. n-Butanol, 60 ml.; pyridine, 40 ml.; distilled water, 30 ml.
2. n-Butanol, 40 ml.; glacial acetic acid, 10 ml.; water, 50 ml.

The mixture is thoroughly shaken. The layers are allowed to separate and are saved separately.

Stains:
1. Aniline hydrogen oxalate reagent. 0.9 ml. of redistilled aniline is shaken with 100 ml. 0.1N oxalic acid solution (used as spray).
2. 0.5% w/v dinitrosalicylic acid in 4% w/v NaOH (used as spray).

Procedure:
1. A small dot is made with a pencil approximately 6 cm. from one end of a strip of chromatography paper (Whatman No. 1). Care must be taken to handle the filter paper with forceps or clean hands.
2. Using a micropipette or a Sahli pipette, 10-20 λ urine are placed on the dot. About 1-2 λ urine are applied at a time to prevent the spot from spreading beyond a 3-4 mm. area. The spot is allowed to dry before the next aliquot is added. This manner of application is followed until the entire 10 or 20 λ urine have been added. The volume of urine depends upon the amount of sugar

present. If less than 0.5% sugar is present, 20 λ urine are used; for 0.5-1% sugar, 10 λ are used; if more than 1% sugar, 5 λ are used.

3. The water-rich stationary phase is placed into two containers at the bottom of the airtight chromatography chamber or tube.

4. The loaded chromatographic strip is carefully inserted into the tube without the strip touching the walls of the tube (Fig. 2-2). The end of the paper having first been placed into a trough within the chamber, the paper is allowed to become saturated by the water vapors of the water-rich phase.

5. The solvent (mobile water-poor phase) is placed into the trough and is allowed to descend the chromato-graphic paper for a distance of approximately 130 mm. (about 2 hr.).

6. The strip is removed from the tube, and the limit of solvent flow is marked with a pencil. The paper is then dried 10 min. at 100°-105° C.

7. The paper is sprayed lightly and evenly with the staining solution. Too much color-developing reagent must be avoided.

8. The paper is then heated at 100°-105° C. for 10 min., and the R_f values are established for the sugars in the urine.

9. Sugars are identified by comparing the R_f values of the unknown with the R_f values obtained from sugar standards (1%) run under identical conditions. (Fig. 2-3.)

$$R_f = \frac{\text{Distance solute spot traveled}}{\text{Distance solvent front traveled}}$$

R_f values:

Glucose	0.31
Fructose	0.38
Galactose	0.28
Lactose	0.14
Xylose	0.50

Since several factors such as temperature, water saturation of mobile phase and of filter paper, filter paper composition, interferring substances, method of chromatography used, etc. slightly influence the R_f value, known controls should always be included in each test.

Quantitative estimation—Benedict method: Into a large test tube, 200 × 25 mm., measure 5 ml. Benedict quantitative

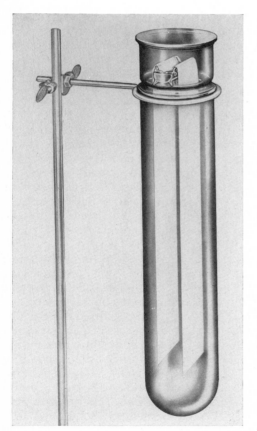

Fig. 2-2. Ring-supported chromatotube with papers. (Courtesy Research Specialties Co., Richmond, Calif.)

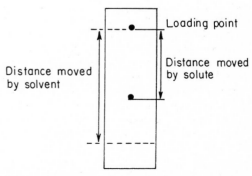

Fig. 2-3. Paper chromatography. Filter paper strip showing method of measuring R_f value.

solution from a burette. Add about 1 gm. sodium carbonate anhydrous (about ¼ tsp.) and a pebble or a glass bead. Heat to boiling and add from a 1 ml. pipette (graduated in 0.01 ml.) the urine which has been filtered and accurately diluted if the qualitative test shows a large amount of sugar. Keep the mixture boiling and determine the amount of urine necessary to cause the disappearance of the last trace of blue color. The urine may be added fairly rapidly in small amounts until a chalklike precipitate is observed, after which it is to be added a drop or two at a time, boiling the mixture thoroughly between each addition. Loss of volume should be restored by adding a few drops of water from time to time. Check determinations should be made.

Reagent:

1. Copper sulfate, CP, fine crystals, 90 gm.
2. Sodium carbonate, crystals (or 500 gm. anhydrous salt), 1000 gm.
3. Sodium or potassium citrate, CP, 1000 gm.
4. Potassium thiocyanate, CP, 625 gm.
5. Potassium ferrocyanide solution, 5%, 25 ml.
6. Distilled water to make 5000 ml.

Dissolve carbonate, citrate, and thiocyanate in about 3500 ml. water by heating and then filter. Dissolve copper in 500 ml. water and pour slowly into the other fluid, stirring constantly. Add the ferrocyanide solution, cool, and dilute to 5000 ml. Weigh the copper accurately and transfer quantitatively; 25 ml. equals 0.05 gm. glucose. Keeps well.

Calculation: One divided by the number of ml. of urine used gives the percentage of sugar (gm./100 ml.) if urine was not diluted. Correction for dilution must be made.

If the sugar is over 2%, make an accurate dilution (1:2 or 1:3) of the urine before proceeding with the tests and make correction in the calculation.

The 5 ml. Benedict quantitative solution is reduced completely by adding 0.01 gm. glucose.

When this method is used for sugars other than glucose, the values equivalent to 5 ml. Benedict solution are as follows: levulose, 0.0106 gm.; galactose, 0.0108 gm.; lactose, 0.0134 gm.; maltose, 0.0148 gm. These values multiplied by 100 and divided by the number of ml. required to reduce the Benedict solution will give the percentage of the sugar (gm./100 ml.).

Report determinations in percentage and also in gm./24 hr.

NOTES: Sucrose is quickly inverted to glucose by yeast at room temperature, giving a strongly positive Benedict test within a few minutes. After fermentation is complete (overnight), the copper reduction test will be negative.

Sucaryl,* a synthetic sweetening agent, does not give the tests for sugar and does not interfere with any of the usual clinical laboratory tests.

GLUCOSE:

Specific enzyme test: The reagent for this test is supplied as test paper (Tes-Tape,† Clinistix†). A specific enzyme, glucose oxidase, oxidizes glucose, forming gluconic acid and hydrogen peroxide; horseradish peroxidase catalyzes the reaction between the hydrogen peroxide and orthotoluidine to form a blue color.[33]

The reagent is nontoxic and stable if protected from strong light. It is specific for glucose and does not give false positive reactions with other sugars or other reducing substances found in the urine. Drugs usually found in the urine do not interfere with the test and do not give false positive reactions, but the presence of large amounts of ascorbic acid will delay or prevent the reaction. The normal pH variation of the urine does not affect the test.

If urine contains glucose, always test for ketone bodies.

Somogyi quantitative test for glucose: This test is based on the caramelization of glucose in a hot alkaline solution. The process produces a yellow to brown color which is quantitative and reproducible and can be compared with the color of standard solutions available in a comparator.‡ This test is not specific for glucose. It is easily and rapidly performed on several specimens at the same time.

---

*Abbott Laboratories, Chicago, Ill.
†Eli Lilly & Co., Indianapolis, Ind.
‡Aloe Scientific Division, Brunswick Corp., St. Louis, Mo.

Reagent:

1. Anhydrous sodium carbonate, 10 gm.
2. Distilled water to make 100 ml.

Procedure: Mix 10 ml. sodium carbonate solution with 1 ml. clear urine in a test tube which is similar to the tubes in the comparator block. The mixture is placed in a boiling water bath for 8 min., and the resulting color is compared with standards in the comparator block.

Fermentation test: Boil urine to kill ferments and microorganisms. Cool and add enough yeast to make a thin emulsion. Mix carefully to avoid absorption of air and pour into a sterile fermentation tube, filling the closed arm. Make two controls as follows. Positive control: add a pinch of glucose to some of the specimen prepared as for the test and place in fermentation tube. Negative control: this is made especially to test for self-fermentation of the yeast. Add yeast to water that has been boiled and cooled and place in a fermentation tube. The fermentation tubes should be cleaned and boiled before use. Stopper the tubes with cotton and incubate for 24 hr. See that there are no air bubbles in the closed arm before tubes are put in incubator. Gas in closed arm indicates a positive test. Results should be discarded if controls fail. This test will be positive with over 0.1% glucose.

If more than 0.5-1% glucose is present, the following quick method (A. P. Mathews) can be used. Boil urine and cool down. To 10 ml. add ¼ cake Fleischmann's yeast, emulsify carefully, and place in test tube in inclined position in water bath at 40°-43° C. The small amount of air enclosed will all come off in a minute in small bubbles. If glucose (or a fermenting sugar) is present, within 5-10 min. numerous small bubbles of gas will rise against the side of the tube. Fermentation is stormy when 3% is present.

This rapid fermentation is useful in getting rid of glucose, an hour's fermentation being sufficient usually. If urine contains glucose only, the Benedict test will be negative after fermentation. If it contains lactose and glucose or pentose and glucose, the Benedict test will be positive after this fermentation. This procedure is useful also in the interpretation of trace reactions, in which a much shorter incubation period of 10-15 min. may be used. Quantitative determinations may be made before and after fermentation to determine the amounts of glucose and lactose or pentose. When reduction is positive after fermentation, test for lactose and pentose.

FRUCTOSE AND PENTOSE:

Benedict modified qualitative test: Place 5 ml. Benedict qualitative reagent in a test tube, add 5 drops urine, mix, and place in water bath at 55° C. for 10 min. Fructose and pentose will reduce the copper reagent.

FRUCTOSE: Levulose (fructose) appears in the urine as a rare disorder of metabolism (idiopathic levulosuria) and with glucose in diabetes mellitus. It may appear after eating large amounts of fruits or honey (alimentary levulosuria) and especially in liver impairment (hepatitis).

Levulose gives a positive Selivanoff test.

Selivanoff test: To 5 ml. reagent add 5 drops urine and heat to boiling. A reddish color and the separation of a red precipitate that is soluble in alcohol indicates the presence of levulose. If glucose is present in large amounts, dilute the urine to make the amount less than 2%.

The test is positive also with mannoheptulose (from the avocado), but fructose is fermentable, whereas mannoheptulose is not.

Reagent: Dissolve 50 mg. resorcinol in 70 ml. water and add 30 ml. concentrated hydrochloric acid.

Fructose is a reducing sugar that can be fermented and is levorotatory; this rotation disappears after fermentation. Paper chromatography and lactosazone formation are other means of identification.

PENTOSE: Pentose occurs in the urine after ingestion of fruits such as cherries (alimentary pentosuria) and as a congenital anomaly of metabolism (idiopathic pentosuria) characterized by inability to metabolize L-xylose. It has no relation to diabetes mellitus. Pentosuria occurs sometimes following the use of carinamide to raise the penicillin blood level.

Bial orcin test: Remove dextrose if present by fermentation and filter. Boil 5 ml. reagent in a test tube, remove from flame, and without further heating add drop by drop with mixing not more than 20 drops of the specimen. A green color indicates the presence of pentose. Add 2 ml. amyl alcohol and shake. Fill tube with water to cause alcohol to separate. The alcohol absorbs the green color.

Reagent:
1. Hydrochloric acid, CP, 100 ml.
2. Ferric chloride solution, 10%, 5 drops
3. Orcin, 0.3 gm.

Glucuronates may give a positive reaction upon continued boiling. Make the **Cole test.** Mix 15 ml. urine with 0.5 gm. Merck blood charcoal, boil, and let stand 10 min., shaking at intervals. Filter. Glucuronates will filter out. Charcoal removes all reducing substances except dextrose, levulose, pentose, and formaldehyde (Urotropin or preservative). Repeat the Bial test with the filtrate.

Aniline test: Remove glucose if present by fermentation and filter. To 2 ml. urine add 2 ml. glacial acetic acid and 5 drops pure (redistilled) aniline. Heat just to boiling and after 2 min. cool and extract with 2 ml. chloroform. Pentose gives a bright red color which is soluble in the chloroform. Sensitivity is 0.03%. Glucose gives an interfering green color if not removed.

Tauber test: To 2.5 ml. reagent add 0.5 ml. urine and mix. Boil 2 min., cool by immersing in water, add 5 ml. distilled water, and mix. Pentose produces a pink to red color.

Reagent:
1. Benzidine, 1 gm.
2. Glacial acetic acid, 25 ml.

GALACTOSE AND LACTOSE:

Mucic acid test: To 50 ml. urine add 12 ml. concentrated nitric acid and boil until volume is about 10 ml. Cool and add 10 ml. water. Let stand overnight. Fine white precipitate of mucic acid crystals indicates the presence of lactose or galactose.

GALACTOSE: Galactose is formed by hydrolysis of lactose. It is converted to glucose in the liver and then is metabolized as glucose with the aid of insulin. The ability of the liver to convert galactose into glucose forms the basis of the galactose tolerance test, a hepatic function test.

Galactosuria occurs as an acquired condition in liver disease and as a congenital disease in infants. In congenital galactosemia there is impaired ability to convert galactose to glucose so that the blood galactose level is elevated and galactose appears in the urine. The basic defect lies in the inability to convert galactose-1-phosphate to glucose-1-phosphate because of a hereditary congenital absence of the enzyme galactose-1-phosphate uridyl transferase. This enzyme is normally present in the red blood cells, which may therefore be used as indicators of galactosemia.

If the disease is allowed to progress, it leads to cirrhosis of the liver, mental retardation, and blindness.

Galactose (galactosuria) can be identified by the mucic acid test, the phloroglucin test, paper chromatography, and osazone crystal formation.

Spot-screening test for galactosemia[36]:
Principle: Whole blood (or for the micromethod, a strip of filter paper with dried capillary blood) is added to a reaction mixture containing alpha-galactose-1-phosphate (Gal-1-P), uridine diphosphoglucose (UDPG), triphosphopyridine nucleotide (TPN), buffer, and saponin. If transferase is present by way of several intermediate steps, beta-glucose-6-phosphate is formed. Glucose-6-phosphate dehydrogenase in the hemolysate oxidizes it to 6-phosphogluconate, which in turn is oxidized to ribulose-5-phosphate. These reactions lead to the reduction of TPN. Reduced TPN fluoresces when activated with long-wavelength ultraviolet light. The reaction mixture is spotted on Whatman No. 1 filter paper and allowed to dry.

Reaction mixture (6 ml.):
1. UDPG sodium salt (6 mg./ml.), 0.2 ml.
2. Gal-1-P dipotassium salt (10 mg./ml.), 0.4 ml.

3. TPN (5 mg./ml.), 0.6 ml.
4. Triacetate buffer (pH 8.0),* 2 ml.
5. Saponin (1%), 0.8 ml.
6. Disodium EDTA (1 mg./100 ml.), 0.03 ml.
7. Distilled water, 1.97 ml.

Technique: Add 0.02 ml. heparinized blood to 0.2 ml. reaction mixture with a pipette which is left in the reaction mixture while it is incubated at 37° C. for 2 hr. The solution is then spotted on Whatman No. 1 filter paper covering an area of 3-15 mm., allowed to dry, and examined under long-wavelength ultraviolet light.

Interpretation: Bright fluorescence indicates a normal specimen or samples from individuals heterozygous for galactosemia or homozygous for the Duarte variant.[37] Blood from homozygous galactosemia patients fails to fluoresce. Heterozygotes for galactosemia and homozygotes for the Duarte variant can be discovered by spotting the filter paper after 1 hr. incubation, at which time they show less fluorescence than normal.

Phloroglucin test (Tollens test): Mix equal parts of urine and hydrochloric acid (specific gravity 1.09 or 50% by volume), add a little phloroglucin, and heat in a boiling water bath.

Galactose, pentose, and glucuronic acid give a red color. Pentose and glucuronic acid give an absorption band in the yellow portion of the spectrum, whereas galactose does not.

A positive mucic acid test rules out all other reducing substances except lactose.

LACTOSE: Lactose appears in the urine of women during lactation and sometimes in the urine of infants, especially during digestive upsets.

Lactose gives a positive Rubner test.

Rubner test: To 10 ml. urine add 2 or 3 gm. lead acetate, shake, and filter. Boil and add 1 ml. strong ammonia. Boil again. Lactose gives a brick-red color with a red precipitate and dextrose, a red solution with a yellow precipitate.

Lactose gives a positive mucic acid test, a negative phloroglucin test (exclud-

ing galactose), and a negative Bial test (excluding pentose).

When the urine is diluted to contain less than 1% lactose, it may be removed with charcoal. (See method in discussion of pentose.)

MALTOSE: This is a reducing sugar that hydrolyzes to glucose. It does not reduce Barfoed reagent. It occurs rarely in urine but may be found with glucose in diabetes.

Barfoed reagent: Dissolve 9 gm. copper acetate in 100 ml. water. Add 1.2 ml. acetic acid, 50%. Mix.

Test: Boil 5 ml. reagent and add 1 ml. urine drop by drop, heating after each addition. Let stand until cool. A red precipitate is positive. Maltose gives a negative test. If maltose is present, the fermentation test produces carbon dioxide, and the osazone test leads to the formation of maltosazones. Lactose also gives a negative Barfoed test, but does not produce carbon dioxide when fermented, forms lactosazones, and gives a positive mucic acid test.

GLUCURONATES: Glucuronates occur in the urine conjugated with aromatic acids, phenols, alcohols, and drugs (aspirin, morphine, sulfonamides, benzoic acid, phenylacetic acid, etc). Glucuronic acid is formed and conjugated in the liver. The glucuronates are not fermentable. They may be removed from the urine by charcoal (**Cole test**).

The clinical significance is twofold: glucuronates are reducing substances and interfere with tests for glucose in the urine, and their presence may be used as an indicator of the detoxifying function of the liver.

NONSUGAR REDUCING SUBSTANCES

Most of these substances give only trace reactions. They are uric acid; creatinine in concentrated urine; preservatives such as chloroform and formalin; drugs such as PAS, terramycin, chloral hydrate, streptomycin, and salicylates; and alkapton bodies. Urines containing over 2% proteins should be rendered protein free by boiling and acidification with acetic acid prior to using the reduction method for sugar.

---

*Tris (81 gm.); distilled water (700 ml.); glacial acetic acid to pH 8.0; and H_2O to 1000 ml.

Uric acid, creatinine, vitamin C (ascorbic acid), and glucuronic acid are weakly reducing and cause difficulties only if present in increased amounts. They can be removed by mixing with charcoal and 0.10 vol. alcohol, followed by filtration. The alcohol prevents the absorption of sugars.

Preservatives such as chloroform and formaldehyde are also nonsugar reducing substances, as are homogentisic acid, penicillin, and streptomycin.

KETONE BODIES

Ketone bodies consist of acetoacetic acid (diacetic acid), beta-hydroxybutyric acid, and acetone. In small amounts these compounds appear normally as intermediary compounds of fat metabolism. Under conditions of depletion of liver glycogen (starvation, diabetes, prolonged vomiting, severe diarrhea in children, von Gierke's disease, high fat diet, and low carbohydrate diet), the oxidation of these compounds of fat metabolism is arrested so that they accumulate in the blood (ketonemia), are excreted in the urine (ketonuria), and lead to a general condition called ketosis. In ketosis, fresh urine contains more acetoacetic acid than beta-hydroxybutyric acid, and both exceed in concentration that of acetone. But on standing the acetoacetic and beta-hydroxybutyric acids decompose, and the concentration of acetone increases.

If urine contains reducing substances, always test for ketone bodies.

Lange nitroprusside test: This is positive with acetone and acetoacetic acid. Dissolve a few crystals of sodium nitroprusside in a few drops of water to a cherry-red color. Add 4 or 5 ml. urine and 0.5 ml. glacial acetic acid. Mix and pour into test tube. Overlay with strong ammonium hydroxide. A purple ring at the line of contact indicates a positive reaction. If positive, make test for acetoacetic acid. Report on basis of 1+ to 4+. One plus is about 1 ml./L.

Rothera nitroprusside test: This reacts with both acetone and acetoacetic acid, being more sensitive for the latter (about 20 times).

To 5 ml. urine add ammonium sulfate to saturation (about 1 gm.) and 2 or 3 drops sodium nitroprusside solution; mix and overlay with strong ammonium hydroxide. A reddish purple ring is positive.

This test has been modified (Wishart) for plasma and may be used as a test for ketosis.

Put 2 drops plasma or serum in a test tube and supersaturate with ammonium sulfate crystals by shaking. Add 2 drops of approximately 5% sodium nitroprusside solution and shake. Add 2 drops strong ammonium hydroxide and shake. Let stand 3 min. A permanganate color indicates a trace; light blue, a moderate amount; and deep blue, a large amount.

NOTE: Phthaleins (as after PSP and BSP tests) and cellulose containers give false positive tests.

Gerhardt ferric chloride test: This is given by acetoacetic acid and certain drugs, but not by acetone. To two thirds of a test tube full of urine, made acid with acetic acid if necessary, add ferric chloride solution (10%) drop by drop until all phosphates are precipitated. Do not add enough to give any color. If color is produced, add more urine, with caution, until the color disappears. Filter and divide filtrate into two parts, one of which is kept as a control. To the other part add more ferric chloride solution. A cherry-red or Bordeaux-wine color is positive and indicates acetoacetic acid or some interfering drug. If positive, measure another portion (10 ml.) of urine, make acid, add an equal volume of water, and boil down in an evaporating dish to about half of the original volume of urine taken (5 ml.). Cool, make up to original volume (10 ml.) with water, precipitate phosphates as before, and filter. To an amount of the filtrate equal to the control add the same amount of ferric chloride used for the other part of the test and compare the three tubes. If color was due to acetoacetic acid, this last tube will be negative or the color will be much paler; if due to a drug, the last tube will be similar to the test made without boiling.

This differential method is based on the fact that acetoacetic acid is oxidized by boiling to acetone which does not give a color reaction with ferric chloride.

Drugs, on the other hand, will not be changed by boiling.

In phenylpyruvic oligophrenia the phenylalanine in the urine gives a dark green reaction with ferric chloride, and in the presence of melanin a black color results.

Some of the drugs that give interfering color reactions are phenols, antipyrin and other coal tar antipyretics, bicarbonates, salicylates, acetates, and cyanates.

Hart test for beta-hydroxybutyric acid: Make urine acid with dilute acetic acid, add an equal volume of water, and boil down to half of the original volume. Cool and make up to the original volume with water. This removes acetone and acetoacetic acid. Divide into two portions and place in test tubes. To one portion add 1 ml. hydrogen peroxide, warm gently, and cool. This changes beta-hydroxybutyric acid to acetone. Make the **Lange test** on each portion. The portion not treated with peroxide should be negative. If beta-hydroxybutyric acid is present in the original specimen, a Lange test on the portion treated with peroxide will be positive.

Urine freed of sugar by fermentation is strongly levorotatory if it contains beta-hydroxybutyric acid.

Acetest and Ketostix: Acetest* (a tablet nitroprusside test) and Ketostix* (a strip nitroprusside test) are specific and accurate in the detection of ketone bodies. Both methods can also be used on serum, and the tablet can be used with whole blood.

Bilirubin

All the tests for bile are tests for bile pigment. Normally bilirubin is formed by the reticuloendothelial system (liver, spleen, and bone marrow) from the heme moiety of the hemoglobin molecule. It is carried in the plasma as free nonconjugated but protein-bound bilirubin to the liver where it is conjugated with glucuronic acid to form bilirubin-diglucuronide, which is excreted into the duodenum as one of the constituents of bile. (Bile consists of bile acids, bile salts, bilirubin, cholesterol, fatty acids, calcium,

*Ames Co., Inc., Elkhart, Ind.

and other substances of lesser importance.) In the intestinal tract the normally present bacteria reduce bilirubin to stercobilinogen and stercobilin. The latter is excreted in the feces, whereas the major portion of the stercobilinogen is absorbed into the portal circulation and excreted into bile and urine. In the urine it is called urobilinogen. After auto-oxidation it gives rise to urobilin. Some bilirubin is also produced outside the reticuloendothelial system from the porphyrin rings of myoglobins and cytochromes.

The kidney does not excrete unconjugated bilirubin but is able to excrete conjugated bilirubin.

The Gmelin, iodine, and Fouchet tests depend on the formation of blue or green compounds when bile pigment is treated with an oxidizing agent.

Gmelin test: Do not filter urine. Pour about 2 ml. urine into a tube and run 1 or 2 ml. yellow nitric acid under the urine. Bile gives a colored ring at the line of contact, green toward the urine, then red, and finally yellow toward the acid. Sensitive to 1:80,000. Thymol may give a similar play of colors, but the green is toward the acid side. Formalin may give a yellow ring. Indican and other pigments may give colored rings but will be unlike those of bile.

Reagent: A small drop of turpentine, a pine shaving, or a piece of tongue depressor placed in nitric acid will give yellow nitric acid.

This test may be applied to filter paper through which large quantities of urine have been filtered (Rosenbach modification). When filter paper is nearly dry, drop yellow nitric acid on it. Bile gives a play of colors with green on the periphery, then red, and yellow nearest the acid. Potassium iodide in urine may give a greenish color and later a bluish color with the filter paper modification.

The filter paper test may be made more sensitive by adding barium chloride to the urine before filtering. Barium chloride, which precipitates phosphates that entrain bile pigment, has been used in various techniques and seems to increase the sensitivity.[38] The following modification has been found most satisfactory.

Harrison's modification of Gmelin test: To about 10 ml. urine add about 1 gm. (¼ tsp.) barium chloride. Mix and filter. Spread the filter paper out and, when partly dry, drop on the precipitate a little Fouchet reagent or yellow nitric acid. A green color of biliverdin is positive and indicates the presence of bile (bilirubin) in the urine.

Fouchet reagent:
1. Trichloroacetic acid, 25 gm.
2. Distilled water, 100 ml.
3. Ferric chloride, 10% aqueous solution, 10 ml.

Watson uses filter paper strips impregnated with barium chloride on which the test is performed.

Franklin method: This method employs tablets of plaster of Paris and Fouchet reagent, both available commercially.*

Fouchet reagent gives an interfering purple color with **salicylates** (sodium salicylate, aspirin). Nitric acid does not do so.

Bile gives a green color with Obermayer reagent, but the color is not soluable in chloroform.

Foam test: Bile gives a yellow color to the foam when the urine is shaken, but the test is not sensitive or specific, being positive with urobilin compounds, acriflavine, and Pyridium.

Iodine test: This should be used when indican and other pigments interfere with the Gmelin test. The urine, acidified with acetic acid if necessary, is run down the side of a test tube under a dilute alcoholic solution of iodine (0.5%). Bile gives an emerald green color which diffuses into the urine. The color is due to a compound of iodine with bile and is not an oxidation product. This test is specific but not as sensitive as the Gmelin test. Sensitive to 1:10,000.

NOTES: It has been recommended that the test for bilirubin be included in every routine urinalysis.[39] A positive test may be the only positive finding in "hepatitis without jaundice."[40] The test has been recommended in the selection of all blood donors.[41]

Ictotest: Ictotest* is the name given to a standardized diazo tablet that acts with bilirubin in the urine to produce a purple color on a test mat within 30 sec.

Removal of bile pigments: Bile that interferes with other tests may be removed by one of several procedures. In the test for indican, bile is usually removed by means of basic lead acetate which also removes other pigments and some of the protein when present, but it will not remove hemoglobin.

In tests for urobilinogen and urobilin, solid calcium hydroxide ($Ca(OH)_2$), 5 gm., is usually preferred because it will remove the bile without removing the urobilinogen or the urobilin. It is usually preferred for removing bile from specimens collected for the PSP test. Mix well and filter through Whatman No. 1 paper.

Three types of jaundice are usually described—obstructive, hepatocellular, and hemolytic. In obstructive jaundice with complete obstruction there is bilirubin without urobilin or urobilinogen in the urine; with partial obstruction, both are present. In hepatocellular jaundice both are present. In hemolytic jaundice urobilin and urobilinogen, without bilirubin, are found in urine.

UROBILIN

Schlesinger test: To 5 ml. urine add 2 or 3 drops Lugol solution and let stand 10 min. to convert the chromogen into pigment. Add 5 ml. saturated absolute alcoholic zinc acetate solution, filter, and examine for a greenish fluorescence. The reaction is more marked after an hour or two.

If bilirubin is present, precipitate with calcium chloride (powder) and filter. Test the filtrate as before.

NOTE: Urobilin gives a yellow tint to the foam if present in a large amount, but does not give the Gmelin test for bile.

Schlesinger reagent: Saturated absolute alcoholic solution of zinc acetate. Grind in mortar. About 2.33 gm./100 ml. This should be freshly made because after about a week the strength is decreased due to the change of zinc acetate

---

*Aloe Scientific Division, Brunswick Corp., St. Louis, Mo.

*Ames Co., Inc., Elkhart, Ind.

to the monoclinic form which precipitates out.

Lugol solution:
1. Iodine, 5 gm.
2. Potassium iodide, 10 gm.
3. Water, 100 ml.

Significance: Urobilin is derived from urobilinogen on exposure to air and light or on addition of Lugol solution. Urobilin is considered identical with stercobilin in the feces. (See discussion of urobilinogen.) Urobilin does not produce color with Ehrlich reagent. The oxidation of urobilinogen to urobilin can be prevented by collecting the urine in a brown bottle containing 100 ml. petroleum ether and 5 gm. anhydrous sodium carbonate. Urobilin can be reduced to urobilinogen with the help of ferrous hydroxide.

Urobilinogen

Qualitative method—Ehrlich benzaldehyde test: Use only fresh urine because the chromogen is changed into pigment on exposure to light. The specimen should be a 2 hr. sample collected between 2 and 4 P.M.

To 10 ml. urine add 1 ml. reagent (Ehrlich benzaldehyde reagent) and let stand about 10 min. A cherry-red color indicates an increased amount of urobilinogen. The trace normally present gives only a very slight color.

Ehrlich dimethylaminobenzaldehyde reagent for urobilinogen:
1. Concentrated hydrochloric acid, 100 ml.
2. Distilled water, 100 ml.
3. *p*-Dimethylaminobenzaldehyde, 4 gm.

When the qualitative test shows an apparent increase of urobilinogen, repeat the test with dilutions of the urine 1:10, 1:20, etc., and report the highest dilution that gives a positive test (Wallace and Diamond). Observe by looking down through the tube held over a white surface. Normally the test is positive in dilutions of 1:20 or less.

NOTES: Formalin or methenamine (Urotropin) interferes with the test.

Acetone or antipyrin may produce a similar color.

If bile is present, precipitate with solid calcium chloride and filter. Test filtrate for bilirubin and, if positive, add more calcium chloride and filter again.

Pyridium, if present, will interfere because of the red color. Make test for urobilinogen on one portion before treating with Lugol solution and on another portion after treatment to convert urobilinogen to urobilin. Use similar amounts of specimen and reagent in each. The difference, if any, represents the amount of urobilinogen present.

Since Ehrlich reagent also gives a red color with indole, always confirm the presence of increased urobilinogen by making the Schlesinger test for urobilin, which is not positive with indole. An indican test will confirm the presence of increased indole.

Porphobilinogen gives a similar red color which, however, is not soluble in chloroform.

The urine of persons receiving para-aminosalicylic acid gives a similar interfering color.

Sulfonamides with a free amino group attached to the benzene ring (sulfanilamide, sulfapyridine, sulfathiazole, and sulfadiazine) and Novocain (procaine hydrochloride) give a greenish yellow color which interferes with the test. Use test for urobilin. (See discussion of test for sulfonamides.)

Quantitative method: See p. 360.

Significance: The chromogen urobilinogen appears in the urine only in traces normally. It is formed in the intestines by the reducing action of bacteria on bilirubin and is absorbed in small part, being chiefly excreted in the feces as urobilin (stercobilin). The absorbed portion is excreted in bile and urine.

Decreased urobilinogen: It is absent in feces and urine of newborn infants (absence of reducing bacteria) and in complete obstruction of the common bile duct. It may be absent after administration of antibiotics or drugs (sulfonamides) that change or destroy the intestinal flora. It is diminished with diminished bile formation (hunger), in incomplete obstruction of the common bile duct, and in acute hepatitis.

Increased urobilinogen: It is increased with increased bile formation, after increased blood destruction as in hemolytic anemias, and after infarctions.

Because of normal diurnal variations a single urine specimen may be negative. In preference to the previously mentioned 2:00 and 4:00 P.M. urine specimen, a 24 hr. urine specimen is advisable. (See discussion of special collection procedures.)

INDICAN

Obermayer test: If bile or other pigments are present, precipitate with basic lead acetate (a penknife point of powder to a test tube of urine) and filter. Calibrate a test tube with marks at 5 ml., 10 ml., and 12 ml. Into this test tube put 5 ml. urine and 5 ml. Obermayer reagent, mix, and let stand for 5 min. Add 2 ml. chloroform and mix by inverting until all of the color is dissolved by the chloroform. Indican gives a blue color. Normally the color is not deeper than sky blue. Add saturated potassium chlorate solution a drop at a time, mixing twice after each addition, and record the number of drops necessary to decolorize. Not over 2 drops are required normally.

Obermayer reagent: Dissolve 2 gm. ferric chloride in a liter of concentrated hydrochloric acid.

Potassium chlorate, saturated aqueous: Crystals 1 part to water 11.5 parts. Or 6.6 gm. anhydrous salt/100 ml. water.

Instead of a blue color, a red or violet color may appear in the chloroform. If the color is red, it may be due to potassium iodide and will disappear upon adding a few drops of strong sodium hyposulfite solution, or it may be due to indigo red, which does not disappear. Indigo red results from oxidation of skatoxyl potassium sulfate and has the same significance as the indigo blue from indican. If the color is violet, it may be due to a mixture of indican and potassium iodide, to the presence of salicyluric acid, or to thymol. The color from these interfering substances disappears after hyposulfite solution. If the chloroform then shows an increase of indican, remove by aspiration the supernatant fluid which contains the interfering substances, wash the chloroform with water twice, and add 5 ml. Obermayer reagent and 5 ml. water.

Then add the potassium chlorate as before.

Formalin and methenamine (Urotropin) prevent the indican reaction, but do not interfere with the potassium iodide reaction.

NOTES: Methylene blue or indigo blue (which may be produced spontaneously by oxidation of indican) may give the urine a greenish or bluish color. Both dyes are soluble in chloroform. To distinguish between these, heat a portion of urine with concentrated hydrochloric acid. Methylene blue is decolorized, and the color returns when the portion is shaken with air (Beddard test[42]).

Methylene blue gives an absorption band in the red portion of the spectrum.

Indigo does not give these tests.

Significance: When protein is decomposed by bacteria, indole and skatol are formed, and these are absorbed, oxidized to indoxyl and skatoxyl, conjugated with sulfuric acid, and excreted as potassium salts. The indoxyl potassium sulfate is indican. Normally there is not more than a trace in the urine. Pathologically it is increased with increased intestinal putrefaction, with diminished peristalsis (high intestinal obstruction), and with protein decomposition anywhere in the body. Indicanuria may be associated with hypercalcemia in a familial disease aptly called **blue diaper syndrome.**[43]

BLOOD: HEMOGLOBINURIA AND HEMATURIA

It is necessary to distinguish between **hematuria** and **hemoglobinuria,** the first being due to the presence of more or less intact red blood cells and the latter to the presence of dissolved hemoglobin. The centrifuged sediment will show red blood cells in the first case and may show hemoglobin casts in the second case but no red blood cells.

Hemoglobinuria

Free hemoglobin in the urine is the result of intravascular hemolysis, but it may also be due to disintegration of red cells in the urine upon standing. In the latter case the centrifuged specimen will contain the red cell envelopes. With the exception of spectroscopy, the tests for hemoglobin in the urine are also positive in hematuria.

Benzidine test—modification for urine: Phosphates, sulfates, urates, and ascorbic acid in the urine may form a milky suspension preventing the benzidine reaction.

Prepare a fresh saturated benzidine solution by mixing benzidine dihydrochloride (as much as would stay on the point of a knife blade) with about 2 ml. glacial acetic acid; add 2 ml. urine and 1 ml. freshly prepared 3% hydrogen peroxide (a 1:10 dilution Superoxol). The intensity and speed of the appearance of the blue color is in direct proportion to the amount of hemoglobin. This method is based on the fact that benzidine is oxidized by hemoglobin in the presence of active oxygen catalytically produced by hemoglobin from hydrogen peroxide.

The reaction with benzidine is very sensitive (1:100,000 dilution or more).

Occultest tablets: Occultest tablets provide a standardized test for occult blood. The test is based on the catalytic properties of hemoglobin. By interaction of tartaric acid and calcium acetate with strontium peroxide, hydrogen peroxide is formed, which is catalytically decomposed by hemoglobin to liberate oxygen which oxidizes orthotoluidine to a blue-colored derivative. This method is also applicable to serum hemoglobin determination. False positive reactions may follow contamination of the specimen with hydrogen peroxide produced by plants and bacteria.

Hemastix reagent strips[44]**:** When the Hemastix reagent strip* is dipped into urine containing hemoglobin, the latter catalyzes the oxidation of orthotoluidine by the peroxide released by the strip by the interaction of water, citrate buffers, and cumene hydroperoxide. The oxidized orthotoluidine is blue.

Spectroscopy: Normal and abnormal hemoglobin compounds can also be identified by spectroscopy. (See p. 103.)

Haptoglobins: Haptoglobin, a serum mucoprotein, unites stoichiometrically with free hemoglobin so that hemoglobin

appears in the urine only after haptoglobin is saturated. Plasma hemoglobin normally does not exceed about 5 mg./ 100 ml., whereas the kidney threshold for haptoglobin is about 150 mg./100 ml. Haptoglobin binds hemoglobin stoichiometrically. Since the haptoglobin-hemoglobin complex is not excreted by the kidneys, hemoglobinuria does not occur until all plasma haptoglobin is saturated (free hemoglobin level of 140 mg./100 ml.). As the hemoglobin-bound haptoglobin is not rapidly replaced, the plasma haptoglobin level falls during continued hemolysis, and free hemoglobin appears in the urine at much lower plasma hemoglobin levels than 140 mg./ 100 ml.

Hemoglobinuria may occur in the following conditions:

1. After incompatible blood transfusion
2. In hemolytic anemias associated with intravascular hemolysis, e.g., due to drugs, chemicals, and parasites (malaria)
3. In severe burns
4. Following poisoning such as from snake venom, spider bites, etc.
5. In paroxysmal nocturnal hemoglobinuria
6. In paroxysmal cold hemoglobinuria

Hemosiderin: Centrifuge the urine and examine the sediment for phagocytes containing a yellowish brown amorphous pigment.

Prussian blue reaction: Stain the sediment by adding a few drops of fresh reagent consisting of equal parts of 2% potassium ferrocyanide and 1% hydrochloric acid. Let stand 10 min. Granules of hemosiderin stain blue.

Hemosiderin is a yellow to brown granular pigment that is an iron hemoglobin derivative. The demonstration of hemosiderin is essentially the demonstration of inorganic iron.

Significance: This pigment contains colloidal ferric iron and occurs in the urinary sediment free and within cells in hemochromatosis and siderosis of the kidney following chronic hemoglobinemias. It is found consistently in the urine in paroxysmal nocturnal hemoglobinuria, in

---

*Ames Co., Inc., Elkhart, Ind.

which it may be present in the absence of acute hemoglobinuria.

Hematuria

The chief causes of hematuria are given in the discussion of urinary sediments (p. 46).

Three-glass test: This test is used to determine in a preliminary way the location and source of pus and blood in the urine of male patients.

Have the patient void and collect the specimen in three containers (urine glasses) without interrupting the flow of urine. Collect small amounts in the first and third containers and most of the voiding in the second container.

Sometimes this method is modified by stopping the flow of urine after the second glass, massaging the prostate and seminal vesicles, and then collecting the third glass.

Observe and record for each portion the relative cloudiness, the type and relative number of shreds grossly, and the relative number of blood and pus cells microscopically.

Make a gram stain on a smear made from a shred.

Significance: Table 2-2 lists the interpretation of the 3-glass test.

MYOGLOBIN

Myoglobin is a ferrous porphyrin similar to hemoglobin, but it has a molecular weight one-fourth that of hemoglobin, 17,000 vs. 68,000 of hemoglobin. Myoglobin is not bound to haptoglobin, its plasma level is low, and it is rapidly excreted by the kidneys.

CAUSES OF MYOGLOBINURIA[45]:
1. **Traumatic myoglobinuria.** It occurs frequently after crush injuries.
2. **March hemoglobinuria.** This appears after severe muscular exercise such as marching. No anemia is present.
3. **Paroxysmal myoglobinuria.** This occurs spontaneously and is accompanied by extreme muscular weakness and cramps. The muscles appear to be sensitive to lactic acid, and myohemoglobin is eliminated in the urine. The condition is seen in horses.
4. **Haff disease.** Myoglobinuria has been described in Germany, apparently due to eating fish and eels that have fed upon by-products (containing resinous acids) of cellulose factories polluting an inlet (Haff). No anemia occurs.

TESTS FOR MYOGLOBINURIA: The routine tests for hemoglobinuria are also positive if the pigment is myoglobin.

Spectroscopy: This test is not very satisfactory because the absorption bands (582 and 542 mμ) are very close to those of oxyhemoglobin. The procedure can be improved by using fluorescent light.

Ammonium sulfate test: In this test 5 ml. urine containing 2.8 gm. ammonium sulfate are centrifuged. Hemoglobin is precipitated, but myoglobin is not since hemoglobin is insoluble in 80% saturated solution of ammonium sulfate.

PORPHYRINS

The porphyrins are complex iron-free cyclic substances that are widely distributed in nature and appear in health as well as in disease. Combined with iron, protoporphyrin forms the pigment fraction of **hemoglobin** and **cytochromes**.

Coproporphyrin (first discovered in feces) and **uroporphyrin** (first discovered in urine) are the chief ones of interest in medicine. Both can be found in feces and urine. There are four main isomers of coproporphyrin and of uroporphyrin, respectively, but only types I and III of each are found in nature.

Porphyrins consist of **four pyrrole rings**

Table 2-2

First glass	Second glass	Third glass	Significance
Diffuse pus	Clear	Clear	Acute urethritis, usually anterior
Pus shreds	Clear	Clear	Subacute or chronic urethritis
Diffuse pus	Diffuse pus	Diffuse pus	Almost invariably infection above the urethra
Clear	Clear	Diffuse pus	Prostatitis, vesiculitis
Pus shreds	Clear	Diffuse pus	Urethritis prostatitis, vesiculitis

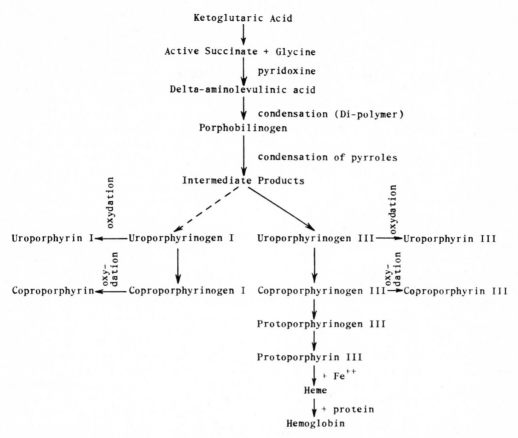

Fig. 2-4. Summary of the steps of biosynthesis of porphyrin derivatives. (Based on Harper: Review of physiological chemistry, ed. 10, Los Altos, Calif., 1965, Lange Medical Publications.)

linked by methene bridges to which various side chains are attached. Porphyrins form complexes with metal ions to produce various compounds such as hemoglobin, an iron porphyrin attached to globin, myoglobin, an iron-containing respiratory pigment occurring in muscle, and cytochrome, an iron-containing transfer agent. Porphyrins are synthesized in the living cell from **glycine** and **active succinate** (succinyl coenzyme A), which is produced from **alpha-ketoglutaric acid.** The first precursor is **delta-aminolevulinic acid** which leads to the formation of **porphobilinogen,** which is converted to **uroporphyrinogen** types III and I. The latter, in turn, are converted to the corresponding **coproporphyrinogens** types III and I. Coproporphyrinogen type III is then further metabolized to form **protoporphyrin-**

ogen type III and finally **heme.** The uroporphyrinogens and coproporphyrinogens under the influence of light form corresponding porphyrins (oxidation products). A porphyrin with symmetric substitution of side chains is classified as type I porphyrin, whereas a porphyrin with asymmetric substitution of side chains is designated as type III porphyrin.

Screening procedure for coproporphyrins and uroporphyrins:

Principle: Coproporphyrins are extracted from urine by ethyl ether and the uroporphyrins are obtained by extraction with ethyl acetate.

Method: Acidify 100 ml. urine with 10 ml. glacial acetic acid, mix, and allow to stand overnight.

Coproporphyrins: Extract the acetic

acid–urine mixture 3 times with 2-3 times the volume of ethyl ether, using a separatory funnel. Combine the ether extracts and wash once with 50 ml. distilled water which is returned to the orginal urine sample. Extract the ether 3 times with 2 ml. 25% aqueous hydrochloric acid. Combine the acid extracts and examine for red fluorescence under ultraviolet light.

Uroporphyrins: Adjust the acidity of the acetic acid–urine mixture to pH 3.0 by adding 1% aqueous hydrochloric acid. Extract the urine 3 times with 1-2 times the volume of ethyl acetate. These extracts are then combined and washed with 50 ml. distilled water. The ethyl acetate extracts are then extracted 3 times with 2 ml. 25% hydrochloric acid. The acid extracts are combined and examined for red fluorescence under ultraviolet light.

Screening test for fecal porphyrins (Dean)[46]: Routine testing for increased porphyrin excretion in stool is more reliable than routine testing for urinary porphyrins as the latter may not be detected in a dilute urine and as there are many false positive reactions (see interpretation).

Technique:
1. Collect a small fragment of stool on a finger stall, glass rod, or wooden stick.
2. Insert stool into a tube containing 2 ml. solvent consisting of equal parts of amyl alcohol, glacial acid, and ether.
3. Stir the solvent until it becomes a light brown color. The liquid is then decanted into a clean test tube.
4. Examine the solution in ultraviolet light in a darkened room or box.
5. The porphyric stool in ultraviolet light will show a brilliant pink fluorescence, persisting even if solvent is diluted several times.
6. If the patient is not porphyric, the solution will be green, gray, or perhaps slightly orange when examined by Wood's light.

Interpretation: A false positive test due to chlorophyll can be separated from a positive test for coproporphyrin and protoporphyrin as follows: add 2 ml. 1.5N HCl to the solvent (step 3), shake the mixture, and allow the acid to settle to the bottom of the tube. Coproporphyrin and protoporphyrin will be in the bottom of the test tube in the HCl, while the chlorophyll will remain in the top of the tube in the ether solution.

A high excretion of coproporphyrins does not necessarily mean that the patient is porphyric; e.g., cancer of colon or stomach may give positive findings.

If a positive screening test is obtained, quantitative stool and urine tests should be carried out if there is any doubt about the diagnosis. Dean reports that if the coproporphyrin is above 30 μg/gm. and the protoporphyrin is above 60 μg/gm. or the combined porphyrin is above 75 μg/gm. dry weight of stool, the possibility of porphyria must be considered. In most adult patients with porphyria variegate, the stool porphyrins are more than 200 μg/gm. dry weight of stool.

Urine screening test for coproporphyrins: Increased excretion of porphyrin in urine is seen in many conditions besides porphyria, e.g., lead poisoning and liver disease. Absence of porphyrin in urine may be found even if fecal porphyrins are positive.

The test is used chiefly as a screening test for lead intoxication.

Technique: To 10 ml. fresh urine in a test tube add 1 ml. of the previous solvent. Invert the tube several times to ensure adequate mixture and extraction. Allow to stand for a few minutes so that the solvent floats to the top. Examine in a dark room with ultraviolet light from Wood's lamp.

Interpretation: If excess porphyrin is present, the ether solution at the top of the test tube will show red fluorescence. In lead poisoning, porphyrin is found in the urine earlier than stippling is seen in the peripheral blood. Excessive porphyrin may be found in the urine even after exposure to lead has been discontinued.

Quantitative determination of urinary coproporphyrins and uroporphyrins[47, 48]:

Principle: Coproporphyrins and uroporphyrins are separated by selective extractions. At pH 4.8 the coproporphyrins are almost completely extracted from aqueous solution with ethyl acetate, while only a small amount of the uroporphyrins is extracted. If the pH is now lowered to 3.0, the uroporphyrins may be extracted with butanol. The porphyrins are then reextracted into 1.5N HCl and their absorbance is measured at 400-410 mμ.

Reagents:

1. Acetate buffer, pH 4.8. Mix 1 vol. glacial acetic acid with 3 vol. water and 4 vol. saturated aqueous solution of sodium acetate.
2. Iodine, 0.005%. Prepare a stock solution of iodine by dissolving 1 gm. iodine in 100 ml. 95% ethyl alcohol. Store in refrigerator. As required for use an aliquot is diluted 1:200 with water.
3. Sodium acetate, 1%. Dissolve 1 gm. anhydrous sodium acetate in water to make 100 ml.
4. Hydrochloric acid, 1.5N. Diluted 128 ml. concentrated hydrochloric acid to 1 L. with water.
5. Ethyl acetate, n-butyl alcohol, and petroleum ether (boiling point, 30°-60° C.) are reagent grade chemicals.

Coproporphyrins:

Procedure: To 100 ml. fresh urine in a separatory funnel add 50 ml. pH 4.8 acetate buffer and 150 ml. ethyl acetate. The mixture is shaken well for 1 min. and the layers are then allowed to completely separate. The lower aqueous layer is drawn off and reserved for uroporphyrin determination. The ethyl acetate phase is washed with 5 ml. portions of 1% sodium acetate solution. The washing procedure is repeated until the washing shows no red fluorescence in ultraviolet light (usually three washings are sufficient).

The washings are added to the reserve aqueous phase containing uroporphyrins. The ethyl acetate solution is then gently shaken with 10 ml. 0.005% iodine solution, and the aqueous layer is drawn off and discarded. The iodine solution should not remain in contact with the ethyl acetate for more than 5 min. in all.

Coproporphyrins are then extracted from the ethyl acetate with 2.5 ml. portions of 1.5N hydrochloric acid until no more fluorescent material is removed, as

shown by examination under ultraviolet light. Usually three extractions will suffice. The HCl extracts are pooled and the final volume is measured.

Absorbance of the acid extract pool is measured in a spectrophotometer with 1 cm. light path against a distilled water blank at 380 mμ, 430 mμ, and 1 mμ intervals between 399 and 404 mμ. The peak absorbance is taken for the calculations. This is usually at 401 mμ.

Uroporphyrins: Concentrated hydrochloric acid is added drop by drop to the aqueous uroporphyrin solution until the pH drops to 3.0 ± 0.2 (narrow-range pH paper or preferably a pH meter). Add 20 ml. n-butanol after transfer to a separatory funnel, and shake the mixture well for 1 min. The phases are allowed to separate and the upper butanol layer is removed for later use. The aqueous layer is extracted with two more 10 ml. portions of butanol. The combined butanol extracts are washed twice with 10 ml. aqueous 0.5% acetic acid, and the wash is discarded. The butanol extract is mixed with 30 ml. petroleum ether and 1 ml. concentrated hydrochloric acid is added. The mixture is shaken well for 1 min. and the layers are allowed to separate. The lower aqueous layer (vol. 7-8 ml.) is drawn off and saved. One more extraction of the organic layer is made with 2 ml. 1.5N HCl. The acid extracts are combined and the final volume measured. Absorbance measurements are taken at 380 mμ, 430 mμ, and 1 mμ intervals between 404 and 408 mμ. The maximum absorbance is taken for the calculation. This is usually at 406 mμ. The reference solution is prepared by extracting the remaining butanol once more with 5 ml. 1.5N hydrochloric acid.

Calculations: For each measurement calculate the corrected absorbance as

$$A(corr) = 2 A(max) - (A380 + A430)$$

where A(max) is the maximum absorbance in the range 400-410 mμ and A380 and A430 are the absorbances at 380 and 430 mμ. Then:

$$\mu g/24 \text{ hr.} = A(corr) \times F \times V \times (T/100)$$

where T is the total volume in ml., V the volume of the acid extract, and F =

8.1 for coproporphyrin and 9.1 for uroporphyrin. Note that A(corr) and V will also be different for the two porphyrins.

If it is suspected that the porphyrin level is very high, observe the urine under ultraviolet light. Urines showing a noticeable fluorescence should be diluted 1:10 with water, i.e., extract the mixture of 10 ml. urine plus 90 ml. water, and make the necessary correction in the calculations.

Coproporphyrin

Formation of coproporphyrin appears to be related to the erythropoietic activity of the bone marrow. Type I coproporphyrin has been found in normal urine, feces, and bile and is increased when there is active blood regeneration (in hemolytic anemias, polycythemia, etc.), following hemorrhage, in infectious hepatitis, and in obstructive jaundice. It is grossly increased in congenital porphyria and porphyria cutanea tarda. Type III has been found in the urine in toxic states, especially in lead poisoning, after sulfonamides, and in acute porphyria (often with porphobilinogen).

In idiopathic coproporphyrinuria, which is rare, large amounts of coproporphyrin III appear in the urine, but without uroporphyrin or porphobilinogen which are characteristic of porphyria.

Normal values: 60-280 μg/24 hr., mainly type I.

Uroporphyrin

Uroporphyrin is found in the urine in congenital porphyria, an inborn error of metabolism (Garrod), and if present in large amounts, it gives the urine a port-wine color. Type I is more common in congenital porphyria. Type III may be found in intermittent acute porphyria.

Uroporphyrin in urine is found normally in traces only; therefore the presence of demonstrable quantities is always pathologic.

Normal values: 5-30 μg/24 hr., mainly type I.

Phosphorus, barbiturates, and alcohol have been reported as causing porphyrinuria.[49] Porphyrinuria has been reported in bromism.[50]

Porphyria

There are two types, both of which may be familial and are characterized by the appearance of uroporphyrins in urine.

INTERMITTENT ACUTE TYPE—PORPHYRIA HEPATICA: This is the most common type and occurs most often in adult women. It is characterized by abdominal and nervous symptoms. Porphyrin is not found in the blood, but is formed apparently by condensation of porphobilinogen after it has been secreted by the kidneys.

The urine contains an increased amount of total coproporphyrins, chiefly type III, and is red at intervals, apparently due to uroporphyrin types I and III or to porphobilin, a pigment of unknown composition. It may be normal in color when voided, becoming dark red upon standing exposed to light and air. The urine contains the chromogen porphobilinogen (colorless and nonfluorescent) which can be easily detected and which is pathognomonic of the disease.

CONGENITAL TYPE—PORPHYRIA ERYTHROPOIETICA: This is usually found in infancy or early childhood and is more common in males. It is characterized by extreme sensitiveness to light, resulting in blistering and scarring of the skin. The urine is continuously red and characteristically contains uroporphyrin type I and a smaller amount of coproporphyrin type I. The porphyrin is found in the blood and becomes deposited in the tissues, especially the bones and the teeth which are stained deep brown. Porphobilinogen is not present in the urine.

Test for porphobilinogen (Watson-Schwartz test[51, 52]): Porphobilinogen gives a red color with Ehrlich p-dimethylaminobenzaldehyde reagent, which is similar to the color due to urobilinogen and indole but differs in solubility.

The method recommended by Watson is as follows:

Fisher's modification of Ehrlich reagent:
1. p-Dimethylaminobenzaldehyde, 0.7 gm.
2. Concentrated HCl, 150 ml.
3. Distilled water, 100 ml.
Keep in dark bottle.

Technique: Shake 5 ml. fresh urine for 30 sec. with 5 ml. Fisher's modification of Ehrlich reagent. Add 10 ml. saturated solution of sodium acetate. Test resulting solution with Congo red paper to a negative (red) reaction. Add sodium acetate if necessary. With porphobilinogen the major color development occurs immediately after addition of Ehrlich reagent; with urobilinogen it occurs after addition of sodium acetate. Shake the solution with 10 ml. chloroform and allow to stand for a few moments. Two layers will separate so that the chloroform forms the lower layer and the water the upper layer. Porphobilinogen remains in the aqueous phase, while urobilinogen and indole are extracted in the chloroform.

The test is positive if the upper (aqueous) layer is red or deep pink and the lower layer (chloroform) is colorless or pale yellow-brown. If the upper (aqueous) layer is pink or red, decant and shake with ½ vol. n-butanol. Red or pink remaining in the aqueous layer is only caused by porphobilinogen.

Interpretation: The reaction of urine with Ehrlich compound is nonspecific. Urobilinogen aldehyde is soluble in chloroform. Porphobilinogen aldehyde is insoluble in chloroform and n-butanol but soluble in water. The aldehyde derivatives of melanogen, serotonin (5-hydroxyindoleacetic acid), and some indoles are soluble in n-butanol and insoluble in chloroform.

Confirmation of the presence of porphobilinogen: The chromogen porphobilinogen changes into the pigment porphobilin, which is reddish brown, and may cause the urine to become reddish, but it does not fluoresce with zinc acetate (Schlesinger test), whereas urobilin does.

When urine (normal color) containing porphobilinogen is acidified and boiled, it becomes dark red, and bands of uroporphyrin and porphobilin are found. Alkali (sodium bicarbonate) prevents the reaction.

The red color due to porphyrins, to porphobilin, to the reaction of porphobilinogen with modified Ehrlich reagent, or to phenolphthalein in alkaline urine is not soluble in amyl alcohol. Uroerythrin, methyl red, and the color due to beets are soluble in amyl alcohol.

The color resulting from indole with Ehrlich reagent can be removed by shaking with petroleum ether, which also removes urobilinogen but not porphobilinogen.

Urobilinogen can be extracted with ethyl acetate before adding Ehrlich reagent, whereas porphobilinogen cannot.

MELANIN

The urine darkens and becomes black upon standing (oxidation), the chromogen melanogen changing into the pigment melanin.

Ferric chloride and bromine water tests:
Principle: Oxidation of the chromogen to the pigment.

Method: To 10 ml. urine add a drop at a time sufficient 10% ferric chloride solution to precipitate all of the phosphates; then add drop by drop enough 10% hydrochloric acid to dissolve the precipitated phosphates. Centrifuge and examine for the gray or black precipitate of melanin. If present, confirm. Decant supernatant fluid and add sodium carbonate (Na_2CO_3) until alkaline to litmus. Melanin precipitate will dissolve. Then add hydrochloric acid (10%) until acid to litmus. If melanin is present, it will be precipitated again as a gray or black sediment when centrifuged.

Bromine water gives a yellow precipitate that turns black.

Thormählen test:
Principle: Sodium nitroprusside is reduced to ferrocyanide (Prussian blue) by the reducing action of melanogen.

Add 2 ml. 5% aqueous sodium nitroprusside solution to 5 ml. urine. Add 2 ml. 25% sodium hydroxide. The urine turns red due to the presence of creatinine. Add 2 ml. glacial acetic acid, and the red color may change to blue-green if melanin is present.

Microscopic examination: Melanin granules may be found in the urinary sediment.

Significance: Melanin occurs with melanotic tumors, especially (or only) with metastasis to the liver.

Differential diagnosis: In alkaptonuria, because of a defect in the amino acid metabolism, homogentisic acid is excreted in the urine and on exposure to air is oxidized to a dark compound (see p. 26).

Test: The addition of an excess of 10% sodium hydroxide darkens urine containing alkapton bodies but does not discolor urine containing melanogen.

PHENOL DERIVATIVES

The urine may be dark upon voiding or only after standing. Color is due to sulfuric acid in conjunction with phenols, etc.

Test: Acidify 200 ml. urine with 50 ml. hydrochloric acid and distill. To the first few ml. of distillate add ferric chloride solution (10%), which gives an amethyst color if phenol derivatives are present.

Significance: These substances occur in increased intestinal putrefaction or with protein decomposition elsewhere in the body and in poisoning with the phenols.

URINARY SEDIMENT[53]

GROSS EXAMINATION

Gross examination may reveal **pus, blood,** and/or **crystals.** If the amount of sediment is too small, reconcentrate specimen by discarding the original supernatant, refilling the tube, and repeating the process two or three times.

MICROSCOPIC EXAMINATION

The specimen must be fresh, though acid urine stored in the refrigerator will preserve almost all cellular elements, crystals, and casts fairly well.[5]

Technique: Mix specimen thoroughly. Fill 15 ml. centrifuge tube to fingerbreadth of top and centrifuge for 3 min. at 1800 rpm. Pour off supernatant fluid by inverting tube without wiping lip of tube. Mix sediment with the small amount of urine that remains in the tube (by holding the top of tube with one hand and striking the bottom of the tube with a finger of the other hand) and pour a drop on a slide. Cover with a cover glass. Faulkner[54] described a rotating Plexiglas stage for microscopic examination of sediments. It appears to be a valuable aid in reducing time and effort required to perform these examinations.

Under subdued light examine with the low-power lens (16 mm.) the entire cover glass area. Casts are most easily found in this way. Turn to the high-power lens (4 mm.) to identify smaller structures (pus and blood cells).

If the amount remaining in the centrifuge tube is about 0.5 ml., the concentration is about 25 times. About 0.05 ml. is usually mounted under the cover glass. Accurate counts may be made in the hemocytometer but are not often necessary. (See discussion of Addis count.)

If urine contains many amorphous urates, mix with equal parts of warm water (not over 60° C.) before centrifuging and correct for the dilution (multiplying by 2 the number of structures observed).

If urine contains many amorphous phosphates and carbonates, add just enough dilute acetic acid to dissolve the amorphous sediment before centrifuging. Too much acid will dissolve the casts.

Staining of sediment[55]

Sternheimer and Malbin developed a gentian violet–safranine stain for urinary sediments. A similar stain called Krystranin* is available commercially.

Appearance of elements stained with Krystranin:

Cellular elements: Squamous cells stain pale purple with dark purple nuclei; renal cells have an orange-purple cytoplasm and dark nuclei; leukocytes are pale pink with purple nuclei; glitter cells stain pale blue; erythrocytes may not stain at all or stain pale pink; yeast cells may stain dark purple or not take the stain at all.

Casts: Hyaline and waxy casts may not stain at all or are pale pink; granular casts have a pink matrix and purple granules; red cell casts are red-purple.

Crystals: They do not stain.

Bacteria: They vary in color.

Spermatozoa: They stain blue.

Trichomonas: They take a pale blue dye; the nucleus is purple.

---

*Scientific Products Division, American Hospital Supply Corp., Evanston, Ill.

Preservation of sediment[56]

Dissolve 6 gm. gelatin in 42 ml. sterile distilled water, heat the solution for 3 min., add 50 ml. glycerin and 2 gm. phenol. Dispense in small amounts and keep frozen in bottles until needed.

Preparation of specimen: Mix 1 small drop of mounting fluid with 1 drop of sediment. One small drop of Sternheimer stain may also be added.

Formed elements may be preserved up to 6 mo., while crystals last from 2 days to 1 mo., depending on their composition.

Leukocytes

In the centrifuged specimen there is usually an occasional leukocyte, not more than 1/hpf in specimens from males and 1-5 in specimens from females and children. Larger numbers, if found consistently, indicate inflammation (pyuria). White corpuscles found constantly in a well-mixed, noncentrifuged specimen are considered evidence of inflammation.

Most of the white cells are granulocytes which may show ameboid movements in a fresh specimen or adopt a spherical, often distended outline in toxic surroundings. Clumping of granulocytes should be noted. The Sternheimer stain differentiates large pale blue so-called renal leukocytes from the smaller pink leukocytes of the lower urinary tract.

White cell casts suggest renal parenchymal infection. A large number of leukocytes will contribute to the protein content of the urine.

Glitter cells: These are altered polymorphonuclear cells, the granules of which show brownian movement. While they can be found in a variety of kidney diseases, they are most closely related to pyelonephritis and to changes in the osmolarity of the urine. The Sternheimer and Malbin gentian violet–safranine stain will stain glitter cells a faint blue.[55]

Blood (erythrocytes)

The causes of hematuria may be grouped as prerenal (purpura, infectious diseases, and drugs), renal (hyperemia, inflammation, malignant tumor, tuberculosis, calculi including sulfonamide crystals, or trauma of the kidney), postrenal (similar lesions of any portion of the tract below the kidney and infestation with *Schistosoma haematobium*), and idiopathic.

Red cells may be evidence of vaginal contamination or may follow catheterization, but with these two exceptions they always represent an important finding. It is of no clinical importance whether they are crenated (as in hypertonic urine) or pale and distended (as in hypotonic urine). They can be stained with the Sternheimer stain.[55] Red cell casts indicate parenchymal renal disease. The presence of red blood cells may be confirmed with Hemastix reagent strip which, depending on the amount of blood, may or may not be positive.

Red cells are highly refractile round yellowish structures that can be distinguished from fat droplets by their color and by the fact that they do not stain with Sudan IV, and from yeast by the addition of dilute acetic acid which dissolves them (Fig. 2-5).

Casts

Casts are cylindric structures with parallel sides and blunt rounded ends. They quickly dissolve in alkaline urine. They are formed in the renal tubules. They

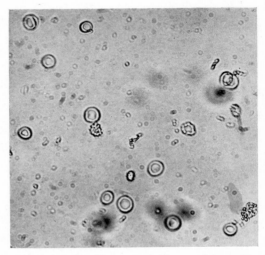

Fig. 2-5. Red cells in urine. (Courtesy Ames Co., Inc., Elkhart, Ind.)

may be present when albumin tests are negative and may be absent temporarily when albumin is present, often occurring in showers. They are composed of a hyaline protein (Tamm-Horsfall protein[57]) matrix (hyaline casts), in which organized structures (blood, pus, renal epithelial cells, bacteria, or fat droplets) or amorphous granules and bile may be incorporated. The former produces red cell casts, pus casts, epithelial casts; the latter produces fine or coarse granular casts and bile casts. If the cellular elements undergo fatty degeneration, fatty casts are formed; if the red cells disintegrate, brown granular hemoglobin casts are formed. Waxy casts are structureless but are more refractile than hyaline casts.

Hyaline casts usually indicate the mildest damage, a few being found after exertion and after palpation of the kidney. **Granular casts** indicate more serious damage. **Very broad casts** are formed in the large collecting tubules and are called **renal failure casts** (Addis[58, 59]). They may be of any type—granular, fatty, etc. **Waxy casts** are rare and are found in amyloid disease and in chronic kidney disease. **Red cell casts** are indicative of glomerular lesions. **Fatty casts** contain fat droplets, varying in size, and are usually accompanied by oval fat bodies. **White cell casts** indicate renal parenchymal infection and are difficult to distinguish from **epithelial casts**. (Figs. 2-6 and 2-7.)

Cylindroids are similar to casts but have one tapering end drawn out like a strand of mucus so that the sides are not parallel. The other end is round. They probably indicate a very mild irritation of the kidney and perhaps represent abortive casts. They may appear prior to the casts and may remain after the casts have disappeared.

Mucous strands: Mucous strands or fibers are present in small numbers normally. Increased numbers are found in chronic inflammation of the urethra and bladder. They cannot be seen grossly like shreds.

Shreds: They consist of a mixture of mucus, pus, and epithelial cells. When mucus predominates, the shreds float on

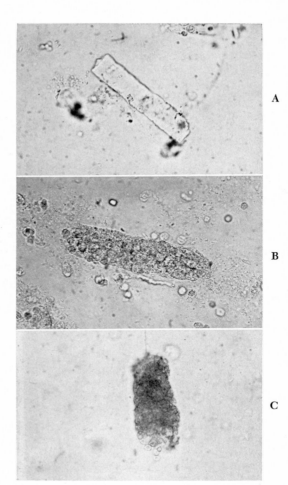

Fig. 2-6. Urinary casts. **A**, Hyaline cast. **B**, White cell cast. **C**, Red cell cast. (Courtesy Ames Co., Inc., Elkhart, Ind.)

the surface; when epithelial cells predominate, they occupy the midzone; and when pus predominates, it draws the shreds down to the bottom of the specimen.

Bacteria

They are of no significance except in fresh or catheterized specimens, when they should be studied by stains and cultures.[58, 59] For special methods of urine culture, see bacteriology section.

Yeast

Upon microscopic examination, double-walled oval to pear-shaped budding organisms, which are smaller than red blood cells, are seen.

Fat and doubly refractile lipids[60]

Fat may be due to contamination from unclean vessels, slides, or lubricants. Fat droplets may be free or appear in degenerated epithelial cells or fatty casts. Fat droplets are usually slightly larger than white cells. Under low-power magnification they appear as dark oval structures. With higher resolution, fat droplets can be recognized which make up the oval structures. Under polarized light

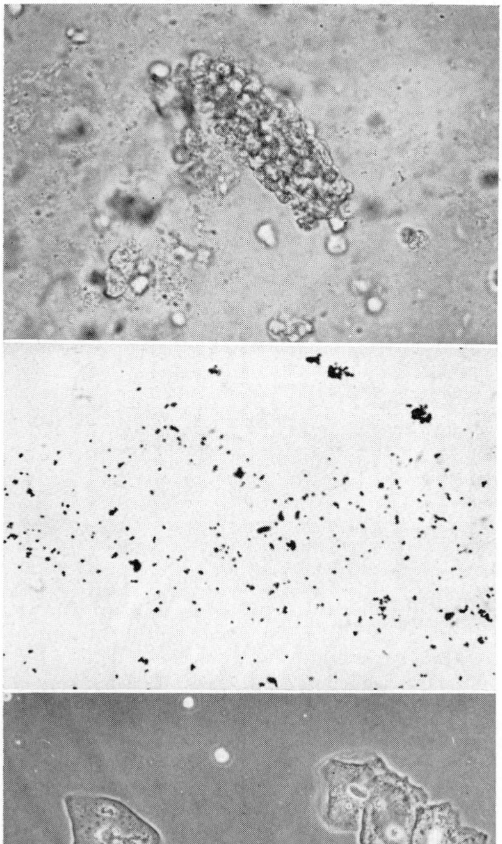

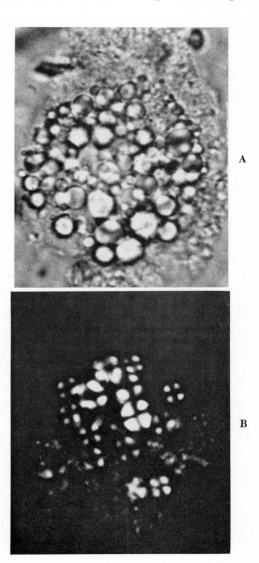

Fig. 2-7. **A,** Pus cast. **B,** Cocci in urine. **C,** Epithelial cells in sediment. **D,** Budding yeast in urine. (Courtesy Ames Co., Inc., Elkhart, Ind.)

Fig. 2-8. Oval fat body viewed under ordinary light, **A,** and under polarized light, **B,** showing Maltese cross patterns. (From Daysog and Dobson: Amer. J. Clin. Path. 39:419, 1963.)

these droplets are doubly refractile, show-ing the Maltese cross pattern (Fig. 2-8). In chyluria the droplets are very small. Some workers[61] believe that staining with Sudan III is satisfactory.

Epithelial cells

Squamous cells: They occur normally in small numbers in urine from males, from the anterior urethra and prepuce, and in large numbers in urine from fe-males, chiefly from the external genitalia.

When present in large numbers, these cells may hide important formed ele-ments; therefore it is necessary to obtain a clean specimen. **Tubular epithelial re-nal cells** are easily confused with white cells, though they often have a promi-nent nucleolus within a centrally located nucleus. The epithelial cells may contain hemosiderin or bile pigment.

Neoplastic cells: A clean or catheterized specimen of urine is mixed with equal amounts of 50% ethyl alcohol immedi-ately after voiding. It is then centrifuged or is allowed to pass through a Millipore filter.* The sediment is smeared on ground glass slides (Dakin or frosted mi-croscope slides†) and immediately fixed in 95% alcohol before drying. The fixed smear or the filter preparation is stained by the Papanicolaou method.

Cells with inclusion bodies: Desqua-mated cells may contain the large inclu-sions of salivary gland virus disease or the small, acid-fast inclusions of heavy metal (lead and bismuth) intoxication.[62]

Semen

Well-preserved spermatozoa are not infrequently found (Fig. 2-9).

Parasites

Animal parasites are rare. Flagellates (*Trichomonas hominis* and *Chilomastix mesnili*), *Schistosoma haematobium*, *Echi-nococcus granulosus*, and filaria may be found (Fig. 2-10). Ova of intestinal para-sites may be present as a contamination, e.g., ova of *Oxyuris vermicularis* (Fig. 2-11).

---

*Millipore Filter Corp., Bedford, Mass.
†Sanders Laboratories, East Rutherford, N. J.

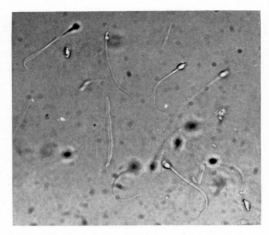

Fig. 2-9. Spermatozoa in urine. (Courtesy Ames Co., Inc., Elkhart, Ind.)

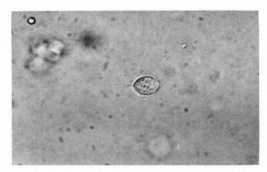

Fig. 2-10. *Trichomonas vaginalis* in urine. (Cour-tesy Ames Co., Inc., Elkhart, Ind.)

Amorphous sediment

Amorphous phosphates, sometimes neutral and amphoteric, are found in al-kaline urines and appear as colorless granular masses. They are soluble in acetic acid, without formation of gas. Granular masses of calcium carbonate are rare and dissolve in dilute acetic acid with effervescence. In acid urines, amor-phous urates appear as very fine gran-ules, usually colored by urinary pigments. The granules appear yellowish micro-scopically and pink grossly.

Occasionally sulfadiazine (and possibly other sulfonamides) will precipitate out as a yellowish gray amorphous sediment instead of crystals. This sediment is not soluble in dilute acetic acid but is soluble in strong acids or alkalies. It may be iden-

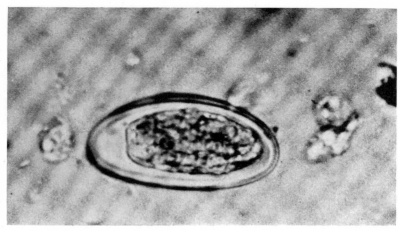

Fig. 2-11. Ovum of *Oxyuris vermicularis* in urine. (Courtesy Ames Co., Inc., Elkhart, Ind.)

tified by the chemical tests for sulfonamides.

Crystals

These are not usually present when urine is voided but form after it cools, either because the urine is supersaturated at the cooler temperature or because changes in the reaction alter the solubilities of the substances. The presence of albumin and other substances often interferes with crystallization.

Crystals are of little clinical significance except cystine, uric acid, and sulfonamide crystals. The importance of the latter has diminished in the last few years. The type of crystal depends largely on the pH of the freshly voided urine.

Crystals in acid urine: **Calcium oxalate crystals** are colorless octahedral, so-called envelope crystals with a highly refractile cross connecting the corners; more rarely they appear as oval spheres or biconcave disks with a dumbbell shape when viewed from the edge. They are soluble in hydrochloric acid and not in acetic acid.

Uric acid crystals are rhombic, usually whetstone-shaped, 6-sided plates, often arranged in rosettelike clusters. Those occurring naturally are stained with urinary pigments and are yellowish or brownish, and in larger clusters they are grossly red like pepper granules. Large numbers of such crystals are often precipitated in the collecting tubules and

in the calices of the kidney during the first week of life, and when passed in the urine, they may be mistaken for blood. Crystals precipitated artificially are colorless. They are soluble in sodium hydroxide and not in acid.

Amorphous urates are red and dissolve when treated with alkali and when heated. The addition of acetic acid or of hydrochloric acid dissolves the urates, which, upon standing, slowly form colorless rhombic crystals of uric acid.

Crystals of the sulfonamides may form in the renal tubules and appear in freshly voided urine which is either acid or alkaline, although conjugated sulfathiazole (acetylsulfathiazole) appears to be more soluble in alkaline urine.[63] Crystals of sulfadiazine and sulfamerazine are likewise thought to be more soluble in alkaline urine.

The sulfonamide crystals are "impure" crystals[64] and are chiefly acetylated derivatives, the crystalline forms depending largely upon the impurities present and differing from those of the chemically pure compounds. The crystals may vary from day to day because of change in the composition of the urine. Free sulfadiazine, because of its low solubility which is even less than the acetyl compound, may also form crystals. Crystals of other free sulfonamides and of acetylsulfanilamide are not likely to be found because of their relatively high solubilities.

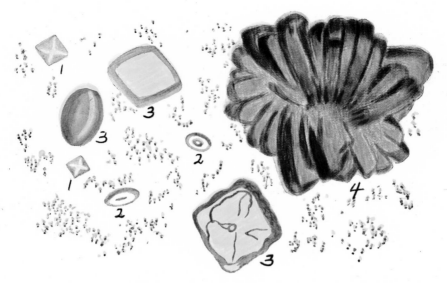

Plate. 1. Crystalline and amorphous sediment in acid urine.

1. Calcium oxalate crystals, typical double envelope forms.
2. Calcium oxalate crystals, unusual oval forms.
Amorphous material is urates.

3. Uric acid crystals.
4. Rosette of uric acid crystals.

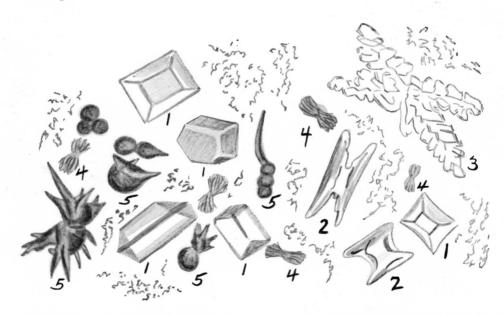

Plate 2. High-power field showing crystalline and amorphous sediment in alkaline urine.

1. Triple phosphate crystals, usual forms.
2. Triple phosphate crystals, dissolving or
poorly formed.
Amorphous material is amorphous phosphates.

3. Triple phosphate crystal, feathery form
produced by rapid precipitation artificially.
4. Calcium carbonate crystals, dumbbell
forms.
5. Ammonium biurate crystals.

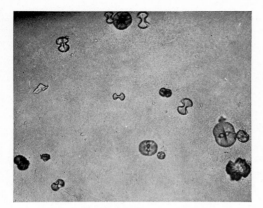

Fig. 2-12. Acetylsulfathiazole crystals. (×100.)

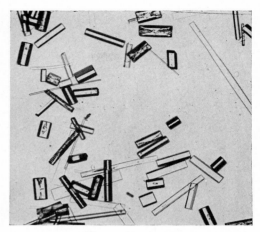

Fig. 2-14. Sulfisoxazole (Gantrisin) crystals. (×100.)

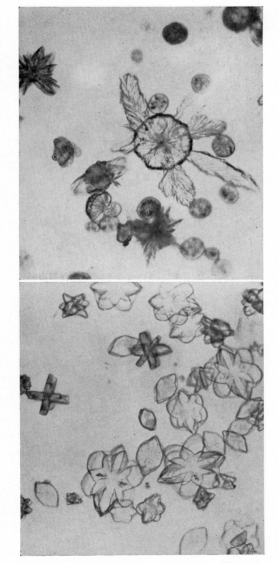

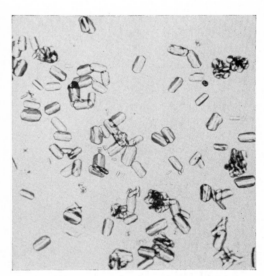

Fig. 2-15. Acetylsulfathiazole crystals. (×100.)

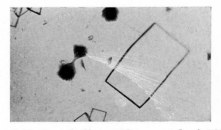

Fig. 2-13. Acetylsulfathiazole crystals. (×100.)

Fig. 2-16. Acetylsulfaguanidine crystals. (×100.)

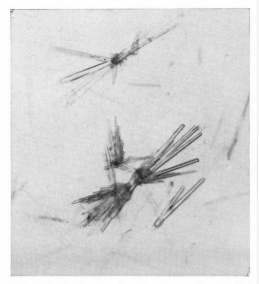

Fig. 2-18. Sulfanilamide (free) crystals. (×100.)

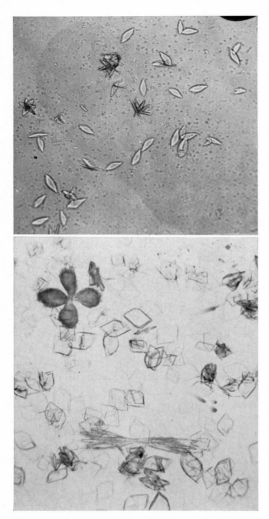

Fig. 2-17. Acetylsulfapyridine crystals. (×100.)

However, the crystals of the different sulfonamides are sufficiently characteristic to permit identification of the form of sulfonamide which has been taken. (Figs. 2-12 to 2-17.)

Free sulfanilamide forms long transparent and colorless rhombic crystals (coarse needles) often arranged in bundles, like fagots (Fig. 2-18). Acetylsulfanilamide forms sheaves and radiating bundles.

Acetylsulfapyridine forms colorless transparent plates, modified to resemble flint arrowheads or small fish or playing card diamonds. Occasionally large somewhat opaque centrally bound sheaves or rosettes of coarse needles are found.

Acetylsulfathiazole forms sheaves of needles with central binding or rosettes and transparent and colorless hexagonal plates, some of which may be modified to resemble whetstones appearing sometimes in rosettes (like colorless uric acid crystals).

Acetylsulfadiazine appears as sheaves of needles with eccentric binding and as assymmetric rosettes resembling shells. Free sulfadiazine appears as large greenish globules covered with needlelike processes and resembles chestnut or chinquapin burs. (Fig. 2-19.) When examined microscopically with reflected light, crystals of sulfadiazine appear pinkish; crystals of other sulfonamides appear white or yellowish.

Acetylsulfaguanidine forms large clear and colorless rectangular plates, often with bulging sides, or sheaves of fine needles somewhat resembling tyrosine crystals.

Succinylsulfathiazole is sparingly absorbed and very soluble so that crystals do not usually appear.

Since sulfonamide crystals may suggest crystals of dicalcium phosphate, uric acid, or tyrosine,[65] a chemical test may be used for identification.

Sulfonamides may precipitate as amorphous granules or very fine crystals dif-

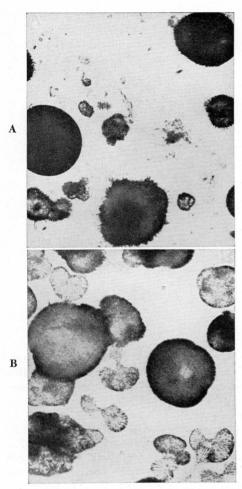

Fig. 2-19. **A,** Crystals of free sulfadiazine. **B,** Crystals of free sulfadiazine and acetylsulfadiazine. (×156.) (From Lehr and Antopol: Amer. J. Clin. Path. **12:**200, 1942.)

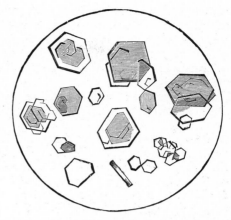

Fig. 2-20. Cystine crystals from patient with cystinuria. (From Gershenfeld: Urine and urinalysis, Philadelphia, 1948, Lea & Febiger.)

ficult to identify except by the chemical test.

The risk of renal chamage due to the deposit of sulfonamide crystals in the kidney tubules may be lessened by alkaline therapy, by maintaining diuresis, and by giving a mixture of the sulfonamides.[66, 67] Higher blood and urine levels result also from the use of mixtures of the sulfonamides.[68] It has been pointed out, however, that the mixture of sulfonamides may cause hypersensitiveness to more than one of the forms used, and the disadvantages may outweigh the advantages.[69]

Cystine crystals are colorless, flat, hexagonal plates with unequal sides. They are not soluble in acetic acid but are soluble in hydrochloric acid or alkali. (Fig. 2-20.)

Chemical test for cystine: Wash crystals with cold water made slightly acid with acetic acid. Suspend in about 2 ml. water and make alkaline with ammonium hydroxide to dissolve crystals. Apply the **Sullivan test** as follows: Add 1 ml. 5% sodium cyanide solution (POISON! Use rubber bulb) and let stand 10 min. Add 0.5 ml. fresh 0.5% 1,2 naphthoquinone-4-sodium sulfonate. Mix and add at once 2.5 ml. 10% anhydrous sodium sulfite in 0.5N sodium hydroxide. Let stand 30 min. and add 0.5 ml. 2% sodium hyposulfite in 0.5N sodium hydroxide. A red color is specific for cysteine or cystine. This test may be applied to protein-free urine.

Tyrosine and leucine: Tyrosine and leucine crystals are rare and indicate serious liver damage. **Tyrosine crystals** appear as fine needles arranged in radiating sheaves. They are soluble in hydrochloric acid or alkali (ammonia) but not acetic acid. **Leucine crystals** appear as oily yellowish or brownish refractile spheroids. They are soluble in alkali but not in dilute acetic acid or in hydrochloric acid. Leucine is soluble in boiling acetic acid, whereas tyrosine is not.

To demonstrate the crystals of tyrosine

or leucine remove albumin (heat, add acetic acid, and filter), evaporate to small volume, adjust one portion to pH 5.8 for leucine and another to pH 6.8-7 for tyrosine. Place in refrigerator and examine for crystals.

Test for tyrosine: Add crystalline precipitate to a few ml. of **Mörner reagent** (formalin 1, water 45, sulfuric acid, 55 parts) and raise to boiling temperature. Tyrosine gives a green color.

Test for leucine: Use the **Salkowski test.** Dissolve **crystals** in a little water and add a small drop of 10% copper sulfate. Leucine gives a blue color that does not disappear upon heating.

Crystals in alkaline urine: Ammonio-magnesium phosphate (triple phosphate) crystals are colorless highly refractile prisms varying in size and presenting 3, 4, or 6 sides, giving the typical coffin-lid and hip-roof forms. They diffract the light so that the edges often appear colored. When the crystals are precipitated artificially, they appear as feathery star-shaped crystals. Dicalcium phosphate crystallizes out when the reaction is near the neutral point, forming slender colorless prisms with one pointed end, often arranged as rosettes or stars (stellar phosphates) or needles. Rarely, in alkaline urine, phosphate forms large irregular flat plates, usually granular, which float on the surface as an irridescent scum. They are soluble in dilute acetic acid without effervescence.

Calcium carbonate crystals are small and dumbbell shaped. They dissolve in dilute acetic acid with effervescence.

Ammonium biurate crystals, so-called thorn apple crystals, are yellowish opaque spheroidal bodies with irregular spines. They dissolve by warming and are soluble in acetic acid, with the formation of colorless uric acid crystals after standing. When sodium hydroxide is added, ammonia is liberated.

Amorphous phosphates are colorless granular masses soluble in acetic acid.

Extraneous structures

Various extraneous structures are often found, e.g., spermatozoa, corpora amylacea, and lecithin granules from con-tamination with semen. Other extraneous substances are numerous and have no significance: molds, fibers of all kinds, fats from lubricants, starch and lycopodium granules, muscle fibers, and fecal contaminations.

ADDIS COUNT[59]

All fluid is restricted for a period of 24 hr. The patient is allowed his usual diet, but fluids are restricted to 200 ml. with each meal (unless the patient has nitrogen retention). Empty the bladder at about 8 P.M., discard this specimen, and collect a 12 hr. specimen of urine, including a specimen at the end of that period. Collect the specimen in a bottle that contains 1 ml. neutral formalin (10%). Avoid excess of formalin which causes precipitation of a formalin-urea complex that is insoluble by usual methods and interferes with the procedure. Obtain specimens from women by catheter.

Mix and measure. Warm a portion carefully to dissolve urates or add just enough acetic acid to dissolve phosphates.

The specific gravity should be 1.022 or higher, and the urine should be acid to preserve formed elements.

Transfer 10 ml. to an Addis tube, a special graduated centrifuge tube with a narrow tip. Centrifuge 5 min. at 1800 rpm. Discard supernatant fluid, adjusting the amount left in the tube to 0.5 ml. (or to some measured amount). Mix and with a pipette mount a portion on a hemocytometer, a special Addis counting chamber, or an Exton counting chamber.[70] Let settle and count all the casts, red blood corpuscles, and white blood corpuscles in the entire ruled area of 9 mm.^{2}

If very numerous, make appropriate dilution before transferring the portion to the counting chamber; if very few, count several preparations.

Calculation: The average for the entire area (0.9 mm.^{3}) divided by 9 and multiplied by 10,000 = number in 1 ml. of the sediment. Multiply by the volume (usually 0.5 ml.) of the sediment, which gives the number contained in the 10 ml. of urine centrifuged. Calculate the number in the 12 hr. specimen by dividing by

10 (or the number of ml. of urine centrifuged) and multiplying by the number of milliliters in the 12 hr. specimen.

Reduced to a formula when X = the number found in the 9 mm.² area, C = the amount centrifuged, S = the volume of the sediment, and V = the 12 hr. volume, then:

$$X \left(\frac{10,000 \times S \times V}{9 \times C} \right) = \text{Number in}$$

12 hr. specimen

Significance: Normally, in the adult about 1000 hyaline casts, 70,000 red blood cells, and 300,000 white blood cells are found in the 12 hr. specimen. More than 9000 casts, 1,000,000 red blood cells, and 3,000,000 white blood cells are definitely abnormal.

In children a somewhat higher normal limit is allowed for casts (10,000), leukocytes (2,000,000), and red blood cells (600,000).

QUALITATIVE ESTIMATION OF ELECTROLYTES

CALCIUM:

Sulkowitch test—a screening procedure: This test is used for rough rapid qualitative analysis of urine calcium.

Specimen: Use aliquot of well-mixed 24 hr. specimen. Random specimens may vary greatly in their calcium contents.

Test: Mix equal parts (about 5 ml. each) of urine and reagent and observe for turbidity.

Reagent: This contains oxalate radicles buffered at such pH that in the test calcium will almost immediately come down as a fine white precipitate.

1. Oxalic acid, 2.5 gm.
2. Ammonium oxalate, 2.5 gm.
3. Glacial acetic acid, 5 ml.
4. Distilled water to make 150 ml.

Method of reporting:
No precipitation
Fine precipitation—normal range
Heavy precipitation

Significance: If there is no precipitate, the serum calcium level is below 7.5 mg./100 ml. (probably from 5-7.5 mg./100 ml.). With the normal range of serum calcium the test shows a moderate amount of turbidity. When the serum level is about 11.5 mg./100 ml. or above, the turbidity is greater and the reaction looks like milk.

If tetany is due to hypoparathyroidism or hypocalcemia, the test is negative since the urine contains no calcium; if it is due to alkalosis (hyperventilation), the test is positive.

After hypoparathyroidectomy the Sulkowitch test can be used to follow the results of therapy, which should bring the zero urine reaction of hypoparathyroidism to the normal fine precipitate. Hypocalcemia of infancy may also be monitored by the Sulkowitch test.

CHLORIDES: Much chloride may be lost by way of the gastrointestinal tract (vomiting, diarrhea) or the skin (sweating), resulting in acute salt depletion.

Fantus test:

Principle: Silver nitrate reacts with the chloride in urine to precipitate silver chloride. Any excess of silver nitrate reacts with potassium chromate to form the reddish precipitate of silver chromate, the appearance of which indicates the end point.

Method: In a test tube place 10 drops urine and 1 drop 20% potassium chromate (K_2CrO_4) solution as indicator. Add drop by drop with the same dropper 2.9% silver nitrate solution until a permanent and distinct color change to a red-brown occurs. The number of drops required to produce the color change expresses the sodium chloride content of the urine in gm./L.

Significance: Normal urine requires from 6-12 drops. In acute salt depletion the amount required may be 1 or 2 drops or less.

QUALITATIVE ESTIMATION OF DRUGS

SULFONAMIDES:

Wood fiber method (lignin or lignocellulose): Wood fiber such as is present in wood pulp paper (newsprint paper and paper toweling) reacts with aniline derivatives[71] (such as the free form of sulfonamides) in a strongly acid medium to form a yellow-orange color. Faint shades of yellow are produced with normal urines due to urea (see Ehrlich method). Urine from patients taking phenacetin may give a pink color,[72] and many other substances (aniline, benzidine, etc.) give positive reactions.

Place a drop of urine on a piece of wood pulp paper, add a drop of 10% hydrochloric acid, and observe for a yellow-orange color, which is a positive reaction. Observe for 15 min. before discarding as negative.

Read light yellow, deep yellow, orange-yellow, and orange colors as 1, 2, 3, and 4+, respectively.

Run a negative control with normal urine (containing no sulfonamide).

QUANTITATIVE URINALYSIS

The following are included in the biochemistry section: quantitative methods for calcium, chlorides, creatinine, creatin, diastase, sulfonamides, total nitrogen, urea nitrogen, and uric acid.

KIDNEY FUNCTION TESTS

Kidney function: The glomeruli excrete a protein-free blood filtrate from which the tubules reabsorb the useful threshold substances (water, glucose, bicarbonate, chloride, phosphate, sodium, potassium, and amino acids). It is estimated that there are in each kidney a million functional units (glomeruli with tubules), only a part of which acts at one time, so that there is a reserve of 60-75%. To produce any effect upon the function the lesion must be diffuse or must involve more

than about two thirds of the kidney tissue. Since the efferent blood vessels of the glomeruli supply the tubules, injury to the glomeruli will also cause injury to the tubules.

The kidney functions are manifold and include the following:

1. Regulation of body water and plasma volume by varying the concentration of the urine
2. Maintenance of the acid-base balance by formation of ammonia, by secretion of free acid, by hydrogen ion exchange, and by reabsorption of bicarbonates and alkaline phosphates
3. Control of electrolyte balance by maintaining optimal concentrations of potassium, calcium, phosphorus, and magnesium in serum (excretion threshold substances)
4. Absorption of substances valuable to the body, e.g., glucose, vitamins, hormones, amino acids, etc.
5. Excretion of waste products (low threshold substances), e.g., urea and creatinine

The glomeruli produce a protein-free ultrafiltrate of the blood plasma with a pH of 7.4 and a specific gravity of 1.010. In the proximal tubules obligatory absorption of high threshold substances takes place independent of water intake and urinary volume. A threshold substance is a substance that is almost completely reabsorbed by the renal tubules when its

Table 2-3. Choice of renal function tests*

Function	Specific measurement	Clinical test
Glomerular filtration	Inulin clearance	Creatinine clearance Urea clearance Plasma urea level
Renal plasma flow	PAH measurement	PSP excretion
Proximal tubular mass	Excretory PAH Tm Reabsorption glucose Tm	PSP excretion
Distal tubular mass	Concentration-dilution Electrolyte balance Acid-base balance Ammonia-forming ability	
Severe tubule damage and/or diguria	(Back diffusion)	Urea clearance Plasma urea level

*From Earle: Amer. J. Med. 9:78, 1950.

concentration in plasma is within normal range. It appears in the urine (is not completely absorbed) when its normal plasma level is exceeded. A high threshold substance is a substance that is almost completely reabsorbed. High threshold substances include glucose, amino acids, creatinine, ascorbic acid, sodium, potassium, magnesium, calcium, phosphate, chlorides, and bicarbonates as well as water. Secretion of phenol red, Diodrast, penicillin, and phenolsulfonphthalein is also accomplished in the proximal tubules. Facultative reabsorption takes place in the distal tubules and varies with varying conditions of water intake, renal circulation, and endocrine influences (antidiuretic hormone). Secretion into the urine of hydrogen ions, ammonia, and potassium also takes place in the distal tubules. Maximal rate at which tubules can accomplish secretion or reabsorption of a substance is called maximal tubular secretion or absorption (Tm). The substances that the kidney excretes as waste materials such as urea, creatinine, and uric acid are not absorbed at all, or only slightly, and are therefore low threshold substances.

Kidney function tests are indicated because urinalysis and blood chemistry tests fail to reflect the extent or the localization of a renal lesion. They are based on the ability of the kidney to excrete nitrogen, salt, water, and dyes. In addition, blood nonprotein nitrogen, urea, uric acid, and creatinine are considered tests of kidney function.

Concentration test (Fishberg): The concentration and dilution tests are easily performed. The concentration test is preferred since there are clinical and physiologic contraindications to the dilution test (heart failure, hypertension, etc.). At 6 P.M. give the patient supper containing not more than 200 ml. of fluid but a high protein content. Allow no other fluid or food until the test is completed. Empty bladder at bedtime and discard urine. Discard urine voided during the night. Collect specimens at 7, 8, and 9 A.M., emptying the bladder each time. Measure and take the specific gravity of each specimen. Subtract 0.003 from the specific gravity for each 1% of albumin present.

The patient should not receive any medication (changes in specific gravity). The total quantity of the urine should also be measured. A well-functioning kidney will produce urine of specific gravity of 1.026 or higher and up to 300 ml. of urine.

Normally the specific gravity of at least one of the specimens will be 1.025 or over; sometimes it is as high as 1.032. With increasing kidney impairment the specific gravity decreases, approaching 1.010, the specific gravity of protein-free blood plasma. Absorption of edema fluid will lower the specific gravity but does not indicate decreased function.

The specific gravity is usually 1.020 before phenolsulfonphthalein excretion is decreased and as low as 1.010 before blood urea nitrogen is elevated.

Edema, sweats, diarrhea, and fever interfere with the water tests.

Phenolsulfonphthalein test: This test measures the secretory activity of the proximal tubules, which excrete 94% of the injected dye that is reversibly combined with plasma albumin. The rate of excretion of the dye in a fixed period is measured. Tubular impairment and decrease in renal plasma flow will affect the dye excretion.

Twenty to 30 min. before beginning the test the patient is asked to drink 2 glasses of water to ensure secretion of urine. Empty bladder and discard specimen. Give 1 ml. of the dye (6 mg.) intravenously. Empty bladder, by catheter if necessary, exactly 15, 30, 60, and 120 min. after injection of dye. Record time of collection and volume of urine and measure dye concentration in each specimen.

Estimation of dye: The volume of each specimen should be at least 40 ml. Filter each entire urine sample into a 1000 ml. volumetric flask. Dilute with distilled water to approximately 500 ml. Add 10 ml. 10% NaOH to each specimen, mix, dilute to 1000 ml., and mix thoroughly. Pour into 15 ml. cuvette and determine percent transmittance at 545 mμ against a water blank. Obtain percent of dye excretion from calibration curve.

Standards for calibration of spectrophotometer:

A. Stock standard. Dilute 5 ml. phenolsulfonphthalein, 6 mg./ml. to total volume of 50 ml. This standard now contains 0.6 mg./ml.

B. Working standards. Dilute 1, 2, 4, 6, and 8 ml. stock standard to about 500 ml. with water and add 10 ml. 10% NaOH to each. Make up to final volume of 1000 ml. and mix. These standards now correspond to 10, 20, 40, 60, and 80% dye excretion, respectively. Determine percent transmittance of each standard against a water blank and prepare a calibration chart from values obtained.

NOTES: Examine the specimen promptly if it is alkaline, or if the determination cannot be made at once, make it acid with acetic acid. Excess alkali causes rapid fading of the color (destruction of dye).

If the urine is bloody, centrifuge, or if blood has hemolyzed, add 1 ml. 10% sodium tungstate solution and 1 ml. ⅔N sulfuric acid. Let stand until the pink color due to blood has disappeared; then filter. If the pink color remains after about 15 min., add more of the sodium tungstate and sulfuric acid in equal parts before filtering. Estimate the dye in the filtrate.

Carinamide inhibits the tubular excretion of PSP.

If bile is present, precipitate with solid calcium hydroxide and filter.

Significance: In normal kidney function, after intravenous injection, 30% of the dye is excreted after 15 min., an additional 15% after 30 min., and an additional 10% after 60 min. so that about 55% is excreted after the first hour and 75% after the second hour. An important use of this method is in testing each kidney separately, when the specimens are collected for 15 min. from ureteral catheters. There should be no leak around catheters into the bladder.

The test is not reliable in acute nephritis. In compensated renal impairment the results may be within the normal range. In uncompensated chronic nephritis without edema the retention is parallel to the impairment of the kidneys and to the nitrogen retention in the blood. Nitrogen retention in the blood begins when the dye excretion is less than 40% in 2 hr., and the excretion of dye practically stops when the nonprotein nitrogen reaches 100 mg./100 ml. In chronic passive congestion, excretion of dye is decreased without increase in blood nitrogen.

Since the liver normally removes some of the dye (25% or more) from the bloodstream, the test is not reliable when liver function is impaired (hepatorenal disease).

Clearance tests[73, 74]

As a means of quantitatively expressing the rate of excretion of a given substance by the kidneys, clearance of the substance is measured. Clearance is the volume of blood or plasma that contains the amount of a given substance excreted in the urine in 1 min. Alternatively, the clearance of a substance may be defined as that volume of blood or plasma cleared of the amount of that substance found in the excretion of urine in 1 min.

Clearance can be mathematically expressed by the following formula which shows clearance to be the amount of excreted substance divided by its plasma concentration:

$$C = \frac{UV}{P}$$

C = clearance (ml./min.)
V = urine flow (ml./min.)
U = urinary concentration (mg./ml.)
P = plasma concentration (mg./ml.)

If a substance is not affected by the tubules at all (neither secreted nor absorbed), the amount found in the urine will equal the amount filtered per minute. The clearance of such a substance, e.g., inulin (which has no threshold), is a measure of glomerular filtration (123 ml./min.). The clearance of a substance completely reabsorbed by the tubules, e.g., glucose, is zero. Substances having clearances greater than zero (glucose) but less than that of inulin are in part reabsorbed by tubules (these include most urinary constituents). Substances having higher clearances than that of inulin are added to the urine by tubular cells (iodopyracet, phenol red, *p*-aminohippurate, and ammonia). The highest clearance is the PAH clearance, the plasma being cleared almost entirely by tubular secretion (about 650 ml./min.). The plasma flow through kidneys (about 700 ml./min.) represents the highest possible clearance.

Significance: Apart from the scientific value of clearance studies, which allow the investigation of the pathogenesis of certain renal and vascular diseases and of the action of drugs, these methods are of value in diagnosis and prognosis. The extent of renal damage can be evaluated, and predominately glomerular lesions can be differentiated from predominately tubular ones. The course of the renal disease can be followed, and the recovery stage can be more clearly determined.

Clearance studies have achieved new importance in the diagnosis of hypertension due to unilateral renal artery disease. On the basis of Goldblatt's experiments (partial occlusion of renal artery produces hypertension in dogs) surgeons have reported cases of hypertension cured by nephrectomy or renal artery enarterectomy. Unilateral renal ischemia, which may lead to curable hypertension, is characterized by excessive reabsorption of water during the passage of the glomerular filtrate down the ischemic tubules. This unilateral water absorption can be studied by comparing the clearance of inulin or *p*-aminohippuric acid (PAH) in the involved and uninvolved kidneys, which are catheterized.

The most recent methods of investigation of unilateral kidney disease employ radioisotope renograms that simultaneously measure the separate function of each kidney. A kidney function dye, which is rapidly excreted and labeled with I^{131}, is injected intravenously. Following the injection of the I^{131}, radiation is detected simultaneously over each kidney area by two scintillation counters.[73, 74]

The following are the most commonly used clearance studies:

Renal plasma flow	Sodium *p*-aminohippurate (PAH) clearance
Glomerular filtration rate	Inulin clearance
	Creatinine clearance
	Urea clearance
Tubular function	Absorption—glucose
	Tm
	Secretion—PAH Tm

RENAL PLASMA FLOW:

Sodium *p*-aminohippurate (PAH) clearance[75]: PAH clearance is almost equal to renal plasma flow since the plasma is cleared of this substance by the kidney in a single passage by way of tubular secretion. Renal plasma flow depends on many extrarenal factors but clinically is used primarily for the study of hypertension. The performance of the test requires intravenous administration of PAH in saline solution at a rapid rate, followed by a sustaining infusion at a slower rate. The urine specimen should be obtained by catheterization. The average normal value for adults is 634 ml. plasma cleared/min./1.73 m.² of body surface.

Method: PAH may be determined by a method similar to that used for sulfanilamides; i.e., it is diazotized and coupled with *N*-(1-naphthyl)-ethylenediamine to give a red-violet color.

Reagents:

1. Acid cadmium sulfate. Dissolve 34.7 gm. crystalline cadmium sulfate ($3CdSO_4 \cdot 8H_2O$) in distilled water. Add 169 ml. 1N sulfuric acid and dilute to 1 L.
2. Sodium hydroxide, 1.1N. Dissolve 45 gm. sodium hydroxide in water to make 1 L. Standardize against known acid and adjust to 1.10 ± 0.05N.
3. Hydrochloric acid, 1.2N. Dilute 110 ml. concentrated hydrochloric acid to 1 L. with water.
4. Sodium nitrite, 0.1%. Dissolve 0.1 gm. sodium nitrite in 100 ml. water. Make up fresh as needed.
5. Ammonium sulfamate, 0.5%. Dissolve 0.5 gm. ammonium sulfamate in 100 ml. water. This solution is stable for about 2 wk. when stored in refrigerator.
6. Coupling reagent. Dissolve 0.1 gm. *N*-(1-naphthyl)-ethylenediamine dihydrochloride in 100 ml. water. This solution is stable several weeks when stored in refrigerator.

7. PAH stock standard. Dissolve 1 gm. sodium *p*-aminohippurate in distilled water to make 1 L. This solution contains 1 mg./ml. A dilution may be made from one of the ampules of the drug used in the test.

8. PAH working standard. Dilute 1 ml. stock standard to 250 ml. with water. This contains 4 μg PAH/ml.

Procedure:

Plasma precipitation and dilution of filtrate: To 2 ml. plasma in a 125 ml. Erlenmeyer flask add 20 ml. water and 6 ml. acid cadmium sulfate and mix well. Add 2 ml. 1.1N sodium hydroxide, stopper, and shake well. Allow to stand 10 min., then filter.

Urine dilution: Measure the volume of each urine specimen into a graduated cylinder, record the volume, then wash the urine into a 250 ml. volumetric flask with distilled water and dilute to the mark. (If volume is over 250 ml. dilute to 500 ml.) In the calculations of the clearance these diluted volumes (250 or 500 ml.) are considered to be the urine volumes of each specimen. The actual measured volumes are for the information of the physician and are to be included in the report.

Make a further dilution of the urine to 1:100 (or 1:50 if the urine was originally made to 500 ml.). This additional dilution is used in the calculation of urinary concentration.

Color development: Set up tubes as follows: blank, 5 ml. water; plasma, 5 ml. filtrate; urine, 5 ml. diluted urine; and standard, 5 ml. working standard. To each tube add 1 ml. 1.2N hydrochloride and mix. Then to each tube add 0.5 ml. sodium nitrite solution and mix well. After 3-5 min. add 0.5 ml. ammonium sulfamate solution to each tube. After an additional 3-5 min. add 0.5 ml. coupling reagent to each tube. Allow to stand for 10 min., then read samples and standards against blank in photometer at 540 mμ.

Calculations: The standard taken contains 4 μg PAH/ml. or 0.40 mg.%.

For plasma on a 1:15 dilution (2 ml. in a total volume of 30 ml.):

For urine on a 1:100 dilution:

$$\frac{\text{OD sample}}{\text{OD standard}} \times 40 = \text{Mg.\% PAH}$$

If the second dilution of the urine is 1:50 instead of 1:100, the factor in the equation is 20 instead of 40.

In the usual formula for clearance:

$$\frac{U}{P} \times \frac{V}{t}$$

U is the urine concentration and P is the plasma concentration in mg.%. V is the total urine volume collected in the time of t minutes. The value of V is taken as that of the first dilution, usually 250 ml.

If the diluted urine specimens give too high readings in the colorimeter, the determination may be repeated using a small aliquot of the diluted urine (making up to 5 ml. with water) and making the appropriate correction in the calculations. Therefore for 2 ml. diluted urine and 3 ml. water, the calculation formula would contain an additional factor of 5/2.

If three urine specimens and two blood samples are received, the first blood sample is used for calculating the clearance with the first urine specimen, the second sample for the third urine specimen, and the average concentration of the two samples for the second urine specimen.

GLOMERULAR FILTRATION RATE[76]: The glomerular filtration rate is determined by measuring the clearance of a completely filtrable substance which is neither absorbed nor excreted by the renal tubules. **Inulin,** a polysaccharide, fulfills this criteria, as does **endogenous creatinine,** though a small portion of the latter is also excreted by the tubules.

Inulin clearance: A priming infusion of inulin given at a rapid rate is followed by a sustaining infusion at a slow constant rate. The urine specimen should be obtained by catheterization. The difficulties associated with the calculation, preparation, and administration of the inulin solution weigh against the clinical use of this test. Clinically the less accurate creatinine clearance is preferred. The average

$$\frac{\text{OD sample}}{\text{OD standard}} \times 0.40 \times 15 = \frac{\text{OD sample}}{\text{OD standard}} \times 6 = \text{Mg.\% PAH}$$

inulin clearance of normal adults is 123 ml./1.73 m.² of body surface.

Method: Inulin is a polysaccharide composed of fructose units. The various methods for the determination of inulin are all based on reactions with fructose obtained by hydrolysis. Glucose also gives some color with the various fructose reagents, but in the method to be described the interference is small because 100 mg.% glucose gives about the same amount of color as 0.4 mg.% inulin. Normal serums also contain small amounts of other chromogenic materials and these may be corrected for by running a serum blank obtained from a blood sample taken before inulin is administered.

Reagents:
1. Indole-3-acetic acid, 0.5%. Dissolve 1 gm. purified indole-3-acetic acid in 200 ml. alcohol. Store in refrigerator.
2. Trichloroacetic acid, 10%. Dissolve 10 gm. trichloroacetic acid in distilled water and dilute to 100 ml.
3. Hydrochloric acid, concentrated.
4. Inulin standard, 0.05 mg./ml. Dry the inulin in a desiccator over calcium chloride. Rub 12.5 mg. with 2-3 drops of water in a 100 ml. beaker until no lumps remain. Rapidly add about 60 ml. distilled water that is nearly at the boiling point. Rinse the solution into a 250 ml. volumetric flask with water, cool, and dilute to volume. This standard can be preserved by saturation with benzoic acid which does not interfere with color reaction.[76]

Procedure: Add 4 ml. 10% trichloroacetic acid to 1 ml. serum or plasma. Add the acid slowly while mixing, let stand for 10 min., and then centrifuge strongly. Urines should usually be diluted 1:100 with water.

To 1 ml. aliquots of filtrate, diluted urine, standard, and water (reagent blank) add 0.2 ml. indole-3-acetic acid reagent and 8 ml. concentrated hydrochloric acid and mix. Place in a 37° C. water bath for 75 min. The temperature of the bath should not be above 37° C. in order to avoid interference from other sugars. After incubation, cool to room temperature and read in colorimeter against reagent blank at 520 mμ. The tubes should be read rather rapidly as the color intensity slowly increases with time.

Calculation:

$$\frac{\text{OD sample}}{\text{OD standard}} \times 0.05 \times D \times \text{Mg.\% inulin}$$

D is the dilution factor (5 for serum filtrates and ordinarily 100 for urine). Hence for serum or plasma

$$\text{Mg.\% inulin} = \frac{\text{OD sample}}{\text{OD standard}} \times 25$$

and for urine (diluted 1:100)

$$\text{Mg.\% inulin} = \frac{\text{OD sample}}{\text{OD standard}} \times 500$$

If the color is too intense, the determination may be repeated using a smaller aliquot or a larger dilution and making the necessary correction in the calculation.

If desired, a serum blank may be run and the value subtracted from the serum inulin levels. No urine blank is needed.

Creatinine clearance (endogenous): The 24 hr. urinary excretion of creatinine and its plasma level are relatively constant, so that a long period of 12-24 hr. can be utilized for the clearance study. The normal range of creatinine clearance is from 100-120 ml./min., or 116-148 L./24 hr./1.73 m.² of body surface.

Technique of 24 hr. clearance: The patient does not need to fast. The entire 24 hr. urine is collected without the aid of a preservative and stored in the refrigerator. (See discussion of urine collection, p. 11.) A serum specimen is obtained in the morning on the day of the test. The urine volume is measured and the creatinine level determined in serum and urine. The previously mentioned clearance formula is used:

$$C = \frac{UV}{P}$$

U = mg./100 ml. creatinine in urine
V = ml. urine excreted/min.
P = mg./100 ml. creatinine in plasma

Correction of clearance to standard 1.73 m.² of body surface (see p. 66):

$$\text{Observed clearance} \times \frac{1.73 \text{ m.}^2}{\text{Observed surface area}} = \text{Corrected clearance}$$

Blood urea clearance: This is the number of milliliters of blood that is cleared of urea per minute.

Principle: Urea produced by the liver is filtered through the glomeruli and partially absorbed by the tubules. The absorption takes place by passive diffusion, which is dependent on the amount of urea, on the urine flow (i.e., the amount of water), and on the state of the tubular epithelium. If the water absorption is increased (low filtration rate), the amount of urea absorbed is also increased, and the clearance is therefore small. If the urine flow is higher than 2 ml./min., the relationship of urea clearance to the filtration rate is nearly constant. The urea clearance thus varies with the urinary flow. An increase in urinary flow from 0-1.5 ml./min. produces an increased clearance, but an increase from 2-8 ml. and more varies the clearance only slightly.[77] When the urinary output is above 2 ml./min., the ratio of blood urea to urine urea is constant and in proportion to the urinary output; when below this "augmentation limit" of 2 ml./min., it is not constant and is in proportion to the square root of the urinary volume. In the former case the clearance is called the maximum clearance (Cm) and in the latter, the standard clearance (Cs). In the standard clearance the usual average urinary output of 1 ml./min. is taken as the standard.

Procedure: The patient must be fasting (no coffee [diuretic] and no protein [blood urea nitrogen]) and is allowed about ½ hr. to drink 4 full glasses of water and 1 hr. to rest. At the end of this period he empties the bladder completely, and the urine specimen is discarded. Urine specimens are then collected at two 30 min. intervals which are accurately timed to the minute. The bladder must be completely emptied each time. Oxalated blood is drawn for blood urea determination in the middle of each period.

Determine the urea concentration of each blood sample. Record the volume of each urine sample, calculate the rate of urine flow for each period as ml./min., and determine the urea concentration of each specimen. In order to accomplish this an aliquot of urine must be diluted so that the concentration of urea will approximate that in a 1:10 blood filtrate. Suggested dilutions are given in Table 2-4.

The analytic procedures required are described earlier in this chapter. Calculate the urea clearance for each period.

The average normal maximum clearance is 75 ml./min. (75% of filtration rate) and is reported as percent of normal (divide clearance by 75 and multiply by 100). The average normal standard clearance is 54 ml./min. (41% of filtration rate) and is also reported as percent of normal.

Calculations:

$$Cm = UV/B$$
$$Cs = U/B \times \text{square root of } V$$
$$U = \text{mg. urine urea/100 ml.}$$
$$B = \text{mg. blood urea/100 ml.}$$
$$V = \text{volume of urine/min.}$$

EXAMPLE:

Blood urea 72 mg./100 ml.
Urine
  First specimen:
    Urea 309 mg./100 ml.
    Amount 146 ml. = 2.43 ml./min.
  Second specimen:
    Urea 564 mg./100 ml.
    Amount 71 ml. = 1.18 ml./min.

$$Cm = \frac{309}{72} \times 2.43 \times \frac{100}{75} = 14\% \text{ of normal}$$

$$Cs = \frac{564}{72} \times \sqrt{1.18} \times \frac{100}{54} = 16\% \text{ of normal}$$

When the volumes of urine vary greatly in amount, duplicates usually do not check, and some investigators recommend mixing the two specimens and running as one specimen.

For very heavy or very thin adults and for children multiply V by 1.73/A (1.73/surface area in m.²). The surface area is estimated from the weight that is usual for a subject of the given height and age rather than from the observed weight (Fig. 2-21). For standard clearance no

Table 2-4

Vol. (ml./min.)	Dilution
0.5-2	1:500
2.0-4	1:250
4.0-8	1:100

Table 2-5. Square roots

Ml./min.	Square root
0.1	0.32
0.2	0.45
0.3	0.55
0.4	0.63
0.5	0.71
0.6	0.78
0.7	0.84
0.8	0.89
0.9	0.95
1.0	1.00
1.1	1.05
1.2	1.10
1.3	1.14
1.4	1.18
1.5	1.23
1.6	1.27
1.7	1.30
1.8	1.34
1.9	1.38
2.0	1.42

correction is necessary for persons between 62 and 71 in. in height; for maximum clearance, correction need not be made for persons between 65 and 69 in.

NOTES: It is **necessary** that the bladder be emptied completely when the test is begun and each time the specimens are collected.

It is **necessary** that the time when the test is begun (the bladder emptied) and the time when each specimen is collected be recorded to the nearest minute since these data enter into the calculation. It is not necessary that the time be exactly 30 min.

Significance: Normally there is a diurnal variation (least in the forenoon) of urea clearance. There is a decrease after arising. No significant change occurs after meals, but a decrease may follow subsistence on a low protein diet. There is a decrease after exercise and an increase after diuretics. Pathologically the blood

urea clearance shows evidence of impairment sooner than the blood urea, the phenolsulfonphthalein test, or the blood creatinine. Usually the clearance is 50% below the normal before the other tests show evidence of impairment. Decreased clearance means either decreased volume of blood passing through the kidney (decompensated heart) or decreased ability to excrete urea.

TESTS FOR TUBULAR FUNCTION:

Tubular absorption: If the clearance of a substance is less than the glomerular filtration rate, this may be due to partial absorption of this substance by the tubules. The absorbed fraction can be calculated from the glomerular filtration rate and the clearance. At high plasma concentration the tubular absorption of certain substances, e.g., **glucose,** becomes constant, representing the **maximal rate of tubular absorption (Tm).** Any excess, e.g., glucose, is excreted in the urine.

Average normal values of maximal tubular absorption of glucose in men (TmG[men]): 300-450 mg./min.

Tubular secretion: If the clearance of a substance is greater than the glomerular filtration rate, it may be assumed that the substance is excreted by the tubules into the urine. Some substances are filtered through the glomeruli **and** excreted by the tubules (PAH); others are filtered, absorbed, and excreted (K, Na); and again others are excreted in their entirety by the tubules (NH_4). At high plasma concentrations the tubular excretion becomes maximal and constant (Tm) and represents the **maximal tubular secretory capacity.** It can be determined by measuring the amount of **PAH** found in the urine corrected for the amount simultaneously filtered through the glomeruli.

Average normal values of maximal tubular secretion of PAH (TmPAH): 80-90 mg./min.

It may appear to be decreased when the specimen of urine is less than about 40 ml. or when the patient has been taking penicillin.

A temporary increase (few weeks) may occur in acute infections in young patients.

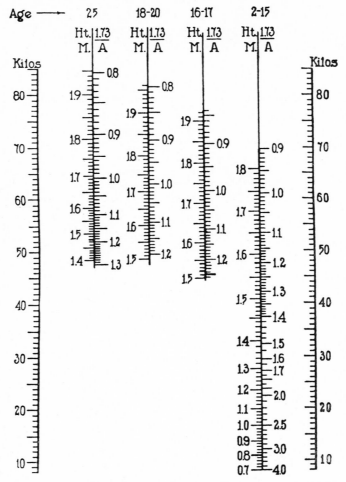

Fig. 2-21. Line chart for calculating for urea clearances the correction for body size in children and in adults with unusual physical structure. The value of $\dfrac{1.73}{A}$ is read off opposite the height of the patient in meters, either on the scale for patients in his age group or on scale 25 for patients of this age or older. The final result is obtained by multiplying the clearance with the figure on the $\dfrac{1.73}{A}$ side. Although these data are not required for urea clearance calculations, this chart in addition permits the estimation of the ideal weight for a patient of a given height in a particular age group. This may be accomplished by drawing a horizontal line from the patient's height to the weight scale on either side of the page. (From Peters and Van Slyke: Quantitative clinical chemistry, methods, Baltimore, 1932, The Williams & Wilkins Co., vol 2.)

URINARY CALCULI[78]

Urolithiasis is often difficult to detect, and it is therefore suggested that the urine of patients with a history of renal colics be filtered through double-thickness gauze.[79]

Urinary calculi are crystalloids em-bedded in a binding substance of mucus and protein which also contains inclusions of bacteria and epithelial cells. Recent methods of x-ray crystallography[80] and polarization microscopy allow determination of the exact chemical composition of the inorganic constituent of urinary calculi. Calculi may consist of calcium oxalate, apatite (calcium phosphate and carbonate), triple phosphates (calcium magnesium, ammonium phosphate, and carbonate), uric acid, and cystine.

Other rarely found substances include cystine and calcium carbonate. Generalized diseases that favor the formation of calculi are hyperparathyroidism (calcium stones) and cystinuria (cystine calculi). A kit for qualitative analysis of urinary calculi is available commercially.*

Analysis of urinary calculi—modified Heller table: Clean and dry. Make record of number, size, shape, color, and consistency. Describe surface (smooth, rough). Cut through the center (bone saw), and describe layers and core, examining them separately when present. Report findings as trace, slight or moderate amount, or "chiefly."

Powder and use a small portion for each test. Make all tests on a microscopic slide, unless otherwise specified, using small drops of reagents.

When filtering is desirable, cut a very small strip of filter paper (3-5 mm. wide and 20 mm. long), place it at the edge of the drop to be filtered, and slant the slide toward the filter. After the paper is wet, touch the lower side of it with a clean glass rod.

Procedure:
1. Heat on platinum foil or platinum wire tightly coiled.
   (a) Does not burn _____ _____ Inorganic material 2
   (b) Does burn _____ _____ Organic material 9
2. Treat a portion with 10% hydrochloric acid.
   (a) Effervesces, gross or microscopic _____ Carbonates 3
   (b) Does not effervesce _____ 4
3. Filter. Add ammonium oxalate, saturated solution (adjust as in 5).
   Calcium oxalate crystals, microscopic _____ Calcium carbonate
4. Heat a portion (on a platinum wire looped concentrically) until red hot,

cool, place on slide, and add 10% hydrochloric acid.
   (a) Effervesces, gross or microscopic _____ Oxalates 5
   (b) Does not effervesce _____ 6
5. Filter. Add ammonium oxalate, saturated solution. Adjust to yellow color with methyl red and phenol red indicators (pH 6.5).
   Calcium oxalate crystals, microscopic _____ Calcium oxalate
6. Dissolve a portion in a drop of concentrated nitric acid. Add a few drops of ammonium molybdate saturated solution and heat. If negative, repeat with ash as in 4.
   A yellow precipitate _____ _____ Phosphates 7 or 8
7. Dissolve a portion in a drop of 10% sodium hydroxide from a small glass rod while testing for liberated ammonia (ammonium chloride fumes) by holding close above the dissolving material the end of another glass rod moistened with hydrochloric acid, or test the portion dissolved in the sodium hydroxide with a drop of Nessler solution (yellow-brown color indicates ammonia).
   (a) Much ammonia _____ _____ Triple phosphates
   (b) Little or no ammonia _____ Calcium and magnesium phosphates
8. Dissolve a portion in a drop of acetic acid; filter and add a drop of ammonia.
   (a) White crystalline precipitate __ _____ Triple phosphates
   (b) White amorphous precipitate __ _____ Calcium and magnesium phosphates
   See note 1.
9. Burns.
   (a) Without flame. Test for urates and uric acid _____ 10
   (b) With flame _____ 13
10. Dissolve a portion in a drop of 10% sodium hydroxide solution; add a drop of uric acid reagent (see blood uric acid).
    (a) Blue color _____ _____ Urates or uric acid 11
    (b) No blue color _____ 12

*G. W. Alban Co., St. Louis, Mo.

Table 2-6. Classification and manifestations of kidney diseases

Type	Urine	Blood	Function	Systemic changes	Prognosis
Acute					
1. Focal glomerular nephritis	Hematuria Moderate albuminuria (trace) Hyaline and granular casts; possibly blood casts Pus, variable amount, normal amount, and normal specific gravity	Normal unless very slight increase in nitrogen	Normal	None	Good
2. Diffuse glomerular nephritis	Oliguria Dark red and cloudy Acid, unless blood makes alkaline High specific gravity (1.020-1.030) Albuminuria (1-1.5 gm./100 ml.) Casts: hyaline, granular, brown granular, and cellular, including blood cell, and epithelial cell casts Blood	Nitrogen retention Urea to 120 mg./100 ml. Uric acid 3-6 mg./100 ml. Creatinine 1-7 mg./100 ml. Anemia	Impairment in proportion to severity	Blood pressure increased Edema present Eyeground changes absent or only slight Anemia	May recover May be fatal May progress to subacute or chronic form
Subacute glomerular nephritis	Intermediate between diffuse and chronic Late in disease there may be polyuria with low fixed specific gravity and small amount of fat and lipoid in epithelial cells	Nitrogen retention increases	More and more impairment	Blood pressure becomes higher Edema present or absent Eyeground changes more marked Moderate to severe anemia	Poor Fatal usually within 2 yr.
Chronic glomerular nephritis					
1. Without edema (diffuse glomerular, with hypertension)	Polyuria; nycturia Pale yellow Clear; no gross sediment Acid reaction Low fixed specific gravity (1.005-1.015) Albuminuria (trace) Casts: hyaline and granular Blood present at times Late in disease: oliguria with low fixed specific gravity Doubly refractile substances in sediment	Nitrogen retention First stage: intermittent Second stage: moderate Third stage: marked and constant; not relieved by diet restriction Albumin-globulin ratio reversed	Impaired At first slight (dye 40%) Second stage: moderate (dye 10-20%) Third stage: severe (dye 0 to trace) Absolute insufficiency	Blood pressure increased Edema absent Eyeground changes absent or present Moderate to severe anemia Heart enlarged Chronic uremia, late	Repeated attacks of acute nephritis Fatal in 2-25 yr.

2. With edema (nephrotic phase of chronic glomerular nephritis)	In general, similar to chronic, but usually smaller amount, with somewhat higher specific gravity, with more albumin and casts, and sometimes with fat and lipoid in epithelial cells and casts. Doubly refractile substances in sediment	Similar to chronic, but when edema prominent, the blood may show findings similar to those in lipoid nephrosis. Hypoproteinemia; increase in $alpha_2$ and beta globulins, hypoalbuminemia	Similar to chronic unless edema interferes with tests	Similar to chronic except for presence of edema. Edema due to 1. Recurrent acute attacks 2. Cardiac failure 3. Combination with lipoid nephrosis	Similar to chronic
Nephrosis 1. Lipoid	Oliguria in proportion to edema. Normal color. Often cloudy. Slightly acid or alkaline. Specific gravity normal to very high. Marked albuminuria (5-20 or 60 gm./L.). Albumin much greater than globulin. Hyaline, granular, and fatty casts. Leukocytes and epithelial cells, both containing fat and lipoids. Free lipoid granules. Occasional blood cell. Doubly refractile crystals	Nitrogen *not* increased. Chlorides *not* increased. Lipoids increased and plasma may appear milky. Cholesterol 0.400-1% (normal about 0.200%). Total protein decreased ⅓-½ (normal 6.5-8.2%). Albumin-globulin ratio changed from 1.5:1 (normal) because albumin decreased and globulin increased, with ratio 1:2 or 1:6	Normal unless edema interferes with tests	Edema marked. No increase in blood pressure. No eyeground changes. B.M.R. low (−19%). Sedimentation velocity of red cells greatly increased. Faulty protein metabolism. More marked in young persons	May recover. Condition may last from months to many years. Some finally develop insufficiency. See chronic, with edema
2. Kidney of toxemia of pregnancy	Lipoid nephrosis but less marked	Nitrogen usually normal or slightly increased. Urea low. Uric acid slightly increased	Normal or slightly impaired	Blood pressure usually increased. Edema present or absent. Eyeground changes present or absent. May have very severe anemia such as addisonian pernicious anemia	Usually good. Some progress to chronic nephritis
3. Amyloid disease	Varies from normal to that of lipoid nephrosis	BUN increased; Congo red test may be positive; plasma protein changes	Insufficiency	Generalized amyloidosis	Death due to primary disease

(*Continued on p. 70*)

Table 2-6. Classification and manifestations of kidney diseases—cont'd

Type	Urine	Blood	Function	Systemic changes	Prognosis
4. Hemoglobinuric (lower nephron syndrome)	Oliguria to anuria Acid Specific gravity low and fixed Albuminuria Hemoglobinuria (or myohemoglobinuria) Hyaline and granular casts Heme casts (breakdown products of hemoglobin) Hemosiderin	NPN, urea, and creatinine increased Phosphorus increased CO_2-combining power of plasma, serum sodium, and chloride decreased	Impaired as in chronic	Blood pressure elevated after second day Edema, especially pulmonary Uremia	Poor if oliguria and hypertension persist
Arteriosclerotic 1. Without insufficiency (benign hypertension)	May be normal (early) Later shows trace of albumin with a few hyaline and granular casts With cardiac failure, findings same as in chronic passive congestion	Normal unless cardiac failure present	Normal unless cardiac failure present	Blood pressure increased Edema absent unless cardiac failure is present Eyeground changes absent or very slight Cardiac dilation, hypertrophy and failure rare	Good unless complicated by cardiac failure
2. With insufficiency (malignant hypertension)	Early, like arteriosclerotic Late, like chronic Differs from chronic: no history of acute attack of nephritis; no recurrent attacks of nephritis Blood pressure is higher Very small amount of albumin in urine	Like chronic	Like chronic	Blood pressure high, usually over 200 mm. Hg Edema absent unless cardiac failure present Eyeground changes marked Cardiac hypertrophy, dilation and failure common Apoplexy common Chronic uremia, late Anemia marked	Bad, but condition may last from few years to decade Fatal in about 6 mo. after absolute insufficiency occurs
Pyelonephritis	Trace of albumin WBC RBC Bacteria	Normal to N retention	Normal to N retention	Pyelitis Cardiac edema	Depends on circulation Uremia

11. Test a portion for ammonia as in 7.
    (a) Much ammonia _____
       _____ Ammonium urate
    See note 2.
    (b) Trace or no ammonia _____
       _____ Uric acid
12. Dissolve a portion (in a crucible) in a little nitric acid. No effervescence. Evaporate to dryness on water bath, yellow residue; add NaOH, orange; heat, red _____ Xanthin
13. Flame is briefly pale blue and has a sharp odor. Dissolve a portion in ammonia, filter, and let evaporate spontaneously.
    (a) Crystals: colorless hexagonal plates _____ Cystine

Dissolve a portion in a drop of 10% sodium hydroxide, add a drop of sodium cyanide solution (5%), and let stand 5 min. Add a drop of sodium nitroprusside solution (saturated). Cystine gives a purple-red color.

NOTE: If the test for calcium is positive, the following test for magnesium should be performed. Ash a small portion, dissolve, and make slightly acid. Saturate a small piece of filter paper with 0.01% alcoholic solution of *p*-nitrobenzene azoresorcinol and dry. Place in the center of this paper a drop of the slightly acid solution to be tested and let dry. Immerse in a dilute solution of sodium hydroxide (about 1%). Magnesium gives a blue spot in the red field. Sensitive to about 0.005 mg. magnesium. Nickel and cobalt give a similar color, and large amounts of ammonium salts and organic matter reduce the sensitivity.

URINARY HORMONES AND METABOLITES[81, 82]

A rigid definition of a hormone is not simple, but most definitions state that hormones are chemical substances originating in discrete endocrine organs and discharged into the bloodstream. Their interaction with appropriate cells produces a characteristic physiologic response. Hormones are one of the major systems for the integration of the physiologic activity of the body (the other being the nervous system). Although various hormones are secreted into the bloodstream, they are present in only very minute quantities and it is often very difficult to separate them from the other blood constituents for analysis. Hormones are excreted in the urine as unchanged hormones and as various metabolites, which may or may not be physiologically active. Because hormones and their metabolites may be found in somewhat higher concentrations in the urine and because it is relatively easier to secure a large urine sample rather than a large blood sample, most hormones are determined in urine, at least in the ordinary clinical laboratory. The methods for most blood determinations are long and tedious and require special apparatus and techniques. The only hormone determination in blood considered to be a routine laboratory procedure is that of the thyroid hormone since the determination of the protein-bound iodine gives a good measure of the amount of circulating thyroid hormone. Most of the other hormones to be discussed are determined in the urine. It is assumed that the amount excreted in the urine is a measure of the amount in the blood, and hence of the amount secreted by the gland. In many instances it is not a specific compound that is measured, but a group of related hormones and metabolites which are assumed to come chiefly from one endocrine gland.

The pituitary gland, which has been called the "master" gland of the body, produces several hormones. At least six hormones are well established: thyroid-stimulating hormone (TSH), follicle-stimulating hormone (FSH), luteinizing hormone (LH), adrenocorticotropic hormone (ACTH), luteotropic hormone (LTH), and growth hormone (GH). There are probably others such as the antidiuretic hormone, oxytocin, and melanocyte-stimulating hormone. Direct determinations of most of these hormones in the blood or urine are well beyond the capabilities of most clinical laboratories. One that is not too difficult is the FSH determination which is measured by a bioassay, measuring the effect of the isolated hormone on the immature rat uterus. This test probably also includes the LH, also known as interstitial cell–stimulating hormone

(ICSH), because both are gonadotropic hormones, i.e., affect the gonads. The determination of FSH may be helpful in determining whether the gonadal insufficiency is primary or due to insufficient stimulation by the pituitary hormones. There is another gonadotropic hormone, the chorionic gonadotropin, which is secreted by the placenta. Its excretion is increased markedly during pregnancy, and the detection of this hormone in urine is used as a test for pregnancy (see p. 89).

Although ACTH cannot be measured directly, an estimate of the function of the pituitary in this regard can often be made by an indirect method. The output of the adrenal cortex depends on, among other things, stimulation by the pituitary ACTH. The adrenal cortex activity can be estimated by measurement of the excretion of adrenal hormone metabolites in the urine. This is discussed more fully in the section on adrenal hormones.

STEROID HORMONES[83]

A large number of hormonal substances, found chiefly in the gonads and adrenal cortex, have a similar basic chemical structure and are known as the steroid hormones. The basic steroid nucleus is as shown:

In the female hormones, estrogens, the methyl group at position 19 is missing (hence these are sometimes known as the C-18 steroids), and the ring A has a benzenoid structure, giving these compounds more acidic properties; therefore they may be separated from the other steroids by extraction with dilute alkali. For the most part the androgenic hormones have the basic structure just shown

and are thus referred to as the C-19 steroids. The adrenocortical hormones and the progesterone derivatives (corpus luteum hormone) have an additional 2-carbon chain attached to carbon 17 and are referred to as the C-21 steroids. Within each group there are usually several different hormones secreted by a given endocrine gland (testes, ovary, adrenal cortex) and often several more chemically similar metabolites are found in the urine. The procedure to determine a single individual compound is quite complicated. Usually a group of similar compounds is assayed together as a class: this is usually sufficient for most clinical purposes. It might also be mentioned that the cholesterol molecule also contains the same steroid nucleus with a longer carbon chain on position 17. Cholesterol is believed to be a precursor in the synthesis in vivo of many of the steroid hormones.

Steroid hormones influence the entire body. They control salt and water metabolism; affect carbohydrate, protein, and fat metabolism; control the development of the primary and secondary sex characteristics; and affect the distribution of hair and development of the muscular and skeletal systems. The physiologic differences of the various hormones result from variations in the nature and position of side chains.

Estrogens

Estrogens and estrogen metabolites have been isolated from the ovaries, placenta, testes, and adrenal cortex. In males and postmenopausal women the total amount of estrogen excreted in the urine is usually less than 15 μg/day, and the determination of such small amounts is technically difficult. In males, estrogen excretion may be increased by estrogen-producing tumors of the adrenal cortex or testes, in cirrhosis when the liver fails to inactivate the estrogens normally produced, and in certain cases of male infertility. In females the estrogen excretion is increased in ovarian tumors. There is a cyclic variation during the menstrual cycle and an enormous increase in pregnancy.

In the normal cycle the excretion may

vary from a low of 10-20 μg/day at the beginning of the cycle to a high of 40-100 μg/day at ovulation. In pregnancy the excretion may rise to near 30 mg./day at term. The chemical determination of estrogens in the urine in the later stages of pregnancy is not difficult. In clinical practice the state of estrogen activity can be estimated from other tests such as the cervical mucus test (fern test), glucose test performed on the vaginal epithelium, cytologic pattern of the desquamated vaginal epithelium, and endometrial biopsy.

Luteal hormones

The corpus luteum of the ovary also produces some hormones. The principal steroid is progesterone which is also a 21-carbon steroid similar to the adrenal steroids. The chief metabolite of this hormone found in the urine is pregnanediol. It is present in quantities of 2-10 mg./day during the latter half of the menstrual cycle. Smaller amounts are found in the earlier part of the cycle, in the urine of men, and in postmenopausal women. The methods for the determination of pregnanediol, usually column chromatography or other methods for separation, are rather complicated and are not ordinarily performed in the usual clinical laboratory. The results of the assays have not proved to be of striking diagnostic value. There is a rise during pregnancy to a peak excretion of 30-100 mg./day, but there are much simpler and more reliable tests for pregnancy. Lower excretion values during pregnancy have been associated with threatened abortion or toxemia of pregnancy, and increased levels of progesterone-like compounds have been found in adrenal hyperplasia.

Androgens

The androgenic hormones have methyl groups at both positions 18 and 19 and an OH or =O group at position 17. Those with the C=O structure at position 17 are the 17-ketosteroids. The most important testicular hormone, testosterone, is actually not a ketosteroid, but a number of its metabolites such as androsterone, dehydroepiandrosterone, and etiocholanolone are ketosteroids found in urine. Thus the

17-ketosteroid concentration will in part represent androgenic activity.

Adrenocortical hormones— corticosteroids

As previously mentioned, corticosteroids have an additional 2-carbon side chain attached to position 17 of the steroid nucleus. They are excreted partially as C-21 steroids and partially as C-17 ketosteroids. A number of methods have been used for the determination of various groups of the corticosteroids. One of the methods presented here involves the change of the corticosteroids into 17-ketosteroids by oxidation; hence the group of compounds determined is known as the ketogenic steroids. These include most of the important corticosteroids and is quite satisfactory for most clinical purposes because the level of ketogenic steroids reflects the adrenal cortex activity quite well.

There is a decrease in ketogenic steroid (and ketosteroid) excretion in Addison's disease, hypopituitarism, Simmonds' disease, and cretinism. An increased level of ketogenic steroid excretion is found in Cushing's syndrome, in precocious puberty due to adrenal hyperplasia, and in physiologic stress (surgery, burns, infectious diseases).

Determination of ketosteroids and hydroxysteroids (ketogenic steroids)[84-87]: Ketosteroids are excreted in the urine chiefly as conjugated sulfates and glucuronates. These are usually hydrolyzed by heating with acid, a method not entirely satisfactory since the acid causes some alteration of the steroids. It is still generally used when only the total ketosteroids are being determined.

After hydrolysis the ketosteroids are extracted from the urine with an organic solvent. Ether is used in the method given here. This solvent has some disadvantages because of its volatility and flammability, but it usually extracts less interfering chromogens and gives less trouble with emulsions during extraction than other solvents. The ether extract is washed with sodium hydroxide solution, which removes some interfering color as well as the estrogens extracted from the urine. The ether is then dehydrated by means of solid sodium hydroxide, filtered, and an aliquot evaporated to dryness for the colorimetric determination.

Steroids having a ketone ($>$ C=O) grouping at position 17 in the molecule (17-ketosteroids) will react with meta-dinitrobenzene in alkaline solution to form a purple-red color. Numerous modifications of the reagents have been used. The ones given here are relatively stable and yield a low blank value. After development of the color (usually 1 hr. or more at room temperature in the dark) the solution is somewhat diluted and read in the colorimeter.

There is usually some interfering brown color present. This can be corrected by various methods. The absorbance can be measured at two or more different wavelengths and an empirically determined correction formula can be used, or the colored solution can be diluted with alcohol, water, and chloroform (or ethylene dichloride) in such proportions that two immiscible layers are formed. The desired ketosteroid color is found in the lower solvent layer; the interfering color in the upper aqueous layer is discarded. If a good spectrophotometer is available, the two-wavelength method is simpler, but if only a filter photometer is available, the extraction method is necessary.

Many of the important adrenocortical steroids and their metabolites have a hydroxyl group and a short carbon chain at position 17 (17-hydroxysteroids) in the molecule $\left(> C\begin{smallmatrix}-OH \\ -CH_3\end{smallmatrix}\right)$. These hydroxysteroids can be oxidized to ketosteroids by the use of sodium bismuthate or sodium periodate. If the urine is first treated with the reducing agent sodium borohydride, the ketosteroids originally present are reduced to compounds that no longer give the color with the reagent even after subsequent treatment with an oxidizing agent. Thus, by successive treatment with borohydride and periodate, the original ketosteroids are eliminated as chromogens and the hydroxysteroids are oxidized to ketosteroids and determined as such (ketogenic steroids). Appreciable amounts of glucose in the urine will interfere, but this can usually be overcome by using larger quantities of the two reagents.

Reagents:

1. Methyl alcohol, purified. To approximately 1200 ml. AR anhydrous methyl alcohol add 2 gm. silver nitrate dissolved in 5 ml. water. Then while stirring add 5 gm. potassium hydroxide dissolved in 25 ml. warm methyl alcohol. Filter under suction through a bed of Celite. Transfer the filtrate to an all-glass still. Distill, discard the first 100 ml. distillate, and collect about 800 ml. of distillate. This purified methyl alcohol is required only for the preparation of the alcoholic potassium hydroxide solution. Elsewhere the regular AR grade may be used.

2. Potassium hydroxide, 4N in methanol. Add 34 gm. potassium hydroxide pellets to 120 ml. purified methanol and dissolve, preferably with the aid of a magnetic stirrer. Filter through hardened paper or centrifuge if necessary and transfer the clear liquid to a polyethylene bottle. Add exactly 2 ml. solution to about 20 ml. water and titrate with standard acid with phenolphthalein indicator. Calculate the normality and dilute to 4.00 ± 0.15N. This reagent is quite stable. A small amount of potassium carbonate may settle out, but this is not harmful.

3. Ethylene glycol monomethyl ether (Methyl Cellosolve). The reagent grade of the solvent may be used without purification. If it gives very high blanks, it may be purified similar to methyl alcohol.

4. Dinitrobenzene, 1%. Dissolve 1 gm. dinitrobenzene (recrystallized from alcohol or special Sigma grade) in 100 ml. Methyl Cellosolve. Store in refrigerator.

5. Sodium hydroxide, 5N. Dissolve 100 gm. sodium hydroxide in water to make 500 ml. This solution need not be standardized.

6. Sodium hydroxide, 1N and 0.1N. Prepare from the 5N solution by appropriate dilutions (1:5 and 1:50).

7. Sulfuric acid, 1N. Add 14 ml. concentrated acid to about 400 ml. water. Cool and dilute to 500 ml.
8. Acetic acid, 25%. Mix 100 ml. glacial acetic acid and 300 ml. water.
9. Acetic acid, 6%. Dilute 30 ml. glacial acetic acid to 500 ml. with water.
10. Sodium borohydride, 10%. Just before use, dissolve 1 gm. sodium borohydride in 10 ml. 0.1N sodium hydroxide solution.
11. Sodium metaperiodate (10%). Just before use, dissolve 2 gm. sodium metaperiodate in 20 ml. water. This solution is near saturation and the salt may dissolve slowly.
12. Steroid stock standard. Dehydro-epiandrosterone is commonly used as a standard for ketosteroids. Dissolve 250 mg. of this steroid in methyl alcohol and dilute to 100 ml. Store in tightly stoppered bottle in refrigerator. One milliliter contains 2.5 mg. of steroid.
13. Working standard. Dilute 2 ml. stock standard to 100 ml. with methyl alcohol. This standard contains 25 μg in 0.5 ml. Store in refrigerator.
14. Ether, AR.
15. Sulfuric acid, 50%. Cautiously add 100 ml. concentrated sulfuric acid to 100 ml. water. Mix and cool.
16. Sodium hydroxide, AR, solid pellets.

General procedure: Measure total volume of a well-mixed 24 hr. urine specimen. Record volume and reserve a few hundred ml. for analysis. Run determinations in duplicate. Perform extractions in 25 × 150 mm. screw-capped tubes with rubber-lined caps. During extraction procedure with ether, keep tubes cooled in ice water or cold, running tap water except during actual manipulations. During warm weather it is helpful to cool the solutions used for washing the ether extract. This is conveniently done by storing bottles of these solutions in the refrigerator. Care must be taken in the evaporation of ether extracts; even a hot plate can ignite high concentrations of ether vapors. The lower aqueous layer is removed from the ether extract in the tubes by means of a 1 ml.

serologic pipette attached with rubber tubing to a source of suction and trap. Suction is controlled by pressure on the rubber tubing at the top of the pipette.

Ketosteroids: To the extraction tube add 7.5 ml. urine and 1 ml. 50% H_2SO_4. Heat in a boiling water bath for 15 min., then cool well. Add exactly 25 ml. ether, cap tightly, and shake for 3 min. Allow the layers to separate while cooling, then remove the lower aqueous layer. Add 5 ml. cold 1N sodium hydroxide solution, cap, and shake for 15 sec. Allow layers to separate and remove lower aqueous layer. Add 20-30 pellets solid sodium hydroxide, cap, and shake at intervals during the next 10 min. Cool well and centrifuge briefly. Filter ether extract through rapid paper, covering top of funnel with watch glass to prevent evaporation. Transfer a 10 ml. aliquot of the filtrate (corresponding to 3 ml. urine) to a 25 × 150 mm. tube. (A larger aliquot may be used if the original total urine volume was over 1500 ml., though in this case it may be advisable to evaporate the ether in portions, adding a second portion to the tube after most of the first has evaporated.) Evaporate the ether on a water bath under a fume hood. CAUTION! No Flame! Dissolve the residue in 0.5 ml. methyl alcohol and again evaporate to dryness on a water bath. Similarly, evaporate a standard of 25 μg steroid in 0.5 ml. alcohol and a blank of 0.5 ml. methyl alcohol. Allow tubes to cool to room temperature before proceeding with color development. Prepare a sufficient quantity of color reagent just before use by mixing 3 vol. 4N alcoholic potassium hydroxide and 4 vol. 1% metadinitrobenzene. Add 0.7 ml. of the mixture to each tube of sample, standard, or blank. After agitating gently to dissolve the residue, allow to stand for 1 hr. at room temperature in the dark. Then add to each tube 5 ml. Methyl Cellosolve and mix. Read standards and samples against blank at 520 and 430 mμ. Calculate the corrected readings for each tube as:

$$\text{Corr. OD} = \frac{\text{OD (520)} - 0.6 \times (\text{OD [430]})}{0.73}$$

NOTES: The corrected OD for the standard should be close (5%) to the uncorrected 520 OD. A lower corrected reading usually indicates faulty reagents. Then:

$$\frac{\text{Corr. OD sample}}{\text{Corr. OD standard}} \times \frac{\mu\text{g standard}}{\text{Ml. urine exct.}} \times$$

$$\frac{\text{Vol. ether added}}{\text{Vol. ether evap.}} = \mu\text{g steroid/ml. urine}$$

Since μg/ml. = mg./L.
Then:

$$\mu\text{g/ml.} \times \text{Volume in L.} = \text{Total mg.}$$
$$\text{ketosteroids excreted}$$

For the aliquots used as given:

$$\frac{\text{Corr. OD sample}}{\text{Corr. OD standard}} \times \frac{25 \times 25 \times \text{urine}}{7.5 \times 10} \times$$

$$\text{Volume in L.} = \text{Total mg. excreted}$$

As an alternative to reading at two wavelengths, proceed as follows: When the color has been developed after standing 1 hr., add to each tube 2.5 ml. Methyl Cellosolve and mix. Add 2 ml. water and mix. Then add 2.5 ml. ethylene dichloride and mix. The reagents must be added in the order given, mixing after each addition. Then agitate strongly and transfer to a smaller test tube and centrifuge at high speed. Remove top aqueous layer completely. If lower layer is not perfectly clear, add a few drops of methyl alcohol. Transfer lower layer to cuvette and read at 520 mμ only. The calculations are the same except that OD at 520 mμ is used without any correction.

Hydroxysteroids (ketogenic steroids): Test urine for sugar with Clinistix or similar test strip. If no more than a trace of sugar is present, proceed as outlined. If more sugar is present, see notes at end of section for necessary modifications. Pipette 7.5 ml. urine to 25 × 150 mm. tube. Check pH and adjust to 6.5-7.5 with short-range paper, using 1N sodium hydroxide or 6% acetic acid as needed. Add a few ml. of ether to aid in reducing foaming, then add 0.9 ml. freshly prepared sodium borohydride solution. Allow the tubes to stand at room temperature for 1 hr. Cautiously add 0.5 ml. 25% acetic acid, adding a few ml. more ether

if necessary to prevent foaming. Allow to stand for a few minutes, check the pH, and add a few drops more of acid if necessary to bring the pH to near 7. Allow to stand for 15 min. with occasional swirling. Add 3 ml. 10% sodium metaperiodate solution and 0.5 ml. 1N sodium hydroxide. Incubate at 37° C. for 1 hr. Add 0.5 ml. 5N sodium hydroxide and incubate for 15 min. more. Cool tubes well, add exactly 25 ml. ether, cap tubes, and shake for 3 min. Remove the lower aqueous layer, It may be necessary to centrifuge briefly at this point to break any emulsion formed on shaking. Gently stir up any white precipitate in the bottom of the tube and remove as much of it as possible along with the aqueous layer. Add 3 ml. 1N sulfuric acid, cap, and shake vigorously. Allow layers to separate while cooling, then remove aqueous layer. Wash the ether layer with 5ml . cold 1N sodium hydroxide solution, shake again for about 15 sec., allow the layers to separate, and remove the lower layer by suction. Add 20-30 pellets of solid sodium hydroxide to the ether. From this point proceed exactly as with the ketosteroids. All final details and calculations are the same.

NOTES: If more than a trace of sugar is present in the urine, proceed as follows: After the addition of the borohydride, allow to stand for 45 min. and add 0.3 ml. 25% acetic acid and about 60-70 mg. more of solid borohydride. Allow to stand for an additional 45 min. Then add 0.5 ml. 25% acetic acid as in the regular procedure and allow to stand for 10 min. More acetic acid may be necessary to bring the pH to 7. After the addition of the periodate, incubate for at least 1½ hr., add an additional 200 mg. periodate after 45 min., and then agitate to dissolve the salt after addition.

Normal values and interpretation: Increases in the ketosteroids are found in testicular or other virilizing tumors and precocious puberty. Decreased levels are found in gonadal agenesis or dysgenesis and in hypothyroidism. A fraction of the ketosteroids measured in the urine also are metabolites of the various hormones secreted by the adrenal cortex; hence changes in the secretion of these hormones will also cause changes in the urinary excretion of ketosteroids. The normal levels of the ketosteroid excretion per day are as follows: birth to 3 yr., less than 1 mg.; 3 to 8 yr., 0.5-2.5 mg.; 12 to 16 yr., 4-9 mg.; adult males, 10-18 mg.; and adult females, 6-15 mg. After the age of about 50 yr., excretion of the ketosteroids begins to decrease and may be only in the range of 4-8 mg./day in either sex after the age of 65. The changes in ketosteroids as reflections of the changes in adrenocortical hormones are included in the discussion of those hormones.

Urinary 17-hydroxysteroids—modified Porter-Silber method[88, 89]: The corticosteroids are excreted as glucuronide conjugates; beta-glucuronidase hydrolyzes these conjugates at the optimum pH 6.8. The corticosteroids are extracted by chloroform. These substances form a yellow chromogen with phenylhydrazine-alcoholic sulfuric acid reagent. A control is run on each urine specimen to compensate for the nonsteroid chromogenic substances present in the urine.

Reagents:

1. Chloroform, reagent grade. If redistilled before use, add 0.1% ethanol to prevent formation of phosgene.
2. NaOH, 0.1N.
3. Absolute ethyl alcohol.
4. Sulfuric acid, 64% (v/v). Add 640 ml. concentrated H_2SO_4 to 360 ml. distilled water.
5. Alcoholic sulfuric acid reagent. Mix 100 ml. 64% sulfuric acid with 50 ml. absolute ethanol.
6. Recrystallized phenylhydrazine hydrochloride. If Baker's phenylhydrazine is used, there is no need for recrystallization. Phenylhydrazine hydrochloride may be twice recrystallized from absolute ethanol and dried in a desiccator over calcium chloride.
7. Phenylhydrazine-alcoholic sulfuric acid reagent. Dissolve 50 ml. recrystallized phenylhydrazine hydrochloride in 50 ml. alcoholic sulfuric acid reagent. This reagent must be freshly prepared before use.
8. Glucuronidase (bacterial) 1000 units/ml. in distilled water. Prepare fresh before use or keep frozen.
9. Phosphate buffer, pH 6.8, 0.5M. Prepare a 1M solution of KH_2PO_4 by dissolving 68 gm. KH_2PO_4 in 500 ml. water. The pH is adjusted to 6.8 by the addition of 100-150 ml. 1N NaOH and diluted to 1 L. in a volumetric flask.
10. Stock standard (1 ml. = 100 μg). Transfer 25 mg. cortisol* (hydrocortisone-alcohol) to a 250 ml. volumetric flask and dilute to volume with absolute ethanol.
11. Working standard (1 ml. = 5 μg). Dilute 5 ml. stock solution to 100 ml. with distilled water.

Procedure: A 24 hr. urine specimen is collected in a bottle containing 10 ml. toluol as a preservative. The total volume is measured and approximately 100 ml. is retained for analysis. To a 100 ml. glass-stoppered cylinder transfer 10 ml. urine, 1 ml. beta-glucuronidase enzyme (1000 units/ml.), 2 ml. 0.5M phosphate buffer, and 1 ml. chloroform.

The reagent blank and standard samples are prepared in like manner by using 10 ml. water and 10 ml. working standard instead of urine. Samples are mixed well and incubated at 37° C. for 18-24 hr. Add to each cylinder 50 ml. chloroform. The contents of the cylinders are mixed by repeated inversion for 30 sec. and then allowed to stand until the organic and aqueous phases have separated. Remove the aqueous supernatant by aspiration. Add 10 ml. 0.1N NaOH to each cylinder and shake for 30 sec. The two phases are allowed to separate and the alkali layer is removed by aspiration. In the same manner the chloroform extracts are washed twice with 10 ml. water. Two 20 ml. aliquots of the chloroform extracts from the blank and the urine are transferred to 50 ml. glass-stoppered cylinders. One 20 ml. aliquot of the standard is transferred to a 50 ml. cylinder. One aliquot of the blank and the unknown serve as the control blank and the unknown control. The other aliquots serve

---

*Sigma Chemical Co., St. Louis, Mo.; Mann Research Laboratories, New York, N. Y.

as the reagent blank, standard, and unknown.

Add 5 ml. alcohol-sulfuric acid reagent to the cylinders containing the control blank and the urine controls. Add 5 ml. phenylhydrazine-alcoholic sulfuric acid to the cylinders containing the reagent blank, standard, and unknowns. The cylinders are tightly stoppered, shaken vigorously for 30 sec., and allowed to stand for 15-20 sec.

Transfer the supernatants from each cylinder to a small cuvette and incubate in a 60° C. water bath for 45 min.

The unknown controls are read against the control blank; the standard and the unknowns are read against the reagent blank at a wavelength of 410 mμ.

Calculations:

$$17\text{-OH corticosteroids (mg./24 hr.)} = \frac{U-C}{S}$$
$$\times 0.005 \times V$$

U = optical density of unknown
C = optical density of control
S = optical density of standard
0.005 = concentration of standard (mg./ml.)
V = volume of urine in ml.

Normal values:
Adults: 10-15 mg./24 hr.
Children: 0-1 yr., 0.5 mg./24 hr.
        1-5 yr., 1-2 mg./24 hr.

Adrenal function tests[90-92]: The adrenal cortex secretes its hormone upon stimulation by the pituitary hormone (ACTH). If the output of the adrenal cortex is low, this may be due to either failure of the pituitary to secrete the necessary ACTH or the failure of the adrenal cortex to respond to the ACTH produced by the pituitary. The administration of exogenous ACTH will aid in differentiating between these two conditions. If the administered ACTH causes a marked rise in the excretion of ketosteroids and ketogenic steroids (in normal individuals the urinary output of ketosteroids may be increased 2-3 times and that of ketogenic steroids 3-4 times), then the original low level is due to the failure of the pituitary to secrete ACTH. If the exogenous ACTH causes little rise in the steroid excretion, the adrenal gland is at fault.

Stimulation test: Collect a 24 hr. urine specimen prior to the test and assay for 17-ketosteroids and 17-hydroxysteroids. On the day of the test start collection of 24 hr. urine specimen at 8 A.M. and begin intravenous drip of saline solution containing 20 units of ACTH. This should be allowed to run for a period of 8 hr. Intramuscular injection of 80 units of ACTH on 2 successive days can also be utilized. The response to the stimulation test is related to the mass of the cortical tissue, the number of units of ACTH, and the sensitivity of the response. A 24 hr. urine specimen is again collected and assayed for 17-ketosteroids and 17-hydroxysteroids.

Suppression test: The theoretic basis for this test is the so-called feedback mechanism. Cortisone derivatives decrease the output of adrenal cortical hormone by depressing the anterior pituitary gland.

A 24 hr. urine specimen is obtained prior to the test. It is assayed for 17-ketosteroids and 17-hydroxysteroids. The test is performed by administering 1 mg. 1-alpha-fluorohydrocortisone, 0.5 mg. Decadron, or 2.5 mg. prednisolone daily for each 3 mg. of 17-hydroxycorticoids in the urine. The dose is divided and given every 6 hr. after meals for 3 days. Then a 24 hr. urine specimen is collected again and assayed for 17-ketosteroids and 17-hydroxysteroids. Table 2-7 summarizes the results obtained in the various adrenal function tests.

Aldosterone

Aldosterone is an adrenal cortical hormone that appears in the urine in amounts up to 15 μg/24 hr. The amount of aldosterone varies with the state of electrolyte balance of the individual. Sodium depletion raises the level, whereas administration of sodium lowers it. These changes are controlled by the extracellular fluid volume rather than by the serum or total body sodium. Administration of potassium also increases the aldosterone level, whereas potassium deficiency lowers it. An increase in aldosterone is referred to as aldosteronism and occurs as primary aldosteronism and secondary aldosteronism.

Primary aldosteronism: In this condi-

Table 2-7. Summary of adrenal function tests

Disease	Hormonal changes in urine		Tests	
	17-ketosteroids	Ketogenic steroids	ACTH stimulation	Cortisone suppression
Cushing's disease (hyperplasia)	± to N	++	+++	50%
Adenoma (unilateral) functioning	++ variable	++variable	KGS + KS variable	None
Carcinoma (unilateral) functioning	++	++	None	None
Adrenogenital syndrome	+++ Dehydroepiandrosterone in urine	Depends on whether due to hyperplasia, adenoma, or carcinoma		
Congenital adrenal hyperplasia	+ Pregnanetriol in urine	+	None	Yes
Addison's disease	Not indicated	Low	None	Not indicated

+ = increased; − = decreased; ± = variable.

tion the high aldosterone excretion is due to adrenal tumors (adenoma and carcinoma). Laboratory findings include normal 17-ketosteroids and 17-OH excretion, low serum potassium, alkalosis, low specific gravity of urine, increased 24 hr. volume of urine, and elevation of serum sodium. The clinical findings are hypertension, weakness, polyuria, and tetany.

Secondary aldosteronism: In this condition the characteristic elevated aldosterone excretion is due to salt depletion, cardiac failure, cirrhosis, pregnancy, and lower nephron nephrosis.

Assay of aldosterone: Because of its importance in the regulation of electrolyte balance, many attempts have been made to find an adequate assay method for aldosterone. The compound is present in the urine in minute amounts representing less than 1% of the total corticosteroid metabolites in the urine. Therefore extremely elaborate methods of separation and purification are required. Most methods use at least one separation by column chromatography, followed by two or more separations by paper or thin-layer chromatography before the final determination. It is evident that the procedure is very tedious and complicated, requires several working days for completion, and can be done only in a well-equipped laboratory.

Catecholamines[93-96]

The adrenal gland consists of the cortex and the medulla. The cortical hormones have been described previously in the discussion of steroids. The adrenal medulla consists of cells that have an affinity for chrome salts and are therefore called chromaffin cells and belong to the chromaffin system. This system embraces not only the adrenal medulla but also the extramedullary chromaffin tissue in the paraganglia. The adrenal medulla produces two pressor amines called epinephrine and norepinephrine which belong to the group of catecholamines. Tumors arising in the adrenal medulla and in the extraadrenal chromaffin tissue are called pheochromocytomas. These tumors, a small percentage of which are malignant, give rise to hypertension, either paroxysmal or sustained, due to their production of these pressor amines.

These pressor substances are found within the red blood cells and serum. In the serum, epinephrine is partially bound to albumin. In the urine, catecholamines appear either free or conjugated to glucuronides. Of the free catecholamines in the urine, 80% are norepinephrine and the remainder are epinephrine. In patients with pheochromocytoma there is an increased excretion of urinary catecholamines.

A number of different procedures have been employed for the determination of catecholamines. These can be classified as biologic, pharmacologic, chemical-colorimetric, and chemical-fluorometric.

The biologic methods employ strips of rabbit aorta and measure the contractile response to urine containing the pressor amines.

The pharmacologic methods involve the measurement of the blood pressure response to epinephrine and norepinephrine blocking agents such as Regitine, histamine, and other substances.

Chemical-colorimetric techniques have proved to be insensitive and somewhat nonspecific when applied to urine.

Physicochemical procedures such as paper chromatography are acceptable methods. The chromatograms have to be examined under ultraviolet light.

Determination of total catecholamines: In this method catecholamines are adsorbed from alkaline urine into activated alumina, eluted with sulfuric acid, and reacted with reagents that produce a fluorescent derivative. The fluorescence is compared with that of standards treated in the same way, using a photofluorometer for quantitation or compared visually with an ultraviolet lamp for semiquantitation. A 24 hr. urine specimen preserved with 1 ml. concentrated H_2SO_4 is required. The patient must abstain from any drugs for 72 hr. before the specimen is collected.

Reagents:
1. Aluminum oxide, chromatography grade. Weigh 2 gm. and transfer to a small graduated cylinder. The weight may be approximated from this volume. Aluminum oxide is washed by shaking 200 gm. in a liter of hot 1N HCl, rinsing free from acid with several changes of distilled water, and drying.
2. Phenolphthalein, 1% solution in ethanol.
3. Sodium hydroxide, 20% solution.
4. Sulfuric acid, 0.20N solution.
5. Sodium bicarbonate, 2% solution. Store in dark.
6. Potassium ferricyanide, 0.25% solution. Store in dark.

7. Ascorbic acid, 2% solution. Stable for 36 hr. in refrigerator.
8. Mixture:
   A. 9 parts 20% NaOH
   B. 1 part 2% ascorbic acid
   This mixture should be centrifuged briefly and prepared just before use.
9. Norepinephrine standard solution. Levophed bitartrate* containing 0.1% norepinephrine base.
10. Working standard, 20 μg/ml. Dilute 0.1 ml. to 5 ml. in distilled water.

NOTES: If the volume of the 24 hr. specimen is greater than 2000 ml., use a 200 ml. aliquot for analysis and correct the result obtained by the appropriate factor. The standards are based on the use of an aliquot of one-tenth the 24 hr. specimen; therefore if a smaller aliquot is used, the result must be corrected accordingly. Usually the test is carried out on an aliquot of a 24 hr. specimen, but in markedly paroxysmal cases a single specimen analyzed after an attack may be more informative.

Procedure: Label four 500 ml. Erlenmeyer flasks No. 1, No. 2, No. 3, and No. 4. Into No. 1 measure one-tenth of a 24 hr. collection of urine; this is the unknown. Into No. 2, No. 3, and No. 4 measure 100 ml. of a normal urine specimen. To No. 2 add 0.3 ml. norepinephrine working standard (20 μg/ml.); this is 100 μg/24 hr. standard. To No. 3 add 0.7 ml. standard; this is 180 μg/24 hr. standard. To No. 4 add 1.1 ml. standard; this is 260 μg/24 hr. standard. Dilute contents of each flask to 200 ml. with distilled water. All subsequent operations are the same for each flask.

Add to each flask 2 gm. aluminum oxide and 0.5 ml. 1% phenolphthalein; then while mixing add drop by drop 20% NaOH until a pink color persists. Continue mixing for about 2 min.; then permit aluminum oxide to settle. The granular aluminum oxide will settle very rapidly but the flocculent precipitate of phosphates will largely remain suspended. Pour off the supernatant fluid and phosphates as completely as possible; then wash the aluminum oxide by adding

---

*Winthrop Laboratories, Inc., New York, N. Y.

about 200 ml. distilled water, mix, allow the aluminum oxide to settle, and pour off the water.

Transfer the aluminum oxide to a 15 ml. centrifuge tube. This can best be accomplished by adding 2-3 ml. water, making a slurry, and sucking this slurry up into a pipette. Centrifuge for 3-4 min. at 1500-2000 rpm. Decant water and drain the centrifuge tube and wipe dry.

Add 5 ml. 0.20N H_2SO_4 to each tube and suspend the aluminum oxide thoroughly with a glass rod. The catecholamines adsorbed on the aluminum oxide are eluted at this stage, so thorough mixing is required.

Centrifuge 2-3 min. at 1500-2000 rpm. Transfer exactly 3 ml. supernatant to a Pyrex tube containing 3.0 ml. 2% Na_2CO_3 and mix. Add 0.5 ml. 0.25% potassium ferricyanide and mix again. After 2 min. add 1 ml. of a mixture containing 9 parts 20% NaOH and 1 part 2% ascorbic acid (this mixture should be prepared just before use) and mix again.

Centrifuge briefly to clarify and transfer supernatant to fluorometer cuvettes and read against water blank or transfer to flat-bottomed nonfluorescent tubes (culture tubes used in bacteriology are satisfactory) and examine tubes for green fluorescence in darkened room under ultraviolet light. This is best accomplished by holding the light under the tubes in a rack in such a manner that each tube is illuminated to approximately the same intensity. Compare intensity of fluorescence of the unknown to that of the standards.

Discussion: Under these conditions preparations from normal urine show faint green fluorescence, whereas those from urine having an abnormally high catechol content show an intense bright green fluorescence. Normal urine can be readily distinguished from urine containing 180 μg or more of catechols/24 hr. The approximate total catecholamines content of the specimen analyzed can be calculated as follows:

$$\text{Total catechols/24 hr.} = \frac{180}{D}$$

where D is the dilution made, or in a

positive test, by diluting the specimen to match the standard.

Quantitative calculations from fluorometric readings: For a quantitative estimation, run a blank, three standards, and the urine sample using the procedure previously described. The samples are then read in a fluorometer using a primary filter at about 394 mμ and a secondary filter at about 530 mμ. The specifications vary with different fluorometers. Holland gives the procedure for the Coleman fluorometer.[*] Usually the instrument is set to zero with a water blank. With the 180 μg standard in the instrument, set the meter at a convenient point, say 50 on the scale. Then read the sample. If the sample is low, adjust the meter if possible with 100 μg standard to give a convenient reading; then read standard, sample, and reagent blank. If the sample is high, adjust the meter so that 260 μg standard and sample both read on scale. Read sample, standard, and reagent blank. Subtract reading of reagent blank from readings of sample and standard, then:

$$\frac{\text{Corr. reading of sample}}{\text{Corr. reading of standard}} \times \text{Conc. of standard} = \text{Conc. of sample in } \mu\text{g/day}$$

Vanillyl mandelic acid (VMA) (3-methoxy-4-hydroxymandelic acid)[97-105]:

VMA is a metabolite of epinephrine and norepinephrine found in the urine in amounts of 10-100 times the amount of pressor amines. Its determination is used as a measure of endogenous secretion of catecholamines. Urinary excretion of VMA is highly elevated in the urine of patients with pheochromocytoma. Because the concentration of VMA in urine is much greater and methods for its determination are simpler and more adaptable to the average laboratory, it is preferred over the more intricate catecholamine determination.

In the method described, acidified urine is treated with Florisil for adsorbance and removal of chromogenic substances. VMA is extracted from the urine with ethyl acetate, subsequently reextracted into alkaline solution, then treated with diazo-

---

[*]Coleman Instruments, Inc., Maywood, Ill.

Table 2-8

	Urine (ml.)	H₂O(ml.)	Working standard (ml.)	Reagent 1	Ethyl acetate (ml.)
Blank		4.0		2 drops	10
Unknown	1	3.0		5 drops	10
Standard		3.8	0.2	2 drops	10

tized *p*-nitroaniline, and reextracted in butanol. The OD of the butanol layer is measured at wavelengths of 540 and 450 mμ.

A 24 hr. urine specimen preserved with 10 ml. concentrated HCl is collected. For 48 hr. before the collection of the specimen the patient must abstain from all medications, coffee, bananas, and substances containing vanilla.

Reagents:

1. Hydrochloric acid, 2N saturated with 1% sodium chloride. Dilute 86 ml. concentrated acid to 500 ml. with water and add 20 gm. NaCl to saturate.
2. Hydrochloric acid, 0.10N saturated with sodium chloride. Dilute 5 ml. concentrated acid to 500 ml. with water and add 20 gm. NaCl to saturate.
3. Potassium carbonate, 5%. Dissolve 5 gm. anhydrous potassium carbonate (K_2CO_3) or 4.6 gm. anhydrous sodium carbonate (Na_2CO_3) in water to make 100 ml.
4. *p*-Nitroaniline. Dissolve 0.5 gm. in 10 ml. concentrated HCl and dilute to 500 ml. with water.
5. Sodium nitrite, 2%. Dissolve 2 gm. in water to make 100 ml. Prepare fresh.
6. Diazotized *p*-nitroaniline. Prepare fresh just before use by mixing 2.5 ml. nitroaniline solution, 7.5 ml. water, and 0.25 ml. sodium nitrite solution.
7. Ethyl acetate, AR.
8. n-Butanol, AR, redistilled.
9. Stock standard solution of VMA. Dissolve 10 mg. 3-methoxy-4-hydroxymandelic acid in 10 ml. water. This solution contains 1000 μg/ml.

It is stable when kept in refrigerator.

10. Working standard. Dilute stock standard 1:10 in water. This solution contains 100 μg/ml. Prepare weekly and keep refrigerated.
11. Florisil* (activated magnesium silicate), 60-100 mesh size.

Procedure: To 10 ml. filtered urine adjusted to pH 2.5-5.5 add 0.5 gm. Florisil. Shake vigorously for 30 sec. and centrifuge. Use the supernatant fluid.

Prepare in duplicate the solutions in Table 2-8 and pipette into 40 ml. round-bottom, narrow-neck centrifuge tubes.

Shake vigorously for 1 min. Add 2.5 ml. reagent 2 and again shake vigorously for 1 min. Centrifuge for 5 min. at 1500 rpm in order to separate the two layers. Transfer 8 ml. of the upper layer (ethyl acetate) to another 40 ml. centrifuge tube and add 5 ml. potassium carbonate. Shake vigorously for 1 min. Centrifuge for 5 min. at 1500 rpm, remove the ethyl acetate (upper layer) by suction, and discard. Transfer 4 ml. of the K_2CO_3 extract to 12 ml. glass centrifuge tubes and add 1 ml. diazotized *p*-nitroaniline. Shake vigorously for 30 sec. and let stand for 1 min. Add 5 ml. butanol, shake again for 30 sec., and centrifuge. Remove the upper layer (butanol extract) carefully.

Read the extracted butanol layer on a photometer at 450 and 540 mμ against the blank of the procedure. The corrected adsorbance (CA) = OD at 540 mμ – OD at 450 mμ.

Calculation:

$$\text{Mg. VMA/24 hr.} = \frac{\text{CA unknown}}{\text{CA standard}} \times 0.02 \times V$$

---

*Floridin Co., Tallahassee, Fla.

where 0.02 is the concentration in mg. of the standard (0.2 ml. 100 μg/ml.) and V is the 24 hr. urine volume in ml.

Normal values and interpretation: The urinary excretion of VMA in the normal adult ranges from 2-14 mg./24 hr. (mean 5.4 ± 3.03). A marked increase is found in functioning pheochromocytoma, with concentrations reaching as high as 150 mg./day.

Serotonin 5-hydroxytryptamine[106-110]

Serotonin is derived from tryptophan, an amino acid, and is excreted as 5-hydroxindolacetic acid. Tryptophan is first oxidized and then decarboxylated to form serotonin (5-hydroxytryptamine). The breakdown occurs through oxidative deamination by the enzyme amino oxidase. Serotonin is produced by the chromaffin cells of the intestines, and therefore under normal circumstances 90-95% is localized in the gastrointestinal mucosa. Small amounts are found in the spleen due to platelet disintegration, and some can be detected in the brain. The small amount found in the blood is essentially due to the serotonin transported by the platelets. Normally only about 1% of dietary tryptophan is used for the production of serotonin. In patients with carcinoid tumors that have metastasized to the liver or lymph nodes, about 60% of the daily tryptophan is diverted by the tumor into the serotonin pathway, leaving less tryptophan available for the formation of niacin and protein. Under these conditions a clinical syndrome is produced called the carcinoid syndrome. This is characterized by skin changes such as flushing and cyanosis, by cardiac signs and symptoms pointing toward involvement of the right heart and lung, by diarrhea, and occasionally by asthma.

The methods described are based on the photometric measurement or visual comparison of the color complex formed by 5-HIAA with nitrous acid and 1-nitroso-2-naphthol.

Reagents:
1. Chloroform, AR.
2. Ether (anhydrous, peroxide-free), AR.
3. Sodium chloride, AR.
4. Ethyl acetate, AR.
5. 2, 4-Dinitrophenylhydrazine. Dissolve 1 gm. in about 160 ml. 2N HCl by heating in boiling water bath. Allow to cool, dilute to 200 ml. with 2N HCl, and filter.
6. Phosphate buffer, 0.5M, pH 7.0. Dissolve 69 gm. sodium phosphate monobasic (NaH_2PO_4) in about 800 ml. water, adjust pH, and dilute to 1 L.
7. 1-Nitroso-2-naphthol reagent, 0.1% in 95% ethanol. Dissolve 100 mg. in 95% ethyl alcohol and dilute to 100 ml.
8. Stock 5-HIAA standard, 1 mg./ml. Dissolve 20 mg. 5-hydroxyindole-3-acetic acid monodicyclohexylammonium salt or 10 mg. 5-HIAA in 10 ml. 0.5M phosphate buffer
9. Working standard, 40 μg/ml. Dilute 1 ml. stock standard to 25 ml. with water.
10. Sulfuric acid, 2N. Carefully add 14 ml. concentrated H_2SO_4 to about 200 ml. water, mix, cool, and dilute to 250 ml.
11. Hydrochloric acid, 2N. Carefully add 43 ml. concentrated HCl to about 200 ml. water, mix, cool, and dilute to 250 ml.
12. Sodium nitrite, 2.5%. Dissolve 2.5 gm. sodium nitrite in water and dilute to 100 ml.
13. Nitrous acid reagent. To 5 ml. 2N H_2SO_4 add 0.2 ml. 2.5% $NaNO_2$. This reagent should be prepared just before use.

Qualitative test: Since 5-HIAA accounts for most of the 5-hydroxyindole material in urine, direct application of the nitrosonaphthol color test, omitting the extraction procedure, provides a simple diagnostic test for malignant carcinoid. This qualitative test is not specific for 5-HIAA and measures all 5-hydroxyindoles; positive tests should be followed by the quantitative determination. Administration of certain drugs may cause interference. Metabolites of chlorpromazine interfere with color formation and patients should abstain from this drug while urine specimens are collected.

Procedure: To test tube containing 0.8

ml. water and 0.5 ml. 1-nitroso-2-naphthol reagent add 0.2 ml. of urine and mix. Add 0.5 ml. nitrous acid reagent and mix again. Let stand at room temperature for 10 min., add 5 ml. ethylene dichloride, and shake once more. The phases should be allowed to separate. In cases of turbidity the tubes should be centrifuged. A positive test is indicated by a purple color in the top layer. Normal might show as a slight yellow color. Assuming an average 24 hr. urine volume of 1000 ml., a purple color will be seen at levels of 5-HIAA excretion as low as 30 mg./24 hr. At high levels the color is more intense and is almost black at levels above 300 mg./24 hr.

Quantitative method: Acidified urine is treated with 2, 4-dinitrophenylhydrazine for removal of interfering keto-acids and extracted with chloroform for removal of indoleacetic acid. The 5-HIAA is then extracted into ether, reextracted into a small volume of phosphate buffer, and reacted with nitrous acid and 1-nitroso-2-naphthol.

A 24 hr. urine specimen preserved with 10 ml. concentrated HCl is required. It is important that patients refrain from taking nonessential medication for 72 hr. prior to urine collection. The specificity of this method is excellent and the only interference is found in *p*-hydroxyacetanilide, which is a fairly insignificant problem because it is present in very minute amounts.

Procedure: To 8 ml. urine in 50 ml. glass-stoppered tube add 8 ml. 2, 4-dinitrophenylhydrazine reagent. Mix and let stand 15-30 min. to permit complete reaction and precipitation. Add 30 ml. chloroform, shake for a few minutes, and centrifuge.

Remove chloroform layer and replace with fresh 30 ml. chloroform and repeat extraction, centrifugation, and removal of chloroform layer. Remove 12 ml. aliquot of the aqueous layer and transfer to 40 ml. glass-stoppered centrifuge tube containing 5 gm. NaCl and 30 ml. ether. Shake for 5 min. and centrifuge. Transfer a 25 ml. aliquot of the ether layer to another 40 ml. glass-stoppered centrifuge tube containing 3.0 ml. 0.5M phosphate buffer (pH 7.0). Shake for 5 min., cen-

trifuge, and remove ether by aspiration. Transfer 2 ml. of aqueous phase into a 15 ml. glass-stoppered centrifuge tube containing 1 ml. of 1-nitroso-2-naphthol reagent and mix. Add 1 ml. nitrous acid reagent, mix, and incubate at 37° C. for 5 min.

Add 8 ml. ethyl acetate and shake to remove yellow pigment in urine extract. After separation of phases, remove ethyl acetate by aspiration and repeat extraction with another 8 ml. portion of ethyl acetate. Remove ethyl acetate, transfer aqueous layer to cuvette, and measure OD at 540 mμ against reagent blank.

Standards are prepared by treating 1, 2, and 4 ml. working standard diluted to 8 ml. with water, exactly as the urine samples. These standards contain 40, 80, and 160 μg 5-HIAA, respectively; or when diluted to 8 ml., 5, 10, and 20 μg/ml. The reagent blank is prepared by treating 8 ml. H_2O in the same manner.

Calculation:

$$\text{Mg. 5-HIAA/day} = \frac{\text{OD unknown}}{\text{OD standard}} \times \text{Conc. of standard} \times \text{24 hr. urine vol.}$$

Normal values and interpretation: Normally small amounts of the serotonin metabolite 5-hydroxyindolacetic acid can be found in the urine. The normal range of excretion is 2-9 mg./24 hr. In the presence of a carcinoid tumor the level rises to 25-1000 mg./24 hr.

REFERENCES

1. Kark, R. M., et al.: A primer of urinalysis, ed. 2, New York, 1963, Harper & Row, Publishers.
2. Kushner, D. S.: J.A.M.A. **195**:119, 1966.
3. Berman, L. B.: G.P. **34**:94, 1966.
4. Cawley, L. P., Sanders, J. A., and Musser, B. O.: Amer. J. Clin. Path. **41**:381, 1964.
5. McIntyre, M., and Mou, T. W.: Amer. J. Clin. Path. **43**:53, 1965.
6. Heyd, C. G.: Ann. Surg. **79**:55, 1924.
7. Mallory, T. B.: Amer. J. Clin. Path. **17**:427, 1947.
8. Menkes, J. H., Hurst, P. L., and Craig, J. M.: Pediatrics **14**:462, 1954.
9. Pfohl, R. A.: Arch. Intern. Med. **116**:681, 1965.
10. Dogramaci, I.: J. Pediat. **30**:6, 1947.
11. Warhol, R. M., Eichenholz, A., and Mulhausen, R. O.: Arch. Intern. Med. **116**:743, 1965.
12. Holmes, J. H.: Workshop on urinalysis and

renal function studies, preworkshop manual, Chicago, 1962, Commission of Continuing Education, American Society of Clinical Pathologists.

13. Holoubek, J. E., Carroll, W. H., Riley, G. M., and Langford, R. B.: J.A.M.A. **153**: 1018, 1953.
14. Howard, T. L.: J. Urol. **46**:241, 1941.
15. Jones, Henry Bence: Philos. Tr. R. Soc. London **1**:55, 1848.
16. Cohen, E., and Raducha, J. J.: Amer. J. Clin. Path. **37**:660, 1962.
17. Naumann, H. N.: Amer. J. Clin. Path. **44**: 413, 1965.
18. Milne, M. D.: Brit. Med. J. **1**:327, 1964.
19. Hargreaves, T.: J. Clin. Path. **16**:293, 1963.
20. Various authors: Brit. Med. Bull. **10**:161, 1954.
21. Khachadurian, A., Knox, W. E., and Cullen, A. M.: J. Lab. Clin. Med. **56**:321, 1960.
22. Siest, D., Siest, G., and Besson, S.: Bull. Soc. Pharm. (Nancy) **51**:19, 1961.
23. Lewis, H. B.: Ann. Intern. Med. **6**:183, 1933.
24. Lane, M. R.: J. Pediat. **58**:80, 1961.
25. Mackenzie, D. Y., and Woolf, L. I.: Brit. Med. J. **1**:90, 1959.
26. Penrose, L. S.: Lancet **2**:949, 1946.
27. McCaman, M. W., and Robbins, E.: J. Lab. Clin. Med. **59**:885, 1962.
28. Wong, P. W., O'Flynn, M. E., and Inouye, T.: Clin. Chem. **10**:1098, 1964.
29. Anderson, J. A., Fisch, R., Miller, E., and Doeden, D.: J. Pediat. **68**:351, 1966.
30. Gentz, J., Jagenburg, R., and Zetterström, R.: J. Pediat. **66**:670, 1965.
31. Brenton, D. P., and Gaull, G. E.: J. Pediat. **67**:58, 1965.
32. Fine, J.: Brit. Med. J. **1**:205, 1967.
33. Eli Lilly & Co.: Physician's Bull. **21**:67, 1956.
34. Sophian, L. M., and Connelly, V. J.: Amer. J. Clin. Path. **22**:41, 1952.
35. Jusie, D., and Fiser-Herman, M.: Clin. Chim. Acta **6**:472, 1961.
36. Beutler, E., and Baluda, M.: J. Lab. Clin. Med. **68**:137, 1966.
37. Beutler, E., Baluda, M., Sturgeon, P., and Day, R.: Lancet **1**:353, 1965.
38. Foord, A. G., and Baisinger, C. F.: Amer. J. Clin. Path. **10**:238, 1940.
39. Konzelman, F. W.: J.A.M.A. **140**:931, 1949.
40. Snell, A. M.: J.A.M.A. **138**:274, 1948.
41. Neefe, J. R.: Ann. Intern. Med. **31**:857, 1949.
42. Beddard, A. P.: Guy's Hosp. Rep. **56**:127, 1902.
43. Drummond, K. N., Michael, A. F., Ulstrom, R. A., and Good, R. A.: Amer. J. Med. **37**:928, 1964.
44. Budinger, J. M., and Cavallo, M.: Amer. J. Clin. Path. **42**:626, 1964.
45. Boroian, T. V., and Atwood, C. R.: J. Pediat. **67**:69, 1965.
46. Dean, G.: S. Afr. Med. J. **34**:745, 1960.

47. Rimington, C.: Biochem. J. **75**:620, 1960.
48. Fernandez, A. A., Henry, R. J., and Goldenberg, H.: Clin. Chem. **12**:463, 1966.
49. Abrahams, A., Gavey, C. J., and Maclagan, N. F.: Brit. Med. J. **2**:327, 1947.
50. Harris, R. S., and Derian, P. S.: Southern Med. J. **42**:973, 1949.
51. Watson, C. J., Taddeini, L., and Bossenmaier, I.: J.A.M.A. **190**:501, 1964.
52. Townsend, J. D.: Ann. Intern. Med. **60**: 306, 1964.
53. Fergus, E. B.: Postgrad. Med. **39**:148, 1966.
54. Faulkner, W. R., and O'Mara, T. F.: Amer. J. Clin. Path. **39**:209, 1963.
55. Sternheimer, R., and Malbin, B.: Amer. J. Med. **11**:312, 1951.
56. Love, B. F., and Petracca, T. R.: Amer. J. Clin. Path. **41**:448, 1964.
57. McQueen, E. G.: Lancet **1**:397, 1966.
58. Addis, T.: Arch. Intern. Med. **30**:378, 1922.
59. Addis, T.: J.A.M.A. **85**:163, 1925.
60. Daysog, A., and Dobson, H. L.: Amer. J. Clin. Path. **39**:419, 1963.
61. Parrish, A. E., and Alpert, L. K.: J.A.M.A. **152**:1713, 1953.
62. Bolande, R. P.: Pediatrics **24**:7, 1959.
63. Schwartz, L., Flippin, H. F., Reinhold, J. G., and Domm, A. H.: J.A.M.A. **117**:514, 1941.
64. Lehr, D., and Antopol, W.: Amer. J. Clin. Path. **12**:200, 1942.
65. Aarons, J. M.: Amer. J. Clin. Path. (tech. sect.) **5**:163, 1941.
66. Lehr, D.: Proc. Soc. Exp. Biol. Med. **58**: 11, 1945.
67. Flippin, H. F., and Boger, W. P.: Virginia Med. Monthly **76**:56, 1949.
68. Lehr, D.: Proc. Soc. Exp. Biol. Med. **64**: 393, 1947.
69. Zeller, W. W., Hirsh, H. L., Sweet, L. K., and Dowling, H. F.: J.A.M.A **136**:8, 1948.
70. Exton, W. G.: J. Lab. Clin. Med. **15**:386, 1930.
71. Runge, S.: Reference in Ztschr. Anal. Chem. **4**:249, 1865. In Hallay, L. I.: Virginia Med. Monthly **69**:334, 1942.
72. Wolman, I. J., Evans, B., and Lasker, S.: Amer. J. Clin. Path. (tech. sect.) **10**:162, 1946.
73. Straffon, R. A., and Garcia, A. M.: J. Urol. **83**:774, 1960.
74. Tubis, M., Posnicl, E., and Nordyke, R. A.; Proc. Soc. Exp. Biol. Med. **103**:497, 1960.
75. Smith, W. W., Finkelstein, N., and Smith, H. W.: J. Biol. Chem. **135**:231, 1940.
76. Dontas, A. S., et al.: Lancet **1**:943, 1966.
77. Renbi, F.: Triangle **4**:301, 1960.
78. Beeler, M. F., Veith, D. A., Morriss, R. H., and Biskind, G. R.: Amer. J. Clin. Path. **41**:553, 1964.
79. Brandt, G.: Acta Chir. Scand. **119**:193, 1960.
80. Lagergren, C., and Ohrling, H.: Acta Chir. Scand. **117**:335, 1959.
81. Young, W. C., editor: Sex and internal

secretions, ed. 3, Baltimore, 1961, The Williams & Wilkins Co.

82. Astwood, E. B., editor: Clinical endocrinology, New York, 1960, Grune & Stratton, Inc.

83. Klyne, W.: The chemistry of the steroids, London, 1957, Methuen & Co., Ltd.

84. Commission of Continuing Education: Workshop on hormone assay, preworkshop manual, Chicago, 1959, American Society of Clinical Pathologists.

85. Commission of Continuing Education: Workshop on hormone assay, technique manual, Chicago, 1959, American Society of Clinical Pathologists.

86. Callow, R. K., and Emmons, C. W., editors: Androgen and adrenocortical hormone group steroids; hormone assay, New York, 1950, Academic Press, Inc.

87. Few, J. D.: J. Endocr. **72:**31, 1961.

88. Silber, R. H., and Busch, R. D.: J. Endocr. **16:**1333, 1956.

89. Porter, C. C., and Silber, R. H.: J. Biol. Chem. **185:**201, 1950.

90. Nabarro, J. D. N.: Brit. Med. J. **5198:**533, 1960.

91. Cope, C. L., and Black, E. G.: Brit. Med. J. **5160:**1117, 1959.

92. Kuhl, W. J., Jr., and Lipton, M. A.: New Eng. J. Med. **263:**128, 1960.

93. Weil-Malherbe, H., and Bone, A. D.: J. Clin. Path. **10:**138, 1957.

94. Henry, R. J., and Sobel, C.: Arch. Intern. Med. **100:**196, 1957.

95. Jacobs, S. L., Sobel, C., and Henry, R. J.: J. Clin. Endocr. **21:**305, 1961.

96. Holland, J. C.: Amer. J. Med. Techn. **25:** 408, 1959.

97. Mahler, D. J., and Humoller, F. L.: Clin. Chem. **8:**47, 1962.

98. Giltow, S. E., et al.: J. Clin. Invest. **39:** 221, 1960.

99. Sunderman, F. W., et al.: Amer. J. Clin. Path. **34:** 293, 1960.

100. Georges, R. J.: J. Med. Lab. Techn. **21:** 126, 1964.

101. Sunderman, F. W., Jr.: Amer. J. Clin. Path. **42:**481, 1964.

102. Pisano, J. J., Crout, J. R., and Abraham, D.: Clin. Chim. Acta **7:**285, 1962.

103. Jacobs, S. L., Sobel, C., and Henry, R. J.: J. Clin. Endocr. **21:**315, 1961.

104. Georges, R. J., and Whitby, L. G.: J. Clin. Path. **17:**64, 1964.

105. Hernandez, A.: Lab. Dig. **29:**10, 1966.

106. Udenfriend, S., Weissbach, H., and Brodie, B. B.: In Glick, D., editor: Methods of biochemical analysis, New York, 1958, Interscience Publishers, Inc., vol. 6.

107. Peart, W. S., Andrews, T. M., and Robertson, J. I. S.: Lancet **1:**577, 1961.

108. Udenfriend, S., Titus, E., and Weissbach, H.: J. Biol. Chem. **216:**499, 1955.

109. Pernow, B., and Waldenström, J.: Lancet **267:**372, 1954.

110. Foreman, R. C.: Ann. Surg. **136:**838, 1952.

Chapter 3

Examination of semen and pregnancy tests

EXAMINATION OF SEMEN

The semen (correctly called ejaculate since it may not contain spermatozoa) is a milky liquid that contains secretions of the prostate and other glands, spermatozoa and some of their precursor cells, epithelial cells, macrophages that are often filled with spermatozoa, and occasional leukocytes, fat droplets, and crystals of fat or of spermine (Fig. 3-1).

Normal values:
Amount: 2.6 ml.
Number: 80,000,000-120,000,000/cm.³
Motility: Progressive decrease at 21° C.

70-90% motile in first hour
70-60% motile in second to fourth hour
60-50% motile in fourth to seventh hour
50-35% motile in seventh to tenth hour
35-25% motile in tenth to fifteenth hour

Morphology: 79-90% normal forms
Lower limits of normal:
Amount: 0.5 ml.
Number: 20,000,000/mm.³
Motility: 40% motile in first hour
Morphology: 60% normal forms

COLLECTION

The physician should instruct the patient how to collect the specimen for examination. Collection should follow a period of abstinence of 4-7 days.

It is usually collected by masturbation or by coitus interruptus into a glass or plastic container. The container should be clean and at body temperature. Condoms, even when thoroughly washed and rinsed, may contain spermicidal agents and should be emptied rapidly into a suitable container. A minute hole made in the condom with a heated needle will not invalidate the test and will make its use acceptable to some religious groups. Exposure of spermatozoa to cold and spermicidal agents reduces the motility. Note the date and exact time when the specimen was obtained.

GROSS EXAMINATION

Make a record of the amount, color, turbidity, and viscosity.

Amount: The average amount is 4-5 ml.

Color and turbidity: In human beings color and turbidity have no relation to spermatozoa contents.

Viscosity: Fresh ejaculate gels, but it liquefies after 10-20 min. Persistence of the gel is abnormal. Examination of semen should not be undertaken until it is liquefied. Viscosity can be tested by drawing out the liquid into a fine strand with a glass rod.

pH: 7.2-7.6.

MICROSCOPIC EXAMINATION

Place 1 drop of semen on a microscope slide to determine whether spermatozoa are present at all and, if present, to judge their motility.

Motility: When the specimen has become liquefied, mount a drop under a cover glass and seal with petrolatum. Insert special eyepiece disk (as for reticulocyte count) and count under the high-power dry lens the motile and nonmotile

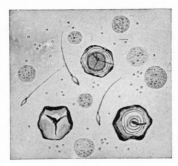

Fig. 3-1. Spermatic fluid showing spermatozoa, corpora amylacea, and lecithin granules. (From Gershenfeld: Urine and urinalysis, Philadelphia, 1948, Lea & Febiger.)

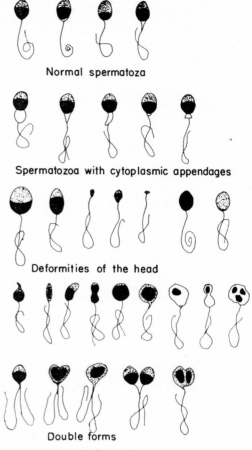

Normal spermatoza

Spermatozoa with cytoplasmic appendages

Deformities of the head

Double forms

Fig. 3-2. Morphology of spermatozoa. (From Vasterling: Praktische Spermatologie, Stuttgart, 1960, Georg Thieme Verlag.)

spermatozoa in two or more areas, reporting the percent of motile forms. Only those that move forward actively are considered motile. Examine at once and at 3, 6, and 24 hr.

Motility depends on the temperature and number of cells. At 37° C. only 50% of the spermatozoa are motile after 3 hr., while at 21° C. 50% are still motile after 7 hr. When the semen is diluted with glucose-Ringer solution (1:10 or 1:20), the motility of the spermatozoa improves. Mixing 1 drop semen with 0.5% yellow eosin (aqueous) will enable detection of dying or dead spermatozoa which are colored yellow. Living spermatozoa do not accept the dye. The degree of activity is important since more active spermatozoa lose their motility faster than sluggish cells.

Spermatozoa count: When the specimen has become liquefied, mix thoroughly and dilute 1:20 with a solution containing 5 gm. sodium bicarbonate, 1 ml. formalin, and 100 ml. distilled water. In a white blood cell diluting pipette, draw semen to mark 0.5 and formalin solution to mark 11.

Let mixture stand until mucus dissolves, shake thoroughly, fill a blood counting chamber, and count as for red cells.

Count one square millimeter area, one large square, and multiply result by 200,000 to obtain number of spermatozoa per milliliter.

Morphology: This is best studied in stained smears, which can be easily prepared from the specimen diluted for the spermatozoa count. Make smears as described for blood and stain with Wright (or Giemsa) stain or by the Gram method. The hematoxylin-eosin staining method is preferred by some. Report the percent of abnormal forms, using the special eyepiece disk and the oil-immersion lens.

The lower the number of spermatozoa, the more abnormal forms occur. The abnormality may be morphologic or tinctorial. Spermatozoa that stain abnormally are potentially abnormal. Of the structural abnormalities, those of the head (very small, very large, etc.) are more important than those involving the tail or neck (Fig. 3-2).

LABORATORY FINDINGS
IN PREGNANCY[1-4]

With a few exceptions, the laboratory findings in normal pregnancy are within the normal range for nonpregnant adults. Significant differences are usually due to some accompanying disease.

Gonadotropic hormone of chorionic origin appears in the blood and urine, yielding positive tests for pregnancy.

The **erythrocyte sedimentation** rate is increased after the third month. There is a slight increase in the **plasma volume** during the second and third trimesters, causing a decrease of about 10-15% in the hemoglobin, the erythrocyte count, and the hematocrit reading. At labor there is moderate **leukocytosis,** which usually disappears during the first week of the puerperium.

The **urine** is increased in volume (25%) during the last trimester and may contain a small amount of albumin (about half the cases). A large amount of albumin suggests a complication. Lactose may appear in the urine at any time during pregnancy but is more likely to be found near term and in the puerperium.

The **blood nonprotein nitrogen** is decreased (20-25 mg.%), with a relatively greater decrease of urea nitrogen (5-10 mg.%). **Cholesterol** is increased near term. The basal metabolic rate is increased.

Coagulation factors in pregnancy: Fibrinogen increases to about 450 mg.% at term. Also increased are the factors II, VII, and IX.

Leukocytic alkaline phosphatase (AP-GL) in pregnancy: Silva and Corbit[5] and others reported a significant elevation of APGL activity during pregnancy, beginning as early as the twentieth day of gestation and returning to normal about 6 wk. postpartum.

Vaginal cytology in pregnancy: The vaginal smear (Papanicolaou stain) shows certain changes at the beginning and at the end of pregnancy that form the basis for cytohormonal evaluation of the patient, and while they do not allow an early diagnosis of pregnancy, they give an indication of its progress and outcome (abortion).[6]

Vomiting of pregnancy: Vomiting occurs in about half the cases of pregnancy, without any abnormal laboratory findings. When it is severe, it is known as pernicious vomiting of pregnancy or hyperemesis gravidarum, and the loss of fluid and the period of starvation may be accompanied by evidences of dehydration (hemoconcentration), of loss of chlorides (alkalosis), and of partial starvation (ketosis).

Preeclampsia and eclampsia: These conditions occur in the last trimester of pregnancy. Eclampsia is the more severe and is characterized typically by hypertension, albuminuria, edema (or excessive gain in weight), convulsions, and coma.

The laboratory findings are not pathognomonic, but are helpful. The following are significant. Oliguria or anuria is frequent. Albuminuria in excess of 0.3 gm. in 24 hr. occurs, with casts, white blood cells, and frequently red blood cells. Usually a large amount of albumin is present. There is a decrease of plasma protein below about 6.5%. Blood uric acid is increased.

PREGNANCY TESTS[7, 8]

All pregnancy tests are designed to detect human chorionic gonadotropin (HCG) in the blood or urine of a pregnant woman.

HCG is present in the tissues, blood, and body fluids whenever there is living placental (chorionic) tissue and can be demonstrated in the urine of pregnant women as early as 10-14 days after conception. It has been demonstrated as early as 2 days after the first missed period. It increases to a peak during the first two months after the first missed period (between the eighth and the twelfth week of amenorrhea), slowly decreases to a constant low level after the sixteenth week, and disappears during the first week after parturition (Fig. 3-3).

Pregnancy tests should be negative 3-4 days after delivery. Of 15 patients with normal deliveries, all had positive pregnancy tests 1 hr. postpartum, 10 patients had negative tests after 24 hr., and the remaining 5 patients had negative tests after 48 hr.[9]

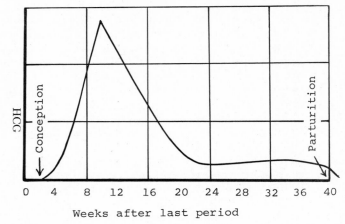

Fig. 3-3. HCG in the urine during normal pregnancy. Curve shows relative amounts in the different weeks.

Within 1 week the pregnancy test should also become negative after the delivery of a mole. After that time a positive test is indicative of a chorionepithelioma or of a persistent mole.

The test is positive also in ectopic pregnancy until the death of the placental tissue.

Variations in HCG level:

Increase: A larger amount of hormone is present in cases of multiple pregnancies, of hydatidiform mole, and of chorioepithelioma, but all three may occur without high titers.

Malignant teratomas (tumors of the ovaries, testis, retroperitoneum, etc.) may contain chorionic elements that give a positive pregnancy test in high dilutions in men and women.

Decrease: In incomplete abortions the titer of HCG is usually low and therefore less sensitive test animals may give a false negative result.

• • •

Pregnancy tests can be divided into two groups:

1. Biologic tests utilize the hyperemic or spermatozoa- and ova-producing effect of HCG on animal gonads, employing such animals as rabbits, mice, rats, frogs, and toads.
2. Immunologic tests are based on the agglutination-inhibition and hemag-

glutination-inhibition principle, using red cells or latex particles sensitized by HCG.

Biologic pregnancy tests

Friedman test: The technique described, which uses serum, is based on the method of Norris and Spink[10] and virtually eliminates death of the animal, which was common formerly.

Technique: Dilute 4 ml. serum with 6 ml. sterile normal saline solution and inject 4 ml. of this mixture into the marginal ear vein of a mature nonpregnant female rabbit. Inject the remaining 6 ml. subcutaneously into the back of the neck. After 48 hr. kill the animal with chloroform anesthesia, do a laparotomy, and examine the ovaries for large hemorrhagic follicles (corpora hemorrhagica) which constitute a positive test (Plate 3). Large follicles with clear yellowish fluid (prolan A-I) are not positive for pregnancy. The hypertrophy of the uterus and tubes, caused by the ovarian follicular hormone, is not positive. Pink areas in large clear follicles are not to be considered positive, but another test should be made later with another specimen.

A negative test will show only unripe follicles with clear fluid. If there are no follicles; if the surfaces of the ovaries are smooth, white, and opaque; and if the ovaries are small, flat, and triangular (not

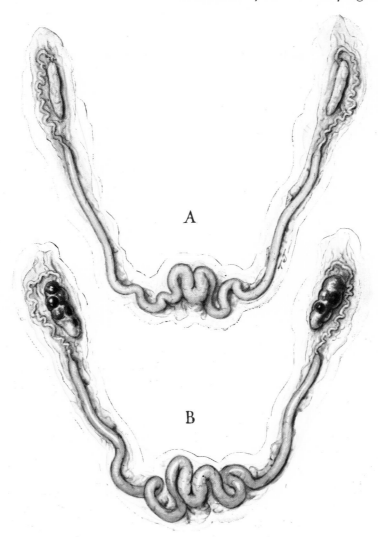

Plate 3. Hormone test for diagnosis of early pregnancy. (From Schneider: Surg., Gynec. Obstet. **52**:56, 1931.)

A. Negative reaction.   **B.** Positive reaction.

cylindric) in cross section, then the ovaries are not sufficiently mature, and the test is not satisfactory.

Female frog (Xenopus laevis) test[11, 12]: The test is sometimes called the Hogben test.

Principle: The mature female carries eggs throughout the year but deposits them only after mating or after injection of pregnancy hormones.

Male frog test (Rana pipiens)[13-15]: The test is best performed with serum. The frogs are kept in the refrigerator.

Procedure: Select two frogs. After they have come to room temperature examine their urine to make sure that it is free of spermatozoa. Inject 4 ml. serum into the peritoneal cavity of each frog. The frog excretes spermatozoa upon injection of serum containing HCG. Examine the urine of each frog for spermatozoa which appear within 1-4 hr. when the test is positive (Fig. 3-4). If none are found at the end of 4 hr., the test is negative.

To obtain urine from the frog, grasp the right hind leg between the index and middle fingers of the left hand, slide the thumb under the abdomen, and insert a capillary pipette into the exposed cloaca. Transfer to a microslide and examine under low-power and high-power dry objectives.

Care of frogs: When received, moisten the frogs with water and place (in crate) in refrigerator for several hours. Check for sex, the male being distinguished by large pigmented thumbs. Transfer to an enamel pan, the bottom of which is covered with water about 1.5 cm. deep. Cover with a perforated top and keep in the refrigerator at 0°-10° C. The frogs will hibernate and require no food. Rinse pan and change water daily. Add chloramphenicol (50 mg./L.) to control "red leg."

For use, transfer frog to a clean dry jar with perforated cover and leave until the frog warms up.

Immunologic pregnancy tests

The techniques used are as follows:
1. Agglutination-inhibition tests (Gravindex*)
2. Hemagglutination-inhibition tests (UCG† and Pregnosticon‡)
3. Precipitation tests (immuno-plate§)

These tests are rapid, sensitive, and accurate. They eliminate the upkeep of animals or the concentration of urine. Some can be used with urine or serum. Most allow a degree of quality control by means of control sera. Several comparative studies of commercially prepared reagents have been published.[16-18] In our hands UCG and Pregnosticon have performed satisfactorily in the diagnosis of pregnancy, even in the early stages.

Principle of agglutination-inhibition and hemagglutination-inhibition tests: These tests utilize an antigen-antibody system. Anti-HCG antibody (antiserum)

---

*Ortho Pharmaceutical Corp., Raritan, N. J.
†Wampole Laboratories, Stamford, Conn.
‡Organon, Inc., West Orange, N. J.
§Hyland Laboratories, Los Angeles, Calif.

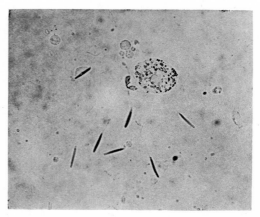

Fig. 3-4. Spermatozoa in urine of *Rana pipiens*.

is prepared by repeated injections of HCG into rabbits. Sheep red cells (UCG, Pregnosticon) or latex particles (Gravindex) coated with HCG are used as antigen. In the presence of anti-HCG antiserum the HCG-coated antigen (red cells or latex particles) will agglutinate and settle out. When urine of a pregnant woman containing HCG is added to the system, HCG neutralizes the antiserum so that it fails to act on the antigen and agglutination of the antigen does not occur. Homogenous settling out of the non-agglutinated antigen represents a **positive test**. The urine of a nonpregnant woman containing no HCG does not inhibit agglutination of the red cells or latex particles by the antiserum. Agglutination therefore represents a **negative test**.

Principle of immuno-plate test: The principle is the same as in the agglutination-inhibition and hemagglutination-inhibition tests, but the antiserum is incorporated in the agar. The antigen-antibody reaction of anti-HCG serum and HCG antigen in the urine of a pregnant woman produces precipitation lines in the agar. As the urine has to be adsorbed with kaolin, the test is somewhat more elaborate than the other techniques.

Technique: Details of the techniques are supplied with the products.

Accuracy of immunologic tests: HCG in urine is stable for 4 mo. at −18° C. At room or refrigerator temperature it is stable for 72 hr.[19] HCG values of 500 I.U.

or less fail to produce a positive immunologic test. Between 500 and 1000 I.U. the test results will be doubtful. A titer of over 1000 I.U. will give a positive test. (Note that the average titer of HCG in normal pregnancy is about 32,000 I.U.) Pituitary luteinizing hormone produces the same reaction as HCG, and in menopausal women it may be present in high enough titer to give a **false positive** pregnancy test. Urine of apparently menopausal women should be "run" undiluted and diluted with equal parts of water. If the patient is pregnant, both specimens will be positive. If there is any doubt, the test should be repeated in 2 wk. Agglutination-inhibition and hemagglutination-inhibition tests are sensitive to detergents and must also be protected from vibrations and temperature changes. The urine must never be warm.

False positive tests have been reported for patients treated with tranquilizers.[20]

Quantitative methods

Biologic quantitative methods are difficult to evaluate because they depend on the sensitivity of the animal and the level of HCG. Immunologic methods compare favorably with HCG assay methods.

Quantitative methods may be used to support a diagnosis of hydatidiform mole or of choriocarcinoma in which the HCG levels are usually elevated. In abortion or in fetal death the levels are low.

For a discussion of the significance of pregnancy tests, see p. 89.

Quantitative Friedman test:

Technique: Use acidified urine. The first rabbit receives an injection of 5 ml. undiluted urine into the marginal ear vein, the second rabbit receives 5 ml. of a 1:10 dilution, and the third rabbit receives 5 ml. of a 1:100 dilution. If the third rabbit shows a positive reaction, a 1:1000 dilution is injected into a fourth rabbit. The rabbits are killed 48 hr. after the injection and the ovaries are examined for corpora hemorrhagica (see p. 91).

Interpretation: A normal pregnancy will give a positive result with the 1:10 dilution. A positive test with the higher dilution suggests a hydatidiform mole or a choriocarcinoma.

Quantitative immunologic slide test[21]:

Technique: The Gravindex slide test is used. Set up eight test tubes and prepare the following dilutions of urine in normal saline solution—undiluted, 1:2, 1:4, 1:8, 1:16, 1:32, 1:64, and 1:128. Add 1 ml. urine to the first tube and 1 ml. saline solution to the other tubes. To the second tube add 1 ml. urine, mix well, and transfer 1 ml. of the mixture to the third tube. Mix and continue transfer until 1 ml. is discarded from the eighth tube. Each dilution should be well mixed in a Vortex stirrer before the next transfer is made. Each dilution is tested with Gravindex. The highest dilution that gives a positive test (no visible agglutination) is the end point.

Interpretation: A titer of 1:64 can be tentatively accepted as the highest titer occurring during normal pregnancy (sixteenth day after last period). A titer of 1:128 or higher is indicative of abnormal pregnancy.

Tamada et al.[22] described a method in which an acetone concentration of urine is used with the Gravindex method in cases of suspected low titer of HCG in disturbed pregnancies during the first trimester.

UCG titration[17]: In this test serum or urine is used and controls are run with each procedure. The urine results are reported in I.U./24 hr. and the serum results in I.U./ml. of HCG. The average value of HCG/24 hr. in normal pregnancy is about 32,000 I.U., with the highest value recorded as 72,000 I.U. In a single case of choriocarcinoma the average HCG concentration is 110,000 I.U. A value of less than 3000 I.U. of UCG/24 hr. from 50-90 days after the last menstrual period is associated with nonviable gestation.

Technique: It is described in detail in the folder accompanying the reagents.

EVALUATION OF PLACENTAL FUNCTION IN ESTABLISHED PREGNANCY

There are three methods for the evaluation of placental function and thus, indirectly, of fetal well-being: amniotic fluid spectrophotometry in Rh sensitization (see p. 276), assay of urinary estriol excretion, and assay of heat-stable serum alkaline phosphatase.

Placental estriol assay

In normal pregnancy urinary estrogen excretion rises constantly until term, when it rapidly falls.[23] If during pregnancy serial determinations of urinary estriol reveal a drop of over 70% of the preceding level, placental insufficiency must be suspected. Gas chromatography is the method of choice.[24]

Heat-stable alkaline phosphatase as index of placental function

The placenta is the major source of a heat-stable isoenzyme of alkaline phosphatase.[25] The total serum alkaline phosphatase is determined first; the serum is then inactivated at 56° C. for 30 min. and assayed as before. A progressive fall of serial values points toward inadequate placental function.

REFERENCES

1. Ducey, E. F.: Amer. J. Clin. Path. **20**:289, 1950.
2. Evans, N., and Krajian, A. A.: Amer. J. Clin. Path. (tech. sect.) **8**:97, 1955 .
3. Brown, T. K.: Amer. J. Obstet. Gynec. **23**:379, 1932.
4. Zondek, B.: J.A.M.A. **108**:607, 1937.
5. Silva, A. R., Jr., and Corbit, J. D., Jr.: Obstet. Gynec. **18**:283, 1961.
6. Nesbitt, R. E. L., Jr., Garcia, R., and Rome, D. S.: Obstet. Gynec. **17**:2, 1961.
7. Tietz, N. W.: Obstet. Gynec. **25**:197, 1965.
8. Thompson, R. B., Mayo, R. W., and Bell, W. N.: Amer. J. Clin. Path. **44**:585, 1965.
9. Mullins, D. F., Jr., Collins, L. R., and Clark, J. R.: J. Med. Ass. Georgia **54**:16, 1965.
10. Norris, J. C., and Spink, J.: Southern Med. J. **46**:919, 1953.
11. Hogben, L. T.: Proc. Roy. Soc. Africa **5**:19, 1930.
12. Hogben, L. T., Charles, E., and Slome, D.: J. Exp. Biol. **8**:345, 1931.
13. Rabau, E., and Szeinberg, A.: J. Clin. Path. **12**:268, 1959.
14. Wiltberger, P. B., and Miller, D. F.: Science **107**:198, 1948.
15. Robbins, S. L., and Parker, F., Jr.: Endocrinology **42**:237, 1948.
16. Coon, B., Mendelow, H., and Dalton, H.: Amer. J. Clin. Path. **42**:215, 1964.
17. Venning, E. H.: Obstet. Gynec. **26**:110, 1965.
18. Thompson, R. B., Mayo, R. W., and Bell, W. N.: Amer. J. Clin. Path. **44**:5, 1965.
19. Noto, T. A., and Miale, J. B.: Amer. J. Clin. Path. **43**:311, 1965.
20. Marks, V., and Shackcloth, P.: Brit. Med. J. **1**:517, 1966.
21. Noto, T. A., Miale, J. B., and Riekers, H.: Amer. J. Obstet. Gynec. **90**:7, 1964.
22. Tamada, T., Taymor, M. L., and Stark, J.: Amer. J. Obstet. Gynec. **95**:249, 1966.
23. Greene, J. W., Duhring, J. L., and Smith, K.: Amer. J. Obstet. Gynec. **92**:1030, 1965.
24. Larsen, A. L., and Engstrom, A. W.: Amer. J. Clin. Path. **46**:352, 1966.
25. Messer, R. H.: Amer. J. Obstet. Gynec. **98**:459, 1967.

Chapter 4

Methods in hematology

THE BLOOD

The blood, which is about one twelfth of the adult body weight (about 85 ml./kg.), consists of a fluid portion, the **plasma,** in which are suspended the **formed elements** (red cells, white cells, and platelets).

Blood formation: Blood cells are first found in the blood islands of the yolk sac, in which the peripheral cells form the walls of the blood vessels (endothelium) and the cells near the center form the primitive blood cells.[1, 2]

Later, blood formation in the embryo occurs in the liver (about the second month), then in the spleen (about the fourth month), and finally in the red bone marrow (about the fifth month).

At birth and for several years thereafter all bones contain hematopoietic marrow. At about 10-14 yr. of age, yellow, fatty (inactive) marrow appears in the distal ends of the shafts of the long bones and then gradually increases from the distal to the proximal ends of the bones until, at about 20 yr. of age, all the hematopoietic marrow in the long bones has been replaced, except in the upper ends of the femur and humerus.

In adults the red marrow is normally confined to the skull, ribs, sternum, scapulae, clavicles, vertebrae, and os innominatum, leaving a considerable reserve of fatty but potentially hematopoietic marrow.

In the infant there is no additional space (reserve) for the development of additional red or hematopoietic bone marrow when increased blood formation becomes necessary so that extramedullary hematopoietic centers arise in the spleen, liver, kidney, and sometimes even in the retroperitoneal adipose tissue. The spleen and liver become enlarged. From the extramedullary centers immature red and white blood cells find their way into the bloodstream, producing a leukoerythroblastic blood picture.

Origin of blood cells: While the origin of the blood cells from a common ancestral tissue (mesenchymal tissue) in the embryo is admitted, there is a lack of agreement in regard to the origin of the blood cells in postnatal life. The monophyletic school holds that all varieties arise through a common primitive stem cell, the hemohistioblast, which is present in all adult hematopoietic tissue, whereas the polyphyletic school holds that there is no such polyvalent stem cell, but that all types of cells arise directly from their own stem cell and have their own separate cycle of development.

The **dualists** describe two series of cells, the lymphoblastic (lymphocytes) and the myeloblastic (granulocytes, monocytes, erythrocytes). The **trialists** describe three series of leukocytes, each having its own stem cell and a different site of origin from the fixed reticuloendothelial tissue—that in the bone marrow producing granular leukocytes, that in lymphoid tissue, lymphocytes, and that in connective tissue, monocytes—and that lining the vascular system of the bone marrow, erythrocytes. They hold that under abnormal conditions the reticuloendothelium at any site may give rise to any variety of cell and that reversion to the embryonic type of blood formation in extramedullary centers (liver, spleen) may occur.

Nomenclature: The committee for clarification of the nomenclature of cells and diseases of the blood and blood-forming organs, sponsored by the American Society of Clinical Pathologists and the American Medical Association, has made recommendations,[3-7] some of the most important of which will be given. The committee recommends the following:

1. Use of the terms "lymphocytic," "granulocytic," "monocytic," "plasmacytic," "erythrocytic," and "thrombocytic" to refer to the respective series of cells
2. Use of the word "leukocyte" to mean any white blood corpuscle or precursor
3. Spelling of leukocyte and other words derived from the same root with the letter *k* and the spelling of neutrophil, eosinophil, etc. without a final *e*
4. For the most undifferentiated cells of each series use the suffix **blast;** for the second stage, use the prefix **pro;** and for the more mature cells, use only the suffix **cyte** except in series showing a fourth stage of immaturity, i.e., in the granulocytic series in which the terms "metamyelocyte" (juvenile cell), "band cell," and "segmented form" are to remain
5. The term "progranulocyte" for the second stage in the granulocytic series (formerly promyelocyte)
6. For the fourth stage in the granulocytic and erythrocytic series the prefix **meta** (metamyelocyte, metarubricyte)
7. Use of new names for the nucleated red cells, the same terms to be applied to both the normoblastic and the megaloblastic series, the latter being designated by the phrase "pernicious anemia type"
8. For the four stages of maturation, beginning with the youngest form, the terms "rubriblast," "prorubricyte," "rubricyte," and "metarubricyte"

NOTE: Rubriblast and prorubricyte in the new terminology refer to cells usually called early and late erythroblasts, re-

spectively. Rubricyte includes the cells usually classified as early (basophilic) and late (polychromatic) erythroblasts. Metarubricyte refers to the mature normoblast with a pyknotic nucleus and older forms with fragmented, partially extruded or partially autolyzed nuclei.

METHODS OF EXAMINATION OF BLOOD

Fresh preparations of blood: This method is useful in studying the shape of the red corpuscles and in searching for extracellular parasites of blood such as filaria, trypanosomes, and spirochetes of relapsing fever *(Borrelia recurrentis)*. It is also useful in the study of the sickle cell trait, Heinz bodies, and intraerythrocytic crystals.

Method: Mount a small drop of fresh blood on a slide under a cover glass, making a very thin preparation, so that the red cells do not tend to form rouleaux.

The other methods of examination of fresh blood include dark-field examination (spirochetes of relapsing fever), phase microscopy, electron microscopy, and fluorescent microscopy.

Phase microscopy: Phase microscopy allows the recognition of structural details not seen by an ordinary microscope since slight differences in refractive index are converted into shades of light and dark. The observer can follow the movement of the white cells and study the living mitochondria and other cytoplasmic structures in health and disease.

Electron microscopy: This method allows magnification of fresh tissue up to 1000 times and of 0.02μ thin section up to 200,000 times. Electron microscopy opened up an entire new field of investigation, allowing visualization of such intracytoplasmic structures as granules, centrosomes, Golgi apparatus, chromosomes, and various inclusions. Some of Bessis' fundamental work in hematologic electron microscopy is contained in his book.[8]

Fluorescent microscopy: This method allows recognition of substances within tissues by their ability to fluoresce. When these substances are hit by invisible ultraviolet light of short wavelength, they absorb this light and are thus excited. In this excited state they emit visible rays of fluorescent light of longer wavelength as long as they are exposed to ultraviolet light. Some tissues fluoresce naturally, whereas others fluoresce only after staining with certain dyes (primary and secondary fluorescence).

Fluorescent technique is extremely sensitive and is able to detect dye concentrations in the order of $1:10^{-18}$.

Fluorescytes: In erythropoietic porphyria, fluorescent erythrocytes and erythroblasts can be seen (fluorescytes).

Fixed bone marrow and blood smears can be stained with acridine orange or with coriphosphine O. In the erythroid series the more mature a nucleus, the more brilliantly will it be stained, whereas the younger the cell, i.e., the less hemoglobin it contains, the more vividly the cytoplasm stains. Heinz bodies can be recognized under ultraviolet light in an air-dried preparation. So far as the white cell series is concerned, living leukocytes have a delicate primary fluorescence which increases as the cell dies. Fluorescent microscopy as well as phase microscopy has been used to show the production of platelets from megakaryocytes.

OBTAINING BLOOD SPECIMENS

Cell counts and hemoglobin results are the same with venous and capillary blood specimens if stasis is prevented. If the hands are cold, they should be warmed before the finger is stuck. If difficulty in puncturing a vein should occur, loosen the tourniquet for a few moments to permit free circulation to be established before drawing the blood. Application of a tourniquet for more than a minute or two will produce significant concentration since plasma fluid will pass from the vessels into the tissues.

Capillary blood: Choose a site free from local circulatory change. The usual site in adults is the finger or the lobe of the ear; in infants it is the great toe or the side of the heel. Cleanse with alcohol and dry. Puncture with a sharp sterile blood lancet. A Bard-Parker knife blade No. 11 is excellent. Hemolets* or other

disposable sterile blood lancets are individually packaged in sterile envelopes and are discarded after being used once. Wipe away the first drop or two of blood and use the subsequent drops.

Venous blood: It has the advantage that tests can be repeated as often as necessary. Venous blood is usually obtained from the median basilic or the median cephalic vein at the elbow. Apply a tourniquet above the elbow and have the patient open and close the hand. Cleanse the site of puncture with 70% alcohol and puncture the vein with a sterile needle and syringe. Enter vein directly with the bevel of the needle upward and use gentle suction. Remove tourniquet before withdrawing the needle, and when the needle is withdrawn, make pressure over the site of puncture with a sterile sponge.

A blood pressure cuff inflated to a level between systolic and diastolic pressures acts as an excellent tourniquet, as does the newly marketed Velket tourniquet.*

BLOOD SPECIMENS FROM INFANTS:

Scalp or jugular veins: In infants, scalp veins may often be found large enough to be entered with the needle. If not, obtain blood from the jugular vein. Wrap the infant in a sheet and fasten it. Let the head hang over the end of a table or bed with the face to one side. The course of the vein runs from the angle of the mandible to the midclavicular region and stands out distinctly when the patient cries.

Longitudinal sinus: The longitudinal sinus may be used before the anterior fontanelle closes (about the eighteenth month). The sinus runs from the anterior to the posterior angle of the fontanelle and is largest at the posterior angle, which is the site of choice. It is not dangerous to obtain blood from this sinus.

Femoral vein: Femoral puncture is performed as follows. The child is held with his legs abducted. The femoral pulse is felt below the inguinal ligament, and a needle is inserted just medially to the pulsating area until it touches the bone.

---

*Scientific Products Division, American Hospital Supply Corp., Evanston, Ill.

*Propper Mfg. Co., Long Island City, N. Y.

It is then slowly withdrawn while suction is being maintained until blood enters the barrel. Apply pressure after the procedure so that no hematoma develops.

• • •

Handle blood gently. Remove the needle and then empty blood in clean dry tube with or without anticoagulant. Gently invert stoppered tube to mix blood and anticoagulant.

Do not rim the clot and do not centrifuge until the clot is well formed.

CHOICE OF ANTICOAGULANTS:

Heparin: Although expensive, it is a good anticoagulant. Swirl 1 or 2 drops around in the test tube to coat the inside with a thin film. Gently invert stoppered tube to mix blood and anticoagulant.

Oxalates: Potassium oxalate shrinks the red blood cells, whereas **ammonium oxalate** produces swelling of the cells. These anticoagulants used alone are therefore not satisfactory, but combined as a **double-oxalate mixture,** they do not affect the shape of the red cells and therefore do not influence the hematocrit.

Double-oxalate mixture:
1. Ammonium oxalate, 1.2 gm.
2. Potassium oxalate, 0.8 gm.
3. Neutral formaldehyde (38% USP), 1 ml.
4. Distilled water to make 100 ml.

Measure 0.5 ml. of this solution into stoppered test tubes. These are dried at room temperature or in an oven at not more than 60° C. The dry mixture is used so as not to dilute the blood.

EDTA: Ethylenediaminetetraacetate (EDTA)* is a satisfactory anticoagulant that can also be used for platelet counts. The dipotassium salt is prepared as a 1% solution in distilled water and a concentration of 0.5 ml./5 ml. blood is used. Since this salt is rather insoluble, 1 drop of a commercial liquid called Prezervol† is used per 5 ml. blood.

Defibrination with glass beads: Add 25 ml. venous blood to a 125 ml. Erlenmeyer flask containing 20 3-4 mm. glass beads. Rotate the flask until the beads are covered with fibrin and cease to make

a rattling noise. Continue for another 2 min. and decant defibrinated blood.

HEMOGLOBIN

Hemoglobin is a conjugated protein (heme + globin). Heme contains iron in the ferrous state and can unite in a loose combination with oxygen to form oxyhemoglobin. About 55% of the red blood cell is hemoglobin.

HEMOGLOBINOMETRY

Numerous methods are available, but they are not all equal in accuracy, ease of performance, and reproducibility.

COLORIMETRIC METHODS: These methods are **not recommended** because of their large percentage of error.

Direct matching: This method is employed in the **Tallqvist** and **Dare** methods. These methods are inaccurate because of the impossibility of matching hemoglobin with artificial standards.

Acid hematin: This technique is used in the methods of **Haden** and **Hausser, Sahli,** and **Newcomber.** These methods are inadequate because of the difficulty of matching acid hematin with colored glass and because of the fact that acid hematin forms a suspension rather than a solution. Complete transformation of hemoglobin into acid hematin takes time; therefore these tests have to be read at a standardized period. Acid hematin is not stable, and its color is affected by the plasma color. Fetal hemoglobin is acid resistant.

Alkaline hematin: The points mentioned in the discussion of acid hematin also apply to alkaline hematin. Fetal hemoglobin is alkaline resistant; therefore this method may give incorrect results in infants as well as in certain hemoglobinopathies.

GASOMETRIC METHODS: These methods are accurate and can be used for standardization of the techniques used routinely. They are based on the amount of gas first bound by hemoglobin and then released and measured.

Oxygen capacity method: The oxygen capacity method measures only oxyhemoglobin, leaving out such hemoglobin derivatives as carboxyhemoglobin, methemoglobin, and sulfhemoglobin. When

---

*Sequestrine, Prezervol, and Versene are commercial preparations of this anticoagulant.
†United Chemical Supply Co., Van Nuys, Calif.

fully converted to oxyhemoglobin, 1 gm. hemoglobin combines with 1.36 ml. oxygen.

Carbon monoxide saturation: Inaccuracies may arise from carbon monoxide dissolved in the plasma and from compounds that readily absorb the gas such as sulfhemoglobin and methemalbumin.

PHOTOMETRIC METHODS: These methods are based on the fact that at specific wavelength the concentration of hemoglobin compounds in solution is proportional to the optical density.

Oxyhemoglobin method: Hemoglobin is transformed into oxyhemoglobin by diluting it with a weak alkaline solution of 0.05% ammonium hydroxide. The maximal absorption is measured at 540 mμ. As mentioned, this method does not measure compounds that are not converted into oxyhemoglobin.

Cyanmethemoglobin method: In 1964 the Technical Subcommittee on Haemoglobinometry of the International Committee for Standardization in Haematology[12] recommended the cyanmethemoglobin method as the method of choice and a cyanmethemoglobin solution as a standard.

Principle: Hemoglobin is converted into cyanmethemoglobin by the addition of a potassium ferricyanide solution. This method measures all hemoglobin derivatives. The pigment, cyanmethemoglobin, and reagents are stable.

Reagent:
Diluent:
Drabkin solution:
1. Sodium bicarbonate, 1 gm.
2. Potassium cyanide, 0.05 gm.
3. Potassium ferricyanide, 0.20 gm.
4. Distilled water up to 1000 ml.

To increase the velocity of the overall reaction the following modification is suggested[13]:
1. Potassium ferricyanide, 200 mg.
2. Potassium cyanide, 50 mg.
3. Potassium phosphate (monobasic), 140 mg.
4. Sterox SE,* 0.5 ml.
5. Distilled water up to 1000 ml.

*A polythiol compound manufactured by Hartman-Ledden Co., Philadelphia, Pa.

Drabkin solution is commercially available as diluent pellets.*

Method using Aculute pellets:
Diluent:
1. Add approximately 100 ml. distilled water to a 250 ml. volumetric flask.
2. Add 1 Aculute diluent pellet.
3. Add distilled water to the calibration mark.
4. Allow to stand for at least 5 min., mixing thoroughly at intervals during this period.

Technique:
1. With a volumetric pipette add exactly 5 ml. Aculute diluent to a clean, dry cuvette.
2. Add exactly 0.02 ml. patient's whole blood (capillary or venous). Use Sahli pipette and rinse pipette several times with the diluted blood. The dilution is 1:251.
3. Mix well and allow cuvette to stand 10 min.
4. Determine the optical density or transmittance of the unknown, using the diluent as the blank. The wavelength should be set at 540 mμ.
5. Find gm.% hemoglobin of the whole blood by referring to a standard curve.

Calibration: A standard solution of cyanmethemoglobin can be obtained commercially.* The concentration of cyanmethemoglobin is given in mg./100 ml. and is usually in the order of 60 mg. hemoglobin/100 ml.

The equivalence of this standard can be calculated as follows:

The dilution employed in the foregoing procedure is 1:251.

$$\text{Equivalence of standard in gm.\% Hb} = \frac{\text{Conc. Hb in standard} \times 251}{1000}$$

Example:

$$\text{Conc. of Hb in standard solution} = 60.5 \text{ mg. Hb/100 ml.}$$

$$\text{Equivalence of standard} = \frac{60.5 \times 251}{1000} =$$

$$12.4 \text{ gm.\%}$$

*Ortho Pharmaceutical Corp., Raritan, N. J.

Having calculated the value of the standard, proceed as follows: Prepare five cuvettes—a blank cuvette containing 6 ml. diluent, No. 1 tube containing 6 ml. undiluted standard, No. 2 tube containing 4 ml. standard plus 2 ml. diluent, No. 3 tube containing 3 ml. standard plus 3 ml. diluent, and No. 4 tube containing 2 ml. standard plus 4 ml. diluent. Determine the transmittance of No. 1 through No. 4, using the blank cuvette as reference. Make a semilogarithmic plot of transmittancies obtained versus the hemoglobin equivalents of each dilution.

Plot the percent transmission on the ordinate (logarithmic scale) and the hemoglobin in gm.% on the abscissa (bottom scale). The hemoglobin equivalent of each dilution is obtained by multiplying the hemoglobin equivalent of the undiluted standard by the appropriate dilution factor, i.e., tube No. 1, 1; tube No. 2, 0.666; tube No. 3, 0.500; tube No. 4, 0.333.

A line connecting the four points (the standard curve) should pass through or come very close to T% = 100. The hemoglobin concentration of unknown bloods can be determined by translating their T% value to hemoglobin concentration on the basis of the curve. For convenience it is advisable to produce a chart listing all possible T% values and their corresponding hemoglobin in gm.%.

SOURCES OF ERROR IN HEMOGLOBIN METHODS:

Errors in sampling:
1. Capillary blood (finger stick, etc.)—inadequate blood flow necessitating squeezing, etc.
2. Venous blood—prolonged stasis and inadequate mixing of blood with anticoagulant and of anticoagulated blood before each test.

Technique and equipment:
1. Unclean (moist) syringes and pipettes, incorrect pipetting, incorrectly calibrated pipettes, inadequate rinsing of pipettes, and blood adhering to the outside of pipettes. Pipettes may have an allowable error of ±2%.
2. Incorrect calibration of the instrument due to incorrect standards or due to errors in the method.

3. The method chosen may be inadequate.

Cleaning of blood pipettes: If necessary, they should be immersed in KOH or NaOH to remove any pigment. They are then cleaned by first aspirating water in adequate amounts, then alcohol, and finally acetone.

The cuvettes used must be thoroughly rinsed and free from fingerprints.

NORMAL HEMOGLOBIN VALUES: The hemoglobin values given in Table 4-1 are calculated from the oxygen capacities given by Peters and Van Slyke[14] and are expressed to the nearest tenth.

Table 4-1

Age	Hemoglobin in gm./100 ml. blood	
	Males	Females
1 day	23.9 ± 3.0	23.9 ± 3.0
2-3 days	21.6 3.0	21.6 3.0
4-8 days	19.4 3.0	19.4 3.0
9-13 days	17.2 3.0	17.2 3.0
2-8 wk.	15.3 3.0	15.3 3.0
3-5 mo.	13.1 ± 2.2	13.1 ± 2.2
6-11 mo.	11.9 2.2	11.9 2.2
1-2 yr.	11.6 ± 1.5	11.6 ± 1.5
3-5 yr.	12.2 1.5	12.2 1.5
6-10 yr.	12.9 1.5	12.9 1.5
11-15 yr.	13.4 1.5	13.4 1.5
16-60 yr.	15.4 1.5	14.2 1.5
60-70 yr.	14.8 1.5	14.2 1.5
Over 70 yr.	14.2 1.5	13.9 1.5

IRON CONTENT METHOD OF WONG (MODIFIED):

Principle[15]*:* The procedure measures the amount of iron present in a measured amount of whole blood without making any corrections for the 1.5% of nonhemoglobin iron present in the total blood iron. The whole blood is digested, and then the color is developed.

In 1 gm. hemoglobin there is 3.47 mg. iron. Therefore to obtain gm. Hb/100 ml. the mg. of iron/100 ml. are divided by 3.47.

Reagents:
1. Hydrogen peroxide, 30%.
2. H_2SO_4, concentrated iron free.
3. Standard iron solution. Dissolve 0.863 gm. clear crystals of ferric ammonium sulfate, $FeNH_4(SO_4)_2 \cdot 12$

H_2O, in 50 ml. H_2O. Add 20 ml. 1:10 dilution of concentrated H_2SO_4. Dilute to 1 L. and mix; 1 ml. equals 0.1 mg. Fe.

Procedure:

1. Pipette 0.5 ml. oxalated whole blood, well mixed, into 50 ml. NPN digestion tubes.
2. Prepare a blank with 0.5 ml. H_2O.
3. Prepare a series of standards with 1, 2, and 3 ml. iron standard.
4. Place 2 ml. concentrated H_2SO_4 in each tube.
5. Insert several glass beads in the tubes.
6. Digest over a small flame until the solution clears and dense white sulfuric acid fumes begin to appear.
7. After about 5 min. of digestion, allow tubes to cool for 30-45 sec. and cautiously add 2-3 drops hydrogen peroxide, 30%. The solution will boil and clear. Hold tube away from face.
8. Continue digestion. Discontinue digestion when the solution is clear and the sulfuric acid volume is constant.
9. Dilute to exactly 50 ml. with distilled water.

Color development:

Reagents:

1. Fresh solution of saturated potassium persulfate.
2. Potassium thiocyanate (approximately 3N). Dissolve 29 gm. potassium thiocyanate (KCNS) in 100 ml. distilled water.

Technique:

1. Transfer 5 ml. digest to cuvette.
2. Add 10 ml. distilled water.
3. Add 0.4 ml. H_2SO_4. Mix and cool to room temperature.
4. Add 1 ml. saturated potassium persulfate.
5. Add 3 ml. KCNS to cuvette, mix, and read optical density at once against digested blank at 480 mμ.

Calculation:

$$\frac{R_u}{R_s} \times 2 \times \frac{100}{0.5} = \text{Mg.\% iron}$$

In this equation the iron standard contains 0.2 mg. iron, and the reading of the standard, R_s, is that obtained for this standard. In most cases this standard will give an optical density closer to that of the unknown than either of the others. If not, the reading and iron content of the standard closest to the unknown should be substituted. The hemoglobin concentration may then be calculated from the iron content as follows:

$$\frac{\text{Mg. iron/100 ml.}}{3.47} = \text{Hb gm./100 ml.}$$

PHYSICAL MEASUREMENTS AS METHODS OF HEMOGLOBIN DETERMINATION:

Specific gravity: The copper sulfate specific gravity method may be used for rapid determination of approximate hemoglobin values.

Hematocrit: The hematocrit value is influenced by the size and shape of the cells as well as by the hemoglobin content.

Refractive index of plasma: Small refractometers* are available which allow direct readings of the specific gravity of plasma (1 drop). If either the specific gravity of whole blood (copper sulfate method) or the hematocrit (micromethod) is known, the hemoglobin can be calculated from line charts, as given in Peters and Van Slyke's book.[14]

SPECTROSCOPIC EXAMINATION OF BLOOD[16]**:** Hemoglobin and hemoglobin compounds such as carboxyhemoglobin, methemoglobin, and sulfhemoglobin can be identified spectroscopically on the basis of the number and position of their absorption bands.

Instrument: The Zeiss-Winkel hand spectroscope† is a satisfactory instrument. It has an illuminated wavelength scale and allows simultaneous viewing of spectra from two samples.

Technique: Collect blood in dry oxalate, prevent hemolysis, and dilute 1:50 with distilled water. Compare absorption bands with Table 4-2 and Fig. 4-1.

CARBOXYHEMOGLOBIN:

Physical characteristics: Carbon monoxide has a greater affinity to hemoglobin

---

*Scientific Products Division, American Hospital Supply Corp., Evanston, Ill.

†Arthur H. Thomas Co., Philadelphia, Pa.

Table 4-2. Absorption spectra

Hemoglobin (Hb) derivative	No. of bands	Wavelengths of bands (mμ)				Reactions and remarks	Controls
		α	β	γ	δ		
Oxyhemoglobin	2	578	540			Addition of some $Na_2S_2O_4$ replaces 2 bands of oxyhemoglobin with single band of reduced Hb	Oxyhemoglobin: add 1 drop blood to 15 ml. water and mix
Reduced Hb	1	556				Photoelectric oximeters provide preferable clinical method of indirectly measuring reduced Hb	Reduced Hb: add 1 ml. blood to 5 ml. distilled water, reduce with addition of some $Na_2S_2O_4$, and mix
Carboxyhemoglobin	2	572	535			Bands are similar to oxyhemoglobin bands but slightly shifted to right (purple side of spectrum); carboxyhemoglobin will resist reduction by $Na_2S_2O_4$; if bands persist after addition of $Na_2S_2O_4$, Hb is carboxyhemoglobin; as there is always some oxyhemoglobin present, single wide band of reduced Hb may also be seen after addition of reducing agent; controls with known oxyhemoglobin, carboxyhemoglobin, and reduced Hb are necessary	Dilute 1 ml. blood in 50 ml. distilled water and saturate with carbon monoxide obtained from commercially available tank
Sulfhemoglobin	1	618				Band disappears on addition of few drops 3% H_2O_2	Dilute blood 1:50 with distilled water; to 5 ml. add 0.9 ml. 0.1% phenylhydrazine hydrochloride and 0.1 ml. water saturated with H_2S gas*
Methemoglobin (neutral)	4	630	578	540	500	Strongest band is at 630 mμ; it disappears on addition of some $Na_2S_2O_4$	Dilute blood 1:50 with distilled water and add crystals of potassium ferricyanide
Methemalbumin (plasma)	1	624				Band disappears after addition of $Na_2S_2O_4$	Confirm by Schumm test
Myoglobin (urine)	2	582	542			Use conversion spectroscope because bands are similar to oxyhemoglobin bands	

*Aitch-Tu-Ess, Henger Co., Philadelphia, Pa.

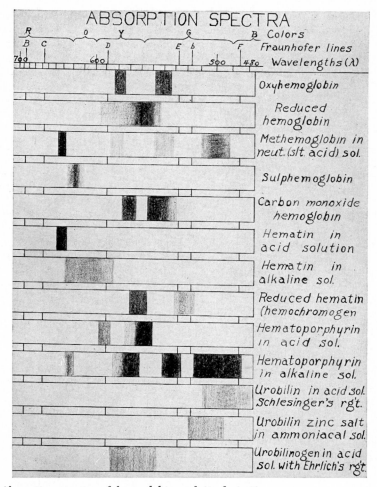

Fig. 4-1. Absorption spectra of hemoglobin and its derivatives.

than has oxygen; therefore when oxyhemoglobin is exposed to carbon monoxide, the latter replaces the oxygen linked to hemoglobin. Carboxyhemoglobin is cherry red. If the patient exposed to carbon monoxide is allowed to breathe normal air, the carbon monoxide is usually rapidly washed out.

Spectroscopic method: The qualitative method in which a simple direct vision spectroscope is used (Table 4-2) can be modified into a very rough quantitative method by means of the Hartridge reversion spectroscope.* It gives two spectra that are close together, one above the

other; but one is reversed. Absorption bands in one can be made collinear with the corresponding bands of the other spectrum by means of a micrometer. A slight shift of one band in one spectrum can thus be evaluated, for instance, the shift of carboxyhemoglobin bands of the spectrum of the unknown blood against the oxyhemoglobin bands of a known sample.

Spectrophotometric method: Spectrophotometric methods for determination of carboxyhemoglobin, methemoglobin, and sulfhemoglobin involve either the measurement of the absorbance at two or more selected wavelengths or the measurement at one wavelength before and

*R. & J. Beck, Ltd., London, England.

after the addition of a compound that changes one component of the system but not the others. Since differences in absorbance of the different hemoglobin derivatives is usually not large and the position of their absorption peaks do not differ greatly, a spectrophotometer must be used that can be read to 0.001 optical density unit (OD) and that has a very narrow bandwidth.

Principle[17, 18]: Dilution of blood in weak ammonium hydroxide solution is treated with a small amount of sodium hydrosulfite to convert the oxyhemoglobin present to hemoglobin without affecting the carboxyhemoglobin. The absorbance is then measured at two wavelengths, 555 and 480 mμ, and the percentage of carboxyhemoglobin is obtained from a calibration curve.

Reagents:
1. Ammonium hydroxide (0.4%). Dilute 14.3 ml. concentrated ammonium hydroxide to 1 L. with distilled water.
2. Sodium hydrosulfite (sodium dithionite, $Na_2S_2O_4$).

Procedure: Dilute 0.05 ml. blood with 10 ml. ammonium hydroxide solution. Mix and allow to stand until hemolysis is complete. Place some of the diluted blood in a spectrophotometer cuvette, add about 10 mg. sodium hydrosulfite, mix by inversion, and read within 30 sec. against a blank of the dilute ammonia at 555 and 480 mμ. Calculate the ratio of OD(555)/OD(480) and determine the amount of carboxyhemoglobin present from a calibration curve.

Determination of calibration curve: Obtain blood specimens (heparinized) from a number of nonsmokers known not to have been recently exposed to carbon monoxide. Pool samples and place about 10 ml. in each of two screw-capped reagent bottles of 500 ml. capacity. Flush out one flask well with 100% oxygen, cap, and rotate through its long axis (e.g., by a roller apparatus) for 30 min. to saturate the blood with oxygen. The other sample is treated similarly with carbon monoxide from a small lecture cylinder available from many laboratory supply houses. (CAUTION! Work with the carbon monoxide under a fume hood with adequate ventilation.) Flush out the carbon monoxide bottle several times with fresh gas during the equilibration period. Then treat the two samples as outlined in the procedure and calculate the ratio. For 100% oxyhemoglobin the ratio OD(555)/OD(480) should be about 3.1, and for 100% carboxyhemoglobin the ratio should be about 1.95. Since the curve is linear, the two points should suffice, but if desired, additional points may be obtained by mixing aliquots of the two blood samples in different proportions. Plot the OD ratio against the percent of carboxyhemoglobin (100% oxyhemoglobin = 0% carboxyhemglobin). A simpler but slightly less accurate method for calibration is to make dilutions of the original blood sample in ammonia, bubble oxygen or carbon monoxide through the solution for 2 min., and then read the spectrophotometer.

Heparinized blood is preferable. All blood specimens should be collected as soon as possible after the presence of carboxyhemoglobin is suspected since over one half of the carbon monoxide in blood may be eliminated in an hour in patients receiving oxygen therapy. Even in subjects breathing air the loss may be as much as 15%/hr. The blood specimens may be kept in well-stoppered tubes in the refrigerator for up to 24 hr. without adverse effects.

Range of values and interpretation: In normal, nonsmoking subjects living in cities under conditions of minimal exposure, 0.25-2% carboxyhemoglobin saturation has been found.[18a] Smokers have saturations of 0.7-6.5%. Those who work with combustion engines in poorly ventilated areas may show an increase in saturation of 4% during a working day, with a final concentration of 6-10%. Blood saturations below 5% are considered normal, and levels below 10% are generally considered not detrimental to normal performance. Some symptoms of carbon monoxide poisoning generally occur with about 15-20% saturation and become severe at around 30%. In fatal cases of carbon monoxide poisoning the saturation range is usually 60-80%, but in some cases death may occur after no more than 40% saturation.

METHEMOGLOBIN[19, 20]:

Spectrophotometric method:

Principle: The characteristic methemoglobin absorption band at 630 mμ in dilute acid solution is almost completely abolished by the addition of sodium cyanide, which converts the pigment to cyanmethemoglobin. The resulting change in absorbance is directly proportional to the concentration of methemoglobin.[18a] To determine the percentage of methemoglobin another portion of the same dilution of the blood is treated with potassium ferricyanide to convert all the hemoglobin to methemoglobin, and the change in absorbance after the addition of cyanide is again measured.

Reagents:

1. Phosphate buffer (M/15, pH 6.6). Dissolve 5.67 gm. anhydrous monopotassium phosphate (KH_2PO_4) and 3.55 gm. disodium phosphate (Na_2HPO_4) in water and dilute to 1 L. Check the pH and adjust if necessary.
2. Phospate buffer (M/60, pH 6.6). Prepare from stock M/15 buffer by diluting 1:4 as required.
3. Potassium cyanide (AR granular).
4. Potassium ferricyanide (AR crystals).
5. Triton X-100 or other nonionic surface-active agent.

Procedure: Wash 0.2 ml. well-mixed blood into 10 ml. M/60 phosphate buffer. Add a small drop of Triton X-100 and mix the solution well by inversion. Allow mixture to stand until hemolysis is complete. If it is not sparkling clear, it is centrifuged. Transfer a portion of the hemolyzed blood to a spectrophotometer cuvette and measure the absorbance at 630 mμ against a blank of the phosphate buffer (A_1). Then add a few milligrams of potassium cyanide to the cuvette and mix by inversion. The absorbance is again measured at 630 mμ (A_2). Identical A_1 and A_2 readings indicate the absence of methemoglobin and the rest of the procedure may be omitted.[18a] To another aliquot of the blood dilution add about 5 mg. potassium ferricyanide, mix the solution well, and transfer to a cuvette. Measure the absorbance at 630 mμ against the phosphate buffer (A_3). Then add a few milligrams of potassium cyanide to the cuvette, mix the contents, and take the reading again at 630 mμ (A_4). Then:

$$\frac{A_1 - A_2}{A_3 - A_4} \times 100 = \text{\%Methemoglobin saturation}$$

To obtain the absolute amount of methemoglobin one must make an independent measurement of the total hemoglobin by the cyanmethemoglobin method. (See also next section on sulfhemoglobin.)

Heparinized venous or arterial blood may be used. Nonhemolyzed specimens may be kept for a few hours in the refrigerator; preferably the analysis should be performed as soon as possible since methemoglobin tends to disappear rather rapidly from drawn blood.

Range of values and interpretation: Small amounts of methemoglobin may be found in the blood of normal subjects; values up to 0.5 gm./100 ml. or 4% saturation have been found in hospital patients not receiving any recognized methemoglobin-inducing drugs. In methemoglobinemia, cyanosis becomes apparent when the saturation reaches about 10-15%. Levels up to 30% saturation may not produce any obvious symptoms. At levels of from 30-45% symptoms such as dyspnea may be observed. Lethargy and semistupor may not occur until levels of about 60%; the lethal level may be above 70%.

SULFHEMOGLOBIN[21-23]:

Spectrophotometric method: Sulfhemoglobin has a characteristic absorption band at 620 mμ, whereas oxyhemoglobin has very little absorbance. The absorbance of the system is measured at 540 and 620 mμ, and the percentage of sulfhemoglobin is calculated from the ratio of absorbances. If methemoglobin is present, it will interfere and a correction must be made for this which complicates the calculations.

Reagents:

1. Phosphate buffer (0.25M, pH 7.4). Dissolve 28.68 gm. disodium phosphate (anhydrous) (Na_2HPO_4) and 6.83 gm. anhydrous monopotassium

phosphate in water to make 1 L. Check pH and adjust if necessary.
2. Potassium cyanide (AR granular).
3. Triton X-100 or other nonionic surface-active agent.

Procedure: Mix exactly 0.20 ml. well-mixed blood with 3.8 ml. phosphate buffer to make a 1:20 solution. Add a small drop of Triton X-100 and mix the solution by inversion. Allow the mixture to stand a few minutes until hemolysis is complete. If the solution is not perfectly clear, it is centrifuged. Transfer a portion of the diluted blood to a 1 cm. spectrophotometric cuvette and measure the absorbance at 634 mμ against the phosphate buffer (A_1). Add a few milligrams of potassium cyanide, and after mixing, measure the absorbance again at 634 mμ (A_2). Now measure the absorbance of the cyanide-containing mixture at 620 mμ (A_3). Dilute 1 ml. solution from the cuvette with exactly 9 ml. water and measure the absorbance of this diluted solution at 540 mμ against a blank of similarly diluted phosphate buffer (A_4).

Calculations:

1. Methemoglobin concentration:

$$\text{MHb gm.\%} = (A_1 - A_2) \times 10.6$$

2. Absorbance corrections:

Corr. $A_{620} = 20 \times A_3 - 0.90 \times \text{MHb}$

Corr. $A_{540} = 200 \times A_4 - 6.88 \times \text{MHb}$

MHb is the methemoglobin concentration in gm./100 ml.

3. Sulfhemoglobin level:

Calculate $R = (\text{Corr. } A_{540})/(\text{Corr. } A_{620})$

Then

$$\%\text{Total Hb as sulfhemoglobin} = \frac{8.76 - 0.144R}{6.26R + 2.86}$$

Note that the factors in the previous equations are valid only for the dilutions given and when the measurements are made in cuvettes of exactly 1 cm. light path.

A somewhat simpler but less exact method is as follows: Dilute 0.1 ml. blood with 10 ml. 2% Sterox SE and add 1 drop 5% potassium cyanide solution. Determine absorbance at 578 and 620 mμ in 1 cm. cuvettes.

Then

$$\%\text{Sulfhemoglobin} = 70 \times \frac{A_{620}}{A_{578}} - 2$$

where A_{620} and A_{578} are the absorbances measured at these wavelengths. This is an approximate method based on data presented by van Kampen and Zijlstra but is accurate enough for many clinical purposes.

Range of values and interpretation: Sulfhemoglobin is not normally found in the body. It is usually formed after the ingestion of certain drugs. The amount necessary to produce cyanosis has been estimated as being from 1-5% by different investigators. Sulfhemoglobinemia following the ingestion of drugs such as acetanilid, phenacetin, and sulfonamide rarely exceeds 10% saturation.

HEMATOCRIT—VOLUME OF PACKED RED CELLS

This test measures the proportion of red blood cells to plasma in the peripheral blood but not in the entire circulation. The **body hematocrit** gives the ratio of total erythrocyte mass to total blood volume.

Definition: The hematocrit reading gives the number of millimeters of packed red cells/100 mm. blood, indicating the volume (%) of packed red cells/100 ml. blood.

The white layer above the packed red cells consists of leukocytes and platelets.

Each 1 mm. represents about 10,000 WBC/mm.[3] blood. In leukopenia and thrombocytopenia the layer will be thin, while in leukocytosis or leukemia it will be of increased thickness.

Wintrobe macrohematocrit method:

Technique: Fill the Wintrobe hematocrit tube to mark 10 with venous blood and anticoagulate by adding 1 drop Versene to 5 ml. blood by means of a hematocrit pipette. Centrifuge at 3000 rpm for 30 min. in a standardized centrifuge which has a sufficient radius to produce a relative centrifugal force of 2.260 *g*, e.g., the Clay-Adams angle-head table model No. CT 1002.

The level of packed cells is read directly from a centimeter and millimeter scale and this figure is multiplied by 10 to give the volume of packed cells/100 ml. blood.

The layers in the hematocrit tube from top to bottom are as follows: plasma, platelets, leukocytes (and nucleated red blood cells), and red blood cells (the younger ones such as reticulocytes are uppermost).

Purpose of hematocrit determination: The hematocrit is used for calculation of blood constants and as a check on the red blood cell count since the hematocrit measures the concentration of red blood cells. As a measure of blood volume it is not always correct.

The packed cell volume is decreased in anemia; it is increased in primary and secondary polycythemia[24] and can be used to determine the necessity of the red blood cell count. If the hematocrit is normal, a red cell count is not indicated. The blood smear must confirm this decision. If the hematocrit is high or low, the red cells must be enumerated.

The hematocrit serves as a rough quality control in hematology in so far as 1 mm. of the hematocrit scale corresponds to 0.34 gm. hemoglobin and to 107,000 RBC/1 mm.³ blood.

Errors in hematocrit determination: See errors in hemoglobin determination and in the use of venous blood.

The type and amount of anticoagulant is critical. Errors in reading must be avoided. Plastic disposable hematocrit tubes are not subject to scratching and to rubbing off of the calibration. Optimal packing of the cells, which is not synonymous with maximal packing, must occur.

The **average error** of the method is ±1.13%. It is therefore one of the most reliable hematologic procedures.

Microhematocrit method:

Technique: Fill two heparinized capillary tubes about two-thirds full with finger blood by capillary attraction and seal the dry end of the tube with molding clay. Centrifuge 2 min. at 12,000 rpm in a centrifuge* provided with a special head for capillary tubes. The sealed end of the capillary tube must touch the rubber ring of the circular platform. The special cover protecting the carrying tray must be screwed on before the centrifuge cover is locked.

After centrifugation, read the volume of packed cells from a scale held against the capillary tube in such a way that the top of the plasma column coincides with the 100% line and the bottom of the packed red cells falls on the zero line.

Capillary tubes are 1.2-1.5 mm. in diameter and 75 mm. long and may be obtained commercially.*

Significance: Because the error of red blood cell counting is in the neighborhood of 8% and the error of the microhematocrit method is about 2%, the latter method has been accepted as a screening method for the detection of anemia and polycythemia. Unless the centrifuge is especially calibrated the degree of packing of red cells produced is different from that of the Wintrobe macromethod.

Normal range:

Infants: 44-62%

Children: 35-37%

Adult males: 40-45%

Adult females: 36-45%

SEDIMENTATION RATE OF RED BLOOD CELLS

Definition: Sedimentation rate is the fall of a red cell column in 1 hr. measured in millimeters.

Factors influencing sedimentation rate: The degree of dilution with the anticoagulant and the height of the column of blood are the most important factors. The greater the **dilution** and the taller the column, the more rapid will be the settling. **Anticoagulants** (except heparin) retard the rate, but this is not significant with the amounts generally used. Anticoagulants should be isotonic. Dry mixture of 4 mg. potassium oxalate and 6 mg. ammonium oxalate/5 ml. blood or 1 drop of Versene/5 ml. blood do not cause shrinkage of the cells.[24] Sodium oxalate solution, 1.1%, is also isotonic.[25] Sodium fluoride retards the rate and is not suitable as anticoagulant. Stasis should be avoided in obtaining the blood be-

---

*Adams autocrit centrifuge, No. CT 2905, Clay-Adams, Inc., New York, N. Y.

*Adams autocrit centrifuge, No. CT 2905, Clay-Adams, Inc., New York, N. Y.

cause it tends to increase the rate. The usual variation in room temperature does not cause appreciable change, though marked variations should be avoided. The temperature of the patient does not seem to be a factor, but the **room temperature** at which the test is performed affects the sedimentation rate.

Food and exercise do not cause significant variations. The test should be completed **within 2 or 3 hr.** after the blood is obtained, during which time the test may be repeated as a check using the same sample of blood after mixing it again. After a longer time there is a marked retardation. The larger the diameter of the tube, the faster is the rate. The tubes must be in a vertical position.

Sedimentation of erythrocytes apparently proceeds in three stages (phases): formation of rouleaux, rapid settling, and final packing.[26] The larger the rouleaux, the more rapid is the rate. Rouleaux formation does not occur with **cells of abnormal shapes** and therefore the sedimentation rate is decreased. In sickle cell disease oxygenation, by decreasing the number of sickle cells, increases the rate, whereas carbon dioxide administration, by increasing the number of sickle cells, decreases the sedimentation rate. The same effect on sickled blood can be produced by taking blood without stasis and then with stasis (application of tourniquet for 6 min.). When the difference in the rates is greater than 20 mm., it is suggested as a positive test for sickle cell anemia.[27]

The number and size of the erythrocytes affect the packing phase. The greater the **anemia,** the more accelerated the sedimentation rate will be; in **polycythemia** the rate is decreased.

Apart from the previously mentioned factors, the sedimentation rate depends on the length and diameter of the tube and on the concentration and composition of serum proteins. Increased fibrinogen and globulins accelerate the sedimentation rate.

Wintrobe method:

Technique: Collect 5 ml. venous blood and place in a test tube with dried potassium and ammonium oxalate or 1 drop Versene. Set up the test within 2 hr. Fill the Wintrobe tube to the 10 cm. mark, stand it in a vertical position, and read the fall of the red cell column at 1 hr. in millimeters. The test should be made at room temperature, between 22° and 27° C. After the sedimentation test has been completed at 1 hr., centrifuge to constant volume for 30 min. at 3000 rpm to pack the cells and to determine their volume.

Normal values for Wintrobe sedimentation rate:

Men: 0-9 mm.
Women: 0-15 mm.
Children: 0-13 mm.

Errors in sedimentation rate: The specimen must be adequately mixed with the correct type and amount of anticoagulant. Delay in setting up the test beyond 2 hr. decreases the sedimentation rate.

The tube must stand in an exact vertical position since even a slight angle of 3 degrees will accelerate the sedimentation rate 30%.

As it is well established that anemia increases the sedimentation rate, correction for the volume of packed cells (hematocrit) is not considered necessary.

Room temperatures below 22° and above 27° C. require temperature correction charts or better temperature control of the procedure by use of a water bath.

Variations in sedimentation rate:

Increase: **Physiologically,** there is a slight increase in young children, during menstruation, and in pregnancy from the third month until about the fourth week postpartum. **Pathologically,** there is an increase in active inflammation, infections, toxemia, cell or tissue destruction, severe anemia, active tuberculosis and syphilis, acute coronary thrombosis, rheumatoid arthritis, and malignancy.

In unruptured acute appendicitis, even when suppurative or gangrenous, the rate is normal, but with abscess or peritonitis the rate increases rapidly.

In rheumatic, gonorrheal, and acute gouty arthritis the rate is increased significantly; in osteoarthritis (hypertrophic arthritis) it may be slightly increased; in nonarticular rheumatism (neuritis, myositis, fibrositis, lumbago, etc.) it is within the normal range.

After operations, due to tissue trauma, the rate is increased for about a week, after which time an increased rate suggests a complication.

The sedimentation rate is increased in all the collagen diseases except diffuse scleroderma. Lipemia interferes, cholesterol and its esters increasing and phospholipids decreasing the rate. A high fibrinogen or globulin content of the serum increases the rate.

Decrease: Clots decrease the rate. They may be detected after the test by emptying the blood on absorbent paper.[28]

There is a decreased rate in the newborn infant, correlated with the decreased fibrinogen of the blood. Hypofibrinogenemia of any cause decreases the rate, as does polycythemia, sickle cell anemia, and congestive failure. Salicylates decrease the sedimentation rate. Cortisone (compound E) and adrenocorticotropic hormone (ACTH) of the anterior lobe of the pituitary gland cause a prompt decrease of the rate in rheumatoid arthritis and in the acute phase of rheumatic fever. A high blood sugar level decreases the rate.

Interpretation: The test is nonspecific and is not diagnostic of any disease, but it is often useful in differential diagnosis and in following individual cases. While the sedimentation rate is normal in many diseases, an abnormal rate indicates some pathologic state rather than a functional disturbance.

In acute disease the change in rate may lag behind the temperature and the leukocytosis for 6-24 hr., reaching the peak after several days; in convalescence the increased rate tends to persist longer than the temperature or the leukocytosis.

BLOOD VOLUME[29-31]

Total blood volume (TBV) is the sum of the red cell volume (RCV) and the plasma volume (PV).

$$TBV = RCV + PV$$

The hemoglobin and hematocrit values are unreliable indicators of the circulating blood volume so that even major blood volume deficits (25%) may remain unsuspected. If the blood volume is not known, intravenous blood may be given either unnecessarily or in amounts either too little or too great.

Indications for blood volume determination

Blood volume determination is indicated in acute bleeding, hypovolemic shock, burns, and postoperative states. In all these conditions the blood volume is decreased, while the hemoglobin and hematocrit values are either normal or increased. In polycythemia vera the blood volume is increased mainly due to a rise in the total red blood cell mass, while in pregnancy it is increased by an increased plasma volume.

Methods of measuring blood volume

Dye-dilution principle: Evans blue dye or others are injected intravenously, and after a period of mixing in the circulation the dye dilution is measured colorimetrically. The dye tags the plasma protein and on the basis of its dilution allows the determination of the circulating plasma volume. On the basis of the hematocrit (vol.% RBC) the total blood volume can be calculated.

$$\text{Blood volume} = \text{Plasma volume} \times \frac{100}{100 - \text{Hematocrit}}$$

Risa for blood volume determination: Human albumin tagged with I^{131} is called radioiodinated serum albumin (human) and is injected intravenously. After a short period (15 or 20 min.) of mixing the plasma volume can be determined on the basis of the dilution principle. The total blood volume can then be ascertained according to the formula given for the dye method.

Volemetron method: The Volemetron* uses prepackaged Risa-I^{131} of a potency of 3-5 μc in a disposable syringe. The Volemetron allows fairly rapid (15 min.) calculation of the blood volume.

Cr^{51} blood volume determination: This method is by far the most dependable because the red blood cell volume of the body does not fluctuate as much as the plasma volume.

---

*Ames Co., Inc., Elkhart, Ind.

Technique: Two methods may be employed. In one, compatible blood bank blood labeled with Cr^{51} is used, while in the other the patient's own tagged cells are used.

Cr^{51} blood volume—ascorbic acid method: Obtain 18 ml. blood and place it in a sterile tube containing 20 μc Cr^{51} as sterile $Na_2Cr^{51}O_4$ and 0.1 ml. heparin (1000 units/ml.). Incubate tube for 45 min. at 37° C., inverting it every 10 min. Add 1 ml. 5% ascorbic acid to the blood and mix well. After incubation the hematocrit is determined on the blood specimen and 5 ml. of the labeled blood is reinjected into the patient. Allowing 20 min. for mixing time in the patient's circulation, blood is withdrawn from the opposite arm and counted. The hematocrit and a plasma count are also obtained. On the basis of a formula the red blood cell mass can be determined.

Normal values for adult males:
Total red cell volume: 24-29 ml./kg.
Total plasma volume: 29-45 ml./kg.
Total blood volume: 56-76 ml./kg.

RED BLOOD CELL COUNT

Principle: All counting methods are based on the dilution of capillary or well-mixed, correctly anticoagulated venous blood with special counting fluids in special counting pipettes. The individual cells are counted in a counting chamber (hemocytometer).

Reagent:
Gowers diluting fluid:
1. Sodium sulfate, 12.5 gm.
2. Glacial acetic acid, 33.3 ml.
3. Distilled water to 200 ml.
This solution prevents rouleau formation in hyperglobulinemic sera.

Technique: Choose a site free from local circulatory change. Cleanse with alcohol and dry. Puncture with sharp sterile blood lancet. Wipe away the first drop or two of blood and use subsequent drops.

In measuring the blood, hold the pipette before the eyes as you would in order to read a line of printing on it and measure accurately.

In mixing the specimen, rotate pipette between fingers and see that the bead is free.

Draw blood to 0.5 mark on red cell diluting pipette with red bead and wipe tip of pipette. Remove excess by touching tip of pipette with fingers. Do not draw far above mark 0.5. Draw up Gowers fluid. Rotate pipette on its long axis horizontally while drawing up diluting fluid. Shake immediately for a few seconds and then mix for 3 min. in a pipette rotor. Discard about one-third, wipe tip, and place the next drop on one side of a double chamber; discard 3 more drops, wipe tip, and place the next drop on the other side of the chamber (Fig. 4-2). Place a special cover glass over the ruled area and deposit the drop of blood close to the edge of the cover slip to allow the blood to flood the counting area by capillary attraction. The moat should not be filled and no air bubbles should be trapped in the preparation. Allow 3 min. for settling.

Count the erythrocytes in both counting chambers. Using the low-power microscopic lens, identify the central large square (No. 5 in Figs. 4-3 and 4-4). In the central square, using the high-power lens, count the erythrocytes in 5 small squares, each of which is bordered by triple lines and is divided into 16 smaller squares. Count from left to right. Of the cells that touch the boundary lines, count all those touching the upper and left-hand

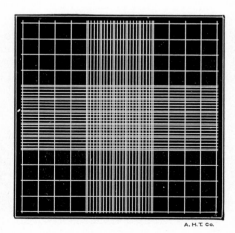

A. H. T. Co.

Fig. 4-2. Improved Neubauer ruling on hemocytometer, showing entire ruled area of 9 mm.². (Courtesy Arthur H. Thomas Co., Philadelphia, Pa.)

lines. Do not count the cells touching the bottom and right-hand lines. This method ensures that no cell will be counted twice. Record the number of cells in each of the 5 groups of 16 smallest squares and add the numbers. The error of this procedure varies from ± 10% to ± 20%.

Calculation: Red cell counts are expressed in units of millions (10^6)/mm.^{3}. The center square occupies 1 mm.^{2}; each

Table 4-3. Dimensions of counting chamber and subdivisions*

Square	Length (mm.)	Area (mm.^{2})	Depth (mm.)	Volume (mm.^{3})
Chamber	3	9	0.10	0.90
1	1	1	0.10	0.10
1A	0.25	0.0625	0.10	0.00625
5A	0.20	0.040	0.10	0.0040

*From Page and Culver: The successor to Thomas Hale Ham's syllabus of laboratory examinations in clinical diagnosis, Cambridge, 1956, Harvard University Press.

of the 25 smaller squares that it contains occupies 1/25 mm.^{2} and each of its 16 smallest squares occupies 1/400 mm.^{2}. A total of 80 (5 × 16) of these smallest squares are counted (Table 4-3).

$$80 \times \frac{1}{400} \text{ mm.}^2 = \frac{1}{5} \text{ mm.}^2$$

(the counted area)

The usual dilution of blood in the red blood cell pipette is 1:200. The depth of the counting chamber is 1/10 mm. The number of erythrocytes/mm.^{3} of blood is calculated as follows:

$$\frac{\text{Counted erythrocytes}}{\text{Counted area} \times \text{Height of chamber} \times \text{Dilution}} =$$

$$\frac{\text{Counted erythrocytes}}{\frac{1}{5} \times \frac{1}{10} \times \frac{1}{200}} =$$

Counted erythrocytes × 10,000 = No. of erythrocytes/mm.^{3} blood

Watch the correction factor in the pipette or do two counts with balanced pipettes (e.g., correction factors of +2 and –2).

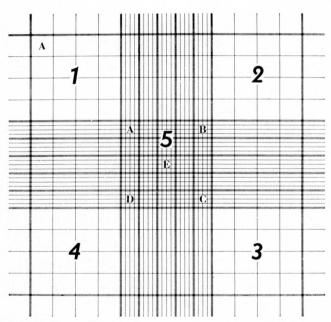

Fig. 4-3. Improved Neubauer ruling for one counting chamber. White cell count is done on the four large corner squares (**1, 2, 3,** and **4**) of each of two counting chambers. Red cell count is done on square **5** (**A, B, C, D,** and **E**) of each of two counting chambers. Platelet count is done on two large corner squares (**1** and **3**) of each of two counting chambers. (From Page and Culver: A syllabus of laboratory examination in clinical diagnosis, Cambridge, 1960, Harvard University Press.)

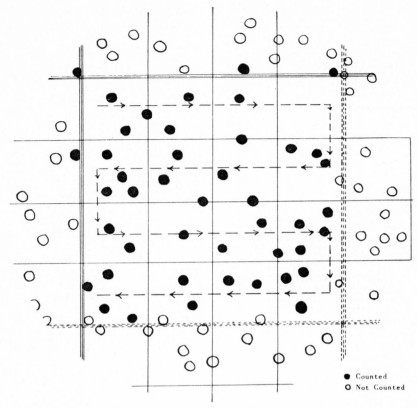

Fig. 4-4. Diagrammatic representation of red cell count. The square shown, comparable to square 5A in Fig. 4-3, is magnified 400 times, using the high-power dry objective of the microscope. The order of counting of the small squares is indicated by the arrows. A red cell is counted only once by counting those within the small square and those touching any line at the left or top but not counting those touching any line at the right or bottom of the small square. By this procedure, all cells touching the triple lines shown as solid lines will be included and all cells touching the triple lines shown as broken lines will be excluded. (From Page and Culver: A syllabus of laboratory examinations in clinical diagnosis, Cambridge, 1960, Harvard University Press.)

Variations of technique in polycythemia and in severe anemias: If the red blood cells are markedly **increased** in number (erythremia, polycythemia), increase the dilution by drawing up blood to the 0.3 mark on the red cell pipette and dilute to mark 101. Count and calculate as before but multiply result by 5/3 since only 3 mm. of the pipette were counted instead of 5 mm. If the number of red blood cells is markedly **diminished** (anemia), decrease the dilution by drawing blood up to 1 mark in the red cell pipette and dilute to mark 101. The dilution is then 1:100. On the basis of this formula the

counted erythrocytes have to be multiplied by 5000 (instead of 10,000).

Errors in red blood cell counting: Red blood cell counts are subject to many errors, such as errors in the equipment, in the performance of the test, and in sampling of the blood. (See sources of error in hemoglobin determination.) The errors of blood sampling, pipetting, and unclean glassware are the same as for hemoglobin determination. Restricted to counting procedures are such defects as inadequate filling or drying up of the counting chamber, dirt in the counting fluid, incorrect enumeration of cells, air

Table 4-4. Average normal blood values at different age levels[*]

	At birth	At 2 days	At 14 days	At 3 mo.	At 6 mo.	At 1 yr.	At 2 yr.	At 4 yr.	At 8-21 yr.
Red cells/mm.³ (in millions)	5.1	5.3	5.0	4.3	4.6	4.7	4.8	4.8	5.1
Hemoglobin									
gm./100 ml.[†]	17.6	18.0	17.0	11.4	11.5	12.2	12.9	13.1	14.1
percentage of normal	113	115	109	73	74	78	83	84	90
White cells/mm.³ (in thousands)	15.0	21.0	11.0	9.5	9.2	9.0	8.5	8.0	8.0
Platelets/mm.³ (in thousands)	350.0	400.0	300.0	260.0	250.0	250.0	250.0	250.0	250.0
Differential smears (percentages)									
Polymorphonuclear neutrophils	45	55	36	35	40	40	40	50	60
Eosinophils and basophils	3	5	3	3	3	2	2	2	2
Lymphocytes	30	20	53	55	51	53	50	40	30
Monocytes	12	15	8	7	6	5	8	8	8
Immature white cells	10	5	—	—	—	—	—	—	—
Percentage of nucleated red cells in total nucleated cells	1-5	2	—	—	—	—	—	—	—
Percentage of reticulocysts in total red cells	2	3	1	0.5	0.8	1	1	1	1

[*]From Blackfan et al.: Atlas of the blood in children, Cambridge, 1944, Harvard University Press.
[†]Hemoglobin in whole blood: value of 15.6 gm./100 ml. equivalent to 100%.

bubbles and fat droplets in the counting area, wet counting chamber, and inadequate mixing of the specimen in the counting pipette.

Cleaning of pipettes: Stained pipettes should be immersed in NaOH, KOH, or cleaning solution overnight. Attach pipette to a suction pump and clean by syphoning through in this order: fresh water, 95% alcohol, acetone, and air. The counting chamber must be gently cleaned after each use.

Electronic counters: The Coulter counter[*] counts the individual red blood cells of a measured volume of diluted blood as they pass through a minute orifice guarded by an electric current flowing between platinum electrodes. The red blood cells, which are poor electrical conductors, passing through the orifice displace an electrically conductive 0.9% saline solution in which they are suspended and thus modulate the electric current. The modulations are amplified and counted. They

depend on the number and size of the cells passing through the orifice. The counter works with an accuracy and reproducibility of about 2%. The electronic counter enumerates red and white blood cells alike, and an error will be introduced if leukocytosis of over 30,000 cells/mm.³ exists. In this case, the result has to be corrected. The electronic counter can also be used in enumerating leukocytes and platelets and accomplishes that with a standard error of 2.8%. (For discussion of the Coulter counter technique, see p. 120.)

Normal values:
Males: 4.5-5.5 million/mm.³
Females: 4.1-5.0 million/mm.³
Children: 4.5-5.5 million/mm.³
Newborn infants: 6.0-8.0 million/mm.³

Variation in number of red blood cells:
Increase—polycythemia: Polycythemia may be temporary and symptomatic (**erythrocytosis**) or idiopathic and progressive (**erythremia**). Temporary polycythemia may be caused by dehydration

[*]Coulter Electronics, Inc., Hialeah, Fla.

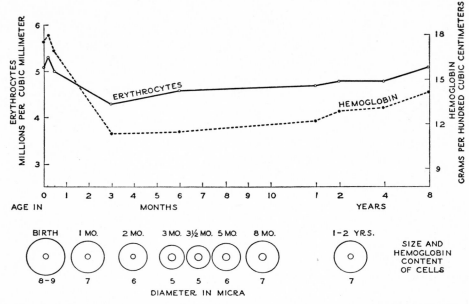

Fig. 4-5. Normal values of erythrocytes and hemoglobin at different age levels. (From Black-fan et al.: Atlas of the blood in children, Cambridge, 1944, Harvard University Press.)

from any cause (fever, loss of fluid, etc.) or from anoxemia (high altitudes, pulmonary and cardiac disease, methemoglobinemia). **Polycythemia vera** (erythremia, Osler-Vaquez disease) is a disease of the erythropoietic tissue characterized by hyperplasia of the bone marrow and enlarged spleen and by the presence in the peripheral blood of increased reticulocytes, platelets, and leukocytes, some of which may be immature. There is a **physiologic erythrocytosis** in newborn infants (Fig. 4-5 and Table 4-4) and in individuals exposed to high altitudes.

Decrease—anemia: A count below 4 million is considered decreased and indicates anemia. A mild anemia, however, may show decreased hemoglobin, with a normal red cell count. Anemias are divided into normocytic, microcytic, and macrocytic anemias.

BLOOD INDICES AND CORPUSCULAR OR BLOOD CONSTANTS[32]

In addition to reporting red blood cells, hematocrit, and hemoglobin in absolute numbers, it is useful at times to express their relationship to each other in the form of ratios, indices, or corpuscular constants. These constants are no more accurate than the figures from which they are derived. The mean corpuscular hemoglobin concentration (MCHC) is probably the most accurate one.

Mean corpuscular volume (MCV)

The mean corpuscular volume is the volume of the average red blood cell of a given sample of blood.

This is calculated as follows:

$$\frac{\text{Vol. packed RBC in ml./1000 ml. blood}}{\text{RBC in millions/mm.}^3} = \text{MCV in } \mu^3$$

The normal average is 87.1 (min. 80 – max. 94) μ^3. This represents the volume of the average red blood cells of a given sample of blood in absolute units.

Mean corpuscular hemoglobin (MCH)

The mean corpuscular hemoglobin is the amount of hemoglobin, by weight, in the average red blood cell of the sample of blood.

The following calculation is used for this determination:

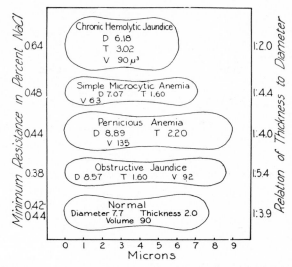

Fig. 4-6. Cross section and measurements of mean erythrocyte in different clinical conditions. (From Haden: Amer. J. Med. Sci. **188**:441, 1934.)

$$\frac{\text{Hb in gm./1000 ml. blood}}{\text{RBC in millions/mm.}^3} = \text{MCH in } \mu\mu g$$

The normal average is 29.5 (min. 27 – max. 32) $\mu\mu$g.

Despite the common use of the term "hyperchromic cells," an individual cell cannot be supersaturated with hemoglobin.

Mean corpuscular hemoglobin concentration (MCHC)

The mean corpuscular hemoglobin concentration is the proportion of hemoglobin (w/v) contained in the average red cell of the sample of blood.

The following calculation is used:

$$\frac{\text{Hb in gm./100 ml. blood}}{\text{Vol. packed cells in ml./100 ml. blood (Hct)}} \times 100 = \text{MCHC in } \%$$

The normal average is 35% (min. 33% – max. 38%).

Value of blood indices

As already pointed out, to be meaningful the corpuscular constants must be based on very accurate determinations of hemoglobin, hematocrit, and red blood cell count. On the basis of corpuscular constants, red blood cells can be characterized as normal in every respect or

as deviating from the norm in volume and/or hemoglobin contents. The deficient states, the anemias, can be classified as macrocytic, normocytic, simple microcytic, and microcytic hypochromic (Fig. 4-6).

	MCV (μ^3)	MCH ($\mu\mu$g)	MCHC (%)
Normocytic cells	80-94	27-32	33-38
Macrocytic anemia	94-160	32-50	32-36
Normocytic anemia	82-92	27-31	32-36
Simple microcytic	72-80	21-24	30-37
Microcytic hypochromic	50-80	12-29	24-30

Determination of the blood constants can also be used as a method of quality control.

Color index

The color index is a rough estimate of mean corpuscular hemoglobin.

$$\text{CI} = \frac{\text{Hb gm./100 ml.}}{\text{RBC in millions} \times 3}$$

The color index is based on percentages rather than on absolute values and it is therefore inaccurate.

Normal values: 0.98-1.1. The color index is diminished in hypochromic anemias and it exceeds 1 in macrocytic anemias.

MEAN DIAMETER OF RED BLOOD CELLS

Price-Jones method: The greatest and smallest diameters of 100-200 RBC of a stained smear of peripheral blood are measured by means of an eyepiece micrometer standardized so that 1 division corresponds to 1μ. The mean of both diameters is plotted on graph paper, the abscissa representing the cell size and the ordinate the frequency in percent. Normal red cells produce a gaussian bell-shaped distribution curve, with the peak at 7-7.5μ. Hemolytic anemias produce a shift to the left of the Price-Jones curve, while pernicious anemia produces a shift to the right (Fig. 4-7).

WHITE BLOOD CELL COUNT

Technique: Draw blood to 0.5 mark on white cell diluting pipette (white bead) and wipe tip of pipette. Draw 0.5% acetic acid or Türk diluting fluid to mark 11. Mix as for red blood cell count. The dilution is 1:20.

Reagent:

Acetic acid (0.5%) or Türk diluting fluid:

1. Glacial acetic acid, 1 ml.
2. Gentian violet (1% aqueous), 1 ml.

3. Distilled water to 100 ml.

Filter before use.

The acetic acid produces hemolysis of all the nonnucleated red cells, but nucleated red blood cells are counted together with the white cells.

Technique: Discard one-third, wipe tip, and place drop on one side of double chamber; discard 2 or 3 drops more, wipe tip, and place next drop on other side of chamber. Allow 3 min. for settling and count 4 corner sq.mm. areas on each of the two preparations. In each large square begin counting (Fig. 4-8) at the extreme upper left, moving toward the right. Count all cells in the upper 4 small quadrants. Then drop down to the lower line of squares and count all the cells, moving back toward the left side. Drop down to the next row of squares and continue. Count the cells that touch dividing lines to the left and above and disregard cells touching the dividing lines to the right and below. The greatest variation should not exceed 12 cells.

Calculation: In each chamber 4 large corner squares are counted, a total of 8 squares. The sum of the numbers of cells counted is multiplied by 25 to give the number of leukocytes per cubic millimeter

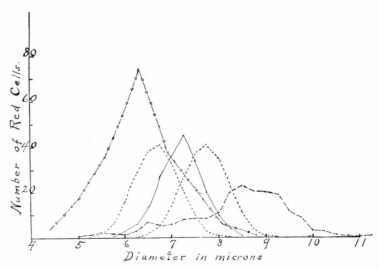

Fig. 4-7. Red cell diameters. o-o-o, Chronic hemolytic jaundice curve superimposed on Price-Jones curves modified by plotting 200 cells. Solid line, the normal mean; dotted lines, the normal range; broken line, a case of pernicious anemia. (Chronic hemolytic jaundice curve from Cheney and Cheney: Amer. J. Med. Sci. **187**:191, 1934; remaining curves from Price-Jones: Red blood cell diameters, London, 1933, Oxford University Press, Inc.)

of blood. The factor 25 is based on the formula described in the red blood cell counting technique.

$$\frac{\text{No. of cells counted} \times \text{Dilution}}{\text{No. of large squares counted} \times \text{Height of chamber}}$$
$$= \text{No. of leukocytes/mm.}^3 \text{ blood}$$

In leukopenia and in leukocytosis the dilution may have to be varied.

For **leukopenia,** use twice the amount of blood for the leukocyte count. Draw blood up to the 1 mark and dilute to the 11 mark, thus diluting 1:10.

For very **high leukocyte counts,** as in leukemia, make the blood dilution in the red cell pipette. If diluted 1:100, multi-

ply by 125; and if the dilution is 1:200, multiply by 250.

If 8 large squares are counted, multiply as follows:

If dilution is 1:10,
    cells counted $\times$ 12.5 = leukocytes/1 mm.^{3} blood
If dilution is 1:20,
    cells counted $\times$ 25   = leukocytes/1 mm.^{3} blood
If dilution is 1:100,
    cells counted $\times$ 125 = leukocytes/1 mm.^{3} blood
If dilution is 1:200,
    cells counted $\times$ 250 = leukocytes/1 mm.^{3} blood

Normal values: It is somewhere around 7000 WBC/mm.^{3}, the generally accepted limits of a normal count being from 5000-11,000 WBC/mm.^{3}. (See discussion of variation in number.)

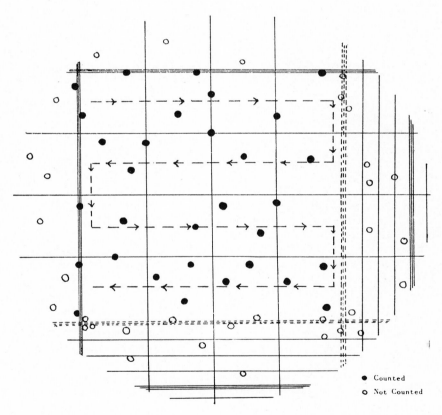

Fig. 4-8. Diagrammatic representation of white cell count. The square shown, comparable to square 1 shown in Fig. 4-3, is magnified 100 times, using the low-power objective of the microscope. The order of counting of the medium-sized squares is the same as that shown in Fig. 4-4. A white cell is counted only once by counting those within the medium-sized square and those touching any line at the left and top but not counting those touching any line at the right and bottom of the medium-sized square. By this procedure all cells touching the triple lines shown as broken lines will be excluded. (From Page and Culver: A syllabus of laboratory examinations in clinical diagnosis, Cambridge, 1960, Harvard University Press.)

VARIATION IN NUMBER OF WHITE BLOOD CELLS: Variation in the total number of leukocytes (the **leukocyte count**) and in the percentage relation of the different types of leukocytes (the **differential count**) is of importance in the diagnosis and prognosis of disease processes.

Total count: The normal range of the leukocyte count in adults is usually given as 3500-12,500, with the generally accepted average range of 5000-11,000/mm.[3]. There is an hourly rhythm, with an early morning low level and a late afternoon (1:00-5:00 P.M.) high peak independent of food.[33] It is probable that taking of food as well as moderate physical or emotional activity will cause a slight increase in the number of leukocytes,[34, 35] but usually the maximum will not exceed twice the minimum count in the normal individual, and the attempt to obtain "basal" leukocyte counts is not practical in clinical work. However, the time of taking the leukocyte count should be recorded.

Increase—leukocytosis: The temporary or symptomatic increase of total leukocytes is called leukocytosis as distinguished from leukemia in which the increase is permanent and progressive. Leukocytosis usually is due to an increase of only one type of cell and is given the name of the type of cell mainly increased, e.g., neutrophilic, lymphocytic, eosinophilic, monocytic, and basophilic. The cause of the increase of the various white cells is discussed under the heading of the involved cells; e.g., lymphocytosis is discussed under the heading of lymphocytes.

Unless stated otherwise, leukocytosis refers to neutrophilic leukocytosis. If the total number of any cell per cubic millimeter is increased, it is called an absolute increase (as **absolute** lymphocytosis, etc.), but if only the percentage is increased, because the other types are decreased, it is a relative increase (as **relative** lymphocytosis).

Leukocytosis under 20,000 is considered slight; to 30,000, moderate; and to 50,000 and over, high.

Leukocytosis can be subdivided according to the cell type involved and according to whether it is physiologic or pathologic.

Physiologic leukocytosis
    Newborn infants, pregnancy, emotional disturbances, sunlight (ultraviolet light), menstruation, and exercise
Pathologic leukocytosis
    Neutrophilic
        Bacterial infections
        Metabolic disturbances—diabetic and uremic coma
        Blood diseases—hemorrhage, granulocytic leukemia, myeloproliferative disorders, and hemolysis
        Drugs—digitalis, mercury, and ACTH
        Tissue breakdown—burns, myocardial infarct, tumors, and gangrene
        Stress—allergies and heat
    Eosinophilic
        Parasitic infections
        Allergies
        Myelogeneous leukemia
        Familial eosinophilia
        Hodgkin's disease and polycythemia
        Subacute infections
    Basophilic
        Granulocytic and basophilic leukemias
    Lymphocytic
        Viral infections—infectious lymphocytosis, mumps, pertussis, infectious mononucleosis, infectious hepatitis, virus pneumonia, and measles
        Bacterial infections—tuberculosis, brucellosis, syphilis, and healing infections
        Blood diseases—lymphatic leukemia, Felty's syndrome, Banti's disease, infectious lymphocytosis, and infectious mononucleosis
        Hormonal diseases—hypothyroidism and hypoadrenalism
    Monocytic
        Virus infections—infectious mononucleosis, chickenpox, and mumps
        Bacterial infections—subacute endocarditis, tuberculosis, and Weil's disease
        Miscellaneous causes—malignant tumors, cirrhosis of liver, Banti's disease, and monocytic leukemia

Leukemoid reaction: In certain diseases the increase of leukocytes is so great or the shift to immature forms so marked that the blood picture suggests leukemia (**the leukemoid blood picture**); e.g., in measles and whooping cough the picture may suggest lymphatic leukemia; and in sepsis, myelocytic leukemia.

Leukocytes in infants and children: The total count in newborn infants varies but is high for the first few days (10,000-20,000 or more). During the first year a count between 9000-11,000 may be considered normal (Fig. 4-9).

At birth there is polymorphonuclear leukocytosis (about 60-70% PMN) which decreases to a low stabilized level about the tenth day, whereas the lymphocytes increase from about 15-55% or more during the same period. Between the third and fifth days, the polymorphonuclear cells and the lymphocytes are about equal in number. After the tenth day there is a gradual increase in the percentage of polymorphonuclear cells and a gradual decrease in the percentage of lymphocytes. Between the third and fifth years the polymorphocytes and the lymphocytes are again about equal in number. Adult values are reached about the tenth year. The normal percentage of polymorphonuclear cells and lymphocytes is given by Wile in Table 4-5.

Decrease—leukopenia:

Definition: Leukopenia is a diminution in the number of circulatory white blood cells. Some acute infections (chiefly those due to virus, protozoa, or bacilli) and many severe infections and intoxications do not cause leukocytosis but may cause a decrease of leukocytes or leukopenia. Most frequently this is due to a decrease

Table 4-5. Normal percentage of polymorphonuclear cells and lymphocytes

Age (yr.)	Polymorpho- nuclear cells (%)	Lymphocytes (%)
Infancy	18-30	70-80
1	35	53
2	38	51
3	42	47
4	47	41
5	52	39
6	52	37
7	53	35
8	54	33
9	55	31
10	60	30

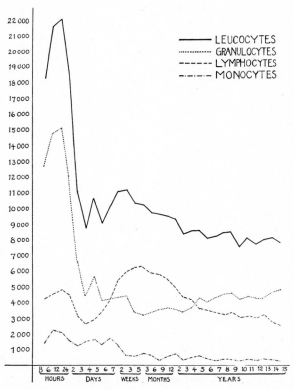

Fig. 4-9. Leukocytes in infancy and childhood. (From Kato: J. Pediat. **7:**7, 1935.)

of neutrophils (neutropenia) which results in relative lymphocytosis.

Leukopenia can be subdivided according to etiology and according to cell type predominantly involved.

The classification according to etiology is as follows:

1. Diminished formation of leukocytes due to a bone marrow defect: radiation effect, effects of drugs and poisons, and aplastic anemia
2. Maturation arrest of white blood cells: agranulocytosis
3. Excessive peripheral destruction of white blood cells: autoimmune antibodies

Following is the classification according to cell type:

Neutropenia
1. Bacterial and parasitic infections: malaria, typhoid fever, brucellosis, and septicemia (overwhelming)
2. Viral infections: measles, hepatitis, poliomyelitis, and mumps
3. Blood diseases: aplastic anemia, agranulocytosis, myelofibrosis, pernicious anemia, and hypersplenism
4. Toxic agents: radiation, cytotoxic drugs, and immune antibodies
5. Hormonal diseases: Addison's disease, thyrotoxicosis, and acromegaly

Eosinopenia
1. Blood diseases: infectious mononucleosis, hyposplenism, aplastic anemia, and pernicious anemia
2. Hormonal influences: Cushing's disease, ACTH administration, epinephrine administration, insulin administration, thyroxin administration, and stress
3. Infections: before recovery stage

Lymphopenia
1. Disease of lymphatic system and blood: Hodgkin's disease and lupus erythematosus
2. Hormones: after the administration of ACTH and cortisone
3. After burns or trauma
4. Chronic uremia

ERRORS IN WHITE CELL COUNTING: The errors in white blood cell counting are similar to the errors enumerated for the red blood cell count; however, because the dilution used is not as great as in the red cell count, the errors are not magnified to the same extent.

CORRECTION OF WHITE BLOOD CELL COUNT FOR NUCLEATED RED BLOOD CELLS: If nucleated red blood cells are present, the white blood cell count has to be corrected because nucleated red blood cells are counted together with the white blood cells. Use the following formula:

$$\text{Corr. WBC count} = \frac{\text{Counted WBC} \times \text{No. of nucleated RBC/100 leukocytes}}{100 + \text{No. of nucleated RBC/100 leukocytes}}$$

The number of nucleated red blood cells is obtained from the differential count.

ERYTHROCYTE AND LEUKOCYTE COUNTING WITH THE COULTER COUNTER: Turn the Coulter counter on and allow several minutes warm-up time.

Sample preparation: Add 0.02 ml. blood containing the correct amount of anticoagulant* (1 drop/5 ml. venous blood) to 10 ml. normal saline solution. Pipettes with an accuracy of 1% should be used and automatic dilutors should provide an automated and accurate method of making dilutions.

From this 1:500 stock solution, the samples for both red and white blood cell counts are prepared.

Red blood count: Dilute 0.01 ml. of 1:500 stock solution with 10 ml. saline solution, giving a 1:50,000 dilution. This dilution is ready for use in the red blood cell count. Because of the coincidence effect, the first three digits of the count on the digital counter should be applied to the conversion chart supplied with the instrument to obtain the corrected red blood cell count. The last two digits are ignored. Add four zeros to the corrected red cell count and report as number of cells/mm.[3].

White blood count: To 3 drops of 10 ml. of the 1:500 stock solution add ZaPonin.† After about 20-30 sec., during which the red blood cells are completely lysed, make the white blood count in the same manner as the red count and read the count directly from the digital and mechanical register.

Counting procedure:
1. With the aperture current and amplifier gain set at the appropriate settings for the type of count being made, and with the threshold also

---

*Sequester-Sol, Cambridge Chemical Products, Inc., Detroit, Mich.

†Coulter Electronics, Inc., Hialeah, Fla.

properly adjusted, place the diluted sample on the platform and immerse the tip of the orifice and the external electrode in the solution.

2. Open the uppermost stopcock momentarily.
3. After mercury in the manometer tube has passed both microswitches (about 2 or 3 sec.), depress the reset button to clear the counting register and to apply current to the aperture circuit.
4. Close the uppermost stopcock.
5. At its completion, note count from the counting register and proceed with next sample.

The aperture current setting (ACS) is set at 5 for the erythrocyte and leukocyte counts. The ACS regulates the height of the pattern on the oscilloscope screen. The response threshold is set at 6 for erythrocytes and at 15 for leukocytes. This is determined by the height of the electric interference and the debris background noise visible at the base of the oscilloscope pattern. The setting must be visible at the base of the oscilloscope pattern and high enough to eliminate the noise but low enough to count the smaller cells. The coincident table for correcting the count according to the probability of more than one cell entering or passing through the orifice simultaneously accompanies the instrument. The coincident factor is so low in leukocyte counts that it is considered negligible.

The leukocyte count may be falsely low in chronic lymphatic leukemia due to the fragility of the lymphocytes. Also, counts over 100,000 WBC are probably inaccurate. Nucleated erythrocytes are enumerated along with leukocytes in the leukocyte count so that a correction must be made when nucleated erythrocytes are observed in the blood smear.

Sources of error:
1. Dilution (due to incorrect pipetting)
2. Dust particles
3. Air bubbles (ZaPonin is a foaming agent)

The orifice must always be kept clean and the plastic valves should be carefully cleaned.

The technologist should avail himself of the course on instrumentation and maintenance offered by Coulter Electronics, Inc. He should keep a good supply of spare parts.

CIRCULATING EOSINOPHIL COUNT

Technique: Draw capillary or oxalated blood to the 1 mark in a white cell pipette. Wipe the tip and draw diluting fluid to mark 11. Repeat same procedure with second pipette. Mix and let stand for 30 min. Shake in mechanical shaker for 30 sec. Expel 4 drops and fill each counting chamber with the contents of one pipette. Count eosinophils in all 9 large squares of each chamber under low power (×100).

Calculation: Dilution 1:10.

$$\frac{\text{No. of eosinophils counted} \times 100}{9} =$$

Eosinophils/mm.[3] blood

Diluting fluid:
1. Propylene glycol, 50 ml.
2. Distilled water, 40 ml.
3. Phloxine (1% aqueous), 10 ml.
4. Sodium carbonate (10%), 1 ml.
5. Heparin sodium, 100 units

Filter before use.

Principle: Phloxine stains the eosinophilic granules red and heparin prevents clumping of white cells that are lysed by the carbonate which spares the eosinophils. The distilled water lyses the red blood cells which are rendered invisible by the propylene glycol.

Normal values: 150-250 eosinophils/mm.[3].

Error in method: There is a large error in the method if the usual **Neubauer counting chamber** is used. To reduce this error Thorn[36, 37] recommends making the eosinophil count in a **Fuchs-Rosenthal counting chamber**, which is 0.2 mm. deep and has a ruling of 16 squares of 1 mm.[2] each. (See basophil count for measurements of chamber.)

Calculation: Dilution 1:10.

$$\frac{\text{No. of eosinophils counted} \times 10}{3.2} =$$

Eosinophils/mm.[3] blood

Speirs[38] has described a special eosinophil counting chamber slide with 4 chambers of 10 mm.[2] each, and each square millimeter is subdivided into 16 small squares. The depth of the chamber is 0.2 mm.

Calculation: Dilution 1:10.

$$\frac{\text{No. of eosinophils counted} \times 10}{8} =$$

Eosinophils/mm.[3] blood

Thorn ACTH test: The Thorn test[39, 40] is based in part on the fact that ACTH produces in 4 hr. a decrease of 50% or more in the eosinophil count in persons with a normally functioning adrenal cortex. It is useful as a diagnostic test in Addison's disease, as a test of adrenal cortex reserve before surgical procedures, and as a test to distinguish functional hypopituitarism from organic disease of the adrenal cortex.

Allow nothing but water after 8 P.M. Make eosinophil count in duplicate the next morning. Give 25 mg. ACTH (25 I.U.) intramuscularly and repeat eosinophil count in duplicate at 4 hr.

Variation in number of eosinophils: See p. 118.

ABSOLUTE BASOPHIL COUNT

Toluidine blue method (Cooper[41]):

Principle: Cetylpyridinium chloride is used to lyse the erythrocytes and to render the basophilic granules insoluble. Aluminum sulfate is used as a mordant to improve the staining qualities of toluidine blue. EDTA prevents platelet agglutination.

Reagents:
1. EDTA (0.1%) in saline solution (disodium salt)
2. Cetylpyridinium chloride (0.5%), 25 ml.
3. Distilled water, 25 ml.
4. Toluidine blue (0.8%) in aluminum sulfate (5%), 20 ml.

Filter before use.

Technique: Add 0.08 ml. solution 1 to test tube (75 × 10 mm.). Add 0.02 ml. finger blood and mix. Add 0.1 ml. solution 2, mix, and stopper. Fill two Fuchs-Rosenthal chambers using a Pasteur pipette. Allow 5 min. for cells to settle.

Fuchs-Rosenthal counting chamber: The use of this chamber has also been suggested for spinal fluid and eosinophil counts. Its measurements are as follows: area 16 mm.[2], depth 0.2 mm., and volume 32 mm.[3].

Formula for undiluted material:

$$\frac{\text{Total count}}{3.2} = \text{Basophils/mm.}^3 \text{ blood}$$

Normal values: 20-50 basophils/mm.[3]; average value 40/mm.[3].

Interpretation: Basophils are seen as purple-red metachromatically stained cells. Other leukocytes, platelets, and red cells do not stain.

Basophils are increased and decreased in a number of conditions which are enumerated on p. 118.

Basophil counts are used to study allergic reactions.[42, 43] Sensitization leads to an increase in the number of basophils which level off when the sensitization has occurred. If the patient is challenged with the same antigen, the count will fall at a rate depending on the type of reaction. Anaphylaxis leads to a rapid fall, while in urticaria the fall is slow. Degranulation of the basophils is responsible for the disappearance of the cells.

Neutral red technique: There are some disadvantages. Eosinophils may also stain, the basophilic granules may be water soluble, and platelet aggregates may interfere with counting.

PLATELET COUNT

There are several techniques available:

Indirect counting method: Platelets are counted in their relationship to red blood cells on fixed smears. This method is least reliable because results depend on the distribution of platelets and the red blood cell count. The permanent record is an advantage since it allows the study of the morphology of the platelets and gives an impression of their number.

The indirect counting method can be used as a rough control of the platelet count. If less than 1 platelet/oil-immersion field is seen, the platelet count will be decreased. If several clumps are visualized, it will be adequate; if more than

25 platelets are observed, the count will be increased.

Direct counting methods: These are the most accurate methods at the present time.

1. Phase microscopy
2. Rees-Ecker
3. Coulter counter

Phase microscopy method of Brecker-Cronkite[44]:

1. Use capillary blood or venous blood obtained by the 2-syringe method (see discussion of blood coagulation technique); the second syringe should be siliconized.
2. Empty blood into siliconized test tube. Keep in refrigerator.
3. Draw blood to 1 mark of two red cell pipettes, and dilute with diluting fluid to mark 101.
4. Shake pipettes for 3 min.
5. Expel first 4 drops and fill both chambers of hemocytometer. Use No. 1 cover slip.

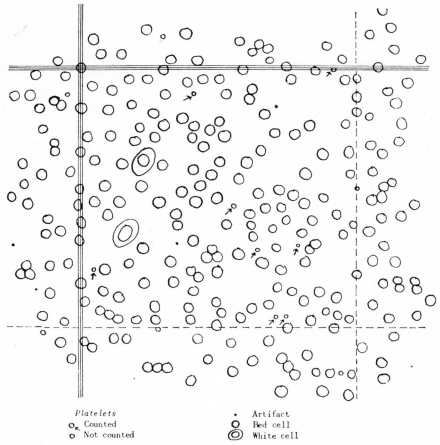

Platelets
○ Counted
○ Not counted

• Artifact
○ Red cell
◎ White cell

Fig. 4-10. Diagrammatic representation of platelet count by the direct method. The medium-sized square shown is comparable to square 1A of the counting chamber, as shown in Fig. 4-3. The magnification is 400 times, using the high-power dry objective of the microscope. A platelet is counted only once by counting those within the medium-sized square and those touching any line at the left and top (solid lines) but not counting those touching any line at the right and bottom (broken lines) of the medium-sized square. The platelet count in this one medium-sized square is 8 (as indicated by the arrows), corresponding to a total of about 250,000 platelets/mm.^{3} or 250×10^3 mm.^{3}. As shown in Fig. 4-3, the platelets are counted and recorded for all medium-sized squares of the two corner squares 1 and 3 of each of two counting chambers. (From Ham: A syllabus of laboratory examinations in clinical diagnosis, Cambridge, 1956, Harvard University Press.)

6. Place hemocytometer in closed petri dish kept humid with moist filter paper in top half. Allow to stand for 15 min.
7. Count platelets by phase microscopy in the central and 4 corner squares of the large central square of the counting chamber as for red blood cell count. The platelets appear as pinkish oval or round structures with small processes.

Calculation:

$$\frac{\text{No. of cells counted} \times \text{Dilution}}{0.004 \times \text{No. squares counted}} =$$
No. of platelets/mm.³ blood

The Brecker-Cronkite method is more accurate than the Rees-Ecker method and is less difficult to perform because of fewer particles that may mimick platelets. If platelets are seen to clump, the procedure must be repeated.

Diluting fluid: Ammonium oxalate, 1%, in distilled water. Store in refrigerator and filter before use.

The direct counting method should always be supplemented by a blood smear, first, to confirm the counted number and, second, to study platelet morphology.

Rees-Ecker method:

1. Draw blood (capillary or venous) that has been aspirated into a siliconized syringe and test tube into a red cell pipette to the 0.5 mark.
2. Draw centrifuged and filtered diluting fluid to the 101 mark.
3. Shake in pipette rotor for 5 min.
4. Expel 4 drops and fill a standard counting chamber (both sides).
5. Allow to stand for 15 min. in closed petri dish kept moist with wet filter paper in top half.
6. Count platelets in finely ruled center area of each chamber. Platelets are bluish and must be distinguished from debris.

Counting technique: See Fig. 4-10.

Calculation: The counted space measures 1 × 1 × 0.1 mm.³. As two such spaces are counted, the platelets in a space of 0.2 mm.³ are enumerated. To obtain the platelets in 1 mm.³ multiply 5 × 200 (the dilution factor) or by 1000.

Diluting fluid:
1. Sodium citrate, 3.8 gm.
2. Neutral formaldehyde (40%), 0.2 ml.
3. Brilliant cresyl blue, 0.1 gm.
4. Distilled water, 100 ml.

Filter and centrifuge for 30 min. Keep stoppered in refrigerator and filter required amount before use.

Errors in method: This method is subject to the same sampling and technical errors as the red blood cell count. Since platelet agglutinates invalidate the count, all glassware must be kept clean so as not to induce clumping.

Platelet count by Coulter counter[45]: Coulter Electronics, Inc., issues a special platelet kit.

Condensed procedure:
1. Aspirate blood into plastic sedimentation tube.
2. Allow sedimentation to occur.
3. Cut tube at either the junction of the red cells and plasma or in the center of the red cell portion.
4. Count platelet suspension on the Coulter counter.
5. Correct count using coincidence and dilution chart and the factor due to excess platelet concentration and hematocrit.

Normal values: 150,000-450,000 platelets/mm.³ blood. For variations, see p. 154.

BLOOD SMEAR

Preparation of smear

SLIDE METHOD: Place a medium-sized drop of blood near one end of a clean slide. Use capillary or fresh venous blood free of any anticoagulant. Place spreader slide in front of drop at an angle of about 45 degrees and allow blood to spread in the angle between the slides. Then, just before the blood has spread quite to the edges, push spreader slide ahead of the drop of blood. Dry at once in air. Label smear. Stain with Wright stain.

Smears of the proper thickness will dry quickly and will appear yellow (not pink) when placed on a white paper. The more acute the angle between the slides and the more slowly the blood is spread, the thinner will be the smear.

COVER GLASS METHOD: Place a small drop of blood (or bone marrow) in the middle of a cover glass held between thumb and forefinger by adjacent corners. Place a second cover glass over the first so that they do not cover each other but so that the second cover glass is rotated 45 degrees on the first. The slides can now be handled by their free corners and pulled apart immediately after the drop of blood has spread between them. Air dry both slides and stain with Wright stain.

Anticoagulants distort white blood cells; therefore only fresh blood should be used for smears. For best results smears should be stained soon after they have dried.

SMEARS OF BUFFY COAT:

Concentration of leukocytes: When leukocytes are scarce (leukopenia, aleukemic leukemia), centrifuge 5-10 ml. defibrinated or heparinized blood and pipette off the plasma (with a little of the adjacent red cell layer) to a Wintrobe sedimentation tube. Centrifuge, discard the plasma, and pipette the leukocyte layer to a concave slide (watch glass or spot plate); prepare smears as for the differential count. Such a preparation is useful in searching for immature cells, for L.E. cells, or for tumor cells, but is not suitable for a differential count because of the uneven distribution of the cells.

It is important to point out that buffy coats in apparently healthy people contain some atypical mononuclear cells and frequently megakaryocytes (or their fragments), metamyelocytes, and myelocytes.[46]

The preparation is best when the blood is gently defibrinated (with a wooden applicator) before clotting has occurred (see p. 208).

Staining techniques

Wright stain:

Method: Make blood film from untreated blood and allow to air dry. Apply Wright stain for 3 min. as fixative, covering slides completely. Add buffer of about the same quantity as the stain and mix by blowing gently on the surface of the stain. Leave for 3-6 min.

Keep slide horizontal and float off scum with distilled water to prevent precipitate from sticking to the slide. Then wash stain off with distilled water until smear is pink and translucent and allow slide to dry by letting edge rest on a blotter. Remove the stain on the back of the slide by cleaning with moistened gauze. The slide may be covered with Permount.*

Reagents:

Buffer solution: Mix 27 ml. M/15 disodium phosphate solution and 73 ml. M/15 monopotassium phosphate solution (pH 6.4). Buffer tablets are commercially available.

Wright stain:

1. Powdered Wright stain (certified), 0.1 gm.
2. Methyl alcohol (acetone free), 60 ml.

Grind stain in mortar, using small portions of the alcohol at a time. Make sure that mortar is clean and dry. Let stand about a week before using, shaking it vigorously each day to promote solution.

Appearance of smear: A well-stained smear will appear pink macroscopically. Microscopically the red blood cells are pink and the white cell nuclei are blue. There should be **no precipitate.** If precipitate forms, it may be due to inadequate or incorrect washing, failure to float off the scum, a dirty slide, dust, or an overconcentrated stain.

Too blue a smear may be due to inadequate washing, too thick a film, overstaining, or excessive alkalinity of water, buffer, and/or stain.

If the smear is **too red,** the pH of the water, buffer, or stain is too acid.

Appearance of cells: Nuclei and basophilic cytoplasmic components are blue, neutrophilic granules are lilac, eosinophilic granules are orange, mast cell granules are deep blue-violet, nucleoli are usually blue-violet, red cells are pink, and cytoplasm of mature monocytes is pale gray-blue.

Giemsa stain:

Method: Fix smear in absolute methyl alcohol for 3-5 min. Wash and place in **diluted Giemsa stain** for 15-30 min. Wash and allow to dry.

---

*Fisher Scientific Co., New York, N. Y.

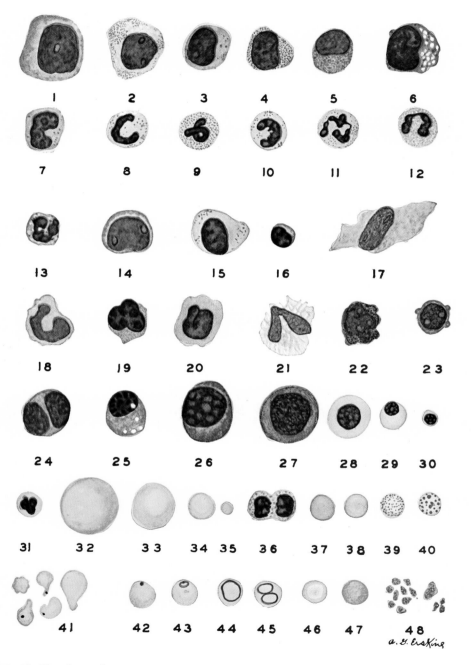

Plate 4. For legend see opposite page.

For intensive staining of material for Donovan bodies, spirochetes, etc., leave in the stain for 1-4 hr.

Reagents:

Dilute Giemsa stain: Dilute 1 ml. stock Giemsa stain with 10 ml. distilled water.

Stock Giemsa stain:

1. Giemsa stain powder, 3.8 gm.
2. Glycerin, 200 ml. at 60° C. for 2 hr.
3. Methyl alcohol (absolute), 312 ml.

A 1% solution of sodium carbonate instead of water intensifies the stain.

Appearance of cells: Similar to Wright stain.

Alkaline phosphatase stain[47]:

Method 1:

1. Make film of fresh blood and air dry.
2. Immerse slide in fixative for 30 sec. at 0° C.
3. Wash in running water for 10 sec.
4. Incubate in substrate mixture for 10 min. at room temperature.
5. Wash in running water for 10 sec.
6. Counterstain with Harris hematoxylin for 3-4 min.

7. Wash in running water for 10 sec. and air dry.
8. Mount.

Reagents:

1. Fixative solution:

   Formalin (36-39% formaldehyde), 10 ml.

   Absolute methyl alcohol, 90 ml.

   Store in freezing unit of refrigerator.

2. Propanediol stock solution (0.2M):

   2-Amino-2-methyl-1, 3-propanediol,* 10.5 gm.

   Distilled water to make 500 ml.

   Store in refrigerator.

3. Propanediol buffer (0.05M, pH 9.75):

   Stock solution propanediol (0.2M), 25 ml.

   Hydrochloric acid (0.1N), 5 ml.
   Distilled water to make 100 ml.

   Store in refrigerator.

_____

*Eastman Kodak Co., Rochester, N. Y.

Plate 4. Blood cells (Giemsa stain; scale 1 mm. = 1μ). (From Frankel and Reitman, editors: Gradwohl's clinical laboratory methods and diagnosis, St. Louis, 1963, The C. V. Mosby Co.)

1. Myeloblast
2. Promyelocyte
3. Neutrophilic myelocyte
4. Neutrophilic myelocyte
5. Eosinophilic myelocyte
6. Basophilic myelocyte
7. Metamyelocyte
8. Band granulocyte
9. Band granulocyte
10. Degenerated band granulocyte
11. Segmented neutrophil
12. Eosinophil
13. Basophil
14. Lymphoblast
15. Large lymphocyte
16. Small lymphocyte
17. Reticuloendothelial cell
18. Monocyte
19. Monocyte
20. Monocyte
21. Endothelial cell
22. Atypical promyelocyte
23. Micromyeloblast
24. Twin-nuclear cell
25. Plasma cell
26. Irritation cell
27. Rubricyte, PA type
28. Metarubricyte, PA type
29. Metarubricyte
30. Metarubricyte
31. Metarubricyte, with nucleus showing karyorrhexis
32. Megalocyte
33. Macrocyte
34. Erythrocyte
35. Microcyte
32-35. Example of anisocytosis
36. Erythroblast with mitotic nucleus
37. Faintly polychromatic erythrocyte
38. Polychromatophilic erythrocyte
39. Basophilic punctation, fine
40. Basophilic punctation, coarse
41. Poikilocytes
42. Marginal granule
43. Ring form of malarial parasite
44 and 45. Cabot rings
46. Erythrocyte showing achromia
47. Hyperchromic erythrocyte
48. Platelets

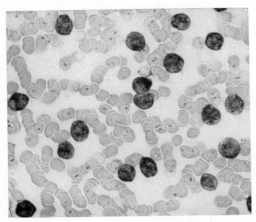

Fig. 4-11. Alkaline phosphatase–positive neutrophils.

Table 4-6

Grade 0	Colorless cytoplasm
Grade 1+	Pale brown cytoplasm; no granules
Grade 2+	Brown cytoplasm; occasional dark granules
Grade 3+	Dark granules
Grade 4+	Black granules

4. Substrate mixture (pH 9.5-9.6):

   Sodium alpha-naphthyl acid phosphate,* 35 mg.
   Fast blue RR,† 35 mg.
   Propanediol buffer (0.05M), 35 ml.

   Filter and use at once.

5. Meyer aqueous hematoxylin:

   Solution A:
   Hematein, 1 gm.
   Ethyl alcohol (90%), 50 ml.

   Incubate 24 hr. at 37° C.
   Solution B:
   Potassium aluminum sulfate, 50 gm.
   Distilled water to make 1 L.

   Mix A and B.
   Place in sunlight for 3-4 wk.

Method 2: A more rapid and easier method employing naphthol AS-MX phosphate concentrate and fast red-violet LB salt has been developed.‡

Interpretation[48]: The granules of segmented and band granulocytes, metamyelocytes, and myelocytes are phosphatase positive and stain from pale brown to black, allowing grading from 0-4+, ac-

cording to the number and color of the granules (Table 4-6).

In the normal blood smear most neutrophils are Grade 0; a few are Grade 1+ to Grade 2+. In infections, in myeloproliferative disorders, and in pregnancy the alkaline phosphatase content of the granules is increased. In acute and chronic myelogenous leukemia the alkaline phosphatase within the neutrophils is decreased.

Peroxidase stain:
Method 1:
1. Add 10 drops solution A to a dry blood smear.
2. After 1.5 min., add 5 drops solution B. Allow to stand for 3-4 min.
3. Wash thoroughly in tap water for 3-4 min.
4. Counterstain with Wright stain.
5. Solution A. Dissolve 0.3 gm. benzidine base in 99 ml. 95% ethyl alcohol. Add 1 ml. saturated aqueous solution of sodium nitroprusside.
6. Solution B. Add 0.3 ml. 3% hydrogen peroxide to 25 ml. distilled water. This solution must be made fresh.

Method 2—simplified myeloperoxidase stain using benzidine dihydrochloride (Kaplow)[49]: Benzidine base is carcinogenic and is difficult to obtain. Benzidine dihydrochloride is less dangerous to handle but its use necessitates a modification of the established method.

Technique: Fix blood or bone marrow slides in 10% formalin-ethanol. Wash for 15-30 sec. in running water and shake off excess water. Place wet slides in incubation mixture for 30 sec. Wash for 5-10 sec. in running water, dry, and examine. The preparation may be recounterstained in 1% aqueous cresyl violet acetate for 1 min. or in freshly prepared Giemsa stain for 10 min.

---

*Dajac Laboratories, Leominster, Mass.
†General Dyestuff Corp., Boston, Mass. (commercial preparation of diazonium salt of 4-benzoyl-2,5 methoxyaniline).
‡Bulletin No. 85, Sigma Chemical Co., St. Louis, Mo.

Reagents:

1. Formalin-ethanol (10%):

   Formaldehyde (37%), 10 ml.
   Ethyl alcohol (absolute), 90 ml.

2. Incubation mixture:

   Ethyl alcohol (30%), 100 ml.
   Benzidine dihydrochloride, 0.3 gm.
   Zinc sulfate ($ZnSO_4 \cdot 7H_2O$) (0.132M, 3.8% w/v), 1 ml.
   Sodium acetate ($[NaC_2H_3]_2 \cdot 3H_2O$), 1 gm.
   Hydrogen peroxide (3%), 0.7 ml.
   Sodium hydroxide (1N), 1.5 ml.
   Safranine O, 0.2 gm.

The reagents should be added in the order listed and mixed well after each addition. Final pH is 6.0 ± 0.05. The solution may be stored in a screw-capped Coplin jar and can be used over and over again for about 6 mo.

Interpretation: Peroxidase-positive cells (Fig. 4-12) contain yellowish green to bluish and brownish green granules, as seen in eosinophils, neutrophilic granulocytes beginning with the promyelocytes, basophils, and most monocytes.

Peroxidase-negative cells are lymphocytes, myeloblasts, plasma cells, reticulum cells, and some monocytes as well as megakaryocytes.

Heinz body stain: See p. 137.

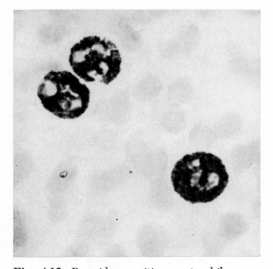

Fig. 4-12. Peroxidase-positive neutrophils.

Stain for siderocytes: See p. 138.

Supravital stain: Slides and cover slips must be washed with alcohol and dried with gauze. Use No. 0 cover slips.

Stock solution:

1. Neutral red, 0.2 gm., in 50 ml. absolute ethyl alcohol, redistilled
2. Janus green, 0.25 gm., in 50 ml. absolute ethyl alcohol, redistilled

Working solution:

1. Janus green, 0.25 ml.
2. Neutral red, 0.8 ml.
3. Absolute ethyl alcohol, 5 ml., redistilled

Method: Flame slides. Allow stain to cover slide. Wipe off edges. Tilt to dry. Put 1 small drop blood or bone marrow on cover slip, put cover slip onto slide (material side down), and seal with nail polish.

Examination of blood smear

Macroscopically, the smear should be pink. Microscopically, under low power, the distribution and staining characteristics of the cells can be judged. An area where the cells just touch each other should be chosen for examination with the oil-immersion lens. If the cells are too crowded, they appear too small, and if they are too widely spaced, they appear too large and hyperchromatic.

The following structures and their characteristics should be examined in a smear:

Red cells (erythrocytes): Study red cells and record the presence or absence of the following qualitative changes:

Size:
1. Normal: normocytes
2. Pathologic: microcytes, macrocytes (megalocytes), anisocytes

Shape:
1. Normal: normocytes
2. Pathologic: poikilocytes, spherocytes, ovalocytes, schistocytes, target cells, sickle cells, teardrop cells, acanthocytes, burr cells

Hemoglobin content (color):
1. Normal: normochromic
2. Pathologic: hypochromia, hyperchromia, polychromasia, anulocytes, basophilic stippling

Maturity:
1. Normal: normocytes
2. Pathologic: nucleated cells, basophilic stippling, reticulocytes (special stain only), Cabot rings and Howell-Jolly bodies, para-

sites, siderocytes (special stain only), crystals in red blood cells, rouleau formation

White cells (leukocytes): Make a differential count. While doing the differential count, study the white blood cells and note the following points:

Number:
1. Leukopenia (decreased)
2. Leukocytosis (increased)

Types and their distribution (leukemoid reactions, i.e., shifts):
1. Normal mature forms
2. Immature forms

Morphologic changes of cytoplasm, nuclei, and granules:
1. Cytoplasm: toxic granulation, toxic vacuolization
2. Granules: Alder's anomaly
3. Nucleus: hypersegmentation, giant forms, pyknotic forms, Pelger-Huët abnormality
4. Inclusions: Auer bodies, Döhle bodies, Hegglin inclusions, Chediak's syndrome

Platelets: State whether platelets are apparently normal, increased, or decreased in number. Note morphology (size and shape).

Differential leukocyte count (Schilling): The Schilling count is the percentile distribution of the various white blood cells. The percentage of each group is based on the total number of leukocytes counted, expressed in percent of 100 leukocytes.

Technique: Starting at the upper edge of the smear, move straight down to the lower edge, then move from left to right and proceed from the lower edge upward. Continue in the same manner until a minimum of 100 cells is classified.

Shift to the left: The increase of young cells in the peripheral blood is called a shift to the left. It is the result of bone marrow stimulation and leads to the appearance of an increased number of band granulocytes, metamyelocytes, and even myelocytes, so that a leukemia-like picture may be produced. If the cells show toxic granulation and other toxic changes, we speak of a degenerative shift as seen in severe infections. If there is no evidence of toxic damage, it is a regenerative shift as seen following hemorrhage.

Shift to the right: The hypersegmented polymorphs of pernicious anemia produce a shift to the right.

Absolute white cell count: This count expresses the absolute number of an individual cell type present in 1 mm.^{3} blood. It is calculated from the percentage distribution and from the total cell count/mm.^{3}.

Example:

Total leukocyte count = 6000
Segmented forms (relative number) = 50%
Absolute number of segmented forms:

$$6000 \times \frac{50}{100} = 3000$$

The relative and the absolute numbers of a given cell type do not express the same thing (Table 4-7). If the relative value of a given cell type is increased, it implies that this cell type is more numerous than normal, but it does not explain whether there is an actual increase in the number of cells or whether there is a decrease of other types of cells.

Examples:

1. Total white blood cell count: 8000 WBC/mm.^{3}
   Differential count:
   Segmented granulocytes, 45%   Absolute
   Lymphocytes, 55%   value of
   Band granulocytes, 2%   lymphocytes:
   Monocytes, 3%   4400
   Impression: Absolute and relative lymphocytosis
2. Total white blood cell count: 4000 WBC/mm.^{3}
   Differential count:
   Segmented granulocytes, 20%   Absolute
   Lymphocytes, 55%   value of
   Band granulocytes, 20%   lymphocytes:
   Monocytes, 5%   2200
   Impression: Relative lymphocytosis

MORPHOLOGY OF HEMATOPOIETIC CELLS

These descriptions of cells are as they appear when stained with Wright stain.

Origin and maturation of blood cells: Maturation is a continuous process and there are intermediate cell forms between the various stages that we accept as being indicative of a certain stage of development.

In general, as the cells of each series mature and become older, they decrease in size, the nuclei occupy relatively smaller portions of the cells and stain more deeply, nucleoli disappear, and the chromatin, at first granular or finely retic-

Table 4-7. Relative and absolute leukocyte values

	Relative value	*Absolute value*
Total leukocytes		6000 - 8000
Myelocytes	0	0
Metamyelocytes	0 - 1	15 - 50
Band granulocytes	2 - 5	150 - 400
Segmented granulocytes	54 - 62	5000 - 6000
Eosinophils	1 - 4	50 - 250
Basophils	0 - 1	15 - 50
Lymphocytes	22 - 30	150 - 300
Monocytes	4 - 8	300 - 650

ular, becomes dense and arranged into characteristic patterns. However, when division is very rapid (acute leukemia), the cells may not have time to regain their usual size before dividing again, and small cells may result (microblasts).

Stem cell (reticulum cell, hemohistioblast):

Size: 15-30μ in diameter; it is relatively small.

Nucleus: It is relatively small and oval with a finely reticular chromatin pattern, producing the appearance of red-violet irregular granules and strands and leaving only very small irregular pink areas of parachromatin. The long axis lies within the long axis of the cell. Blue, round, poorly delineated nucleoli can be found. They are 0-3 or 4 in number.

Cytoplasm: It is large in amount, pale to dark blue, and contains azurophilic granules.

Hemocytoblast:

Size: 10-20μ in diameter.

Nucleus: It is large, oval or round, pink-purple, and contains a fine chromatin network with small regular pink interstices. There is no chromatin clumping.

Erythropoiesis

Normal erythropoiesis occurs in the **bone marrow.** Under pathologic conditions (hemolytic anemias, bone marrow replacement by fibrous tissue, etc.) the call for blood is met by other reticuloendothelial organs, e.g., liver, spleen, etc., where **extramedullary hematopoiesis** leads to the formation of blood.

Normoblastic erythropoiesis takes place in health when an ample supply of the

building stones of red blood cells is available. If folic acid and/or vitamin B_{12} are missing, **megaloblastic erythropoiesis** will take over or occur side by side with normoblastic development.

Progressive maturation and aging are accompanied by a gradual decrease in the size of the cell and of the nucleus, with deeper staining of the chromatin, which becomes more homogeneous, and by the appearance of more hemoglobin in the cytoplasm, provided that iron is available. When there is a deficiency of iron, the cells mature but fail to acquire the normal amount of hemoglobin (hypochromic anemias).

Pronormoblast (rubriblast):

Size: 12-20μ in diameter.

Nucleus: It is large, round to oval, and contains 0-2 light bluish nucleoli. The chromatin forms a delicate network, giving the nucleus a reticular appearance and allowing only tiny dots of pink parachromatin to shine through the interstices. There is some clumping of chromatin, mainly around nucleoli.

Cytoplasm: There is a narrow rim of dark blue cytoplasm, less than seen in the myeloblast and more condensed than in the myeloblast or the promyeloblast. There may be a perinuclear halo.

Basophilic normoblast (prorubricyte):

Size: 10-16μ in diameter.

Nucleus: It is round or oval and smaller than the pronormoblastic nucleus. The chromatin is denser and coarser and the strands are thicker. Usually no nucleoli are seen. The parachromatin is arranged in irregular small pink dots.

Cytoplasm: There is a slightly wider

ring of deep blue cytoplasm than in the pronormoblast.

Polychromatophilic normoblast (rubricyte):

Size: 8-10μ in diameter.

Nucleus: It is small (smaller than in the basophilic normoblast) and has a thick membrane and coarse strands of chromatin condensed into masses in some areas. There is no nucleolus. The para-chromatin forms pink, small, irregular areas in the interstices.

Cytoplasm: As the nucleus is somewhat shrunken, there is a wider band of cytoplasm. It has a lilac (polychromatic) tint because of beginning hemoglobinization.

Orthochromic normoblast (metarubricyte):

Size: 7-10μ in diameter.

Nucleus: It is small, central, or eccen-

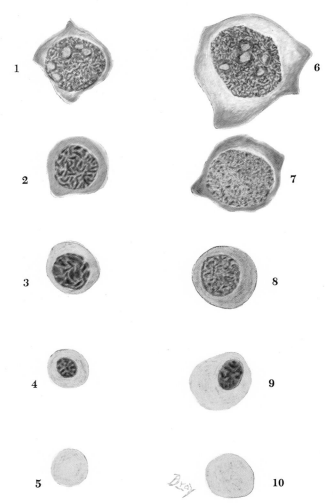

Plate 5. Red blood cell series.

From normal bone marrow
1. Rubriblast
2. Prorubricyte
3. Rubricyte
4. Metarubricyte
5. Erythrocyte

From bone marrow of pernicious anemia
6. Rubriblast, pernicious anemia type
7. Prorubricyte, pernicious anemia type
8. Rubricyte, pernicious anemia type
9. Metarubricyte, pernicious anemia type
10. Macrocyte

tric with condensed homogeneous structureless chromatin.

Cytoplasm: A wide rim of red cytoplasm surrounds the shrinking nucleus. The entire cell is somewhat smaller than the preceding one.

Nuclear degeneration: When the nucleus disappears atypically or incompletely, as it often does in pernicious anemia, myelocytic leukemia, and very severe anemias, it may leave a remnant of the nuclear membrane, forming a **Cabot ring,** or it may break up and leave small spheroidal pyknotic portions known as **Howell-Jolly bodies.**

VARIATIONS IN NORMOBLASTS:

Multinucleated normoblasts: Failure of cytoplasmic division leads to the formation of normoblasts with 2-4 or even more nuclei. Such cells may occur in pernicious anemias and in erythroleukemia. In erythroleukemia the nuclei contain nucleoli and the cytoplasm may vary from deep blue to lavender because of beginning hemoglobinization.

Small normoblasts: Unusually small cells may occur in iron-deficiency anemia and in erythroleukemia.

Erythrocyte:

Size: About 7.5μ in diameter and 2μ thick.

Nucleus: The cell is nonnucleated.

Cytoplasm: Biconcave orange cytoplasm that has a paler staining center occupying one third of the cell area.

MEGALOBLASTIC ERYTHROPOIESIS: Megaloblasts are not present in the normal bone marrow, their appearance being due to a deficiency in vitamin B_{12} and/or folic acid. They mature in a manner similar to the members of the normoblastic series, but each stage differs morphologically from its normoblastic counterpart. The differences lie in the size of the cell and nuclei as well as in the nuclear-cytoplasmic dissociation, implying that the nucleus and the cytoplasm do not mature in parallel but rather nuclear maturation lags behind cytoplasmic hemoglobinization. As the megaloblastic cells mature, these differences become more marked so that the diagnosis of megaloblastic erythropoiesis can be made by recognizing the orthochromic megaloblast. The cells of this series are either called various types of megaloblasts or are classified by their corresponding rubriblastic title with the suffix pernicious anemia (PA) type.

Promegaloblast (rubriblast, PA type):

Size: 20-30μ in diameter.

Nucleus: It is round or oval and larger than that of the corresponding normoblastic cell. The chromatin is arranged in small delicate masses and bands that produce an open, somewhat stippled appearing network surrounding prominent areas of pink parachromatin. Large pale nucleoli are seen surrounded by chromatin.

Cytoplasm: The cytoplasmic-nuclear ratio is greater than in the corresponding normoblast. The cytoplasm is basophilic and shows some purple mottling.

Basophilic megaloblast (prorubricyte, PA type):

Size: 18-25μ in diameter.

Nucleus: It is round or oval in size and the chromatin pattern is very similar to that of the promegaloblastic nucleus. Nucleoli are difficult to see or may be absent.

Cytoplasm: The cytoplasmic ring is wider than in the promegaloblast. It is basophilic and shows some purple mottling.

Polychromatophilic megaloblast (rubricyte, PA type):

Size: 16-20μ in diameter.

Nucleus: The coarse chromatin network with irregular pink chromatin is similar to the pattern of the basophilic megaloblastic nucleus. The nucleus is usually eccentric and the nucleoli are difficult to see or absent.

Cytoplasm: There is a large, ovoid area of lilac to pink-gray cytoplasm.

Orthochromic megaloblast (metarubricyte, PA type):

Size: 12-15μ in diameter.

Nucleus: The chromatin is condensed and devoid of parachromatin and of nucleoli. The nucleus is usually eccentric.

Cytoplasm: It is red because of hemoglobinization. The cytoplasmic-nuclear ratio greatly exceeds that of orthochromic normoblasts.

Megalocyte:

Size: 9-12μ in diameter.

Nucleus: None present.

Cytoplasm: Dark red because it lacks the central area of clearing characteristic of the normal erythrocyte. Megalocytes of PA type are characteristically ovoid or pear shaped.

Variation of erythrocytes in stained smear

VARIATION IN SIZE: The normal range includes a few cells as small as 6μ in diameter and a few as large as 9μ in diameter.

Anisocytosis: Various sizes of cells are present. On the basis of their diameters, cells are divided into macrocytes, megalocytes, and microcytes.

Macrocytes: Cells are larger than 9μ in diameter. They may be due to B_{12} or folic acid deficiency or they may be young red cells that can be stained for reticulocytes. They are found in megaloblastic anemias, cirrhosis, and hemolytic anemias (Fig. 4-18).

Megalocytes: Cells measure 12-16μ in diameter and are usually due to folic acid or B_{12} deficiency.

Microcytes: Cells measure less than 6μ in diameter. They are due to deficiency of iron or other necessary building material.

VARIATION IN STAINING:

Anulocytes: They are thin cells with low hemoglobin which is represented only by a thin stained ring surrounding a large central space (Fig. 4-13).

Hyperchromasia: The hemoglobin content of the individual cell, which is thicker than normal, is high. The entire cell stains deep pink, lacking the usual

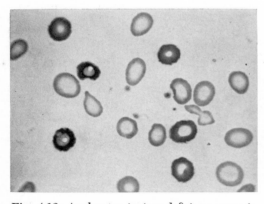

Fig. 4-13. Anulocytes in iron-deficiency anemia.

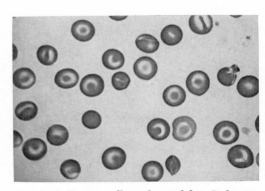

Fig. 4-14. Target cells in hemoglobin-C disease.

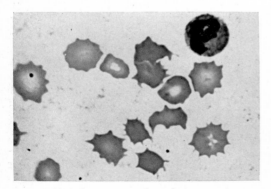

Fig. 4-15. Pyknocytes in hemolytic anemia.

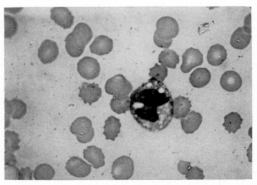

Fig. 4-16. Burr cells in hemolytic anemia.

central pallor. Spherocytes and megalocytes are hyperchromic cells (Fig. 4-21).

Hypochromasia: When hemoglobin is greatly decreased, the central pale area increases in size and becomes more prominent (see discussion of anulocytes).

Polychromasia: When young erythrocytes appear in the peripheral blood, they stain bluish pink. They are usually larger than normal cells, and when stained with methylene blue, they are seen to be reticulocytes. They have the same significance as reticulocytes and indicate active blood regeneration. These younger cells appear to be more subject to injury than the more mature ones and often show fine or coarse blue-staining granules (basophilic stippling or punctate polychromatophilia). They appear frequently in severe anemias and in lead poisoning (Fig. 4-22).

Target cells (leptocytes[50]**):** They have a hemoglobin-free, clear zone between the well-stained center and the stained periphery (Fig. 4-14). An occasional target cell may be found in the normal smear. They are frequently seen in obstructive jaundice, in hypochromic anemia, in sickle cell anemia, in Cooley's anemia, and after splenectomy. The target cells are thinner than normal erythrocytes and are more resistant to hypotonic salt solution (Fig. 4-14).

VARIATION IN SHAPE: The normal erythrocytes are uniform in shape, appearing as circular disks in fixed smears.

Acanthocyte[51]**:** It is a malformed erythrocyte that is somewhat similar to a pyknocyte (Fig. 4-15). It is shrunken, irregular in outline, and has thorny projections. It is found in thrombotic microangiopathy and in some congenital anomalies.

Burr cells[52-53]**:** Burr cells, with one or more spiny projections, are found in uremia, carcinoma of the stomach, and bleeding peptic ulcer. They are to be distinguished from crenated cells which appear in larger numbers per field and have smaller, more numerous, and more uniform projections (Fig. 4-16). Crenated cells are artifacts due to drying of an inadequate blood smear.

Elliptocytes: Oval cells are found in certain normal individuals as an inherited trait (ovalocytosis or elliptocytosis) and usually have no relation to anemia or other disease (Fig. 4-17). Rarely are they associated with hemolytic anemia. Oval macrocytes are characteristic of pernicious anemia (Fig. 4-18).

Poikilocytes: The cells assume abnormal and often bizarre shapes. Pear-shaped, raquet-shaped, or pessary-shaped cells can be seen (Fig. 4-19). These changes are characteristically found in severe hemolytic anemias.

Sickle cells: The tendency of the red cells to be sickle shaped (sicklemia, drepanocytosis) is an inherited trait found in about 7% of the Negro population and probably confined to that race (Fig. 4-20). About 1 out of 15 persons having this trait develops a severe hemolytic anemia (sickle cell anemia)—the homozygous form. The heterozygous form, which usually is not accompanied by anemia, is called sickle cell trait. The hemoglobin of sickle cell trait is a mixture of normal adult hemoglobin (A) and sickle cell hemoglobin (S); that of sickle cell anemia is sickle cell hemoglobin only (see p. 174).

Spherocytes: Small spheroidal cells (Fig. 4-21) are characteristic of congenital spherocytosis but are also seen in acquired hemolytic anemias, in some hemoglobinopathies, and in ABO erythroblastosis. They have a smaller than normal diameter and lack the normally present central area of clearing. They contain a normal amount of hemoglobin.

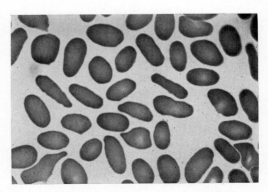

Fig. 4-17. Elliptocytes in congenital elliptocytosis.

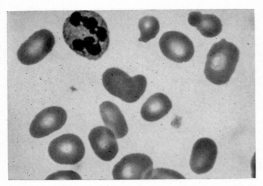

Fig. 4-18. Oval macrocytes and hypersegmented polymorph in pernicious anemia.

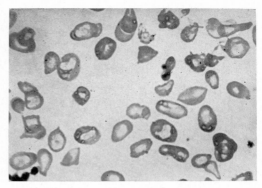

Fig. 4-19. Poikilocytes in thalassemia major.

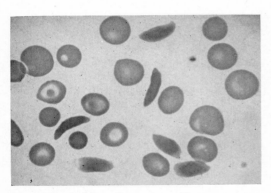

Fig. 4-20. Sickle cells, target cells, macrocytes, and spherocytes in sickle cell anemia.

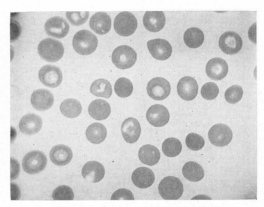

Fig. 4-21. Spherocytes in congenital spherocytosis.

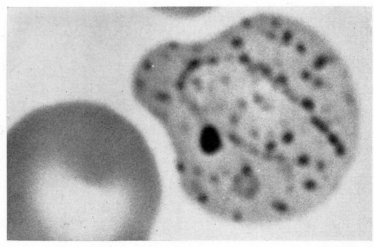

Fig. 4-22. Basophilic stippling, Cabot ring, diffuse basophilia, and Howell-Jolly body. (Courtesy Dr. L. W. Diggs.)

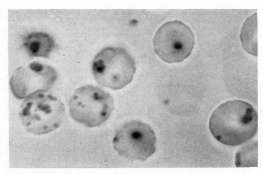

Fig. 4-23. Heinz bodies in normal blood (fewer than 5 Heinz bodies/RBC). (Courtesy Dr. L. W. Diggs.)

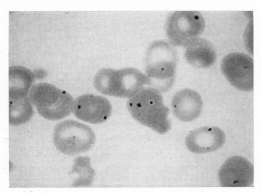

Fig. 4-24. Siderocytes in sideroachrestic anemia. (Courtesy V. Minnich.)

The globoid shape renders them prehemolytic so that the osmotic fragility test reveals increased fragility (Fig. 4-21).

ERYTHROCYTIC INCLUSIONS[54]:

Basophilic stippling: Basophilic stippling (Fig. 4-22) is the name given to basophilic granules appearing in red blood cells in cases of disturbed erythropoiesis, as seen in lead poisoning and severe anemias.

Cabot rings: They are purple, thin, small rings within erythrocytes. They are artifacts (Fig. 4-22).

Heinz bodies: They do not stain with Wright stain but can be seen by phase microscopy in the wet preparation. When they are stained with cresyl violet, the light microscope reveals purple, round, oval, or irregular granules varying in size from 1-2μ (Fig. 4-23). There may be one

or several, usually peripherally distributed. They occur in primaquine-sensitive type of drug-induced hemolytic anemia and are also seen in thalassemia and after splenectomy. The hemolytic effect was first noted in Negroes following the administration of primaquine for the treatment of malaria. The erythrocytes, hemolyzed by drugs, which normally have no action on red blood cells, have a genetically determined congenital deficiency of glucose-6-phosphate dehydrogenase that leads to abnormal oxidation of glucose and to failure to reduce oxidized glutathione. Reduced glutathione is necessary for the protection of hemoglobin from the toxic action of drugs. The production of Heinz bodies is associated with drug sensitivity and methemoglobin formation.[20] This drug sensitivity can be diagnosed by determination of the glucose-6-phosphate dehydrogenase contents of the red blood cells. Heinz body anemias have been described in premature and full-term newborn infants.[28]

Staining technique:
1. Mix equal parts of 1% crystal violet in normal saline solution and of oxalated blood in a test tube.
2. Incubate for 15 min.
3. Place 1 drop of the mixture on a cover slide and turn it over onto a microscope slide, allowing the liquid to spread into a thin film.
4. Blot the excess and rim the preparation with nail polish.

Howell-Jolly bodies: Howell-Jolly bodies are chromatin-rests that stain blue and are often seen together with nuclear remnants as evidence of rapid blood regeneration, which also leads to the production of Cabot rings (Fig. 4-22).

Malaria pigment: Malaria produces two kinds of granules of denatured hemoglobin, Schüffner's dots *(P. vivax)* and Maurer's dots *(P. falciparum)*. The latter are coarse and dark (see p. 497).

Siderocytes,[55] **Pappenheimer bodies,**[56, 57] **and sideroblasts:**

Siderocytes: Iron-containing granules that give the Prussian blue reaction can be demonstrated in some erythrocytes (siderocytes). With Wright stain the granules appear bluish purple (Fig. 4-

24). They are not visible in unstained blood, are not related to the granules in reticulocytes or in punctate basophilia, and are not related to Howell-Jolly bodies. The granules may be extruded into the plasma.[31] Normally the number of siderocytes is small (0.5-3.0%), but it increases in hemolytic types of anemia, following phenylhydrazine treatment of polycythemia vera, and after splenectomy. In the treatment of pernicious anemia the siderocytes (8-14%) decrease in number more rapidly than the reticulocytes increase. They appear whenever there is a defect in hemoglobin formation and indicate abnormal iron utilization.

Heilmeyer described a group of primary refractory anemias which he called sideroblastic or siderachrestic anemias that are characterized by defective iron utilization and by the appearance of numerous siderocytes and sideroblasts.

Sideroblasts: They are normoblasts (bone marrow) that show stainable iron granules which may vary from fine dust-like particles to coarse, irregular deposits. They occur in the same conditions in which siderocytes are found.

Ringed sideroblasts: Stainable iron in the form of very fine particles surrounds the entire nucleus of normoblasts. They are found in pernicious anemia, in lead poisoning, after treatment with antimetabolites, and in rare primary anemias such as idiopathic sideroblastic anemia (acquired) and its hereditary form.

In the bone marrow the number of sideroblasts is dependent on the serum iron level. If the serum iron level is normal, 20-40% can be found. If the iron level rises, the number of sideroblasts increases, as in hemolytic anemias, pernicious anemia, and hemochromatosis. It may reach the level of 70%. In iron deficiency the sideroblasts disappear. Their absence is a reliable criterion of **iron-deficiency** anemia.

Iron stain:

Technique: Allow blood or bone marrow smears to dry and cover with a freshly prepared solution of Prussian blue reagent for 30 min.

The water and all glassware must be iron free.

Prussian blue reagent:

1. Potassium ferrocyanide, 4 gm.
2. Distilled water, 20 ml.

Add concentrated hydrochloric acid until a white precipitate is formed, filter reagent, and stain for 30 min. Counterstain after washing with dilute safranine for 2-3 sec.

Interpretation: The granules stain blue. The counterstain is red.

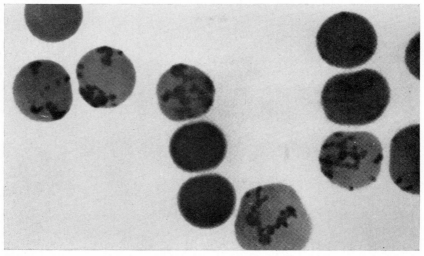

Fig. 4-25. Reticulocytes. (From Merker: Zyto- und Histochemie der Hämatologie, Berlin, 1963, Springer-Verlag.)

Reticulocytes: Reticulocytes (Fig. 4-25) are young red blood cells, some of which appear as macrocytic polychromatic cells (gray-blue) on smears stained with Wright stain, and if stained with supravital dyes, they exhibit a blue-staining reticulum. The latter can be graded into four stages because it varies in appearance from a coarse network to finest dots. In younger reticulocytes the reticulum is coarser, more filamentous, and plentiful. In older reticulocytes the reticulum may be replaced by a single dot. The reticulum is made of ribonucleic acid, and on electron microscopy it is seen to have a mitochondrial pattern. If marrow reticulocytes are released into peripheral blood, they often contain nuclear remnants in addition to a heavy reticulum.

Variation in number of reticulocytes:

Increase: Reticulocytes are increased after hemorrhage, with a peak on the fifth to the tenth day, and after splenectomy.

A very marked increase occurs in hemolytic anemias (congenital spherocytosis, sickle cell anemia, erythroblastosis).

After specific treatment of anemias, the increase may be used as an index of the effectiveness of the treatment and as a therapeutic diagnostic test. After adequate doses of iron in iron-deficiency anemia, the rise in reticulocytes may exceed 15-20% (Fig. 4-26), and in the treatment of pernicious anemia with B_{12}, the increase of reticulocytes is usually well correlated with the therapeutic response (Fig. 4-27). The increase is delayed by transfusions.

Decrease: Reticulocytes are decreased when the bone marrow becomes depressed from toxic injury (irradiation, chronic infection), and they are very scarce in aplastic anemia. In pernicious anemia in relapse, reticulocytes are decreased.

Staining of reticulocytes:

Technique: Mix 1 drop of **new methylene blue N** staining solution with 1 drop fresh or oxalated blood in a test tube, mix, and allow to stand for 10 min. Or first draw the stain (filtered) to mark 1 and then the blood to the same mark. Draw both into the pipette bulb, mix in a white blood cell diluting pipette and let stand 10 min.

Whichever method is used, mix again and make thin smears that are allowed to air dry. The cells must be evenly distributed and should not be crenated.

Stain:

1. New methylene blue N,* 0.5 gm.
2. Potassium oxalate, 1.6 gm.
3. Distilled water, 100 ml.

Let stand several days and filter. It keeps well. Filter before use.

Reticulocyte count: With the oil-immersion lens, count the number of reticulated red cells per thousand red cells and express the result in percentage, i.e., /100 RBC. All cells that contain a blue-staining reticulum or even just a fragment or granule of it are counted as reticulocytes. The reticulum of young cells is heavy, while older cells may only show a single small granule.

It is at times more meaningful to express reticulocyte response as the number of reticulocytes/mm.[3] of whole blood rather than as percent of circulating red blood cells.

Normal values and significance: The normal value for adults is under 2%

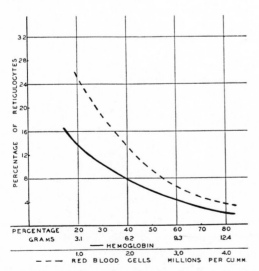

Fig. 4-26. The expected reticulocyte rise in iron-deficiency anemia following administration of iron, showing the relation of the response to hemoglobin and red cell levels. (From Heath: Arch. Intern. Med. **51**:459, 1933.)

*Burrell Corp., Pittsburgh, Pa.

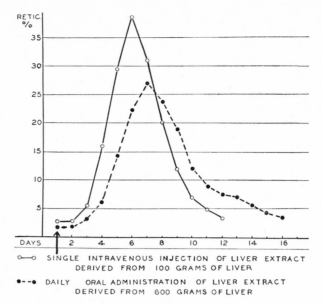

Fig. 4-27. Average reticulocyte response in pernicious anemia to liver extract by single injection (13 cases) and by uniform oral daily doses (20 cases). Average red cell count 1.2 million/mm.³. (From Minot: Trans. Ass. Amer. Physicians **49**:287, 1934.)

(usually 0.1-0.8%); for children, 0.5-4%; for infants, 2-5%.

Absolute count: The normal values are 20,000-60,000/mm.³.

The number of reticulocytes is a good index of the erythropoietic activity of the bone marrow.

White blood cell

There are three series (types) of leukocytes: myelocytic (granulocytic), lymphocytic, and monocytic. The origin of these cells has been mentioned in the discussion of the origin of blood cells.

Myeloid (granulocytic) series

The cells of this series develop in the bone marrow.

Stem cell (reticulum cell, hemohistioblast): For description see p. 131.

Myeloblast:

Size: 15-20μ in diameter.

Nucleus: The nucleus, which occupies more than half the cell, is pale with an indistinct outline and contains several nucleoli with indistinct margins. The chromatin is finely granular. There is a small amount of pink parachromatin.

Cytoplasm: The cytoplasm is nongran-

ular and stains deep blue and is lighter next to the nucleus.

Auer body: The cytoplasm of a few myeloblasts may contain one or more rods that stain red and are known as Auer bodies. These may also be found in monoblasts but never in lymphoblasts. When present, they are helpful in the diagnosis of acute leukemias.

Promyelocyte:

Size: 14-25μ in diameter.

Nucleus: The nucleus may be round, oval, or lobulated, the chromatin is somewhat coarser, and the nucleoli are less well defined.

Cytoplasm: The promyelocyte is larger than the myeloblast because of the relatively larger amount of bluish cytoplasm, which lacks the perinuclear clearing of the myeloblast. A few coarse granules may be present in the cytoplasm or over the nucleus. They may be neutrophilic, basophilic, eosinophilic, or azurophilic.

As the promyelocyte matures, it becomes smaller, the nucleoli disappears, the cytoplasm loses its basophilia and the azurophilic granules. When the nucleus loses the nucleoli, the cytoplasm develops characteristic granules (neutrophilic, eosinophilic, basophilic), and the cell becomes a **myelocyte.** Generally, most of the myelocytes acquire neutrophilic granules and become neutrophilic myelocytes which, becoming older, are the polymorphonuclear granulocytes of normal blood. In like manner the eosinophils and the basophils are formed from the eosinophilic and the basophilic myelocytes.

Myelocyte:

Size: 15-18μ in diameter.

Nucleus: The myelocyte has a round eccentric nucleus with coarse chromatin, and the nucleoli are absent. There is a small amount of pale blue parachromatin.

Cytoplasm: The cytoplasm is light blue to pink and may contain azurophilic, neutrophilic, eosinophilic, or basophilic granules which are coarse in the younger cell and become finer as the cell matures.

As the cells become older, they become smaller (12-16μ in diameter), the cytoplasm appears more crowded with granules, and the nucleus stains more deeply and becomes first indented and then lobulated. When the indentation is half the diameter of the nucleus, the cell is known as a **metamyelocyte.**

Metamyelocyte:

Size: 12-16μ in diameter.

Nucleus: The chromatin in the nucleus tends to become condensed into irregular thick and thin areas characteristic of the older forms. The nucleus is central or eccentric and slightly indented. The nuclear membrane is thick and heavy.

Cytoplasm: The cytoplasm is abundant, pale or pink, and contains numerous specific granules (neutrophilic, eosinophilic, basophilic).

Band granulocyte:

Size: 10-15μ in diameter.

Nucleus: The nucleus becomes elongated and rod shaped (stab, staff), often bent in the shape of the letter C, E, U, V, S, or W. It is not segmented. The chromatin is thick, coarse, and contains a small amount of pale blue parachromatin.

Cytoplasm: It contains specific granules.

Segmented granulocyte:

Size: 10-15μ in diameter.

Nucleus: It is central or eccentric, with heavy, thick chromatin masses and a small amount of parachromatin. It is divided into several (3-4) lobes connected to each other by delicate chromatin bridges.

Cytoplasm: It is abundant, slightly eosinophilic or colorless, and contains specific granules. The basophilic granules may overlie the nucleus.

Sex difference in nuclei: A sex difference has been noted in the pattern of the nucleus of the mature neutrophil[58, 59] and eosinophil.[59] In the female about 1 in 38-60 segmented neutrophils will have a solid nuclear appendage shaped like a **drumstick** attached by its narrow segment to one of the main lobes. This structure has not been found in the blood of the male. The irregular tags, clubs, and pale racquet bodies sometimes found extending from the nuclear lobes in blood from males must be distinguished from the typical drumstick appendage.

Moore and Barr[60] reported a sex difference in most somatic cells, the **sex chromatin** being planoconvex in shape and situated adjacent to the inner surface of the nuclear membrane.

In man there are 46 chromosomes (Fig. 4-28). They consist of 22 pairs of **autosomes** and 2 **sex chromosomes.** All chromosomes are diploid, with the exception of the chromosomes of the mature germ cell which are haploid.

Sex chromosomes: The female cell (Fig. 4-29) is characterized by a pair of

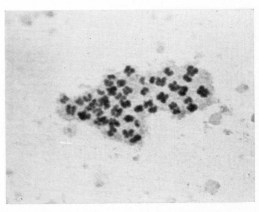

Fig. 4-28. Chromosomes in white cell of culture.

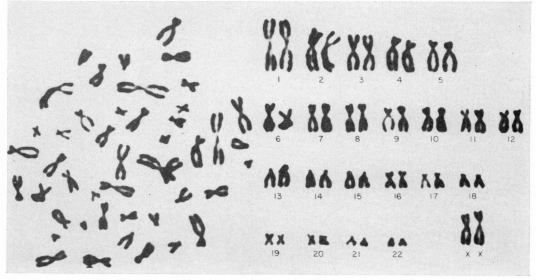

Fig. 4-29. Human karyotype (female).

like (XX) sex chromosomes, whereas the male cell has a pair of unlike (XY) sex chromosomes. The chromatin bodies just described represent the second X chromosome and are therefore not seen in the male cells. The recognition of the sex chromatin within the cell is helpful in the investigation of conditions in which the chromosomal sex differs from the anatomic sex. These conditions are (1) gonadal dysgenesis (Turner's and Klinefelter's syndromes), (2) true hermaphroditism, and (3) superfemale.

Turner's syndrome is due to ovarian agenesis or dysgenesis, whereas **Klinefelter's syndrome** is due to testicular agenesis or dysgenesis. Both conditions are associated with physical abnormalities as well as with sterility. The chromatin pattern in Turner's syndrome is XO, whereas in Klinefelter's syndrome it is XXY.

In true **hermaphroditism,** in which the sex glands contain components of both ovary and testis, the chromosomal sex pattern is a mixture of XX and XY.

The chromosomal pattern of the superfemale is XXX.

Methods of nuclear sexing: The methods of nuclear sexing include **skin biopsy, buccal smear,** and **peripheral blood smear.**

The tissue technique employs the usual hematoxylin-eosin stain. The peripheral blood smear is satisfactory when stained with Wright stain.

The Papanicolaou technique can be employed to stain buccal or vaginal smears. Best results are obtained with 2% orcein–acetic acid stain.

Orcein–acetic acid stain:

Technique: The slides are rapidly fixed in either 95% alcohol or equal parts of ether and absolute ethyl alcohol. After fixation the procedure is as follows.

Procedure:

1. Run slide through 50% ethyl alcohol (ROH) (5 dips) and distilled water (5 dips).
2. Place slide in aceto-orcein stock stain for 5 min.
3. Wash for 10 sec. with distilled water in gentle wash-bottle stream.
4. Dehydrate in 50, 70, 80, and 95% ROH (5 dips each).
5. Stain in fast green stock stain for 1 min.
6. Wash in 95, 100, and 100% ROH-xylene (5 dips).
7. Place in xylene for 5 min.
8. Mount.

Reagents:

Aceto-orcein stock:

1. Orcein, 1 gm.
2. Glacial acetic acid, 45 ml.

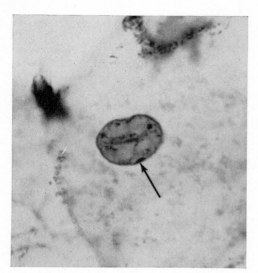

Fig. 4-30. Sex chromosome in epithelial cell.

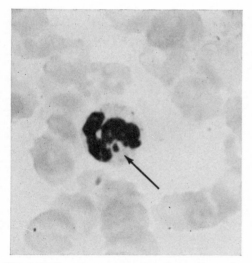

Fig. 4-31. Sex chromosome in polymorphonuclear leukocytes.

3. Distilled water, 55 ml.

Heat acid on hot plate to 80°-85° C. Be sure to use asbestos pad. Add orcein, shaking rapidly or using a mechanical stirring rod. Gradually add this solution to the distilled water (room temperature), stirring constantly. Stopper flask and bathe in cold running water, shaking to cool solution. Filter (No. 1 filter paper) and store in brown Coplin jar with screw top. Stain improves with age.

Fast green stock:
1. Fast green, 0.03 gm.
2. 95% ROH, 100 ml.

Add fast green stain to the alcohol and stir to dissolve.

Leukocyte culture technique: Modifications of cell culture technique allow the culture of blood or bone marrow and analysis of human chromosomes at metaphase. Abnormal **karyotypes** have been described in the following **hematologic conditions:** hemophilia, leukemia, Gaucher's disease, and irradiation effect.

A commercially prepared kit* is available which contains a basic tissue culture medium, TC-199, with phytohemagglutinin, antibiotics, and serum added. Detailed directions are contained in the kit. Methods are described in the books by Yunis,[61] and by Eggen.[62]

Outline of technique: The patient is requested to fast for 3-4 hr. Venous blood (10 ml.) is obtained in a sterile heparinized syringe. The needle is then capped and the syringe is inverted and allowed to stand at room temperature for 3 hr. until the plasma-leukocyte layer separates. This layer is then added to the culture medium. The culture is incubated at 37° C. for 72 hr. and at the end of this period the mitoses are arrested in the metaphase by the addition of colchicine. The culture is then reincubated for an additional 6 hr. at 37° C. Following this it is centrifuged in a conical centrifuge tube for 10 min. at 800 rpm. The supernatant is discarded and the separated cells are washed in warm Hanks solution.* To produce swelling of the cells, they are incubated for another 10 min. at 37° C. in a small amount of supernatant rendered hypotonic by the addition of warm water. The leukocytes are then separated by centrifugation and fixed by the addition of a freshly prepared mixture of 1 part acetic acid and 3 parts methanol. After 30 min. of fixation and short centrifugation, 1 drop of sediment is deposited on a clean refrigerated microscope slide which is then momentarily flamed and air dried. Several slides are prepared. They are stained with dilute Giemsa stain and

---

*Difco Laboratories, Detroit, Mich.

examined under the microscope. The cells that show well-isolated and defined chromosomes are photographed. The microphotographs are then enlarged, printed on paper, and the chromosomes are cut out and arranged into a karyotype pattern.

Each chromosome is characterized by its overall length, by the length of its arms, and by the position of its centromere. Each chromosome has an identical mate within the nucleus, with exception of the two sex chromosomes in the male cell, which are not identical.

PATHOLOGIC FORMS OF SEGMENTED POLY-MORPHS:

Alder's anomaly or Reilly bodies: Alder's anomaly is a rare hereditary anomaly characterized by coarse, dark, azurophilic granules in the cytoplasm of white cells, especially the polymorphs. Patients with **gargoylism** show similar granules in their leukocytes, which are often referred to as Reilly bodies.

Basket cell: The remnants of the degenerated nucleus appear as a loosely woven network.

Chediak-Higashi syndrome[63]: See Fig. 4-32. The neutrophils show pale large inclusions resembling Döhle bodies. The granules are prominent, more pronounced than in toxic granulation. The lymphocytes may contain deep red granules. The monocytes, basophils, and platelets show no abnormality. The anomaly of the neutrophils is part of a hereditary syndrome that includes albinism, abnormal skin pigmentation, repeated infections, hepatosplenomegaly, and ultimately leads to anemia, neutropenia, thrombocytopenia, and early death.

Döhle or Amato bodies[64]: With Wright stain they are seen as blue-staining cytoplasmic inclusions. They are round, oval, or irregular and lie close to the periphery of the cell. They vary from the size of cocci to about 2μ in diameter (Fig. 4-33). They are found in severe infections, Chediak's syndrome, May-Hegglin anomaly, and normal pregnancy.

Hypersegmented forms: Large forms with many nuclear lobules (6-10) and with large reddish granules are often found in pernicious anemia. Similar cells may also occur as a congenital abnormality or in infections.

Jordans' anomaly[65]: Jordans described fat-containing vacuoles in granulocytes of patients with progressive muscular dystrophy.

Malignancy associated changes (MAC): Thin and threadlike nuclear excrescences

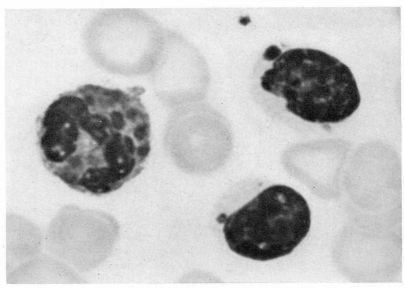

Fig. 4-32. Chediak-Higashi syndrome (peripheral blood). (Courtesy Dr. L. W. Diggs.)

have been reported in granulocytes of patients with carcinoma.[66]

May-Hegglin anomaly[67]: The cytoplasm of neutrophils may show pathologic changes apart from the previously mentioned toxic granulation and Döhle bodies. Hegglin described inclusions in the polymorphonuclear cells that are similar to Döhle bodies but are also found in monocytes and lymphocytes. Hegglin inclusions are associated with abnormal **giant platelets**. Döhle bodies are similar to the inclusions found in Chediak's syndrome. Hegglin's anomaly is of no clinical significance.

Pelger-Huët anomaly: It is characterized by marked condensation of nuclear chromatin in all white cells and by decreased lobulation of the neutrophils so that most polymorphs are bilobed or band forms (Fig. 4-34). The abnormality is either congenital or acquired (pseudo Pelger-Huët anomaly).

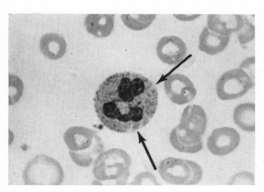

Fig. 4-33. Döhle bodies.

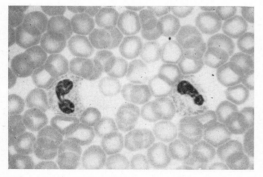

Fig. 4-34. Pelger-Huët anomaly, congenital. (Courtesy V. Minnich.)

The Pelger-Huët anomaly is important for two reasons: First, it should not be mistaken for a severe shift to the left. Second, the acquired form is seen in such blood diseases as chronic myelogenous leukemia, acute leukemia, myeloid metaplasia, and agranulocytosis. In the acquired form the cell may contain Döhle bodies.

Pyknotic cell: The nucleus becomes smaller and denser so that the chromatin bridges between the nuclear segments disappear, leaving several small balls of dense chromatin.

Snapper-Scheid bodies: They are inclusions that appear in the cytoplasm of myeloma and plasma cells after therapy with amidine drugs.

Smudge cell: When any type of leukocyte becomes markedly degenerated, the cytoplasm may disappear, leaving a naked nucleus that stains poorly and somewhat reddish and shows no characteristic chromatin pattern. Smudge cells are found only rarely in normal blood and in chronic myelocytic leukemia, but in large numbers in acute myeloblastic and lymphoblastic leukemia and chronic lymphatic leukemia. They may be artifacts.

Toxic granulation: In severe infections and toxic states, most marked in pneumonia and septicemia, the cytoplasm contains large dark-staining granules (toxic granules) and often vacuoles. When toxic granulation is marked, peroxidase-positive granules are scarce or absent (Fig. 4-35).

VARIATION IN NUMBER OF POLYMORPHONUCLEAR LEUKOCYTES:

Increase—leukocytosis:

Physiologic leukocytosis: It is seen in the first few days of life, in the last month of pregnancy, at parturition, after prolonged cold baths, and after sunlight (ultraviolet rays).

Pathologic leukocytosis: Pathologically, the most frequent leukocytosis is seen in acute pyogenic infections in which the degree depends upon the severity of the infection and the patient's resistance. The total number parallels the patient's ability to react, whereas the degree of shift toward the younger cells (in the Schilling differential count) is more in proportion to the severity of the infection.

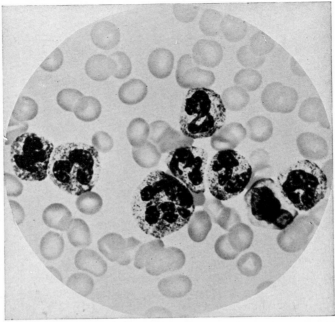

Fig. 4-35. Acute lobar pneumonia. Toxic granules in all segmented and nonsegmented poly-morphonuclear neutrophils. Note anisocytosis of the leukocytes and also large polymorpho-nuclear neutrophils. (Jenner-Giemsa stain.) (From Kugel and Rosenthal: Amer. J. Med. Sci. **183:**657, 1932.)

Other causes of leukocytosis are marked hemorrhage (with peak at 10 hr. and lasting 3-4 days), trauma or tissue injury (postoperative, with peak at about 6 hr. and lasting 4-5 days), malignant disease, especially of the gastrointestinal tract, liver, and bone (metastasis), toxins (uremia, coma, eclampsia), drugs (ether, chloroform, quinine, pentnucleotide), serum sickness, circulatory diseases (coronary thrombosis, dehydration), tissue necrosis (infarct, gangrene), myeloproliferative disorders, and leukemia.

Decrease—leukopenia: Leukopenia occurs during the course of or following severe infections that depress the bone marrow, virus infections, or hypersplenism. Bone marrow depression is produced by drugs, antimetabolites, benzene, heavy metals, radiation, etc. It also occurs in the course of blood diseases: agranulocytosis, acute leukemias, pernicious anemia, aplastic anemias, bone marrow failure, reticuloendothelioses, multiple myeloma, etc.

EOSINOPHILS:

Maturation of eosinophils: These cells of the myelocytic series acquire in the myelocyte stage large red-staining granules which are uniform in size. The immature granules are often black to gray. The mature granules are large and seldom overlap the nucleus. The eosinophilic cells are fragile and easily release their granules.

Eosinophils mature in the same manner as the neutrophils, but most of the eosinophils in the normal blood contain nuclei with only two lobular masses. In the differential count all the eosinophils are placed in one group, except the eosinophilic myelocytes which are counted separately since they have a greater significance, being found only in leukemia or leukemoid blood pictures in the peripheral blood.

Mature eosinophil:

Size: 16μ in diameter.

Nucleus: It is bilobed and contains dense chromatin masses.

Cytoplasm: It is densely filled with granules so that its pale blue color can only be appreciated if the granules escape.

Normal variation: Normally there are about 2-5% eosinophils in the peripheral blood, giving an absolute count of 40-200 eosinophils/mm.[3] of blood. The normal eosinophil count is lowest in the morning and then rises from noon till after midnight. Repeated eosinophil counts should be performed at about the same time in the afternoon.

Increase—eosinophilia[68]:

1. Diseases of the blood-forming organs. Included in this category are myelocytic leukemia, eosinophilic leukemia, (up to 85%), following splenectomy (10%), and erythremia (Vaquez-Osler disease).

2. Allergic conditions. This category includes asthma and hay fever (15-30%), urticaria, eczema, Henoch's purpura, favism, arachnidism, reactions to tuberculin serum and foreign proteins, and sometimes angioneurotic edema.

3. Parasitic diseases (10-30%). Especially important in this category are the diseases due to *Trichinella* and filaria and the most common cestodes, trematodes, and nematodes. The eosinophilia does not depend so much upon the type of parasite as upon the sensitized state of the patient. *Trichinella* may produce eosinophilia of 75-85%.

4. Skin diseases. Psoriasis, eczema, pemphigus, and scabies are the important diseases in this category. The degree of eosinophilia is more in proportion to the extent of the involvement than to the type of disease.

5. Certain infectious diseases. In this category are scarlet fever, erythema multiforme, and pyogenic infections (during convalescence known as postfebrile eosinophilia).

6. Familial eosinophilia. This is a rare condition in which the eosinophils vary in number but may be numerous (up to about 60%).

7. Other conditions, some of which may be due to allergy. In this category are such varied conditions as reaction to camphor (9%), digitalis, and arsenic, malignant disease (about half the cases), Hodgkin's disease (about 15% of the cases), penicillin therapy (20-30%),[69] tropical eosinophilia, Loeffler's syndrome,[70, 71] and repeated irradiation therapy.

Decrease—eosinopenia: Eosinophils are decreased (hypoeosinophilia) or absent (aneosinophilia) in acute infections and in marked intoxications (uremia). They disappear early in pyogenic infections when there is an increase in the total leukocyte count with a marked shift to the left. They are decreased after the administration of ACTH (if the adrenal glands are functioning), after administration of cortisone, or in hyperadrenalism (Cushing's syndrome). (See Thorn test.) They are decreased after stress (burns, postoperative states, severe infections, etc.) and in disseminated lupus.

BASOPHILS:

Maturation of basophils: These cells in the myelocytic stage acquire dark purple-staining granules that are spheroid and vary in size, the larger ones appearing much darker. The granules are not numerous, and they tend to be peripherally arranged.

Mature basophil: Basophils are somewhat smaller than eosinophils, measuring 10-12μ in diameter. The granules often overlie the nucleus but do not fill the cytoplasm as completely as the eosinophilic granules do. They are peroxidase negative. The nucleus is indented in several places, giving rise to a cloverleaf pattern.

The cytoplasm is pale blue to pale pink.

Function: The blood basophils are at least functionally related to their morphologically similar connective tissue counterpart, the tissue mast cell.[72, 73] Both have the same function of storing and producing heparin, histamine, and serotonin.

Increase: An increase occurs in myelocytic leukemia, basophilic leukemia, myeloproliferative disorders (e.g., polycythemia vera), and hypersensitivity states.

Decrease: There is a decrease following

steroid therapy, in stress (e.g., myocardial infarct and bleeding peptic ulcer), in immediate hypersensitivity reactions (e.g., urticaria and anaphylactic shock), and in hyperthyroidism.

Mast cell (tissue basophil): It is normally never found in the peripheral blood and only rarely seen in the normal bone marrow.

Size: 20-25µ in diameter.

Nucleus: It is usually round and almost completely covered by granules.

Cytoplasm: It can hardly be seen because of the large, numerous, closely packed, deeply blue-staining granules which differ from the granules of basophils in size, number, insolubility in methyl alcohol, and in their metachromatic-staining reaction with toluidine blue.

Increase: An increase in tissue mast cells has been reported in macroglobulinemia, rheumatoid arthritis, mast cell leukemia, anaphylaxis, and hypoadrenalism. They are also increased in lymphomas invading the bone marrow and, at times, in urticaria pigmentosa.

Lymphocytic series

MATURATION OF LYMPHOCYTES: Lymphocytes develop in the lymphoid organs of the body such as the thymus, lymph nodes, tonsils, gastrointestinal tract (appendix), and spleen.

Lymphoblast:

Size: The youngest cell of this series, the lymphoblast, is a large cell (15-20µ in diameter).

Nucleus: The ovoid nucleus occupies more than half the cell; the chromatin is more coarsely reticular than that of the myeloblast and is somewhat more dense around the periphery, making the nuclear outline distinct; 1 or 2 nucleoli, usually well outlined, are present. Motility gives rise to characteristic hand mirror shapes.

Cytoplasm: The cytoplasm is nongranular and stains blue.

Prolymphocyte:

Size: The prolymphocyte, or immature large lymphocyte, is usually 15-18µ in diameter.

Nucleus: The large nucleus is ovoid and often shows remnants of the nucleoli; the chromatin tends to become condensed

into a mosaic pattern, the denser chromatin not being sharply marked off from the lighter staining pale blue parachromatin. As these cells mature, this blocking of the chromatin becomes more pronounced, and the nucleus stains more deeply as the cells become smaller.

Cytoplasm: The cytoplasm may show azurophilic granules.

Mature lymphocyte: It is customary to class lymphocytes that are larger than a polymorphonuclear cell as large lymphocytes and the smaller cells as small lymphocytes.

Large lymphocytes:

Size: 12-16µ in diameter.

Nucleus: The dense round, oval, or slightly indented nucleus is centrally or eccentrically located. Its chromatin is dense, clumped, and fuses imperceptibly with the pale blue parachromatin.

Cytoplasm: Abundant gray to pale blue cytoplasm in which 30-60% contains a few azurophilic granules.

Small lymphocytes:

Size: 9-12µ in diameter.

Nucleus and cytoplasm: The cytoplasm forms a narrow rim around the nucleus, which is similar to that of the large lymphocyte.

FUNCTION:

Immunocyte[74, 75]: Lymphocytes, together with the plasma cells and reticulum cells, belong to the immunocyte complex. Small lymphocytes are immunologically competent cells capable of interacting with antigen and initiating a primary immune response. The latter is evidenced by a peripheral lymphocytosis and the appearance of plasmacytoid cells. Lymphocytes do not form antibodies, but they may be responsible for the storage of immunologic experience (immunologic memory) so that a second contact with the antigen elicits an accelerated and increased response. The plasma cells are the source of antibodies and immunoglobulins.

PATHOLOGIC FORMS OF LYMPHOCYTES:

Virocytes (infectious mononucleosis cells, atypical lymphocytes, Türk cells, Downey cells): Virocytes are described in detail in the discussion of infectious mononucleosis (p. 188), but it should be emphasized that they may occur in many other virus diseases such as viral hepatitis, viral pneumonia, and viral upper respiratory tract infections. Virocytes may also be found in apparently healthy children. In differential counts in children they are not reported unless they exceed 10% of all lymphocytes. Virocytes have many features of the **transformed lymphocytes** appearing in stimulated lymphocytic cultures.

Size: Up to 16μ in diameter. Both the nucleus and cytoplasm are larger than in the small lymphocytes.

Nucleus: It is usually indented, oval, kidney-shaped, at times round, and often slightly eccentric. Its shape varies from cell to cell. The nuclear membrane is thick, the chromatin pattern is coarse, lymphocytic, or at times lighter and more delicate, resembling the monocytic nucleus.

Cytoplasm: It is usually increased in amount and basophilic, but at times it is deep blue and represented only by a thin rim. It may or may not contain azurophilic granules and vacuoles. There is often a perinuclear halo. The cell margins are irregular, often with pseudopods.

Lymphocytoid cell (plasmacytoid cell):
Size: 10-16μ in diameter.

Nucleus: It is eccentric and may have the pattern of a lymphocytic or plasmacytic nucleus. The parachromatin is pale blue and fuses with the coarse chromatin strands.

Cytoplasm: It may contain azurophilic granules and is usually more abundant than in the small lymphocytes. It may be mottled, pale, or dark blue.

These cells are seen in macroglobulinemia and are probably more closely related to plasma cells than to lymphocytes. The cells may well be an expression of activity of stimulated transformed lymphocytes.

Transformed lymphocyte, pyroninophilic cell, and lymphocyte culture[76-78]**:** Lymphocytes can be grown in tissue culture by a method that is similar to the peripheral blood culture method used for chromosome studies. Small lymphocytes grown in tissue culture remain small lymphocytes until stimulated by the addition of phytohemagglutinin, antigens, or other means. When thus stimulated, they transform into large cells, the nuclei of which are enlarged and contain a fine reticular chromatin pattern and nucleoli. The cytoplasm is deeply basophilic and there may be a perinuclear halo. The plasmacytoid type of stimulated cell is strongly basophilic, and because it stains heavily with pyronin (a red basic dye staining ribonucleic acid), it is called a pyroninophilic cell. The transformed lymphocytes are ameboid and may resemble blast cells, infectious mononucleosis cells, virocytes, or plasmacytoid cells. It can be shown that these cells produce immunoglobulins. This transformation into actively growing immunoglobulin-producing cells is impaired in cultures of lymphocytes of Hodgkin's disease, lymphatic leukemia, lymphocytosis, or some cases of agammaglobulinemia. Increased response has been noted in sarcoidosis. The culture method is one of a series of tests to determine **histocompatibility** of recipient and donor, aiding in the selection of donors for tissue grafts. The test is based on the observation that lymphocytes from an unrelated individual added to a lymphocyte culture stimulate the production of up to 3% of transformed lymphocytes. Lymphocytes from siblings react together less strongly; from fraternal twins they do not react.

Chromosomal analysis of lymphocyte cultures of individuals exposed to radiation may prove to be one of the most sensitive tests for radiation injury.

Türk cell: It resembles the prolymphocyte, showing an opaque deep blue cytoplasm without granules but usually with vacuoles and a rather pale reddish nucleus with a coarse reticular chromatin pattern and remnants of nucleoli. It is considered to be a transformed lymphocyte.

Rieder cell: It is similar to a lymphoblast except that it has a notched, lobulated, or segmented nucleus. It occurs in acute lymphatic leukemia.

Vacuolated lymphocyte: PAS-positive vacuoles have been described in lymphocytes of patients with lipidoses.[78a]

VARIATION IN NUMBER OF LYMPHOCYTES:

Normal values: Normal blood contains about 21-35% lymphocytes with only an occasional large lymphocyte, except in children.

Increase—lymphocytosis: An increase

may be **relative** or **absolute** or both. A relative increase (over 40%) occurs in those cases in which there is neutrophilic leukopenia. Absolute lymphocytosis (an increase in the total number) occurs in childhood, whooping cough, infectious mononucleosis, infectious lymphocytosis, lymphatic leukemia, brucellosis, typhoid fever, syphilis, hypogammaglobulinemia, agammaglobulinemia, hepatitis, herpes zoster and simplex, chickenpox, mumps, German measles, and chronic exposure to irradiation.

There is a slight increase in rickets and scurvy and in convalescence from pyogenic infections. There is an increase, with monocytes, in most protozoan diseases.

Smith reported several cases, usually associated with upper respiratory infection and characterized by absolute lymphocytosis (normal lymphocytes), for which he suggested the name **acute infectious lymphocytosis**. Finucane and Philips[79] report 21 cases in children from 1½-5½ yr. of age. The leukocytes ranged from 22,500-120,000 with 62-97% lymphocytes. The duration of the leukocytosis was from 2½-7 wk. Eosinophilia usually appeared as the total count decreased. Absence of anemia helps to distinguish this disease from leukemia.

Most of the **viral upper respiratory infections** (Coxsackie virus, myxovirus, etc.) are associated with lymphocytosis.

In **chronic lymphatic leukemia**, leukemic phase, there is a marked relative and absolute increase of lymphocytes (100,000-200,000/mm.³, with 90% or more of lymphocytes). The more acute the leukemia, the larger is the number of immature lymphocytes.

Decrease—lymphopenia: A relative decrease in number occurs in myelocytic leukemia, in Hodgkin's disease, neutrophilic leukocytosis, lupus erythematosus, and early acute irradiation syndrome.

Monocytic series

Monocytes are histiocytic reticulum cells that probably originate from the fixed reticulum cell component of the various organs of the reticuloendothelial system such as bone marrow, spleen, liver, and lymph nodes.

MATURATION OF MONOCYTES:

Monoblast:

Size: 15-30µ in diameter.

Nucleus: It is round, oval, or at times notched and indented. The chromatin pattern may resemble that of a **myeloblast (Naegeli type)** in which delicate blue to purple stippling with regular pale pink or small blue parachromatin areas is seen. On the other hand, the chromatin pattern may resemble that of a **reticulum cell (Schilling type)** in which an irregular network of strands and granules with irregular masses of parachromatin occurs. The nucleoli are pale, blue, large, and round. There are 3-5 in number.

Cytoplasm: It is often relatively large in amount, contains a few azurophilic granules, and stains pale blue or gray. The cell border is irregular, with pseudopods and indentations.

The cytoplasm filling the nuclear indentation is often lighter in color than the surrounding cytoplasm.

Motility is characteristic, several pseudopodia being extended in different directions at the same time.

With Wright stain the monoblasts are difficult to distinguish from myeloblasts, and this distinction will at times depend on the company they keep, i.e., on the type of mature cell they are associated with. The cytoplasm may contain Auer bodies, which are crystalline, periodic acid–Schiff positive structures that always indicate leukemia. (See p. 140.)

Promonocyte:

Size: 15-25µ in diameter.

Nucleus: The nucleus is large, ovoid, convoluted, and indented. The chromatin forms a loose, open network.

Cytoplasm: The gray-blue cytoplasm contains prominent azurophilic granules.

Monocyte:

Size: 14-20µ in diameter.

Nucleus: It is kidney-shaped or round, often lobulated with 2 or more lobes, and at times folded at the periphery. The chromatin network consists of coarse, loose threads producing areas of thickening at their junctions. The parachromatin is distributed in irregular spaces, giving the nucleus an almost transparent appearance.

Cytoplasm: It is abundant, gray-blue,

and may be vacuolated. It contains azurophilic dust.

The cells of this series are actively motile and phagocytic.

Normal values: 4-8%.

Increase—monocytosis[80]:

Hematologic disorders:
Monocytic leukemia
Myeloproliferative disorders
Lymphomas
Multiple myeloma

Bacterial infections:
Tuberculosis
Collagen diseases
Ulcerative colitis
Regional enteritis

Phagocytic monocytes: Phagocytic monocytes (**macrophages**) may be found in small numbers in the peripheral blood in many conditions such as severe infections, lupus erythematosus, hemolytic anemias, agranulocytosis, thrombocytopenic purpura, etc. The so-called **Tart cell** (named after a patient) is at times a monocyte containing an engulfed nucleus. The **Ferata cell** is a phagocytic cell frequently, but not constantly, seen in subacute bacterial endocarditis. Phagocytic cells are normally found in the bone marrow.

Endothelial cell

Lining cells of blood and lymph vessels resemble phagocytic monocytes and usually appear in clumps in smears of bone marrow and peripheral blood. Groups of endothelial cells resemble syncytial masses.

Size: 20-30μ in length.

Nucleus: It is round or oval, eccentric, and contains fine chromatin arranged in delicate threads. There is a single blue nucleolus.

Cytoplasm: It is bluish gray, surrounds the nucleus, and then extends into drawn out, elongated, and at times irregular and indistinct shapes. It often contains phagocytosed material.

Plasma cell series

Origin: The origin of plasma cells has not been agreed upon. They are probably derived from reticulum cells and/or lymphocytes. Various transitional forms can be seen which have been named lymphoid reticulum cells, lymphoid plasma cells, or lymphocytoid cells. Such intermediate forms can be seen in bone marrow in macroglobulinemia and in peripheral blood in infectious mononucleosis and hepatitis (virocytes and atypical lymphocytes).[81]

In lymphocyte cultures (see p. 149), transition of small lymphocytes to immunologically active, large transformed lymphocytes can be seen. It has been reported that some of these cells also transform into macrophages and plasma cells.

Maturation of plasma cells:

Plasmablast:

Size: 8-20μ in diameter.

Nucleus: It is round or oval and the chromatin is bluish purple and arranged in a fine chromatin network with some clumping. In general the nucleus resembles the reticulum cell nucleus. The blue nucleoli are difficult to see although there may be up to 6 present.

Cytoplasm: The nongranular cytoplasm is moderate in amount, light blue, and may be mottled.

Proplasmacyte:

Size: 15-25μ in diameter.

Nucleus: The round or oval nucleus is eccentric and contains a coarse reticulum chromatin network. Parachromatin spaces are irregular. Nucleoli are still visible.

Cytoplasm: There is abundant deep blue, nongranular cytoplasm, which shows a perinuclear clear zone called hof. There may be peripheral cytoplasmic dissolution.

Plasmacyte (plasma cell):

Size: 14-20μ in length.

Nucleus: It is eccentric and small. The condensed chromatin forms clumps that may be concentrated in the periphery of the nucleus, creating the so-called cartwheel pattern which is best seen in tissue sections or in bone marrow smears.

Cytoplasm: It is dark blue and ovoid. There is usually a clear zone close to the nuclear membrane. The cytoplasm is nongranular but may contain vacuoles.

In bone marrow smears these vacuoles are frequently seen to be filled with opalescing, rounded, small bodies that may at times be slightly eosinophilic. They are called **Russell bodies.** If the cytoplasm is completely filled with pale blue globoid bodies, the cell is called a **grape cell.** Protein crystals may also be seen in the cytoplasm as well as in the nucleus.

FUNCTION OF PLASMA CELLS: The occasional plasma cell found in peripheral blood is probably inactive, whereas its counterpart in bone marrow is responsible for the production of gamma globulins and thus for the production of antibodies. Pathologic conditions associated with **hypergammaglobulinemia** usually show an increase in bone marrow plasma cells, whereas hypogammaglobulinic states usually show a diminution or absence of these cells.

INCREASE: Plasma cells are increased in measles and German measles and markedly increased in plasma cell leukemia. They may be increased in serum sickness and infectious mononucleosis. Occasional plasma cells may be found in chronic infections and in allergy. In **macroglobulinemia** the bone marrow shows a curious mixture of plasma cells, lymphocytes, and intermediate forms.

PATHOLOGIC FORMS: The pathologic plasma cells produce abnormal proteins such as paraproteins, macroglobulins, cryoglobulins, and mucopolysaccharides containing proteins such as amyloid and paramyloid.[82]

In **multiple myeloma** the significant cells (myeloma cells) suggest atypical and immature plasma cells. The increase is found in bone marrow only.

Inclusions that stain blue with Wright stain are found in the cytoplasm of plasma cells following treatment of multiple myeloma for 3-4 wk. with stilbamidine. The inclusions may remain for months after treatment has been discontinued.

In the bone marrow the plasma cells are often binucleated and trinucleated.

DIFFERENTIAL DIAGNOSIS: In bone marrow smears, osteoblasts may be mistaken for single plasma cells and osteoclasts for groups of these cells.

Megakaryocytic series and platelet formation

Platelet formation occurs in the bone marrow and lungs from megakaryocytes.

Megakaryoblasts:
Size: 15-30μ in diameter.

Nucleus: There may be a single large oval or kidney-shaped nucleus with a fine reticulum chromatin network and several pale blue nucleoli which are difficult to see. This type of nucleus is rare. More frequently megakaryoblasts contain chains of 2-4 nuclei.

Cytoplasm: It forms a bluish irregular ring around the nucleus. The periphery shows cytoplasmic projections and pseudopodia-like structures. The cytoplasm is devoid of granulations and it is often surrounded by platelets.

Promegakaryocyte:
Size: 20-50μ in diameter. It is much larger than the megakaryoblast.

Nucleus: It is large, indented, polylobulated, and rarely multinucleated. The chromatin appears as coarse, heavily stained strands and may show some clumping. Nucleoli are present.

Cytoplasm: There is a large amount of finely granular basophilic cytoplasm and early azurophilic granules. There may be platelets surrounding the cell.

Megakaryocyte:
Size: 30-100μ in diameter. It is the largest cell found in the bone marrow. Functionally two types can be distinguished, the platelet-producing (active) megakaryocyte and the nonplatelet-producing (inactive) megakaryocyte. The normal bone marrow contains 1-2 megakaryocytes/hpf.

Active megakaryocyte:
Size: As before.

Nucleus: It is plump, multilobulated, indented, and at times multinucleated, the nuclei being arranged in chains or rings. The nuclei may partially cover each other. The chromatin is in heavy clumps. Nucleoli are not visible.

Cytoplasm: A large amount of polychromatic cytoplasm produces pseudopodia-like projections and contains aggregates of azurophilic granules surrounded by pale halos. These structures give rise to platelets at the periphery of the megakaryocytes. The line of cleavage goes through the hyaline cytoplasm of the halo so that the granular mass becomes the platelet center.

Inactive megakaryocyte:
Size and nucleus: As before, although

the nucleus may be very irregular and bizarre.

Cytoplasm: It is polychromatic but free of azurophilic granules and aggregates. It may show peripheral vacuolization.

Megakaryocytes in peripheral blood: Megakaryocytes or fragments of these cells may appear in the peripheral blood in myelogenous leukemia, leukoerythroblastic anemias (extramedullary hematopoiesis), and polycythemia vera. Megakaryocyte blood counts[83] reveal from 1-100 megakaryocytes/5 ml. blood.

Variation in number of megakaryocytes:

Increase: An increase of megakaryocytes accompanies megakaryocytic leukemia, myelogenous leukemia, polycythemia vera, idiopathic thrombocytopenic purpura, hypersplenism, and splenic infarcts.

Decrease: A decrease of megakaryocytes is seen in toxic bone marrow depression, heat stroke, pernicious anemia, acute leukemia, some forms of aplastic anemia, myelofibrosis, and multiple myeloma.

Differential diagnosis of megakaryocytes: Megakaryocytes must be distinguished from other multinucleated giant cells found in the bone marrow such as osteoclasts, multinucleated plasma cells, multinucleated erythroblasts, Reed-Sternberg cells, and giant reticulum cells (polykaryocytes).

Reed-Sternberg cell: It is about the size of a megakaryocyte and the differentiation may offer some difficulty in tissue sections, but in the bone marrow it is easily distinguished.

Nucleus: There are usually 2 large ovoid and notched nuclei with a heavy, irregular chromatin network and with 1-2 large, pale blue nucleoli.

Cytoplasm: There is a large amount of pale blue and at times vacuolated cytoplasm lacking granulation.

Polykaryocyte: It may be a phagocytic reticulum cell containing phagocytosed nuclei, or it may be the result of fusion of histiocytic monocytes which is one of the explanations offered for the giant cells seen in bone sections of hyperparathyroidism.

Variation in morphology of megakaryocytes:

Degenerating megakaryocyte: The nuclei are transformed into pyknotic lobulated masses. The cytoplasm is absent, leaving naked nuclear masses, or it is represented by a thin basophilic rim.

Abnormal megakaryocytes: **Hyperlobulated** forms with large nuclei containing prominent nucleoli are seen in megakaryocytic leukemia, a form of myelogenous leukemia. Hyperlobulation is also seen in pernicious anemia, the vitamin B_{12} deficiency of which leads to the formation of a nucleus with a fine, reticulated chromatin pattern which is similar to that found in megaloblasts. These abnormal forms fail to produce platelets.

In idiopathic thrombocytopenic purpura the megakaryocytic cytoplasm is hyaline, agranular, and vacuolated.

Thrombocytes (platelets): Platelets are detached portions or fragments of the cytoplasm of mature megakaryocytes found in the bone marrow and in the lung. They are small hyaline structures from one-fourth to one-half the size of an erythrocyte and have ragged edges. They stain pale blue and contain azurophilic granules that tend to collect near the center. They are very fragile and tend to clump together in large masses and to degenerate. Each platelet contains a **central chromomere** surrounded by a **hyalomere.** By means of their adhesive faculty (pseudopodium formation and spreading), they can adhere to an injured vessel wall, and during the ensuing process of agglutination they release serotonin (vasoconstriction) and various factors necessary for the production of thromboplastin (first phase of clotting). They also play a role in clot retraction.[84-86]

Platelets live for only a short time (3-5 days) and are destroyed by the reticuloendothelial cells of the spleen.

Normal values: The normal platelet count is from 250,000-400,000/mm.³, depending upon the method used.

Variation in number of platelets:

Increase—thrombocytosis and thrombocythemia: The count may reach several million and the condition may be associated with a tendency to clotting as well as to bleeding.

PATHOLOGIC: Pathologic thrombocytosis

may occur in polycythemia vera, in malignant tumors, in chronic myelogenous leukemia, after splenectomy, and in splenic atrophy, myelosclerosis, and megakaryocytic leukemia.

PHYSIOLOGIC: Physiologic thrombocytosis occurs in pregnancy, during menstruation, following hemorrhage and exercise, and after adrenaline injection.

Decrease—thrombocytopenia: The decrease becomes critical when it reaches 50,000 platelets/mm.[3], at which level the prothrombin consumption test becomes shortened and, clinically, bleeding follows minor trauma. At a level of 20,000 platelets/mm.[3] spontaneous bleeding may occur.

Thrombocytopenia may be classified as follows:

I. Amegakaryocytic thrombocytopenia
   A. Due to bone marrow damage:
      Congenital absence of megakaryocytes
      Aplastic anemia due to marrow failure or due to drugs and infections
      Involvement of bone marrow by tumor or leukemia (acute)
      Radiation effect
II. Megakaryocytic thrombocytopenia
   A. Due to disturbance of platelet formation (ineffective thrombocytopoiesis):
      Pernicious anemia
      Paroxysmal nocturnal hemoglobinuria
      Hegglin's anomaly
      Aldrich's syndrome
   B. Due to excessive destruction of platelets (nonimmune sequestration):
      Hemangiomas
      Hypersplenism
      Septicemia (gram-negative organisms)
      Microangiopathic thrombocytopenia
      Defibrination syndrome
      Heat stroke
   C. Due to excessive platelet destruction by immune mechanisms (immunologic thrombocytopenia):
      Idiopathic
      Symptomatic
         Drug induced
         Posttransfusion
         Neonatal
         Viral infections
         Systemic lupus erythematosus
         Lymphoproliferative disorders
         Hemolytic anemia

Variation in morphology of platelets: In qualitative deficiencies the platelets vary markedly in size and configuration. Numerous giant forms make their appearance and there is poor differentiation of the chromomere and loss of granulation with diffuse basophilia. Qualitative platelet deficiencies are seen in thrombasthenia (Glanzmann) and thrombocytopathia.

NONHEMATOLOGIC CELLS IN THE PERIPHERAL BLOOD SMEAR

Nonhematologic cells found in the peripheral blood include the following: (1) parasitic cells, as in malaria and *Bartonella* infestation, etc., which are considered in the discussion of parasitic hemolytic anemias, (2) fungal cells, as in infection with *Histoplasma capsulatum*, which is included in the discussion of mycology, and (3) tumor cells.

Tumor cells in peripheral blood[87]

Since carcinoma spreads by lymphatic and hematogenous routes, tumor cells may be found in peripheral blood. Concentration methods have been devised that utilize Millipore filters* and enzymes.

RED BLOOD CELL PATHOLOGY

Anemia, the deficiency of red blood cells and/or hemoglobin, requires careful laboratory investigation to determine its cause and thus its treatment.

Classification of anemia

No classification of anemia is entirely satisfactory. The division into **primary anemia,** for which the cause is not known, and **secondary** or **symptomatic anemia,** for which the cause is known, is not adequate.

Morphologic classification: This classification is based on the size of the erythrocytes and their hemoglobin content (the hematocrit). Wintrobe divides the anemias into four groups: (1) macrocytic, characterized by erythrocytes with mean corpuscular volume larger than normal and mean corpuscular hemoglobin (content) greater than normal, but with hemoglobin concentration not above normal; (2) simple microcytic, characterized by erythrocytes with mean corpuscular volume smaller than normal and mean corpuscular hemoglobin (con-

---

*Millipore Filter Corp., Bedford, Mass.

tent) less than normal, but the hemoglobin concentration normal; (3) hypochromic microcytic, characterized by erythrocytes with mean corpuscular volume less than normal and both mean corpuscular hemoglobin (content) and mean corpuscular hemoglobin concentration less than normal; (4) normocytic, characterized by erythrocytes with normal mean corpuscular volume and hemoglobin content (Table 4-14, p. 113).

Erythrokinetic evaluation: It is based on quantitative measurements of red cell production and red cell destruction and has been made possible by the introduction of radioactive isotope methods.

Red cell production: Red cell production can be evaluated by the reticulocyte count, by red cell utilization of radioiron, and by plasma iron turnover as well as by the erythroid-myeloid ratio in the bone marrow.

Red cell destruction: Red cell destruction can be evaluated by measuring fecal urobilinogen and red cell survival.

The erythrokinetic approach to the diagnosis of anemias stresses the site of the defect—whether it is premarrow, marrow, or postmarrow in origin.

MACROCYTIC ANEMIAS

CLASSIFICATION: Macrocytic anemia may be divided into two groups: **megaloblastic,** characterized by megaloblastic hyperplasia of bone marrow (pernicious anemia, sprue, idiopathic steatorrhea, megaloblastic anemia of infancy and of pregnancy), and **nonmegaloblastic** (liver disease, hypothyroidism, hemolytic anemia).

Megaloblastic anemias:
Hereditary constitutional megaloblastic anemia
  Pernicious anemia—absence of intrinsic factor
Symptomatic megaloblastic anemia
  Malabsorption syndrome—vitamin B_{12} and folic acid deficiency
  Primary: tropical sprue, idiopathic steatorrhea, and celiac disease
  Secondary: regional ileitis, small intestinal resection, blind loops, chronic pancreatitis, diverticula, stomach resection, gastric carcinoma, and hypothyroidism
  Nutritional (diminished supply of folic acid or vitamin B_{12}): kwashiorkor, goat's milk anemia, and inadequate diet (vegetarians)

  Increased utilization: pregnancy, infancy, fish tapeworm (*Diphyllobothrium latum*), pathologic intestinal flora, blind loop operations, small bowel strictures and diverticula, and leukemia
Liver disease
Drugs: anticonvulsants—Dilantin, Amytal, Seconal, Rutonal, and folic acid antagonists

Nonmegaloblastic anemias:
Liver disease
Hypothyroidism
Hemolytic anemias

MACROCYTIC ANEMIA DUE TO ABSENCE OF INTRINSIC FACTOR (PERNICIOUS ANEMIA)

Hematopoietic principle: Pernicious anemia is due to a deficiency of the hematopoietic principle that is normally formed in the stomach by the interaction of the **intrinsic factor** secreted by the gastric mucosa and the **extrinsic factor** supplied in meat protein and other foods. It is absorbed from the small intestines and stored in the liver. In pernicious anemia the chief deficiency is the absence of the intrinsic factor. The hematopoietic principle is necessary for the maturation of megaloblasts, and when it is absent, megaloblasts persist in the bone marrow and produce macrocytes via megaloblastic maturation.

Vitamin B_{12} is the extrinsic factor, and **absorbed** vitamin B_{12} is synonymous with the hematopoietic principle.

The intrinsic factor is produced by the hydrochloric acid–secreting cells of the stomach. Its nature is not known.

Pernicious anemia is characterized by the following:
1. Deficiency of vitamin B_{12} (or of folic acid) leads to interference with normal cell maturation (mitotic activity) due to disturbance of ribonucleic and deoxyribonucleic acid synthesis.
2. Atrophy of the gastric mucosa is responsible for the absence of intrinsic factor so that vitamin B_{12} is not absorbed.
3. A hemolytic component is responsible for a shortened survival time of the red cells so that the free bilirubin in the serum and the urobilinogen in urine and feces are increased.

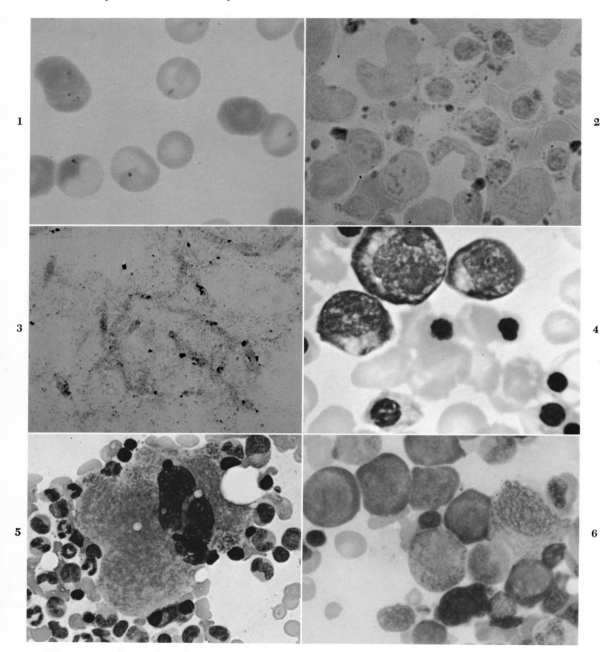

Plate 6. Red blood cell pathology.

1. Siderocytes in peripheral blood in sidero-achrestic anemia, Prussian blue stain. (Courtesy V. Minnich.)
2. Ring sideroblasts in bone marrow in sideroachrestic anemia, Prussian blue stain.
3. Hemosiderin casts in urinary sediment in paroxysmal nocturnal hemoglobinuria, Prussian blue stain. (Courtesy V. Minnich.)
4. Hemolytic disease of the newborn (erythroblastosis fetalis), peripheral blood, Wright stain.
5. Normal bone marrow, Wright stain.
6. Megaloblasts in bone marrow in pernicious anemia, Wright stain.

Laboratory findings:

Hematologic findings:

1. Blood: reduction of red cells and hemoglobin.
2. Reticulocytes: low.
3. Red cell survival time: shortened.
4. Smear: shows anisocytosis, macrocytosis, poikilocytosis, hyperchromia, polychromasia, and basophilia.
5. White cells: hypersegmented neutrophils, giant neutrophils, shift to the right, and leukopenia with relative lymphocytosis.
6. Platelets: reduced (thrombocytopenia).
7. Bone marrow: erythroid hyperplasia, megaloblastic type (Plate 6). An abnormal delay in mitotic activity of the erythroblasts is followed by diminution in the number of normoblasts and abnormal hemoglobinization of the erythroblasts. The myelocytes show abnormal granulation and giant forms, and the polymorphonuclear leukocytes are hypersegmented and large. The megakaryocytes are diminished, and many abnormal forms are seen. There is usually an increase in reticulum cells and in stainable iron.

Nonhematologic findings:

1. Stomach: histamine-fast achlorhydria; abnormally large cells are seen in cytologic preparations.
2. Serum: decreased vitamin B_{12} level, elevated iron, free (nonconjugated) bilirubin increased, uric acid increased, haptoglobin diminished, prothrombin low, and **lactic acid dehydrogenase** increased.
3. Urine: increased urobilinogen and urobilin, aminoaciduria (taurine increased), increased formiminoglutamic acid excretion (if folic acid deficiency), decreased vitamin B_{12} excretion, and decreased uropepsin.

Methods of detecting B_{12} deficiency:

Assay of B_{12} concentration in serum:
Microbiologic assay[88]: Test sera are added to cultures of B_{12}-dependent microorganisms such as *Euglena grazilis* or *Lactobacillus leishmanii*. The amount of B_{12} in the serum is estimated by comparing the growth produced in the serum-containing culture with the amount of growth produced by control cultures containing known amounts of B_{12}.

Normal serum B_{12} level: 140-900 $\mu\mu g/$ml.

In pernicious anemia the level is usually 80 $\mu\mu g/$ml.

Radioactive B_{12}:

URINARY EXCRETION OF Co^{60}-B_{12} (METHOD OF SCHILLING)[89]: When radioactive vitamin B_{12} is administered orally to a normal individual, it is absorbed and about 15% is excreted in the urine if at the same time the blood is saturated with nonradioactive vitamin B_{12} administered intramuscularly so that the radioactive vitamin B_{12} is not utilized by the body. Patients with pernicious anemia, who lack the intrinsic factor, are unable to absorb Co^{60}-B_{12}, which is therefore excreted in the feces and not in the urine. If the test is repeated with Co^{60}-B_{12} plus intrinsic factor, vitamin B_{12} will be absorbed from the bowel and excreted in the urine.

Hematologic response to treatment: Specific treatment with vitamin B_{12} changes the megaloblastic erythropoiesis to normoblastic erythropoiesis in about 3 days and is followed by a rise in reticulocytes, hemoglobin, and mature erythrocytes and by a fall in plasma iron, serum bilirubin, and fecal urobilinogen. It does not restore secretion of hydrochloric acid or of the intrinsic factor.

MACROCYTIC ANEMIAS DUE TO FOLIC ACID DEFICIENCY

1. Megaloblastic anemia of pregnancy —cause unknown
2. Megaloblastic anemia of childhood —pure milk diet, goat's milk disease, and celiac disease
3. Anticonvulsant drugs—interference with folic acid metabolism
4. Therapy with folic acid antagonist—interference with nucleic acid synthesis
5. Macrocytic hemolytic anemia
6. Macrocytic anemia due to liver disease

Methods of detecting folic acid deficiency:

Assay of folic acid concentration in serum[90]: A folic acid coenzyme, 5-methyl-tetrahydrofolic acid, present in normal serum, is diminished in folic acid deficiency and is microbiologically active for *L. casei.*

Normal serum folic acid levels *(L. casei)*: 5.9-21 mμg/ml.

Folic acid deficiency levels *(L. casei)*: less than 4 mμg/ml.

Determination of formiminoglutamic acid (FIGLU) in urine[91]: FIGLU is a metabolic product of histidine metabolism that is normally metabolized to glutamic acid with the help of tetrahydrofolic acid (THFA). In folic acid deficiency, THFA is not available and FIGLU is found in the urine in increased amounts. The sensitivity of the test can be increased by the histidine-loading technique.

The folate level may also be determined in the red cells.[92]

MICROCYTIC ANEMIAS AND MICROCYTIC HYPOCHROMIC ANEMIAS

CLASSIFICATION ACCORDING TO ETIOLOGY:
Iron deficiency
Infection
Pyridoxine deficiency
Sideroachrestic hypochromic anemias
Thalassemia
Hemoglobin variants
Lead poisoning

IRON-DEFICIENCY ANEMIA

This anemia is closely linked to iron metabolism.

Iron metabolism: Alimentary iron is converted to ionized ferric iron in the stomach where it is reduced to ferrous iron (Fig. 4-36). Iron absorption depends on several factors, some of which are not definitely known. It depends on the food article, on the iron content of the depot organs, and on the activity of the bone marrow. In the process of absorption the iron is oxidized to the ferric state and bound to an alpha$_2$ globulin, **apoferritin,** the iron complex of which is called **ferritin.** After absorption the iron circulates in the plasma bound to a beta globulin called **transferrin** or **siderophilin.** This protein is normally only one-third saturated with iron. By means of the bloodstream the iron is transported to the **storage depots** such as bone marrow, liver, and spleen. Most of the iron is utilized for hemoglobin synthesis. A small amount is incorporated into enzymes and myoglobin. Excess iron is stored as ferritin, which does not stain with Prussian blue, and as **hemosiderin,** which gives the Prussian blue reaction. Most of the alimentary iron is excreted in feces. A small amount of iron is lost in urine, sweat, and desqua-

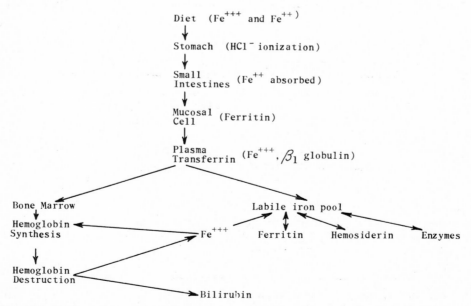

Fig. 4-36. Outline of iron metabolism.

mating mucosal and cutaneous cells. Parenterally administered iron is not excreted.

Causes: The causes of iron deficiency include insufficient intake (inadequate diet in childhood), inadequate absorption (chronic gastrointestinal diseases), increased demand (pregnancy, childhood, etc.), blood loss (physiologic, as in the menses, and pathologic, as in hemorrhage and hemolysis), and abnormal intrinsic iron metabolism (pulmonary hemosiderosis, sideroachrestic anemia).

Insufficient intake is one of the frequent causes of iron-deficiency anemia in children, especially at the age of about 3-6 mo. and again at the end of the first or second year. This iron-deficiency anemia is more marked in premature children.

Laboratory findings:
Hematologic findings:
1. Hemoglobin and red blood cell count decreased, hypochromasia, microcytosis, anulocytosis, occasional target cells, and anisocytosis
2. Reticulocytes: decreased
3. Osmotic fragility: normal to decreased
4. Platelets and white cells: usually normal
5. Serum iron: low
6. Serum iron-binding capacity: increased
7. Bone marrow: increase in basophilic normoblasts; absence of stainable iron (see p. 138)

Nonhematologic findings:
1. Gastric achlorhydria; epithelial changes

ANEMIA OF INFECTION

The serum iron level is as low as it is in true iron-deficiency anemia, but the serum iron-binding capacity is also diminished (in iron-deficiency anemia it is increased).

PYRIDOXINE (VITAMIN B_6)-DEFICIENCY ANEMIA

This hypochromic anemia is characterized by a high serum iron and by its lack of response to treatment with iron. The tryptophan tolerance test helps to substantiate the diagnosis.

SIDEROACHRESTIC HYPOCHROMIC ANEMIAS

These anemias are due to interference with the hemoglobin synthesis whereby iron cannot be utilized although it is present in adequate amounts. The serum iron level is high, and siderocytes and sideroblasts are increased (Plate 6).

Classification: This anemia is classified into primary and secondary forms. In the latter group fall several of the anemias mentioned under the heading of normocytic hemolytic anemias, such as thalas-

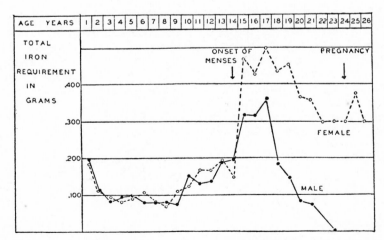

Fig. 4-37. Annual iron requirements for growth, menstruation, and pregnancy. (From Heath and Patek: Medicine **16:**267, 1937.)

semia, lead poisoning anemia, and the anemia of vitamin B_6 deficiency.

NORMOCYTIC ANEMIAS

CLASSIFICATION ACCORDING TO ETIOLOGY:
According to their etiology, normocytic anemias can be classified as follows:

Hemolytic anemias
Anemias due to blood loss (up to 3 mo.)
Aplastic or hypoplastic anemias
Myelophthisic anemia
Anemia of pregnancy
Anemia of infection
Anemia of uremia (kidney diseases)
Anemia of endocrine disturbances

HEMOLYTIC ANEMIAS

COMMON FEATURES OF ALL HEMOLYTIC ANEMIAS AND METHODS OF INVESTIGATION:
The basis of all hemolytic anemias is the increased rate of blood destruction and the shortened life-span of the red blood cells.

Laboratory investigation therefore centers on the following:

1. **Diagnosis of anemia, excessive hemolysis, and bone marrow response:**

   Complete blood count, with careful attention to morphology of red cells
   Osmotic fragility of red blood cells
   Serum bilirubin, haptoglobin determinations, and methemalbumin
   Urine urobilinogen, hemosiderin, and hemoglobin
   Fecal urobilinogen
   Bone marrow examination
   Red cell survival in patient

2. **Diagnosis of the cause of anemia:**
   Once the anemia has been established as hemolytic in type, its cause should be investigated on the basis of the following classification:

On the basis of their **etiology,** hemolytic anemias can be classified into those due to intracorpuscular defects and those due to extracorpuscular defects.

Due to intracorpuscular defects
   Hereditary spherocytosis
   Hereditary elliptocytosis
   Thalassemia
   Hemoglobinopathies
   Paroxysmal nocturnal hemoglobinuria
   Enzyme-deficiency hemolytic anemias
   Hereditary (congenital) nonspherocytic hemolytic anemia

Due to extracorpuscular defects
   Antibodies: isoimmune and autoimmune
   Infections: bacterial, viral, and parasitic
   Toxins: snake venom
   Physical agents: burns
   Hypersplenism
   Symptomatic: secondary to other diseases such as lymphomas, lupus erythematosus, etc.

Hemolysis: There are two main methods of red cell destruction: extravascular breakdown and intravascular breakdown. Usually both occur, but one or the other predominates.

Extravascular destruction: The dying red cells are phagocytosed by the macrophages of the reticuloendothelial system of the bone marrow, spleen, liver, lung, etc. and are destroyed so that their hemoglobin is set free. Hemoglobin is broken down into its components:

Heme (Fe + Protoporphyrin) + Proteins (globin)

The iron is carried to the depot organs and is reutilized. The porphyrin moiety is converted into free nonconjugated bilirubin. The latter is conjugated in the liver to glucuronic acid and excreted as conjugated bilirubin into the intestine, where, by the action of bacteria, it is converted into urobilinogen and then partly reabsorbed and excreted as urinary urobilinogen. It is partly retained in the feces to be excreted as fecal urobilinogen.

Intravascular breakdown: Hemoglobin liberated within the blood vessels is bound to plasma proteins called **haptoglobins,** which have a special affinity to hemoglobin. If a large amount of free hemoglobin is present, the serum has a pink tinge, and the condition is called **hemoglobinemia.** The haptoglobin-hemoglobin molecule is taken up by the reticuloendothelial system, where the hemoglobin is split in the same way as in extravascular destruction. If the free hemoglobin exceeds 140 mg./ 100 ml., the haptoglobin-binding capacity is saturated so that free hemoglobin appears in the serum (hemoglobinemia) and in the urine (**hemoglobinuria**). The renal threshold for hemoglobin depends on the haptoglobin level. Some of the free plasma hemoglobin becomes oxidized and unites with albumin to form **methemalbumin,** which colors the plasma brown.

Hematologic findings: There is usually a marked reduction in the number of red blood cells, with a corresponding lowering of the hemoglobin value so that a **normocytic normochromic anemia** results. If there are many reticulocytes present, the anemia may be macrocytic.

The white blood cells show a moderate **leukocytosis,** with a shift to the left.

Platelets: They are increased.

Blood smear: Anisocytosis and poikilocytosis with anisocytosis are characteristic of hemolytic anemias. Some of the abnormal cells have a characteristic morphology.

Spherocytes: Spherocytes are small (microspherocytes) round cells occurring in both acquired and congenital hemolytic anemias. They represent a prehemolytic state, being easily hemolyzed in hypotonic saline solution. (See Fig. 4-21, p. 136.)

Burr cells: They are irregularly shaped red blood cells with spinous projections. (See Fig. 4-16.)

Reticulocytosis: In all hemolytic anemias the stimulated erythroblastic activity of the bone marrow leads to the release of many young erythrocytes, which in the Wright-stained smear appear as macrocytes and in the smear treated with supravital dyes are seen to contain the reticulum of reticulocytes. A normal reticulocyte count does not rule out a hemolytic process. (See discussion of marrow compensation and also Fig. 4-25.)

Schistocytes: They are fragmented cells of very irregular shapes and sizes. (See Fig. 4-24.)

Anisocytosis and poikilocytosis: The presence of the above-mentioned cells imparts to the smear the appearance of an irregularity in size and shape of cells which is highly suggestive of a hemolytic process. (See Fig. 4-19.)

Red cell inclusions: Many of the inclusions described before (p. 137) can be seen in hemolytic processes. They are Heinz bodies (special stain needed), Howell-Jolly bodies, Cabot rings, and nuclear remnants.

Normoblasts and erythroblasts: In cases of marked erythroid hyperplasia of the bone marrow, nucleated red cells are released into the peripheral circulation.

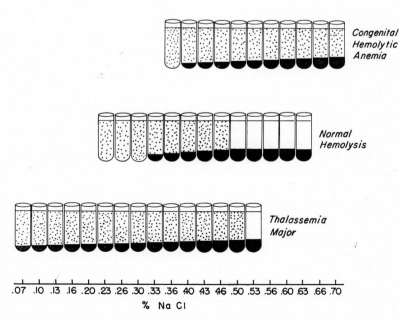

Fig. 4-38. Osmotic fragility of erythrocytes (method of Sanford).

Osmotic fragility: The red blood cell is surrounded by a semipermeable membrane that allows exchange of water and electrolytes. If the red cell is placed in a hypotonic saline solution, osmotic equilibrium will be established by drawing water into the cell which then swells. In hypertonic saline solution the cell will lose water and shrink. Many variables such as age, temperature, oxygen saturation, etc. affect osmotic fragility measurements. Osmotic fragility measurements should be strictly standardized, and a normal control should be run with each test. Spherocytes represent one of the stages the red cell goes through when exposed to hypotonic saline solution. Naturally occurring spherocytes therefore exhibit an increased tendency to hemolysis.

Screening test for increased fragility:
Tube 1: 1.0 ml. of 0.85% saline solution
Tube 2: 0.1 ml. of 0.50% saline solution

To each tube add 0.1 ml. oxalated blood. Mix and centrifuge.

Result: If hemolysis occurs in tube 2, the osmotic fragility of the test cells is probably increased.

Fragility test (method of Sanford): See Fig. 4-38.

Technique: Arrange a series of 12 small test tubes (10 × 75 mm.) in a rack and number them from 25-14, inclusive. Set up one series for the test blood and one series for the normal control blood.

From a capillary pipette, place in each tube the number of drops of 0.5% salt solution indicated by the number on the tube. Hold pipette at same angle to ensure uniform drops.

With the same pipette, rinsed thoroughly, add to each tube the number of drops of distilled water required to make the volume in each tube 25 drops and mix.

Puncture vein with sterile hypodermic needle and syringe and place 1 drop from the needle into each of the tubes. Mix and let stand at room temperature for 2 hr.

Examine for initial hemolysis and for complete hemolysis. The percentage of salt in each tube is obtained by multiplying its number by 0.02.

Record the percentage salt solutions

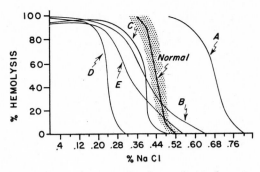

Fig. 4-39. Osmotic fragility of erythrocytes (method of Dacie). **A,** Hereditary spherocytosis; **B,** thalassemia major; **C,** thalassemia minor; **D,** hemoglobin-E disease; **E,** hemoglobin-E thalassemia. (From Frankel and Reitman, editors: Gradwohl's clinical laboratory methods and diagnosis, St. Louis, 1963, The C. V. Mosby Co.)

showing initial hemolysis and complete hemolysis. Always run a normal blood for control.

Normal values: Initial hemolysis occurs in 0.44 or 0.42% and is complete in 0.34% normal saline solution.

Fragility test (method of Dacie): This method (Fig. 4-39), which is the best of a number of procedures, has been well described by Dacie.[93] Blood is diluted in hypotonic saline solution and buffered to pH 7.4 with phosphates. A series of tubes is prepared, each containing a different concentration of saline solution. After standing at room temperature, the hemolyzed (ghost) cells are removed by centrifugation, and the degree of hemolysis in each tube is determined spectrophotometrically on the basis of free hemoglobin.

Reagents:
1. Stock solution (osmotically equivalent to 10% saline solution):

   NaCl, 180 gm.
   Na_2HPO_4, 27.31 gm.
   $NaH_2PO_4 \cdot 2H_2O$, 4.86 gm.
   Distilled water up to 2000 ml.
2. Working solution: 1% working solution is made by diluting the stock solution 1:10 with normal saline solution. Prepare 50 ml. each of the following dilutions by diluting with distilled water and keep in blood bank refrigerator (4° C.).

0.85%	42.4 ml. of 1% solution
0.75%	27.5 ml. of 1% solution
0.65%	32.5 ml. of 1% solution
0.60%	30.0 ml. of 1% solution
0.55%	27.5 ml. of 1% solution
0.50%	25.0 ml. of 1% solution
0.45%	22.5 ml. of 1% solution
0.40%	20.0 ml. of 1% solution
0.35%	17.5 ml. of 1% solution
0.30%	15.0 ml. of 1% solution
0.20%	10.0 ml. of 1% solution
0.10%	5.0 ml. of 1% solution

Technique: Set up 12 tubes containing 5 ml. each of the various dilutions of saline solution. Obtain heparinized venous blood and add 0.05 ml. to each tube, mixing immediately. Allow tubes to stand for 30 min. at room temperature. Mix again and centrifuge at 2000 rpm for 5 min. Separate supernatant and read in colorimeter at 545 mμ the degree of hemolysis, using the supernatant from 0.85% saline solution as blank and the supernatant from 0.1% saline solution as 100%.

Recording the results of osmotic fragility test: Draw a fragility curve by plotting on graph paper the %hemolysis in each tube against the corresponding concentration of salt solution. In normal persons an almost symmetric sigmoid curve results (Fig. 4-39).

Normal range of osmotic fragility:

0.30% saline solution	97-100% hemolysis
0.35% saline solution	90-99% hemolysis
0.40% saline solution	50-95% hemolysis
0.45% saline solution	5-45% hemolysis
0.50% saline solution	0-6% hemolysis
0.55% saline solution	0% hemolysis

In disease, deviations from the curve occur (Fig. 4-39).

Interpretation of fragility tests:

1. Increased osmotic fragility: Osmotic fragility is increased in hemolytic anemias (common denominator: spherocytes). In congenital spherocytosis the initial hemolysis occurs in 0.47-0.48% and is complete in 0.41% normal saline solution.

2. Decreased osmotic fragility: There is decreased osmotic fragility in thalassemia, sickle cell disease, Hb-C disease, iron-deficiency anemia, and jaundice (liver disease) in newborn infants (common denominator: thin

red blood cells and target cells). In chronic obstructive jaundice, hemolysis occurs in 0.39-0.40% normal saline solution and is complete in 0.31% saline solution.

Rapid micromethod for recording red cell osmotic fragility: Danon[94, 95] developed the following method: Insert a dialyzing cell, containing 0.075 ml. of a 1:10 dilution of whole blood in isotonic saline solution, into a test tube of distilled water. Place the test tube into a colorimeter with a recorder. The degree of hemolysis is proportional to the increasing transparency of the red cell suspension. The increasing light transmission can be recorded as a function of time, yielding an osmotic fragility curve. This method requires less than 1 drop of blood and from 6-10 min. Its use has been suggested to determine the degree of deterioration of stored blood bank blood after 21 days.

Osmotic fragility after incubation at 37° C. for 24 hr.: The blood used should be sterile. It is defibrinated by shaking with glass beads.

Technique: Add 2 ml. defibrinated blood to two sterile screw-capped test tubes and incubate at 37° C. for 24 hr. Mix the two samples and determine osmotic fragility by the method of Dacie.

Normal range of osmotic fragility after 24 hr. incubation at 37° C.:

0.20% saline solution	95-100% hemolysis
0.30% saline solution	80-100% hemolysis
0.35% saline solution	75-100% hemolysis
0.40% saline solution	65-100% hemolysis
0.45% saline solution	55-95% hemolysis
0.50% saline solution	40-85% hemolysis
0.55% saline solution	15-70% hemolysis
0.60% saline solution	0-40% hemolysis
0.65% saline solution	0-10% hemolysis
0.70% saline solution	0-5% hemolysis
0.75% saline solution	0% hemolysis
0.85% saline solution	0% hemolysis

Significance: The red blood cells of hereditary spherocytosis, when incubated, show a greater increase in osmotic fragility than do normal cells. Osmotic fragility after incubation is also increased in nonspherocytic hemolytic anemia in which the osmotic fragility is normal.

Autohemolysis screening test: Distribute about 5 ml. blood (without hemolysis) into three tubes. Place one tube in the incubator at 37° C., leave one tube at room temperature, and place one tube in the refrigerator. Incubate for 24 hr. In paroxysmal nocturnal hemoglobinuria, hemolysis occurs in the tube incubated at room temperature and at 37° C.

Quantitative autohemolysis test:

Equipment and reagents: All equipment must be sterile.

1. 20 ml. syringe
2. 125 ml. Erlenmeyer flask containing 20 glass beads (3-4 mm. in diameter)
3. 10% glucose
4. Six 5 ml. screw-capped vials

Technique: A control test using normal blood should be run parallel with the unknown blood.

Obtain 20 ml. venous blood under sterile conditions. Separate 3 ml. and allow to clot to obtain preincubation serum. The rest of the blood is defibrinated in an Erlenmeyer flask. Add 2 ml. sterile defibrinated blood to each of six screw-capped 5 ml. vials. To three of the vials add 0.1 ml. 10% glucose to reduce autohemolysis. Incubate all six vials at 37° C. for 24 hr. After that time, mix bottles gently and incubate for another 24 hr. After 48 hr., if there is no contamination, pool each pair of bottles. Determine hematocrit and centrifuge specimen to obtain supernatant serum. The amount of hemolysis is estimated by measuring the amount of hemoglobin in the serum. Dilute the serum 1:25 or 1:50 in cyanmethemoglobin diluent and use the cyanmethemoglobin method for hemoglobin determination. A corresponding dilution of the preincubation serum is used as blank and a 1:100 or 1:200 dilution of whole blood in diluent is used as standard.

$$\% \text{Hemolysis} = (D_2 - D_3) \times \text{Dilution of serum} \times \frac{100 - \text{Hematocrit}}{D_1 \times \text{Dilution of blood}}$$

D_1 = OD of diluted whole blood
D_2 = OD of diluted serum after incubation
D_3 = OD of preincubation serum

Normal range: Lysis at 48 hr. is 0.4-4.5% without glucose and 0.03-0.4% with glucose.

Significance of increased autohemolysis: Increased autohemolysis with glucose

is seen in congenital and in most acquired hemolytic anemias and in paroxysmal nocturnal hemoglobinuria.

Mechanical fragility: In hemolytic anemias the mechanical fragility of the red blood cells is increased.

Technique: The test cells are hemolysed by shaking with glass beads and the degree of hemolysis is compared with that of normal red blood cells under similar circumstances. The test is not considered routine laboratory procedure. It is described by Dacie and Lewis.[96]

Normal range: 2-5% hemolysis.

Significance: Spherocytes, sickle cells, and agglutinated cells show increased susceptibility to mechanical trauma.

Tests on serum:

Serum bilirubin: There is elevation of the free nonconjugated bilirubin (indirect van den Bergh value).

Serum hemoglobin: In some hemolytic anemias the serum hemoglobin is elevated (hemoglobinemia).

Test for hemoglobinemia using Hematest reagent tablets[97]:

PRINCIPLE: The colorless orthotoluidine present in the solution of Hematest reagent acts as an oxygen acceptor. Hemoglobin and some of its degradation products possess properties comparable to those of peroxidase enzymes and, accordingly, liberate active oxygen from hydrogen peroxide. The orthotoluidine is then oxidized to a blue reaction product.

PROCEDURE:

1. Measure 10 ml. Hematest reagent into a pair of 19 × 150 mm. Coleman colorimeter tubes.
2. Add 0.02 ml. serum with a micropipette. Be sure to rinse carefully by drawing the solution up into the pipette and expelling it. Mix the tube by inversion. Prepare another tube containing 0.02 ml. standard (equivalent value 15 mg./100 ml.) and carry through the rest of the procedure.
3. In exactly 8 min. measure the optical density of %T using the 630 mμ wavelength.

CALCULATION: Convert photometer reading of unknown to concentration of unknown using standard curve or calculate concentration of unknown from optical densities of unknown and standard (which has been processed with unknown) as follows:

$$\frac{\text{OD of unknown}}{\text{OD of standard}} \times \text{Conc. of standard} =$$

$$\text{Conc. of unknown}$$

STANDARDIZATION: Pipette the following volumes of the dilute hemoglobin standard (100 mg./100 ml.) into 100 ml. volumetric flasks:

Dilute hemoglobin standard (ml.)	Water (ml.)	Equivalent concentration (mg./100 ml.)
5	100	5
10	100	10
15	100	15
25	100	25
50	100	50

Use 0.02 ml. of these solutions in place of the serum in step 2 of the procedure. The photometer readings are plotted against equivalent concentrations to obtain the standard curve.

NORMAL VALUES: 0-15 mg./100 ml. (sample collected in Vacutainer tube).

REAGENTS AND STANDARDS:

HEMATEST REAGENT: Thoroughly crush 4 Hematest reagent tablets and add 100 ml. distilled water. Mix thoroughly by shaking 3-4 min. Allow to stand 30 min. Filter through a Buechner funnel using Whatman No. 40 filter paper, double thickness. This reagent is not stable and should be discarded when it becomes discolored. Store in the refrigerator.

STANDARD HEMOGLOBIN SOLUTION: Wash 2-3 ml. whole blood three times with 0.9% sodium chloride. Lyse red cells by freezing and thawing. Dilute to approximately 10 gm./100 ml. hemoglobin and determine the exact hemoglobin content by the cyanmethemoglobin method. Prepare a dilute standard solution of 100 mg./100 ml. by diluting the stock appropriately. For example, if the stock is 10 gm./100 ml., pipette 1 ml. into 100 ml. volumetric flask. Make up volume with distilled water.

NOTES: Unknowns with values more than 100 mg./100 ml. should be repeated on diluted amounts. Unknowns with values less than 15 mg./100 ml. should be repeated using larger amounts of specimen and sufficient Hematest reagent to make 10 ml.

Serum haptoglobins: In hemolytic processes they are decreased.

Haptoglobins are a family of plasma proteins that move electrophoretically with alpha$_2$ globulins, are capable of uniting with hemoglobin, and are inherited according to the mendelian system. When united with hemoglobin, the haptoglobin-hemoglobin complex migrates electrophoretically with the beta$_1$ fraction. Free hemoglobin can be found between the beta and gamma fractions. Note that haptoglobin fails to bind myoglobin.

Quantitative serum haptoglobin determination:

Principle: Haptoglobin binds hemoglobin to form a stable compound, the haptoglobin-hemoglobin complex. It contains peroxidase which splits hydrogen peroxide and thus oxidizes benzidine and guaiacol from the colorless reduced form to the colored form.

There are two methods: (1) the electrophoretic method[98] and (2) the chemical method measuring the haptoglobin concentration in relation to its peroxidase activity.[99]

Electrophoretic method: This method is based on the fact that, when serum containing free hemoglobin and hapto-hemoglobin undergoes electrophoresis and is then stained for peroxidase activity, two bands are seen. The one further away from the application point represents the hemoglobin-haptoglobin combination, whereas the band closest to the application point represents free hemoglobin. A series of test tubes is prepared, each one containing 0.1 ml. serum. To these test tubes hemoglobin solutions increasing in concentration by increments of 10 mg.% are added. These mixtures are then subjected to electrophoretic action and stained for peroxidase activity. The last strip, which shows only one band of the hemoglobin-haptoglobin complex, represents the highest hemoglobin concentration in which the entire hemoglobin is taken up by the haptoglobin. The concentration of haptoglobin in the serum is expressed as the largest amount of hemoglobin in mg.% that the serum is capable of binding.

Normal values: Normal serum binds from 100-125 mg.% hemoglobin.

Variations: In the first 4 mo. of life there exists a **physiologic ahaptoglobinemia.** After this period, adult values are encountered.

In pathologic conditions the haptoglobin level is **elevated** in inflammatory conditions and is often directly proportional to the intensity of the inflammatory process and to the sedimentation rate.

In severe liver disease and in hemolytic processes, **ahaptoglobinemia** is frequently encountered, but there is always **hypohaptoglobinemia.**

Methemalbuminemia:

Spectroscopy: The bands are faint.

Schumm test: Cover serum or plasma with ether and add 0.1 vol. saturated solution of yellow ammonium sulfide, mix, and examine spectroscopically. In the presence of methemalbumin a positive Schumm test will show a sharp band at 558 mμ.

Urine tests: The urobilinogen is usually increased.

Tests for urinary hemosiderin, hemoglobin, and urobilinogen are described on pp. 37-39. In hemolytic anemias free hemoglobin may be present in the urine and the sediment may contain hemosiderin, which may be seen to encrust shed epithelial cells and casts on examination of the sediment.

Hemoglobinuria must be distinguished from the rarer myoglobinuria (see p. 40).

Fecal urobilinogen: In hemolytic anemias it is increased.

Technique: It is described on p. 453.

Bone marrow examination for type of response to hemolysis:

Erythroid hyperplasia: Marked erythroid hyperplasia involving all red cell precursor forms is present. The marrow hyperplasia may expand the marrow cavities and produce characteristic radiologic findings. The marrow hyperplasia has been classified into **effective** and **ineffective erythropoieses** as well as into compensated, decompensated, and dyseryth-

ropoietic hyperplasia. **Compensated** hyperplasia implies that the bone marrow produces an adequate number of cells to counteract the lytic process so that no anemia develops. **Decompensated** erythroid hyperplasia implies that the bone marrow production of red cells is inadequate to counterbalance the red blood cell destruction so that anemia results. The **dyserythropoietic** bone marrow is unable to respond to the call for increased red cell production.

Crises in hemolytic anemias: The term implies a sudden rapid drop in the blood count. In hemolytic anemias three types of crises may occur. If the exhausted (dyserythropoietic) bone marrow is suddenly not able to respond to the call for additional red blood cells, this sudden bone marrow failure is called **aplastic** or a **regenerative crisis.** Other forms of crisis are the **hemolytic crisis** characterized by a sudden increase in hemolytic activity and the **thrombotic crisis** that occurs in sickle cell anemia.

Red cell survival time: The normal lifespan of red blood cells is 120 days ± 20.

Ashby technique: Red cell survival can be measured by the Ashby technique of differential agglutination which requires the administration of compatible donor cells that nevertheless differ in type from those of the recipient. O cells, for instance, can be transfused into A, B, and AB recipients.

Isotope technique (transfusion method): Isotope methods allow not only the measurement of the survival time of the patient's own cells in his own circulation but also localization of the site of destruction as well as examination of their behavior in a recipient other than the patient. Red cells can be tagged with Cr[51]. The use of tagged red cells allows the following three experiments:

1. Injection of the patient's own tagged cells into the patient
2. Injection of the patient's tagged cells into a normal compatible recipient
3. Injection of tagged normal compatible donor cells into the patient

Depending on the behavior of the cells in these three circumstances, it can be established whether the hemolytic anemia

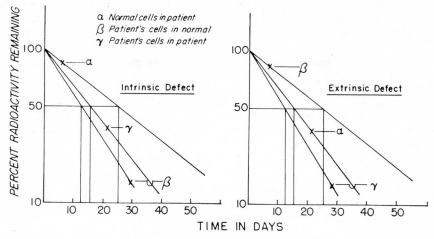

Fig. 4-40. Survival of red blood cells labeled with Cr[51] in transfusion studies. Normal half-time is about 25 days.

is intrinsic, extrinsic, or a mixture of both (Fig. 4-40).

HEMOLYTIC ANEMIAS DUE TO INTRACORPSULAR DEFECTS

Hereditary spherocytosis (congenital hemolytic jaundice, acholuric jaundice)

This is a hereditary disease transmitted as a mendelian dominant. The red cells have a shortened survival time due to an intrinsic defect as yet not identified. Various enzymatic and lipid deficiencies have been shown to exist. Splenectomy does not cure the basic disease but removes the site of hemolysis.

Hematologic findings: If the hemolytic process is compensated, there may be no anemia, but the blood smear will show spherocytes and an increased number of reticulocytes. If the hemolysis is more pronounced, anemia will result and the markedly increased number of reticulocytes will lead to a mixture of spherocytes and macrocytes. The MCHC may be elevated. The white cells and the platelets are not remarkable. The bone marrow is not diagnostic.

The osmotic fragility is markedly increased so that hemolysis may start at 0.7% saline solution. If there is any doubt, the osmotic fragility should be determined after incubation at 37° C. for 24 hr.

This method is of value in testing the asymptomatic members of the patient's family.

Serum findings: As in all hemolytic anemias, the indirect van den Bergh value is increased.

Urine and feces: The urobilinogen and stercobilinogen are increased.

Hereditary elliptocytosis

This is a condition in which red blood cells are oval. Usually the condition is asymptomatic. In normal blood smears, up to 1% of the cells may be elliptocytes (ovalocytes). The disease is transmitted as a mendelian dominant character.

Thalassemia (Cooley's anemia, Mediterranean anemia)[100]

This disease is the result of a biochemical change in the hemoglobin molecule. The thalassemia gene interferes with the synthesis of adequate amounts of hemoglobin A and with the incorporation of iron. It is transmitted as a mendelian dominant autosomal character. In the homozygous form it produces a severe disease called **thalassemia major**, whereas in the heterozygous form it produces a disease varying in intensity called thalassemia minor.

Thalassemia major:

Main laboratory findings: Most of the above-mentioned signs of hemolysis and red cell regeneration.

BLOOD SMEAR: It shows striking aniso-cytosis and poikilocytosis, emphasized by schistocytes, target cells, basophilic stippling, nucleated red cells, and reticulocytes (see Fig. 4-19). The smear is reminiscent of a severe microcytic hypochromic anemia, but when stained for free iron, siderocytes are found (the high plasma and bone marrow iron is also a differential diagnostic point). There may be a leukemoid type of leukocytosis. The platelets are normal. The cells are hypochromic so that the MCV is greatly reduced. The MCHC is only slightly reduced or normal. This relationship of MCV to MCHC suggests thalassemia rather than iron deficiency.

OSMOTIC FRAGILITY: Target cells are thinner than normal red cells and are therefore more resistant to hypotonic saline solutions, exhibiting a decreased osmotic fragility. Their mechanical fragility, on the other hand, is increased. In hypotonic saline solution the hemolysis begins at about the normal level but fails to be complete even below 0.1% concentration of saline solution. (See Fig. 4-38.) Note that severe iron-deficiency anemia will also show a decreased osmotic fragility.

HEMOGLOBINS: They are a mixture of normally occurring hemoglobins, but in abnormal amounts.

The hemoglobin in thalassemia major is a mixture of hemoglobins A, A_2, and F. The alpha-chain type of thalassemia major has a low A_2, while the beta-chain type has an elevated A_2. In beta-chain thalassemia, hemoglobins A_2 and F are relatively increased. The fetal hemoglobin (Fig. 4-41) may vary from 15-90% of the total hemoglobin, and hemoglobin A may vary from 20-80%. Hemoglobin A_2 will be found to be raised when compared to hemoglobin A rather than to the total hemoglobin (A + F). Hemoglobin F is demonstrated by the alkali denaturation method, while hemoglobin A_2 requires starch block, starch gel, agar gel, or cellulose acetate electrophoresis in Tris buffer.

In alpha thalassemia the hemoglobin is mainly hemoglobin Barts, with minimal amounts of hemoglobins A and F and some H. Electrophoretically, both hemoglobins Barts and H move fast. Hemoglobin H denatures easily within red cells and produces inclusions that can be stained with brilliant cresyl blue (see p. 134).

Thalassemia minor:

Laboratory findings: The anemia is slight, but there is anisocytosis and poikilocytosis. Target cells (Fig. 4-14, p. 134) may be very prominent. Hypochromia and osmotic resistance are the same as in thalassemia major. The morphologic changes far exceed the alterations expected from the mild degree of anemia. The high serum iron and the stainable iron in the bone marrow distinguish it from iron-deficiency anemia. The hemoglobins are a mixture of hemoglobins A, A_2, and variable amounts of F (Fig. 4-42). The hemoglobin A_2 always exceeds the normal level (2.0-2.5%), varying from 4-5%.

Thalassemia in combination with abnormal hemoglobins: Thalassemia may be found combined with hemoglobins S, C, E, and J. The thalassemia combinations must be differentiated from heterozygous forms of hemoglobin S, C, and E disease (A-S, A-C, A-E). In the latter conditions hemoglobin A exceeds the abnormal hemoglobins in amount, while in thalassemia combinations the abnormal hemoglobins predominate.

Hemoglobinopathies

Hemoglobin consists of a heme component and a protein moiety. The macrocytic (vitamin B_{12}-deficiency) and microcytic (iron-deficiency) anemias are essentially due to interference with the heme component. In the hemoglobinopathies an abnormality of the protein component exists, and the heme portion is unaffected. This abnormality is genetically controlled and is characterized by changes in the amino acid composition of the globin portion (alpha, beta, and gamma chains). There are three normally occurring varieties of hemoglobin: **hemoglobin F** (fetal hemoglobin), **hemoglobin A** (adult hemoglobin), and **hemoglobin A_2**. At birth most of the hemoglobin is hemoglobin F, but by the end of the first year of life only about 1% of the fetal hemoglobin can be detected. The abnormal hemoglobins are named by capital letters, more or less in order of their discovery. About 70 abnormal hemoglobins are known at the present time.

LABORATORY INVESTIGATION OF ABNORMAL HEMOGLOBINS[101]:

1. Fetal hemoglobin
   (a) Alkali denaturation
   (b) Agar gel electrophoresis (pH 6.0)
   (c) Kleihauer method
2. Hemoglobin electrophoresis
   (a) Paper electrophoresis
   (b) Starch gel or starch block electrophoresis
   (c) Agar gel electrophoresis
   (d) Cellulose acetate electrophoresis
   (e) Microzone method
3. Ferrohemoglobin solubility

Fetal hemoglobin:

Significance of fetal hemoglobin: In newborn infants 50-80% of the hemoglobin is fetal in type. It disappears during

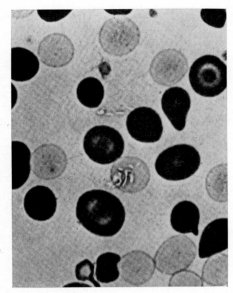

Fig. 4-41. Thalassemia major. (From Kleihauer: Zyto- und Histochemie in der Hämatologie, Berlin, 1963, Springer-Verlag.)

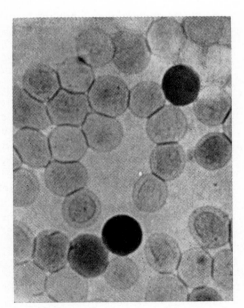

Fig. 4-42. Thalassemia minor. (From Kleihauer: Zyto- und Histochemie in der Hämatologie, Berlin, 1963, Springer-Verlag.)

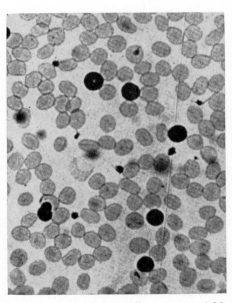

Fig. 4-43. Hemoglobin-F cells in maternal blood in fetal-maternal transfusion. (From Kleihauer: Zyto- und Histochemie in der Hämatologie, Berlin, 1963, Springer-Verlag.)

the first 4 mo. of life, leaving a residual of about 4% until the age of 2½ yr. It may persist for longer periods in anemic children, e.g., in hereditary spherocytosis. In adults 0.5-1.7% of the hemoglobin is fetal in type. Increased amounts of fetal hemoglobin are found in adults in thalassemia major (Fig. 4-41) and minor (Fig. 4-42) and in the various combinations of thalassemia with hemoglobins S, C, E, etc., in hereditary persistence of fetal hemoglobin, erythroleukemia, aplastic anemia, Fanconi-type anemia, hereditary spherocytosis, and in fetal-maternal transfusion (Fig. 4-43).

Methods for fetal hemoglobin:

Alkali denaturation method for fetal hemoglobin:

Principle: Under the conditions of the test, alkali converts adult hemoglobin to alkaline hematin within a period of 1 min. Alkaline hematin is not soluble and precipitates. Fetal hemoglobin resists alkali denaturation and remains in solution. The amount of fetal hemoglobin is expressed as a percentage of the initial total hemoglobin.

Reagents:
1. Exactly 1/12N KOH solution. To 10 ml. of exactly 1N KOH add 110 ml. distilled water. The final pH should be 12.7. Keep the solution in the refrigerator.
2. Acidified ammonium sulfate solution. To 800 ml. 50% saturated ammonium sulfate solution add 2 ml. concentrated HCl (prepare a saturated solution of ammonium sulfate and dilute 400 ml. with 400 ml. distilled water and add 2 ml. concentrated HCl).

Test: Pipette 1.6 ml. 1/12N KOH solution into a small test tube. Note time and add 0.1 ml. hemoglobin solution. Mix by blowing up and down with the pipette six times. In exactly 60 sec. add 3.4 ml. acidified ammonium sulfate solution. Mix by inverting and filter immediately through Whatman No. 44 filter paper. If not clear, refilter. Pink color in the filtrate denotes abnormal amount of hemoglobin F. Colorless filtrate denotes that the amount of hemoglobin F is normal or only slightly increased. Read the optical density of the filtrate in a spectrophotometer at 540 mμ, using distilled water as blank. This is the OD of fetal hemoglobin. Add 0.02 ml. hemoglobin solution to 5 ml. distilled water and read optical density at 540 mμ, using distilled water as blank.

Calculation:

$$\% \text{Hb-F} = \frac{\frac{1}{5} \text{ OD of filtrate}}{\text{OD of original Hb solution}} \times 100$$

The dilution of the fetal hemoglobin is 1:51 and that of the untreated hemoglobin is 1:251. The ratio is 51:251 or about 0.20 (⅕).

Normal values: In normal adults 0.5-1.7% of the hemoglobin is of fetal type.

NOTE: Hemoglobin Barts, which occurs in thalassemia, is also alkali resistant.

Abt-Downey test[102]: It is based on the alkali denaturation of fetal hemoglobin found in feces and gastric contents of bleeding newborn infants and serves to differentiate it from maternal blood.

Test: Mix the material with water about 1:10 to lyse the red cells. Centrifuge the mixture, separate the pink supernatant, and filter. Mix 1 ml. 1% sodium hydroxide with 5 ml. hemoglobin solution. After 2 min. incubation at room temperature, examine. Adult hemoglobin changes from pink to light brown, while fetal hemoglobin remains pink. Controls of mother's and infant's blood specimens are advisable.

Starch gel, starch block, or agar gel electrophoresis: Paper electrophoresis is not suitable to separate fetal and adult hemoglobins when the usual barbital or Tris buffers are used. This separation can be achieved by starch gel, starch block, and agar gel electrophoresis. Paper electrophoresis may be employed if the method of Schilling is used.[103]

Demonstration of fetal hemoglobin in the red blood cell by the acid dilution method of Kleihauer:

Principle: If air-dried and fixed blood smears are treated with citric acid phosphate buffer (McIlvaine), pH 3.3, at 37° C., the hemoglobin A is dissolved out of the red cells, while hemoglobin F, which is acid resistant, remains in the cells and can be stained.

Reagents:

1. McIlvaine citric acid phosphate buffer (pH 3.3):

   Citric acid monohydrate, 1.5016 gm.
   Disodium phosphate (Na_2HPO_4), 0.8094 gm.
   Distilled water, 100 ml.

2. Acid hematoxylin
3. Erythrosin B,* 1% aqueous solution

Technique: Fix blood smears in 80% ethyl alcohol for 5 min. Elute smears in Copling jar filled with buffer, warmed to 37° C., for 3 min. Leave Copling jar in water bath and remove slide momentarily every minute, mix buffer, and reinsert slide. Rinse in running water. Stain with acid hematoxylin for 3 min. Stain with erythrosin B for 3 min. Wash and mount with Permount.* Run a normal and newborn control.

Interpretation: The hemoglobin-A cells are recognizable as ghost cells, while the hemoglobin-F cells are bright red.

Application: This method has several areas of application (Figs. 4-41 to 4-43):

In hematologic disorders it allows evaluation of the quantity as well as the distribution of hemoglobin F in the red blood cells. Each red cell may contain either hemoglobin A or hemoglobin F or a mixture of both, as seen in the "intermediate" cells in newborn infants. The hemoglobin F is irregularly distributed in such conditions as thalassemia, hereditary spherocytosis, and erythroleukemia, some cells containing hemoglobin A or some abnormal hemoglobin, other cells containing hemoglobin F, and others containing a mixture of both. In hereditary persistence of fetal hemoglobin all cells contain hemoglobin F.

In the area of obstetrics and gynecology the Kleihauer method can be used to identify fetal cells in the maternal blood in cases of fetal-maternal bleeding which may be the cause of anemia in the newborn infant or of sensitization (e.g., Rh) of the mother. In cases of maternal vaginal bleeding at term or in rectal bleeding of the newborn infant the acid dilution method can be used to decide whether

the fetus is contributing to the mother's bleeding in the first case or whether the infant has ingested maternal blood in the second case.

Wilson et al.[104] attempted to improve the Kleihauer method, which at times results in inadequate differentiation of the adult and fetal cells. Their method, using ferricyanide, gives better differentiation but is complex and the reagents are unstable.

Hemoglobin electrophoresis[105]: The various hemoglobins differ in the speed with which they travel in an electric field on paper. In a Veronal buffer solution of pH 8.6 on paper the order will be as follows: Closest to the starting point is B_2 and then follows C, E, E_2, O, S, D, L, T, G, Q, A_1, A_3, M, F, K, J, N, H, and I. Some of the hemoglobins overlap so that complete separation by paper electrophoresis alone is not possible. Better separation can be achieved by using starch block or gel, agar gel, or cellulose acetate media or by altering the buffer.

Whatever method is used, the migration distances of the unknown hemoglobin are compared with the distances of various known hemoglobins which are included in the run. The latter can be obtained commercially in lyophilized form.* They are reconstituted with water or with TEB buffer (pH 9.1).†

Techniques:

Preparation of hemoglobin solution: Collect 3-5 ml. venous blood and put into tube containing an anticoagulant. Wash red cells three times with normal saline solution. Draw off saline and add 1.6 vol. distilled water to the cells. Mix and add approximately ⅕ vol. toluene. Shake vigorously for 5 min. Centrifuge at 2500-3000 rpm for 30 min. Suction off toluene and white layer. Filter hemoglobin solution. If the solution is not clear, centrifuge or filter again. The hemoglobin solution should be adjusted to about 10 gm. hemoglobin/100 ml. by adding distilled water.

---

*Fisher Scientific Co., New York, N. Y.

---

*Hyland Laboratories, Los Angeles, Calif.
†Tris(hydroxymethyl)aminomethane, 16.1 gm.; Na_2-EDTA, 1.56 gm.; boric acid, 0.92 gm.; and distilled water, 1000 ml.

Paper electrophoresis: The Beckman electrophoresis system or any other hanging strip method is satisfactory.

Buffers:

1. For preliminary classification of hemoglobin use **standard barbiturate buffer** (pH 8.6, ionic strength 0.05):

   Sodium diethylbarbiturate, 10.3 gm.
   Diethylbarbituric acid, 0.9 gm.
   Distilled water to 1 L.

   Spinco B-2 buffer is satisfactory if prepared as directed and then 500 ml. diluted with 250 ml. distilled water.

2. For demonstration of hemoglobin A_2, differentiation of hemoglobins C and E, and separation of hemoglobins S and F use **Tris buffer** (pH 8.9):

   Tris (hydroxymethyl) aminomethane, 50.4 gm.
   Ethylenediaminetetraacetic acid, 5 gm.
   Boric acid, 3.8 gm.
   Distilled water to 1 L.

3. For distinguishing hemoglobin C from hemoglobin E and some of the rarer fast hemoglobins from one another use **phosphate buffer** (pH 6.5, ionic strength 0.1):

   KH_2PO_4, 3.11 gm.
   $Na_2HPO_4 \cdot 2H_2O$, 1.87 gm.
   Distilled water to 1 L.

Method: The Whatman No. 3 MM strips are marked in the middle and 10-15μ of unknown and control hemoglobin solutions are applied with a wire sample applicator along the penciled line. The strips are already in position in the chamber and are wetted with buffer. Electrophoresis is allowed to proceed for 16 hr. at 190 volts. At the end of the time the strips are dried immediately in a preheated (120°-130° F.) oven. Staining is not necessary.

Micromethod for starch gel electrophoresis of hemoglobin[106]: This method is excellent for hemoglobin typing because it allows well-defined separation in about 80 min. or less.

Reagents:

1. Stock buffer (pH 8.8):

Tris (hydroxymethyl) aminomethane, 30.25 gm.
Ethylenediaminetetraacetic acid, 3.0 gm.
Boric acid, 2.3 gm.
Distilled water to 1000 ml.

2. Gel buffer:

   Dilute 1 part of stock buffer with 2 parts of distilled water.

3. Electrode chamber buffer (pH 8.2):

   Boric acid, 18.5 gm.
   Sodium hydroxide, 2.5 gm.
   Distilled water to 1000 ml.

   Add a few crystals of bromphenol blue to the buffer to visualize the borate front during the electrophoresis.

4. Starch: Hydrolyzed starch for gel electrophoresis (13.3 gm./100 ml. of gel buffer) may be obtained commercially.*

Preparation of gel: Mix 200 ml. gel buffer and 26.6 gm. hydrolyzed starch in 500 ml. Pyrex suction flask, cook, and degas. The gels are molded into clear plastic trays, 23 cm. in width, and divided into 8 even channels 10 cm. in length and 3 mm. in depth.

Technique: The hemoglobin solution is introduced into the gels by means of a 2 × 20 mm. strip of Whatman No. 3 MM filter paper inserted in cuts made with a razor blade. The hemoglobin-impregnated strips are laid on the blade and the cut is made vertically approximately 3 cm. from the cathodic end of the gel. Electric connections with the gels are made with heavy wick papers (Spinco-Beckman 319329). The starch is covered with a glass plate and the entire equipment is cooled during the run.

Cellulose acetate electrophoresis[107]: This method allows the detection of hemoglobin F in small amounts and separation of hemoglobin A_2 even in the presence of hemoglobin S. The hemoglobin A_2 separation correlates well with the values obtained with starch block electrophoresis.

Agar gel electrophoresis[108]: This system serves as a rapid screening method since

---

*Fisher Scientific Co., New York, N. Y.

all hemoglobin types may be separated and A₂ quantitated. For more refined separation, acrylamide gel electrophoresis and starch gel electrophoresis are desirable.

Reagents and apparatus:
1. Spinco electrophoretic system (Model R).
2. Stock barbital buffer (pH 8.6, ionic strength 0.075).
3. Working barbital buffer (pH 8.6, ionic strength 0.05). Dilute stock solution (2 parts of stock buffer to 1 part of water).
4. Glycine.
5. Agar gel. Dissolve by gently boiling 300 mg. Agarose* in 25 ml. working barbital buffer and 25 ml. H_2O. (Avoid excessive evaporation as this concentrates the buffer salts.) Add 0.7 gm. glycine and mix well.
6. Fixative solution (8% v/v glacial acetic acid–methanol solution). Dissolve 40 ml. acetic acid in 460 ml. methanol.
7. Thiazine stain (1% w/v aqueous thiazine solution). Dissolve 5 gm. thiazine red R† in 500 ml. distilled water and add 50 ml. glacial acetic acid.
8. Destaining solution (2% v/v aqueous acetic acid solution).
9. Sodium chloride (0.85%).
10. Toluene.

Procedure:
1. Preparation of hemolysate (see p. 171): Collect 5 ml. blood in EDTA and separate the cells from the plasma. In addition to the patient's hemolysate, prepare an Hb AA control and an Hb F control. An Hb AS control is also desirable. Adjust the hemoglobin concentration to approximately 5 gm.% with distilled water. Electrophoretic separation appears to be better at this hemoglobin concentration.
2. Coat film strips with 5 ml. agar gel and allow to harden.
3. Place strips on electrophoretic cell and inoculate 1.5 cm. to the cathode with 3 μL. of hemolysates, using the "stripper."
4. Allow to migrate at 150 volts for 120 min.
5. Fix, dry, and stain as for protein electrophoresis, except increase fixation time to at least 40 min. or until all glycine is removed.
6. When dry, scan in Analytrol* and calculate the percentage of the different hemoglobin fractions.

Microzone method: This method is described in Beckman Technical Bulletin, RM*TB-006, August, 1964, Stanford Industrial Park, Palo Alto, Calif., Spinco Division, Beckman Instruments, Inc.

FURTHER IDENTIFICATION OF ABNORMAL HEMOGLOBINS:

Hemoglobins S and D: The mobility of hemoglobin S coupled with the absence of sickling suggests hemoglobin D. Hemoglobins S and D can be separated by the ferrohemoglobin solubility test and by the Itano solubility test.

Ferrohemoglobin solubility test[109, 110]: The ferrohemoglobin solubility test and Itano solubility test are based on the low solubility of hemoglobin S in its reduced form.

Reagents:
1. Phosphate buffer:

   KH_2PO_4, 16.9 gm.
   K_2HPO_4, 21.7 gm.
   Distilled water up to 100 ml.

2. Sodium dithionite: $Na_2S_2O_4$, 20 mg.
3. Barbiturate buffer: same as used for serum protein electrophoresis
4. Normal saline solution

Technique: Wash 1 ml. oxalated blood three times in normal saline solution. After final wash, discard supernatant, add 2 vol. Veronal buffer for electrophoresis, mix, and freeze overnight in deep freeze. Allow to thaw in refrigerator and add 20 mg. $Na_2S_2O_4$ to 1.8 ml. phosphate buffer and 0.2 ml. hemoglobin solution. Mix and allow to stand for 15 min. Filter through Whatman No. 5 paper. Prepare a second preparation by adding 20 mg. $Na_2S_2O_4$ to 3.8 ml. buffer and add 0.2 ml. of the

---

*Bausch & Lomb, Rochester, N. Y.
†Allied Chemical Corp., New York, N. Y.

*Spinco Division, Beckman Instruments, Inc., Palo Alto, Calif.

first filtrate. Mix and read optical density at 415 mμ.

Control: Dilute 0.1 ml. original hemoglobin solution in 20 ml. saline solution.

Calculation:

$$\text{Solubility } \% = \frac{\text{OD test}}{\text{OD control}} \times 100$$

Significance: Solubility of hemoglobin S is very low. Solubility of hemoglobins A, F, and D is 90% or over.

Hemoglobin H: Intercytoplasmic inclusion bodies in red blood cells will confirm the diagnosis of hemoglobin H.

Hemoglobin H inclusion method: Incubate 2 parts blood with 1 part 1% cresyl blue in saline solution. After ½ hr. of incubation, red cells show inclusions in wet preparations and dried films.

Hemoglobins A$_2$ and E: Hemoglobins A$_2$ and E are indistinguishable by paper electrophoresis with Veronal buffer, but there are quantitative differences. Hemoglobin A$_2$ in thalassemia trait does not exceed 15% (normally it is less than 4%), while hemoglobin E usually amounts to at least 20%. Starch and agar gel electrophoresis may be used to separate hemoglobin A$_2$.

Hemoglobins A$_2$ and C: Hemoglobins A$_2$ and C cannot be distinguished on the basis of their electrophoretic position, but quantitatively they differ since hemoglobin A$_2$ never exceeds 6%, while hemoglobin C in A-C disease comes close to 50%.

Sickle cell disease: Sickle cell disease is due to the presence of hemoglobin S which is genetically determined (mendelian dominant). The homozygous disease is called **sickle cell anemia (disease)**, whereas the heterozygous condition is called **sickle cell trait.**

Sickle cell anemia: The homozygous form is a disease occurring in about 0.2% of American Negroes. There is a high infant and child mortality, and of the persons with this disease who survive the early years, very few reach 25 yr. of age. Clinically, the disease is characterized by enlargement of the liver and spleen (in later years the spleen contracts and fibroses), by the appearance of leg ulcers, and heart disease. In addition to the two types of crises occurring in all hemolytic anemias, i.e., hemolytic and aplastic, which rarely occur in sickle cell disease, there occur thrombotic crises that lead to infarctions in various organs. These crises are due to the vascular occlusion produced by the interlocking of sickle-shaped cells. In sickle cell anemia the hemoglobin is almost pure hemoglobin S (always over 70%); a moderate amount of hemoglobin F may be present. In sickle cell trait, hemoglobin S and hemoglobin A can be identified, hemoglobin S being usually below 50%. Hemoglobin S differs markedly from hemoglobin A in many respects. Reduced hemoglobin S, which is difficult to dissolve, not only gels into sickle-shaped crystalloid structures (tactoids) but also increases the viscosity of the blood.

Laboratory diagnosis of sickle cell disease:

Hematologic findings: Sickling is produced by the reduction of oxygen.

SODIUM METABISULFITE METHOD: Dissolve 1 sodium metabisulfite tablet (0.2 gm.)* in 10 ml. distilled water, prepared fresh each time. Mix 1 or 2 drops sodium metabisulfite solution with 1 drop blood, cover with cover glass, allow to stand for 15 min., and examine microscopically for sickling, using high-power dry lens.

INTERPRETATION: If **sickle cell disease** is present, sickling will occur in 15 min. If it fails to occur, rim slide with nail polish and allow to stand up to 24 hr. at room temperature. In **sickle cell trait** it may take that long for sickling to appear.

Electrophoresis of hemoglobin S: In sickle cell anemia the hemoglobin S exceeds hemoglobin F in amount. Hemoglobin A is absent. Hereditary persistence of high hemoglobin-F levels may prevent sickling and anemia in sickle cell disease (hemoglobins F and S). Hemoglobin S must be distinguished from hemoglobin D of the same motility by the ferrohemoglobin solubility test; the reduced hemoglobin S is almost insoluble.

Sickle cell trait: Hemoglobin electrophoresis reveals a combination of hemoglobins A and S, hemoglobin A exceeding hemoglobin S in amount.

Urinary findings: In sickle cell trait the

---

*Aloe Scientific Division, Brunswick Corp., St. Louis, Mo.

specific gravity of the urine is low, and aminoaciduria and hematuria are also present.

Combinations of hemoglobin S: The sickle cell gene is frequently combined with other abnormal hemoglobin genes such as sickle cell–thalassemia, sickle cell–hemoglobin C disease, and sickle cell–hemoglobin E disease.

Other hemoglobin variants:

Hemoglobin C: It may be inherited in the homozygous or in the heterozygous form associated with thalassemia or with hemoglobin S. In the homozygous form, target cells and intraerythrocytic hemoglobin crystals are seen.

Hemoglobin D: It has the same electrophoretic motility as hemoglobin S; its reduced form is easily soluble.

Hemoglobin H: Cells with hemoglobin H show inclusion bodies when stained with cresyl blue.

Hemoglobin M: It is associated with a hereditary form of methemoglobinemia but not with any hemolytic anemia. It is included here because its abnormal behavior is probably due to some globin abnormality.

Methemoglobinemia

Methemoglobin is an abnormal hemoglobin that firmly links to oxygen and thus, by shifting the oxyhemoglobin dissociation curve to the left, prevents the red cells from giving up oxygen so that anoxia and cyanosis are produced. The latter is characteristically out of proportion to the meager clinical findings (absence of evidence of heart or lung disease). The normal bivalent hemoglobin iron is oxidized to the trivalent form. In normal red cells there is an enzyme system (DPNH-methemoglobin reductase) that prevents the oxidation of hemoglobin to methemoglobin and is able to reduce normally formed methemoglobin to hemoglobin.

Classification of methemoglobinemia:

Toxic: The reductase system may be poisoned by the following:
Nitrates in food (spinach) or in drinking water
Aniline dyes in garments or marking inks
Acetylsalicylic acid
Sulfonamides, etc.

Congenital:
Due to hemoglobin M, which spontaneously oxidizes to methemoglobin at twice the rate of normal hemoglobin
Due to an inherited reductase deficiency, a recessive trait

Tests for methemoglobinemia: Spectroscopic or spectrophotometric methods are available (see p. 105).

Paroxysmal nocturnal hemoglobinuria (PNH)

This is a rather uncommon disease that is characterized by paroxysmal attacks of nocturnal hemoglobinuria (Plate 6) associated with the presence of pancytopenia, i.e., anemia, leukopenia, and thrombocytopenia. The disease is caused by at least two factors: (1) intraerythrocytic abnormality and (2) a plasma factor. However, the actual cause of the disease is still unknown. The erythrocytic defect is an enzymatic defect in the acetylcholinesterase activity. The plasma factor may be related to a complement-properdin-magnesium system, or it may be in the nature of an antibody or related to a thrombin-plasma factor system. The anemia is hemolytic. The red cells appear to be sensitive to the increase of carbon dioxide that occurs during sleep and lowers the pH of the plasma. The plasma is darker in the morning than during the rest of the day because of the hemolysis.

Acid-serum test (Ham): Defibrinate 10 ml. patient's blood in an Erlenmeyer flask containing 10 glass beads 3-4 mm. in diameter. Centrifuge the defibrinated specimen to separate the serum. The remaining cells are washed three times in normal saline solution and then used to prepare a 50% suspension of the washed cells in normal saline solution. Acidify 0.5 ml. serum by adding 0.05 ml. 0.2N HCl acid. Set up control using 0.5 ml. unacidified serum. Add 1 drop 50% suspension of patient's washed cells to each serum. Incubate at 37° C. for 1 hr. Centrifuge. If the cells are from a patient with paroxysmal nocturnal hemoglobinuria, marked hemolysis will occur after 15 min. Run a parallel test with normal cells.

Autohemolysis screening test: See p. 163.

Thrombin test (Crosby): Defibrinate

10 ml. patient's blood in Erlenmeyer flask containing 10 glass beads. Handle normal control blood the same way. Decant the blood and centrifuge to separate the serum. The cells are then washed three times in normal saline solution and the saline decanted after the last wash. The cells are then stored in refrigerator.

Number four tubes from 1-4 and place them in 37° C. water bath. Add to each tube 0.5 ml. normal saline solution and 0.05 ml. 0.2N HCl. To tubes 1 and 2 add 1 drop patient's cells and to tubes 3 and 4 add 1 drop normal control blood. To tubes 2 and 4 add 0.05 ml. topical thrombin solution* containing 50 units of thrombin.

Incubate all tubes at 37° C. for 15 min. Centrifuge for 2 min. at 1000 rpm and examine supernatant for hemolysis.

Significance: No hemolysis should occur with normal blood (tubes 3 and 4). In paroxysmal nocturnal hemoglobinuria, hemolysis occurs in tubes 1 and 2, and it will be greater in tube 2 than in tube 1.

Enzyme-deficient hemolytic anemias[111]

In this group are included the hemolytic anemias produced by the action of certain drugs (such as sulfanilamide, acetanilide, phenacetin, primaquine, phenylhydrazine, etc.) and of certain plants (such as the fava bean) in susceptible individuals. The cause of these anemias lies in the following hereditary enzyme deficiencies of the erythrocytes:

Glucose-6-phosphate dehydrogenase (G-6-PD) deficiency
Glutathione reductase (GSSG-R) deficiency
Reduced glutathione deficiency (GSH)
Pyruvate kinase deficiency
Diphosphoglyceromutase deficiency
Adenosine triphosphatase (ATPase) deficiency
Triose phosphate isomerase deficiency

The anemia produced by drugs in susceptible individuals is called drug-induced hemolytic anemia or primaquine-sensitive type of anemia because it was first investigated during World War II when some American Negroes developed hemolytic anemias following antimalarial treatment with 8-aminoquinolines.

These anemias are grouped under the heading of congenital nonspherocytic

hemolytic anemia. The autohemolysis test of Dacie mentioned on p. 164 was formerly used to classify these anemias into two types, depending on the presence (type 2) or absence (type 1) of increased hemolysis after the addition of glucose. These anemias are also called Heinz body anemias since some are characterized by the production of these red cell inclusions.

Congenital nonspherocytic hemolytic anemia

There is usually a history of jaundice and anemia dating back to infancy, both varying markedly in intensity from case to case and often related to drug administration. The smear may show pyknocytosis, macrocytosis, and reticulocytosis. The osmotic fragility is normal but is often increased after incubation at 37° C. for 24 hr. (see p. 163).

Screening tests for glucose-6-phosphate dehydrogenase deficiency: Various tests have been described in which red cells are hemolyzed in an environment of glucose-6-phosphate, TPN, and a receptor dye.

G-6-PD spot test (Fairbanks and Beutler)[112]: This test is commercially available as a kit.*

Technique: Anticoagulated blood is centrifuged and the packed cells are added to phosphate-treated DEAE (diethylaminoethyl cellulose or Whatman DE 81) paper on both sides with a Pasteur pipette to fill the printed circle. To elute the hemoglobin, immediately insert paper in distilled water for 20 min. When all the hemoglobin has been eluted, dissolve the reagents in the reagent vial and develop color by adding the spot test reagent to the spot on the paper. If G-6-PD is present, the spot turns purple within 2 min. If the enzyme is absent, little or no color change occurs.

Micromethod for detection of erythrocyte G-6-PD deficiency[113]: As many of the patients are children or infants, this method is especially useful.

Preparation of reagents:
1. Krebs-Ringer-phosphate buffer solution (pH 7.4):

---

*Parke, Davis & Co., Detroit, Mich.

*Calbiochem, Los Angeles, Calif.

0.9% NaCl (0.154M), 100 parts
1.15% KCl (0.154M), 4 parts
1.22% $CaCl_2$ (0.11M), 3 parts
3.82% $MgSO_4 \cdot 7H_2O$ (0.15M), 1 part
0.1M phosphate buffer (pH 7.4), 20 parts

2. Methylene blue solution (10M). Dissolve 100 mg. methylene blue chloride in 25 ml. distilled water.

Staining solution (prepared fresh each day):

1. Krebs-Ringer-phosphate buffer (pH 7.4), 10 parts
2. Methylene blue solution, 2 parts
3. 5% glucose solution in 0.9% saline solution, 1 part

Equipment:

1. Heparinized microhematocrit tubes (75 × 1.5 mm.)
2. Critocap* or clay
3. Microfuge
4. 37° C. incubator
5. Cover slips and glass slides

Procedure: Capillary blood is collected in a microhematocrit tube; one end is closed with a Critocap and the tube is centrifuged for 5 min., after which the Critocap is removed and the red cell column transferred by capillary attraction to a second hematocrit tube. The buffy coat and the plasma layer are left behind. The microhematocrit tube containing the red cell column is then dipped into a small test tube which holds the staining solution, and by capillary attraction an amount equal in volume to the red cell column is allowed to enter. The microhematocrit tube is then placed horizontally, with the ends open, in a 37° C. incubator for 2½-4 hr. At the end of the incubation period the tube is broken in the middle and cover slip smears are prepared, air dried, and mounted. The slides can then be examined under low magnification at a convenient time.

Result: Smears from normal individuals will contain approximately 10% red cells (7.8-16.9%) stained varying intensities of blue, while cells from patients with G-6-PD deficiency will not be stained at all or only faintly (0.0-0.2%).

It is important to use equal parts of staining solution and red cells because if disproportionate amounts of staining solution are employed a nonspecific staining of cells will occur.

***Methemoglobin reduction test of Brewer**[114]:*

Principle: Hemoglobin is oxidized to methemoglobin by sodium nitrate. In the presence of methylene blue, a dye, the methemoglobin is reduced to hemoglobin. In this reduction TPNH is utilized through the methemoglobin reductase system. In the normal, mature erythrocyte G-6-PD initiates the process by which TPN is reduced to TPNH. Cells deficient in G-6-PD generate inadequate amounts of TPNH and methemoglobin is not reduced.

Reagents:

1. Anticoagulant: 0.5 mg. heparin/1 ml. blood. Perform test within 1 hr.
2. 0.18M sodium nitrate and 0.28M dextrose solution:

   Dextrose, 5 gm.
   Sodium nitrate, 1.25 gm.
   Distilled water, 100 ml.

3. 0.0004M methylene blue chloride solution:

   Methylene blue chloride, trihydrated, 0.15 gm.
   Distilled water, 1000 ml.

Incubation tubes: Screw-top glass vials measuring 10-15 mm. internal diameter.

1. Normal reference tube: no reagent
2. Positive reference tube: 0.1 ml. sodium nitrite–dextrose solution
3. Unknown sample tube: 0.1 ml. sodium nitrite–dextrose solution; 0.1 ml. methylene blue solution

Method:

1. Add 2 ml. blood (normal, unknown, or known control) to both positive and normal reference tubes. Mix by inverting 15 times. Do not shake.
2. Add 2 ml. patient's blood to unknown sample tube and mix as before.
3. Incubate all three tubes at 37° C. for exactly 3 hr.
4. Mix tubes by inversion and test.
5. Add 10 ml. distilled water to three glass tubes of equal diameter.
6. Transfer 0.1 ml. from each incubated tube into one of the distilled water

---

*Scientific Products Division, American Hospital Supply Corp., Evanston, Ill.

tubes and mix by blowing through transfer pipette.

7. Within 2-10 min. after the transfer (dilution), compare the color of the unknown sample test tube visually with the colors of the positive and normal reference tubes.

Interpretation: In individuals with the full expression of the trait over 70% of methemoglobin remains after incubation. In normal individuals less than 5% persists.

Normal: The color in the diluted unknown sample tube is clear red, similar to that in the normal reference tube.

G-6-PD deficiency, full expression (hemizygous males, homozygous females): The color in the diluted unknown sample tube is dark gray or brown, similar to that in the positive reference tube.

G-6-PD deficiency, intermediate expression: The color in the diluted unknown sample varies from red to brown, according to the degree of expression of the enzyme defect.

Detection of glucose-6-phosphate dehydrogenase deficiency in heterozygotes[115]: Severe glucose-6-phosphate dehydrogenase deficiency is usually seen in males and its detection offers few problems. As the trait is sex-linked (X chromosome) and shows variable penetrance, several genotypic classes are found in females, normal and abnormal heterozygotes as well as homozygotes. The diagnosis of heterozygosity in the female is difficult to make with the tests available and is best accomplished by genetic family studies. A recent survey suggests that the methemoglobin reduction test (Brewer) is 80% successful in detecting heterozygotes.

Screening procedures for glucose-6-phosphate dehydrogenase deficiency, pyruvate kinase deficiency, and glutathione reductase deficiency using fluorescence (Beutler)[116]:

Principle of the procedures: Minute quantities of reduced pyridine nucleotide (TPNH) fluoresce when activated with long-wave ultraviolet light. The test for glucose-6-phosphate dehydrogenase (G-6-PD) deficiency is based on the reduction of oxidized pyridine nucleotide (TPN). The tests for pyruvate kinase (PK) deficiency or for glutathione reductase

(GSSG-R) deficiency are based on the oxidation of reduced pyridine nucleotide (DPNH). Blood is added to a reaction mixture, incubated at room temperature, spotted on filter paper, allowed to dry, and examined for fluorescence under ultraviolet light.

Fluorescence spot test for glucose-6-phosphate dehydrogenase:

Method: Glucose-6-phosphate in the reaction mixture is oxidized to 6-phosphogluconate, and triphosphopyridine nucleotide (TPN) is reduced to triphosphopyridine (TPNH) if G-6-PD is present. TPNH fluoresces when activated by ultraviolet light.

Reaction mixture:

1. Glucose-6-phosphate (0.01M), 0.1 ml.
2. TPN (0.0075M), 0.1 ml.
3. Saponin (Mann), 1%, 0.2 ml.
4. Potassium phosphate buffer (pH 7.4, 0.25M), 0.3 ml.
5. Distilled water, 0.3 ml.

Test: 0.02 ml. heparinized or EDTA anticoagulated blood is added to 0.2 ml. reaction mixture and allowed to incubate at room temperature for 5 min. At the end of this period a spot is made on Whatman No. 1 filter paper. The spot will fluoresce under ultraviolet light if normal G-6-PD activity is present, and it will fail to do so if the blood is G-6-PD deficient. A base line spot may be applied before the incubation is started.

Fluorescence spot test for pyruvate kinase:

Method: Pyruvate kinase leads to the formation of pyruvate and adenosine triphosphate in the reaction mixture. The pyruvate is reduced to lactate by the lactate dehydrogenase in the blood and at the same time the reduced diphosphopyridine nucleotide (DPNH) is oxidized to diphosphopyridine nucleotide (DPN), which does not fluoresce. There is therefore gradual loss of fluorescence.

Reaction mixture:

1. Phospho(enol)pyruvate (PEP), tricyclohexyl ammonium salt (0.15M), neutralized,* 0.03 ml.
2. ADP (0.03M), neutralized,* 0.1 ml.

---

*Neutralized to pH 7-8 with pH paper, using approximately 0.2N NaOH.

3. DPNH (0.015M), neutralized,* 0.1 ml.
4. $MgSO_4$ (0.08M), neutralized,* 0.1 ml.
5. Potassium phosphate buffer (pH 7.4, 0.25M), 0.05 ml.
6. Distilled water, 0.62 ml.

Test: Centrifuge heparinized or EDTA anticoagulated blood, remove plasma and buffy coat, and add 4 vol. physiologic saline solution to prepare a 20% red blood cell suspension. Add 0.02 ml. red blood cell suspension to 0.20 ml. reaction mixture. Apply control spot on filter paper (Whatman No. 1) and allow mixture to incubate at 37° C. for 30 min. and apply second spot. If pyruvate kinase is present, the original fluorescence will have disappeared, while it persists in pyruvate kinase–deficient samples.

Fluorescence spot test for glutathione reductase:
Method: Oxidized glutathione (GSSG) in the reaction mixture is reduced to GSH in the presence of glutathione reductase. At the same time TPNH is oxidized to TPN. TPNH fluoresces under ultraviolet light, while TPN does not. There is therefore a gradual loss of the fluorescence.

Reaction mixture:
1. GSSG (0.003M), 0.1 ml.
2. TPNH (0.015M), 0.1 ml.
3. Potassium phosphate buffer (pH 7.4, 0.25M), 0.6 ml.
4. Saponin (Mann), 1%, 0.2 ml.

Test: Add 0.02 ml. heparinized or EDTA anticoagulated blood to 0.20 ml. reaction mixture. Spot filter paper every 15 min. and compare disappearance of fluorescence with control test. In glutathione reductase deficiency the fluorescence fails to disappear.

Quantitative assay of G-6-PD: A method has been described by Ellis and Kirkman.[117]

Glutathione stability test[118]**:** When blood of individuals deficient in G-6-PD is incubated with acetylphenylhydrazine, a rapid decrease in glutathione levels occurs.

Heinz bodies: In toxic hemolytic ane-

mias due to the action of compounds such as phenylhydrazine, naphthalene, nitrobenzene, etc. Heinz bodies are produced in the red blood cells. They can also be found following splenectomy.

In the primaquine-sensitive type of anemia the red blood cells develop Heinz bodies under the influence of a great number of drugs that normally do not initiate hemolytic episodes. These anemias are mentioned in the section on enzyme-deficient anemias (p. 176).

Congenital Heinz body anemia that is not related to drug administration has also been described. In some instances Heinz body formation is associated with the production of methemoglobin (see p. 175).

Heinz bodies are irregularly shaped, deep purple inclusions within red cells. They vary from minute structures to 2μ globoid bodies which are frequently arranged peripherally.

Heinz body test:
Reagents:
1. Methyl violet, 0.5 gm.
2. Saline solution, 100 ml.

Technique: In a white cell counting pipette, mix equal volumes of capillary blood and dye. Allow it to stand for 15 min., make a smear with the mixture, and examine for Heinz bodies under oil immersion.

Interpretation: Normal red cells may contain 1-2 Heinz bodies. Cells deficient in G-6-PD contain over 5 Heinz bodies.

HEMOLYTIC ANEMIAS DUE TO EXTRACORPUSCULAR DEFECTS—ACQUIRED HEMOLYTIC ANEMIAS

Introduction to immunohematology: Immunohematology embraces all disease complexes that arise from the action of autoantibodies on the hematopoietic system of the individual and includes the following: (1) autoimmune hemolytic anemia due to antierythroid antibodies, (2) autoimmune thrombocytopenia due to antiplatelet antibodies, and (3) autoimmune leukopenia due to antileukocytic antibodies. Various combinations of these antibodies may occur.

Autoantibodies: Autoantibodies are antibodies that react with the individual's own tissues. Similar to all other anti-

---

*Neutralized to pH 7-8 with pH paper, using approximately 0.2N NaOH.

bodies, these antibodies are **immune gamma globulins.** If they react best at low temperature (4° C.), they are called **cold autoantibodies** (19S, IgM); they usually act best in a saline medium. If they act best at body temperature (37° C.), they are called **warm antibodies** (7S, IgG); they act best in a high molecular protein medium and are demonstrable with the Coombs technique. This division is not always clear-cut since each one of these antibodies may be bivalent (complete or saline acting) or univalent (incomplete or high molecular medium acting). If complement and/or properdin is available, they may be **hemolyzing.** Various theories have been advanced as to the circumstances that lead to the formation of antibodies against the individual's own cells: (1) the blood cells may be altered immunologically by the action of bacteria, viruses, enzymes, drugs, etc.; (2) they may be altered immunologically by the presence of abnormal proteins in the serum (e.g., cirrhosis); (3) the antibodies may be the result of abnormally functioning cells (e.g., abnormal proteins produced by lymphoblasts).

Autoimmune hemolytic anemias[119]

In **idiopathic** autoimmune hemolytic anemia, as the name implies, the underlying cause is not known. It may have to do with an abnormal ability of the patient to produce antibodies in response to relatively minor antigenic stimulation.

Symptomatic autoimmune hemolytic anemias frequently accompany lymphomas, lymphatic leukemia, infectious mononucleosis, macroglobulinemia, collagen diseases such as lupus erythematosus, virus diseases such as hepatitis and virus pneumonia, ovarian tumors, and cirrhosis.

Hematologic findings: They are the same as in any hemolytic anemia. The anemia is frequently the macrocytic type and shows moderate reticulocytosis, occasional spherocytes, siderocytes, normoblasts, and polychromatic cells. The osmotic fragility will depend on the number of spherocytes. Autohemolysis is excessive, and the blood samples may show autoagglutination. The sedimentation rate

is increased, showing an ill-defined zone between plasma and red cell mass consisting of reticulocytes. White blood cells and platelets may be normal or depressed. Acute hemolytic episodes are usually accompanied by leukocytosis.

Nonhematologic findings: The findings in the urine and serum are the same as in any hemolytic anemia. The serum frequently contains autoantibodies that are able to act on all human red blood cells, similar to isoantibodies. Investigation of autoantibodies necessitates the following steps:

Serologic investigation of autoimmune hemolytic anemia*:

1. Establish the existence of sensitizing (red blood cell coating) antibodies with the direct quantitative antiglobulin test (Coombs test), using anti-gamma and anti-nongamma globulin sera.

2. Establish the nature of the antibodies. Are they warm or cold? A positive anti-gamma globulin test points toward warm antibodies coating the red cells, while a positive nongamma globulin test is suggestive of cold antibodies.

3. Determine their specificity. If a warm antibody appears to be present, elute the antibody from the red blood cells and confirm its existence by the indirect Coombs test, using trypsinized and nontrypsinized red cells of known antigenic composition (Hemantigen† or Selectogen‡). Confirm the adequacy of the eluate by repeating the direct Coombs test on the eluted cells—it should be negative or only weakly positive. If the eluate contains a warm antibody, determine its exact specificity by the use of a panel of cells in albumin medium (by the Coombs technique). In hemolytic anemias the most frequently found antibodies are cold antibodies that act best in saline solution.

---

*For further details of method, see discussion of blood banking.
†Chas. Pfizer & Co., Inc., New York, N. Y.
‡Ortho Pharmaceutical Corp., Raritan, N. J.

4. If a cold antibody appears to be present, proceed as follows: Is the antibody directed against the patient's own cells (isoantibody)? Is it directed against all types of red cells (autoantibody)? Is it directed against human and animal red cells (heteroantibody)?

5. Determine the titer. Normally occurring cold agglutinin titers do not exceed 1:32. A titer of 1:64 is pathologic. Usually in hemolytic anemias the cold agglutinin titer is very high (between 4000 and 128,000) and falls with increasing temperature. The red cell agglutination is reversible at 40° C.

Detection, titration, and determination of thermal amplitude of cold, complete, saline-acting antibodies or of incomplete albumin-acting antibodies:

Technique: Set up 13 test tubes (12 × 75 mm.) and label 1-12 and control. Add 0.1 ml. saline solution to each tube except the first. Add 0.1 ml. serum to tubes 1 and 2. Mix contents of tube 2 and transfer 0.1 ml. to tube 3. Mix and transfer as before. Discard 0.1 ml. from tube 12. Add 0.1 ml. 2% suspension of group O red cells in saline solution to each tube and shake. The control tube contains only saline solution and red cell suspension. Incubate for 2 hr. at room temperature (20° C.). Centrifuge. Dislodge red cell button and read macroscopically for agglutination.

The dilutions are 1:1, 1:2, 1:4, 1:8, 1:16, 1:32, 1:64, 1:128, 1:256, 1:512, 1:1024, and 1:2048. The saline titer is the highest dilution showing agglutination. After reading the titer at room temperature, resuspend cells in all the tubes by shaking the rack and place in refrigerator for 2 hr. at 4° C. Read again before cells can warm up. Shake rack and place in water bath for 2 hr. at 37° C.

By substituting 20-22% albumin for saline solution the test can be used for incomplete antibodies and the direct Coombs test can be done on all nonagglutinated cells, after washing them three or four times with saline solution. The antiglobulin titer is the highest dilution giving agglutination.

Cold agglutinins[120]:

Determine specificity: Wiener described an anti-I specificity of cold agglutinins but noted that I-negative cells are also agglutinated at 4° C. The majority of cold agglutinins are of anti-I type, but anti-H or anti-O types have also been found.

Determine hemolytic activity:

TYPES OF HEMOLYSINS: According to their dependency on temperature and pH, three types of hemolysins can be distinguished:

1. Biphasic type
2. Monophasic type, with or without acid
3. Warm type, with or without acid

The pathologic cold agglutinins are acid cold hemolysins. The reaction is monothermal and does not require the biphasic temperature arrangement described for the Donath-Landsteiner test. The hemolysis is most marked at pH 6.6-7.0 and usually ceases when the pH rises to 8.0 or falls to 6.0.

Warm hemolysins are uncommon and are similar to the acid cold hemolysins except that they unite optimally with red cells at 37° C.

Screening test for cold hemolysins of monothermal types excluding Donath-Landsteiner hemolysins: Set up seven test tubes (75 × 10 mm.). Prepare 50% suspension of washed group O red blood cells in saline solution or 5% suspension of trypsinized or PNH red cells in saline solution. Deliver red cells directly into serum.

Tube 1	0.5 ml. patient's serum 0.05 ml. 0.2N hydrochloric acid 0.05 ml. 50% group O cell suspension
Tube 2	0.25 ml. patient's serum 0.25 ml. normal serum 0.05 ml. 0.2N hydrochloric acid 0.05 ml. 50% group O cell suspension
Tube 3 (control)	0.5 ml. patient's serum 0.05 ml. 50% group O cell suspension
Tube 4 (control)	0.5 ml. normal serum 0.05 ml. 0.2N hydrochloric acid 0.05 ml. 50% group O red cell suspension
Tube 5	0.25 ml. patient's serum 0.25 ml. 5% suspension of group O trypsinized red cells of PNH cells
Tube 6	0.125 ml. patient's serum 0.125 ml. normal serum

0.25 ml. 5% suspension of group O
trypsinized red cells or of PNH
cells

Tube 7   0.25 ml. normal serum
(control) 0.25 ml. 5% suspension of group O
trypsinized red cells or of PNH
cells

The tubes are incubated for 1 hr. at room temperature (20° C.), at 4° C., and at 37° C. In the latter case all equipment and material should be warmed to 37° C. prior to the test. Centrifuge gently and inspect for lysis.

Results: In immune hemolytic anemias, hemolysis is seen in the tube of acidified patient's serum (pH 6.5-7.0), and no lysis is observed in the unacidified tube (pH 8.0). Trypsinized red cells and paroxysmal nocturnal hemoglobinuria red cells are more sensitive to hemolysis than normal red cells. Normal serum is added to ensure adequate amounts of complement.

Detection of Donath-Landsteiner hemolysin, biphasic type: This antibody occurs in paroxysmal cold hemoglobinuria and differs from the high-titer monophasic hemolysin in that it is biphasic, acts in nonacidified serum, and readily lyses normal red cells. The term "biphasic" implies that the hemolysin and the complement are bound to the red cells at low temperature (0°-10° C.), but hemolysis does not occur until 15°-30° C. is reached. Complement is needed for lysis. The patient's own red cells or group O cells may be used for the test.

Technique: In a syringe warmed to 37° C. collect 5 ml. patient's blood and allow to clot in a 37° C. water bath. Separate the serum in a centrifuge tube surrounded by a 37° C. water jacket.

Prepare a 50% suspension of normal group O cells washed in saline solution. In each of two test tubes place 1 ml. of washed cells and 9 ml. of patient's serum. Mix and place 1 tube immediately into crushed ice at 0° C. for 30 min. Place the other tube in a water bath at 37° C. After 30 min. remove the first tube from ice and deposit it in the 37° C. water bath for 1 hr. Centrifuge both tubes at 1000 rpm for 2 min. and examine serum for hemolysis.

Results: In paroxysmal nocturnal hemoglobinuria the serum of the chilled suspension should contain free hemoglobin. The serum of the clot kept at 37° C. should be free of hemolysis. In paroxysmal cold hemoglobinuria the serum of the chilled and then warmed tube contains free hemoglobin. Repeat a negative test with a mixture of 50% patient's serum and 50% normal serum to ensure adequate amounts of complement.

Interpretation: Biphasic cold hemolysins occur in syphilitic paroxysmal hemoglobinuria.

Hemolytic anemias due to isoantibodies

There are two types of hemolytic anemias due to isoantibodies—erythroblastosis fetalis and hemolytic transfusion reactions.

Erythroblastosis fetalis or hemolytic disease of the newborn (HDN)

Erythroblastosis fetalis is a hemolytic anemia of the fetus and newborn infant and is due to the action of antierythrocytic isoantibodies that are transferred across the placenta from the mother to the fetal circulation. The maternal antibodies are produced in response to fetal cells which escape into the maternal circulation and contain antigens which the mother lacks. Though erythroblastosis due to Rh incompatibility was the first form to be described, ABO erythroblastosis is more common, but less dangerous. Any fetal antigen that the mother lacks may be responsible for erythroblastosis. The fetal hemolytic process leads to jaundice, release of toxic free bilirubin, and an anemia which may be severe enough to cause fetal heart failure with edema (hydrops fetalis). Unless the mother has been stimulated to produce antibodies by parenteral administration of blood prior to the first pregnancy, erythroblastosis fetalis usually does not involve the first child.

Rh erythroblastosis: Many factors determine the incidence of erythroblastosis: (1) constitutional factors that determine the ease with which an individual can be sensitized, (2) the antigenicity of the antigen (e.g., D is more antigenic than C, and c is more antigenic then E or e), (3) the paternal genotype (heterozygosity or homozygosity for the antigen) affects the incidence of erythroblastosis, and (4) the ABO type of the fetal red blood cells which on one hand may be responsible for the production of ABO erythroblastosis, but on the other hand may protect the baby from Rh erythroblastosis.

Production of anti-Rh antibody: Most of the clinical Rh sensitizations in the Rh-negative group are due to the presence of anti-Rh_o. Considering that 85% of the Caucasian population is Rh_o positive and 15% is Rh_o negative, about 13% of all marriages would be between Rh_o-positive husbands and Rh_o-negative wives; yet erythroblastosis occurs not oftener than once in about 300-1000 births.

If the father is homozygous (RhRh), all of his children will be Rh positive and susceptible to the disease; if he is heterozygous (Rhrh), one half of the children should be Rh negative and escape the disease. About five times as many cases of erythroblastosis occur when the father is homozygous. Fortunately, all who are susceptible do not develop erythroblastosis. The Rh-positive cells may not pass through the placental barrier; the mother may not be sensitized even if such passage does occur (anergy).

It has been estimated that some leakage of blood from the fetus to the mother through the placenta occurs in all pregnancies, maximally during delivery. Repeated pregnancies with Rh-positive fetuses may be necessary to raise the anti-Rh titer sufficiently high to cause erythroblastosis.

Hematologic picture: See Plate 6. In the newborn infant the demonstration of a hemolytic anemia, usually macrocytic, with a rising count of nucleated red blood cells and with leukocytosis including eosinophils and a few immature leukocytes (promyelocytes and myelocytes) suggests erythroblastosis. The presence of over 10 nucleated red blood cells/100 white blood cells is very suggestive of erythroblastosis, but may be found in normal but immature infants.

Serologic and biochemical findings: The diagnosis of HDN may be confirmed by a high serum bilirubin, by the incompatibility of the bloods of the mother and child (or husband), by demonstration of the presence in the infant's blood of a specific isohemolysin capable of hemolyzing the infant's red blood cells, or by demonstrating sensitized red blood cells of the infant by the direct Coombs test.

Cord bilirubin: The cord blood bilirubin level of the normal mature newborn infant averages about 2 mg.%. The level increases to about 6 mg.% at 24 hr. and to about 7 mg.% (3-13 mg.%) at 48 hr., decreasing after the second day.[121, 122] In healthy premature infants the level for the first 2 days is about normal but it continues to rise for the next 2 days. In erythroblastosis the cord blood level is high (2.1-10.3 mg.%), averaging about 5 mg.%, and the level increases more rapidly and to a higher peak than normal, even to 40 mg.% by the third day.[121, 122]

An initial cord blood level above 3 mg.% usually and above 6 mg.% nearly always is evidence of erythroblastosis. A high or rapidly increasing level is indication for exchange transfusion in order to prevent kernicterus (cerebral jaundice), which is not so likely to occur with a level below 20 mg.%, but is quite likely with a level at or above 20 mg.%.

The **serologic aspects,** including **exchange transfusion,** are discussed on p. 276.

ABO erythroblastosis

ABO erythroblastosis may result from the immunization of a group O mother by agglutinogens A and B of the fetal red blood cells. The theoretic basis for this immunization is the C factor which is shared by the antigens A and B, but which is absent in antigen O. The C factor is not related to the Rh antigen C. The immunized mother with group O blood may thus develop immune anti-A or rarely anti-B antibodies which are capable of traversing the placenta and producing erythroblastosis in infants with group A, B, and AB blood. The normal isoantibodies anti-A and anti-B do not pass the placenta.

For laboratory investigation of ABO erythroblastosis, see p. 278.

Hemolytic transfusion reactions

A hemolytic reaction will occur if antibodies are present in the donor's plasma which are active against the recipient's red cells.

Hematologic picture: Within 24 hr. a very rapidly progressing hemolytic anemia makes itself noticeable by a rapid drop in hemoglobin, hematocrit, and number of red blood cells associated with hemoglobinemia and hemoglobinuria. The latter may lead to anuria and uremia. For laboratory investigation of hemolytic transfusion reactions, see p. 263.

Toxic hemolytic anemias

In this group there are hemolytic anemias produced (1) by the action of exogenous agents on nonenzyme-deficient red blood cells and (2) by the action of endogenous agents.

The **exogenous agents acting on normal red blood cells** are such substances as phenol derivatives, lysol, aniline dyes, nitrobenzene, amyl nitrite, and mushroom and snake venoms.

Hematologic picture: There may be an initial leukocytosis, which later gives way to leukopenia. The degree of hemolysis and the reparative response will be in direct relationship to the degree of toxicity.

Lead poisoning (plumbism): The anemia in lead poisoning may be acute or chronic. It has all the characteristics of a hemolytic anemia, but there are certain features that are characteristic.

Basophilic stippling consists of numerous fine to coarse dark dots scattered throughout the cytoplasm of red cells or confined to the periphery. Their presence indicates young, damaged red cells (see p. 137).

Urine examination: Because of the interference with the porphyrin metabolism, coproporphyrins are increased in stool and urine, and delta-aminolevulinic acid levels are augmented. The lead level in urine and blood is elevated.

For screening tests for coproporphyrins in feces and urine, see p. 42.

Endogenous agents producing hemolytic anemias occur in uremia and following extensive burns and may lead to the production of burr cells and schistocytes.

Infectious toxic agents are responsible for the hemolytic anemia accompanying many bacterial infections such as those produced by hemolytic streptococci, staphylococci, *Clostridium perfringens*, pneumococci, and cholera bacilli. Parasitic infections such as malaria, kala-azar, Oroya fever, and bartonellosis are frequently causes of hemolytic episodes.

Bartonellosis: In active infections the causative organism, *Bartonella bacilliformis*, can be found in the red blood cells of patients who have a progressive, frequently macrocytic hemolytic anemia associated with fever (Oroya fever) and a skin eruption (verruga peruana). Incidence of the human infection is confined to Peru, Colombia, and Ecuador.

APLASTIC ANEMIAS

Definition: Aplastic anemia can be defined as an idiopathic pancytopenia resulting not only from marrow insufficiency but from a collapse of all hematopoietic activity. Myelofibrosis and myelosclerosis, which also lead to marrow failure, stimulate the production of blood in extramedullary hematopoietic centers.

Etiology:

1. **Idiopathic.** In most patients the cause remains unknown.
2. **Constitutional.** Hereditary factors determine the development of the anemia in later years. Into this group fall the congenital hypoplastic anemia of Diamond-Blackfan and the anemia seen in Fanconi syndrome.
3. **Secondary.** These anemias follow therapy by radioactive isotopes, ionizing radiation, or antimetabolites. They may also follow therapy by almost any drug, which in susceptible patients may produce bone marrow depression. Some drugs are especially noted for this effect, e.g., thiouracil, gold, aminopyrine, and phenylbutazone. It is difficult to incriminate any one drug, as usually more than one is administered, and the role of the primary disease for which the drugs are given must also be considered.

Hematologic findings: There is a severe normochromic anemia associated with leukopenia and thrombocytopenia. The differential count shows lymphocytosis and anisocytosis and poikilocytosis of the red cells. The reticulocytes are diminished as a result of the depressed erythropoiesis.

Bone marrow: There is marrow insufficiency, as evidenced by a paucity of hematopoietic cells, moderate lymphocytosis, and slight plasmacytosis. The marrow may be hypercellular and erythroblastic in some areas, but in others it will be acellular.

Nonhematologic findings: The serum iron is elevated and the urine may contain an abnormal amino acid pattern.

MYELOPROLIFERATIVE DISORDERS

In the group of myeloproliferative disorders a number of diseases are included that may or may not be related, at times overlap, and have the following features in common: (1) their etiology is unknown; (2) they originate in erythropoietic cells, either in the bone marrow or in extrameduallary sites such as liver and spleen; (3) they are characterized by the proliferation of one or the other or of all elements occurring in the bone marrow; and (4) the proliferation is progressive, irreversible, and malignant. The benign forms of bone marrow proliferation, the cause of which is usually known and which represent temporary leukemoid reactions, are not included in the category of myeloproliferative disorders.

Classification
Chronic types
  Polycythemia vera
  Myelosclerosis with myeloid metaplasia
  Chronic granulocytic leukemia
  Chronic erythemic myelosis (Heilmeyer)
  Thrombocytosis and thrombocythemia
Acute types
  Acute erythremic myelosis (di Guglielmo's disease)
  Acute granulocytic leukemia

POLYCYTHEMIA

Polycythemia is a term used to describe an increase in the number of circulating erythrocytes, above 6 million/mm.³.

CLASSIFICATION:
Polycythemia vera (erythremia, Vasquez-Osler disease)
Secondary polycythemia (anoxic erythrocytosis)
Symptomatic polycythemia
Relative polycythemia (hemoconcentration, dehydration)

Polycythemia vera (erythremia)[123]

Laboratory findings:
Peripheral blood: The red blood cell count is elevated, varying from 7-9 million/mm.³ or even higher. The hemoglobin level is raised, but usually lags behind the red cell count so that the cells are hypochromic. The erythrocytosis is accompanied at times by a pronounced leukocytosis, which may vary from 10,000-15,000/mm.³ but may reach much higher levels. The platelets are also increased, reaching levels of about 1 million/mm.³.

The **differential count** reveals a shift to the left of the myeloid elements and often an increase in basophils and eosinophils. The lymphocytes are always relatively, and often absolutely, decreased. The alkaline phosphatase contents of the segmented forms is increased. This increase occurs in no other forms of polycythemia. The red cells may show some anisocytosis, poikilocytosis, and hypochromasia. The polychromasia roughly corresponds to the reticulocytosis seen with vital dyes.

The **hematocrit** is markedly increased, reflecting the increase in the total blood volume, in particular in the red cell volume, as the plasma volume remains normal. The viscosity of the blood is increased and the sedimentation rate slowed to almost 0-1 mm. Hypercoagulability of the blood is often associated with a bleeding tendency. The oxyhemoglobin saturation is normal.

Serum: The increased uric acid level reflects the stimulated nucleic acid metabolism. No increased amounts of erythropoietin can be demonstrated.

Bone marrow: It is hyperplastic, the hematopoietic elements crowding out the adipose tissue. All hematopoietic components are increased, though characteristically the emphasis is on megakaryocytes and on erythroblasts. The stimulation of myelocytes and of promyelocytes, though present, is less marked.

Table 4-8. Laboratory tests in differential diagnosis of polycythemia

Laboratory test	Relative polycythemia (hemoconcentration)	Erythrocytosis (secondary polycythemia)	Erythemia (polycythemia vera)
Number of red blood cells	Increased	Increased	Increased
Immature red blood cells	None	None	Occasionally
Number of white blood cells	Increased	Increased	Increased
Hemoglobin	Increased	Increased	Increased
Hematocrit	Increased	Increased	Increased
Red cell mass	Normal	Normal	Increased
Plasma mass	Decreased	Normal or decreased	Normal or decreased
Number of platelets	Increased	Normal	Increased
Oxyhemoglobin saturation	Normal	Decreased	Normal
Uric acid	Normal	May be increased	Increased
Bone marrow	Normal	Erythroid hyperplasia	Hyperplasia of all hematopoietic elements
Basal metabolism (apart from thyroid dysfunction)	Normal	Normal	Increased
Sedimentation rate	Increased	Normal	Decreased
Serum iron	Normal	Increased	Decreased
Plasma iron clearance and turnover	Normal	Normal	Accelerated
Leukocyte alkaline phosphatase	Normal	Normal	Increased
Erythropoietin[124]	Normal	Increased	Normal

Secondary polycythemia (anoxic erythrocytosis)

It is a response to extrinsic or intrinsic oxygen lack. **Lack of extrinsic oxygen** occurs at high altitudes and physiologically in utero. **Intrinsic lack of oxygen** occurs in chronic lung and heart diseases. Congenital heart disease is particularly prone to lead to erythrocytosis. Methemoglobinemia, especially the congenital form, leads to an increase in red blood cells.

Blood picture: Secondary polycythemia shows only the increase in red blood cells, their number being usually below 8 million/mm.³. The oxygen saturation is reduced. The bone marrow shows erythroid hyperplasia only.

Symptomatic polycythemia

Erythrocytosis not associated with any form of anoxemia has been described in association with tumors such as hypernephroma, uterine fibroids, cardiac myxoma, and cerebellar hemangioblastoma. There are numerous reports associating various types of kidney disease with erythrocytosis, suggesting the possibility that an increased production of erythro-

poietin is responsible for the increase in red cells. Erythrocytosis of cerebral origin can be seen in encephalitis, Cushing's syndrome, and brain tumors.

Polycythemia may accompany peptic ulcers and may be the initial manifestation of aplastic anemia, of myelosclerosis, and of leukemia.

Hematologic findings: They are similar to the findings in secondary polycythemia.

Relative polycythemia (hemoconcentration)

This is a pseudopolycythemia due to water loss or inadequate water supply. It may follow chronic diarrhea or vomiting and may accompany abnormal water retention as seen in edema.

Laboratory findings: The oxygen saturation is normal and the plasma volume is always decreased.

Myelofibrosis or myelosclerosis with myeloid metaplasia (myelophthisic anemia)

The disease begins insidiously, usually after 40 yr. of age, as a slowly progressing anemia. It is characterized by progressive loss of hematopoietic marrow elements due to progressive fibrosis, focal at first and later generalized, and enlargement of the liver and spleen due to extramedullary hematopoiesis.

Hematologic findings:

Peripheral blood: There is a normochromic normocytic anemia which may vary in severity, though the early stages may be polycythemic. The red cells show anisocytosis and poikilocytosis and frequently "tear-drop" cells can be identified. Nucleated red cells are often numerous, exceeding the number usually seen in chronic myelogenous leukemia, which is mimicked by the leukocytosis and shift to the left occurring in myelophthisic anemia. The leukocytosis may hover around 15,000-20,000, but it may reach values of 50,000-100,000. The differential count shows a pathologic shift to the left with myelocytes, occasional myeloblasts, and juvenile and band cells. Fragments of megakaryocytes are seen in combination with increased and often abnormally shaped platelets. The platelet count may reach 1 million.

Bone marrow: The aspirate is difficult to obtain and the small amount of material, when smeared, shows lack of hematopoietic elements, fibrous strands, and often masses of platelets accompanying megakaryocytes and reticulum cells. The myeloid elements disappear before the erythroid cells vanish. The diagnosis should be confirmed by surgical bone biopsy.

Serum findings: In myelosclerosis the serum iron is elevated.

Differentiation from chronic granulocytic leukemia: In chronic granulocytic leukemia the alkaline phosphatase in the leukocytes is uniformly low, while in myelophthisic anemia it is normal to high, though it must be stated that occasionally it may be low. In myelosclerosis the number of normoblasts in the peripheral blood exceeds the number seen in myelogenous leukemia. The hypercellular marrow of leukemia is in contrast to the acellular marrow of sclerosis, but marrow sclerosis may be initiated by a hypercellular marrow and myelogenous leukemia may exhibit marrow fibrosis. Repeated marrow aspirations from various sites at various times may be necessary to arrive at a correct diagnosis. The serum iron in leukemia is often low. An increase in basophils and in eosinophilic myelocytes is in favor of granulocytic leukemia.

MARBLE BONE DISEASE (ALBERS-SCHÖN-BERG): This disease, which is also known as osteopetrosis, osteofibrosis, and diffuse osteosclerosis, has its beginning before birth (hereditary) and is usually recognized in childhood. Spontaneous fractures are common.

The blood picture is the same as that just described. The progressive sclerosis of the bones leads to splenic and hepatic enlargement due to the development of extramedullary hematopoiesis.

WHITE BLOOD CELL PATHOLOGY

AGRANULOCYTOSIS

Definition: This is a blood disease characterized by the disappearance or marked diminution of neutrophils from the peripheral blood.

Classification:

Congenital forms

Neonatal agranulocytosis (transient, due to transplacental transmission of maternal antileukocytic antibodies)

Chronic benign granulocytopenia of childhood

Acquired forms

Immunoagranulocytosis—drugs, infections (bacterial and viral), infectious mononucleosis, atypical pneumonia, hypersplenism (Felty's syndrome), and lupus erythematosus

Bone marrow depression—aplastic anemia, myelofibrosis, irradiation, and cytotoxic drugs

Etiology: The cause in most cases is not known (idiopathic), but drugs and agents that produce hypersensitiveness or injure the bone marrow are frequently responsible (amidopyrine, sulfonamides, dinitrophenol, aminopterin, phenylbutazone, chloramphenicol, thiouracil, chlorpromazine, pyribenzamine, gold preparations, acetazolamide, arsenicals, benzene), irradiation, or overwhelming infection.

Hematologic findings:

Blood: The leukocyte count is low, usually less than 1500/mm.[3]. The polymorphonuclear cells are absent or markedly diminished. Eosinophils are also absent or reduced in number, while lymphocytes and monocytes show a relative and/or absolute increase. The platelets and red blood cells are normal.

Bone marrow: In the aplastic type, leukopoietic activity has ceased, but in most cases there is a maturation arrest at the promyelocytic level. In all cases the marrow is hypocellular. The erythroid elements and the megakaryocytes are not involved.

Differential diagnosis: The picture of agranulocytosis may be produced by the early stages of infectious mononucleosis and acute leukemia.

INFECTIOUS MONONUCLEOSIS

Acute infectious mononucleosis[125] or glandular fever[126] is usually considered to be a viral infection. It is associated with a wide variety of clinical manifestations, depending upon the organs or systems chiefly affected. It is a generalized disease usually characterized by lymphadenopathy, fever, and abnormal lymphocytes in the peripheral blood.

Laboratory findings

BLOOD: There is usually a moderate to, at times, pronounced leukocytosis (10,000-30,000 WBC/mm.^{3}) and lymphocytosis. Rarely normal white counts are encountered, but occasionally an initial leukopenia is noted which may mimic the picture of agranulocytosis. The red blood cell and platelet counts are within normal limits, though thrombocytopenia accompanied by petechiae and hemolytic anemia may be encountered. The differential count shows over 50% pathologic lymphocytes which are called Downey cells, virocytes, or infectious mononucleosis cells. Three types are described. Type I is called plasmacytoid lymphocyte since the oval, round, or indented nucleus contains clumped chromatin. The cytoplasm is deep blue and often vacuolated. This cell is probably the reactive lymphocyte of Türk (Türk cell). Type II is called monocytoid lymphocyte since the adult nucleus has a coarse chromatin network, is indented, and surrounded by a large amount of pale, grayish blue cytoplasm

which usually lacks azurophilic granules. The cytoplasm is fragile and is often drawn out into projections between accompanying red cells. Type III somewhat resembles a large lymphoblast, with a coarse arrangement of chromatin. The cytoplasm may be deeply basophilic and may be vacuolated. Azurophilic granulation may be increased in infectious mononucleosis cells, and about 1% of the cells may contain immature nuclei with finely stippled chromatin.

The classification of these cells serves no clinical purpose. Similar cells called **virocytes** can be found in many virus diseases such as hepatitis, upper respiratory virus infections, measles, virus pneumonia, and herpes zoster and simplex.

Infectious mononucleosis type of cells have been reported after splenectomy[127] and after pulmonary and cardiac surgery (extracorporeal circulation). Serum disease, which is no longer seen, used to give rise to infectious mononucleosis type of cells. See discussion of transformed lymphocytes in culture, p. 149.

SPINAL FLUID: Central nervous system involvement may lead to lymphocytosis of the spinal fluid.

BONE MARROW: It is usually hyperplastic, often normal, but frequently infiltrated by the infectious mononucleosis cells.

SERUM FINDINGS[128]:

Heterophil antibodies: Heterophil antibodies for sheep red cells are found in about 60% of cases. The reaction may become positive between the fourth and tenth day and will show a rising titer. A negative test does not exclude infectious mononucleosis. Other diseases besides infectious mononucleosis may give a slight to moderate rise in the heterophil titer.

Normal individuals (83%) may have a titer of 1:28 or lower. After antitoxin administration, in virus diseases and lymphoproliferative disorders, and after administration of blood group–specific substances the titer may rise to 1:896. In cases of infectious mononucleosis the titer is usually greater, reaching its peak in about 10 days or 2 wk., and may go from 1:224-1:7168 or higher. The agglutination

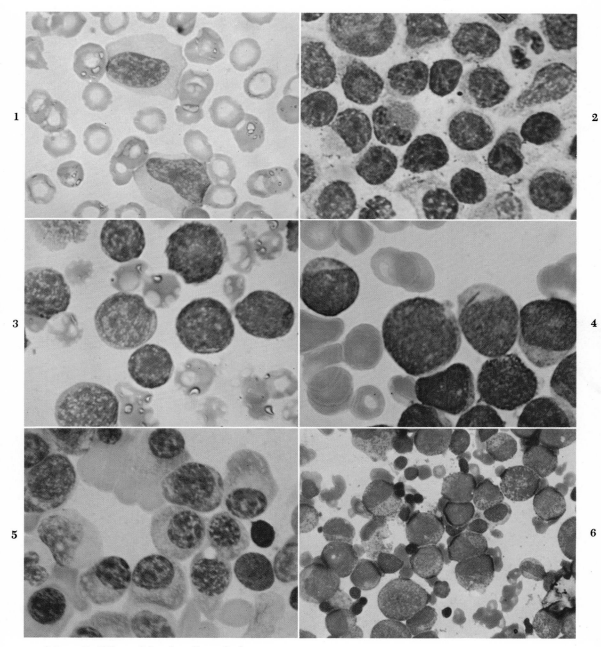

Plate 7. White blood cell pathology.

1. Infectious mononucleosis cells in peripheral blood, Wright stain.
2. Lymphocytes of chronic lymphatic leukemia in bone marrow, Wright stain.
3. Lymphoblasts of acute lymphatic leukemia in bone marrow, Wright stain.
4. Monomyeloblastic leukemia, Auer body in blast cell, Wright stain.
5. Multiple myeloma cells in bone marrow, Wright stain.
6. Bone marrow in agranulocytosis, absence of segmented granulocytes, metamyelocytes, and band granulocytes, Wright stain.

may persist after clinical and hematologic recovery.

Heterophil agglutination—routine or presumptive (Paul-Bunnell test):

Principle: The presence and the titer of heterophil antibodies in human serum are discovered by adding sheep red blood cells to varying dilutions of human serum.

Technique: Inactivate the patient's serum and a normal control serum for 30 min. at 56° C. Set up 12 tubes (75 × 10 mm.) for each serum. Into the first tube place 0.4 ml. saline solution (0.9%) and into each of the others, 0.25 ml. Place 0.1 ml. inactivated serum into the first tube; mix and transfer 0.25 ml. to the second tube, etc., discarding 0.25 ml. from the eleventh tube, leaving the twelfth tube for control without serum. The serum dilutions are 1:5, 1:10, etc. Add 0.1 ml. 2% washed sheep cells (see Notes) to each tube, mix well, and leave at room temperature 2 hr. Final dilutions are 1:7, 1:14, 1:28, 1:56, 1:112, 1:224, 1:448, 1:896, 1:1792, and 1:3584.

Let tubes stand at room temperature for 2 hr. Shake tubes gently to resuspend cells and read for agglutination with the naked eye. The titer is the highest dilution that gives agglutination.

NOTES: Keep the sheep blood in the refrigerator (2°-10° C.). Keeps 4 wk. in Alsever solution.

Alsever solution:
1. Glucose, 20.5 gm.
2. Sodium citrate, 4.2 gm.
3. Trisodium citrate, 8 gm.
4. Citric acid, 0.55 gm.
5. Distilled water, 1000 ml.

Before use the cells must be washed well with large amounts of normal saline solution. Washed cells are not stable.

Interpretation: See above.

Differential test for infectious mononucleosis (differential absorption test—Davidsohn)[129-131]**:**

Principle: Heterophil antibodies are of several types: (1) a normally occurring Forssman antibody, (2) a serum disease antibody that may follow the administration of horse serum, and (3) the infectious mononucleosis antibody. As the antigens reacting with the nonspecific heterophil antibodies occur in certain animal organs, differential absorption of these antibodies differentiates infectious mononucleosis antibodies from the Forssman type. The infectious mononucleosis antibody is not completely absorbed by the guinea pig kidney, while the noninfectious mononucleosis antibodies are. Boiled beef red cells completely absorb the infectious mononucleosis antibody but incompletely absorb the Forssman type.

Indications: Whenever virocytes are found in the peripheral blood and the presumptive test is of low titer. As already stated, many virus diseases, especially hepatitis, infectious lymphocytosis, measles, etc., may hematologically mimick infectious mononucleosis.

Since only the differential test is specific for infectious mononucleosis, some laboratories routinely perform the presumptive test and the test with guinea pig kidney absorbed serum at the same time.

Technique:

Absorption: Guinea pig kidney antigen and beef red cells are commercially available.

Set up two test tubes (10 × 75 mm.). Into one place 1 ml. of well-shaken suspension of guinea pig kidney, and into the second one place 1 ml. of well-shaken suspension of beef cell antigen.

Add 0.2 ml. of inactivated serum (56° C. for 30 min.) to each tube. Shake the tubes well and let stand for 3 min. Then centrifuge at 1500 rpm for 10 min. With a Pasteur pipette transfer the clean supernatant to two test tubes.

Test: Set up two rows of 10 test tubes each (10 × 75 mm.) and add 0.25 ml. of saline solution to all tubes except the first tube in each row. To the first two tubes in the first row add 0.25 ml. serum absorbed with guinea pig kidney. Mix the second tube. To the first two tubes in the second row add 0.25 ml. of serum absorbed with beef cell antigen. Mix the second tube. Transfer 0.25 ml. of well-mixed mixture of the second tube in each row to the third tube, mix, and continue transfer until 0.25 ml. is discarded from the last tube.

Add 0.1 ml. of a 2% suspension of washed sheep cells to each tube, shake,

Table 4-9. Differential test for infectious mononucleosis

| | Absorption of heterophil antibodies (sheep cell agglutinins) | |
	Guinea pig kidney	Beef red cells
Infectious mononucleosis	Incompletely (50-75%) absorbed; the titer should not drop more than 3 tubes	Completely absorbed; the titer will drop over 4 tubes
Other diseases such as virus diseases, lymphoproliferative disorders, etc.	Completely absorbed	Completely or incompletely (35%) absorbed
Normal sera	Completely absorbed	Completely or incompletely (35%) absorbed

and allow to stand for 2 hr. at room temperature. Shake the tube to resuspend cells and read for agglutination with naked eye.

The final serum dilutions are 1:7, 1:14, 1:28, 1:56, 1:112, 1:224, 1:448, 1:896, 1:1792, and 1:3584.

Interpretation: See Table 4-9.

Rapid slide test for infectious mononucleosis (Monospot slide test)[132]: The basic principles of the absorption steps are comparable to the Davidsohn differential test. The material for the test is available in a kit that contains the necessary instructions.*

Ox cell hemolysin test: Ericson[133] finds that the ox cell hemolysin test is more sensitive than the Paul-Bunnell test and that the results can be obtained within 1 hr. The titer remains high during the first year after the infection.

Technique: Inactivate serum at 56° C. for 30 min. Prepare serial dilutions of 0.5 ml. serum in 0.85% sodium chloride containing 0.1 gm. $MgSO_4$/L. To each tube add 0.5 ml. 1:15 dilution of complement and 0.5 ml. 2% suspension of beef cells. Incubate tubes at 37° C. in water bath for 15 min., centrifuge, and compare with a 50% hemolysis standard.

Tests with papain-treated sheep erythrocytes (modification of Wöllner enzyme test II):

Principle: Wöllner described the principle in 1956 and Robinson and Smith[134] developed a screening test in 1966. Infectious mononucleosis serum absorbed

*Ortho Pharmaceutical Corp., Raritan, N. J.

with papain-treated sheep cells will fail to agglutinate these cells but will continue to agglutinate untreated sheep red cells.

Comparison of serologic tests for infectious mononucleosis: Davidsohn compared five tests—presumptive test, differential test, Wöllner enzyme test I (not mentioned here), Wöllner enzyme test II, and beef hemolysin test—and came to the conclusion that the beef hemolysin test and the Wöllner enzyme test II were valuable aids to the presumptive and differential tests.

Complications of infectious mononucleosis

Liver involvement: Liver involvement produces a picture which in most cases is indistinguishable from that of acute infectious hepatitis. The confusion is aggravated by the fact that cells of the infectious mononucleosis type may be seen in viral hepatitis (indication for the Davidsohn differential test).

Central nervous system: There is pleocytosis of the spinal fluid.

Hematologic complications: They have already been alluded to—leukopenia, hemolytic anemia, and thrombocytopenia.[135, 136]

SYSTEMIC LUPUS ERYTHEMATOSUS (S.L.E.)[137, 138]

Disseminated lupus erythematosus is an acute and chronic systemic disease, the cause of which is not known. It is usually classed with the collagen diseases which include periarteritis nodosa, diffuse scleroderma, dermatomyositis, and according to some, rheumatic fever and rheumatoid arthritis. The most constant laboratory findings occur in blood and urine.

Hematologic findings:
1. Normocytic normochromic anemia
2. Leukopenia
3. Thrombocytopenia
4. Demonstration of the L.E. cells

Nonhematologic findings:
1. Hypergammaglobulinemia
2. Increased sedimentation rate
3. False positive serologic tests for syphilis
4. Positive flocculation tests
5. Proteinuria

Hematologic findings

Over 50% of patients have a normocytic normochromic anemia associated with leukopenia and slight thrombocytopenia. The anemia is partly hemolytic and partly due to bone marrow depression. The sedimentation rate is moderately increased.

Bone marrow[139]: In the early stages it is hyperplastic, but as the disease progresses it becomes hypoplastic and more and more fibrous and adipose.

Serologic tests

In lupus erythematosus various antinuclear antibodies appear that are directed against nucleoproteins, DNA, or nuclear constituents. They are immune gamma globulins. The blood clot, slide test, and fluorescent antibody methods are tests for antinuclear antibodies.

Blood clot method for L.E. cells:

Technique: Allow 10 ml. venous blood to clot in a test tube. After 2 hr. decant serum and set it aside for the slide screening test. With a pestle, grind clot through a fine stainless steel wire gauze (40 meshes/in.) and collect defibrinated blood in a white evaporating dish. Discard the fibrin adherent to the screen and distribute the sieved portion into Wintrobe sedimentation tubes. Centrifuge at 1000 rpm for 10 min. Discard serum and transfer buffy coat with a Pasteur pipette to a slide. Make cover slide preparations from a small amount of buffy coat. Stain with Wright stain and examine for L.E. cells.

L.E. cells: The L.E. cell is usually a neutrophilic granulocyte that has phagocytosed, homogenized nuclear material which has lost its original basophilia (Fig. 4-44). This phenomenon is due to antinuclear antibodies directed against nucleoprotein. The formation of L.E. cells is accompanied (1) by the production of

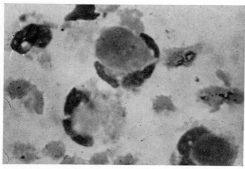

Fig. 4-44. L.E. cells from patient with disseminated lupus erythematosus. Concentration of leukocytes of the peripheral blood. (Wright stain.) (×1000.)

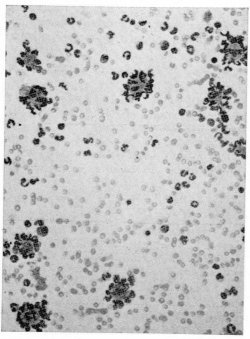

Fig. 4-45. Rosettes in positive L.E. test. (From Haserick: J.A.M.A. **146**:16, 1951.)

free L.E. bodies, which are homogenized, swollen nuclei that have lost their basophilia, and (2) by the production of rosettes, which are polymorphonuclear cells arranged around a central L.E. body.

Interpretation: A positive L.E. test should show frequent L.E. cells accompanied by L.E. bodies and rosettes (Fig. 4-45). L.E. cells are rarely seen in other diseases except in rheumatoid arthritis, scleroderma, and some drug reactions. In general the cell is considered to be specific for lupus erythematosus, though it may not be found in some established cases and may also be suppressed by ACTH and cortisone therapy. Several methods should be tried before a negative result is reported. The L.E. test is positive in 75-80% of patients with L.E.

Tart cells: These cells must not be interpreted as L.E. cells. They are polymorphonuclear cells that have phagocytosed nuclei which retain their chromatin pattern.

Fluorescent antibody test:
Reagents:
1. Buffered saline solution
2. Fluorescent anti-human gamma globulin

Technique:
1. Prepare a thin smear of a small drop of normal peripheral human blood on about one third of a clean microscope slide and air dry.
2. Fix 10 min. in 95% ethanol and air dry.
3. Mark an area of the smear near the feathered tip with a grease pencil. On the marked area allow 1 drop of the patient's test serum to react for 30 min. in a moist chamber. (Controls should be done simultaneously on other slides.)
4. Rinse the slide with phosphate-buffered saline solution, pH 7.4-7.8, from a squeeze bottle. Then gently swing the slide back and forth two or three times in a Copling jar of buffered saline solution and allow it to stand for 10 min. Finally, dip the slide in distilled water to remove salt and air dry.
5. Place 1 drop of fluorescent anti-human gamma globulin on the marked

portion of the smear and allow to react for 30 min. in a moist chamber.
6. Repeat the cycle of washing, step 4.
7. Mount cover slips with buffered glycerol, pH 7.4-8.0.

Result: Examine the slide with a fluorescence microscope.

A serum is considered positive if the nucleus of nucleated cells fluoresces more brightly than does the cytoplasm. Known positive controls are run as a check on the fluorescent reagent. The whole nucleus evenly stained is most typical of L.E. The DNA pattern seen in acute stages shows the periphery of the nucleus most brilliantly.

The test is positive in 95-100% of patients with L.E., but antinuclear antibodies are also found in 3% of males, ages 20-60 yr., 7% of females in the same age group, and in almost 50% of individuals over 80 yr. old.

Rapid slide test (L.E. test*): This test employs a reagent prepared from polystyrene latex and nucleoprotein. Positive and negative controls as well as directions come with the test. It is positive in about 30% of patients with L.E.

Nonhematologic investigation

Serum electrophoresis: The gamma globulin is elevated, and in acute stages the alpha$_2$ globulin may be increased. Hypoalbuminemia is seen in 50% of patients.

Urine examination: About 50% of all patients show renal involvement. Proteinuria, pyuria, and casts are the most frequent findings.

Autoimmune reactions in addition to the L.E. test: In about one third of all patients with L.E. the test for the rheumatoid factor is positive. In one tenth of all patients the serologic tests for syphilis with cardiolipins is falsely reactive. In about 5% of patients who have evidence of an autoimmune hemolytic anemia the direct Coombs test is positive.

Flocculation tests: The cephalin flocculation and thymol turbidity test are positive because of the disturbance of the albumin-globulin ratio in L.E.

---

*Hyland Laboratories, Los Angeles, Calif.

LEUKEMIAS

The leukemias are characterized by a purposeless, malignant proliferation of the blood-forming tissues, each type of leukemia (granulocytic, lymphocytic, monocytic) showing the greatest activity in the tissue producing the respective cell type. Leukemia, which is fatal, may run an acute or a chronic course. The total white cell count is increased except in remissions and in aleukemic leukemia. The percentage of the cells of the involved series is usually more than 80%.

In acute leukemia, blast cells predominate. Occasionally only blast cells and their mature counterparts, without any intervening forms, are found in the blood smear, a picture which Naegeli described as hiatus leukemicus.

The bone marrow, even in aleukemic leukemia, reflects the nature of the leukemia, except in some cases of chronic lymphatic leukemia where it may be normal.

Acute leukemias

GENERAL CONSIDERATIONS:
LABORATORY FINDINGS:

Blood count: In 50% of cases there is a leukopenia in the early stages; in the remaining 50% there is a moderate to advanced leukocytosis. In the early stages the red cell count may be normal, but characteristically there is a severe normochromic or hypochromic anemia. As the platelet count is always markedly reduced, its combination with leukopenia and anemia produces the picture of the pancytopenia of aplastic anemia. Acute monocytic leukemia is noted for temporarily masquerading as aplastic anemia.

Blood smear: In the majority of acute leukemias the pathologic blood cells can be identified in the peripheral blood smear. In some cases their exact identification is difficult. The distinguishing features of blast cells are outlined in Table 4-10. Helpful in the evaluation of blast cells is the "company they keep," the type of mature cell accompanying the blast forms. In addition to the peroxidase reaction, other cytochemical investigations may shed some light on the nature of blast cells. The PAS stain for glycogen is strongly positive in leukemic lymphoblasts, slightly positive in monoblasts, and usually negative in myeloblasts and stem cells. The blast cells of erythroleukemia are also PAS positive, while normal erythroblasts (including erythroblasts in polycythemia vera) are PAS negative.

Bone marrow: In the fully developed disease the normal marrow elements are almost completely replaced by immature white cells varying from stem cells to blast forms. The myeloid, erythroid, and megakaryocytic cells are suppressed. In early stages of an acute leukemia the blast cells may have to be searched for.

Sedimentation rate: It is markedly accelerated; it may reach 100 mm./hr.

SPECIFIC ACUTE LEUKEMIAS:

Acute granulocytic leukemia: The predominant cell type is the myeloblast, which can be recognized by the features tabulated in Table 4-10. Auer bodies may be present and there may be attempts at differentiation toward promyelocytes and myelocytes. In some cases the myeloblasts are unusually small. The peroxidase stain may be positive even if myeloblasts appear to predominate. Megakaryocytes and red cell precursors are markedly reduced.

Acute monocytic leukemia (Naegeli type): In the peripheral smear the predominating cell is the monocyte or monoblast, often with Auer bodies. In the bone marrow the picture is more pleomorphic as the monocytes are accompanied by myeloblasts and promyelocytes.

Acute monocytic leukemia (Schilling type): In the peripheral blood, monocytes in various stages of development are seen. Various transition forms to histiocytes are seen in the blood as well as in the bone marrow. The blast forms in the bone marrow are monoblasts. Megakaryocytes and erythroid elements are depressed.

Acute lymphocytic leukemia: The peripheral smear shows lymphoblasts alternating with a variable number of lymphocytes. In the bone marrow the normal marrow elements are replaced by lymphoblasts so that there is a marked reduction in erythroid elements and megakaryocytes.

Erythroleukemia (di Guglielmo's dis-

Table 4-10. Distinguishing features of myeloblasts, lymphoblasts, and monoblasts (Wright stain)*

Characteristic	Myeloblast	Lymphoblast	Monoblast
Cell size (μ)	10-18	10-18	12-20
Cell border	Even	Even	Irregular, pseudopods
Shape of nucleus	Oval	Oval	Indented, lobular
Nuclear membrane	Fine, smooth	Coarse	Fine, delicate
Nuclear chromatin	Fine, even, delicate, little condensation	Moderately coarse, some condensation	Fine, lacy, no condensation
Nucleoli	2-5	1-2	2-5
Cytoplasm	Blue	Blue	Grayish blue
	No granules	No granules	Granules
Differentiation	Promyelocytes	Lymphocytes	Monocytes
Peroxidase	+	−	±

*From Cartwright: Diagnostic laboratory hematology, ed. 3, New York, 1963, Grune & Stratton, Inc.

ease): In the early stages the peripheral blood may show the features of a macrocytic anemia that may resemble pernicious anemia because of the diminution in platelets and white cells. If the latter are increased, the picture may suggest a macrocytic hemolytic anemia. In the well-developed case, myelocytes, promyelocytes, and myeloblasts appear in the peripheral blood accompanied by normal and abnormal nucleated red cells and by a diminished number of platelets.

In the bone marrow, quite different from other acute leukemias, there is marked erythroid hyperplasia with megaloblasts and erythroblasts, again suggesting pernicious anemia. These erythroid forms soon become bizarre, multinucleated, giant in size, and often show severe nuclear-cytoplasmic dissociation. As the disease progresses, myeloblasts and promyelocytes appear in increasing numbers.

Chronic leukemias

GENERAL CONSIDERATIONS:
LABORATORY FINDINGS:

Hematologic findings: There is generally a slight to moderate anemia that is normocytic and normochromic. There is a moderate to severe pathologic (not reactive) leukocytosis that exhibits a shift to the left. The bone marrow shows quantitative and qualitative changes, depending on the type of leukemia. The sedimentation rate is increased and the hem-

atocrit shows a prominent white cell column.

Nonhematologic findings: The basal metabolic rate is elevated in the absence of thyroid disease. In the urine and serum the uric acid level is increased.

SPECIFIC CHRONIC LEUKEMIAS:
Chronic myelogenous leukemia:

Laboratory findings: The peripheral blood usually shows a marked leukocytosis (up to 500,000 WBC/mm.[3]) and only a slight anemia. The smears reveal representatives of all granulocytic forms and their precursors. A characteristic increase in basophils and eosinophils may be noted. Platelets are often increased and at times accompanied by fragments of megakaryocytes. Occasional metarubricytes are seen. As the disease progresses, the platelets decrease.

Cytochemically the absence of alkaline phosphatase activity in granular leukocytes is characteristic, while the peroxidase reaction is strongly positive.

Bone marrow: It shows myeloid metaplasia with a shift toward younger forms, often associated with some depression of the erythroid elements. The megakaryocytes initially may be increased. Basophils and eosinophils may be prominent. In the late stages myeloblasts may appear in large numbers.

Differential diagnosis: The separation of benign leukocytosis from chronic myelogenous leukemia may be difficult. In myelogenous leukemia the total white blood cell count is usually higher and the leukocytic alkaline phosphatase reduced, while the number of normoblasts in the peripheral blood is only moderate. In leukocytosis the findings are usually just the opposite. The differentiation from myelophthisic anemia may have to rest on the red cell morphology, on the increased number of nucleated red cells, and on the increased leukocytic alkaline phosphatase seen in the latter disease.

Chronic lymphatic leukemia:

Lymphoproliferative disorders: Dameshek includes chronic lymphatic leukemia among the lymphoproliferative disorders, which also embrace infectious mononucleosis, lymphomas, and macroglobulinemia.

Laboratory findings:

Peripheral blood: It shows a pure lymphocytic leukocytosis which is moderate compared to that in myelogenous leukemia. It does not usually exceed 10,000-20,000 WBC/mm.[3]. Anemia does not appear until late in the course of the disease. The platelets are normal in number, but as the disease progresses they diminish. The blood smear reveals apparently mature lymphocytes alternating with atypical younger forms and with distorted smudged cells.

Bone marrow: Bone marrow aspiration reveals infiltration by apparently mature and immature lymphocytes. In the early stages it may be normal or exhibit an increased number of lymph follicles.

Serology: The abnormal lymphocytes may be responsible for the production of abnormal antibodies, which may lead to autoimmune hemolytic anemias or thrombocytopenias. They may be responsible for positive L.E. tests or for reactive serologic tests for syphilis. Various types of abnormal proteins can be detected in the serum such as macroglobulins or cryoglobulins.

PROLIFERATIVE DISORDERS OF PLASMA CELLS AND LYMPHOCYTES WITH PROTEIN ABNORMALITIES

They are diseases that are associated with proliferation of plasma cells and lymphocytes and with the production of abnormal serum proteins.

In this group are multiple myeloma, light-chain disease, macroglobulinemia of Waldenström, heavy-chain disease, monoclonal gammopathies of Waldenström (plasmacytic dyscrasias), agammaglobulinemia, hypogammaglobulinemia, infectious mononucleosis, and chronic lymphatic leukemia.

Multiple myeloma

Multiple myeloma is due to malignant proliferation of functioning myeloma cells which are anaplastic plasma cells. The myeloma cells form bone-destroying tumors, and may break through the bone

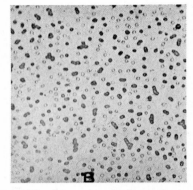

Fig. 4-46. Blood smear, multiple myeloma, showing rouleaux in thin areas. (From Foord and Randall: Amer. J. Clin. Path. **5**:532, 1935.)

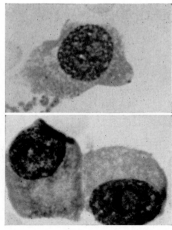

Fig. 4-47. Myeloma cells from bone marrow, case of multiple myeloma. (Wright stain.) (×1000.)

cortex into soft tissues and into the blood-stream.

HEMATOLOGIC FINDINGS:

Blood: Over 80% of patients have an **anemia,** which is usually severe, though it may fluctuate. It is mainly due to depression of the hematopoietic marrow by the tumor rather than replacement.

The **white cell count** shows a leukopenia which terminally, in about 25% of cases, gives way to a leukocytosis with a shift to the left. In about 23% of cases the differential count periodically shows plasma cells. Usually there are about 4% of these cells, but in plasma cell leukemia they predominate. They resemble normal plasma cells rather than myeloma cells. Characteristically the blood smear shows rouleaux formation (Fig. 4-46) due to an increase in gamma globulin which produces evenly spaced small collections of red cells arranged side by side in one direction.

The **platelets** may be normal, though thrombocytopenia occurs in over 50%.

The **sedimentation rate** is markedly increased; in over 60% it is 100 mm./hr.

Hemorrhagic tendencies are seen in about 10% of cases. There are many factors that may contribute to hemorrhage: thrombocytopenia is the least important. Many of the normal clotting factors are absorbed by the abnormal plasma proteins and there may be some increased fibrinolytic activity.

Bone marrow: In typical cases the bone marrow is permeated by masses of myeloma cells.

Myeloma cell (Fig. 4-47): See discussion of plasmablasts, p. 151.

Nucleus: It is large, eccentric, and the chromatin network is fine, resembling a reticulum cell, or it may be coarser and more mature; but it is seldom arranged in clumps as in mature cells. One or more nucleoli are seen and multinucleated forms are common. There is usually some nuclear-cytoplasmic dissociation, the nucleus appearing younger than the cytoplasm.

Cytoplasm: There is a large amount of pale to dark blue cytoplasm that may show a perinuclear clear zone. Vacuoles may be present but no granules. If these vacuoles are numerous, the cell is called a **morula cell (Mott cell),** and if they extend into the cytoplasmic edge and stain bluish with Wright stain, the cell is designated as a **grape cell.** The myeloma cell, similar to the plasma cell, may show Russell bodies (fuchsinophilic inclusions) and they may also be present in the nuclei.

In addition to myeloma cells (rarely excluding them), there may be plasmacytoid and histiocytoid lymphocytes.

NONHEMATOLOGIC FINDINGS:

Urine: Seldom is any other form of proteinuria other than Bence Jones proteinuria found. This protein has a low molecular weight and escapes through intact glomeruli. The urinary calcium level may be elevated. Bence Jones protein casts may be seen in the sediment.

Serum: The serum calcium is elevated. If there is much kidney involvement, the blood urea nitrogen will rise. As in all lymphomas, the uric acid level is high.

Myeloma proteins in serum: In multiple myeloma 52% of patients exhibit hyperglobulinemia as diagnosed by paper electrophoresis. In most cases it is due to an increase in gamma globulins. Beta and alpha hypergammaglobulinemias, as seen by paper electrophoresis, are rare.

Gamma globulins and immunoglobulins (Ig): By immunoelectrophoresis the normal gamma globulin can be divided into four major classes of normal immunoglobulins capable of reacting with antigens. They are (1) immunoglobulins G, forming 71% of all immunoglobulins; (2) immunoglobulins A, forming about 22% of all immunoglobulins; (3) immunoglobulins M, the normally occurring macroglobulins; and (4) immunoglobulins D (Fig. 4-48 and Table 4-11).

Corresponding to each normal immunoglobulin there exists an abnormal counterpart of so-called paraproteins occurring in proliferative disorders of plasma cells and lymphocytes. These paraproteins are (1) the gamma-G myeloma protein, (2) the gamma-A myeloma protein, (3) the macroglobulins of Waldenström, and (4) the Bence Jones protein. Using paper electrophoresis, these pathologic proteins appear to be more homogeneous—pro-

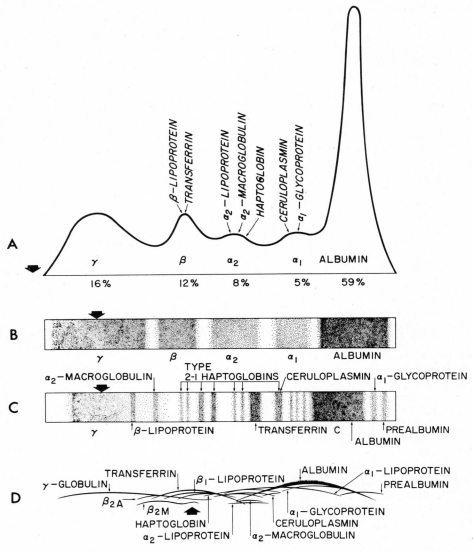

Fig. 4-48. Schematic comparison of Tiselius, **A,** paper, **B,** starch gel, **C,** and immunoelectrophoresis, **D,** of serum in Veronal buffer (pH 8.6). The broad vertical arrow represents the starting point in each case. Nomenclature: γ-globulin = IgG; β_2-A = IgA; β_2-M = IgM. (From Putman. In Neurath, editor: The proteins, New York, 1965, Academic Press, Inc., vol. 3, p. 153.)

ducing a single sharp spike (**monoclonal gammopathy**)—than the normal gamma globulins. All immunoglobulins have in common a group of polypeptide chains, the L or **light chains,** and differ from each other on the basis of their H or **heavy chains.** The composition of these chains is genetically determined. The nor-

mal individual is polyclonal and has all the necessary genes to make all varieties of L and H chains. In the case of pathologic paraproteins, asynchronous production of large amounts of L chains leads to formation of Bence Jones protein and to **light-chain disease.** Asynchronous production of H chains leads to **heavy-chain**

Table 4-11. Immunoglobulins (Ig)

Class	Electrophoretic mobility	Pathologic counterpart	Sedimentation constant	Approximate molecular weight	Total globulin (%)	Serum concentration (gm./100 ml.)	Carbohydrate content (%)
IgG	γ	γ-G myeloma globulin	7S	150,000	71	0.8-1.5	3
IgA	Slow β	γ-A myeloma globulin	7S (7S-15S)	150,000 and multiples	22	0.056-0.193	10
IgM	Between γ and β	Waldenström macroglobulin	19S	900,000-1,000,000	0.7	0.039-0.117	10
IgD	Between γ and β	Bence Jones proteins	2S	22,000	0.2	—	0

disease. Synchronous production of excessive L and H chains is responsible for the various myeloma proteins just mentioned.

Laboratory diagnosis of myeloma paraproteinemia:

Urine: Examine for Bence Jones protein (see p. 20).

Serum: Examine for paraproteins by paper electrophoresis and by immunoelectrophoresis. Paper electrophoresis (see p. 324) will establish the diagnosis of hyperglobulinemia and whether beta or gamma in type. Immunoelectrophoresis will separate the various myeloma paraproteins: 7S gamma-G myeloma protein is seen in about 70% of cases and γ-A myeloma protein in the remainder. In addition, macroglobulins and micromolecular paraproteins (Bence Jones proteins) can be identified. Ultracentrifugation can be used to confirm the presence of macroglobulins.

Immunoelectrophoresis[140]:

Principle: Immunoelectrophoresis is carried out in two steps. The first step is the electrophoretic separation of the serum proteins. Serum is deposited in an antigen well cut into buffered agar. After the electrophoretic separation in gel is completed, a long narrow trough is cut into the gel layer parallel to the long axis of the preparation and at a distance from the electrophoretic pattern. Immune serum is added to the trough. The preparation is incubated in a humid atmosphere and at constant temperature, allowing the immune serum to diffuse into the gel toward the electrophoretically separated proteins, each of which also diffuses radially from its original position. Arc-shaped precipitation lines occur wherever and whenever the diffusing antibodies meet homologous antigens. The location of the precipitation lines identifies the antigen.

Reagents and apparatus:

Spinco electrophoretic system (Model R*):

Veronal buffer solution (pH 8.6, ionic strength 0.05): This is made by diluting the Spinco buffer B-2, which has a pH of 8.6 and an ionic strength of 0.075 with 1 part of distilled water to 2 parts of buffer.

Agar buffer (0.75%): Dissolve 375 mg. Agarose in 50 ml. Veronal buffer by bringing the solution slowly to a boil. To prevent bacterial growth, sodium azide (0.5 gm.) is added to make a 1% solution (w/v).

Photographic film base: DuPont Cronar polyester photographic film base P-40B leader, unperforated, 35 mm.

Preparation of film leader agar-coated immunoelectrophoretic strips: Polyester 35 mm. photographic film leader is cut into 16 cm. lengths and placed on a glass plate which covers a pattern showing the relationship of antisera and antigen wells. The strips are held in position with masking tape and then covered evenly with

---

*Spinco Division, Beckman Instruments, Inc., Palo Alto, Calif.

4 ml. of warm agar-buffered solution. One such design plate is available commercially as Immuno-gel Board.* Microhematocrit tubes are placed in position to match the design for antisera troughs. They rapidly sink into the agar before it hardens and are removed after the gel has solidified. The antigen well is cut with a 13-gauge needle, ground off flush at the tip, and attached to suction.

Antisera: They are commercially available.†

Staining solutions: Amido black 10-B (10 gm.) is dissolved in 100 ml. of glacial acetic acid and made up to 1000 ml. with distilled water. Strips are decolorized in aqueous 2% acetic acid. One percent tannic acid solution for 10 min. is used instead of staining prior to photography.

Technique: The agar-coated strips are placed in the electrophoretic cell, the antigen is added to the central well of the strip, and electrophoresis is continued for 30-45 min. at 200 volts. After electrophoresis the strips are removed and placed in a moist chamber. The antiserum is placed in the trough with disposable calibrated pipettes.‡ The strips are kept in a moist chamber from 24-48 hr. Precipitation bands begin to appear after 6 hr. After the completion of the diffusion the strip is inserted into the tannic acid solution and then photographed using darkfield illumination§ and a Polaroid camera. The strip may also be stained.

Cryoglobulinemia

Cryoglobulins: They are proteins that precipitate or gel at 5° C. and redissolve on warming to 37° C. They occur not only in multiple myeloma but also in macroglobulinemia, lupus erythematosus, and leukemia. They are mainly responsible for the rouleaux formation of red cells in cases of multiple myeloma and may interfere with typing at room temperature as all cells type out AB positive and Rh positive. They increase the viscosity of the blood and may interfere with red blood

cell counts in Hayem fluid, with the sedimentation rate determination, with the hematocrit, and with electrophoresis.

Test for cryoglobulins:

Technique: Allow venous blood to clot in a 37° C. water bath. Centrifuge and transfer 5 ml. of serum to blood bank refrigerator, 4°-5° C. Examine for gel or precipitate after 30 min. and then daily for several days. If precipitate forms, warm it in 37° C. water bath to bring it into solution.

Interpretation: See above.

Macroglobulinemia

MACROGLOBULINS: They are paraproteins with a molecular weight of over 1 million. Small quantities of macroglobulins are found in the normal serum, but they may be abnormally increased in multiple myeloma and lymphomas. They are characteristically increased in **macroglobulinemia of Waldenström.** They are associated with a hemorrhagic diathesis.

LABORATORY DIAGNOSIS: The sedimentation rate is markedly accelerated.

Peripheral blood: The differential count may show a slight lymphocytosis with plasmacytoid cells.

Bone marrow examination: There is an increase in lymphocytes, almost giving the impression of chronic lymphatic leukemia, except that there is a rich admixture of plasma cells, plasmacytoid, and histiocytoid lymphocytes. The red cells and megakaryocytes are not affected. Tissue mast cells may be increased.

Screening tests:

Euglobulin (Sia test): Normal serum proteins diffuse throughout water, while some paraproteins are precipitated because of the reduction of the electrolyte contents.

Technique: Allow 1 or 2 drops of serum to fall into a test tube filled with distilled water.

Interpretation: In macroglobulinemia a heavy white precipitate forms. Not all macroglobulins give a positive test. The diagnosis must be confirmed by the ultracentrifugation pattern or by immune electrophoresis. The sedimentation constant of macroglobulins is 17-32S.

Formol-gel test: When serum globulin is increased, formalin will cause the se-

---

*HCS Corp., Wichita, Kansas.
†Hyland Laboratories, Los Angeles, Calif.
‡Drummond Microcaps, Drummond Scientific Corp., Philadelphia, Pa.
§May be obtained from HCS Corp., Wichita, Kansas.

rum to gel. This test has been used as a presumptive test for kala-azar, multiple myeloma, monocytic leukemia, lymphopathia venereum, and other conditions characterized by hyperglobulinemia.

Technique: Add 1 drop formalin (40% formaldehyde) to 1 ml. serum, mix, and observe at room temperature.

Interpretation: Globulin is increased if a gel is formed within 30 min.

Electrophoresis: Paper or gel electrophoresis will show hypergammaglobulinemia, possibly with a monoclonal peak. Immunoelectrophoresis and the ultracentrifugation pattern will identify macroglobulins.

Amyloid

Amyloid and paramyloid: These paraproteins are deposited in the tissues in cases of multiple myeloma. For special stains, see tissue section.

Agammaglobulinemia and hypogammaglobulinemia

This is a condition in which the gamma globulins are low or absent or, if present, their immune globulin components are depressed or altered. This defect leads to a markedly increased susceptibility to infection, often produced by organisms and fungi that do not normally produce disease.

Classification:
1. Congenital form.
2. Acquired form: It may occur in the course of infections.
3. Symptomatic form: Hypogammaglobulinemia and agammaglobulinemia may accompany proliferative diseases of lymphocytes, plasma cells, and reticulum cells such as lymphomas, macroglobulinemia of Waldenström, multiple myeloma, amyloidosis, etc.

Laboratory diagnosis:

Serum: Paper, gel, and cellulose acetate electrophoresis reveal depression or almost complete absence of gamma globulins. The remaining protein fractions are normal or increased.

Immunoelectrophoresis: It will show absence of normal immunoglobulins.

Peripheral blood: The anemia and leukocytosis reflect the susceptibility to infections. In the absence of infection the blood picture is one of leukopenia exhibiting lymphopenia and eosinopenia.

Bone marrow: It shows absence of plasma cells and transformed lymphocytes.

NOTE: There may be difficulty in reverse typing of the blood of a patient with agammaglobulinemia.

Infections

Patients suffering from plasma-, lympho-, and myeloproliferative disorders are very prone to bacterial and fungal infections. In the acute leukemias and in chronic granulocytic leukemia this is probably related to granulocytic dysfunction or to treatment with antimetabolites. In lymphomas, chronic lymphatic leukemia, and multiple myeloma the increased susceptibility is in part due to decreased immunologic responsiveness.[141]

STORAGE DISEASES

Histiocytosis X: This term embraces three related conditions of unknown etiology that vary from the benign localized eosinophilic granuloma involving certain bones or soft tissues to the generalized chronic Hand-Schüller-Christian disease of young children to the rapidly fatal Letterer-Siwe disease of infants and newborn babies. The first has no hematologic manifestation.

Hand-Schüller-Christian disease: The blood picture is not characteristic and only in the late stages of the disease does it show evidence of myelophthisic anemia. The bone marrow preparation, especially if obtained from the skull, shows characteristic lipid-laden cells.

Letterer-Siwe disease: The blood picture shows an anemia and thrombocytopenia with a leukocyte level varying from leukopenia to leukocytosis. The bone marrow aspirate shows proliferation of malignant reticulum cells.

Niemann-Pick disease: Bone marrow aspiration reveals lipid-laden foam cells. The peripheral blood may show a slight anemia with leukocytosis. The serum may show increased levels of cholesterol and lipids.

Gaucher's disease: Bone marrow aspiration is characterized by the presence of

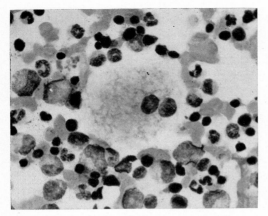

Fig. 4-49. Gaucher cell in bone marrow.

Gaucher cells (Fig. 4-49) which are large cells with pyknotic small eccentric nuclei and a large amount of clear, fibrillary cytoplasm. The blood picture frequently shows a hypochromic anemia which may progress to a myelophthisic type of anemia. There is a leukocytosis with a relative lymphocytosis.

BONE MARROW EXAMINATION

Bone marrow examination is performed for several reasons: (1) as an aid in diagnosis, (2) to study response to therapy, (3) to assess marrow function, and (4) to help in prognosis.

The main hematologic indications are (1) red blood cell disorders, which include macrocytic anemias, microcytic anemias (iron stain), normocytic and aplastic anemias; (2) white blood cell disorders, which include leukemias, leukemoid reactions, and agranulocytosis; (3) platelet disorders, which include primary and secondary thrombocytopenic purpura; and (4) multiple myeloma, metastatic carcinoma, myelosclerosis, and myelofibrosis.

Other indications are bacterial infections (culture), parasitic infections (diagnosis), and storage diseases.

Contraindication: Hemophilia.

CHOICE OF SITE OF MARROW ASPIRATION: Adults: Sternum, iliac crest, and spinous processes

Children: Iliac crest and spinous processes

Infants: Tibia

During the first few years of life all the marrow is red. At about 5-7 yr. of age fat appears and progressively replaces the red marrow until about 18-20 yr. of age, after which red marrow is found only in the vertebrae, the ribs, the sternum, the skull, the scapulae, the clavicles, the innominate bones, and to a slight extent in the proximal epiphyses of the femur and humerus.

METHODS OF OBTAINING MARROW SPECIMEN: Specimens may be obtained by puncture, trephine, Silverman needle, or surgery.

Sternal puncture technique: With the patient in a supine position, locate the sternomanubrial junction at the level of the second rib attachment. Shave the area if necessary and paint with disinfectant. Infiltrate the puncture site, which is usually in the midline of the sternum at the level of the second interspace, with 2% Novocain, including skin, subcutaneous tissue, and periosteum. Using a sterile, dry bone marrow biopsy needle, puncture the anterior bony plate of the sternum with pressure and a very slight rotary movement. When the marrow cavity is entered, the operator experiences a "give." Remove the stylet from the needle and with a dry plastic 10 ml. syringe aspirate 0.5-1 ml. of marrow. The syringe may be heparinized. Place the aspirate into a large watch glass (5-6 cm. in diameter), drain the blood off into a second watch glass, and make cover slip preparations of the marrow particles that adhere to the glass surface, picking up with a white cell counting pipette. The remainder of the aspirate is fixed in formalin or Zenker fixative for tissue sections.

In apparent failure (dry tap), sufficient material is often obtained for a few smears if they are made directly from the material in the needle. If the stylet is not inserted, except for the skin penetration, a small button of material plugging the needle will be found which is suitable for sectioning.

Trephine technique (Turkel needle): The site is chosen and prepared as previously described. Penetrate the skin with the needle, making sure that the stylet is in place. As soon as the needle touches the outer table of the sternum, position the needle at a right angle to the bone, and keeping one finger on the stylet, rotate the needle between two fingers to drill a small opening. Aspiration of marrow and preparation of slides are the same as before.

Table 4-12. Differential count of normal bone marrow—adults

	%
Reticuloendothelial cells	0-1
Myeloblasts	0-2
Promyelocytes	1-5
Myelocytes	
Neutrophilic	5-25
Eosinophilic	0-3
Basophilic	0-0.5
Metamyelocytes	10-20
Band granulocytes	15-30
Neutrophilic granulocytes	10-25
Eosinophils	0-5
Basophils	0-0.5
Lymphocytes	5-20
Monocytes	0-3
Plasma cells	0-5

	per 100 WBC
Nucleated RBC	
Rubriblasts	1-5
Prorubricytes	1-6
Rubricytes	5-25
Metarubricytes	2-20
Myeloid: erythroid ratio	3-8:1
Megakaryocytes	1-2 or more per high-power dry field

Bone marrow biopsy using a Silverman needle: With this instrument a small biopsy of the medullary bone can be obtained which is used to make touch preparations and is then fixed prior to decalcification and processing as tissue. After the bone biopsy is obtained an aspiration needle may be inserted through the outer cannula of the Silverman needle, which is left in place, to provide bone marrow smears.

Surgical method: The surgical method in which a button of bone with the marrow is removed requires operating room technique. It is indicated for the confirmation of the diagnosis of myelofibrosis, myelosclerosis, aplastic anemia, granulomatous lesions, etc.

STAINING OF SMEARS AND OF TOUCH PREPARATIONS: Wright stain and Prussian blue stain are used routinely. Giemsa stain, alkaline phosphatase, and PAS stains are used for special cases.

EXAMINATION OF BONE MARROW SMEARS: The smears should be screened under the low-power microscope to discover areas that are thin, well stained, and allow recognition of the individual cell types. Scanning of the smear also allows judging the distribution of the hematopoietic marrow versus the fatty component and recognition of clumps of tumor cells, granulomas, or other large pathologic cells, e.g., Gaucher cells. Several preparations should be scanned before one field of one of the smears is selected

Table 4-13. Normal values for children*

	Control figures for various age groups									
	1-2 mo.	*3-12 mo.*	*1-2 yr.*	*3-4 yr.*	*5-6 yr.*	*7-8 yr.*	*9-10 yr.*	*11-12 yr.*	*13-14 yr.*	*15-16 yr.*
Myeloblasts	1.6	1.9	0.7	1.4	1.8	1.0	1.4	1.1	1.2	1.3
Progranulocytes	5.6	1.8	3.4	3.2	3.2	1.8	2.0	1.7	1.1	1.9
Myelocytes	18.1	16.7	13.3	15.9	17.2	17.4	16.5	15.31	16.4	16.8
Metamyelocytes	25.6	23.9	21.8	22.0	22.9	23.4	26.1	22.2	21.6	23.2
Band and segmented cells	9.3	7.2	14.1	16.4	12.6	12.3	10.9	12.2	12.2	13.3
Pronormoblasts	0.8	0.6	0.8	0.4	0.5	0.4	0.3	0.2	0.4	0.5
Basophilic normoblasts	1.9	2.1	1.2	1.0	1.2	1.7	1.6	1.8	1.3	2.2
Polychromatophilic normoblasts	12.6	14.5	19.5	16.4	17.3	19.4	19.1	21.8	18.3	15.1
Orthochromic normoblasts	1.6	2.5	2.1	1.2	3.6	3.4	2.4	2.7	3.1	2.5
Lymphocytes	19.7	25.4	19.3	18.6	17.5	13.6	13.6	16.0	18.0	17.4
Myeloid:erythroid ratio	5.5	3.5	2.5	3.4	2.8	2.6	2.9	2.3	2.7	3.3

*From Miale: Laboratory medicine—hematology, ed. 3, St. Louis, 1967, The C. V. Mosby Co.

for examination under oil immersion and for the differential count. Scanning of several slides is important since the distribution of some cells (e.g., tumor cells) may be irregular, and if a bone marrow lymph node has been aspirated, one or two smears may give an erroneous impression of lymphatic leukemia. A minimum of 300 cells should be counted. It cannot be overemphasized that an experienced observer should scan the slides since a count of even 500 cells may be misleading.

EVALUATION OF BONE MARROW SMEARS:

1. Changes in the **erythroid-myeloid ratio** and in the distribution and number of the various cell types. The erythroid-myeloid ratio is the ratio of the total number of erythroid elements to the total number of myeloid elements.
    (a) Erythroid hyperplasia: anemias (iron deficiency, B_{12} and folic acid deficiency, hemolytic), polycythemia vera
    (b) Erythroid hypoplasia: anemias (aplastic, myelophthisic, pure red cell), leukemia, lymphoma, multiple myeloma
    (c) Myeloid hyperplasia: leukocytoses (leukemias, leukemoid reactions, myeloproliferative disorders)
    (d) Myeloid hypoplasia: aplastic anemia, leukemia, multiple myeloma
    (e) Lymphoreticulocytic hyperplasia: leukemia, marrow lymph nodes, macroglobulinemia, multiple myeloma, lymphoproliferative disorders
2. The presence of cells which are not normally found: tumor, multiple myeloma, histiocytosis
3. The presence of parasites: malaria, histoplasmosis, leishmaniasis
4. Iron deposits: normal—in amount and distribution; decreased—iron-deficiency anemia; increased—hemolytic anemias, cirrhosis, hemochromatosis, sideroblastic anemias

CELLS PECULIAR TO BONE MARROW

Reticuloendothelial elements:

Stromal cell:

Nucleus: It is large, round to ovoid, and has a fine, loose chromatin pattern and a single pale blue nucleolus.

Cytoplasm: There is a large amount of poorly defined cytoplasm with irregular edges and various inclusions such as fat, pigments, cell fragments, etc. The color varies from pale gray-blue to lavender-gray.

Sinusoidal cell:

Nucleus: Same as in stromal cells but with an eccentric nucleolus.

Cytoplasm: There is usually a small syncytium present. The large amount of cytoplasm is usually drawn out into an elongated structure with poorly defined boundaries. It contains inclusions of pigments and cell fragments.

Reticulum cells, plasma cells, and **tissue mast cells** are described on pp. 131 and 151.

Osteoblast: These cells are most frequently seen in the bone marrow of children under physiologic conditions, and pathologically, they may accompany osteoblastic metastatic carcinoma cells.

Nucleus: It is ovoid to round with a very fine, closely meshed chromatin network. It contains several bluish nucleoli and is eccentrically placed so that it appears to be almost outside the cell.

Cytoplasm: There is a large amount of bluish ovoid cytoplasm that contains lav-

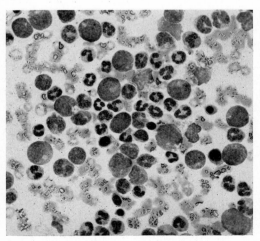

Fig. 4-50. Normal bone marrow.

ender-colored areas of clearing away from the nucleus. There are no inclusions or granulations.

Osteoclast: These cells may accompany metastatic carcinoma cells of osteolytic lesions and are seen in aspirations of brown tumors of hyperparathyroidism (osteitis fibrosa cystica). Only portions of these very large cells are usually found. Osteoclasts differ from megakaryocytes in having many unconnected nuclei of approximately the same size, each containing a nucleolus. Osteoclasts do not form platelets.

Nucleus: It is a large, irregularly outlined giant cell with numerous (up to 30) nuclei, which are similar to the osteoblastic nuclei, each nucleus containing a not easily discernible nucleolus.

Cytoplasm: It is bluish gray, delicate, and often filled with lavender granulations.

BONE MARROW IN DISEASE

In the preceding section the important bone marrow findings of most blood diseases are mentioned. In general it is unwise to base a hematologic diagnosis on bone marrow material alone without consulting peripheral smears and the history. There are some exceptions to this statement as some diagnoses can be made readily on the basis of bone marrow material, e.g., multiple myeloma, acute leukemia, and storage diseases.

Many hematologic diagnoses can be made without the aid of a bone marrow examination, though it often helps to substantiate the diagnosis. There are instances in which a bone marrow examination should be performed, e.g., pancytopenia, leukopenia, lymphocytosis, unexplained anemias, and macrocytic anemias.

COAGULATION OF BLOOD[142]

Hemostasis, the arrest of bleeding, depends on two main factors: functionally intact blood vessels and adequate blood coagulation.

As a cause of bleeding, vascular defects by far exceed in frequency coagulation defects or circulating anticoagulants. The onset of bleeding is always associated with a vascular defect, and a defective clotting mechanism is responsible for the continuation of the bleeding. In health, the freely flowing blood within the blood vessels is the result of intact blood vessel walls and of an equilibrium established by the various clotting factors and their antagonists.

The ultimate aim of blood clotting is the formation of fibrin. Fibrin formation is accomplished by the interaction of two systems: an intrinsic system, in which factors present only in the blood itself take part, and an extrinsic system, in which tissue factors such as tissue thromboplastin also take part.

The extrinsic system initiates the clotting mechanism, whereas the intrinsic system is responsible for definite hemostasis. After the formation of one or two intermediate products, both processes, intrinsic and extrinsic, follow a similar pathway to the formation of fibrin.

SCHEME OF MECHANISM OF COAGULATION

The outline in Fig. 4-51 is markedly simplified as it is now believed that each clotting factor is activated by the activated form of its predecessor.[143]

PHASES OF COAGULATION: Coagulation

Table 4-14. Clotting factors

International nomenclature	Synonymous names
I	Fibrinogen
II	Prothrombin
III	Tissue thromboplastin (tissue extract)
IV	Calcium
V	Labile factor, accelerator globulin, proaccelerin
VII	Stable factor, proconvertin
VIII	Antihemophilic factor (AHF), antihemophilic globulin (AHG), hemophilic factor A
IX	Plasma thromboplastin component (PTC), Christmas factor, hemophilic factor B
X	Stuart-Prower factor
XI	Plasma thromboplastin antecedent (PTA), hemophilic factor C
XII	Hageman factor (HF), contact factor
XIII	Fibrin-stabilizing factor
	Platelet factors, phospholipids

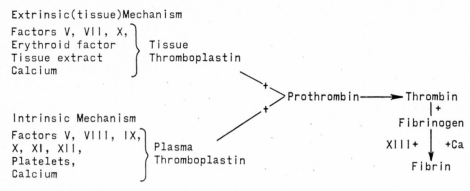

Fig. 4-51. Simplified scheme of blood coagulation.

can be visualized as occurring in three phases.

First phase: (1) **Plasma thromboplastin** production: In this reaction the following factors are involved: surface factors, plasma factors XII, XI, IX, VIII, and X, platelet phospholipids, V, and calcium. The intrinsic thromboplastin is produced within 4-5 min., is labile, and disappears within 1 hr. (2) **Tissue thromboplastin** production: It involves a tissue factor and plasma factors VII, X, and V and calcium. The extrinsic and/or intrinsic thromboplastin activates prothrombin— the second phase of the clotting mechanism.

Second phase: Conversion of prothrombin to thrombin by action of thromboplastin generated in the first phase.

Third phase: Conversion of fibrinogen to fibrin by thrombin produced in the second phase. It is aided by calcium and by factor XIII. After the fibrin clot is formed it retracts, and after a certain period of time it is dissolved by the fibrinolytic system of the blood. The latter two phenomena are at times classified as phase IV.

CHARACTERISTICS OF CLOTTING FACTORS:
For the presence of a given factor in serum or plasma, fresh or stored, and for adsorbability by $BaSO_4$ or by $BaCO_3$, $Al(OH)_3$, and $Ca_3(PO_4)_2$, see Table 4-15.

Factor I (fibrinogen): Fibrinogen is a globulin that is not present in serum and is precipitated by 23-45% ammonium sulfate. It is present in fresh and in stored oxalated plasma in concentrations of 250-400 mg./100 ml. It is formed in the liver and probably in the bone marrow and is the precursor form of fibrin.

Factor II (prothrombin): Prothrombin is a globulin that is precipitated by 50% ammonium sulfate and is present in fresh and in stored plasma (20 mg. or 350 units/ml.) but not in serum. It is consumed in the clotting process so that normal serum contains only a trace of factor II. Vitamin K is essential for the production of prothrombin by the liver and probably by the lung. Prothrombin shares this dependence on vitamin K with factors VII and IX. Prothrombin is converted to thrombin by the action of thromboplastin (1 unit prothrombin to 1 unit thrombin).

Factor III (thromboplastin): Two types of thromboplastin are distinguished —tissue thromboplastin and plasma thromboplastin. The first acts within seconds and for its formation requires tissue extract and factors V, VII, and X. The latter requires several minutes for its production, and factors V, VIII, IX, X, XI, XII, platelets, and calcium are necessary for its formation. Thromboplastin is required for the conversion of prothrombin to thrombin.

Factor IV (calcium): Calcium ions are necessary for the formation of thromboplastin. Many anticoagulants used in the laboratory base their action on the removal of calcium. Clinically, diminution of plasma calcium may occur after massive transfusions or after exchange trans-

Table 4-15. Coagulation factors present in fresh and aged plasma, in serum, and in BaSO₄ adsorbed plasma

Factor	Fresh normal plasma*	Aged normal plasma*	Normal serum*	Adsorbed normal plasma†	BaSO₄ eluate*	Absorbed serum†
Fibrinogen (I)	+	+	0	+	0	0
Prothrombin (II)	+	+	0	0	+	0
Factor V	+	0	0	+	0	0
Factor VII	+	+	+	0	+	0
Factor VIII	+	0	0	+	0	0
Factor IX	+	+	+	0	+	0
Factor X	+	+	+	0	+	0
Factor XI	+	+	+	±	+	+
Factor XII	+	+	+	±	+	+
Factor XIII	+	+	+	+	+	0

*+ = factor present; 0 = factor absent.

†+ = factor not absorbed (present in plasma or serum); 0 = factor adsorbed (not present in plasma or serum); ± = factor slightly adsorbed.

fusions if citrated blood is used instead of heparinized blood.

Factor V (labile factor): Factor V is activated by thrombin to its active form, which was formerly called factor VI. It is consumed during the clotting mechanism and is not affected by Dicumarol or vitamin K administration, but is diminished in severe liver disease. It is inactivated by heating to 58° C. and is precipitated by 33% ammonium sulfate. It is present in fresh and in citrated plasma but not in serum.

Factor VII (stable factor): This factor is produced in the liver with the aid of vitamin K. It is present in fresh and in stored oxalated plasma and in serum. In the neonatal period it is diminished. Dicumarol administration produces a reduction of factor VII (and of factors II and IX).

Factor VIII (antihemophilic factor): This is a globulin that is necessary for the formation of plasma thromboplastin. Its production in the liver, lung, and kidneys is controlled by the hemophilia genes. It is present in fresh plasma and absent in serum. It is not stable in plasma for more than 24 hr.

Factor IX (plasma thromboplastin component): This factor is present in plasma and serum, is dependent on vitamin K, and is stable.

Factor X (Stuart-Prower factor): This factor is similar to factor IX and is involved in the production of thromboplastin. It is also present in plasma and serum.

Factor XI (plasma thromboplastin antecedent—PTA): This is a factor present in plasma and serum; it is stable during blood storage.

Factor XII (Hageman factor): This factor is activated by glass and has to do with the initiation of blood clotting in glass containers. It is required for the initiation of clotting by surface contact and appears to have some indirect enhancing effect on fibrinolysis.

Factor XIII (fibrin-stabilizing factor)[144]: It is a serum factor that enzymatically stabilizes the linkage between the fibrin monomers of the blood clot. In its absence the clot is weak and in vitro is soluble in concentrated solutions of urea (5M) in which normal clots are insoluble.

Platelets: Platelets have to do with the initiation of blood clotting, during which process they undergo viscous metamorphosis and release phospholipids necessary for coagulation. Platelets also have to do with the retraction of the clot once it is formed and with the integrity of the walls of small blood vessels. Four platelet factors have been described; of these, factor III is the most important.

COLLECTION OF BLOOD FOR
COAGULATION TESTS

Two-syringe method: A clean needle puncture is required to prevent tissue juice (tissue thromboplastin) from reaching the blood sample. Discard the first syringe after aspiration of 2 ml. blood and without removing the needle attach a second plastic syringe and obtain the specimen by gentle traction. Disposable needles should be used.

Glassware: All glassware, test tubes, and syringes must be soaked in sulfuric acid dichromate for 12 hr., even if new, and then washed with detergent and rinsed several times in distilled water. It is advisable to use disposable plastic syringes and test tubes that can be discarded after each use.

Siliconizing of glassware:
Reagent: Siliclad* (1%).

Test tubes should be filled with the silicone solution, pipettes immersed in a cylinder containing the solution, and plungers and barrels of syringes immersed in the liquid. After 10 sec. of coating, rinse well in tap water and follow by distilled water. Dry in oven.

NOTE: Water should have a flat meniscus in a well-coated test tube.

Reasons for using siliconized glassware: Blood clots more rapidly in a dry glass tube than in a siliconized tube. The more glass contact there is, the shorter will be the clotting time. This "glass activation" involves factors XI and XII and occurs whenever plasma is exposed to glass. Siliconizing glassware minimizes the glass-activation factor.

BLOOD DERIVATIVES AND REAGENTS USED IN
COAGULATION PROCEDURES

Patient's plasma: Add 4.5 ml. blood to 0.5 ml. 0.1M sodium oxalate. Mix by inversion. Centrifuge at 1500 rpm for 5 min. and aspirate plasma. As factor V is labile, store in refrigerator not longer than 2 hr. A 1:10 dilution with saline solution is obtained by adding 0.1 ml. plasma to 0.9 ml. saline solution.

Adsorbed normal plasma: Obtain plasma as above and add 0.4 ml. aluminum hydroxide gel (Amphojel*) to 2 ml. plasma. Mix for 5 min. and then centrifuge at 3000 rpm for 3 min. Separate plasma and transfer to refrigerator because of the instability of factor V. The one-stage prothrombin time on the adsorbed plasma should be over 60 sec. If the plasma is refrigerated, it should be used within 2 hr., or it may be distributed into small aliquots and frozen.

Aged normal plasma: Collect plasma as above and incubate at 37° C. for 24 hr. Store it in aliquots at –20° C. The prothrombin time on the plasma should be over 60 sec.

Normal serum: Obtain blood by venous puncture and allow it to clot in a water bath at 37° C. for 4 hr. Centrifuge, separate serum, and allow it to stand at room temperature for 24 hr.

Platelet-rich plasma: Add 9 vol. whole blood to 1 vol. 3.8% sodium citrate using siliconized glassware. The mixture is inverted several times and then centrifuged at 1500 rpm (500 *g*) for 15 min. The supernatant, platelet-rich plasma, is separated.

Platelet-poor plasma: Blood is collected as for platelet-rich plasma and centrifuged at 3000 rpm for 20 min. The supernatant, platelet-poor plasma, is then separated.

Anticoagulants:
1. Calcium chloride (0.025M), 2.27 gm./1000 ml. distilled water
2. Sodium oxalate (0.1M), 13.4 gm./1000 ml. distilled water
3. Sodium citrate (0.1M), 32.34 gm./1000 ml. distilled water
4. EDTA (1%), 1 gm./100 ml. 0.7% saline solution

Defibrination with glass beads: Add 25 ml. venous blood to 125 ml. Erlenmeyer flask containing 20 3-4 mm. glass beads. Rotate flask until beads are covered with fibrin and cease to make a rattling noise. Continue for another 2 min. and decant defibrinated blood.

Thrombin: Dissolve the contents of one vial Parke Davis topical thrombin (5000 NIH units/ml.) in 10 ml. saline solution to obtain a stock solution of 500 units/

---

*Clay-Adams, Inc., New York, N. Y.

*Wyeth Laboratories Division, American Home Products Corp., Philadelphia, Pa.

ml. Dilution of this stock solution 1:50 with normal saline solution gives a concentration of 10 units/ml.

INVESTIGATION OF THE BLEEDING PATIENT

Prior to the laboratory investigation of the patient, detailed personal and family histories should be obtained, including previous episodes of bleeding, allergies, liver disease, etc. The clinical examiner should pay special attention to the presence of petechiae, which are suggestive of thrombocytopenia, to the presence of ecchymoses, which are suggestive of coagulation factor defects, and to the size of the liver, spleen, and lymph nodes.

The laboratory investigation should follow a given outline:

1. Tests for vascular function: bleeding time, tourniquet test
2. Tests of platelets function and quantity: clot retraction, platelet count, serum prothrombin time, thromboplastin generation test, bleeding time
3. Tests for overall clotting ability: clotting time, recalcified plasma coagulation time, thrombin time
4. Tests of phase III: fibrinogen level, fibrinolysins
5. Tests of phase II: plasma prothrombin time (extrinsic system)
6. Tests of phase I: thromboplastin generation test, partial thromboplastin, serum prothrombin time (intrinsic system)
7. Tests for circulating anticoagulants

TESTS FOR VASCULAR FUNCTION

BLEEDING TIME: The bleeding time depends upon a number of factors, chiefly the number and functional activity of platelets, ability of the tissue juice to initiate or accelerate clotting, elasticity of the skin, and tonus of the capillaries.

Bleeding time is not coagulation time.

The **methods for measuring bleeding time** are the Duke method and the Ivy method.

Duke method: Cleanse the earlobe well with 75% alcohol. With a sterile Bard-Parker blade 11, make a 5 mm. deep stab into the earlobe, which is steadied by a microscope slide held against it posteri-orly. The point of the blade should just touch the slide. The blood must flow freely and the lobe must not be squeezed. As soon as the puncture is made, start a stopwatch and every 30 sec. blot the blood with a piece of filter paper without ever touching the surface of the lobe.

Normal Duke bleeding time: 3-5 min.; upper limit 7 min.

Ivy method: Apply a sphygmomanometer cuff to the patient's upper arm and, inflating it to 40 mm., maintain this pressure. With a sterile Bard-Parker blade 11, make a 4 mm. deep incision in the skin of the forearm, which has been cleaned with 75% alcohol and stretched between the thumb and forefinger. Avoid superficial veins. Start a stopwatch and blot the bleeding point with filter paper every 30 sec. by just touching the tip of each drop. The wound must not be touched.

Normal Ivy bleeding time: Upper limit 5-6 min.

The Ivy method is the method of choice because the pressure and the incision can be fairly well standardized. The area also allows multiple testing and easier control of bleeding should it become excessive.

Interpretation: Bleeding time is prolonged in thrombocytopenia, thrombasthenia, von Willebrand's disease, thrombocytopathia, and plasma factor deficiencies, if severe.

NOTE: In hemophila A and B, bleeding may occur from the puncture wound 24 hr. after the test even though the bleeding time may be normal.

CAPILLARY FRAGILITY TEST (TOURNIQUET TEST, RUMPEL-LEEDE TEST): Mark any petechiae already present on the hand or forearm. Apply the blood pressure cuff to the upper arm and inflate to 80 mm. Hg and leave it at this pressure for 5 min. Remove the cuff and examine forearm, hand, and fingers for petechiae. A 5 cm. circle is outlined and the petechiae are graded as follows:

Grade	Petechiae
1 +	0-10
2 +	0-20
3 +	20-50
4 +	50 and over

Interpretation: A positive test indicates weakness of the capillary walls. It is positive in thrombocytopenia, thrombasthenia, vascular purpura, scurvy, and senile purpura. If petechiae are present prior to the performance of the test, there is no need to proceed with the test.

TESTS FOR OVERALL CLOTTING ABILITY
COAGULATION TIME (CLOTTING TIME)

Principle: If tissue thromboplastin is prevented from entering the blood by the 2-syringe method, then the whole blood clotting time is a measure of the time required to form intrinsic thromboplastin (Fig. 4-51). The test is so insensitive that only severe defects of any one factor will significantly affect the result.

Lee-White method: Place three tubes in a 37° C. water bath. Obtain 5 ml. blood from a vein in a plastic syringe, using the 2-syringe method and the usual aseptic technique. Place 1 ml. of blood into each of three clean, dry, 13 × 100 mm. test tubes by removing the needle and allowing the blood to run down the side of the tubes. Start a stopwatch as the blood enters the first tube. Gently tilt the third (last) tube to receive the blood every 30 sec. until the blood in it clots; the second tube is then done in the same manner; last, the first tube is tilted until no flow of blood is observed on tilting. The coagulation time is the time required for the blood to clot in the last tube.

Normal values: The normal clotting time by this method is 7-15 min. A clotting time over 15 min. is abnormal. If siliconized tubes are used, the clotting time is 25-45 min.

Note that the Lee-White clotting time must be carefully standardized as it is dependent on such factors as temperature, size of tubes used, frequency and angle of tilting, amount of blood in tube, etc.

Interpretation: The whole blood clotting time is increased in severe deficiencies of factors I, II, V, and VII-XII, circulating anticoagulants, and hyperheparinemia. At best the test is only a rough measure of coagulability and the prothrombin time and prothrombin consumption time are far better tests for the above-mentioned factors. If the blood fails to clot, the diagnosis is afibrinogenemia or hyperheparinemia. If the clotting time is markedly prolonged, moderate to severe hemophilia is the most likely cause. Mild hemophilia and thrombocytopenia do not affect the clotting time. The main value of the test is in the control of heparin therapy. The tubes may be held for observation of clot retraction and lysis and for serum prothrombin time determination.

Control of heparin therapy: The whole blood clotting time test is used to control heparin therapy. The test should be performed 3½-4 hr. after the last injection. If the result is greater than twice the normal value, the test should be repeated ½ hr. before the next dose of heparin is due.

Clot timers: Their action is based on the fact that changes in the surface tension and viscosity occur during clotting which interfere with electric conductivity.

Coagulation time of recalcified plasma (plasma clotting time):

Principle: Plasma recalcification time is the time required for a fibrin clot to appear in recalcified plasma. The blood specimen is first prevented from clotting by removing calcium with a known amount of sodium oxalate. Calcium is then added in the form of a known quantity of calcium chloride to start the clotting mechanism.

As tissue juice is kept out of the clotting system, clotting is dependent on the factors that control the formation of intrinsic thromboplastin (p. 206) and on the concentration of prothrombin and fibrinogen. The recalcification time is a more sensitive test of clotting time than the whole blood clotting time.

Procedure: Use 2-syringe method for obtaining blood.

Add 4.5 ml. blood to 0.5 ml. 0.1M sodium oxalate. Mix well, centrifuge at 3000 rpm in an angle centrifuge for 20 min., and remove plasma. By high centrifugation many platelets are sedimented so that a platelet-poor plasma is obtained, which makes the test relatively independent of platelet function. Repeat the same procedure on normal control blood.

Add 0.2 ml. platelet-poor plasma to a

test tube and warm in 37° C. water bath for 1 min.

Add 0.1 ml. 0.025M sodium chloride by forcibly blowing it into the tube and start timer immediately. Time the fibrin formation by gently tilting the tube every 30 sec. and observing it for clot formation.

Repeat procedure using a normal control.

Normal values: Platelet-poor plasma (high centrifugation) will clot in 120-180 sec. Platelet-rich plasma (low centrifugation, 5 min. at 1000 rpm) will clot in a shorter time (80-120 sec.).

Significance: The test is useful for the diagnosis of hemophilia, a disease in which both high and low centrifuged specimens show a prolonged recalcification time.

TESTS FOR CLOTTING FACTOR DEFECTS

The role the various factors play in some of the tests to be described is summarized in Table 4-16.

TESTS OF PHASE III OF COAGULATION

In phase III of the clotting mechanism, fibrinogen is converted to fibrin with the help of thrombin. After its formation the **clot retracts** and later is **lysed** by a proteolytic enzyme, plasmin. Defects in phase III are defects in fibrin formation.

The **clot retraction** is a function of platelets, while the **lysis** is an expression of the fibrinolytic system, of the adequacy of fibrinogen, and of its polymerization to fibrin.

Tests of platelet function and quantity

Clot retraction—character of blood clot: The separation of the blood clot from the wall of the test tube is normally observed after 1 hr. and is complete after 2 hr., at which time the clot is approximately 50% of the original blood volume.

The clot retraction may be measured on the basis of the amount of serum expressed.

Method: Transfer 2 ml. blood to test tube which is placed in a water bath at 37° C. Do not disturb the blood for 1 hr. At the end of 1 hr. examine for clot retraction from the sides of the tube. Retraction is considered complete when the clot separates from three sides.

Semiquantitative method of clot retraction: Decant the expressed serum and measure the amount. The percentage of expressed serum can be calculated as follows:

Table 4-16. Requirements of common coagulation tests*

	Fibrin-ogen	Pro-throm-bin	Factor V	Factor VII	Factor VIII	Factor IX	Factor X	Factor XI	Factor XII	Plate-lets
Extrinsic system										
Prothrombin time test	+	+	+	+			+			
Intrinsic system										
Clotting time test	+	+	+		+	+	+	+	+	
Prothrombin consumption test		+	+		+	+	+	+	+	+
Thromboplastin generation test			+		+	+	+	+	+	(+)†
Partial thromboplastin time test	+	+	+		+	+	+	+	+	

*From Goulian: Ann. Intern. Med. **65:**782, 1966.
†In a common form of the test, platelets are replaced by a lipid substitute.

$$\%\,\text{Expressed serum} = \frac{\text{Vol. of expressed serum}}{\text{Vol. of whole blood} \times 100}$$

Normal values: The clot will retract from three sides in 1-2 hr. and express 45-60% serum.

Observation for fibrinolytic activity: Continue incubation of clot and observe at 1, 2, 4, and 24 hr. of incubation. A normal clot will not disintegrate within 24 hr. Excessive fibrinolytic activity will cause the clot to dissolve or acquire a worm-eaten appearance.

Significance: Clot retraction is directly proportional to the number and functional activity of platelets, though an undue rise in the number of platelets may not shorten the clot retraction time. Other factors are temperature, pH, fibrinogen, thrombin, calcium, and glucose. Clot retraction is inversely proportional to the fibrinogen contents and the red cell mass.

Poor clot retraction is present in thrombocytopenia (less than 50,000 platelets/mm.[3]), thrombocytopathia, and increased red cell mass.

Test for platelet adhesiveness (Salzman method)

Principle: Most tests depend on the adherence of platelets in whole blood to glass surfaces. Salzman[165] collects patient's blood directly into a glass bead filter.

Technique: Collect blood sample with siliconized 20-gauge needle in a 7 ml. Vacutainer* tube containing Na_2-EDTA. This sample passes through a glass bead filter which is siliconized except for the glass beads and the polyvinyl tubing.

Collect control sample from the opposite arm in the same type of Vacutainer.

Perform platelet counts on both blood samples.

Result: The difference between the counts in the test and control samples is expressed as a percentage of the control count and represents the platelet adhesiveness.

• • •

Other platelet tests such as platelet count, serum-prothrombin time, tourni-quet test, bleeding time, and thromboplastin generation test are discussed elsewhere.

Fibrinogen deficiency and fibrinolysis[145-147]

FIBRINOGEN DEFICIENCY TESTS:

1. Rapid screening methods, necessitated by the urgency of the clinical situation: Fibrindex* and Fi-Test†.
2. Fibrinogen titer: a semiquantitative test for clottable fibrinogen.
3. Biochemical method: does not measure clottable fibrinogen only.

Fibrindex:

Principle: When added to plasma containing fibrinogen, thrombin produces clotting. Thrombin (human) for this test is available commercially.

Method: Add 1 ml. physiologic saline solution to the ampule of dried thrombin (Fibrindex). Dissolve and mix. This solution will not keep longer than 6 hr. Make tests at room temperature.

Into one small test tube (10 × 75 mm.) place 2 drops plasma from the patient's oxalated blood, and into another tube place 2 drops plasma from oxalated normal blood for control.

To each tube add 2 drops thrombin solution and start stopwatch immediately.

Mix gently; then tilt the tubes back and forth and record in seconds the time of clotting in each tube.

Significance: Normal plasma, like the control, begins to clot after 5-10 sec., and after 30-60 sec. the clot is firm (without serum) and sticks to the wall of the tube.

No clot will form in the absence of fibrinogen, and in hypofibrinogenemia only a small clot will form, which may dissolve. Heparin or other antithrombins will also prevent clotting.

Fi-Test: It is a rapid slide test based on the agglutination of fibrinogen-coated red blood cells by latex-antihuman fibrinogen reagents.

Fibrinogen titer:

Principle: Serial dilutions of plasma are clotted with thrombin. The titer is the highest dilution in which a fibrin clot

---

*Becton, Dickinson & Co., Rutherford, N. J.

*Ortho Pharmaceutical Corp., Raritan, N. J.
†Hyland Laboratories, Los Angeles, Calif.

can be seen, and it is related to the fibrinogen concentration and indirectly to the presence of circulating anticoagulants.

Technique: Add 1 ml. saline solution to each of four small test tubes. Add 0.5 ml. patient's plasma to the first tube, mix, and transfer 0.5 ml. of the mixture to the second tube and so on. Plasma dilutions are 1:3, 1:9, 1:27, and 1:81. Repeat procedure with normal control plasma. Place all tubes in a 37° C. water bath for 3 min. Add 0.1 ml. undiluted thrombin to each tube and mix. Incubate for 15 min. Examine each tube by tilting for the presence or absence of a clot. The titer is the highest dilution in which a fibrin clot can be seen.

Interpretation: The titer of normal plasma is at least 1:27, usually higher. The quality of the clot should be compared with that of the control clot.

PLASMA THROMBIN TIME: See p. 214.

Quantitative fibrinogen determination: See section on clinical chemistry.

FIBRINOLYSIS: It is generally assumed that under physiologic conditions a minimal amount of intravascular clotting takes place, which is opposed by a proteolytic enzyme—plasmin (fibrinolysin) (Fig. 4-52). It is derived from its circulatory precursor plasminogen (profibrinolysin) upon surface or tissue injury activation.

Pathologic stimulation of the fibrinolytic system leads to hyperplasminemia, with consequent degradation of fibrin and fibrinogen into split products and, at

times, destruction of factors V and VIII; both events may lead to hemorrhage.

Screening tests for excessive fibrinolysis

Fibrinolysin is unstable at room temperature. Whole blood should be stored at 37° C. and plasma should be placed in the refrigerator. The tests should not be delayed.

Whole blood clot lysis time: The clot, obtained by the Lee-White method or the clot retraction test, is kept in the 37° C. water bath for 24 hr. Increased fibrinolytic activity is evidenced by partial or complete lysis of the clot within 24 hr. Factor XIII deficiency will produce a similar picture of excessive lysis.

Control: Refrigerate part of the specimen at 4° C. The clot should remain firm.

This test is relatively insensitive, but if positive it has clinical significance.

Screening tests to distinguish between plasma factor defect or circulating anticoagulants: A prolonged clotting time of whole blood may be due to a severe plasma factor defect (afibrinogenemia or hypofibrinogenemia) or due to circulating anticoagulants.

Technique: Add to 0.1 ml. patient's blood (or plasma) 0.1 ml. normal plasma. If the normal plasma corrects the prolonged clotting time of a patient's blood, the defect lies in one of the clotting factors. If the addition of normal plasma fails to shorten the clotting time significantly, a circulating anticoagulant is prob-

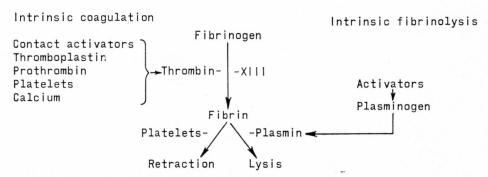

CLOT FORMATION AND FIBRINOLYSIS

Fig. 4-52. Scheme of clot formation and fibrinolysis.

Table 4-17. Serial dilution of patient's plasma and normal plasma mixture

Tubes	1	2	3	4	5	6
Patient's citrated plasma (ml.)	1.0	0.8	0.6	0.4	0.2	0
Normal citrated plasma (ml.)	0	0.2	0.4	0.6	0.8	1.0
Dilutions of patient's plasma		4.5	2.5	2.5	1.5	

ably responsible for the prolonged clotting time.

Diluted plasma clot lysis:

Principle: This test is more sensitive than the whole blood clot lysis. Inhibitors are diluted but not completely inhibited.

Set up six test tubes (13 × 100 mm.) marked 1-6 and prepare serial dilutions of patient's plasma with normal plasma as in Table 4-17.

Mix plasma mixtures and add 0.1 ml. thrombin (10 units/ml.) to each tube. Mix, incubate at 37° C., and examine for fibrin clots, which should form within a few seconds. Tubes 1 and 6 are controls. Examine hourly up to 12 hr. for zones of lysis which indicate the presence of fibrinolysin. Lysis within 12 hr. indicates increased lytic activity.

Control: A duplicate set of patient's plasma dilutions should be made with 1% epsilon aminocaproic acid in saline solution, which counteracts the effect of fibrinolysis.

Euglobulin clot lysis[148]: Collect blood in plastic test tubes containing dried ammonium oxalate. Centrifuge at 1500 rpm for 5 min. to separate plasma.

Add 8 ml. distilled water and 0.15 ml. 1% acetic acid to 0.5 ml. plasma to precipitate the euglobulin. Centrifuge at 2500 rpm, pour off supernatant fluid, and dissolve in 0.5 ml. borate buffer. Add 0.2 ml. euglobulin solution to 0.1 ml. of a mixture of equal parts of 100 units thrombin and 0.025M $CaCl_2$.

The resulting clot is observed for complete lysis.

Normal values: About 300 min. or longer before normal lysis occurs. Strong lysis, 60 min. or less. Increased lytic activity, 120 min.

Fluorometric assay of fibrinolytic activity: The use of thrombolytic agents in thromboembolic vascular disease requires a rapid assay method of increased clot-lysing plasma activity. Genton et al.[149] described a method of plasma assay using fluorescein-labeled clots.

Test for circulating anticoagulant

Plasma thrombin time[150]: The thrombin time test detects qualitative or quantitative fibrinogen changes and is useful for the demonstration of inhibitors of the thrombin-fibrinogen reaction.

Principle: Plasma is clotted by thrombin, and the time taken is dependent on the amount and quality of fibrinogen and on inhibitors. Fibrinolytic activity may not only destroy fibrin but also attack fibrinogen.

Reagents:

1. Thrombin. Dissolve the contents of one vial of Parke Davis topical thrombin (5000 NIH units/ml.) in 10 ml. saline solution to obtain a stock solution of 500 units/ml. A 1:1000 dilution of the stock solution will have a concentration of 0.5 units/ml. The addition of 0.1 ml. of this dilution will clot 0.1 ml. plasma in 11-14 sec. (working solution of thrombin).

2. Patient's citrated plasma.

Technique: Incubate plasma and thrombin working solution in a 37° C. water bath for 3 min. Thereafter, keeping the tubes in the water bath, add 0.1 ml. test plasma to 0.1 ml. working solution of thrombin and start timer immediately upon addition of plasma. Time clot formation. The method is suitable for automatic clot timers. **Repeat test with normal plasma.** Also inspect the quality of the clot and compare it with the control clot. A feeble clot is indicative of low fibrinogen.

Interpretation: Prolongation of the thrombin time of the patient's serum over that of the control is due to the

Table 4-18. Clotting time mixtures

Reagents	Tubes	1	2	3	4	5	6
Normal plasma		0.1	0.1	0.1			
Test plasma					0.1	0.1	
Protamine sulfate							0.1
(0.5% in saline solution)			0.1			0.1	0.1
Toluidine blue							
(0.1% in distilled water)				0.1			
Dilute thrombin							
(10 units/ml.)		0.1	0.1	0.1	0.1	0.1	0.1

presence of antithrombins, heparin, or heparin-like circulating substances or is due to qualitative and/or quantitative changes in fibrinogen (fibrinogen level below 100 mg./100 ml.).

Correction of prolonged thrombin time: This correction can be attained by either protamine sulfate or toluidine blue (substances with heparin-neutralizing properties) if heparin is responsible for the prolonged plasma thrombin time.

Technique: See Table 4-18.

Plasma antithrombin test[151]: The plasma thrombin time may not detect small amounts of heparin, of heparin-like substances, or of fibrinolysins. Titration of the plasma with decreasing amounts of thrombin will detect small amounts of anticoagulants.

Reagent: Diluted thrombin. The stock thrombin solution of 500 units/ml. (see plasma thrombin time) is diluted 1:50 with normal saline solution to obtain a concentration of 10 units/ml. (working solution).

Technique: Set up two sets of six test tubes in a 37° C. water bath. Prepare serial twofold dilutions of the working solution of thrombin by setting up five tubes numbered 2-6, containing 1 ml. normal saline solution each, and by adding 1 ml. working solution of thrombin to tube 2, mixing well, and then transferring 1 ml. of the tube 2 mixture to tube 3, etc. Discard 1 ml. of mixture of the sixth tube. Add 0.1 ml. test plasma to one set of six tubes, and add 0.1 ml. normal plasma to the other set of six tubes. To the first tube of the test plasma set add 0.1 ml. working thrombin solution (10 units/ml.) and time the clot formation. Repeat procedure for each thrombin

dilution, using normal plasma in one tube and test plasma in the other. Keep all tubes in a 37° C. water bath while performing the test. An automatic clot timer may be used.

If the test plasma contains antithrombin or fibrinolysin, a prolongation of the clotting time over the normal will occur in one of the dilutions.

The presence of antithrombin will also lead to a prolongation of the one-stage prothrombin time.

Causes of abnormal tests of phase III

1. **Platelet dysfunction:**
   Quantitative defect
   Qualitative defects (thrombasthenia)
2. **Fibrinogen deficiency**
3. **Excessive fibrinolysis:**
   Excessive activator
   Excessive plasmin
   Both excessive

TESTS OF PHASE II OF COAGULATION

In phase II, prothrombin is converted to thrombin with the help of thromboplastin (intrinsic or extrinsic) and calcium. The defects in phase II are defects in thrombin formation.

One-stage prothrombin time (Quick):

Definition: It is the clotting time obtained when an excess of thromboplastin and optimum calcium are added to oxalated plasma under standardized conditions. Under these conditions the clotting time is a function of the prothrombin concentration. The prothrombin time is essentially a test for the formation of extrinsic thromboplastin—(tissue extract + factors V, VII, and X in the presence of calcium, Fig. 4-51). The extrinsic thromboplastin thus produced acts on prothrombin to form thrombin, which in turn leads to the formation of a fibrin ,lot. Factors VIII, IX, XI, and XII and platelets do not enter into the formation of extrinsic thromboplastin.

It must be noted that factor V deteriorates in oxalated blood (but not in citrated blood) and this decay may therefore prolong the prothrombin time if the specimen is collected in oxalate. The prothrombin time will remain constant if the specimen is kept in the refrigerator for not longer than 2 hr. If the blood specimen is allowed to stand over 4 hr. at room temperature or at refrigerator temperature, the prothrombin time of oxalated blood will be prolonged, while the citrated plasma time will be shortened.

Technique: To 0.5 ml. 0.1M sodium oxalate or sodium citrate in a graduated tube add exactly 4.5 ml. venous blood to the 5 ml. mark. Centrifuge at 1500 rpm for 5 min. Aspirate the plasma into a clean tube and place in a 37° C. water bath or refrigerate if the test cannot be performed immediately. Into a test tube (12 × 75 mm.) pipette 0.1 ml. thrombo-plastin and 0.1 ml. 0.025M calcium chloride and allow to incubate for at least 10 min. in a 37° C. water bath. If the thromboplastin used has calcium chloride already added, use 0.2 ml. of this reagent. Blow 0.1 ml. warmed plasma into the thromboplastin-calcium mixture and simultaneously start stopwatch. Leave mixture in water bath for 5-6 sec., then remove tube, wipe the outside, and tilt gently back and forth against a diffuse light until the very earliest fibrin strand can be detected, which denotes the end point. Control with lyophilized normal control plasma is essential.

Normal range: 12-14 sec.

Methods of reporting:

1. **Prothrombin time reported in seconds.** This method reports the patient's plasma time and the control plasma time in seconds.

2. **Prothrombin reported as percentage concentration.** The result of the prothrombin time (time in seconds) can be expressed as a percentage concentration by referring to a hyperbolic calibration curve (Fig. 4-53) which expresses the relationship

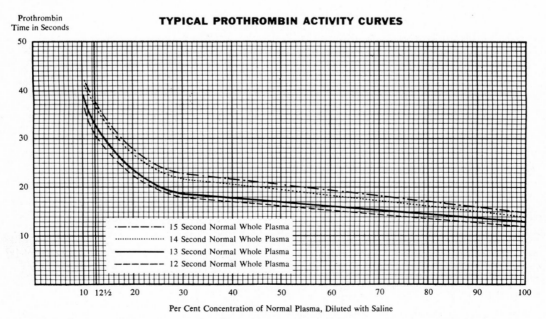

TYPICAL PROTHROMBIN ACTIVITY CURVES

Prothrombin Time in Seconds

- ·—·—·—·— 15 Second Normal Whole Plasma
- ·············· 14 Second Normal Whole Plasma
- ———— 13 Second Normal Whole Plasma
- – – – – 12 Second Normal Whole Plasma

Per Cent Concentration of Normal Plasma, Diluted with Saline

Fig. 4-53. Typical prothrombin activity curves. (Courtesy Warner-Chilcott Laboratories Division, Warner-Lambert Pharmaceutical Co., Morris Plains, N. J.)

of concentration of prothrombin to clotting time.

Preparation of dilution curve for prothrombin concentration in plasma:

Principle: Various dilutions of normal oxalated plasma are made with saline solution and the prothrombin time of each of these dilutions is determined so that a prothrombin dilution curve can be constructed. If the patient's prothrombin time in seconds is known, the corresponding prothrombin concentration can be read off the curve. The clotting time of the normal control plasma determines which curve is used.

Dilution of normal plasma with saline solution decreases the concentration of factor V, fibrinogen, prothrombin, and factor VII. If prothrombin-free plasma ($BaSO_4$ adsorbed plasma) is used as diluent, a slightly differently sloped curve is obtained since barium sulfate plasma contains factor V and fibrinogen, and these factors therefore remain constant in the various dilutions. As the concentrations of prothrombin and factor VII are the only factors that will vary in these various dilutions, the barium sulfate adsorbed plasma method more closely reflects the changes occurring in the plasma in coumarin-type therapy. Nevertheless, most laboratories prefer the saline dilution method.

Technique: Use lyophilized plasma with a prothrombin activity of 12-13 sec. or 100%. Label four tubes: 100%, 50%, 25%, and 12.5%. Add 4.5 ml. saline solution to the first tube and 1 ml. saline solution to the other three. Pipette 0.5 ml. normal plasma into the first tube, mix well, and prepare twofold dilutions in the remaining tubes by transferring 1 ml. of the mixture in the first tube to the second tube. Mix again and transfer 1 ml. of the mixture. Do at least three prothrombin time determinations on the five samples and plot clotting time versus prothrombin activity on graph paper (Fig. 4-53).

Quality control of prothrombin time[152]: Two prothrombin time ranges should be controlled: the therapeutic range and the normal range.

Control determinations should be run in duplicate at the beginning, middle, and end of each run of tests and with each "stat" request. They should fall within ±1 sec. of the normal control and within ±2 sec. of the 20% control. The control results should be charted daily to provide a constant check on test conditions and their accuracy.

Therapeutic range: A 20% dilution, 1 part control plasma and 4 parts normal saline solution, is suggested. The range should be between 20 and 29 sec.

Normal range: It should fall between 12 and 14 sec.

The factors enumerated in the section on quality control also apply to the prothrombin time. The controversy regarding the type of diluent used in the preparation of the dilution curves and regarding the type of thromboplastin used in the test make standardization of the prothrombin time difficult.

Significance: Vitamin K is necessary for the formation of the vitamin K–dependent clotting factors by the liver: factors VII, IX, and X and prothrombin. In the adult this vitamin is normally supplied by the diet and by bacterial action in the intestines. The vitamin is fat soluble and is absorbed from the intestines, together with lipids, with the aid of bile. It is not stored in appreciable amounts.

Causes of prolonged one-stage prothrombin time:

1. **Deficiencies of prothrombin and factors VII and X:**
   Hereditary
   Liver disease
   Coumarin drugs
   Newborn infants
   Vitamin K deficiency
2. **Deficiency of factor V:**
   Hereditary
   Liver disease
   Leukemia
   Purpura fulminans
3. **Circulating anticoagulants**

Liver disease: If the liver parenchyma is severely damaged, the liver is unable to synthesize the vitamin K–dependent factors even if adequate amounts of the vitamin are available.

Coumarin drugs: The administration of Dicumarol or other coumarin derivatives

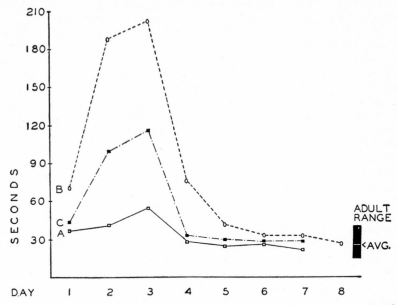

Fig. 4-54. Average prothrombin time (Quick) in the newborn infant. **A,** 14 cases with clotting time not over 5 min.; **B,** 9 cases with clotting time over 5 min.; **C,** average of all cases. (From Bray and Kelley: Amer. J. Clin. Path. **10**:154, 1940.)

interferes with the function of vitamin K in the liver and thus with the production of the vitamin K–dependent blood factors: prothrombin and factors VII, IX, and X. The coumarin drugs are therefore used to lower the coagulability of blood in patients with thromboembolic phenomena. After the administration of Dicumarol, factor VII is suppressed first for 1 or 2 days and then prothrombin, followed by factors IX and X.

Prothrombin time in newborn infants: In newborn infants the maternal supply of vitamin K is largely used up in 3-5 days and a decrease of prothrombin (hypoprothrombinemia) occurs before the intestinal flora necessary for the production of vitamin K is established. The prothrombin time is very variable, tending to be within the normal adult range (method of Quick) on the first day, rising to a peak, which is definitely higher than the normal adult range, between the second and the fifth days (usually the third day), and falling within the normal adult range after the fifth day (Fig. 4-54).

Vitamin K deficiency: Failure to absorb the fat-soluble vitamin occurs in external

biliary fistula and in obstructive jaundice because of the absence of bile from the intestinal tract and in sprue and related diseases because of the inability to absorb fat. Sterilization of the intestinal flora by antibiotics leads to diminished vitamin K supply because of the disappearance of the normal flora. As already stated, severe liver disease interferes with the utilization of vitamin K.

Evaluation of the one-stage prothrombin time—correction studies: If fibrinogen is normal and if there is no abnormal antithrombin present, the clot formation in the one-stage prothrombin time depends on several factors. The main ones are prothrombin and factors V and VII, while factor X is of less significance. The diminution of one factor may be masked by the adequacy of the remaining factors, whereas a slight diminution of two factors may unduly prolong the one-stage prothrombin time.

If it is necessary to determine the main cause of a prolonged prothrombin time, **substitution studies** should be performed.

Correction studies of one-stage prothrombin time: Prepare the following mixtures and do one-stage prothrombin time determinations.

1. 0.9 ml. patient's plasma plus 0.1 ml. stored serum (supplies factor VII)
2. 0.9 ml. patient's plasma plus 0.1 ml. fresh BaSO$_4$ adsorbed plasma (supplies factor V)
3. 0.9 ml. patient's plasma plus 0.1 ml. stored oxalate plasma (supplies prothrombin)

Whichever of the added factors corrects the originally prolonged prothrombin time can be considered the factor primarily responsible for the prolongation.

Serum corrects factor VII deficiency, adsorbed plasma corrects factor V deficiency, and plasma corrects deficiencies of factors II, V, and VII.

Other methods for determining the prothrombin time:

Fibrometer: The Fibrometer* is an electric coagulation timer which, with the help of electrodes, determines the end point of a clotting procedure.[153, 154]

Micromethod: Miale[155] described a micromethod in which capillary blood is used.

Prothrombin and proconvertin method (P and P method): In the modified P and P test the patient's plasma is diluted 1:10 to reduce the effect of antithrombin and to increase the sensitivity of the procedure. The patient's plasma is diluted with barium sulfate adsorbed plasma which contains fibrinogen and factor V so that the test becomes insensitive to changes in these two factors of the test plasma. On the other hand, it is sensitive to changes in the vitamin K–dependent factors (prothrombin and factors VII, IX, and X). The test may also reflect prothrombin time changes sooner than the one-stage method. If the patient's citrate or oxalate plasma cannot be tested within 2-4 hr., the P and P method is preferred because it compensates for the disappearance of factor V on standing. It can also be used for patients receiving heparin therapy.

The method consists of the following steps. The diluted plasma, with the help of a special optimal thromboplastin mixture, activates the prothrombin-thrombin

*Baltimore Biological Laboratory, Baltimore, Md.

reaction. The amount of thrombin formed is tested on a fibrinogen substrate. The calculation of the prothrombin contents of the test plasma is based on the assumption that 1 unit of thrombin is formed from 1 unit of prothrombin, and 1 unit of thrombin will clot a standard fibrinogen solution in 15 sec.

Thrombotest method: Coumarin therapy depresses prothrombin and factors VII, IX, and X; it does not affect factor V. The one-stage prothrombin time does not measure factor IX as it is a measure of extrinsic thromboplastin formation in which factor IX has no part. The special dilute thromboplastin reagent for the thrombotest, developed by Owren and Aas, containing factor V and fibrinogen, allows the performance of a reproducible test sensitive to all vitamin K–dependent factors: II, VII, IX, and X. The test can be adapted for the Fibrometer and also allows a capillary blood method.

ANTICOAGULANT THERAPY

HEPARIN AND DICUMAROL: Therapeutically, heparin and Dicumarol are widely used as anticoagulants.

Heparin: The action of heparin in prolonging the coagulation time is more or less immediate and of short duration. It is given parenterally because it is not active when given orally. It is an antithrombin, antithromboplastin, and antiprothrombin. Its effect, therefore, is followed by determining the coagulation time of whole blood rather than the prothrombin time.

Heparin therapy is controlled to keep the coagulation time of whole blood about twice normal by the Lee-White method.

Heparin interferes with the one-stage prothrombin time and prolongs the clot retraction. It inhibits coagulation in vivo and in vitro.

Dicumarol: It is the cause of spoiled sweet clover disease (hemorrhagic disease) in cattle and acts slowly. Its effect is not manifest until after 10 hr., becoming marked in 2-5 days. It has a cumulative action that may persist for 10-14 days after the last dose. Dicumarol delays or prevents the formation of the vitamin K–dependent factors, and its activity can be followed by the prothrombin time determination. Dicumarol therapy[132] is usually so controlled that the prothrombin time is kept at about twice normal.

Dicumarol does not effect the clot retraction and the whole blood clotting time is not prolonged until the prothrombin time falls to 10% activity.

TESTS OF PHASE I OF COAGULATION

Phase I of clotting involves platelets, the Hageman factor, and the various plasma factors that generate the plasma thromboplastin. Some of the tests mentioned are a measure of the platelet's participation in the thromboplastin formation (production of phospholipids) and of the activity of factors V, VIII, IX, and X provided the tests of phase II are normal.

Serum prothrombin time (prothrombin consumption test)[156]:

Principle: The amount of thrombin formed by the interaction of prothrombin and thromboplastin is a measurement of the concentration of prothrombin since 1 unit of thrombin will be produced by 1 unit of prothrombin. Thus the amount of thrombin produced can be taken as a measure of the amount of prothrombin present, though there is evidence that the reaction is not truly stoichiometric in nature due to the presence of factors V and VII.

During normal clotting, thromboplastin converts all plasma prothrombin to thrombin. If thromboplastin is deficient, only a portion of prothrombin will be converted, leaving residual prothrombin in the serum. The prothrombin consumption test measures the residual prothrombin in the serum by the Quick one-stage method. It is an indirect test for the adequacy of the intrinsic thromboplastin formation.

Method: Obtain blood (preferably in fasting state) by venipuncture, using 2-syringe method, and put 2 ml. in a small test tube (100 × 12 mm.). Place tube in water bath at 37° C. and let clot.

Remove the tube 60 min. after clotting. Ring once, centrifuge for 1 min. at high speed, remove serum from clot, and return serum to water bath. Make a prothrombin time determination on the serum

immediately. The determination is made in the same manner as the original plasma method of Quick, except 0.1 ml. deprothrombinized rabbit plasma is added to supply fibrinogen.

In a test tube (100 × 12 mm.) put 0.1 ml. barium sulfate adsorbed plasma, 0.1 ml. thromboplastin solution, and 0.1 ml. 0.025M calcium chloride solution (2.77 gm./L.) and place in water bath at 37° C. until warm. Add, also warmed, 0.1 ml. serum, which should be blown from the pipette into the other reagents. Start a stopwatch and record time of clotting.

Run tests in duplicate and run a normal control each time.

Normal values: If the prothrombin consumption time is measured 1 hr. after clotting, the normal is over 30 sec. Values below 25 sec. are abnormal (Table 4-19).

Impaired consumption time (shortened serum prothrombin time): A decreased value indicates a deficiency in any factor responsible for intrinsic thromboplastin generation: V, VIII, IX, X, XI, XII, platelets, or the presence of a circulating anticoagulant.

Partial thromboplastin time (PTT)[157-159]: This is a general screening test of the coagulation mechanism, but it is especially useful for the investigation of deficiencies involving the factors that make up the intrinsic thromboplastin.

Principle: The patient's plasma provides all the factors for clotting (see Table 4-15) except calcium (removed by oxalate or citrate). Calcium and a platelet factor reagent (or a partial thromboplastin) are added to the patient's fresh plasma and the time of clot formation is noted. Partial thromboplastin is a crude cephalin extract which does not clot hemophilic blood as

Table 4-19. Prothrombin consumption time in seconds

	Minutes after clotting			
	15	*30*	*45*	*60*
Normal	10	15	25	35
Hemophilia	11	11	11	11
Thrombocytopenic purpura	9	10	12	15
Hypoprothrombinemia	30	35	45	55

rapidly as normal plasma, hence the name partial. Complete thromboplastin such as tissue extract used for the one-stage prothrombin time reacts with factors V, VII, and X and prothrombin; the partial thromboplastin reacts with all coagulation factors except factor XII and platelet factor. The test must be performed with controls. When performed in conjunction with the prothrombin time, it will distinguish phase I, II, and III deficiencies. An abnormal PTT and a normal prothrombin time indicate a phase I deficiency, while an abnormal PTT and PT indicate a phase II or III deficiency.

The addition of kaolin particles renders the test more consistent because the kaolin provides optimal contact activation, thereby minimizing the influence of other surfaces such as test tubes, etc.

Technique of PTT (kaolin activated)[160]:
1. Obtain 5 ml. venous blood by the 2-syringe method.
2. Add 4.5 ml. blood to 0.5 ml. special anticoagulant solution immediately after step 1. Mix by gently tilting and inverting. Do not shake.
3. Centrifuge at 2000 rpm for 10 min. Transfer plasma to another tube and store at 2°-10° C. until ready for testing, which must be done within 4 hr.
4. Resuspend the reconstituted partial thromboplastin by filling and expelling from a pipette and immediately add 0.1 ml. to a prewarmed 10 × 75 mm. test tube.
5. Add 0.1 ml. of the test plasma, mix by giving the tube a sharp shake, and incubate at 37° C. for 3 min. Time accurately with stopwatch.
6. Add 0.1 ml. prewarmed calcium chloride using a prothrombin pipette, start stopwatch, and give tube a sharp shake to mix.
7. At about 30 sec. remove the tube from the water bath and gently tilt back and forth, not faster than once per second. Stop the watch at a final gel formation, not at the point of partial coalescence of kaolin.
8. Repeat the test upon another aliquot of the specimen and report the average of the two tests.
9. Run two control tests.

Micromethod: A micromethod, using the Miale micropipette, is also available.

Normal values: 30-45 sec.

Prolonged PTT (kaolin activated): Any PTT of 50 sec. or over is considered prolonged. Deficiencies of clotting factors of all three phases, with the exception of deficiencies of factor VII and of platelet factor, produce an abnormally long PTT. If the one-stage prothrombin time is normal, an abnormally prolonged PTT indicates a phase I deficiency, usually of factors VIII or IX.

Differential partial thromboplastin time[160]: Classical hemophilia (factor VIII deficiency) may be differentiated from Christmas disease (factor IX deficiency) by performing a **differential PTT,** using commercially obtained factors VIII and IX (Hyland AHF reagent and Hyland PTC reagent).

Principle: The differential PTT is performed by mixing one of the above-mentioned correcting reagents with the patient's plasma, partial thromboplastin, and calcium chloride solution and noting the time of clot formation. The test is then repeated using the other correcting reagent. The test is then run a third time using normal saline solution as a control in place of either of the two correcting reagents.

Technique: See technique of PTT. After step 4 add 0.1 ml. AHF reagent and then continue with step 5.

Repeat test using the PTC reagent after step 4, and finally repeat test using normal saline solution in place of the correcting reagents.

Interpretation: About 83% of phase I disorders are due to factor VIII deficiency—classical hemophilia. The prolonged PTT of these patients is almost completely corrected by the AHF reagent, with little correction by the PTC reagent.

About 14% of phase I disorders are due to factor IX deficiency (Christmas disease or hemophilia B). The prolonged PTT of these patients will be almost completely corrected by the PTC reagent.

The rare factor XI deficiency will reveal a partial correction of the PTT with either reagent since both reagents contain some factor XI.

Thromboplastin generation test (TGT)[161, 162]:

Principle: The thromboplastin generation test is essentially a one-stage prothrombin test, but the thromboplastin added is not tissue (brain) extract. It is intrinsic plasma thromboplastin, formed by the interaction of the patient's plasma factors: platelets, $Al(OH)_3$ adsorbed plasma (factors V and VIII), serum (factors VII, IX, X, XI, XII), and calcium. The formation of the intrinsic thromboplastin is the first phase of the TGT.

In the second phase at regular intervals small amounts of the thromboplastin reaction mixture are added to platelet-poor plasma (contributing fibrinogen and prothrombin) containing calcium. The combination of thromboplastin and platelet-poor plasma and calcium leads to fibrin (clot) formation. The more thromboplastin is formed in the first phase, the shorter will be the recalcification time of the second phase.

Under these circumstances the mixture will produce a clotting time of 10 sec. or less after 5 min of incubation at 37° C. If the thromboplastin generation is defective, the clotting time may exceed 12 sec., or though it may be shorter, it will be delayed beyond the 6 min. of incubation time. In the case of defective thromboplastin generation the cause can be traced to one of the three main components of the system—serum, adsorbed plasma, or platelets—by substituting for each, one at a time, a normal control. Thus the activity of the patient's fraction can be compared with the activity of a normal control. For instance, by substituting a suspension of normal platelets for the unknown platelets, it can be determined whether the platelet function of the unknown blood is responsible for the abnormal TGT. Normal blood fractions are available commercially and are marketed as TGTR.*

Technique: It is described in detail in the leaflet accompanying the reagents.

Hicks-Pitney modification of TGT (kaolin modification)[150]:

This is a rapid, simplified modification of the TGT which allows routine screening.

Principle: Diluted test plasma (providing all factors necessary for intrinsic thromboplastin formation) is recalcified in the presence of a platelet substitute. At regular intervals aliquots of the recalcified plasma are added to a normal platelet-poor plasma substrate (providing prothrombin and fibrinogen) in the presence of calcium. The amount of thromboplastin generated by the patient's plasma is then determined by a series of one-stage prothrombin times. As the concentration of thromboplastin in the patient's plasma increases, the prothrombin time becomes progressively shorter.

The reproducibility of the test is improved by preincubation of the plasma with kaolin.

Reagents:
1. Platelin*
2. Diagnostic Plasma*
3. Calcium chloride (0.025M)
4. Sodium oxalate or citrate (0.1M)
5. Sodium chloride (0.85%)
6. Kaolin suspension

Preparation of reagents:
1. Reconstitute the Platelin by adding 2.5 ml. distilled or deionized water to the vial. Shake to ensure dispersion of the fine suspension.
2. Reconstitute the Diagnostic Plasma by adding 0.5 ml. distilled water. Swirl gently to dissolve. For multiple determinations the large-sized vial may be used. Reconstitute with 2.5 ml. distilled water.
3. Dilute the patient's plasma to 10% by adding 0.1 ml. patient's plasma to 0.9 ml. 0.85% saline solution warmed to 37° C. in water bath. Add 0.1 ml. kaolin suspension and start stopwatch. Leave in water bath. Testing should be started exactly 5 min. after dilution.

Equipment: Place the following in a water bath at 37° C.: test tube containing diluted patient's plasma, test tube con-

---

*Warner-Chilcott Laboratories Division, Warner-Lambert Pharmaceutical Co., Morris Plains, N. J.

*Warner-Chilcott Laboratories Division, Warner-Lambert Pharmaceutical Co., Morris Plains, N. J.

taining Platelin, test tube containing 2 ml. 0.025M calcium chloride, empty test tube, four prothrombin time tubes, each containing 0.1 ml. 0.025M calcium chloride, and test tube containing Diagnostic Plasma.

The entire test is done in a 37° C. water bath. Two timers are required: one to measure the overall incubation period and the other for the individual prothrombin time determinations.

Technique:

1. Into the empty test tube, pipette in rapid succession 0.2 ml. each of Platelin, dilute patient's plasma, and 0.025M CaCl$_2$. Start the incubation timer simultaneously with the addition of the CaCl$_2$. This is the generation mixture.
2. At 3 min. 45 sec., remove 0.1 ml. generation mixture and blow into one of the tubes containing 0.1 ml. 0.025M calcium chloride. Do **not** stop the incubation timer.
3. At 4 min., blow 0.1 ml. Diagnostic Plasma into the tube containing 0.1 ml. each of generation mixture and calcium. Simultaneously, start the second timer and time the clot formation exactly as in the prothrombin time test.
4. At 5 min. 45 sec., repeat step 2.
5. At 6 min., repeat step 3.
6. At 7 min. 45 sec., repeat step 2.
7. At 8 min., repeat step 3.
8. At 9 min. 45 sec., repeat step 2.
9. At 10 min., repeat step 3.

When enough plasma thromboplastin has been generated to clot the Diagnostic Plasma in 7-12 sec. or less, stop the incubation timer and terminate the test.

NOTE: If a clot forms in the generation mixture tube at any time during the test, remove it to prevent interference with pipetting. Do **not** stop the incubation timer (a clot in the generation mixture has no bearing on the test).

Interpretation: The shortest clotting time obtained using normal plasma should lie between 7 and 12 sec. and should be reached in 4 min. In defects in phase I of coagulation the shortest clotting time obtained using the patient's plasma will exceed the control by over 5 sec. and will require over 6 min.

Causes of prolonged tests of phase I:

Defective formation of intrinsic thromboplastin:

1. **Deficiency of factor VIII:**
   Hemophilia A
   von Willebrand's disease
2. **Deficiency of factor IX:**
   Hemophilia B (Christmas disease)
   Vitamin K deficiency
      Newborn infants
      Liver disease
      Malabsorption
      Antibiotics
      Coumarin drugs
3. **Deficiency of factor XI:**
   Hemophilia C
4. **Deficiency of platelets:**
   Thrombocytopenia
   Thrombopathy
5. **Circulating anticoagulants**

HEMORRHAGIC DISEASES[163]

According to the nature of the main defect, hemorrhagic diseases can be subdivided into those due to (1) vascular defects, (2) coagulation factor defects, (3) circulating anticoagulants, and (4) platelet defects.

They may also be classified into congenital (hereditary) or acquired defects. The congenital hemorrhagic disorders are usually due to one single defect, while the acquired forms often have more than one, though multiple congenital deficiencies have been described.

Congenital (hereditary) hemorrhagic disorders:

1. Factor I deficiency: hypofibrinogenemia and afibrinogenemia
2. Factor II deficiency: congenital hypoprothrombinemia
3. Factor V deficiency: Owren's disease
4. Factor VII deficiency
5. Factor VIII deficiency: hemophilia A and von Willebrand's disease
6. Factor IX deficiency: hemophilia B (Christmas disease)
7. Factor X deficiency
8. Factor XI deficiency: hemophilia C
9. Factor XII deficiency
10. Factor XIII deficiency

11. Platelet deficiency and deficiency of factor III (thrombocytopathia); deficiency of adhesiveness (von Willebrand's disease); and deficiency of glycolysis (Glanzmann's thrombasthenia)
12. Circulating anticoagulants: hyperheparinemia

Acquired hemorrhagic disorders:
1. Factor I deficiency: fibrinolysis, hypofibrinogenemia, and defibrination syndrome
2. Factors II, VII, IX, and X deficiency: vitamin K deficiency and oral anticoagulants
3. Factor V: liver disease
4. Blood vessel diseases: vitamin C deficiency and platelet deficiency
5. Circulating anticoagulants: dysproteinemia, hyperheparinemia (shock, anaphylaxis), and fibrinolysins (endotoxins)

HEMORRHAGIC DISEASES DUE TO VASCULAR DEFECTS

Vascular defects are twofold: increased permeability (vitamin C deficiency) and increased fragility (congenital and acquired—related to platelet deficiency or deficiency of plasma factors).

The purely vascular purpuras include hereditary hemorrhagic telangiectasia and pulmonary hemosiderosis.

Vitamin C deficiency (scurvy): In this disorder there is a defect in the ground substance which leads to defective endothelial cement substance. The latter defect is responsible for the increased vascular permeability.

Characteristically the bleeding is in the periosteum and gums. While scurvy is rare, subclinical cases may be seen in bottle-fed infants.

Purpura senilis: This is a common form of purpura appearing in older debilitated patients who have petechiae and ecchymoses in the skin of the back of hands and feet.

Increased vascular fragility: Increased vascular fragility is present in the purpura that occurs in old age, after cortisone administration, during menopause, in the course of infections, in the course of endocrine disturbances such as Cushing's disease, and in toxemias such as diabetes and uremia. The allergic type of vascular purpura has received special attention and is called Schoenlein-Henoch purpura.

Schoenlein-Henoch purpura: Synonymous names for this condition are **allergic purpura** and **nonthrombocytopenic purpura.** It is a disease characterized by an urticaria-like skin eruption, cutaneous petechiae, gastrointestinal symptoms, and joint involvement.

Purpura fulminans: There is extensive diffuse hemorrhage into the soft tissues of the extremities. It often follows infections and may be related to a factor V deficiency.

Hereditary hemorrhagic telangiectasia: There may be bleeding from congenital vascular malformations which may be visible, e.g., in the nose.

Waterhouse-Friderichsen syndrome: It represents severe capillary damage due to meningococcal septicemia, though it may also be seen in streptococcal and pneumococcal infections.

Laboratory findings in vascular defects:
1. Bleeding time: prolonged
2. Coagulation time: normal
3. Clot retraction: normal
4. Tourniquet test: positive
5. Prothrombin time: normal
6. Prothrombin consumption time: normal
7. PTT: normal
8. Platelets: normal

HEMORRHAGIC DISEASES DUE TO COAGULATION FACTOR DEFECTS

FACTOR I: FIBRINOGEN DEFICIENCY AND FIBRINOLYSIS[145-147]: Factor I deficiency may be congenital or acquired (defibrination syndrome).

Congenital hypofibrinogenemia and afibrinogenemia: Complete absence of fibrinogen in congenital or constitutional afibrinogenemia is associated with a bleeding tendency from birth and episodes of severe and widespread bleeding. The blood is incoagulable. In congenital hypofibrinogenemia or fibrinogenopenia the fibrinogen is greatly decreased, and the bleeding tendency develops later. Clotting is slow and is usually only partial.

Acquired hypofibrinogenemia (defibrination syndrome): It may complicate surgical procedures on lung, heart, prostate, and uterus and may follow obstetric conditions such as abruptio placentae, amniotic fluid embolism, and prolonged retention of a dead fetus. It is seen in malignant tumors of prostate, pancreas, and stomach and in hematologic conditions such as acute myelogenous leukemia, multiple myeloma, Rh sensitization, transfusion of mismatched blood, and massive transfusions.

It may be due to excessive utilization of fibrinogen by extensive and widespread clotting, inadequate fibrinogen production in advanced liver disease, fibrinolysis or interference with the polymerization of fibrinogen molecules.

Laboratory investigation: See fibrinogen determination and screening tests for fibrinolysis, p. 212.

Factor II deficiency:

Hypoprothrombinemia: There are two types—congenital and acquired. The acquired form, as stated previously, follows vitamin K deficiency, parenchymal liver disease, and therapy with anticoagulants.

Acquired hypoprothrombinemia is one of the causes of hemorrhagic diathesis of the newborn infant, who may develop rectal bleeding, but may also bleed from other areas. This condition is due to the inability of the fetal liver to produce prothrombin from vitamin K. There is also a marked depression of factor VII.

Laboratory diagnosis: The one-stage prothrombin time is prolonged, while the prothrombin consumption time is normal.

Factor V deficiency: It may be congenital or acquired in severe liver disease. The one-stage prothrombin time is prolonged.

Factor VII deficiency: It occurs as a mendelian-dominant congenital defect and in acquired form in severe liver disease and after coumarin therapy. It may be associated with other plasma factor defects that give abnormal PTT.

Factor VIII deficiency:

Hemophilia A: Hemophilia A is a hereditary disease transmitted as a sex-linked recessive character that leads to defects which remain the same from generation to generation. It affects men almost exclusively and is transmitted by females who are usually unaffected. The disease is due to a defect in the antihemophilic globulin. Clinically, the disease may vary from an almost asymptomatic slight depression of factor VIII to a severe hemorrhagic disease due to almost complete absence of the factor. Factor VIII deficiency leads to abnormal formation of thromboplastin.

Factor IX deficiency:

Hemophilia B (Christmas disease): Hemophilia B is due to factor IX deficiency, which interferes with the thromboplastin generation.

From the point of view of therapy it is noteworthy that factor IX is stable in stored plasma, while factor VIII is not.

Laboratory diagnosis of hemophilias:
1. Coagulation time: prolonged (depends on severity of disease)
2. Bleeding time: normal
3. Prothrombin time: normal
4. Prothrombin consumption time: abnormal
5. Thromboplastin generation test: abnormal

von Willebrand's disease[164]: This disease affects both sexes and is, according to some reports, quite common. In this disorder there is a defect in the AHG associated with defective adhesiveness of platelets, which leads to prolonged bleeding time. Morphologically and numerically the platelets are normal (see p. 153).

Factor XI deficiency: This is a congenital disorder inherited by a recessive autosomal gene which causes bleeding only in the homozygous form and is restricted to patients of Jewish extraction.

Factor XII deficiency: The absence of bleeding tendency is in contrast with the abnormal clotting tests in glass tubes.

Factor XIII deficiency[166]: The picture is the opposite from the one produced by factor XII deficiency. There is a clinical bleeding tendency associated with normal routine coagulation tests.

Hemorrhagic diseases due to circulating anticoagulants

Each phase of blood clotting is subject to the action of inhibitors. Under physiologic conditions they maintain the blood in the fluid state and counteract coagulation factors formed in excess. Under pathologic conditions they may lead to bleeding. Circulating anticoagulants may be directed against the deficient factor as in some cases of hemophilia. They may appear in dysproteinemias, e.g., macroglobulinemia and multiple myeloma.

1. Inhibitors of phase I: antithromboplastin, antifactor VIII factor, antitissue thromboplastin, and antifactors V and VII substances
2. Inhibitors of phase II: antithrombin, heparin plus cofactor which acts as antithrombin, and fibrinogen (adsorbs thrombin, thus acting as antithrombin)
3. Inhibitor of phase III: fibrinolysin

Hyperheparinemia: Congenital and acquired forms of hyperheparinemia are recognized. The acquired form may follow shock and may be seen in allergies, collagen diseases, thermal and irradiation burns, liver disease, leukemia, and malignant tumors.

Fibrinolysis: See discussions of afibrinogenemia, hypofibrinogenemia, and fibrinolysis assay.

HEMORRHAGIC DISEASES DUE TO PLATELET DEFECTS

The defect may lie in the number or in the quality of the platelets or both. It may be hereditary or acquired.

The platelet's functions are many. They have to do with the integrity of the endothelial lining of blood vessels, as evidenced by bleeding that occurs if the platelet number falls below 20,000 platelets/mm.[3]. Platelets also have to do with the initiation, continuation, and retraction of the blood clot.

Qualitative platelet defects usually do not cause spontaneous bleeding but are responsible for posttraumatic and postoperative bleeding. The prolonged bleeding time is a common denominator of all qualitative platelet defects. These defects may be associated with clotting factor defects as seen in thrombocytopathic hemophilia and in thrombosis-fibrinolysis syndrome.

Qualitative platelet defects

Thrombasthenia (Glanzmann)[167-169]: In this condition there are a number of en-zymatic platelet defects that lead to defective glycolysis, defective platelet fibrinogen, and impaired clot retraction. The number of platelets is normal but there is marked variation in size as seen in the blood smear. In addition there is absence of normal granularity that is replaced by a diffuse basophilia. The platelets appear singly rather than in the normal aggregates.

Laboratory diagnosis: The bleeding time is prolonged and clot retraction is defective.

Thrombocytopathia (von Willebrand's disease)[170]: It may be hereditary or acquired.

Hereditary form: In this condition there is a defect in the release or contents of phospholipids of the platelets that can be discovered by an abnormal thromboplastin generation test. The clot retraction is normal. The platelet count is normal and in the blood smear the platelets are not altered morphologically. The plasma shows AHG deficiency and the platelets are characterized by inadequate adhesiveness (see p. 212).

Acquired form: It may accompany polycythemia vera, uremia, myeloproliferative disorders, and macrocytic anemias.

Laboratory diagnosis: Bleeding time is prolonged. Prothrombin consumption is abnormal. PTT and TGT are abnormal. Platelet adhesiveness is abnormal.

May-Hegglin type of thrombocytopathia, thrombasthenia, and thrombocytopenia: In this congenital disease, which also involves the white blood cells (see p. 154), the platelets are morphologically abnormal in size and shape. There is an absence of normal granularity and the platelets are numerically diminished. The bleeding time is prolonged. Clot retraction and prothrombin consumption are abnormal.

Defects in number of platelets

DECREASE IN NUMBER OF PLATELETS:

Congenital thrombocytopenia[171]: This is a rare disorder that is due to a familial hereditary disposition to produce antiplatelet antibodies.

Acquired thrombocytopenia: The causes are enumerated on p. 154.

Immunologic thrombocytopenic purpura (ITP)[172]:

Peripheral blood: There is a diminution in the number of platelets to a level below 10,000 platelets/mm.[3]. The platelets are morphologically not altered, and unless there is bleeding the red and white cells are not remarkable.

Bone marrow: The megakaryocytes are increased in number and may show some shift to the left so that there is a relative increase in immature forms. Many show morphologic changes and nuclear-cytoplasmic dissociation. Giant forms are seen that have a blue hyaline, homogenous, and at times peripherally vacuolated cytoplasm devoid of granulations. They fail to produce platelets or give rise to only a few. The giant forms alternate with small promegakaryocytes that have abnormally lobulated nuclei and deep blue cytoplasm. The nuclei often show hyperchromatism and irregular lobulation.

Platelet survival studies: The patient's platelets are labeled with Cr[51] and their life-span within the patient's circulation is determined. In immunologic thrombocytopenia the life-span is always shortened. In acute cases it may be shortened to a few hours, while the life-span of normal platelets varies from 8-10 days.

Antiplatelet factor: Harrington, in 1951, proved by experiments on himself that in immunologic thrombocytopenia a factor was present in the plasma which produced thrombocytopenia when transfused into normal recipients. This factor has not been identified by the immunologic methods available at the present time.

Test for detection of platelet antibodies in serum: Osterberg published the following method[173]:

1. Take 7 ml. fresh O-negative versenated blood and centrifuge 10 min. at 1000 rpm.
2. Withdraw platelet-rich plasma and recentrifuge at 2400 rpm for another 10 min. Discard supernatant, leaving a platelet button.
3. Wash platelets three times in 0.85% saline solution and then suspend in 2 ml. saline solution by gentle inversion for 5 min. Use Parafilm to cover tube.
4. Centrifuge at 500 rpm for 5 min. to remove large platelet clumps. Use suspension immediately.
5. Obtain fasting blood specimen and allow to undergo firm clot retraction. Centrifuge serum for 10 min. at 3000 rpm to remove remaining platelets. Incubate 0.2 ml. test serum with 0.2 ml. platelet suspension for 1 hr. at 37° C.
6. At the same time run a control, using 0.2 ml. 0.85% saline solution and 0.2 ml. platelet suspension.
7. Perform platelet counts on control and patient specimens. A decrease of platelets of 50% or more in the patient specimen as compared to the saline control represents a significant decrease.

Coagulation studies: The bleeding time is prolonged but not as much as in the thrombocytopathias. The clotting time is normal, but the clot retraction is poor, which can be demonstrated visually by thromboblastography. The heparin tolerance and the prothrombin consumption tests are abnormal.

Thrombotic microangiopathy (thrombotic thrombocytopenic purpura)[174]: This is a rare generalized disease characterized by the development of multiple small thrombi in the arterioles of various organs.

Blood picture: There is a progressive hemolytic anemia with thrombocytopenia and leukocytosis. The reticulocyte count is elevated in response to the hemolysis. The blood smear reveals erythrocytes which show great variation in size and shape so characteristic of hemolytic anemias, emphasized by the presence of burr cells, schistocytes, and angular microspherocytes. (Fig. 4-15, p. 134.)

Thrombocytopenia associated with hemangiomas: This condition occurs in newborn babies and infants and is accompanied by anemia and hemorrhagic diathesis.

INCREASE IN NUMBER OF PLATELETS:

Thrombocythemia (thrombocytosis): It may be primary or secondary (Fig. 4-55).

Primary form: The platelet count may reach several millions/mm.[3]. The increase in platelets leads to a tendency to thromboses as well as to hemorrhagic diathesis.

Table 4-20

Defect	Blood or blood fractions
Acute blood loss	Stored blood, fresh blood, plasma, dextran
Thrombocytopenia	Platelet concentrates, fresh blood
Hypofibrinogenemia and afibrino-genemia (fibrinolysins)	Fresh blood, fibrinogen, lyophilized plasma, stored blood (fresh)
Hypoprothrombinemia	Fresh blood, stored blood (fresh), lyophilized plasma
Factor V deficiency	Fresh blood, fresh frozen plasma
Factor VIII deficiency	Fresh blood, fresh frozen plasma, lyophilized plasma, stored blood (fresh), antihemophilic globulin
Hemophilia B	Fresh blood, antihemophilic globulin, fresh frozen plasma, lyophilized plasma
Liver disease	Fresh blood, fresh frozen plasma, albumin
Dicumarol bleeding	Stored blood (fresh), vitamin K₁, fresh blood
Agammaglobulinemia	Fresh blood, gamma globulin, stored blood
Heparin bleeding	Protamine sulfate

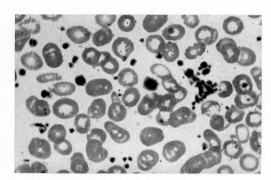

Fig. 4-55. Thrombocythemia.

The bleeding and clotting times may be abnormal.

Blood findings: The blood smear reveals masses of variously sized platelets, often accompanied by fragmented megakaryocytes. There may or may not be a leukocytosis. The bone marrow shows numerous clumps of megakaryocytes.

TRANSFUSION THERAPY
OF COAGULATION DEFECTS

Since the laboratory may be responsible for procuring the necessary blood factors, a short list of the defects and the blood or blood fractions used in their correction is given in Table 4-20.

REFERENCES

1. Maximow, A. A.: Physiol. Rev. **4**:533, 1924.
2. Bloom, W., and Bartelmez, G. W.: Amer. J. Anat. **67**:21, 1940.
3. First report: Amer. J. Clin. Path. **18**:443, 1948.
4. Second report: Amer. J. Clin. Path. **19**:56, 1949.
5. Third report: Amer. J. Clin. Path. **20**:562, 1950.
6. Fourth report: Amer. J. Clin. Path. **20**:571, 1950.
7. Fifth report: Amer. J. Clin. Path. **20**:574, 1950.
8. Bessis, J. B. M.: Hematologie, Paris, 1958, Masson & Cie.
9. Sunderman, F. W.: Amer. J. Clin. Path. **43**:9, 1965.
10. Beeler, M. F., Deupree, R. H., and Goheen, E. M.: Amer. J. Clin. Path. **44**:203, 1965.
11. Skendzel, L. P., and Copeland, B. E.: Amer. J. Clin. Path. **44**:245, 1965.
12. Technical Subcommitteee on Haemoglobinometry of the International Committee for Standardization in Haematology: Blood **26**:104, 1965.
13. Van Kampen, E. J., and Zijlstra, W. G.: Advances Clin. Chem. **8**:141, 1965.
14. Peters, J. P., and Van Slyke, D. D.: Quantitative clinical chemistry; methods, Baltimore, 1932, The Williams & Wilkins Co., vol. 2.
15. Mason, E. C., and Adarraga-Elizarin, A.: J. Clin. Path. **16**:604, 1963.
16. Sunderman, F. W.: Amer. J. Clin. Path. **40**:227, 1963.
17. Klendshoj, N. C., Feldstein, M., and Sprague, A. L.: J. Biol. Chem. **183**:297, 1950.
18. Gettler, A. O., and Freimuth, H. C.: Amer. J. Clin. Path. **11**:603, 1940.
18a. Sunderman, F. W., and Sunderman, F. W., Jr.: Hemoglobin: its precursors and metabolites, Philadelphia, 1964, J. B. Lippincott Co.
19. Evelyn, K. A., and Malloy, H. T.: J. Biol. Chem. **126**:655, 1938.
20. Bodansky, M.: Pharmacol. Rev. **3**:144, 1951.
21. Silver, D., Brown, I. W., and Eadie, G. S.: J. Lab. Clin. Med. **48**:79, 1966.

22. Van Kampen, E. J., Zijlstra, W. G.: Advances Clin. Chem. **8**:187, 1965.
23. Brandenberg, R. O., and Smith, H. L.: Amer. Heart J. **42**:582, 1951.
24. Heller, V. G., and Paul, H.: J. Lab. Clin. Med. **19**:777, 1934.
25. Graff, S., and Clark, H. T.: Arch. Intern. Med. **48**:808, 1931.
26. Cutler, J. W.: New Internat. Clin. **3**:62, 1940.
27. Winsor, T., and Burch, G. E.: Amer. J. Med. Sci. **207**:152, 1944.
28. Montgomery, L. G.: Amer. J. Clin. Path. (tech. sect.) **7**:115, 1943.
29. McClenahan, J. B., Yamauchi, H., and Roe, B. B.: J.A.M.A. **195**:356, 1966.
30. Gray, S. J., and Sterling, K.: J. Clin. Invest. **29**:1604, 1950.
31. Birkeland, S.: Acta. Chir. Scand. **253**: (supp.):64, 1960.
32. Wintrobe, M. M.: J. Lab. Clin. Med. **17**: 899, 1932.
33. Sabin, F. R., et al.: Bull. Hopkins Hosp. **37**:14, 1925.
34. Current Comment: J.A.M.A. **101**:1240, 1933.
35. Editorial: J.A.M.A. **126**:914, 1944.
36. Harley, J. D., and Maver, M. A.: Blood **16**:1722, 1960.
37. Barrett, A. M.: J. Path. Bact. **46**:603, 1938.
38. Stats, D., Rosenthal, N., and Wassermann, L. R.: Amer. J. Clin. Path. **17**:585, 1947.
39. Roche, M., Thorn, G. W., and Hills, A. G.: New Eng. J. Med. **242**:307, 1950.
40. Thorn, G. W., Forsham, P. H., Prunty, F. T. G., and Hills, A. G.: J.A.M.A. **137**: 1005, 1948.
41. Cooper, J. R., and Cruickshank, C. N. D.: J. Clin. Path. **19**:402, 1966.
42. Shelley, W. B., and Parnes, H. M.: J.A.M.A. **192**:108, 1965.
43. Katz, H. I., Gill, K. A., Baxter, D. L., and Moschella, S. L.: J.A.M.A. **188**:351, 1964.
44. Brecher, G., Schneiderman, M., and Cronkite, E. P.: Amer. J. Clin. Path. **23**:15, 1953.
45. Bull, B. S., Schneiderman, M. A., and Brecher, G.: Amer. J. Clin. Path. **44**:678, 1965.
46. Efrati, P., and Rozenszajn, L.: Blood **16**: 1012, 1960.
47. Kaplow, L. S.: Amer. J. Clin. Path. **39**: 439, 1963.
48. Schmidt, D. Z.: Amer. J. Med. Sci. **465**: 113, 1966.
49. Kaplow, L. S.: Blood **26**:215, 1965.
50. Hattersley, P. G.: J.A.M.A. **189**:997, 1964.
51. Mier, M., Schwartz, S. O., and Boshes, B.: Blood **16**:158, 1960.
52. Bell, R. E.: Brit. J. Haemat. **9**:552, 1963.
53. Harley, J. D., and Maver, M. A.: Blood **16**: 1722, 1960.
54. Barnes, A., Jr.: J.A.M.A. **198**:151, 1955.
55. A symposium on sideroblastic anemia: Brit. J. Haemat. **11**:41, 1965.
56. Hall, R., and Losowsky, M. S.: Brit. J. Haemat. **12**:334, 1966.
57. Petz, L. D., Goodman, J. R., Hall, S. G., and Fink, D. J.: Amer. J. Clin. Path. **45**: 581, 1966.
58. Davidson, W. M., and Smith, D. R.: Brit. Med. J. **2**:6, 1954.
59. Tenczar, F. J., and Streitmatter, D. E.: Amer. J. Clin. Path. **26**:384, 1956.
60. Moore, K. L., and Barr, M. L.: Brit. J. Cancer **9**:246, 1955.
61. Yunis, J. J.: Human chromosome methodology, New York, 1965, Academic Press, Inc.
62. Eggen, R. R.: Chromosome diagnostics in clinical medicine, Springfield, Ill., 1965, Charles C Thomas, Publisher.
63. White, Z. G.: Blood **28**:143, 1966.
64. Abernathy, M. R.: Blood **27**:380, 1966.
65. Rozenszajn, L., Klajman, A., Yaffe, D., and Efrati, P.: Blood **28**:258, 1966.
66. Johnston, B., Mayhood, M. E., Arthur, T. E., and Brady, J.: Acta Cytol. **11**:304, 1967.
67. Buchanan, J. G., Pearce, L., and Weatherley-Mein, G.: Brit. J. Haemat. **10**:508, 1964.
68. Donohugh, D. L.: Calif. Med. **104**:421, 1966.
69. Lyons, C.: J.A.M.A. **123**:1007, 1943.
70. Current Comment: J.A.M.A. **133**:776, 1947.
71. Loeffler, W.: Beitr. Klin. Erforsch. Tuberk. **79**:368, 1932.
72. Frederick, R. E., and Maloney, W. C.: Blood **14**:571, 1959.
73. Riley, J. F.: Mast cells, Edinburgh, 1959, E & S Livingstone, Ltd.
74. Mellors, R. C.: Blood **27**:871, 1966.
75. Craddock, C. G., et al.: Ann. Intern. Med. **64**:687, 1966.
76. Lowenstein, L., and Bain, B.: Vox Sang. **2**:305, 1955.
77. Zmijewski, C. M., and Amos, D. B.: Vox Sang. **11**:377, 1966.
78. Harris, R., et al.: Brit. Med. J. **1**:509, 1966.
78a. Spiegal-Adolf, M., Bairo, H. W., Coleman, H. S., and Szekeley, E. G.: In Aronson, S. M., and Volk, B. W., editors: Cerebral sphingolipidoses, New York, 1962, Academic Press, Inc., p. 129.
79. Finucane, D. L., and Philips, R. S.: Amer. J. Dis. Child. **68**:301, 1944.
80. Maldonado, J. E., and Hanlon, D. G.: Mayo Clin. Proc. **40**:248, 1965.
81. Bessis, C. M.: Lab. Invest. **10**:1040, 1961.
82. Rebuck, J. W., and Lo Grippo, G. A.: Lab. Invest. **10**:1068, 1961.
83. Melamed, M. R., Clirrton, E. E., Mercer, C., and Koss, L. G.: Amer. J. Med. Sci. **252**:301, 1966.
84. Seegers, W. H.: Advances Enzym. **16**:23, 1955.
85. Johnson, S., Monto, R. W., Rebuck, J. W., and Horn, R. C., editors: Blood platelets, Boston, 1961, Little, Brown & Co.
86. Ferguson, J. H.: Lipoids and blood platelets, Chapel Hill, N. C., 1960, University of North Carolina Press.

87. Roberts, S., et al.: Ann. Surg. **154**:362, 1961.
88. Anderson, B.: J. Clin. Path. **17**:14, 1964.
89. Schilling, R. F., Clatanoff, D. V., and Korst, D. R.: J. Lab. Clin. Med. **45**:926, 1955.
90. Chanarin, I., and Berry, V.: J. Clin. Path. **17**:111, 1964.
91. Mohamed, S. D., and Roberts, M.: J. Clin. Path. **19**:37, 1966.
92. Hoffbrand, A. V., Newcombe, B. F. A., and Mollin, D. L.: J. Clin. Path. **19**:17, 1966.
93. Dorland, G. A., and Worthley, U.: J. Lab. Clin. Med. **20**:1122, 1935.
94. Danon, D., Frei, Y. F., Rimon, A., and Ammon, B. D.: Transfusion **4**:339, 1964.
95. Danon, D.: J. Clin. Path. **16**:377, 1963.
96. Dacie, J. V., and Lewis, S. M.: Practical hematology, ed. 3, New York, 1963, Grune & Stratton, Inc., p. 144.
97. Hands, G. E., Cassell, M., Ray, R. N., and Chaplin, H., Jr.: J. Lab Clin. Med. **56**:486, 1960.
98. Kauder, E., and Mauer, A. M.: J. Pediat. **59**:286, 1961.
99. Veneziale, C. M., and McGurckin, W. F.: Mayo Clin. Proc. **40**:751, 1965.
100. Lehmann, H.: Acta Haemat. **36**:256, 1966.
101. Schulman, I.: Med. Clin. N. Amer. **46**:93, 1962.
102. Abt, L., and Downey, W. S., Jr.: J. Pediat. **47**:6, 1955.
103. Schilling, R. W., and Klein, G. C.: Amer. J. Clin. Path. **44**:662, 1965.
104. Wilson, H., Nakai, H., and Landing, B.: Stain Techn. **35**:205, 1960.
105. Lehman, H., and Ager, J. A. M.: Laboratory detection of abnormal hemoglobins, The Association of Clinical Pathologists, Broadsheet No. 33 (new series) May, 1961.
106. Marsh, C. L., Jolliff, C. R., and Payne, L. C.: Amer. J. Clin. Path. **41**:217, 223, 1964.
107. Marengo-Rowe, A. J.: J. Clin. Path. **18**:790, 1965.
108. Cawley, L. P.: Workshop manual on electroporesis and immunoelectrophoresis, Chicago, 1966, American Society of Clinical Pathologists.
109. Itano, H. A.: Arch. Biochem. **47**:108, 1963.
110. Goldberg, C. A. J.: Clin. Chem. **3**:1, 1957.
111. Beutler, E.: Seminars Hemat. **2**:91, 1965.
112. Fairbanks, V. F., and Beutler, E.: Blood **20**:591, 1962.
113. Oski, F. A., and Growney, P. M.: J. Pediat. **66**:90, 1965.
114. Brewer, J. G., Tarlov, A. R., and Alving, A. S.: J.A.M.A. **180**:386, 1962.
115. Stamatoyannopoulas, G., Papayannopoulou, T., Bakopoulos, C., and Motulsky, A. G.: Blood **29**:87, 1967.
116. Beutler, E.: Blood **28**:553, 1966.
117. Ellis, H. A., and Kirkman, H. N.: Proc. Soc. Exper. Biol. Med. **106**:607, 1961.
118. Beutler, E.: J. Lab. Clin. Med. **49**:84, 1957.
119. Schwartz, R. S., and Costea, N.: Seminars Hemat. **111**:2, 1966.
120. Schubothe, H.: Seminars Hemat. **111**:27, 1966.
121. Allen, F. H., Jr., and Diamond, L. K.: J.A.M.A. **155**:1209, 1954.
122. Hsia, D. Y., Allen, F. H., Jr., Diamond, L. K., and Gellis, S. S.: J. Pediat. **42**:277, 1953.
123. Miescher, P. A.: Seminars Hemat. **33**:175, 1966.
124. Rosse, W., Waldeman, T. A., and Cohen, P.: Amer. J. Med. **34**:76, 1963.
125. Sprunt, T. P., and Evans, F. A.: Bull. Hopkins Hosp. **31**:410, 1920.
126. Pfeiffer, E.: Jahrb. Kinderh. **29**:257, 1889.
127. Rosenberg, A., and Van Slyck, J.: Ann. Intern. Med. **63**:965, 1965.
128. Davidsohn, I., and Lee, C. L.: Amer. J. Clin. Path. **41**:115, 1964.
129. Davidsohn, I.: J.A.M.A. **108**:289, 1937.
130. Davidsohn, I.: Amer. J. Dis. Child. **49**:1222, 1935.
131. Davidsohn, I.: Amer. J. Clin. Path. **5**:455, 1935.
132. Lee, C. L., and Davidsohn, I.: Scientific Exhibit, ASCP-CAP, Sept., 1967.
133. Ericson, C.: Acta Med. Scand. **166**:225, 1960.
134. Robinson, L., and Smith, H.: J. Clin. Path. **19**:339, 1966.
135. Fekete, A. M., and Kerpelman, E. J.: J.A.M.A. **194**:158, 1965.
136. Stone, G. E., and Redmond, A. J.: Amer. J. Med. **34**:541, 1963.
137. DuBois, E. L., and Tuffanelli, D. L.: J.A.M.A. **190**:104, 1964.
138. Miescher, P. A., and Riethmüller, D.: Seminars Hemat. **2**:1, 1965.
139. Burkhardt, R.: Seminars Hemat. **2**:29, 1965.
140. Cawley, L. P., et al.: Clin. Chim. Acta **12**:105, 1965.
141. Scharff, M. D., and Uhr, J. W.: Seminars Hemat. **2**:47, 1965.
142. Goulian, M.: Ann. Intern. Med. **65**:782, 1966.
143. Davie, E. W., and Ratnoff, O. D.: Science **145**:1310, 1964.
144. Loewy, A. G., et al.: J. Biol. Chem. **236**:262, 1961.
145. Rosner, F., and Ritz, N.: Arch. Intern. Med. **117**:17, 1966.
146. Johnson, A. J., and Newman, J.: Seminars Hemat. **1**:401, 1964.
147. Sherry, S.: Gastroenterology **51**:901, 1966.
148. Iatridis, S. G., and Ferguson, J. H.: Thromb. Diath. Haemorrh. **6**:411, 1961.
149. Genton, E., Fletcher, A. P., Alkjaersig, N., and Sherry, S.: J. Lab. Clin. Med. **64**:313, 1964.
150. Hardisty, R. M., Ingram, G. I. C., and Sharp, A. A.: Laboratory investigation and control of the defibrination syndrome, The Association of Clinical Pathologists, Broad-

sheet No. 48 (new series replacing No. 19), 1964.

151. Eichelberger, J. W., Jr.: Laboratory methods in blood coagulation, New York, 1965, Harper & Row, Publishers.
152. Brooks, R. A., and Copeland, B. E.: Amer. J. Clin. Path. **42:**221, 1964.
153. Wyle, C. R. R., and Fraser, C.: J. Clin. Path. **18:**372, 1965.
154. Miale, J. B.: Amer. J. Clin. Path. **43:**475, 1965.
155. Miale, J. B., and Winningham, A. R.: Amer. J. Clin. Path. **33:**214, 1960.
156. Quick, A. J.: Amer. J. Clin. Path. **45:**105, 1966.
157. Goulian, M., and Beck, W. S.: Amer. J. Clin. Path. **44:**97, 1965.
158. Proctor, R. R., and Rapaport, S. I.: Amer. J. Clin. Path. **36:**212, 1961.
159. Quick, A. J., and Geppert, M.: Amer. J. Clin. Path. **40:**465, 1963.
160. Hyland reference manual of coagulation procedures, Los Angeles, 1964, Hyland Laboratories.
161. Miale, J. B.: Laboratory medicine—hematology, ed. 3, St. Louis, 1967, The C. V. Mosby Co.
162. Workshop on Techniques in Blood coagulation, revised manual, Chicago, 1960, American Society of Clinical Pathologists.
163. Gollub, S., and Ulin, A. W.: Ann. N. Y. Acad. Sci. **115:**1, 1964.
164. Blombäck, M., Jorpes, J. E., and Nilsson, I. M.: Amer. J. Med. **34:**236, 1963.
165. Salzman, E. W.: J. Lab. Clin. Med. **62:**724, 1963.
166. Fisher, S., Rikover, M., and Naon, S.: Blood **28:**34, 1966.
167. Friedman, L. L., et al.: Mayo Clin. Proc. **39:**908, 1964.
168. Pittman, M. A., Jr., and Graham, J. B.: Amer. J. Med. Sci. **247:**293, 1964.
169. Nachman, R.: J. Lab. Clin. Med. **67:**411, 1966.
170. Karaca, M., and Stefanini, M.: J. Lab. Clin. Med. **67:**237, 1966.
171. Harms, D., and Sachs, V.: Acta. Haemat. **34:**30, 1965.
172. Baldini, M.: New Eng. J. Med. **274:**1245, 1301, 1360, 1966.
173. Osterberg, M. M.: Flor-Ocular (Florida Div. ASMT) **13:**6, 1965.
174. Allanby, V. D., Huntsman, R. G., and Sacher, L. S.: Lancet **1:**237, 1966.

Chapter 5

Blood groups, blood typing, and crossmatching*†

ANTIGENS AND ANTIBODIES

Antigens: An antigen is a substance, protein or nonprotein, which, when introduced parenterally into an animal, causes the production of an antibody which reacts specifically with that antigen. An antibody is a substance (protein) produced in the serum as a result of antigenic stimulation that reacts specifically with the antigen (or closely related antigens) in a manner that is directly visible or can be rendered visible. The blood group substances are mucopolysaccharides composed of carbohydrates and polypeptides and are thought to be arranged on or immediately below the surface of red blood cells. They act as antigens, and the antibodies to these antigens are the blood group antibodies. A haptene cannot stimulate antibody formation, but it can react with an antibody.

Antibodies[3]: They are gamma globulins, or immunoglobulins, which are divided into the following groups: IgG, IgA, IgM, IgD, and IgE (γ-G, γ-A, γ-M, γ-D, and γ-E) (Table 5-1). Antibodies can be named according to different characteristics. Some damage red blood cells and are hemolysins (interacting with complement and/or properdin), others

agglutinate red blood cells and act as agglutinins. Not all antibodies act under the same conditions. Some act only in a saline medium and are called complete antibodies, whereas others act only in a high protein medium and are named incomplete antibodies. Again, others appear not to act until the red blood cells have been treated with enzymes (trypsin, papain, etc.) to remove the most superficial red cell coats.

γ-M antibodies: They are the naturally occurring antibodies that are the result of unavoidable exposure to group-specific substances. They differ physicochemically from other antibodies: they agglutinate red cells optimally in saline medium and act more strongly at low temperatures (4°-20° C.). They are high molecular weight antibodies (macroglobulins and euglobulins) with a sedimentation constant of 19S. They are first produced (primary) in the process of immunization. They are cold agglutinins, isohemagglutinins, and naturally occurring antibodies.

γ-G antibodies: They are also called univalent (though all antibodies are probably bivalent), conglutinating, blocking, incomplete, or coating antibodies. They are thermostable and appear later in the course of immunization after a second exposure to the antigen (secondary). The univalent antibodies tend to coat their specific cells when brought in contact with them in saline medium, but they do not clump them. When high molecular proteins are added, the univa-

---

*In this chapter **boldface** type is used for blood factors and their corresponding antibodies, regular type for agglutinogens and phenotypes, and *italics* for genes and genotypes.

†Standard references for the student are *Technical Methods and Procedures of the American Association of Blood Banks*[1] and Mollison's *Blood Transfusion in Clinical Medicine.*[2]

Table 5-1. Summary of characteristics of antibodies[4]

Characteristics	IgM antibody	IgG antibody	IgA antibody	IgD antibody	IgE antibody
Classification and synonyms	Agglutinating, precipitating, complete, bivalent antibody (agglutinins, precipitins)	Conglutinating, incomplete, univalent, coating antibody	Complete and incomplete antibodies	—	Reagin
Optimum medium	Saline	Albumin	Saline	Saline	Saline
Sedimentation constant	19S	7S	7, 10, 13S	7S	—
Effect of heat (56° C. for 3 hr.)	Thermolabile	Thermostable	Thermostable	Thermostable	Thermostable
Molecular weight	Approximately 1,000,000	Approximately 150,000	150,000 (monomer)	150,000	—
Reaction with complement, production of hemolysis	Does not fix complement, does not produce hemolysis	Fixes complement, may produce hemolysis	Does not fix complement	—	—
Location by electrophoresis	Gamma, fast, or beta	Gamma, slow	Slow, beta	Between gamma and beta	Between gamma and beta
Behavior in relation to placenta	Held back	Passes through	Held back	Held back	Held back
Effect of type-specific substance	Neutralization	None	Partial	—	—
Role in erythroblastosis	Minor	Major	Minor	—	—
Optimum temperature for activity*	5°-25° C.	37° C.	5°-25° C.	—	—

*Not necessarily true.

lent antibodies cause the cells to clump. The γ-G antibodies act best at 37° C. and agglutinate red cells suspended in protein medium. They are low molecular weight antibodies with a sedimentation constant of 7S. They are the antibodies to viruses and bacteria and of passive immunization of the newborn infant.

The placenta is able to transmit 7S gamma globulin but retains 19S gamma globulins.

γ-A antibodies: They are present in secretions (parotid, saliva) and in serum, e.g., antithyroid.

Complement (C'): Complement is a globulin consisting of several components $(C'_1-C'_9)$ present in normal serum. It is thermolabile and is nonspecifically involved in some antigen-antibody reactions by being adsorbed by the sensitized antigen. In combination with some antibodies, e.g., immune anti-**A** or immune anti-**B**, it may be hemolytic. Heating serum to 56° C. for 30 min. inactivates C'. Storage at 4° C. maintains its activity for 24-48 hr., while freezing at –50° C. preserves it for 2 mo. The addition of 1 drop of fresh serum or 2 drops of stored serum to an antigen-antibody reaction guarantees adequate complement levels.

Heparin and EDTA are anticomplementary.

Antigen-antibody reaction: Antigen-antibody reaction occurs in two phases: (1) the antibody combines with the antigen, thus sensitizing the antigen (e.g., red cells), and (2) the sensitized antigen is agglutinated or lysed with the help of complement.

At times special systems have to be used to prove sensitization, e.g., the addition of Coombs serum or treatment of red cells with proteolytic enzymes.

Antigen-antibody reaction is dependent on several factors:

1. Antibody:
   (a) Concentration and avidity: The concentration of the antibody is related to the occurrence of a prozone—failure of agglutination to occur in the face of excess antibody.
   (b) Type of antibody: Does it require complement?
   (c) Temperature: Most testing is done at room temperature at approximately 20° C. even though some antibodies act best at 4° C. and others at 37° C.
2. Antigen: Not all antigens are equally strong. Some are naturally weak and others may be weakened by age, disease, storage, or presence of other antigens. Homozygosity strengthens an antigen.
3. Medium: Reaction occurs in saline or albumin medium and in the presence of complement, etc.
4. Technical factors: Incubation period, temperature, and centrifugation.

ANTIGLOBULIN TEST (COOMBS TEST)[5, 6]: The test is based on the agglutination of human red cells sensitized by gamma globulin antibodies by the use of antihuman gamma globulin serum prepared in rabbits. The antiglobulin serum may be specific for γ-G globulin or it may also act on nongamma immunoglobulins, which are frequently complement dependent.

Two test procedures, which are essentially similar, will be described. The direct Coombs test detects red cells sensitized in vivo, while the indirect Coombs test detects red cells sensitized in vitro.

Direct antiglobulin test (direct Coombs test):

Principle: The test directly demonstrates the sensitization of red cells that has occurred in vivo.

Method:
1. With a wooden applicator transfer a small amount of red blood cells from the clot (preferred) or from blood containing anticoagulant to a large amount of saline solution.
2. Centrifuge at 3400 rpm in Sero-Fuge for 15 sec. until the cells are packed.
3. Decant saline solution completely, wiping mouth of tube.
4. Repeat the washing two more times, adding a small amount of the saline solution at first and mixing well to suspend the cells; then add more saline solution by washing it down the sides of the tube.
5. Add saline solution to the washed cells to make a 2% suspension.
6. To 2 drops of this suspension add 1 drop Coombs serum and proceed according to the directions received with the serum.
7. Spin in Sero-Fuge at full speed for 15 sec.
8. Gently dislodge the cell button and observe for agglutination, both macroscopically and microscopically.

Interpretation: Agglutination indicates a positive Coombs test, proving that the red cells are sensitized.

Indications for direct Coombs test:
1. Diagnosis of erythroblastosis fetalis
2. Diagnosis of autoimmune hemolytic anemias
3. Diagnosis of transfusion reaction due to incompatible blood

Indirect antiglobulin test (indirect Coombs test):

Principle: The serum antibody is bound to suitable red cells in vitro and this sensitization is then demonstrated by the direct Coombs technique. Two procedures are required: first, incubation of the serum with red cells of selected (known) types in order that the cells may become sensitized by (coated with) the antibody if present and, second, testing the cells for sensitization by the application of the direct Coombs test.

Method:

1. To 1 drop serum add 1 drop 2% suspension of selected red cells in saline solution.
2. Incubate for 15-30 min. in water bath at 37° C. Some antibodies (anti-**Duffy**, anti-**Kidd**) may require longer.
3. Wash cells three times in large amounts of normal saline solution in Sero-Fuge at 3400 rpm for 15 sec. each.
4. Prepare 2% suspension of washed cells.
5. Label test tube and place 1 drop anti-human globulin serum into tube and add 1 drop 2% red cell suspension.
6. Mix and centrifuge at 3400 rpm for 15 sec.
7. Gently shake tube and examine for agglutination, both macroscopically and microscopically.

Interpretation: The presence of agglutination indicates a positive Coombs test and thus the presence of antibodies in the serum capable of acting with the test cells.

Indications for indirect Coombs test:

1. Crossmatching to detect incompatibility
2. Detection and identification of irregular antibodies
3. Detection of antigens such as Rh, Kell, Duffy, and Kidd

Choice of cells for indirect Coombs test: It is recommended that two different test cells be used: (1) group O, type Rh_1Rh_1 (CDe/CDe) and (2) group O, type Rh_2Rh_2 (cDE/cDE).

One cell sample should be Kell positive. The homozygosity of the factors increases the sensitivity of the test cells.

Group O red cells of these Rh phenotypes, which in addition contain a number of known blood group factors, are commercially available (Selectogen I and II*).

Washing cells for Coombs tests: The washing must be rapid and thorough.

After the third wash the supernatant must not show any evidence of protein precipitation if an equal volume of 25% sulfosalicylic acid is added.

Controls of Coombs test:

1. The antiglobulin serum should be checked daily against red cells weakly sensitized with anti-Rh_o (D), a γ-G type antibody, and against red cells sensitized with anti-**Le** or anti-**Fy**, complement-dependent non-gamma globulins.
2. Sensitized cells may also be added to a negative Coombs reaction, in which case they should be clumped by the Coombs serum not being utilized. A very weakly positive Coombs test may leave enough Coombs serum free to give a positive control test similar to the truly negative Coombs test.

Preparation of sensitized control cells:

1. Prepare a 2% suspension of washed Rh_o-positive cells in saline solution.
2. Dilute 1 part anti-Rh_o slide typing serum with 9 parts normal saline solution.
3. Prepare a mixture of 0.5 ml. 2% cell suspension and 0.5 ml. diluted anti-Rh_o serum.
4. Incubate for 30 min. at 37° C.
5. Wash cells well three times in normal saline solution and prepare 2% suspension.
6. Use 1 drop cell suspension plus 1 drop Coombs serum.

For negative control use Rh_o-negative (rh) cells (cde) in this procedure. Coated reagent red blood cells are commercially available as Checkcell.*

Sources of error in Coombs technique:

False negative test:

1. The smallest amount of protein neutralizes the Coombs serum:
   (a) Dirty test tube or pipette
   (b) Inadequate washing of red cells
   (c) Contact with fingers
2. Lack of antibody present on red cells:
   (a) Insufficient incubation
   (b) Incubation at a temperature at which the antibody is not active

---

*Ortho Pharmaceutical Corp., Raritan, N. J.

*Chas. Pfizer & Co., Inc., New York, N. Y.

(c) Delay in reading the test, allowing the antibody to be eluted off the red cells

(d) Improper storage, causing test cells to lose reactivity

3. The serum is inactive due to improper storage or has been omitted.

4. Complement-dependent antibodies require complement that may not be available in plasma.

5. The wrong concentration of cells is used.

False positive test:

1. Presence of heavy metal ions and silica in saline solution used
2. Bacterial contamination due to improper storage of saline solution
3. Hypertonicity of saline solution used
4. High-titered, incomplete cold agglutinins
5. Test cells giving positive direct antiglobulin (Coombs) test
6. Presence of Wharton's jelly in cord blood—must be washed four or more times with saline solution
7. High reticulocyte count[7]
8. Inadequately absorbed Coombs serum
9. Contaminated glassware
10. Hyperglobulinemia
11. Penicillin antibody[8]

Coombs technique with enzyme-treated cells: Treatment of red blood cells with proteolytic enzymes increases the sensitivity of the method in which they are used. The enzymes employed are trypsin, bromelin, ficin, papain, or activated papain. Follow the manufacturer's directions. Bromelin is marketed under the trade name Bromelase solution.*

There are antibodies that can be detected by the indirect Coombs technique but that fail to react with enzyme-treated cells (K, Fy^a, etc.).

Nongamma globulin–antiglobulin test (gamma globulin neutralization test, complement antiglobulin test): By the addition of human gamma globulin, Coombs serum can be neutralized so that it will fail to react with gamma globulin type antibodies. The remaining Coombs

*Dade Reagents, Inc., Miami, Fla.

serum fraction (the neutralized serum) contains nongamma globulin–antiglobulin fractions such as anti-alpha and anti-beta globulin that can be inactivated by the addition of human alpha and beta globulins. The so-called neutralized Coombs serum acts with complement and is active against the complement-binding antibodies such as immune anti-**M**, anti-**Le**^{a}, anti-**Le**^{b}, anti-**Lu**^{a}, anti-**Lu**^{b}, anti-**A**, and anti-**B** and is specific for one of the fractions of complement (C_1). There are commercial Coombs sera, called widespectra sera, that are active against gamma and nongamma globulins.

BLOOD GROUP SYSTEMS

Related blood factors are collected into blood group systems that are inherited independently of each other.

ABO BLOOD GROUPS AND ABO TYPING

The blood group substances are genetically determined and inherited as mendelian characteristics. There are three allelic genes (A, B, and O) that determine four blood groups as follows: group O, genotype *OO*; group A, genotypes *AA* and *AO*; group B, genotypes *BB* and *BO*; and group AB, genotype *AB*.

In 73.5% of Caucasians and in 58.5% of Negroes these factors are also present or absent (in conformity with the ABO group of red cells) in the saliva, gastric secretions, urine, and tissue, together with a substance called the H substance.

Depending on which blood group antigen is on the red blood cell, the reciprocal antibody is found in the plasma (serum). The groups are named according to the antigen present on the red cell (Table 5-2).

Table 5-2

Agglutinogen (antigen present on cell)	Agglutinin (antibody present in serum)	Designation of blood group
O	Anti-**A**, anti-**B**	O
A	Anti-**B**	A
B	Anti-**A**	B
AB	None	AB

The serum always contains the isoagglutinins for which there are no corresponding agglutinogens in the red cells (Landsteiner's rule).

The following incidence is usually given for white persons in the United States: group O, 45%; group A, 40%; group B, 10%; and group AB, 3%.

ABO blood grouping

The following two tests should be made:

1. **Determination of cell group** by testing red cells with antisera of known type.
2. **Determination of serum group** by testing serum with red cells of known type.

CELL GROUPING:

Slide method:

1. Mark a glass microslide A on left and B on right and identify with number or name of blood being tested. Divide slide by marking through center with a wax pencil.
2. Place 1 drop anti-**A** serum in the square marked A and 1 drop anti-**B** serum in the square marked B.
3. With the aid of a wooden applicator or pipette and using finger blood or clotted, oxalated, or citrated whole blood, place a small amount of the blood specimen (not greater than one-half the volume of serum used) next to each drop of antiserum.
4. Mix with separate applicator sticks.
5. Tilt slide backward and forward and observe for macroscopic agglutination. Do not warm slide.
6. Interpret red cell group according to Table 5-3.

Agglutination will occur within a few seconds except in the case of weak A and AB cells. Agglutination of A_2, A_3, A_2B, and A_3B cells may be only partial (mixed field reaction). The maximal time is 2 min.

Test tube method:

1. Use 10 or 12 × 75 mm. test tubes. Mark one test tube A and a second test tube B and write number or name of blood on each tube.
2. Place 1 drop anti-**A** serum in tube A and 1 drop anti-**B** serum in tube B.
3. Prepare a 2-4% saline suspension of red cells that have been washed once. Add 1 drop to each tube.
4. Mix by shaking and centrifuge at 1000 rpm for 15 sec.
5. Gently dislodge the red cell button and observe for agglutination by viewing with the low-power objective of the microscope.
6. Interpret the red cell group according to Table 5-3.

SERUM GROUPING[9-11]:

Test tube method:

1. Mark one test tube A and a second test tube B and write number or name of blood on each tube.
2. Place 2 drops serum to be tested in each tube.
3. Add 1 drop freshly prepared 2-4% saline suspension of known group A cells to tube marked A and 1 drop freshly prepared 2% saline suspension of group B cells to tube marked B.
4. Mix by shaking and centrifuge at 3400 rpm for 15 sec.
5. Gently dislodge button and observe for agglutination or hemolysis. Hemolysis may occur if an immune

Table 5-3. Method of cell grouping*

Reaction of red cells with test sera			Designation of blood group
Anti-**A**	Anti-**B**	Group O	
−	−	−	O
+	−	+	A
−	+	+	B
+	+	+	AB

*+ = agglutination; − = no agglutination.

Table 5-4. Serum grouping*

Reaction of serum with test cells			Designation of blood group
A	B	O	
+	+	−	O
−	+	−	A
+	−	−	B
−	−	−	AB

*+ = agglutination; − = no agglutination.

antibody is present, if noninactivated serum is used, and if 1 hr. incubation at room temperature is used instead of centrifugation.

6. Interpret reverse grouping according to Table 5-4.

In reading, avoid hard shaking as this may break up light agglutination that may be due to a weak serum antibody.

In infants anti-**A** and anti-**B** antibodies are not well developed and reverse grouping may fail to confirm the cell grouping.

DISCREPANCIES BETWEEN CELL AND SERUM GROUPING[9-11]: If discrepancies between cell and serum grouping occur, repeat both tests with fresh reagents, paying careful attention to technique.

Wash patient's cells in saline solution and test with patient's serum for auto-antibodies. Test for subgroups of A. Test serum for atypical antibodies.

Subgroups of A and AB

Cells that are agglutinated rapidly and completely with anti-**A** serum are designated A_1 or A_1B, respectively. Cells that react more weakly and less rapidly with the same serum are classified as A_2 and A_2B, respectively, or as A_3, A_4, etc.

For routine blood bank work the subgroups of A need not be determined, but they must be investigated if difficulties arise in ABO cell or serum typing.

TESTING FOR SUBGROUPS A_1, A_2, AND A_3: **Antisera:**

Absorbed anti-A serum: B group serum contains two agglutinins—α and α_1. Agglutinin α_1 agglutinates red cells containing agglutinogen A_1 and does not react with agglutinogen A_2. On the other hand, agglutinin α reacts almost equally well with agglutinogens A_1 and A_2. When suitable B serum is absorbed with A_2 blood cells, the agglutinin α is absorbed, whereas the α_1 is not much affected and remains active. Therefore when absorbed B serum is used for subgrouping of A and AB bloods, agglutination indicates the presence of A_1 cells (subgroup A_1 or A_1B) and absence of agglutination indicates A_2 cells (A_2 or A_2B).

Anti-A$_1$ lectin: Another method of detecting A subgroups is the use of lectin (extract of the plant *Dolichos biflorus*),

which agglutinates only A_1 cells. Lectin reacts more strongly than absorbed anti-A serum.

Group O serum and anti-C[12]: The serum of group O individuals contains, in addition to the anti-**A** and anti-**B** agglutinins, an agglutinin that is called anti-**C** and is directed against a **C** factor shared by agglutinogens A and B. The anti-**C** is important for two reasons:

1. It traverses the placental barrier more readily than naturally occurring anti-**A** and anti-**B** and appears to be the antibody most often involved in ABO hemolytic disease of the newborn.

2. It reacts strongly with weak A subgroups, allowing the recognition of very low-grade group A individuals, variously designated as A_x, A_4, or A_0. The red cells of these individuals failing to react with anti-**A** and anti-**B** sera would be classified as group O if it were not for the fact that they are agglutinated by group O serum. The agglutination appears to be the result of the anti-**C** isoagglutinin present in group O serum reacting with the blood factor **C** in the A cells.

Anti-H lectin (Ulex europeus[13]): It reacts preferentially with red cells of group O, group A_2, and group A_2B (in that order) and less well with A or B cells. Wiener postulates that all normal individuals are homozygous, genotype *HH*, for a gene that determines the H substance and that the *H* and the *ABO* genes compete for the same substrate. The plant anti-**H** reagent is similar in specificity to anti-**H** cold agglutinin which may be found in normal sera and is often found in bloods of type A_2, A_3, and A_x.

Cell grouping of subgroups A_1, A_2, and A_3: See Table 5-5.

Technique: Follow manufacturer's instructions accompanying these antisera.

ATYPICAL COLD ANTIBODIES IN THE A_1 AND A_2 SUBGROUPS: About 2% of the A_2 subgroup and about 25% of the A_2B subgroup contain atypical cold agglutinins of anti-A_1 activity. The appearance of these cold agglutinins may lead to difficulties in ABO typing. For instance, the

Table 5-5. Cell grouping of subgroups A_1, A_2, and A_3 with known sera*

Cell type	Anti-A	Anti-B	Anti-A_1	Group O serum	Anti-H
A_1	4+	−	4+	4+	−
A_2	3-4+	−	−	4+	2+
A_3	2+ mf	−	−	4+	4+ mf

*+ = agglutination; − = no agglutination; mf = mixed field agglutination (agglutination accompanied by many nonagglutinated cells).

Table 5-6. Serum grouping of subgroups A_1, A_2, and A_3 with known cells*

Serum of group	O cells	A_1 cells	A_2 cells	B cells
A_1	−	−	−	+
A_2	−	−	−	+
A_3	−	−	−	+

*+ = agglutination; − = no agglutination.

Table 5-7. Antigens and antibodies of the ABO system[14]

Group (agglutinogens)	Agglutinins usually present	Agglutinins that may be present
A_1B	None	Anti-H
A_2B	None	α_1 (25-30%)
A_1	β	Anti-H
A_2	β	α_1 (1-2%)
B	α, α_1	Anti-H
O	α, α_1, β, anti-C	None

serum of subgroup A_2B will agglutinate A_1 cells by means of its anti-A_1 cold agglutinin. Retyping of the A_2B cells with anti-A_1 serum and repeating the original typing at 37° C., at which temperature the cold agglutinins are inactivated, will establish the cells as belonging to group A_2B (Tables 5-7 and 5-8).

Specific cold agglutinins are more likely to occur in certain blood types, for instance, anti-A_1 in A_2 individuals (rare), anti-H in A_1 and A_1B individuals, anti-P in P-negative subjects, and anti-M in infants (rare).

Some of the cold antibodies detected in reverse grouping of A, B, or AB patients can be identified by the degree (strong, weak, or not at all) to which they preferentially agglutinate test cells at room temperature or better at 15°-18° C.

Subgroups of A weaker than A_3[15]: Weaker subgroups of A such as A_x, A^h_m, etc. fail to react with anti-A serum but react with group O serum that contains anti-C. They also react with anti-H serum.

Table 5-8. Identification of nonspecific cold agglutinins of anti-A_1, anti-H, and anti-I

Test cell	Anti-A_1 in A_2 subjects	Anti-H in A_1 subjects	Anti-I	Nonspecific cold agglutinins
A_1 Rh negative	4+	+	4+	4+
A_2 Rh negative	−	3+	4+	4+
B Rh negative	(4+ due to natural anti-B)	(4+ due to natural anti-B)	4+	3+
O Rh negative	−	4+	4+	4+
O cord blood	−	4+	−	4+
Patient's cells	−	−	− to 4+	4+

Table 5-9. Cell grouping of subgroups A weaker than A_3 with known sera[*]

Cell type	Anti-A	Anti-B	Anti-A_1	Group O serum	Anti-H
A_x	$\pm$ or $-$	$-$	$-$	2+	4+
A_m	$-$	$-$	$-$	$-$	$-$
A^h_m	$-$	$-$	$-$	2+	$-$
A_{el}	$-$	$-$	$-$	$-$	$+$

[*]$+$ = agglutination; $-$ = no agglutination; $\pm$ = weak agglutination.

Table 5-10. Serum grouping of subgroups of A weaker than A_3 with known cells

Cell type	A_1 cells	A_2 cells	B cells	O cells	Antibody in eluate	Blood group substance in saliva of secretors
A_x[16]	$-$ or $+$	$-$	$+$	$-$	Anti-A	H
A^h_m[17]	$-$	$-$	$+$	$-$	Anti-A	A, H
A_{nd}[18]	$-$	$-$	$+$	$-$	Anti-A	A, H
A_{el}[18]	$-$	$-$	$+$	$-$	Anti-A	H

Table 5-11. Cell grouping with known antisera[*]

Cell type	Anti-A	Anti-B	Group O serum	Anti-H
B_1	$-$	$\pm$	$\pm$	$-$
B_3	$-$	$\pm$	$+$ mf	$+$
B_x	$-$	$\pm$	$\pm$	$+$
B_w	$-$	$-$	$\pm$	$+$

[*]$+$ = agglutination; $-$ = no agglutination; $\pm$ = weak agglutination; $\pm$ = very weak agglutination; mf = mixed field agglutination.

As these cells also fail to react with anti-**B** serum, they appear to be group O on cell grouping. Serum grouping (Table 5-10) will reveal the absence of agglutinin anti-**A**, which is normally found in group O blood.

Identification of some of the cells that do not react with anti-**A** serum is aided by the examination of the eluate. Group A cells adsorb anti-**A** antibody in the same way as group B cells adsorb anti-**B** antibody. The antigenically strong cells do not readily part with the adsorbed substance, but weak subgroups readily give it up so that it can be removed by elution. If the eluate contains anti-**A**, it identifies the cell as presumably belonging to group A.

Identification of the group substances in the saliva of secretors may further help in the identification of weak A subgroups (see p. 253).

ALTERED ANTIGENS[19, 20]:

Pseudo-B antigen[21]: Several authors have described the development of a form of B antigen in group A_1 individuals as an acquired character. It is thought to be due to bacterial enzymatic action in vivo.

Ag and Bg: They are weakened A and B antigens as described in leukemia.

VARIATIONS WITH AGE: The A antigen may be weak in old age and in infants up to the age of 6-12 mo., prior to which time A_1 cells often react like A_2 cells, except for failure to react with anti-**H**.

Subgroups of B[22]

They are B_1, B_3, B_x, and B_w (Tables 5-11 and 5-12).

Errors in red cell and reverse typing

1. Outdated test cells, test sera, or methods
2. Weak antigens due to the presence of subgroups, e.g., A_3, A_x, etc.; due to late formation of antigens as in newborn infants; due to suppression of the *ABO* genes (Bombay

Table 5-12. Serum grouping with known cells*

Cell type	O cells	A₁ cells	A₂ cells	B cells	Antibody in eluate	Blood group substance in saliva of secretors
B₁	−	+	+	−	Anti-**B**	B, H
B₃	−	+	+	−	Anti-**B**	H
Bₓ	−	+	+	−	Anti-**B**	B, H
Bᵥ	−	+	+	−	Anti-**B**	B, H

*+ = agglutination; − = no agglutination.

blood)[23] so that the cells do not react with anti-**A**, anti-**B**, and anti-**H** serum though the serum contains anti-**A**, anti-**B**, and anti-**H** agglutinins; or, last, due to weakening of the red cell receptors in such conditions as acute leukemia, etc.

3. Presence of abnormal cold agglutinins
4. Hypogammaglobulinemia or agammaglobulinemia
5. Chimeras
6. Fetal-maternal hemorrhage with transient neutralization of maternal isoagglutinins
7. Technical mistakes such as drying and heating of slides
8. Weak antibodies as they may occur in old age (70-80 yr.) and in newborn infants[24]
9. Inadequate training of technicians, failure to follow directions, and prolonged observation
10. Blood of wrong patient because of inadequate identification of patient or test tube or because of negligence
11. Omission of reverse typing
12. Use of "old" blood, blood that was not refrigerated, lysed blood, or a wrong concentration of red cells
13. Failure to obtain a fresh specimen and to retype it every time the patient is to receive blood
14. Bacterial contamination

BLOOD CHIMERAS[25]

Red cell chimerism is the phenomenon of two genetically different red cell populations being present in the same organism. It is thought that the organism fails to develop antibodies against the acquired red cell population because of the development of immunologic tolerance. This tolerance is acquired by an organism if it is persistently exposed to a foreign antigen during embryonic life. Two types of red cell populations have been reported in bovine and very rarely in human twins, each twin tolerating the red blood cells of the other.

RH BLOOD GROUPS AND RH BLOOD GROUPING
Rh factor

This antigen (agglutinogen), discovered by Landsteiner and Wiener,[26] was named Rh because the red blood cells containing it agglutinated with antiserum produced by injecting rabbits with the washed red blood cells of the monkey *Macaca rhesus*. The original antiserum reacted only with the Rh₀ factor which is present in about 85% of the white population, irrespective of sex, age, and presence of other agglutinogens. It is absent in about 15% of the white population, in about 10% of the Negro population, and in a much smaller percentage of American Indians, Australian aborigines, and Chinese, among whom erythroblastosis is rare.[27] The incidence of **Rh₀**-negative types among the Japanese is very low (less than 1%). See Table 5-13.

The factor corresponding to the original rhesus factor is called Rh₀ (D). The red cells that contain the Rh₀ (D) factor are called Rh positive, and the red cells that do not contain the **Rh₀** factor are called Rh negative. The term "Rh factor" without qualification means **Rh₀** (D) and Rh positive means **Rh₀** (D) positive.

In human blood there exist several factors related to the original rhesus factor. Originally four Rh factors, **Rh₀** (D), rh′

Table 5-13. Representative data on the racial distribution of the eight Rh types[*]

Ethnic group	Approximate frequency (%) of Rh blood types							
	rh	rh'	rh''	rh$_y$	Rh$_o$	Rh$_1$	Rh$_2$	Rh$_z$
Caucasoids (N. Y. C.)[1]	13.5	1.0	0.5	0.02	2.5	53.0	15.0	14.5
Negroids								
N. Y. C.[2]	7.5	1.5	0	0	45.0	25.0	15.5	5.5
Africa[3]	3.75	0.75	0	0	70.0	15.0	9.0	1.5
Puerto Ricans[4]	10.1	1.7	0.5	0	15.1	39.1	19.6	14.0
Chinese[5]	1.5	0	0	0	0.9	60.6	3.0	34.4
Japanese[6]	0.6	0	0	0	0	51.7	8.3	39.4
Filipinos[7]	0	0	0	0	0	87.0	2.0	11.0
Mexican Indians[8]	0	0	0	0	1.1	48.1	9.5	41.2

[*]Modified from Wiener: Amer. J. Clin. Path. **16:**477, 1946.
[1]Wiener et al.; Unger et al.; Levine.
[2]Wiener et al.; Levine.
[3]Hubinont et al.
[4]Torregrosa.
[5]Wiener et al.
[6]Waller and Levine; Miller and Taguchi.
[7]Simmons and Graydon.
[8]Wiener et al.

Table 5-14. Scheme of the eight Rh types[*][†]

	Rh$_o$-*negative types*				Rh$_o$-*positive types*		
		Reactions with serum				Reactions with serum	
Designation	Anti-rh'	Anti-rh''	Anti-Rh$_o$	Designation	Anti-rh'	Anti-rh''	Anti-Rh$_o$
rh	−	−	−	Rh$_o$	−	−	+
rh'	+	−	−	Rh$_1$	+	−	+
rh''	−	+	−	Rh$_2$	−	+	+
rh$_y$	+	+	−	Rh$_z$	+	+	+

[*]From Wiener: Dade County Med. Ass. Bull. **20:**20, 1949.
[†]The types are named after the Rh blood factors (and agglutinogens) present in the red cells, Rh$_1$ being short for Rh$_o$rh' (or Rh'$_o$) and Rh$_2$ short for Rh$_o$rh'' (or Rh''$_o$). Similarly, rh$_y$ is used in place of rh'rh'' and Rh$_z$ in place of Rh$_1$Rh$_2$ (or Rh'$_o$Rh''$_o$).

(C), **rh''** (E), and **rh**^{w} (C^w), and two Hr factors, **hr'** (c) and **hr''** (e), were described. At the present time, according to Wiener, 10 agglutinogens are known to exist. The **agglutinogen** represents a molecular characteristic of the red cell surface and the **blood factors** are its serologic specificities defined by the use of antisera (Tables 5-14 and 5-15).

The capital letter R in **Rh$_o$** is chosen to emphasize its serologic importance. The factors **rh'** and **rh''** have small letter r's to indicate their lesser clinical importance. The symbol Hr is chosen to indicate the reciprocal relationship to Rh.

Wiener's nomenclature and theory of multiple alleles[28]: Wiener uses separate terms for the **agglutinogen,** for the gene-determined antigen entity, and for the various **factors** that represent the specific serologic manifestations, the extrinsic attributes, of the agglutinogen molecule. For instance, the gene R^z determines the agglutinogen Rh$_2$, which has the blood factors **Rh$_o$**, **rh''**, and **hr'**. To account for the eight Rh types (rh, rh', rh'', rh$_y$, Rh$_o$, Rh$_1$, Rh$_2$, Rh$_z$), it is necessary to postulate a unit agglutinogen containing several factors inherited by corresponding allelic genes. Eight allelic genes (r, r', r'', r^y, R^o, R^1, R^z, R^z) lead to 36 possible genotypes and 27 phenotypes (Tables 5-13 to 5-16).

In Table 5-14 the first four types are Rh negative with anti-Rh$_o$ serum and can be identified with three antisera:

anti-Rh$_0$, anti-rh', and anti-rh''. The second group of four types is Rh positive.

The originally described rhesus factor, **Rh$_0$**, is the most important as it is the most common cause of Rh sensitization.

Fisher's nomenclature: See Tables 5-17 and 5-18. Fisher introduced the letters C, D, and E for the various Rh antigens and the symbols c, d, and e for the allelomorphic antigens.

The equivalents are as follows:

$$Rh = D$$
$$rh' = C$$
$$rh'' = E$$
$$d$$
$$hr' = c$$
$$hr'' = e$$

Fisher uses the terms "agglutinogen," "antigen," and "factors" interchangeably. According to his theory, there are three Rh antigens, which he calls agglutinogens D, C, and E. For each of these agglutinogens there exists a corresponding antithetical antigen called d, c, and e. The three pairs of Rh antigens are determined by three corresponding pairs of allelic genes—Dd, Cc, and Ee—that are closely linked. One set of these pairs of Rh genes is inherited from each parent: C or c, D or d, E or e, so that there are three genotypes for each antigen, e.g., DD, Dd, and dd—homozygous for D, heterozygous for D, and homozygous for d. There are three places (loci) on each chromosome where one, and only one, of each corresponding pair of antigens or genes (Dd,

Table 5-15. Rh-Hr agglutinogens—their genes and blood factors

Gene symbols		Agglu-tinogen symbols	Serologic specifications (blood factors)
Wiener	Fisher-Race		
r	cde	rh	hr', hr'', hr
r'	Cde	rh'	rh', rh^G, rh$_i$, hr''
r''	cdE	rh''	rh'', hr'
r^y	CdE	rh$_y$	rh', rh'', rh^G
R^o	cDe	rh$_o$	Rh$_o$, rh^G, hr', hr'', hr
R^1	CDe	Rh$_1$	Rh$_o$, rh', rh^G, rh$_i$, hr''
R^2	cDE	Rh$_2$	Rh$_o$, rh'', rh^G, hr'
R^z	CDE	Rh$_z$	Rh$_o$, rh', rh'', rh^G

Table 5-16. Wiener's Rh-Hr nomenclature for Rh-Hr blood types

8 Rh phenotypes				20 Rh-Hr phenotypes				36 corresponding genotypes
	Reactions with				Reactions with			
Designation	Anti-Rh$_o$	Anti-rh'	Anti-rh''	Designation	Anti-hr'	Anti-hr''	Anti-hr	
rh	−	−	−	rh	+	+	+	rr
rh'	−	+	−	rh'rh	+	+	+	r'r
				rh'rh'	−	+	−	r'r'
rh''	−	−	+	rh''rh	+	+	+	r''r
				rh''rh''	+	−	−	r''r''
rh$_y$	−	+	+	rh'rh''	+	+	−	r'r''
				rh$_y$rh	+	+	+	r^{y}r
				rh$_y$rh'	−	+	−	r^{y}r'
				rh$_y$rh''	+	−	−	r^{y}r''
				rh$_y$rh$_y$	−	−	−	r^{y}r^y
Rh$_o$	+	−	−	Rh$_o$	+	+	+	R^{o}R^o, R^{o}r
Rh$_1$	+	+	−	Rh$_1$rh	+	+	+	R^{1}r, R^{1}R^o, R^{o}r'
				Rh$_1$Rh$_1$	−	+	−	R^{1}R^1, R^{1}r'
Rh$_2$	+	−	+	Rh$_2$rh	+	+	+	R^{2}r, R^{2}R^o, R^{o}r''
				Rh$_2$Rh$_2$	+	−	−	R^{2}R^2, R^{2}r''
Rh$_z$	+	+	+	Rh$_1$Rh$_2$	+	+	−	R^{1}R^2, R^{1}r'', R^{2}r'
				Rh$_z$rh	+	+	+	R^{z}r, R^{z}R^o, R^{o}r^y
				Rh$_z$Rh$_1$	−	+	−	R^{z}R^1, R^{z}r', R^{1}r^y
				Rh$_z$Rh$_2$	+	−	−	R^{z}R^2, R^{z}r'', R^{2}r^y
				Rh$_z$Rh$_z$	−	−	−	R^{z}R^z, R^{z}r^y

Cc, and Ee) is located, and the arrangement of these chromosomes in pairs, one from each parent, determines the Rh type. Eight possible combinations of three genes exist for each chromosome. At each locus the antigens may be homozygous (ee, DD, etc.) or heterozygous (Ee, Dd, etc.). With two chromosomes, this makes possible 36 genotypes and 27 phenotypes (8 homozygous and 19 heterozygous). The genotypes are expressed as fractions, each integer representing one parent's genes.

Table 5-17. Fisher-Race linked gene theory

Genes	Antigens
cde	cde
CDe	CDe
cdE	cdE
CdE	CdE
cDe	cDe
CDe	CDe
cDE	cDE
CDE	CDE

For example, type rh (always homozygous) is $\dfrac{dce}{dce}$. Rh$_1$ homozygous is $\dfrac{DCe}{DCe}$. Rh$_1$ heterozygous is $\dfrac{DCe}{dce}$.

There are six antisera corresponding to the six antigens, called anti-D, anti-d, anti-e, etc.[29]

There is increasing evidence that Fisher's theory fails to explain many facets of the Rh-Hr complex. The anti-d antiserum, predicted by Fisher and reported by some authorities,[30] has actually never been found. Certain factors, e.g., C and e, appear to be inherited together so that the Rh gene must be considered to be an entity rather than a complex of separable genes.

Wiener's nomenclature of the Rh-Hr blood types has a precise scientific basis, allowing a logical arrangement of the various types, and readily fits into recent serologic developments. The CDE notations have been mentioned in this section only because many European books and journals as well as typing sera labels continue to use them.

Table 5-18. Comparison of two methods of designating Rh-Hr antibodies and their corresponding blood factors

	Wiener		Fisher-Race	
	Antibodies	Blood factors	Antibodies	Blood factors
1.	Anti-rhesus / Anti-Rh$_o$	**Rh$_o$ and $\mathfrak{Rh}_o$**	Anti-D	D and D″
2.	Anti-rh′	rh′	Anti-C	C
3.	Anti-hr′	hr′	Anti-c	c
4.	Anti-rh″	rh″	Anti-E	E
5.	Anti-hr″	hr″	Anti-e	e
6.	Anti-rh^{w1}	rh^{w1}	Anti-C^w	C^w
7.	Anti-hr	hr	Anti-f or anti-ce	f or ce
8.	Anti-rh$_i$	rh$_i$	Anti-Ce	Ce
9.	Anti-rh$_{ii}$	rh$_{ii}$	Anti-cE	cE
10.	Anti-rh	rh	Anti-CE	CE
11.	Anti-rh^x	rh^x	Anti-C^x	C^x
12.	Anti-hr^v	hr^v	Anti-V or anti-ce^s	V or ce^s
13.	Anti-hr^H	hr^H	No equivalent term	
14.	Anti-rh^{w2}	rh^{w2}	Anti-E^w	E^w
15.	Anti-rh^G	rh^G	Anti-G or anti-C + D	G
16.	Anti-Rh^A	**Rh^A**	No equivalent term	
17.	Anti-Rh^B	**Rh^B**	No equivalent term	
18.	Anti-Rh^C	**Rh^C**	No equivalent term	
19.	Anti-Rh^D	**Rh^D**	No equivalent term	
20.	Anti-hr^S	hr^S	No equivalent term	
21.	Anti-Hr	**Hr**	Anti-C + c + E + e + f	

Rh typing

Slide test with slide or rapid tube anti-Rh$_o$ (D): The testing serum contains blocking antibodies that agglutinate Rh$_o$-positive cells in the presence of concentrated protein. The required protein concentration can be attained by doing the typing in plasma with 6-8% protein or in bovine albumin, which provides a preferable concentration of 25-30%. The cells should be suspended in plasma or serum to give a concentration of 40-50%. Anemic blood must be concentrated to this hematocrit level by centrifugation of the oxalated specimen and by discarding the necessary amount of plasma.

An Rh viewing box should be used, the electric bulb of which keeps the plate temperature between 45°-50° C., allowing the test slide to reach a temperature of 37°-39° C. during the 2 min. required for the test.

Since some cells may react with the albumin alone, an albumin control must be included with each test.

Method:
1. Label slide and place 1 drop slide test serum on it.
2. On a second labeled slide place 1 drop albumin for the control test.
3. To each slide add 2 drops 40-50% suspension of red cells in serum or plasma.
4. With separate applicator sticks mix each suspension and spread over an area of about 2 × 4 cm.
5. Place both slides on the viewbox and tilt slowly back and forth, observing for agglutination, which should occur within 2 min.

Interpretation: The cells are Rh$_o$ positive if the antiserum produces agglutination and if it is absent on the albumin slide. If the albumin control is positive, repeat the test with saline-agglutinating antiserum and do a direct Coombs test.

The cells are Rh$_o$ negative if agglutination fails to occur.

Tube test with slide or rapid tube anti-Rh$_o$ (D): Follow directions accompanying the typing sera.

Method:
1. Label one test tube and add 1 drop slide antiserum.
2. Label a second tube and add 1 drop albumin as a control.
3. Add to each tube 1 or 2 drops 2-4% suspension of red cells in saline solution or serum according to directions. An applicator stick dipped into the red cells may be used provided the amount of transferred blood corresponds to a 2-4% concentration.
4. Mix and centrifuge.
5. Dislodge sediment and observe for agglutination, both macroscopically and microscopically.

Interpretation: See previous interpretation.

Tube test with saline-agglutinating anti-Rh$_o$ (D): Follow manufacturer's directions.

Method:
1. Label a 75 × 10 mm. test tube and place 1 drop saline-agglutinating antiserum in it.
2. Add 1 drop 2% suspension of freshly washed red cells in saline solution.
3. Mix and place in a 37° C. water bath for 15-60 min. according to directions.
4. Centrifuge at 3400 rpm for 15 sec. or according to directions.
5. Gently dislodge sedimented cells and examine for microscopic agglutination.

Interpretation: Agglutination indicates that the blood cells are **Rh$_o$** positive and absence of agglutination indicates that they are **Rh$_o$** negative.

Errors in Rh$_o$ typing:

False positive tests: They may be due to drying (the observation period exceeding 2 min.), rouleaux formation, or autoagglutination.

False negative tests: They may be due to old red cells (only fresh cells should be used), wrong concentration of red cells, hemolysis, inadequate mixing of red cells, old typing sera, or incorrect temperature. The blood cells are of the Rh$_o$ variant type or the rare type rh^G.

They may also be due to the presence of blocking antibodies in a high enough titer to prevent typing of the cells even with incomplete antibody serum in a high protein medium.

Anti-Rh testing sera: They are of two

types: The saline-agglutinating antibodies agglutinate red cells suspended in saline solution only. The albumin-acting antibodies do not act in saline medium but require a high molecular environment. When added to saline-suspended cells, they coat the red cells without clumping them (blocking) and render them inagglutinable by saline-acting antibodies.

Anti-Rh antibodies: There are no anti-**Rh** antibodies present in the serum of normal individuals. They may appear as immune antibodies following sensitization due to pregnancy, miscarriage, and administration of incompatible blood. They are of two types (Table 5-18). The 19S antibodies agglutinate red cells suspended in saline medium, while the 7S antibodies require a high molecular medium. In saline medium they coat the red cells without clumping and render them inagglutinable by saline antibodies.

Tests for anti-Rh antibodies: Since the problem is to determine the presence or absence of any type of anti-Rh antibody, the test is carried out with pooled Rh-positive and Rh-negative cells, the antigenic makeup of which is known. Rh agglutinins are detected by their ability to agglutinate cells suspended in saline solution, and Rh-blocking antibodies by their ability to agglutinate cells suspended in high protein medium. If both occur together, the Rh agglutinins can be destroyed by heating the serum at 58° C. for 5 min. For the detection of certain antibodies the use of the Coombs technique and enzyme-treated cells is necessary. The identification of Rh antibodies is discussed under the heading of antibody identification (see p. 267).

Determination of Rh phenotypes and genotypes

Determination of the phenotype: See Table 5-19. The phenotype is the visible or detectable sum of traits of an individual. The traits may be physical, serologic, biochemical, etc. With the combined use of Rh and Hr antisera a number of phenotypes can be determined. The exact number will depend on the number of different antisera available and used. If, for instance, the test cells are tested with five antisera—anti-$\mathbf{Rh_o}$ (D), anti-**rh′** (C), anti-**rh″** (E), anti-**hr′** (c), and anti-**hr″** (e)—as many as 18 phenotypes can be distinguished in Caucasians. For example, a positive reaction with all five antisera describes the phenotype Rh_1Rh_2 (CcDEe). If, in another example, all reactions are positive except anti-**hr″** (e), the phenotype will be Rh_zRh_2 and in Fisher's nota-

Table 5-19. Determination of some Rh phenotypes from typing results*

Antisera					*Phenotype*	
anti-$\mathbf{Rh_o}$ *(D)*	*anti-***rh′** *(C)*	*anti-***rh″** *(E)*	*anti-***hr′** *(c)*	*anti-***hr″** *(e)*	*Rh-Hr*	*CDE*
+	+	−	+	+	Rh_1rh	CcDee
−	−	−	+	+	rh	ccdee
+	+	−	−	+	Rh_1Rh_1	CCDee
+	+	+	+	+	Rh_1Rh_2	CcDEe
+	−	+	+	+	Rh_2rh	ccDEe
+	−	−	+	+	Rh_o	ccDee
+	−	+	+	−	Rh_2Rh_2	ccDEE
−	+	−	+	+	rh′rh	Ccdee
−	−	+	+	+	rh″rh	ccdEe
+	+	+	−	+	Rh_zRh_1	CCdEe
+	+	+	+	−	Rh_zRh_2	CCDEe
−	+	+	+	+	rh_yrh	CcDEE
+	+	+	−	−	Rh_zRh_z	CcdEe
−	+	+	−	+	rh_yrh'	CCDEE
−	+	+	+	−	rh_yrh''	CCdEE
−	+	+	−	−	rh_yrh_y	CcdEE

*From Technical methods and procedures of the American Association of Blood Banks, ed. 4, Chicago, 1966, American Association of Blood Banks.

tion CcDEE since absence of **hr″** (e) implies a double dose of E.

Determination of the probable genotype: See Table 5-20. The genotype of an individual is his full set of genes, representing the gene combination inherited from each parent. In Fisher's nomenclature the two sets are separated by an oblique stroke.

The above-mentioned phenotypes are inherited by at least eight allelic genes so that there are 36 theoretically possible genotypes corresponding to the 18 phenotypes. The most probable genotype is derived from a chart enumerating the frequency of various genotypes within a given population (Table 5-21). The gene combination occurring with the highest frequency represents the most probable genotype. The determination of the probable genotype allows deductions as to whether an individual is homozygous or heterozygous for a given factor. Such considerations may be important in the investigation of paternity and erythroblastosis fetalis. If, for instance, the phenotype is Rh_1Rh_1 (CCDee), the most probable genotype is R^1R^1 (CDe/CDe), but it may also be R^1r' (CDe/Cde).

Variants of the Rh factor (D^u, weak Rh_0)

Certain Rh_0-positive cells (about 1%) fail to be agglutinated by otherwise potent anti-Rh_0 (anti-D) serum, but after

Table 5-20. Estimation of Rh genotypes from the phenotype (Caucasians)*

Phenotype	Most probable genotype		Other possible genotypes	
Rh-Hr	Rh-Hr	CDE	Rh-Hr	CDE
Rh_1rh	R^1r	CDe/cde	R^0r'	CDe/cDe
			R^0r'	cDe/Cde
rh	rr	cde/cde		
Rh_1Rh_1	R^1R^1	CDe/CDe	R^1r'	CDe/Cde
Rh_1Rh_2	R^1R^2	CDe/cDE	R^1r''	CDe/cdE
			R^2r'	cDE/Cde
			$R^zr‡$	CDE/cde
			$R^zR^0‡$	CDE/cDe
			$R^0r^y‡$	cDe/CdE
Rh_2rh	R^2r	cDE/cde	$R^zR^0†$	cDE/cDe
			R^0r''	cDe/cdE
Rh_0	R^0r	cDe/cde	$R^0R^0†$	cDe/cDe
Rh_2Rh_2	R^2R^2	cDE/cDE	R^zr''	cDE/cdE
rh'rh	r'r	Cde/cde	None	None
rh″rh	r″r	cdE/cde	None	None
Rare combinations				
Rh_zRh_1	R^zR^1	CDE/CDe	R^zr'	CDE/Cde
			R^1r^y	CDe/CdE
Rh_zRh_2	R^zR^2	CDE/cDE	R^zr''	CDE/cdE
			R^2r^y	cDE/CdE
rh_yrh	$r^yr†$	CdE/cde	$r'r''$	Cde/cdE
Rh_zRh_z	R^zR^z	CDE/CDE	R^zr^y	CDE/CdE
rh_yrh'	r^yr'	CdE/Cde	None	None
rh_yrh''	r^yr''	CdE/cdE	None	None
rh_yrh_y	r^yr^y	CdE/CdE	None	None

*From Technical methods and procedures of the American Association of Blood Banks, ed. 4, Chicago, 1966, American Association of Blood Banks.
†Most probable genotype in Negroes.
‡These genotypes can be distinguished by the use of anti-hr (f).

Table 5-21. Approximate frequency of Rh-Hr phenotypes and genotypes*

2 Rh phenotypes			12 Rh phenotypes					28 Rh-Hr phenotypes					55 genotypes†
Designation	Approximate frequencies in N.Y.C. whites (%)	Reaction with anti-Rh₀ (or anti-rhesus)	Designation‡	Approximate frequencies in N.Y.C. whites (%)	Anti-rh'	Anti-rh''	Anti-rh^w	Designation	Approximate frequencies in N.Y.C. whites (%)‖	Anti-hr'	Anti-hr''	Anti-hr	
Rh negative	15	−	rh	14.4	−	−	−	rh	14.4	+	+	+	rr
			rh'	.46§	+	−	−	$rh'rh$	.46	+	+	+	$r'r$
								$rh'rh'$	.0036	−	+	−	$r'r'$
			rh'^w	.004	+	−	+	rh'^wrh	.004	+	+	+	r'^wr
								rh'^wrh'	.00006	−	+	−	r'^wr' or $r'^wr'^w$
			rh''	.38	−	+	−	$rh''rh$	.38	+	+	+	$r''r$
								$rh''rh''$	.0025	+	−	−	$r''r''$
			rh_y	.01	+	+	−	$rh'rh''$	.006	+	+	−	$r'r''$
								rh_yrh	.008	+	+	+	r^yr
								rh_yrh'	.0001	−	+	−	r^yr'
								rh_yrh''	.0001	+	−	−	r^yr''
								rh_yrh_y	.000001	−	−	−	r^yr^y
			rh^w_y	.00005	+	+	+	rh'^wrh''	.00005	+	+	−	r'^wr''
								rh^w_yrh'	.000001	−	+	−	r'^wr^y

Rh-Hr type	Freq (%)	Rh₀	rh'	rh''	hr'	hr''	Rh type	Freq (%)	Genotypes
Rh positive	85	+							
Rh₀	2.1	+	−	−	+	+	Rh₀	2.1	R^0R^0 or R^0r
Rh₁	50.7	+	+	−	+	+	Rh₁rh	33.4	R^1r, R^1R^0, or R^0r'
		+	+	−	−	+	Rh₁Rh₁	17.3	R^1R^1 or R^1r'
Rh$^w_1$	3.3	+	+	−	+	+	Rh$^w_1$rh	1.6	$R^{1w}r$, $R^{1w}R^0$, or R^0r^{1w}
		+	+	−	−	+	Rh$^w_1$Rh₁	1.7	$R^{1w}R^1$, R^1r^{1w}, or $R^{1w}r'$; $R^{1w}R^{1w}$, or $R^{1w}r^{1w}$
Rh₂	14.6	+	−	+	+	+	Rh₂rh	12.2	R^2r, R^2R^0, or R^0r''
		+	−	+	+	−	Rh₂Rh₂	2.4	R^2R^2 or R^2r''
Rh$_z$	13.4	+	+	+	+	+	Rh₁Rh₂	12.9	R^1R^2, R^1r'', or R^2r'
		+	+	+	+	+	Rh$_z$rh	.2	R^zr, R^zR^0, or R^0r^y
		+	+	+	−	+	Rh$_z$Rh₁	.2	R^zR^1, R^zr', or R^1r^y
		+	+	+	+	−	Rh$_z$Rh₂	.07	R^zR^2, R^zr'', or R^2r^y
		+	+	+	−	−	Rh$_z$Rh$_z$	.0004	R^zR^z or R^zr^y
Rh^w_z	.6	+	+	+	+	+	Rh$^w_1$Rh₂	.6	$R^{1w}R^2$, $R^{1w}r''$, or R^2r^{1w}, or R^zr^{1w}
		+	+	+	−	+	Rh^w_zRh₁	.008	$R^{1w}R^z$, $R^{1w}r^y$, or R^zr^{1w}

*From Wiener and Wexler: An Rh-Hr syllabus, the types and their applications, ed. 2, New York, 1963, Grune & Stratton, Inc.

†This table does not include genes R^{zw} and r^{yw}, which appear to be very rare.

‡In this table Rh₁ is used as a short designation for Rh'₀; Rh₂ is short for Rh''₀; rh$_y$ is short for rh'; rh$_z$ is short for rh''; and Rh$_z$ is short for Rh₀'''.

§The reduction in the frequency of type rh' as compared with that given in earlier charts can be attributed to recognition of bloods of type Rh₁ (containing Rh₀ variant), which are now included in type Rh₁ instead of rh'. The agglutinogens Rh₀, Rh₁, and Rh₂, and their corresponding genes R^0, R^1, and R^2, are not given here because this would serve unnecessarily to complicate the chart by increasing the number of possible genotypes to 91. Also, no attempt is made to include certain rare exceptional bloods such as those lacking both factors hr' and hr', and/or lacking both hr'' and hr'', etc.

‖Based on the estimated gene frequencies, $r = .38$, $r' = .006$, $r'' = .005$, $r^y = .0001$, $r'^w = .005$, $r'' = .006$, $r'^y = .00005$, $R^0 = .027$, $R^1 = .41$, $R^2 = .15$, $R^z = .002$, and $R^{1w} = .02$.

exposure to **Rh₀** (D) antibodies, these cells will give a positive reaction if treated with Coombs serum. They contain the $\mathfrak{Rh}_0$ (Dᵘ) antigen, which may vary in activity, so that some strong variants can be detected with potent anti-**Rh₀** serum, but the agglutination is slow to appear and is usually fine. Weak variants are agglutinated only by an occasional anti-D serum. Variants of Dᵘ are antigenic if injected into an **Rh₀**-negative (d) patient.

Two types of Dᵘ are recognized, the so-called hereditary type (Dᵘce/dce), which is transmitted as a weak D, and the gene interaction type (DCe/dCe), which is the result of suppression of D by gene C on the opposite chromosome. Donors and recipients with Dᵘ type blood of either kind are classified as Rh-positive individuals.

Dᵘ occurs more commonly in Negroes and is rare among Caucasians.

Wiener uses the symbol $\mathfrak{Rh}_0$ for the entire group of high- and low-grade variants. $\mathfrak{Rh}_0$, like the factor Rh₀, may occur alone or together with rh′, rh″, or both. To account for agglutinogens $\mathfrak{Rh}_0$, $\mathfrak{Rh}_1$, and $\mathfrak{Rh}_2$, the existence of three additional allelic genes has been postulated: $\mathfrak{R}^0$, $\mathfrak{R}^1$, and $\mathfrak{R}^2$.

Intermediate genes have also been described for factors **rh′** and **rh″**.

Test for Rh₀ variants:

1. Label test tube and add 1 drop anti-**Rh₀** (D) serum for slide testing, which (according to the manufacturer's instructions) can be used for the indirect antiglobulin technique.
2. Add 1 or 2 drops (according to directions) 2% saline suspension of red cells that have been washed once.
3. Mix and incubate at 37° C. for 30 min. or according to directions.
4. Label a second tube control and add 1 or 2 drops of the same cell suspension.
5. Wash both cell suspensions carefully with at least three changes of large amounts of saline solution in preparation for the antiglobulin test.
6. Remove all saline solution and 1 or 2 drops of antiglobulin serum to

each tube or follow instructions. Mix.
7. Centrifuge at 3400 rpm for 15 sec.
8. Dislodge the packed cells gently and observe for agglutination, both macroscopically and microscopically.

Interpretation: If the routine slide or tube test is negative or weakly positive and if the control is negative (a direct Coombs test), agglutination indicates that the patient has the Rh₀ variant.

If the routine slide and tube tests are negative and if the previous test and the control are negative, the blood is Rh negative.

If the control direct Coombs test is positive, the previous test is invalid and the cause of the positive Coombs test should be investigated.

All apparently Rh-negative persons should be tested for Dᵘ with the indirect Coombs test.

Combination of Rh₀ (D) and hr′ (c): About 80% of Rh₀-positive individuals are hr′ positive, whereas the remaining 20% are hr′ negative. Since hr′ is second in importance to Rh₀ as an antigen, all Rh₀-positive female recipients of childbearing age and all patients who will need multiple transfusions should be checked for hr′.

Factors Rhᴬ, Rhᴮ, Rhᶜ, and Rh^D31: Wiener described a case of erythroblastosis fetalis in which the mother was **Rh₀** positive (not an intermediate Rh₀) but her serum contained an anti-**Rh₀**-like antibody that failed to clump her own cells, but otherwise gave all the expected reactions of an anti-**D** antibody. To explain this occurrence Wiener suggested that the blood of Rh₀-positive individuals has associated with Rh₀ factor a series of factors: **Rhᴬ, Rhᴮ**, etc. In rare cases if one or more of these factors are missing, an individual may become sensitized to the missing factor.

OTHER BLOOD GROUP SYSTEMS
MNSU system[32, 33]

When certain immune sera from rabbits injected with human red blood cells are treated with certain samples of human red blood cells to absorb completely the agglutinins α and β, the sera still contain agglutinins that act upon the red blood cells of some bloods of all four groups: O, A, B, and AB.

Antigens: The agglutinogens in these red blood cells are called M and N. They are found in red cells but not in body fluids or secretions.

Three phenotypes are distinguished: M, N, and MN. The types can be determined at birth. About 50% of the white population are type MN; 30%, M; and 20%, N.

Another factor, S, has been found that is associated with the M and N agglutinogens, each of the three types being either S positive (about 55%) or S negative (about 45%). The positive is designated S and the negative s. This gives six phenotypes: MS, Ms, MNS, MNs, NS, and Ns.

Antibodies of MNSU system: Anti-M may occur spontaneously as cold agglutinin, acting best at 4° C. It may also be formed as an immune antibody following multiple transfusions and very rarely during pregnancy.

Anti-N is much less frequent than anti-M and is also a cold agglutinin, acting best at 4° C., at which temperature it will agglutinate M cells. Anti-N is rarely an immune antibody.

Anti-S may occur is a natural antibody but most frequently it is an immune antibody following frequent transfusions. It may also be responsible for hemolytic disease of the newborn. It acts best at temperatures over 22° C.

Anti-s is very rare and is best demonstrated by the antiglobulin technique.

Anti-U is rare and can best be demonstrated by the antiglobulin technique.

The existence of other antibodies that are fairly common but of little clinical significance complicate the MNSU system.

P and Jay (Tj[a]) system[34]

Antigens: The P_1 antigen that is found in about 74% of English people varies considerably in strength and this variation is inherited. The P_1-negative state is classified as P_2.

The Tj[a] factor belongs to the P blood group system and its relationship to the P system can be seen in Table 5-22. Sanger postulated the existence of three

Table 5-22. P system

Anti-P_1	Anti-P_1 and P_2 (Anti-Tj[a])	Anti-p^K	Phenotype	Genotype
+	+	−	P_1	P_1P_1
+	+	−		P_1P_2
+	+	−		P_1p
−	−	−	P_2	P_2P_2
−	−	−		P_2p
−	−	−	p	pp
+*	+*	+	p^K	p^Kp^K
+*	+*	+		p^Kp

*May contain anti-p^K.

allelic genes, P_1, P_2, and p, at the P locus. P_1 determines the agglutinogens P and Tj[a], P_2 determines the agglutinogens of P-negative blood, P_2 and Tj, while p determines the agglutinogens of Tj[a]-negative blood. The antigen p^K is genetically independent of the P_1 and P_2 genes.

Antibodies: Anti-P_1 is a commonly occurring natural antibody that acts best at low temperatures and may then agglutinate P_1 and P_2 cells.

Anti-P_1 and P_2 (anti-Tj[a]) and anti-p^K are hemolytic antibodies occurring naturally in some P-negative (p) people and may react with p^K cells.

Kell (K) system[35]

Antigens: Within the Kell system there are at least seven antigens: Kell **K**, Cellano **k**, Penny **Kp**[a], Rautenberg **Kp**[b], Sutter **Js**[a], and Matthews **Js**[b]. The McLeod type requires further identification.

Nine percent of the English population are Kell positive, having the genotype *KK* or *Kk*. Ninety-one percent are Kell negative.

Antibodies: Anti-**K** is a relatively common immune antibody usually following transfusions since Kell closely follows **Rh**$_0$ (D) and **hr'** (c) in effectiveness as antigen. The probability that a Kell-negative patient will develop anti-**K** antibodies following transfusion with **K**-positive blood is about 1:10.

Duffy (Fy) system

Antigens: Antigens are found in about 66% of the English population, being

Table 5-23. Frequency of Duffy genotypes and phenotypes

		Frequency (%)	
Phenotype	Genotype	Caucasians	Negroes
Fy(a + b −)	Fy^aFy^a	17	9
Fy(a + b +)	Fy^aFy^b	49	2
Fy(a − b +)	Fy^bFy^b	34	22
Fy(a − b −)	$FyFy$	0	68

present in the homozygous form (Fy^aFy^a) in about 17% and in the heterozygous form (Fy^aFy^b) in 49% (Table 5-23). Sixty-eight percent of Negroes are Duffy negative, being of the type Fy(a–b–), while 22% are of phenotype Fy(a–b+). The absence of both Fy^a and of its allele Fy^b is explained on the basis of a third gene, Fy. The Fy antigen is easily destroyed by proteolytic enzymes.

Homozygous (Fy^aFy^a) cells are more strongly agglutinated than heterozygous cells (dosage effect).

Antibodies: Anti-**Fy**^{a} is a fairly common immune antibody that is demonstrated best at 37° C. by the indirect antiglobulin technique. As it is easily eluted, it is advisable to use homozygous test cells and to wash the cells rapidly prior to the performance of the Coombs test.

Anti-**Fy**^{b} is a rare antibody that also requires the indirect Coombs technique for its demonstration. Enzyme treatment of the cells is not indicated as it may inhibit the indirect antiglobulin reaction.

Lewis (Le) system

The Lewis system (Table 5-24) is primarily a system of water-soluble antigens found in body fluids and secretions such as saliva. The presence or absence of the Lewis substance in secretions is determined by a pair of allelic genes, Le and le. If the Lewis substance is present in the serum, the red cells acquire it by adsorption on their surface.

Secretion of ABH substance and the Lewis system[36-38]

The Lewis substance and the ABH blood group substance are derived from a common precursor, mucopolysaccharide. The Lewis genes, Le and le, and the ABH secretor genes, Se and se, are inherited independently of each other but compete for the common precursor substance. The ABH secretor genes govern the secretion of the H substance into body fluids (together with A and/or B) in line with the ABO group of red cells. The interplay of the genes for the Lewis substance and for the H substance leads to the formation of four secretor types designated as as Les Sec, Les nS, nL Sec, and nL nS. The presence of the Lewis substance is indicated by Les and its absence by nL, while the presence of H substance is designated as Sec and its absence as nS (Table 5-24). Secretors of the Lewis and ABH substances are determined by testing the saliva for the presence or absence of the Lewis and H substances. The frequency of salivary secretors cannot readily be confirmed by the examination of the red cells with anti-Le^a serum because of the variation in the adsorption of the secretor substance by the cells. Because of the common origin of the Lewis and H substances it is reasonable that nonsecretors of ABH substances (Les nS) have larger amounts of the Le substance in their body fluids than have ABH secretors (Les Sec). Individuals of secretor type Les nS therefore usually have red cells that readily react with anti-**Le** serum and that are designated as Le$_1$. Red cells less reactive with anti-Lewis serum are designated as Le$_2$, while nonreactive cells are labeled le.

TYPING RED CELLS FOR LEWIS TYPE:
Reagent:
Ficinated red cells:
1. Wash cells twice with saline solution.
2. Mix 4 parts washed packed red cells with 1 part 1% solution of ficin.
3. Allow to stand for 1 hr. at 37° C.
4. Wash once with saline solution.
5. Prepare 2% suspension of ficinated cells.

Technique:
First stage:
1. Add 1 drop anti-**Lewis** serum to 1 drop ficinated cells in a small test tube.
2. Allow to stand at 37° C. for 1 hr.

3. Gently dislodge sediment and read reaction.

Interpretation: Agglutination indicates type Le_1 cells.

Second stage:
1. Wash nonagglutinated cells four times with saline solution.
2. Centrifuge and add 1 drop anti-human globulin serum to sediment.
3. Centrifuge 1 min. at low speed.
4. Dislodge sediment and read.

Interpretation: Cells agglutinated after the second stage are of type Le_2; cells that are not agglutinated are type le.

The most reliable method to determine the Lewis type is the testing of saliva as well as red cells.

Wiener describes a two-part test performed on saliva: (1) for Lewis substance and (2) for H substance.

A titration method using ficinated red cells is suggested as the method of choice because it is more sensitive than the one-tube test method described.

Lewis antigens in infants: All newborn infants type as Le(a–b–). The antigens do not appear in the red cells for several weeks and then 80-90% are Le(a+). After 2 yr. of age retyping shows approximately 20% to be Le(a+), the adult frequency.

Antibodies:

Anti-Le^a (Le$_1$): It may occur spontaneously in ABH secretors who are Lewis negative, Le(a–b–). The antibody is a saline agglutinin, 19S reacting best at room temperature or lower only with type Le_1 cells. The immune anti-Le_1 antibody of the incomplete variety (7S) reacts best at 37° C. with cells of type Le_1 and Le_2. The latter antibody is detected by the indirect antiglobulin test and the agglutinated red cells may have a stringy appearance when spread on a slide. When fresh complement is present in the system, the antibody is hemolytic.

Anti-Le^b: It may be found in secretors of type Les Sec who have Lewis and H substances in their saliva as well as the hybrid substance of Lewis and H called Le^b (Le^H).

Anti-Le^x: It is an antibody containing a mixture of anti-Le^a and anti-Le^b. It will react with all cells except those of phenotype Le(a–b–).

Tests for Lewis antibody:
Technique for detecting complement binding with anticomplement globulin serum (two-stage antiglobulin test)*:
Lewis antibodies bind complement, act as hemolysins, and require fresh serum. According to Mollison, the most reliable test for Lewis antibodies is the two-stage antiglobulin test.

Principle: In the first stage the red cells are incubated with EDTA-treated antibody, allowing them to take up the serum antibody. The cells are then washed and treated with fresh normal serum to allow uptake of complement.

Reagents:
1. Anti-gamma globulin that has anticomplement (C') globulin activity
2. EDTA solution:

   K_2H_2 EDTA, 4.45%

   NaOH, 0.3%

   Mix, dispense 0.1 ml. amounts into tubes, and dry at 37° C. Each tube will contain 4 mg. EDTA to treat 1 ml. serum.
3. Group O red cells of known Le_1, Le_2, and le types.

Method: Mix 4 vol. EDTA-treated serum with 1 vol. 20% suspension of red cells and incubate in a water bath at 37° C. for 1½ hr. Then wash cells three times and incubate with 2 vol. fresh serum for 15 min. at 37° C. before finally washing and treating with the antiglobulin serum.

Wiener suggests the ficinated-cell agglutination method and the ficinated-cell antiglobulin technique for the identification of anti-Lewis antibodies.

Test for blood group substances in saliva (test for ABH secretor status):
Principle: The blood group substance in the saliva neutralizes antiserum that is added to the saliva, which then fails to agglutinate type-specific test cells. An individual is a secretor or nonsecretor depending on the presence or absence of soluble blood group substances in the body fluids.

Saliva: Collect about 5 ml. saliva and

---

*The discussion of this technique is from Mollison: Blood transfusion in clinical medicine, ed. 4, Philadelphia, 1967, F. A. Davis Co.

Table 5-24. Lewis types*

	Saliva					Blood				
	Frequency (%)		Group-specific substances present in saliva†			Designation		Reactions of red cells with‖		
Designation	Cauca-sians‡	Negroes§	Le	H	Le^H	Recom-mended	Commonly used	Anti-Le (anti-Le^x)	Anti-Le₁ (anti-Le^a)	Anti-Le^H (anti-Le^b)
Les nS	23.1	18.6	+	−	−	Le₁	Le(a + b −)	+	+	−
Les Sec	73.5	58.5	+	+	+	Le₂	Le(a − b +)	+	−	+
nL Sec	2.8	17.0	−	+	−	le	Le(a − b −)	−	−	−
nL nS	0.6	5.9	−	−	−					

*From Wiener: Amer. J. Clin. Path. **43**:388, 1965.
†+ = presence of the respective substance, as shown by inhibition of the corresponding antiserum; − = no substance present, i.e., inhibition does not occur in the tests.
‡England (McConnell).
§Charleston, W. Va. (Ceppellini and associates).
‖+ = agglutination; − = no agglutination.

destroy its enzymes by boiling in a water bath for 20 min.

Centrifuge at high speed until the supernatant is clear. Place into another test tube or into a series of test tubes, which can be frozen (−20° C.).

Control: As the H substance is usually used as the indicator of the secretor state, control saliva of an H secretor and of an H nonsecretor must be used.

Antiserum: An anti-**H** lectin is used, the sensitivity of which is increased by diluting it, usually 1:4, with saline solution to give a 2+ macroscopic agglutination with the test cells. To test for H substance alone is usually sufficient.

Technique:
1. Label test tubes and add 1 drop diluted antiserum.
2. Add 1 drop saliva to each test tube and incubate at room temperature for 10 min.
3. Add 1 drop 2% saline suspension of O cells that have been washed once to all tubes. The O cells are chosen because they contain more H substance than A or B cells.
4. Mix and incubate at room temperature for 30 min.
5. Centrifuge at 3400 rpm for 15 sec.
6. Gently dislodge cell button and observe for macroscopic agglutination.

Interpretation: Agglutination of red cells in this test is found in nonsecretors provided the control is positive. Lack of agglutination signifies secretors since the blood group substance in the saliva neutralizes the antiserum.

Kidd (Jk) system

Antigen: About 75% of Caucasians are Kidd positive, 25% of genotype Jk^aJk^a and 50% of genotype Jk^aJk^b (Table 5-25). The homozygous cells show a marked dosage effect.

Antibodies: Anti-**Jk**^{a} and anti-**Jk**^{b} are isoimmune antibodies best discovered by the indirect antiglobulin test. They are complement-binding antibodies that require fresh human serum to be added to the antiglobulin test during the incubation period. The lability of the complement is responsible for the apparent instability of the antibody.

Table 5-25. Phenotypes and genotypes of the Kidd system

Phenotype	Genotype	Frequency (%)	
		Caucasians	Negroes
Jk(a + b −)	Jk^aJk^a	25	57
Jk(a + b +)	Jk^aJk^b	50	34
Jk(a − b +)	Jk^bJk^b	25	9
Jk(a − b −)	$JkJk$		

Table 5-26. Phenotypes and genotypes of Lu system

Phenotype	Genotype	Frequency (%)
Lu(a + b −)	Lu^aLu^a	0.15
Lu(a + b +)	Lu^aLu^b	7.5
Lu(a − b +)	Lu^bLu^b	92.3

Lutheran (Lu) system

Antigens: About 8% of Caucasians are Luᵃ positive (Table 5-26).

Antibodies: Most anti-**Lu** antibodies are natural (complete 19S) antibodies that do not pass the placenta and react in saline medium at room temperature. Anti-**Lu**ᵃ characteristically produces agglutination evidenced by many large agglutinates among nonagglutinated cells.

Anti-**Lu**ᵇ is a rare antibody that may be complete, acting best at room temperature and in saline solution, or it may be of the immune type (incomplete), acting best at 37° C. in high protein medium.

Diego (Di) system

The antigen **Di**ᵃ is found in 5-15% of Japanese and Chinese and in 36% of certain South American Indians. It is not found at all in the Caucasian population.

Low-incidence antigens

Some blood groups are confined to one person or family and are not related to the known blood group systems. Such factors are **Wr**ᵃ, **Be**ᵃ, **S**ʷᵃ, etc. Patients suffering from lymphoproliferative disorders may form antibodies to these rare antigens.

High-incidence antigens

Antibodies to the high-incidence blood factors appear to react with most blood samples. In this group belong the previously described anti-**U**, anti-**Tj**ᵃ, anti-**H**, anti-**k**, anti-**Lu**ᵇ, and anti-**Jk**. Anti-**Vel**, anti-**I**, and anti-**Ge** are the antibodies to antigens Vel, I, and Ge, which belong to separate groups.

If serum reacts with all cells except the patient's own cells, an antibody for a high-incidence factor may be present, a mixture of anti **Le**ᵃ and anti-**Le**ᵇ, or several other antibodies.

Ii system[39]

Antigens: With very few exceptions the red cells of adults have factor **I** but lack **i**. The few rare adults of type **i** lack factor **I** but have factor **i** instead. In newborn infants the factor **I** is still undeveloped and blood factor **i** is present. In adults the factors **I** and **i** behave as though they were reciprocally related; but on the basis of the erratic distribution of these factors in monkeys, Wiener concludes that they fall into the group of heterophile antigens.

Antibodies: Anti-**I** may occur as cold antibody in acquired hemolytic anemia even in **I**-positive subjects and as natural antibody in **I**-negative individuals.

Anti-**i**[40] has been reported as cold antibody in acquired hemolytic anemia, malaria, infectious mononucleosis, and cirrhosis. Anti-**i** reacts strongly with cord blood and with the rare adult **i**-positive blood.

BLOOD GROUPING TESTS IN DISPUTED PATERNITY

The Medico-Legal Committee of the American Medical Association has approved the use of ABO, MN, and Rh-Hr grouping as the basis for investigating disputed paternity. In the hands of quali-

Table 5-27. Exclusion of paternity by ABO groups*†

Phenotype of putative mother	Phenotype of putative father			
	O	A	B	AB
O	A, B, **AB**	B, **AB**	A, **AB**	O, **AB**
A	B, AB	B, AB	None	O
B	A, AB	None	A, AB	O
AB	**O**, AB	**O**	**O**	**O**

*From Wiener, and Wexler: Heredity of the blood groups, New York, 1958, Grune & Stratton, Inc.

†Find the phenotypes of the putative father and mother at the top and side columns of the tables and locate the box at which these intersect. In the box are given the groups not possible in children of the mating; groups given in **boldface** type represent children for whom **maternity** is excluded.

Table 5-28. Exclusion of paternity by M and N types[*][†]

Phenotype of putative mother	Phenotype of putatitive father		
	M	N	MN
M	MN, N	M, N	**N**
N	**M**, N	M, MN	**M**
MN	**N**	**M**	None

[*]From Wiener, and Wexler: Heredity of the blood groups, New York, 1958, Grune & Stratton, Inc.

[†]Find the phenotypes of the putative father and mother at the top and side columns of the table and locate the box at which these intersect. In the box are given the types not possible in children of the mating; types given in **boldface** type represent children for whom **maternity** is excluded.

fied experts other systems may also be used. The first three systems have an efficiency of approximately 55% in detecting false claims of paternity.

SERUM PROTEIN GROUPS

At the present time there are six groups of hereditary serum proteins known that are transmitted by allelic genes similar to the red cell groups. Methods used in blood grouping fail in the identification of the serum groups that require immunoelectrophoretic techniques.

These systems are as follows:
1. Haptoglobins (discussed in the hematology section)
2. Transferrin (also discussed in the hematology section)
3. Gc group system[41]
4. Gm group system[42]

Table 5-29. Exclusion of paternity by **Rh-Hr** blood types[*][†]

Phenotype of putative mother		1 rh Rh_0	2 rh'rh Rh_1rh	3 rh'rh' Rh_1Rh_1	4 rh''rh Rh_2rh
1	rh Rh_0	2, 3, 4, 5, 6a, 6b, 7, 8, 9	3, 4, 5, 6a, 6b, 7, 8, 9	1, 3, 4, 5, 6a, 6b, 7, 8, 9	2, 3, 5, 6a, 6b, 7, 8, 9
2	rh'rh Rh_1rh	3, 4, 5, 6a, 6b, 7, 8, 9	4, 5, 6a, 6b, 7, 8, 9	1, 4, 5, 6a, 6b, 7, 8, 9	3, 5, 6b, 7, 8, 9
3	rh'rh' Rh_1Rh_1	1, 3, 4, 5, 6a, **6b**, 7, 8, 9	1, 4, 5, 6a, 6b, 7, 8, 9	1, 2, 4, 5, 6a, **6b**, 7, 8, 9	1, 3, 4, 5, **6b**, 7, 8, 9
4	rh''rh Rh_2rh	2, 3, 5, 6a, 6b, 7, 8, **9**	3, 5, 6b, 7, 8, 9	1, 3, 4, 5, 6b, 7, 8, 9	2, 3, 6a, 6b, 7, 8, 9
5	rh''rh'' Rh_2Rh_2	1, 2, 3, 5, 6a, **6b**, 7, 8, 9	1, 2, 3, 5, **6b**, 7, 8, 9	1, 2, 3, 4, 5, **6b**, 7, 8, 9	1, 2, 3, 6a, **6b**, 7, 8, 9
6a	rh'rh'' Rh_1Rh_2	1, 3, 5, 6a, **6b**, 7, 8, 9	1, 5, **6b**, 7, 8, 9	1, 2, 4, 5, **6b**, 7, 8, 9	1, 3, **6b**, 7, 8, 9
6b	rh_yrh Rh_zRh_0	2, 3, 4, 5, 6a, 7, 8, 9	3, 4, 5, 6a, 8, 9	1, 3, 4, 5, 6a, 6b, 8, 9	2, 3, 5, 6a, 7, 9
7	rh_yrh' Rh_zRh_1	1, 3, 4, 5, 6a, 7, 8, 9	1, 4, 5, 6a, 8, 9	1, 2, 4, 5, 6a, 6b, 8, 9	1, 3, 4, 5, 7, 9
8	rh_yrh'' Rh_zRh_2	1, 2, 3, 5, 6a, 7, 8, 9	1, 2, 3, 5, 8, 9	1, 2, 3, 4, 5, 6b, 8, 9	1, 2, 3, 6a, 7, 9
9	rh_yrh_y Rh_zRh_z	1, 2, 3, 4, 5, 6a, 7, 8, 9	1, 2, 3, 4, 5, 6a, 8, 9	1, 2, 3, 4, 5, 6a, 6b, 8, 9	1, 2, 3, 4, 5, 6a, 7, 9

[*]From Wiener, and Nieberg: J. Forensic Med. **10**:6, 1963.
[†]**Boldface** figures represent phenotypes of children for whom **maternity** is excluded. This Table is to be negative, necessarily all **Rh_0**-positive children are excluded. The phenotypes corresponding to the code

5. Ag group system[43]
6. Lp group system[44]
7. Ld group system[45]

Numbers 5 and 6 are β-lipoprotein systems.

Precipitating isoantibodies against some of these have been found following pregnancy and following multiple transfusions, especially in patients with thalassemia.

Some of these groups can also be used in the investigation of disputed paternity.

LEUKOCYTE AND PLATELET GROUPS[46]

Some antigens are common to red cells, platelets, and white cells. Most of these are in the ABO group. Other antigens are found only on platelets, on white cells, on both, and/or also in tissue. Two platelet groups are recognized that are confined

to platelets. One antigen is present only on lymphocytes, but the majority of antigens are common to platelets, granulocytes, and lymphocytes. Four such systems are now recognized. Antibodies to leukocytes or platelets may be demonstrated by the antiglobulin consumption test.[47]

BLOOD DONOR SELECTION

A donor card should be made out on every donor. It must contain the donor's name, age, home and business address, sex, telephone number, occupation, and date of donation.

Donors should be between the ages of 21 and 60 yr. If they are over 60 they should have a physician's consent. Fasting is not necessary, but a wait of 3-4 hr. after a fairly heavy meal is required.

Phenotype of putative father					
5 rh″rh″ Rh_2Rh_2	6a rh′rh″ Rh_1Rh_2	6b rh_yrh Rh_zRh_0	7 rh_yrh' Rh_zRh_1	8 rh_yrh'' Rh_zRh_2	9 rh_yrh_y Rh_zRh_z
1, 2, 3, 5, 6a, 6b, 7, 8, 9	1, 3, 5, 6a, 6b, 7, 8, 9	2, 3, 4, 5, 6a, 7, 8, 9	1, 3, 4, 5, 6a, 7, 8, 9	1, 2, 3, 5, 6a, 7, 8, 9	1, 2, 3, 4, 5, 6a, 7, 8, 9
1, 2, 3, 5, 6b, 7, 8, 9	1, 5, 6b, 7, 8, 9	3, 4, 5, 6a, 8, 9	1, 4, 5, 6a, 8, 9	1, 2, 3, 5, 8, 9	1, 2, 3, 4, 5, 6a, 8, 9
1, 2, 3, 4, 5, 6b, 7, 8, 9	1, 2, 4, 5, 6b, 7, 8, 9	1, 3, 4, 5, 6a, 6b, 8, 9	1, 2, 4, 5, 6a, 6b, 8, 9	1, 2, 3, 4, 5, 6b, 8, 9	1, 2, 3, 4, 5, 6a, 6b, 8, 9
1, 2, 3, 6a, 6b, 7, 8, 9	1, 3, 6b, 7, 8, 9	2, 3, 5, 6a, 7, 9	1, 3, 4, 5, 7, 9	1, 2, 3, 6a, 7, 9	1, 2, 3, 4, 5, 6a, 7, 9
1, 2, 3, 4, 6a, 6b, 7, 8, 9	1, 2, 3, 4, 6b, 7, 8, 9	1, 2, 3, 5, 6a, 6b, 7, 9	1, 2, 3, 4, 5, 6b, 7, 9	1, 2, 3, 4, 6a, 6b, 7, 9	1, 2, 3, 4, 5, 6a, 6b, 7, 9
1, 2, 3, 4, 6b, 7, 8, 9	1, 2, 4, 6b, 7, 8, 9	1, 3, 5, 6a, 6b, 9	1, 2, 4, 5, 6b, 9	1, 2, 3, 4, 6b, 9	1, 2, 3, 4, 5, 6a, 6b, 9
1, 2, 3, 5, 6a, 6b, 7, 9	1, 3, 5, 6a, 6b, 9	2, 3, 4, 5, 6a, 7, 8	1, 3, 4, 5, 6a, 8	1, 2, 3, 5, 6a, 7	1, 2, 3, 4, 5, 6a, 7, 8
1, 2, 3, 4, 5, 6b, 7, 9	1, 2, 4, 5, 6b, 9	1, 3, 4, 5, 6a, 8	1, 2, 4, 5, 6a, 6b, 8	1, 2, 3, 4, 5, 6b	1, 2, 3, 4, 5, 6a, 6b, 8
1, 2, 3, 4, 6a, 6b, 7, 9	1, 2, 3, 4, 6b, 9	1, 2, 3, 5, 6a, 7	1, 2, 3, 4, 5, 6b	1, 2, 3, 4, 6a, 6b, 7	1, 2, 3, 4, 5, 6a, 6b, 7
1, 2, 3, 4, 5, 6a, 6b, 7, 9	1, 2, 3, 4, 5, 6a, 6b, 9	1, 2, 3, 4, 5, 6a, 7, 8	1, 2, 3, 4, 5, 6a, 6b, 8	1, 2, 3, 4, 5, 6a, 6b, 7	1, 2, 3, 4, 5, 6a, 6b, 7, 8

applied only to matings in which at least one of the parents is Rh_0 positive. Where both parents are Rh_0 numbers are given in the marginal headings, e.g., 1 is the code number for phenotypes rh and Rh_0.

Medical history:
1. Reject if there is history of:
   (a) Malaria
   (b) Syphilis
   (c) Viral hepatitis
   (d) Close contact with viral hepatitis within 6 mo.
   (e) Brucellosis
   (f) Coronary artery disease, severe hypertension, or rheumatic fever (either recently or significant cardiac damage from remote attack)
   (g) Active tuberculosis
   (h) Diabetes mellitus
   (i) Pregnancy, now or within past 6 mo.
   (j) Infections of upper respiratory tract:
       (1) Occasional but recent: 1 wk. free of disease
       (2) Frequent: 3 mo. free of disease
   (k) Bleeding tendency
   (l) Allergies if actively present for 1 wk. (reject all asthmatics)
   (m) Major surgical operation within 6 mo.
   (n) Tattoos (danger of hepatitis)
   (o) Alcoholism and drug addiction (danger of hepatitis)
   (p) Immunization with animal sera or vaccines or live viruses for 1-2 wk.
   (q) Infectious mononucleosis until completely recovered
   (r) Convulsions
2. Judgment of physician desirable and recommended if history of:
   (a) Fainting associated with previous donations
   (b) Jaundice not from hepatitis
   (c) Tuberculosis
   (d) Signs or symptoms of possible heart disease
   (e) Recent weight loss

Medical examination:
1. Reject if:
   (a) Weight below 110 lb. (50 kg.)
   (b) Temperature above 99.6° F.
   (c) Systolic blood pressure below 100 mm. Hg or above 200 mm. Hg
   (d) Diastolic blood pressure above 100 mm. Hg or below 50 mm. Hg
   (e) Hemoglobin below 12.5 gm./100 ml. for female donors; below 13.5 gm./100 ml. for male donors
   (f) Hematocrit below 37% for female donors; below 40% for male donors
   (g) Pulse below 50 or above 110/min.

Blood collection: Blood is obtained under sterile conditions by phlebotomy and is collected in plastic bags by the gravity method or in glass bottles by the vacuum method. Bags or bottles contain about 125 ml. acid-citrate-dextrose isotonic anticoagulant solution (trisodium citrate, citric acid, dextrose, water) per about 450 ml. blood.

CROSSMATCHING

The crossmatch consists of a series of tests performed with the blood of the prospective recipient of a blood transfusion and the blood of the proposed donor (or donors). The purpose is to detect any possible incompatibility between the recipient's serum and the donor's red cells (**major crossmatch**) and between the donor's serum and the recipient's erythrocytes (**minor crossmatch**) that might lead to a transfusion reaction.

An incompatible crossmatch is recognized by agglutination or lysis of the donor's or the recipient's red cells at any phase of the crossmatch, which need not be continued then unless (1) for study of the behavior of the antibody, (2) the agglutination is due to cold agglutinins, or (3) the "least incompatible" blood is being searched for as in cases of autoimmune hemolytic anemia.

An incompatible crossmatch may be due to an error in typing of donor or recipient, an error in the identification of the specimen, or atypical antibodies in either donor or recipient blood.

A compatible crossmatch is recognized by the absence of agglutination or lysis. The latter must be recognized as it may so reduce the number of available red cells as to prevent the recognition of agglutination. The crossmatch is preceded by the serologic tests necessary to type (ABO, Rh, and any other factor that appears to be indicated) the donor and the recipient.

SCREENING OF DONOR AND RECIPIENT FOR ATYPICAL ANTIBODIES

If there is enough time, donor and recipient should be screened for atypical antibodies in advance of the transfusion. **Screening of the donor** may reveal serum antibodies that would not be detected unless the recipient has the corresponding antigen. The antibody may also react with the blood of one of the other donors. **Screening of the recipient** may also uncover atypical antibodies in advance of the transfusion so that ample time may be available to find compatible blood. Prescreening is not a substitute for the minor crossmatch that uncovers errors in the ABO typing which prescreening fails to do. Screening does replace the minor crossmatch when O blood is administered to AB patients since the minor crossmatch will always be incompatible.

METHODS OF CROSSMATCHING

The crossmatch procedure used must be such as to detect different types of antibodies, saline-acting antibodies, high protein medium–acting antibodies, and antibodies recognizable only with the antiglobulin technique. Crossmatching should therefore be done by at least four different approaches: in saline solution at 22° and 37° C., in high protein medium, and by the indirect antiglobulin technique.

Crossmatching technique

Recipient's blood: It must be fresh, less than 24 hr. old, and not hemolyzed. After each transfusion a fresh specimen must be obtained. The ABO and Rh_o type should be ascertained, and if time allows, the blood should be tested for atypical antibodies and autoagglutinins.

Donor's blood: ABO and Rh_o type-specific blood is chosen. Screening for atypical antibodies is advisable if time allows. Note expiration date and examine plasma for evidence of hemolysis. Retest pilot tube and make sure that it matches the

bottle. The exact Rh phenotype should be known, especially if the blood is Rh_o negative.

Step 1—saline crossmatch at 22° C. (room temperature):

NOTE: In practice, steps 1 and 3 are set up at the same time.

1. Place 2 drops recipient's serum in a test tube marked RS (for major crossmatch) and 2 drops donor's serum in a test tube marked DS (for minor crossmatch).
2. Add 2 drops 2% saline suspension of donor's cells to tube marked RS and 2 drops 2% saline suspension of recipient's cells to tube marked DS. Allow to stand at room temperature for 15 min. Serum-suspended cells may be used instead of saline suspensions.
3. Mix and centrifuge at 3400 rpm for 15 sec.
4. Dislodge the cells gently.
5. Observe macroscopically and microscopically for agglutination and hemolysis.

Step 2—saline crossmatch at 37° C.:

1. If there is no agglutination in the previous procedure, mix the tube contents and incubate at 37° C. for 30 min.
2. Centrifuge immediately at 3400 rpm for 15 sec.
3. Dislodge cells gently and observe macroscopically and microscopically for agglutination or lysis.

Step 3—protein crossmatch[48]:

1. Place 2 drops recipient's serum in a test tube marked RS and 2 drops donor's serum in a test tube marked DS.
2. Add 2 drops 5% serum suspension of donor's cells to tube marked RS and 2 drops 5% serum suspension of recipient's cells to tube marked DS.
3. Mix and add 2 drops 22% albumin.
4. Mix and centrifuge immediately so as to forestall a prozone reaction.
5. Observe for agglutination or hemolysis.
6. If there is no reaction, incubate for 30 min. at 37° C.
7. Centrifuge immediately at 3400 rpm for 15 sec.

8. Examine macroscopically and microscopically for agglutination or hemolysis.
9. If there is no reaction, continue with the antiglobulin test.

Step 4—antiglobulin crossmatch:

1. If there is no reaction in the protein crossmatch, continue to use the same cells.
2. Wash the red cells at least three times in normal saline solution, filling the tube with saline solution each time and mixing the cells well.
3. Add 1 or 2 drops antiglobulin serum according to manufacturer's instructions.
4. Centrifuge at 3400 rpm for 15 sec.
5. Examine macroscopically and microscopically for agglutination.

Interpretation of steps of the crossmatching procedure

Step 1: Agglutination or hemolysis in the saline procedure at 22° C. will detect:

1. ABO incompatibility, often due to incorrect typing
2. Cold agglutinins or autoagglutinins
3. Saline-acting antibodies such as anti-**M**, anti-**N**, anti-**S**, anti-**Lu**, anti-**P**, and anti-**Le** (hemolysis)

Step 2: The saline crossmatch at 37° C. detects:

1. Saline-acting anti-**Rh-Hr** antibodies
2. Some anti-**M**, anti-**N**, and anti-**S** antibodies
3. Some anti-**K** and anti-**Le** antibodies (hemolysis)

Agglutination produced by cold agglutinins will disappear or diminish.

If difficulties arise in the saline crossmatch:

1. Retype and reverse type the donor's and recipient's blood specimens for ABO and determine **Rh-Hr** types.
2. Test for cold agglutinins and autoagglutinins.
3. Suspect anti-**Le** if hemolysis occurs.

Step 3: The high protein crossmatch at 37° C. detects:

1. Most anti-**Rh-Hr** antibodies
2. Some anti-**M**, anti-**N**, and anti-**S** antibodies
3. Some anti-**Le** antibodies (hemolysis)

It serves as the initial step of the antiglobulin test.

If difficulties arise in the high protein crossmatch:

1. Retype and Rh-Hr phenotype patient and donor.
2. Test serum of recipient if major crossmatch is involved or serum of donor if minor crossmatch is involved on panel of test cells.
3. Employ all methods of testing: saline, albumin, antiglobulin, and enzyme techniques.
4. If hemolysis is noted, suspect anti-**Le**.
5. Test for autoagglutinins.

Step 4: The antiglobulin crossmatch detects:

1. Almost all anti-**Rh-Hr** antibodies
2. Most immune antibodies

It is the only method to detect anti-**Fy**, anti-**Jk**, and most anti-**K** antibodies.

If difficulties arise in the antiglobulin crossmatch:

1. Test the serum of the recipient if the major crossmatch is involved and of the donor if the minor crossmatch is involved on panel of cells.
2. Crossmatch several donors and note frequency of incompatibility.

The percentage of incompatible crossmatches produced by specific antibodies are as follows: anti-**K**, 10%; anti-**Le**^{a} (Le$_1$), 20%; anti-**Fy**^{a}, 65%; anti-**Jk**^{a}, 75%; and anti-**Le**, 95%.

See whether donor's direct Coombs test is positive. If it is, screen his serum for atypical antibodies. If the serum is negative when tested against selected cells or panel of cells, elute antibody off red cells and test eluate on panel of cells. All four techniques (saline, albumin, antiglobulin, enzyme) should be used.

NOTE: Even the most carefully performed crossmatch will not detect all possible sources of incompatibility.[49]

Emergency crossmatching procedures

In an extreme emergency (a matter of life or death when no blood substitute is available) group O, Rh-negative blood may be released without typing the patient or crossmatching. This procedure is not recommended as a routine and is potentially dangerous, but under the circumstances of an extreme emergency it can be the lesser of two evils.

In emergencies that allow only a minimal amount of time for typing and crossmatching (mass casualties), anti-**A** serum may be used to group patients into those who react with anti-**A** (groups A and AB) and those who do not react (groups O and B). The slide test should be used for Rh typing. Rh-specific blood of group A is administered to patients of groups A and AB, and group O blood to patients of groups O and B. The advantage of this approach lies in the speed of the typing procedure and in the fact that the two most common blood groups, A and O, are used to satisfy all blood needs.

Even in emergencies blood should not be administered without some type of crossmatching procedure. The fastest procedure (which does not detect every type of incompatibility) consists of mixing 2 drops patient's plasma with 1 drop donor's blood on a tile. Mix, tilt back and forth, and read after 2-3 min. If compatible, confirm results by regular crossmatching procedure. If incompatible, do not release blood.

If more time is available, do saline solution and high albumin crossmatches and issue the blood if both are compatible, but proceed with antiglobulin crossmatch. Should the latter prove to be incompatible, the patient by then will have received only a small amount of blood (less than 50 ml.), an amount that is usually not followed by serious transfusion reactions.

Choice of blood
For transfusions

ABO and Rh type-specific blood compatible by all crossmatching procedures should be chosen unless clinical indications demand otherwise. In emergencies low-titer O blood may be issued to A or B recipients, but it should not be given to group AB individuals as either A or B blood is preferable to O blood if group-specific blood is not available.

It may not be possible to satisfactorily crossmatch a patient with acquired hemolytic anemia characterized by a positive direct and indirect antiglobulin test. Type-specific blood should be issued.

For exchange transfusions[50]

Irrespective of the type of erythroblastosis (Rh or ABO), blood for exchange transfusions must be compatible with the serum of the mother. In Rh erythroblastosis in which the mother is Rh negative, Rh-negative blood compatible with the mother should be chosen. If the mother and the baby are of the same ABO blood group, that blood group is preferred. If they differ in their ABO blood group, group O blood should be selected. It should be of low anti-**A** and anti-**B** titer. If the antibody is anti-c (**hr′**), the chosen blood must be homozygous C (type Rh_1Rh_1). In ABO erythroblastosis the Rh type of the transfused blood should be that of the baby.

There is at least one report of massive intravascular sickling after exchange transfusion with sickle cell trait blood.[51] In general, sickle cell trait blood is considered safe for transfusions to patients with the exception of erythroblastotic infants and sickle cell anemia patients in crisis.

The universal donor

The safety with which group O blood can be administered to individuals of other than group O depends not only on the titer of the saline-acting anti-**A** and anti-**B** antibodies but, even more important, on the presence of immune anti-**A** or anti-**B** antibodies, which cannot be neutralized by the addition of group-specific substances.

Group O blood should only be used for group O recipients. In emergencies, for exchange transfusions in the newborn infant, and if the patient's group cannot be ascertained, group O blood may be issued, provided that there is no high-titer antibody present. Generally, O blood is considered safe if the titer of both isoagglutinins is less than 1:50.

Screening test for high isoagglutinin titer of group O blood:
1. Dilute donor's serum 1:50 in saline solution by adding 0.1 ml. serum to 4.9 ml. saline solution.

2. Label one test tube A and one B. To each add 0.1 ml. diluted serum.
3. Add 0.1 ml. 2% suspension of A cells to tube A and 0.1 ml. 2% suspension of B cells to tube B.
4. Mix and allow to incubate at room temperature for 15 min.
5. Centrifuge at 3400 rpm for 15 sec.
6. Gently dislodge cell button and observe macroscopically for agglutination.

Interpretation: If agglutination occurs in either tube, the titer is higher than 1:50 and the blood cannot be considered to be of low titer. The saline agglutinin (rM) titer does not necessarily reflect the albumin (rG) antibody titer, which may be the more important titer since it is able to pass the placenta.

Screening test for immune anti-A and anti-B (neutralization test):

Blood group–specific substances A and B (Witebsky substance): These A and B substances are used to neutralize the anti-A and anti-B isohemagglutinins of group O blood. One unit (vial) is sufficient to reduce the anti-A and anti-B in 500 ml. O blood to at least one fourth of its original titer.

The A and B specific substances, however, are ineffective against immune anti-A and anti-B so that they may not prevent transfusion reaction. There is also evidence that they are antigenic.

A- and B-specific substances are found in the saliva and in the gastric juice of some individuals (called secretors) as well as in the red blood cells and tissues. They are found widely distributed in both plants and animals. The commercial products are made chiefly from the gastric mucosa of hogs and horses, the former containing highly potent A but no B and the latter containing both A and B and, rarely, pure B.

Method:

Reagent: Blood group–specific substances A and B have the capacity to combine specifically with anti-A and anti-B isoagglutinins, thus preventing these antibodies from agglutinating A and B cells.

1. To 0.2 ml. serum add 0.2 ml. blood group–specific substances A and B.

2. Add 3.6 ml. saline solution, producing a dilution of 1:20.
3. Mix and incubate at room temperature for 5 min.
4. Test 2 drops neutralized serum on 2 drops 2% suspension of A cells in saline solution in a test tube marked A.
5. Repeat the same procedure with B cells in a tube marked B.
6. Mix and allow to incubate at room temperature for 10 min.
7. Centrifuge at 3400 rpm for 15 sec. and examine grossly and microscopically for agglutination.
8. If agglutination occurs in either tube, repeat procedure with serum neutralized by the addition of 0.8 ml. group-specific substance A and B to 0.2 ml. serum.

Interpretation: Lack of agglutination indicates absence of γ-M (or γ-G) anti-A and anti-B antibodies in dangerous amounts, while agglutination proves the presence of nonneutralizable antibodies. In the latter case the blood should not be issued to other than group O individuals.

BLOOD STORAGE AND "STORAGE LESION"

Blood must be stored in a special blood storage refrigerator that operates between 1° and 6° C., is well lighted, and is attached to an automatic temperature-recording device equipped with an alarm system. The suggested temperature is 4° C.

There is a 21-day limit on storage of blood bank blood that is meant to assure the survival of at least 70% of the transfused cells 24 hr. after transfusion. During storage the clinically most important change in the plasma is the gradual rise in the **potassium** concentration, which may rise from an initial level of from 4-7 mEq./L. to 32 mEq./L. or over after 21 days. The other plasma changes are of less importance. There is a slight lowering of the pH associated with some accumulation of lactic acid. There is also about a 1% hemolysis of the red cells, some increase in ammonia, and a loss of glucose and sodium, the latter into the red cells. The blood components that are least stable are the white cells, platelets, and coagulation factors II, V, and VIII.

TRANSFUSION REACTIONS

The term "transfusion reaction" is usually restricted to untoward reactions occurring during a transfusion or shortly afterward and does not include such long-term deleterious effects as the transmission of hepatitis or such immediate results as acute congestive heart failure.

It cannot be overemphasized that the generally accepted indications for transfusion therapy should be strictly adhered to since every transfusion entails a certain risk. Whenever a transfusion reaction occurs, the transfusion must be discontinued at once.

Transfusion reactions can be divided into hemolytic and nonhemolytic.

Nonhemolytic reactions

Nonhemolytic reactions include allergic reactions, febrile reactions, and bacterial reactions.

Allergic reactions: They are the most common and at the same time the least severe reactions. Antihistaminics and cortisone should not be added to the blood, but rather administered to the patient directly.

Febrile reactions: The use of disposable equipment and strict adherence to blood bank regulations, such as never allowing a blood bottle to be contaminated or exposed to room temperature for any length of time except at the time of transfusion, have gone a long way to eliminate febrile reactions. Some reactions may be due to antileukocyte antibodies or unknown reactions. Others may be due to antileukocyte or antiplatelet antibodies or unknown antigens in the donor's blood. The use of leukocyte and platelet-poor blood or of packed cells may be suggested to prevent febrile reactions.

As a febrile reaction cannot be differentiated from a hemolytic reaction in its early stages, it must be treated as one. See discussion of hemolytic transfusion reactions.

Bacterial reactions: They are usually due to a break in technique and are preventable. The bacteria are usually gram-negative rods that are able to multiply at 4° C. The patient's reaction is often severe and anaphylactoid in nature or characterized by profuse bleeding.[52]

Hemolytic reactions

Hemolytic reactions are the most serious and carry a mortality varying from 10-30%. They are due to the destruction of red blood cells by antibodies in the plasma of the donor or recipient. The severity of the reaction will somewhat depend on the amount of blood transfused and on the type and avidity of the antibody. In a patient under anesthesia, unexplained oozing from the operative wound may be the first sign of a reaction.

The earliest clinical manifestations may be chills, fever, pain in the back and the chest, pallor, sweating, feeling of oppression, and fall in blood pressure with an increase in pulse rate.

There are some hemolytic transfusion reactions that are **latent** or **delayed** but are nevertheless due to an antigen-antibody reaction. An unexpected rapid fall of the patient's red cell count following transfusion may indicate hemolysis of the donor's red cells and can be confirmed by the determination of the levels of serum hemoglobin, indirect bilirubin, and fecal urobilinogen.

Serious hemolytic transfusion reactions result in hemoglobinemia, methemalbuminemia, hemoglobinuria, hyperbilirubinemia (3-6 hr. after transfusion—jaundice), leukopenia followed by leukocytosis, appearance of immune antibodies, absence of the expected rise of the red cell count or even anemia, and possibly lower nephron nephrosis.

Investigation of hemolytic reaction

Any type of reaction during or after a blood transfusion should be reported to the laboratory, and it is the technologist's duty to investigate each report. As soon as a reaction occurs the transfusion should be stopped at once, and the blood bottle, pilot tubes, and identification tags should be brought to the laboratory with a completed form stating the reason for the return of the bottle. As soon as a transfusion reaction is reported, clotted, oxalated, and heparinized blood and urine should be obtained from the patient. Repeat posttransfusion samples are obtained 5-24 hr. and 3 and 5 days after the transfusion. No further transfusion should be given.

It is good blood bank practice to store each patient's pretransfusion sample in the blood bank refrigerator for 2 wk. After a hemolysis transfusion reaction the post- and pretransfusion samples are studied together.

Laboratory evidence of hemolytic transfusion reaction is as follows:

1. Hemoglobinemia. Compare color of pretransfusion and posttransfusion sera. Posttransfusion serum may be pink. Examine serum spectroscopically or with the benzidine test for free hemoglobin.
2. Methemalbuminemia. Methemalbuminemia may color the plasma brown and can be recognized spectroscopically (see p. 102).
3. Haptoglobin level. The decrease in haptoglobin is a sensitive indicator of hemolysis.
4. Bilirubinemia. The indirect van den Bergh reaction is the procedure of choice. Maximal elevations of bilirubin are often found after 5 hr. and may disappear after 24 hr.
5. Comparison of pretransfusion and posttransfusion hemoglobin and hematocrit levels. After 48-74 hr. each completed transfusion should raise the hemoglobin level by 1.5 gm.% and the red blood cell level by 500,000 cells. In case of a hemolytic transfusion reaction the expected rise will not take place and there may be a rapid drop in the red cell count.
6. Urine examination. Look for evidence of hemoglobinuria, oliguria, and hemoglobin casts.
7. Blood chemistry. Obtain blood urea nitrogen level as a base line for future comparison.

If a hemolytic reaction has occurred, the following steps should be taken:

1. Investigate the record keeping for the possibility of incorrect labeling or of a mix-up in blood bottles. Also investigate the patient's name, room number, location of bed, and hospital number.
2. Make sure that the following blood samples are available: (a) pretransfusion samples of patient and donor blood, (b) pilot tubes of all bloods administered, (c) bottle blood of all bloods administered, (d) immediate posttransfusion sample of patient's blood, and (e) delayed (3-6 days later) sample of patient's blood.
3. Examine 2% saline suspension of patient's blood for mixed blood appearance, e.g., the appearance of small clumps of agglutinated cells (donor's) within even suspension of recipient's red blood cells.
4. Retype donor's and recipient's blood, including Rh subgroups, if indicated.
5. Crossmatch blood from each pilot tube as well as blood taken directly from the bottles used in the transfusions with the patient's serum taken from the pretransfusion and posttransfusion blood clots.
6. Perform Hemantigen* test, using patient's serum to detect atypical antibodies. Use antiglobulin technique with or without enzymes.
7. Perform Panocell* test, employing antiglobulin technique with or without enzymes, to identify the atypical antibodies found in the Hemantigen test.
8. Perform direct antiglobulin test on patient's cells to discover antibodies coating the red cells but not present free in the serum. Note that antiglobulin test may not detect anti-**A** and anti-**B** antibodies.

DANGERS OF TRANSFUSIONS
Single transfusions

The following untoward conditions may occur:

1. Formation of immune antibodies to red cells, white cells, and platelets
2. Formation of immune antibodies to clotting factors
3. Temporary arrest of erythropoiesis

---

*Knickerbocker Laboratories, New York, N. Y.

4. Transfusion reactions
5. Overloading of circulation due to speed or excessive volume of transfusion
6. Transmission of disease—hepatitis, malaria, infectious mononucleosis, etc. (syphilis cannot be transmitted by stored blood)
7. Hemosiderosis and posttransfusional hemochromatosis
8. Thrombophlebitis

Massive transfusions

During massive transfusions the following difficulties may develop:
1. Fall in level of clotting factors (fibrinogen, calcium, platelets)
2. Increase in anticoagulants (heparin, fibrinolysins)
3. Increase in potassium as donor's cells release their potassium
4. Citrate toxicity and fall in ionized calcium
5. Overloading of circulation

BLOOD AND BLOOD COMPONENTS IN CLINICAL USE

Fresh blood transfusions: Use of blood less than 12 hr. old is indicated in hemophilia A, thrombocytopenic purpura, and erythroblastosis fetalis.

Blood bank blood transfusions: The main indications are as follows:
1. Surgical shock due to blood loss, burns, or operative procedures
2. Chronic and acute blood loss
3. Preparation for operation
4. Bleeding following heparin and Dicumarol therapy (factors II and IX are relatively stable in stored blood)

Massive transfusions: Massive transfusions are often needed in vascular surgery and when extracorporeal circulation or exchange transfusions are used. There is some evidence that before large quantities of stored blood are to be given it should be warmed to body temperature.[53]

Packed cells: Packed cells allow the administration of blood without a rapid change in blood volume. They are indicated when the cardiac reserve of the patient is low and in severe anemias.

Plasma transfusions[54]**:** Plasma is available in liquid and in dried or frozen form and can be administered as a single unit that is obtained from one donor or as pooled plasma obtained from several (8) donors. Pooling increases the danger of serum hepatitis. Plasma should be group specific. It may contain immune anti-**A** and anti-**B** antibodies. Plasma is indicated in the treatment of burns, lower nephron nephrosis, when blood is not immediately available, and in hemophilia. Storage of pooled liquid plasma at 30°-34° C. for 6 mo. or longer diminishes the risk of hepatitis. Single donor fresh frozen plasma is used for the treatment of hemophilia A because it contains factor VIII.

Platelet transfusions[52]**:** Platelet transfusions temporarily control thrombocytopenic bleeding in acute leukemias and in idiopathic thrombocytopenia and may be used prior to surgery.

Blood-derivative transfusions: Albumin (25%), which in 100 ml. units is equivalent to 500 ml. citrated plasma, is used in the treatment of burns, erythroblastosis, and hypoproteinemia. There is no danger of transmission of hepatitis.

The use of fibrinogen is indicated in hypofibrinogenemia and in fibrinolysis.

Plasmaphoresis[54a]**:** The introduction of plastic equipment allows the bleeding of a donor, separation of the plasma, and autotransfusion of the red cells. The donor must meet the standard blood bank requirements and have an adequate serum protein level, which can be ascertained by the rapid refractometer method (see p. 101). Two units of platelet-rich plasma (1000 ml.) can be obtained almost weekly from a single donor. The packed cells are returned to the donor within a short period of time through an attachment to the donor set (Fenwal plasmaphoresis set*). Platelet-rich plasma may be used to concentrate platelets or it may be administered as such whenever platelet transfusion is indicated.

DETECTION AND IDENTIFICATION OF BLOOD GROUP ANTIBODIES

The detection and identification of blood group antibodies is important in the following instances:

---

*Fenwal Co., Morton Grove, Ill.

1. In the serum of multiparous women, with or without a history of erythroblastosis
2. In the serum of blood donors
3. In the serum of recipients of blood transfusions
4. In the eluate to identify antibodies in erythroblastosis fetalis and in acquired hemolytic anemia

SCREENING TESTS FOR ANTIBODIES: The procedures are the same as used for crossmatching.

1. Test cells suspended in saline solution are mixed with serum.
2. Albumin-suspended cells are mixed with serum.
3. The indirect antiglobulin technique is employed.
4. The cells are treated with one of the proteolytic enzymes.

An **autoagglutinin control** must always be included. The patient's ABO group and subgroup and Rh-Hr type should be known so that certain antibodies can be excluded.

Procedure: It is recommended that two different test cells be used: (1) group **O**, Rh_1Rh_1 (CDe/CDe), and (2) group **O**, Rh_2Rh_2 (cDE/cDE).

One cell sample should be Kell positive. The homozygosity of the factors increases the sensitivity of the test cells.

Individual group O cells of the abovementioned Rh-Hr phenotypes are commercially available. They also contain a number of blood group factors that are identified and known to cause hemolytic transfusion reactions and hemolytic disease of the newborn.

Saline tube method:

1. Label two tubes No. 1 and No. 2 according to the cell groups used and place 2 drops patient's serum into each tube.
2. Add 2 drops 2% saline suspension of cells No. 1 to tube No. 1 and repeat procedure with cells No. 2 or follow directions accompanying the cells.
3. Mix and incubate at room temperature for 15 min.
4. Centrifuge at 3400 rpm for 15 sec.
5. Examine for agglutination and hemolysis.

6. If there is no reaction, incubate the tubes at 37° C. for 30 min.
7. Centrifuge at 3400 rpm for 15 sec.
8. Examine for agglutination or hemolysis.

If the saline test is negative, proceed with the albumin test. If the test is positive as evidenced by agglutination or hemolysis, it will detect saline-acting atypical antibodies that react at room or body temperature. In this category they are the antibodies to factors **A, B, H, M, N, S,** and **P.** Some examples of anti-**Le,** anti-**K,** and anti-**Rh** may also react. The agglutination of cold agglutinins should diminish or disappear at 37° C.

Albumin test:

1. Label two test tubes No. 1 and No. 2 according to the cell groups used and place 2 drops serum into each tube.
2. Add 2 drops 2-5% suspension of No. 1 cells to tube No. 1 and repeat procedure with cells No. 2 or follow directions accompanying the test cells.
3. Mix and add 2 drops 22% bovine albumin to each tube.
4. Mix and centrifuge at 3400 rpm for 15 sec.
5. Examine for agglutination and hemolysis.
6. Resuspend cells if there is no reaction and incubate cells for 30 min. at 37° C.
7. Centrifuge at 3400 rpm for 15 sec.
8. Examine for agglutination or hemolysis.

If there is no reaction, continue with the antiglobulin test. If hemolysis or agglutination is present, the test is positive and will suggest the presence of albumin-acting atypical antibodies reacting best at 37° C., such as anti-**Rh**$_0$ (D), anti-**hr'** (c), anti-**rh''** (E), some anti-**Lewis,** some anti-**M,** and some anti-**P** antibodies.

Antiglobulin test[55]:

1. If there is no reaction in the albumin test, wash the cells well in large amounts of normal saline solution.
2. Add 2 drops antiglobulin serum or as recommended by the manufacturer.

Table 5-30. Approximate frequencies of certain blood factors

Blood factors	Approximate frequency (%)		Blood factors	Approximate frequency (%)	
	Caucasians	Negroes		Caucasians	Negroes
M	78	75	K	10	2
N	72	77	k	99	98
S	54	29	Fy^a	66	11
s	88	90	Fy^b	83	24
U	100	98+	Fy	100	34
P$_1$	79	94	Jk^a	76	91
P (Tj)	Almost 100	Almost 100	Jk^b	73	43
			Le$_1$	22	22
Lu^a	8	4	Le^H	72	55
Lu^b	92	96	Le	94	78

Table 5-31. Characteristics of certain blood group antibodies*

Antibody	Preferred method or medium for detection	Optimal temperature range (°C.)
Anti-A Anti-A$_1$ Anti-B Anti-H	Saline	4°-20°
Anti-Rh Anti-hr	High protein, antiglobulin	37°
Anti-K Anti-k	Antiglobulin	37°
Anti-Fy^a Anti-Fy^b	Antiglobulin	37°
Anti-Jk^a Anti-Jk^b	Antiglobulin (anti-non-gamma and complement needed)	37°
Anti-Le^a	Saline, antiglobulin (anti-nongamma and complement needed)	20°-37°
Anti-Le^b	Saline	4°-20°
Anti-Lu^a	Saline	20°-37°
Anti-Lu^b	Saline, antiglobulin	20°-37°
Anti-M Anti-N	Saline	4°-20°
Anti-S	Saline, antiglobulin	20°-37°
Anti-s	Antiglobulin	37°
Anti-U	Saline, antiglobulin	37°
Anti-P$_1$	Saline	4°-15°
Anti-P (Tj)	Saline	20°-37°

*From Hyland reference manual of immuno-hematology, Los Angeles, 1964, Hyland Laboratories, p. 100.

3. Centrifuge at 3400 rpm for 15 sec.
4. Examine for agglutination.

Agglutination will indicate the presence of atypical antibodies acting best at 37° C. in high protein medium and detected best by the antiglobulin technique, such as anti-**K**, anti-**Duffy**, anti-**Kidd**, and anti-**Lewis** antibodies. Anti-**Rh** antibodies also react by the antiglobulin technique. Anti-**Lewis** and anti-**Kidd** antibodies may produce hemolysis.

IDENTIFICATION OF ANTIBODIES: The screening test will detect the presence of atypical antibodies but it will not identify them. Identification is accomplished by testing the serum against a panel of cells of known antigenic composition under the circumstances that gave a positive screening test. If the serum reacted more strongly in saline solution at room temperature, it should be tested against the panel of cells in saline solution at room temperature. If the antiglobulin screening test was positive, the antiglobulin method must also be chosen for the panel cells.

The panel of cells is composed of group O cells selected from many donors and tested for the various antigens. They are commercially available as Identigen.*

Technique: The patient's own cells must be tested parallel to the panel cells. The techniques used are similar to the crossmatching techniques except that the cells are known reagent cells and the serum is that of the patient. The cells

*Ortho Pharmaceutical Corp., Raritan, N. J.

Table 5-32. Antibodies encountered in crossmatching*†

Antibody	Approximate frequency in crossmatch	Optimum temperature of reaction (°C.)	Type of crossmatch Saline tube	Type of crossmatch High protein Tube	Type of crossmatch High protein Slide	Type of crossmatch Indirect Coombs	Approximate % blood (white) compatible with antibody	Relation to human disease (HTr, hemolytic transfusion; EF, erythroblastosis fetalis)	Comments
1. Anti-**B**	Almost universal	5-20	Good	Good	Poor	No need	85	HTr-EF	Natural antibody—immune forms; may be hemolytic
2. Anti-**A**	Almost universal	5-20	Good	Good	Poor	No need	55	HTr-EF	Natural antibody—immune forms; may be hemolytic
3. Anti-**Rh**$_0$ (D)	1 in 400	37	Poor	Good	Good	Often no need	16	HTr-EF	Most common immune antibody; enzyme enhanced
4. Anti-**Rh**$_0$′ (D + C)	1 in 600	37	Poor	Good	Good	Often no need	15	HTr-EF	**rh**′ (C) alone is rare—combination frequent; enzyme enhanced
5. Autoantibody	1 in 2000	37	Poor	Fair	Fair	Good	0	?	Acquired hemolytic anemia, lupus; occasionally specific (anti-**hr**′, anti-**hr**′′, anti-**c**, anti-**e**)
6. Cold agglutinin	1 in 2000	5	Good	Good	Poor	No need	0	?	Viral pneumonitis; reacts with all cells
7. Anti-**hr**′ (c)	1 in 5000	37	Fair	Good	Good	Often no need	20	HTr-EF	Most common immunization in Rh-positive persons
8. Anti-**rh**′′ (E)	1 in 6000	37	Poor	Good	Good	Often no need	80	HTr-EF	Common immunization in Rh-positive persons; enzyme enhanced
9. Anti-**hr**′ + **rh**′′ (c + E)	1 in 6000	37	Poor	Good	Good	Often no need	19	HTr-EF	Combination occurs in Rh_1Rh_1 (CDe/CDe); enzyme enhanced
10. Anti-**A**$_1$	1 in 10,000	5	Good	Good	Poor	No need	64	HTr ?	Natural antibody occurs in A_2 and A_2B donor and recipient
11. Anti-**K** (Kell)	1 in 15,000	37	Poor	Poor	Fair	Good	92	HTr-EF	Potent antibody in erythroblastosis fetalis
12. Anti-**Rh**$_0$′′ (D + E)	1 in 15,000	37	Poor	Good	Good	Often no need	15	HTr-EF	Combination found in Rh-negative (rh) persons (cde/cde)
13. Anti-**Le**$_1$ (Lewis)	1 in 20,000	20	Good	Good	Fair	Often no need	77	HTr-EF ?	Natural antibody—complex system; may be hemolytic; enzyme may enhance

Antibody	Occurrence	Temp.					Titer	HTr	Remarks
14. Anti-Fy^a (Duffy)	1 in 20,000	37	Poor	Poor	Fair	Good	35	HTr-EF	Acquired by transfusion and pregnancy; enzyme may destroy
15. Anti-P	1 in 20,000	5-20	Good	Good	Poor	Often no need	25	HTr ?	Natural—weak—often at refrigerator temperature
16. Anti-M	1 in 30,000	20-37	Good	Good	Fair	Often no need	22	HTr	Natural—rarely immune; enzyme destroys
17. Anti-Rh$_0$'' (C+D+E)	1 in 30,000	37	Poor	Good	Good	Often no need	14	HTr-EF	Acquired antibodies in the Rh-negative person
18. Anti-Jk^a (Kidd)	1 in 30,000	37	Poor	Poor	Good	Good	25	HTr-EF	Acquired; enzyme enhanced
19. Anti-rh' (C)	1 in 50,000	37	Fair	Good	Good	Often no need	33	HTr-EF	Acquired—rare in Rh-negative person as single antibody
20. Anti-hr'' (e)	1 in 100,000+	37	Fair	Good	Good	Often no need	2	HTr-EF	Acquired by transfusion and pregnancy in Rh$_2$Rh$_2$ (cDE/cDE)
21. Anti-S	1 in 100,000+	20-37	Good	Good	Fair	Often no need	45	HTr-EF	Natural or acquired; MN system; reacts more often with M or MN cells
22. Anti-rh$^w_1$ (C^w)	1 in 100,000+	37	Fair	Good	Good	Often no need	98	HTr ?	Acquired; "pure" anti-rh$^w_1$ (anti-C^w) in type Rh$_1$Rh$_1$ or type Rh$_1$rh
23. Anti-k (Cellano)	1 in 100,000+	37	Poor	Poor	Fair	Good	0.2	HTr-EF	Acquired; factor allelic to **K**
24. Anti-Jk^b (Kidd)	Occurrence extremely rare	37	Poor	Poor	Poor	Good	25	HTr ?	Acquired—enzyme enhanced; factor allelic to Jk^a
25. Anti-Fy^b (Duffy)	Occurrence extremely rare	37	Poor	Poor	Poor	Good	17	HTr	Acquired—enzyme may destroy; factor allelic to Fy^a
26. Anti-Lu^a (Lutheran)		20-37	Good	Good	Poor	Often no need	92	?	Acquired—enzyme may destroy
27. Anti-hr (f)		37	Fair	Good	Good	Often no need	35	?	Acquired—positive with cells of individuals having gene r or gene R^0
28. Anti-N		20-37	Good	Good	Poor	No need	28	HTr ?	Natural—enzyme destroys

*Modified from Dade Reagents, Inc, Miami, Fla.

†Low-frequency factors such as **Be^a**, **Becker**, **Ca^a**, **Gr**, **Jobbins**, **Levay**, **Mi^a**, and **R$_m$** react with family members and rarely anyone else (private antigens). High-frequency factors such as **I**, **Vel**, **Yt^a**, and **Kp^b** react with almost all cells tested (public antigens). Reactions given are those usually found and recorded. Antibodies made by different persons may react differently, e.g., one person's anti-**Le** may react in saline solution; another Le^a may be detected only by indirect Coombs test; likewise with anti-**S**, etc.

Table 5-32. Antibodies encountered in crossmatching—cont'd

Antibody	Approximate frequency in crossmatch	Optimum temperature of reaction (°C.)	Saline tube	High protein Tube	High protein Slide	Indirect Coombs	Approximate % blood (white) compatible with antibody	Relation to human disease (HTr, hemolytic transfusion; EF, erythroblastosis fetalis)	Comments
29. Anti-s		37	Poor	Poor	Poor	Good	11	HTr ?-EF	Acquired; related to MN system; factor allelic to S
30. Anti-Le^H		20	Fair	Fair	Poor	Often no need	22	?	Le^H reactions are reliable with A$_2$ and O cells—difficult to type bloods for this
31. Anti-U		37	Poor	Fair	Fair	Good	0	HTr-EF	Acquired only by S-negative, s-negative person; compatible donor rare and only Negro blood
32. Anti-Tj^a	← Occurrence extremely rare →	20-37	Good	Good	Poor	No need	0	? Miscarriages	Natural; related to P system
33. Anti-Vel		37	Poor	Poor	Poor	Good	0	HTr	Only about 4 in 10,000 fail to react
34. Anti-H		5	Good	Good	Poor	No need	0	?	Rare as strong antibody—also reacts most strongly with group O and A$_2$ cells; anti-H inhibited by saliva of secretor; anti-O not inhibited by saliva
35. Anti-Lu^b (Lutheran)		20-37	Good	Good	Poor	No need	0.2	?	Rare; existence only recently proved
36. Anti-He (Henshaw)		20	Good	Good	Poor	No need	100	EF	Related to MN system; reacts with a few Negro bloods
37. Anti-Di^a (Diego)		37	Poor	Poor	Poor	Good	100	EF	Corresponding factor found in South American Indians and Orientals
38. Anti-Wr^a (Wright)		37	Fair	Fair	Fair	Often no need	100	HTr ?-EF	May be natural; antibody may be frequent; reported often in anti-E serum
39. Anti-Ven		37	Poor	Poor	Poor	Good	100	EF	Reacts only with family
40. Anti-Hu (Hunter)		20-37	Good	Good	Fair	No need	100	?	Related to MN system; reacts only with 21% Negro bloods

have to be tested in saline solution at room temperature (22° C.), at 37° C., in albumin at 37° C., and by the antiglobulin technique. If necessary, they may have to be treated with proteolytic enzymes. Each test may have to be performed at 4°, 22°, and 37° C.

Procedure: With the red cell panel a list of the cells and their antigenic composition is supplied. After the reaction of the patient's serum with the reagent cells is completed, an attempt is made to identify the antibody in the serum on the basis of the list giving the antigenic composition of each cell group used in the test. Starting with cell group 1, all the antigens that fail to react with the patient's serum are crossed out not only in the column of cell group 1 but also in the columns of all the other cells that contain them. The procedure is repeated with cell group 2 and continued with the remaining cell samples. By this process of elimination there will only be one or two antigens left that have not been eliminated and that may correspond to the antibody in the patient's blood.

The correctness of the answer can be confirmed by studying the following:

1. Behavior of the antibody (Table 5-31)
2. Frequency with which it occurs, producing positive reactions with random blood samples (Table 5-30)
3. Presence or absence of hemolysis
4. Strength of reaction in various media (Table 5-32)

It may also be possible to adsorb the antibody from the serum with suitable test cells and thus confirm its identity.

Absorption of antibodies[56]

Principle: The antibody or antibodies present in the serum are removed from the serum by adsorption onto red cells that have the corresponding antigen or antigens.

Use of absorption:

1. Absorption of the serum in the preparation of an eluate
2. Separation of antibodies in a mixture of antibodies on the basis of the antigen and the temperature at which the antibodies react

3. Removal of unwanted antibodies and cold agglutinins

Technique:

1. Select cells that are homozygous for the antigen and wash the cells thoroughly in normal saline solution six to eight times to remove any residual serum. If the antibody is a nonspecific cold antibody, the saline solution should be warmed to 37° C. After the last wash the cells are drained well.
2. Mix 1 vol. packed cells with 1 vol. serum. A wide tube should be used to increase the contact area between the cells and the serum. If the antibody is weak, the amount of serum may be increased.
3. Place mixture in water bath, the temperature of which depends on the type of antibody to be adsorbed.
4. Centrifuge. Mix in centrifuge cups that may have to be prechilled to 4° C. or warmed to 37° C.
5. Remove serum rapidly and test serum for complete adsorption by bringing it in contact with suitable test cells. The direct antiglobulin test should be positive when the adsorbing cells are tested.

Elution of antibodies[55]

Elution is the removal of adsorbed antibody from coated cells.

Use of elution:

1. To identify the antibody in hemolytic disease of the newborn
2. To identify the antibody in acquired hemolytic anemia
3. To investigate transfusion reactions
4. To separate and identify antibodies in a mixture
5. To demonstrate weak variants of group A or B (see pp. 238 and 240)

Heat elution technique:

1. Wash the cells well in normal saline solution six to eight times at 4° C. to remove any unabsorbed antibody.
2. Repeat the direct antiglobulin test on the packed cells to see that the coating antibody is still present. The last saline wash may also be tested for the presence of the antibody with

suitable cells. The last wash should be negative for the antibody.

3. Add an equal volume of saline solution or 6% albumin of group AB serum to the packed cells and mix.
4. Place mixture in 56° C. water bath for 7-10 min., agitating constantly.
5. Centrifuge immediately in preheated (56° C. water bath) centrifuge cups. At high speed, pack cells in as short a time as possible.
6. Remove supernatant fluid (eluate) immediately.
7. Treat supernatant eluate as unknown serum and test against known cells.

Titration of antibodies

Principle: The titer is the relative amount of antibody present in the serum and it is determined by making serial twofold dilutions of the unknown serum and testing it against saline- and albumin-suspended cells of suitable type. The amount of these cells added to each tube is constant.

Precautions in titration procedures: Serologic titrations are subject to many variables and it is important to adhere to certain guidelines.

The test cells should preferably be from an individual homozygous for the antigen concerned. For repeat titrations a constant supply of these cells should be available.

To prevent carry-over of test serum, fresh clean pipettes should be used in making each dilution.

Serum specimens should be frozen for direct comparison with subsequent specimens and should be retitrated parallel with the repeat specimen.

Saline titration:
Technique:
1. Label 10 small test tubes as follows: 1, 2, 4, 8, 16, 32, 64, 128, 256, 512, and control, representing dilutions of serum that are as follows: undiluted, 1:2, 1:4, 1:8, 1:16, 1:32, 1:64, 1:128, 1:256, and 1:512.
2. With a 1 ml. pipette graduated in 0.1 ml. divisions, pipette 0.1 ml. saline solution into all tubes except the first.
3. Using a 0.2 ml. pipette, pipette 0.1 ml. serum in tubes 1 and 2.

4. Mix well tube 2 contents three times with a clean pipette and discard pipette. With a second clean pipette, transfer 0.1 ml. from tube 2 to tube 3, mix, and discard pipette.
5. Continue in this manner, using a fresh pipette for each dilution and discard 0.1 ml. from tube 512.
6. The control tube contains saline solution only. The 0.1 ml. removed from tube 512 may be saved for further dilutions.
7. With a 1 ml. pipette add 0.1 ml. 5% suspension in saline solution of washed red cells to each tube including the control.
8. Shake tubes to mix thoroughly, and incubate at 37° C. for 30 min. or at the temperature required for the particular antibody.
9. Centrifuge at 3400 rpm for 15 sec.
10. Gently dislodge sedimented cells and examine for agglutination, beginning observation with tube 512 and then down the line. This procedure prevents misinterpretation of prozoning in the first two or three tubes.
11. The titer of the serum is the reciprocal of the highest dilution showing distinct 1+ agglutination.
12. The nonagglutinated and weakly agglutinated cells are washed in saline solution three or four times in preparation for the antiglobulin test. The antiglobulin titer is expressed in the same way as the saline titer.

Albumin titration: The technique is the same as that for saline titration except that in step 2, 22% albumin is substituted for the saline solution and in step 7 the 5% suspension of red cells is prepared in 22% albumin.

The albumin titration can also be converted into a Coombs titration technique.

Enzyme titration:
Enzyme methods: The commonly used enzymes are papain, ficin, trypsin, and bromelin. These enzymes increase the reactivity of some systems but destroy others. The increased sensitivity of the red cells can lead to false positive reactions.

Choice of enzymes: **Trypsin** increases the reactivity with anti-**Rh** antibodies and also with anti-**A**, anti-**B**, anti-**P**, and anti-**Lewis** antibodies. It is not the enzyme of choice for antibodies of the **MNS** and **Duffy** system, though by the indirect antiglobulin technique anti-**Duffy** serum reacts well with trypsin-treated cells.

Papain treatment increases the sensitivity of the reaction with anti-**Rh** antibodies, anti-**Lewis,** and anti-**P** antibodies. Papain probably destroys M, N, and Duffy antigens.

Ficin produces a reaction similar to those produced by trypsin and papain and increases the sensitivity of reaction with anti-**Rh,** anti-**P,** and anti-**Lewis** antibodies and can also be used for anti-**Kell** and anti-**Kidd** antibodies. Similar to papain, it destroys M, N, S, and Duffy antigens.

Bromelin is similar in its action to the previously mentioned enzymes.

The enzyme preparations are commercially available and the manufacturer's instructions should be followed for the various tests.

Bromelin method of Pirofsky-Mangum[57]**:**
Reagents:
1. Sorensen buffer (M/15, pH 5.5):
   Solution A:
   KH_2PO_4 (anhydrous), 9.08 gm.
   Distilled water to 1 L.
   Solution B:
   NA_2HPO_4 (anhydrous), 9.47 gm.
   Distilled water to 1 L.
2. Bromelin powder
Store solutions A and B at 4° C. but mix at room temperature. To attain pH 5.5 add 4 ml. solution B to 96 ml. solution A.

Preparation of reagents:
1. Add 90 ml. saline solution and 10 ml. Sorensen buffer (pH 5.5.) to 0.5 gm. bromelin powder.
2. Add 0.1 gm. sodium azide as bactericidal and fungicidal agents.
3. Store in small test tubes. The solution is stable for 1 mo. at 4° C. and for 4-5 mo. at −20° C.

Procedure for detection of serum antibodies using bromelin[58]*:*
1. Place 2 drops serum in a small test tube.

2. Add 1 drop 4% saline suspension of unwashed test cells.
3. Add 1 drop bromelin solution.
4. Mix and incubate at room temperature for 15 min.
5. Centrifuge at 3400 rpm for 15 sec.
6. Gently dislodge cell button and observe for microscopic agglutination.

White cell antibodies (leukoagglutinins)[59]

Leukoagglutinins are probably responsible for some nonhemolytic transfusion reactions and can be prevented by administering buffy coat–poor blood. Because of the fact that after the rejection of a graft the patient develops group-specific leukocyte antibodies, it is possible that leukocyte antigens and transplantation antigens are related and that study of the leukocyte antigens may shed light on tissue antigens. See discussion of transformed lymphocytes.

White cell–agglutinating antisera are produced in a number of laboratories but leukoagglutination is difficult to interpret because of the nature of the antigen.

Platelet antibodies[59]

It has been shown that there is a relationship between nonhemolytic fever-chill transfusion reactions and the presence of platelet antibodies. The development of platelet antibodies may follow repeated transfusion of whole blood or transfusion of platelets.

COLD AGGLUTININS

Cold agglutinins occur in *Mycoplasma pneumoniae* infections, lymphatic leukemia, hemolytic anemias, and liver diseases. They are autohemagglutinins, causing the agglutination of the patient's own corpuscles at temperatures usually ranging from 0°-20° C., occasionally at room temperature, and very rarely at 30°-37° C. They may agglutinate the red cells of all blood groups. Typically the reaction is reversible, disappearing at body temperature.

Cold antibodies are complete antibodies that are frequently nonspecific in the sense that they act on an antigen common to all red blood cells, but they may have blood group specificity such as anti-**M,** anti-**A**, anti-**N**, anti-**I**, anti-**P**, anti-**H**, and anti-**Rh.**

They are gamma globulins with a sedimentation constant of 16-19S. If they are hemolytic, they interact with complement best at an acid pH of 6.3, binding of the complement and lysis of the red cells occurring at the same time (monothermic hemolysins). The bithermic Donath-Landsteiner cold hemolysin is a special type of cold agglutinin that unites with the red blood cells at 4° C., but hemolysis occurs at 15°-40° C. Cold agglutinins occur in the plasma as well as being attached to the cells, and if present in high titer, they may interfere with the antiglobulin test and with blood grouping at room temperature.

They may lead to spontaneous clumping of the red cells if brought in contact with their own serum or with typing sera. The cells will appear to be group AB, Rh positive, but because of the cold agglutinins in the serum they will reverse type as group O cells. Even if the cold agglutinins do not agglutinate their own cells, they may agglutinate some of the test cells used in reverse typing. Cold agglutinins such as anti-**Rh,** anti-**M**, anti-**P**, etc. will interfere with reverse typing if the test cells contain the corresponding antigens.

Despite the fact that cold agglutinins interfere with typing and crossmatching, their existence can be ignored in transfusion therapy since there is evidence that antibodies which act in vitro at low temperature do not cause harm at 37° C.

Handling of blood when cold agglutinins are present

1. Confirm presence of cold agglutinins.
2. Absorb the patient's serum and use washed red cells and absorbed serum for ABO grouping and for crossmatching.
3. Titer the antibody if indicated.
4. Identify the cold agglutinins after elution.

Test for cold autoagglutinins: Confirm the presence of cold autoagglutinating agglutinins by washing the patient's cells in saline solution and by adding his own serum to his washed cells in a test tube. If agglutination occurs, warm the tube in a water bath to see whether the degree of agglutination lessens.

If cold agglutinins are present, carry out typing procedures at 37° C. If this is not satisfactory, the cold agglutinins must be absorbed from the serum by the patient's own cells in the cold. The serum can then be used for typing as the other antibodies are not altered.

Absorption of cold agglutinins: At the bedside have an ice bath and a portable 37° C. water bath.

1. Obtain a blood specimen, half of which is immediately inserted into ice and allowed to clot. The other half is oxalated and immediately incubated at 37° C.
2. Allow the iced specimen to continue clotting in a refrigerator for about 30 min., after which time it is centrifuged in a refrigerated centrifuge or in iced centrifuge cups. Immediately remove serum from the clot. Remove plasma from the oxalated specimen.
3. Wash the oxalated cells three times in 37° C. saline solution, using warmed centrifuge tubes.
4. Prepare a 2% suspension of these cells in saline solution and use these cells for typing.
5. Test the serum against the red cell suspension to see whether the cold agglutinin was removed in the initial incubation.
6. If residual antibody remains, add 1 vol. serum to 1 vol. washed patient's cells and place in ice bath for 2 hr. Shake every 30 min.
7. Centrifuge in refrigerated centrifuge, remove serum, and retest with 2% suspension of patient's cells.
8. Repeat procedure if cold antibody activity is still present.

Elution of cold antibody: Have an ice bath and portable water bath at the bedside.

1. Obtain venous blood and divide into two test tubes, one with and the other without anticoagulants.
2. Insert tube without anticoagulant into water bath (37° C.), allow to

clot, and centrifuge in tubes surrounded by 37° C. water jackets. Remove serum.

3. Place the tube with anticoagulant into ice water bath, centrifuge in tubes surrounded by ice water, and remove plasma. Wash the red cells several times with saline solution at 4° C.

4. After the last washing add an equal volume saline solution to the packed red cells.

5. Mix well and incubate at 37° C. for 30 min.

6. Prepare **eluate No. 1** by centrifuging in tubes surrounded by cuffs of 37° C. water. Remove the eluate immediately.

7. Wash the red cells three times in saline solution at 37° C. and do a direct antiglobulin test. A negative test indicates that the antibody has been completely eluted.

8. If the test is positive, incubate a mixture of equal parts of packed red cells and saline solution at 56° C. for 10 min. Mix the specimen every 3 or 4 min.

9. Centrifuge in tubes surrounded by water at 56° C.

10. Immediately remove **eluate No. 2.**

11. Repeat direct antiglobulin test.

12. Test eluate and serum obtained in step 3 on a panel of cells.

Titration of cold antibody: See p. 272.

HEMOLYTIC DISEASE OF THE NEWBORN (HDN) OR ERYTHROBLASTOSIS FETALIS[60]

The hematologic manifestations are discussed under hemolytic anemias. Erythroblastosis fetalis is a fetal hemolytic anemia due to an antibody transmitted from the mother to the fetus via the placenta and directed against one of the antigens of the fetal red cells. The fetal red cells by their escape into the mother's circulation stimulate the formation of the maternal antibody.[61]

Immunization of the mother may be due to pregnancy or incompatible blood transfusion.

In every pregnancy there exists the possibility of immunologic maternal-fetal incompatibility that is not restricted to Rh incompatibility, as the mother may develop antibodies in her serum to any fetal blood factor that her red cells lack. The basis for the isoimmunization of pregnancy is the transplacental escape of fetal erythrocytes into the maternal circulation. By the elution method of Kleihauer, fetal cells can be demonstrated in the maternal blood in ratios of 1:1,000,000 or more (see p. 170).

Incidence of HDN: Irregular antibodies can be found in the mother's serum in about 3% of all pregnancies. According to Mollison, the overall incidence of erythroblastosis fetalis is about 1 in 180 pregnancies, 12% of which end in intrauterine death.

Anti-**Rh**$_0$ (D) is the most common antibody responsible for HDN encountered in the maternal serum. Next in decreasing frequency are anti-**hr'** (c), anti-**rh''** (E), anti-**Fy**, and anti-**Jk**.

Moreover, in the near future erythroblastosis fetalis due to sensitization to **Rh**$_0$ may become even rarer. The administration of γ-G immunoglobulin to Rh factor for the prevention of active immunization of Rh-negative mothers at risk has proved to be successful in preventing future antibody formation, so that these mothers in subsequent pregnancies give birth to unaffected Rh-positive infants.[62]

Prenatal studies in HDN

This involves the performance of certain tests on the blood of the mother and father and on the amniotic fluid.

The technique of the serologic methods is described in the section on antibody identification.

Maternal testing

The purpose of the investigation of the mother's serum is to detect, identify, and titer irregular antibodies that react with the father's red blood cells.

Grouping and typing of the mother's red cells: If the mother is A, B, or AB and the Rh type is positive, the probability of maternal sensitization is remote. If, in addition, the screening for circulating irregular antibodies is negative, no further work-up is required.

If, however, the maternal group is O

and/or the Rh is negative, the possibility of ABO or Rh sensitization exists.

Screening for maternal antibodies: The screening tests should be performed when the patient is first seen during the pregnancy and then again around the thirty-eighth week.

The most important antibodies are the 7S or immune globulins that are able to cross the placenta. The 19S saline-acting globulins do not cross the placenta and are therefore not involved in hemolytic disease of the newborn.

Agglutination of the pooled cells indicates the presence of an irregular antibody in the mother's serum, against one or more of the antigens of the pooled cells.

Specific antibody identification: Once an irregular antibody is detected, its specificity is established by the use of a panel of cells of known antigenic composition, employing the same method that gave optimal results in the screening tests.

Titration of antibody[63]: If an irregular antibody is found, it should be repeatedly titrated during the last 3 mo. of pregnancy to see whether it is rising or staying on an even keel.

The serum from the previous titration should be saved and frozen and run in parallel with the repeat specimen. Titration should be carried out using a single cell population containing the homologue antigen for the antibody in the mother's serum. The titer should be determined in saline solution and albumin and by the antiglobulin and, if necessary, enzyme technique.

Paternal testing

The purpose is to demonstrate any maternal-paternal group incompatibility.

Grouping and typing of the father's cells: If it is known that the mother has or has had irregular antibodies, complete phenotyping of the father is indicated in order to determine his most likely genotype. If the father is homozygous for the antigen causing the antibody in the mother's serum, the baby and all future babies will carry it on their red cells. If, on the other hand, he is heterozygous for this antigen, there is a 50% chance that the fetal cells will not inherit it.

Fetal testing

The purpose is to evaluate the destruction of fetal erythrocytes by the examination of the amniotic fluid. The fluid is obtained by amniocentesis.

Examination of amniotic fluid[64]

Bevis and Walker reported increased bilirubin pigment in the amniotic fluid of erythroblastotic fetuses, which reflected the intravascular fetal hemolysis and correlated well with the level of cord hemoglobin. The pigment, which is not excreted by the mother (as is the fetal serum bilirubin), is apparently acquired by the amniotic fluid during its circulation through the fetal gastrointestinal tract. The pigment on spectrophotometric analysis of the amniotic fluid has a distinct peak at 450 mμ.

Spectrophotometric analysis of amniotic fluid: The aspirated amniotic fluid is placed in a brown container, which in turn is protected by a lightproof container. Exposure to light rapidly denatures the pigment. The specimen may be kept at room temperature but must be protected from light. It should be examined as soon as possible. If the specimen is turbid and/or bloody, it should be centrifuged and filtered immediately to prevent lysis of the red blood cells. If still too turbid, it is diluted with distilled water to allow light transmission in an acceptable range. A spectral absorption curve is drawn by plotting the readings obtained at approximately 10 mμ wavelength intervals from 350-360 mμ. Distilled water is the blank. Normally a straight line can be drawn through several of the points. The bilirubin pigment produces a "hump" in the curve (Fig. 5-1). The hump is maximal at 450 mμ. The amount of deviation is measured and reported as the difference between the expected and plotted curves at 450 mμ. If the specimen has been diluted, a correction must be made for the dilution. The deviation of the abnormal curve is graded according to Freda in optical density

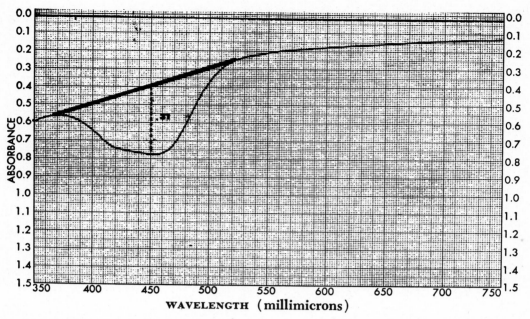

Fig. 5-1. Amniotic fluid spectrophotometric scan on a linear scale, demonstrating a typical "bilirubin hump." A heavy line projected from 375-525 mμ demonstrates the approximate course of the amniotic fluid scan in the absence of bilirubin. An upright (broken) line drawn at 450 mμ shows the deviation of this bilirubin peak from normal, in this case 0.37. (From Queenan: Clin. Obstet. Gynec. 9:491, 1966.)

units at 450 mμ from 1+ to 4+. Grades of 3+ and 4+ indicate severe fetal distress and imminent death, respectively.

$$1+ = 0.0\text{-}0.2 \text{ OD}$$
$$2+ = 0.2\text{-}0.35 \text{ OD}$$
$$3+ = 0.35\text{-}0.7 \text{ OD}$$
$$4+ = 0.7 \text{ OD and greater}$$

A linear amniotic absorption curve is only obtained in the latter months of pregnancy (thirty-fourth week).

Dissolved hemoglobin (fetal or maternal) produces a peak at 415 mμ (oxyhemoglobin), thus increasing the apparent deviation at 450 mμ. If both bilirubin and oxyhemoglobin are present, Liley uses a correction factor that is 5% of the deviation at 415 mμ.

Quantitative chemical examination of the amniotic bilirubin also gives satisfactory results.[65, 66]

Fetal blood accidentally obtained by amniocentesis allows the determination of fetal blood groups, the performance of a direct Coombs test, and an evaluation of the number of normoblasts in the blood smear.

The amniotic cells may show presence or absence of Barr bodies.[67]

Analysis of the amniotic fluid allows selection of cases for intrauterine transfusion.

Intrauterine transfusion[68]: Group O, Rh-negative blood is used. At birth the infant may type Rh negative and have a negative direct antiglobulin test if the intrauterine transfusion is successful.

Postnatal studies (newborn testing)

The investigation and evaluation of the jaundice and anemia of HDN are discussed in the hematology and biochemistry sections.

The presence of atypical antibodies in the mother's serum does not of itself allow a diagnosis of HDN. It is only presumptive evidence. Diagnostic evidence requires the proof of sensitization of the infant's red cells by the direct antiglobulin technique.

Typing, grouping, and antiglobulin testing of the red cells of the newborn infant

Cord blood: It should be collected at the time of delivery from the umbilical vein of the segment of cord attached to the placenta. The cord should not be squeezed so that the blood remains free of Wharton's jelly. The latter can cause false agglutination. The cells should be washed at least two times with sterile normal saline solution.

Capillary blood: If cord blood is not available, the baby's heel is incised with a No. 11 Bard-Parker blade and the blood collected in several micro blood collecting tubes that are then sealed with Critocaps.

Antiglobulin test: Agglutination of the infant's cells by the direct antiglobulin technique indicates sensitization of the red cells by antibodies. In Rh HDN the agglutination is usually strong, while in ABO HDN the agglutination is weak or absent. Even in Rh HDN it may be negative after intrauterine transfusion, and very occasionally even in nontransfused HDN. If the direct antiglobulin test is negative and hemolytic disease of the newborn is strongly suspected, the test should be repeated with a number of antiglobulin sera in varying dilutions after carefully washing the cells.

The specificity of the antibody of the baby's red cells can be discovered by eluting the antibody and then testing it on a panel of cells. This step is necessary if the mother's serum is not available or if it contains multiple antibodies.

If the direct Coombs test (antiglobulin test) is positive, the following tests should be performed on the blood: ABO and Rh typing, hemoglobin concentration, bilirubin concentration, complete blood count (paying special attention to the number of normoblasts and the presence or absence of spherocytes), and a reticulocyte count.

HDN can be excluded if maternal serum can be crossmatched with the baby's cells by the indirect antiglobulin, albumin, and enzyme techniques.

Typing and grouping of infant's cells: In Rh HDN the cells are usually Rh_0 positive. Very rarely they type as Rh_0 negative because of the presence of blocking maternal antibodies or because the antibody is not anti-Rh_0 but, for instance, anti-hr' (c).

The ABO group should be confirmed with group O serum. Reverse serum grouping is not performed as the natural antibody level in newborn infants is too low. In ABO HDN the ABO group is either A or B but never O. A_1 cells may temporarily type as A_2 cells.

Exchange transfusions

The choice of blood is governed by two rules:

1. The blood for exchange transfusion must be compatible with the serum of the mother. If the mother is Rh negative, the donor's blood must be Rh negative.
2. If the mother and baby are of the same ABO blood group, that blood group should be used. If they differ, group O cells should be chosen.

If the mother's serum is not available, use an eluate of the baby's cells for the crossmatch and identification of antibody. If the antibody is anti-Rh_0 (D), use Rh_0-negative blood; if it is anti-**hr'** (c), use type Rh_1Rh_1 blood (DCe/DCe); if it is anti-**A**, use group O blood with low anti-A titer; if it is anti-**B**, use group O blood with low anti-B titer; and if it is anti-**K**, use donor blood compatible with eluate or with mother's blood.

ABO HEMOLYTIC DISEASE OF THE NEWBORN

The hematologic features are discussed in the hematology section.

Laboratory diagnosis

Tests on mother's blood:

ABO grouping: The mother is almost always group O and rarely subgroup A_2.[68a]

Rh typing: The mother is usually Rh positive.

Screening for immune anti-A, anti-B, and anti-C antibodies:

1. Determine titer of saline-agglutinating anti-**A** or anti-**B** (at 22° and 37° C.) and antiglobulin titer.
2. Examine for IgG anti-**A** or anti-**B**

after neutralizing the natural anti-**A** or anti-**B**.

Tests on infant's blood:

ABO grouping: The infant is group A or B, never O. He may be group AB if the mother is subgroup A₂.

Rh typing: The infant is usually Rh positive.

Direct Coombs test: It is usually negative or only weakly positive.

Examination of eluate of fetal cells for immune anti-A or anti-B antibodies: The modified direct antiglobulin test is used.[69]

Attempt to detect red cell sensitization: Use the antiglobulin consumption test.

Tests on father's blood:

ABO grouping: The father is group A, B, or AB.

Rh typing and genotyping: Not contributory. Crossmatching the father's cells with maternal serum produces agglutination.

GLOSSARY OF BLOOD BANKING TERMS

absorption Method of removing antibodies from a serum by treatment with red cells. An absorbed serum is one from which antibodies have been removed by adsorption.

adsorption Attachment of antibody onto the red cells.

agglutination Clumping of red cells due to the presence of an agglutinogen on the red cell surface and the action of a corresponding antibody.

agglutinin An antibody demonstrable by agglutination tests.

agglutinogen An antigen that stimulates the production of agglutination.

AHF Antihemophilic factor (factor VIII).

Table 5-33. Comparison of ABO and Rh hemolytic disease of the newborn*

	Hemolytic disease of newborn due to:	
	Rh incompatibility	*ABO incompatibility*
In infant:		
Jaundice	Severe	Mild to moderate
Hemoglobin concentration	Low	Frequently normal to high
Anemia	Moderate to severe	Slight to moderate
Saline fragility of erythrocytes	Normal	Increased
Spherocytes	Absent	Present
Nucleated red cell increase	Moderate to marked	Mild to moderate
Reticulocyte increase	Mild to moderate	Marked
Direct Coombs test	Positive	Weakly positive or negative
Eluate of infant's cells	Contains Rh antibodies	Contains anti-**A** or anti-**B** and/or anti-**C**
Witebsky test	Usually positive with albumin	Usually positive with serum
Munk-Andersen test	Often negative	Positive
Indirect Coombs test with cord (infant's) serum	Positive with cells of appropriate Rh type	Positive with A₁ or B cells
Incidence	About 1 in 300 deliveries	May be considerably greater than Rh incompatibility
Occurrence in firstborn	Unlikely	Likely
Exchange transfusion	Usually needed	Frequently unnecessary unless bilirubin increases
Group and type of blood or packed cells to be used for exchange transfusion	Mother and infant of same ABO group: use their ABO group, mother's Rh type. Mother and infant of different ABO groups: use low-titer group O, mother's Rh type	Use low-titer group O, infant's Rh type
In mother:		
Hemolysins	No anti-**Rh** hemolysins	Anti-**A** and/or anti-**B** hemolysins present
Indirect Coombs test with mother's serum	Positive with cells of appropriate Rh type	Positive with A₁ or B cells after neutralization of isoagglutinins
Prognosis for future infants of sensitized mothers	Poor when infant has Rh factor to which mother is sensitized	Usually good

*Modified from Hyland reference manual of immunohematology, Los Angeles, 1964, Hyland Laboratories, p. 91.

allele (allellomorph) Genes (one to several) that occupy the same position (locus) on paired homologous chromosomes and that determine alternative characteristics or variants of the same class of inherited characteristics. Normally only one gene of an allelic pair is transmitted to the offspring. It may be either dominant or recessive to its allele. In the general population there may be multiple alleles for one locus, but one individual has only two genes on one locus, which have an allelic relationship to each other. Allelic genes are responsible for differences in genotypes.

anamnestic reactions Exaggerated response to the injection of an antigen that occurs in a subject previously immunized to the same antigen.

antibody A specifically reacting substance produced by the body in response to the introduction of an antigen. Antibodies are gamma globulins.

antigen A substance that, when introduced into the body, generally only stimulates the formation of antibodies if the individual lacks the introduced substance.

antigenic determinant That portion of the antigen molecule that reacts in a specific and demonstrable way with an antibody.

antigenicity Ability of an antigen to stimulate antibody production.

antiglobulin Anti-human globulin (antiglobulin serum) prepared by immunizing animals with purified human gamma globulin.

atypical antibody An antibody not regularly present in the plasma.

autoagglutinin Agglutinating antibodies reactive with the individual's own red cells. They usually also clump red cells from all other persons.

autoantibody Antibodies reactive with the individual's own red cells.

autologous Belonging to the individual himself.

autologous transfusion Transfusion in which the patient is transfused with his own blood.

autosomal chromosome (autosome) Nonsex chromosome or somatic chromosome.

autotransfusion See autologous transfusion.

avidity of an antibody Degree of affinity between an antibody and the corresponding antigen or blood factor, as demonstrated by speed and intensity of agglutination.

Barr body See sex chromosome.

bivalent antibody M (IgM) antibody; 19S antibody.

blocking antibody Antibody that coats red cells without agglutinating and prevents the subsequent reaction with saline agglutinins directed against the same antigen. *See* incomplete antibody.

blood factor One of the multiple serologic specificities of an agglutinogen on the surface of a red cell; an extrinsic attribute of the agglutinogen molecule.

blood grouping Classification of blood specimen into groups (or types) on the basis of the blood factor or agglutinogens that they contain.

chromatin Nuclear substance made of DNA.

chromatin positive Nuclei that contain two or more X chromosomes, as shown by presence of a Barr body. If they contain only one, or none, the individual is chromatin negative.

chromosome Intranuclear body that has a strong affinity to basic dyes. Genetically it can be considered a linear arrangement of genes. In all body cells the chromosomes are double (diploid) except in the sex cells after maturation (ova and spermatozoa), which contain a single set of chromosomes (haploid).

chromosome aberration Abnormal number or configuration of chromosomes.

cold agglutinins Agglutinin reacting best in the cold (4° C.).

complement Thermolabile complex of proteins present in fresh normal serum that causes lysis of red cells which have combined with their specific antibodies.

complete antibody An antibody that acts in saline solution.

Coombs serum See antiglobulin serum; bivalent antibody.

crossing over Exchange of chromosome segments of homologous chromosomes.

deoxyribonucleic acid Nuclear material responsible for genetic information.

diploid A double number of chromosomes of the somatic cell and of the sex cells before their division.

dominant Behavior of a gene that completely suppresses its allelic gene. Intermediate dominance implies a lesser degree of gene expression as seen in the heterozygous form in comparison to the homozygous form.

dosage effect Difference in strengths of the activity of an antigen in the homozygous and the heterozygous state.

eluate Liquid containing eluted antibodies.

elution Reverse of adsorption; antibodies adsorbed onto red cells are freed into solution.

gene Smallest unit of inheritance carried on chromosomes and composed of DNA, with specific genetic function arranged in linear fashion. The location of the gene is called its locus.

genotype Gene complement of an individual. Genotype symbols are paired. The capital letter usually indicates dominance over the small-lettered recessive gene.

globulin A protein fraction in the serum.

haploid Cells bearing a single set of chromosomes, the normal complement of gametes (ova or spermatozoa).

hemoglobin Oxygen-carrying red pigment of the red cells.

hemolysin An antibody that causes hemolysis of red cells in the presence of complement.

hemolysis Liberation of hemoglobin from red cells.

heteroagglutinin An agglutinin directed against antigens found in another species.

heterospecific pregnancy Pregnancy in which the maternal serum contains anti-A and anti-B antibodies incompatible with the fetal red cells, e.g., group O mother, group A fetus.

heterozygous Structurally or functionally dissimilar members of a gene pair on corresponding loci of corresponding chromosomes.

homologous blood Blood with the same ABO group.

homologous chromosomes Pair of matching chromosomes.

homologous serum jaundice Hepatitis caused by a virus contained in transfused human blood or blood derivatives.

homozygous Identical gene pairs on corresponding loci of paired chromosomes.

immunization Process that leads to the production of an antibody in response to an antigenic stimulus.

inactivation of serum Heating of serum at 56° C. for 30 min. to destroy the heat-labile portions of the complement.

incomplete antibody An antibody that adheres to the surface of red cells suspended in saline solution but fails to agglutinate them. *See* blocking antibody; univalent antibody.

isoagglutinin An agglutinin that reacts with antigens from animals in the same species.

linked genes Genes located together on the same chromosome so that they tend to be inherited together.

locus Location of a gene on a chromosome.

lyophilization Rapid freezing and dehydration of a biologic substance in a vacuum.

lysis Disruption of cells.

meiosis Cell division that produces mature sex cells with half the number of chromosomes possessed by the original cells.

mitosis Cell division that produces daughter cells with the same number of chromosomes as the original cells.

mutation Out-of-line change in genetic material that may involve a gene, a chromosome segment, or the number of chromosomes.

nonsecretor Person who does not have water-soluble A, B, or H substances in his body fluids.

panagglutinin An agglutinin that clumps red cells of all individuals.

panel of cells Set of reagent red blood cells of known antigenic composition.

phenotype Total characteristics of an individual that can be observed.

plasma Liquid portion of unclotted blood.

proteolytic enzyme An enzyme that catalyzes the digestion of protein.

prozone Phenomenon in which signs of an antigen-antibody reaction fail to occur at a lower dilution of the antibody, but do occur with higher dilutions.

recessive gene A gene is recessive in relation to its allele if its existence is not evident. It can express itself only in the homozygous state.

rouleaux formation Pseudoagglutination of red cells giving the appearance of stacks of coins.

saline solution Isotonic sodium chloride solution.

saline antibody Complete antibody. *See* bivalent antibody.

secretor Person who possesses water-soluble A, B, or H substances in his body fluids.

sensitization Immunization.

sensitization of red cells Antibody is attached to the red cell surface.

serum Fluid portion of clotted blood. Plasma without fibrinogen.

sex chromatin (Barr body) Planoconvex mass of chromatin seen in the nuclei of genetically normal females (XX) applied to the inner aspect of the nuclear membrane.

sex chromosome Genes that determine the sex of the individual. They may be homologous or nonhomologous. The male (XY) is nonhomologous (heterogametic), while the female (XX) is homologous (homogametic).

somatic chromosome *See* autosomal chromosome.

specificity Ability of an antibody to react with a particular antigen or antigens to the exclusion of others.

thermal amplitude Temperature range of activity of an antibody.

titer Reciprocal of the highest dilution of a serum that gives a distinct (1+) reaction in a titration.

titrate Procedure to determine the concentration of a specific antibody by testing serial (usually doubled) dilutions of the serum against agglutinable red cells.

univalent antibody G (IgG) antibody; 7S antibody.

warm antibody An antibody reacting at 37° C. better than it does at lower temperatures.

wash Successive centrifugation of cells in large volumes of saline solution to free them of all but insignificant traces of serum or plasma.

REFERENCES

1. Technical methods and procedures of the American Association of Blood Banks, ed. 4, Chicago, 1966, American Association of Blood Banks.
2. Mollison, P. L.: Blood transfusion in clinical medicine, ed. 4, Philadelphia, 1967, F. A. Davis Co.
3. Seminar on advanced technics in blood banking, Sixteenth Annual Meeting of the American Association of Blood Banks, Detroit, Mich., Nov. 5, 1963.
4. Schmidt, R. P.: Seminar on advanced technics in blood banking, Sixteenth Annual Meeting of the American Association of Blood Banks, Detroit, Mich., Nov. 5, 1963, p. 19.
5. Pollack, W., Hager, H. J., and Hollenbeck, L. L., Jr.: Transfusion 2:17, 1962.
6. Treacy, M.: Seminar on advanced technics in blood banking, Sixteenth Annual Meeting of the American Association of Blood Banks, Detroit, Mich., Nov. 5, 1963, p. 25.
7. Fayen, A. W., and Miale, J. B.: Amer. J. Clin. Path. 39:645, 1963.

8. Clayton, E. M., Altschuler, J., and Bove, J. R.: Amer. J. Clin. Path. **44**:648, 1965.
9. Clear, J.: Seminar on the ABO blood group system, Los Angeles, Calif., 1966, p. 55.
10. Melonas, K., and Heustess, M. B.: Seminar on the ABO blood system, Los Angeles, Calif., 1966, p. 63.
11. McQuire, D.: Seminar on the ABO blood group system, Los Angeles, Calif., 1966, p. 43.
12. Wiener, A. S., and Ward, F. A.: Amer. J. Clin. Path. **46**:27, 1966.
13. Wiener, A. S., Moor-Jankowski, J., and Gordon, E. B.: Int. Arch. Allerg. **29**:82, 1966.
14. Wiener, A. S.: Blood groups and transfusion, ed. 3 (reprint), New York, 1962, Hafner Publishing Co., Inc., Chapter 12.
15. Gammelgaard, A.: On rare weak A antigens (A₃, A₄, A₅, and Aₓ) in man, Washington, D. C., 1964, Walter Reed Army Institute of Research, Walter Reed Army Medical Center.
16. Yokoyama, M., and Plocinik, B.: Vox Sang. **10**:149, 1965.
17. Solomon, J. M., Waggoner, R., and Leyshon, W. C.: Blood **25**:4, 1965.
18. Sturgeon, P., Moore, B. P. L., and Weiner, W.: Vox Sang. **9**:214, 1964.
19. Burns, W., Friend, W., and Scudder, J.: Surg. Gynec. Obstet. **120**:757, 1965.
20. Levine, P., et al: Blood **10**:1100, 1955.
21. Marsh, W. L.: Vox Sang. **5**:387, 1960.
22. Bennett, M. H., et al.: Vox Sang. **7**:579, 1962.
23. Bhatia, H. M., and Sanghvi, L. D.: Vox Sang. **7**:245, 1962.
24. Hostrup, H.: Vox Sang. **8**:557, 1963.
25. Van der Hart, M., and Van Loghem, J. J.: Vox Sang. **12**:161, 1967.
26. Landsteiner, K., and Wiener, A. S.: Proc. Soc. Exp. Biol. Med. **42**:223, 1940.
27. Peterson, O. L., Ham, T. H., and Finland, M.: Science **97**:167, 1943.
28. Wiener, A. S.: Blood groups and transfusion, ed. 3 (reprint), New York, 1962, Hafner Publishing Co., Inc., p. 253.
29. Race, R. R., Sanger, R., and Selwyn, J. G.: Nature(London)**166**:520, 1950.
30. Waller, R. K., Sanger, R., and Bobbitt, O. B., Jr.: Brit. Med. J. **1**:198, 1953.
31. Wiener, A. S., and Geiger, J.: Exp. Med. Surg. **15**:75, 1957.
32. Levine, P., and Wong, H.: Amer. J. Obstet. Gynec. **45**:832, 1943.
33. Wiener, A. S.: Amer. J. Clin. Path. **16**:477, 1946.
34. Kortekangas, A. E., et al.: Vox Sang. **10**:385, 1965.
35. Stroup, M., MacIlroy, M., Walker, R., and Aydelotte, J. V.: Transfusion **5**:309, 1965.
36. Walker, R. H.: Seminar on the ABO blood group system, Los Angeles, Calif., 1966, p. 17.
37. Wiener, A. S.: Amer. J. Clin. Path. **43**:388, 1965.
38. Watkins, W. M., and Morgan, W. T. J.: Vox Sang. **4**:97, 1959.
39. Wiener, A. S., Moor-Jankowski, J., Gordon,
E. B., and Davis, J.: Amer. J. Phys. Anthrop. **23**:389, 1965.
40. Rubin, H., and Solomon, A.: Vox Sang. **12**:227, 1967.
41. Hirschfeld, J., and Beckmann, L.: Acta Genet. **10**:48, 1960.
42. Vierucci, A.: Vox Sang. **10**:82, 1965.
43. Buetler, R.: Vox Sang. **10**:736, 1965.
44. Berg, K.: Vox Sang. **12**:71, 1967.
45. Berg, K.: Vox Sang. **10**:513, 1965.
46. Dausset, J., and Tangun, Y.: Vox Sang. **10**:641, 1965.
47. Steffen, C.: J. Lab. Clin. Med. **55**:9, 1960.
48. Griffiths, J. J., Frank, S., and Schmidt, R. P.: Transfusion **4**:461, 1964.
49. Walker, P. C., Jennings, E. R., and Monroe, C.: Amer. J. Clin. Path. **44**:193, 1965.
50. Allen, F. H., Jr.: Transfusion **6**:101, 1966.
51. Veiga, S., and Vaithianathan, T.: Transfusion **3**:387, 1963.
52. Medal, S. L., Gonzales, C. R., Manura, R., and Dominguez, T. J. L.: Vox Sang. **6**:170, 1961.
53. Leading article, Lancet **1**:1193, 1966.
54. National Research Council Report: J.A.M.A. **195**:171, 1966.
54a. Kliman, A., and Lesses, M. F.: Transfusion **4**:469, 1964.
55. Stroup, M., and MacIlroy, M.: Transfusion **5**:184, 1965.
56. Stroup, M.: Seminar on advanced technics in blood banking, Sixteenth Annual Meeting of the American Association of Blood Banks, Detroit, Mich., Nov. 5, 1963, p. 65.
57. Pirofsky, B., and Mangum, M. E.: Proc. Soc. Exper. Biol. Med. **101**:49, 1959.
58. Gerard, M., Sr.: Amer. J. Clin. Path. **43**:487, 1965.
59. Baudanza, P.: Seminar on advanced technics in blood banking, Sixteenth Annual Meeting of the American Association of Blood Banks, Detroit, Mich., Nov. 5, 1963, p. 101.
60. Oski, F. A., and Naiman, J. L.: Erythroblastosis fetalis, hematologic problems in the newborn, Philadelphia, 1966, W. B. Saunders Co., p. 136.
61. Woodrow, J. C., and Finn, R.: Brit. J. Haemat. **12**:297, 1966.
62. Freda, V. J., and Gorman, J. G.: Science **151**:828, 1966.
63. Crawford, J. W., Cameron, C., and Walker, C. H. M.: Lancet **1**:887, 1966.
64. Little, B., McCutcheon, E., and Desforges, J. F.: New Eng. J. Med. **274**:332, 1966.
65. Gambino, S. R., and Freda, V. J.: Amer. J. Clin. Path. **46**:198, 1966.
66. Bower, D., and Swale, J.: Lancet **1**:1009, 1966.
67. Steele, M. W., and Breg, W. R., Jr.: Lancet **1**:383, 1966.
68. Editorial: J.A.M.A. **196**:148, 1966.
68a. Wiener, A. S.: Personal communication, 1968.
69. Pollack, W., Reiss, A. M., and Treacy, M.: Vox Sang. **3**:442, 1958.

Chapter 6

Clinical chemistry

There are many factors that influence the chemical composition of blood and other body fluids in disease. One general factor includes those instances of increases in blood constituents due to alterations of permeable membranes in the excretory organs such as the lungs, kidneys, and liver. The accumulation of nitrogenous waste products in certain forms of nephritis and the hyperbilirubinemia associated with liver disease are examples of retention brought about by such processes. In other instances, alterations in blood constituents may be due to changes in the rate of formation or in the use of these constituents. The accumulation of glucose in the blood of diabetic individuals due to a metabolic derangement in the use of this substance is an example. Furthermore, the administration of drugs may alter the concentration of some blood constituents.

Without multiplying examples, it is evident that knowledge of the concentrations of the various blood constituents (and also of other body fluids such as cerebrospinal fluid, urine, etc.) is a very important aid to the physician not only in diagnosis but also in evaluating the results of therapy. Since the success or failure of the physician's efforts and even the life of the patient may depend on accurate determinations of the blood levels of the important constituents and the transmission of these data to the physician in time for them to be of greatest use to him, the need for accuracy and speed in the analysis cannot be overemphasized. However, except for an emergency, accuracy should never be sacrificed for speed. The patient's welfare is as much a trust of the laboratory technician as of the supervising physician.

During the past 20-30 yr. there has been an enormous development in laboratory methods and techniques. Constituents for which no satisfactory tests were available a few years ago are now routinely determined in the clinical laboratory. Many new methods have been developed and improvements are being made constantly. Many methods are available for the commonly determined constituents. Some of these, however, may require special equipment. In the following sections we have endeavored to give one or two methods for each of these constituents which we believe to be the most satisfactory for the general clinical laboratory from the point of view of accuracy and simplicity. This does not imply that other equally satisfactory methods may not be available or that those given are the best for every purpose. Every method has its limitations, but we have endeavored to give those of general applicability.

In the discussion of the specific details of the various procedures or tests, mention may be made of an apparatus or other component made by a particular manufacturer. This does not mean that products of other manufacturers may not be equally satisfactory. Since it is impractical to mention all possible sources of supply, we have generally mentioned a type that is readily available as a guide to the exact kind of material or apparatus desired. The same is true of reagent chemicals; we may mention that the chemical from a certain manufacturer gives a very low blank. Other brands may also give a low blank, but we have not been able to test all of them and merely mention one that we have found satisfactory.

COLLECTION OF BLOOD SPECIMENS[1, 2]

In the analysis of blood constituents the first consideration is collection of the specimen. Even if this is not done by the laboratory technician, he should be familiar with the technique and principles involved. The different chemical tests will require different types of specimens, i.e., clotted blood or blood containing a particular anticoagulant or preservative. Usually venous blood is used. Sometimes small amounts of capillary blood from the fingertip or earlobe will be satisfactory, and very rarely arterial blood may be required. For some tests a small amount of hemolysis may not be of great importance, whereas in other tests it must be scrupulously avoided. It is best to develop a technique that will keep hemolysis at a minimum at all times. The technician must be familiar with these factors to advise others as to the type of sample required, even if he does not actually draw the specimen himself.

Venous blood may be obtained by the use of a hypodermic syringe and a 20- or 21-gauge needle. If many samples are to be drawn, it may be convenient to use the commercially available evacuated blood collecting tubes (such as Vacutainers*) obtainable from most laboratory supply houses. This method of securing blood samples eliminates the trouble involved in cleaning the syringes. If glass syringes are used, they must be thoroughly dried before use to prevent hemolysis due to traces of water. Disposable plastic syringes may also be used. When blood is being transferred from the syringe to a test tube or other container, the needle should be removed first and the blood should not be forced out too vigorously, as this will also cause some hemolysis. Special attention should be given to ade-

quate sterilization of needles in order to guard against spread of viral hepatitis. Needles should be sterilized by autoclaving for 30 min. at 15 lb. pressure. Another way in which this danger can be eliminated, particularly if adequate sterilization facilities are not available, is through the use of disposable needles that can be used once and then discarded. This also eliminates the necessity of sharpening needles.

Anticoagulants: Either whole blood or plasma may be required for many tests. This necessitates the use of an anticoagulant to prevent clotting. Not all anticoagulants are equally satisfactory for every test. Some may interfere with the chemical reactions of a given test. **Heparin** is an excellent anticoagulant but is more expensive than other chemicals used for this purpose. The amount required depends upon the potency of the product and should be stated on the vial. **Potassium oxalate** is a commonly used anticoagulant. It is generally used when oxalate is required since it is more soluble than sodium or lithium salts; 20 mg. of potassium oxalate is sufficient for 10 ml. of blood. This may be added to the collection tubes as 0.1 ml. of a 20% solution which is then dried at a temperature of not over 100° C. (high temperatures may decompose the oxalate). Alternately, one can make up a small "spoon," which may be a short section of plastic rod with a handle and a small hole drilled into it and adjusted so that when the hole is filled with finely powdered potassium oxalate and is leveled off it will contain approximately 20 mg. of the salt. The use of commercially available evacuated containers that are furnished with a number of different anticoagulants eliminates the trouble of preparing the tubes. A large excess of anticoagulant may interfere with some chemical tests. When the tubes are prepared, care should be taken to avoid a large excess.

Another anticoagulant that is sometimes used is **disodium salt of ethylenediaminetetraacetic acid.** This is sold under a variety of trade names. It is somewhat less generally applicable than oxalate. About 10 mg. is required for 10 ml. of

*Becton, Dickinson & Co., Rutherford, N. J.

blood. When a powdered anticoagulant is used, care must be taken to ensure that it is thoroughly mixed with and dissolved in the blood as soon as possible after the blood is added to the tube.

A special anticoagulant is a **0.1M solution of sodium oxalate**, which is made by dissolving 1.34 gm. of reagent grade sodium oxalate in water to make 100 ml. This is used to secure blood plasma for **prothrombin time** determinations. In this procedure 4.5 ml. of blood is added to 0.5 ml. of the oxalate solution.

Preservation of blood samples: Many constituents of blood may change more or less rapidly in concentration on standing, particularly at room or elevated temperatures. A conspicuous example of this is blood glucose. On standing at room temperature, the glucose in whole blood may be metabolized to the extent of 5% or more per hour. The loss is less at lower temperatures, and blood samples may be kept for several hours without great loss if they are immediately chilled in an ice bath and kept at this temperature. (Merely placing the tubes in the refrigerator may not be satisfactory since cooling may be very slow, particularly if several tubes are placed together in a small container.) For blood sugar determinations in which there is to be some delay before analysis, it is best to add a preservative that will inhibit glycolysis. **Thymol** and **fluoride** have been used for this purpose. Fluoride is generally simpler to use. Fluoride has some anticoagulant properties in itself, but relatively larger amounts are required than for oxalate. A mixture of 15 mg. of potassium oxalate and 25 mg. of sodium fluoride is a satisfactory amount. Because of solubility considerations this cannot be added as a solution which is then dried, but must be added as 40 mg. of an intimate mixture of 3 parts of powdered potassium oxalate and 5 parts of powdered sodium fluoride from a spoon calibrated to deliver this amount. Evacuated tubes containing both fluoride and oxalate are available commercially. **Fluoride will inhibit enzyme action;** therefore it cannot be used when any such reaction is involved (except amylase or urease if the fluoride is not over 2 mg./ml. of blood).

However, most enzymatic determinations are made on serum in which no anticoagulant is used. If the glucose determination involves preparation of a protein-free filtrate and the first step in this is the dilution and laking of the blood, the determination may be delayed at this point. Glycolysis in the hemolyzed blood is low provided that the blood has been diluted at least 1:10.

Other changes may also occur in blood if left standing, e.g., changes in phosphate due to hydrolysis of organic phosphate esters, changes in lipids due to lipolysis, and changes in chloride due to shifts of chloride between cells and serum. Accordingly, it is best to begin analysis as soon as possible after the blood has been drawn. If serum or plasma is to be used for analysis, it should be separated from the cells or clot as soon as possible. (However, at least 30 min. should be allowed for complete clotting at room temperature.) After separation, serum or plasma can usually be kept for a somewhat longer time without deterioration. For most tests including some enzymes, serum or plasma may be kept for a few days in the refrigerator; for most enzymes, the serum may be kept for several days if frozen. If the serum is frozen, one must be certain that the material is completely thawed and well mixed again before use. Special precautions for preservation or collection of samples are given in connection with the particular test involved.

COLORIMETERS

Quantitative analysis of many substances is based on the production of a colored solution by a chemical reaction in such a way that the intensity or depth of the color may be used as a measure of the concentration of the substance being determined. The theoretic relationship between the concentration of the color-producing molecular species and the intensity of the color is known as **Beer's law.** Like many laws of physics it is usually stated in mathematical form, but for our purposes we need only two deductions from the general formula. The first is that if the same proportion of light is absorbed by passage through two different solutions then $C_1L_1 = C_2L_2$, where C_1 and C_2 are the concentrations of the colored substance in the two solutions and L_1 and L_2 are the lengths of the light paths through the two solutions.

Visual colorimeter: The previous equation is the basis on which the Duboscq visual colorimeter operates. Two colored solutions (sample and standard) are compared by varying the length of the light path through one of the two solutions until the intensity of the light absorbed by the two solutions appears to be equal. Then the above-mentioned relation will hold and it may be written as $C_1/C_2 = L_2/L_1$. The instrument suffers from a number of disadvantages and is rarely used except for some specialized purposes. It has a rather narrow range since the accuracy is small when the ratio of L_1 to L_2 is less than ½ or more than 2. Visual comparison of color involves considerable subjective error since two technicians will often obtain different readings.

Photoelectric colorimeter: Most laboratories now use one of several types of photoelectric colorimeters in which the intensity of light is measured by electronic means, thus eliminating the personal error. In the discussion of the general nature of these instruments a few elementary facts may be mentioned. It may be recalled that white light can be broken up into the familiar violet-blue-green-yellow-orange-red spectrum seen in the rainbow. The different portions of the spectrum may be identified by the wavelengths of the light, which are usually measured in units of 10^{-9} m. This unit has been designated as a **millimicron** (**mμ**), but recently additional prefixes have been adapted for the metric units and the unit mμ should now be designated as a **nanometer (nm.)**. Numerically the units are the same (i.e., 1 mμ = 1 nm.) but the latter designation is preferred, although it has not yet come into general use. The wavelength of visible light ranges from approximately 400 nm. for violet to 700 nm. for red. A colored solution appears blue by transmitted light because it absorbs more light at the red end of the spectrum and transmits more

of the blue. Accordingly, if we wished to measure the concentration of the colored substance, we could, in general, do this more accurately by using light that is more strongly absorbed (in the previous example, red light). The light of the desired wavelength is obtained either by the use of a glass or other type of optical filter that will allow light of only a certain narrow range of wavelengths to pass (electrophotometer, photoelectric colorimeter) or by means of a prism or diffraction grating that splits the light into the spectrum and only the desired wavelength is allowed to pass through the solution to be measured (spectrophotometer). The latter method is more convenient. By means of a wavelength scale one can select the desired wavelength within the range of the instrument and hence the instrument can be adapted to new procedures without the expense of purchasing new filters. Also, from a theoretic point of view, it is better to measure the color with as narrow a range of wavelengths as possible. This is more readily done with a spectrophotometer type of instrument. The interference type of filters that are available do have a narrow bandwidth, but they are quite expensive.

By measuring the absorbance of the solution to be analyzed at different wavelengths and plotting the results, one obtains an absorption curve that indicates at which wavelength the absorption is greatest. This is usually the wavelength selected for measurement, although there are exceptions that will be mentioned later.

The source of light in most instruments is an incandescent tungsten lamp. The light intensity must be kept as constant as possible and most circuits include a constant-voltage transformer or other electronic voltage-regulating device. If the line voltage to the laboratory is subject to marked fluctuations, it is almost essential to use a voltage regulator if one is not supplied with the instrument. A storage battery is used with some colorimeters as a constant-voltage source for the lamp. Although this gives a relatively constant voltage, the maintenance of the storage battery requires a certain amount of extra effort.

The other essential part of a photoelectric colorimeter is a device for measuring light intensity. This usually consists of some sort of photocell or phototube that delivers a small current proportional to the intensity of the light falling on it and the current is then measured. In most instruments the current is measured with a sensitive microammeter, either directly or after electronic amplification. In some instruments the light intensity is read directly on the meter scale; in others a potentiometric balance method is used in which the photocurrent is balanced out and the result is read on a calibrated dial. The instruments usually have a scale calibrated in percent transmission from 0-100. The scale is linear in that a reading of 100% means that twice as much light is striking the photocell as when the reading is 50%. The nature of the light absorption process as indicated by Beer's law is such that the relationship between the concentration of the colored substance and the percent transmission is nonlinear. Mathematically the relation is

$$2 - \text{Log} \ (\%T) = KC$$

where %T represents the percent transmission, C is the concentration of the colored substance, and K is a constant, the value of which depends upon the wavelength of the light used, the light path, and other factors that are always kept the same during the series of measurements. The expression $2 - \log \ (\%T)$ is the optical density (OD) or absorbance (A) and is directly proportional to the concentration. This makes the former much more convenient for computation. Some photometers have an optical density scale as well as a percent transmission scale (with 100% transmission equal to 0 OD). For instruments not having this scale a conversion table can be used (Table 6-1).

If Beer's law held exactly, the optical density would be strictly proportional to the concentration over a very wide range of concentrations. This is not entirely true except for the most precise instruments.

Table 6-1. Conversion table, percent transmittance-optical density

Transmission (%)	*Optical density*	*Transmission (%)*	*Optical density*
1	2.000	51	0.2924
2	1.699	52	0.2840
3	1.523	53	0.2756
4	1.398	54	0.2676
5	1.301	55	0.2596
6	1.222	56	0.2518
7	1.155	57	0.2441
8	1.097	58	0.2366
9	1.046	59	0.2291
10	1.000	60	0.2218
11	0.959	61	0.2147
12	0.921	62	0.2076
13	0.886	63	0.2007
14	0.854	64	0.1939
15	0.824	65	0.1871
16	0.796	66	0.1805
17	0.770	67	0.1739
18	0.745	68	0.1675
19	0.721	69	0.1612
20	0.699	70	0.1549
21	0.678	71	0.1487
22	0.658	72	0.1427
23	0.638	73	0.1367
24	0.620	74	0.1308
25	0.602	75	0.1249
26	0.585	76	0.1192
27	0.569	77	0.1135
28	0.553	78	0.1079
29	0.538	79	0.1024
30	0.523	80	0.0969
31	0.509	81	0.0915
32	0.495	82	0.0862
33	0.482	83	0.0809
34	0.469	84	0.0757
35	0.456	85	0.0706
36	0.444	86	0.0655
37	0.432	87	0.0605
38	0.420	88	0.0555
39	0.409	89	0.0505
40	0.398	90	0.0458
41	0.387	91	0.0410
42	0.377	92	0.0362
43	0.367	93	0.0315
44	0.357	94	0.0269
45	0.347	95	0.0223
46	0.337	96	0.0177
47	0.328	97	0.0132
48	0.319	98	0.0088
49	0.310	99	0.0044
50	0.301	100	0.0000

Limitations of the instruments such as stray light and nonlinearity of the response of the photocell and the milliammeter cause deviations. Also, it can be shown that the percentage errors are much greater at very high or very low optical densities. It is best to adjust the concentrations so that the readings for most samples fall between 30 and 70% transmittance, or 0.15 and 0.55 OD.

In practically all colorimetric procedures the substances being determined, e.g., glucose, uric acid, cholesterol, etc., are not themselves colored or are only slightly so, but they form a colored compound through a series of often complex chemical reactions. The amount of color formed is then dependent upon the concentrations of the reagents as well as other conditions such as the time and temperature of heating or incubation. Hence in comparing the concentration of the unknown sample with that of a standard of known concentration, the sample and standard should preferably be run at the same time to ensure that the conditions for color development and measurement are the same for both. Standards should be run with each set of analyses to avoid errors caused by changes in the conditions mentioned. The use of precalibrated charts that are often supplied with the instruments can lead to very serious error and their use is strongly condemned by most workers in the field of clinical chemistry. MacFate and associates[3] stated that in relying on factory calibration of colorimeters one becomes liable for errors from improper calibrations in addition to becoming dependent on methods that may be outmoded or nonspecific.

We have found variations between different instruments of the same make in regard to stray light, wavelength calibration, and linearity of response of the photocell, all of which will cause deviations from precalibrated charts and serious errors in the final analysis.

Often the reagents themselves will give a certain amount of color to the final solution, even when none of the substance being determined is present. This is the **reagent blank.** In such circumstances the instrument may be set to 100% transmittance or 0 OD with the blank solution containing all of the reagents, but none of the substance being determined. This is treated under the same conditions as the samples and standards. Preferably the conditions should be adjusted so that the color due to the blank is minimal. If readings are made in terms of optical density, both samples and blank can be read against water (or other solvents) and the reading of the blank subtracted from that of the sample before calculation. As mentioned earlier, photometric readings are usually made at the wavelength at which the absorption of the sample solution is greatest. But if the reagents themselves produce colors that are considerably different from those produced by the sample, it may be convenient to read at the wavelength where the difference between the sample and blank is greatest instead of the wavelength where the absorption of the sample solution is greatest.

Calculations with photometric readings[4]**:** There are several methods that may be used in the calculations of concentrations from photometric readings. From Beer's law we have $C = K \cdot A$ (what follows C refers to concentrations, with subscripts to denote sample, standard, etc., and A denotes absorbance, OD, with subscripts). From this we find

$$\frac{C_1}{A_1} = \frac{C_2}{A_2} \text{ or } C_2 = \frac{C_1}{A_1} \times A_2$$

where subscript 1 refers to the standard and subscript 2 refers to the sample. If one is determining a number of samples with the same standard, it is often convenient to calculate $C_1/A_1 = K$, which is constant for a given standard determination, and $C_2 = K \times A_2$. If several standards of different concentrations are run, then the K values calculated from the different standard readings would be the same if Beer's law held exactly. If they are not exactly the same, one could use an average value. If Beer's law is not obeyed, this is usually indicated by the fact that the K values increase with increasing concentrations. For example, concentrations of 1, 2, and 3 mg.% might give absorbances of 0.125, 0.236, and

0.333, which would give K values of 8.0, 8.5, and 9.0, respectively.

In such a determination the K value for the standard having the reading closest to a particular sample is used, i.e., the K of 8.0 for absorbances of less than 0.18, 8.5 for absorbances between 0.18 and 0.28, and 9.0 for absorbances above 0.28.

It is important to check each procedure for conformance to Beer's law. Deviations will vary from procedure to procedure and with different instruments. Usually conditions are chosen so that conformance is good over the most important range of values. If there are marked deviations, this is usually mentioned in the procedure and one must then run more standards.

In the formulas given, C theoretically refers to the actual concentrations in the colorimeter cuvette, which may be quite different from the initial concentrations in the samples. If the standard and sample are treated exactly the same in regard to dilution, addition of reagents, etc., then in the calculations we can use the original concentration of the standard and obtain the concentration in the sample directly. For example, if a sample for glucose determination is diluted 1:10 (as in the preparation of a protein-free filtrate) and 1 ml. of the dilution is added to a definite quantity of reagents to develop the color, and if a standard containing 100 mg.% glucose is similarly diluted and 1 ml. is also added to the same quantities of reagents, we could take C_1 in our formula to be 100 mg.% to calculate the sample concentration directly. Usually one does not dilute the standard each time but prepares a larger quantity of the standard which actually contains 10 mg.% glucose even though it may be termed a 100 mg.% equivalent standard (it is assumed that the sample is always diluted 1:10).

If the standard and sample are diluted differently or are made up to different final volumes for the colorimetric readings, these facts must be taken into account in the calculations. In such instances it may be more convenient to take C_1 as the actual concentration of standard in the aliquot added or in the final cuvette volume, and then multiply by the factors for the dilution of the sample and standard.

Another way of calculating the results is to run a series of standards and plot the concentration of the standards against the absorbance on linear cross-section paper or against the percent transmission on semilog paper and draw a smooth curve through the points (straight line if Beer's law holds and readings are accurate). One can then read off the concentrations corresponding to other absorbances from the curve. If the standard gives slight differences from day to day because of varying conditions, one would need a number of curves or make a correction in some other way.

It is often convenient to make the readings in terms of percent transmittance. This is a linear scale on most instruments.

$$C_2 = C_1 \times \frac{A_2}{A_1}$$

Or in terms of %T:

$$C_2 = \frac{C_1 \ (2 - \text{Log } \%T_2)}{(2 - \text{Log } \%T_1)}$$

If these ratios are calculated in terms of %T, one could easily prepare a chart for the concentrations for different values of %T when the standards have a given value. The calculations are laborious but need be done only once.

In regard to calculations one other point might be mentioned. In Table 6-1, 50% T = 0.301 OD and 49% T = 0.310 OD. The difference of 1% T corresponds to a relative difference of 3% in the OD and consequently in the concentration. Even with the best instruments it is difficult to read more accurately than $\frac{1}{4}$% T, which would correspond to about 1% variation in concentration. Since there are many other sources of error in addition to the colorimeter reading, it appears that most results could not be accurate to within less than 1% at best. Consequently it is usually not necessary to report more than three significant figures in the results. It is meaningless to report a result as 136.27 mg.% when with the routine method one could just distinguish between 136 and 137 mg.%; therefore the result should be reported as 136 mg.%.

FLAME PHOTOMETRY[5]

When the atoms of a number of chemical elements are introduced into a nonluminous flame, they emit light of definite wavelengths characteristic of the particular element involved. This is illustrated by the yellow light seen when sodium salt is introduced into the flame of a Bunsen burner. Within certain limits the amount of light emitted is proportional to the amount of the element in the flame. It is also dependent upon the temperature of the flame and is influenced by the amount of gas and air or oxygen introduced. These conditions must be carefully controlled. The wavelength of light characteristic of the element being determined is isolated by means of an appropriate prism, grating, or filter arrangement similar to those used in spectrophotometry. The intensity of the emitted light is measured with a photocell. Comparison is made with the light emitted when a standard solution is used in place of the unknown.

The ratio between the concentration and the light emitted may be linear only over a short range. This must be considered when making the required dilution of the sample. The presence of one element in the solution may interfere with the light emission by another element, particularly if the former is present in a much higher concentration. This is sometimes compensated for by adding a large excess of the first element to all dilutions of standards, samples, and blanks so that the effective concentration of this element is substantially the same in all solutions.

The details of operation differ considerably from instrument to instrument. Some instruments use ordinary commercial gas, while others require bottled propane gas. Some use compressed air and others require oxygen. Some instruments use the internal standard principle. An element not ordinarily present in biologic samples (usually lithium) is added to the standard, samples, and blank dilutions in the same concentration. Two photocells are used with appropriate filters. One photocell measures the (red) light emitted by lithium and the other measures the light emitted from the element being determined (i.e., the yellow light from sodium). The outputs from the photocells are balanced against each other. In theory the fluctuations in flame temperature or aspiration rate should affect the emission of sodium and lithium equally, and this would balance out and not affect the reading based on the sodium concentration. Not all instruments use this principle, but it is helpful in reducing the errors from fluctuations in the flame intensity. Some of the photometers give a direct reading or employ a calibrated meter scale, while in others the balance is made by a potentiometric arrangement and the concentration is read from a calibrated dial. In all instruments the sample of serum or other body fluid is diluted to a rather low concentration with water or other solutions, usually with the addition of a nonionic wetting agent. Sodium and potassium can be determined on the same dilution of serum in many instruments.

The exact details of operation differ sufficiently from instrument to instrument that they will not be discussed here. The general outline presented should be helpful in understanding the operation of any flame photometer.

ATOMIC ABSORPTION SPECTROPHOTOMETRY[6]

In recent years a new method has been introduced for determining low concentrations of metallic elements in biologic material. This is known as atomic absorption spectrophotometry. The principles on which this instrument are based are closely related to those of emission flame photometry. The basic difference is that in emission flame photometry we measure the light emitted by a small fraction of the sample atoms injected into a hot gas flame (emission of energy), while in atomic absorption spectrophotometry (AAS) we measure the light absorbed by a much greater number of atoms that are never excited enough to become luminous (absorption of energy).

In atomic absorption spectrophotometry the sample is sprayed into a flame and atomized. A light beam at one of the characteristic wavelengths of the element to be analyzed is directed through the flame, into a monochromator, and onto a detector. The detector measures the final intensity of the beam. The amount absorbed by the flame is proportional to the concentration of the element in the sample. Since each metallic element has its own characteristic absorption wavelength, a different source lamp is used for each element.

Atomic absorption is presently used for the determination of calcium, magnesium, sodium, potassium, copper, zinc, iron, lead, cadmium, thallium, chromium, mercury, nickel, bismuth, cobalt, manganese, and strontium in biologic material.

Operating procedures for atomic absorption equipment are very similar to those used for emission flame photometry. Details of operation for the various instruments on the market vary considerably.

At present the instruments are too costly for the average clinical laboratory, but with the modifications and simplifications that come with use it is possible that within a short time these instruments will become as common in clinical laboratories as flame photometers are today. Before the introduction of flame photometry, sodium and potassium determinations in blood were done infrequently because of the tediousness of the chemical methods; today these procedures have become routine. The introduction of atomic absorption spectrophotometry may greatly influence the routine analyses of other metallic elements in body fluids.

FLUOROMETRY[7]

Some chemical compounds have the property of absorbing light energy and then reemitting some of this energy in light of a longer wavelength than the light originally absorbed. This phenomenon is known as **fluorescence**, and it can be used as a method of analysis. Commonly the exciting light is ultraviolet or near ultraviolet in the range of 250-450 nm., and the emitted light is of a longer wavelength. If a solution containing a fluorescent substance is illuminated with ultraviolet light, the fluorescent molecules will emit light of a longer wavelength.

By using a light filter that will transmit the fluorescent light but not the original exciting light, the amount of fluorescence can be measured with a photocell. This light will be proportional to the amount of the fluorescent substance present. It will also depend upon the intensity of the exciting light and geometry of the apparatus. These factors must be kept constant. Since it is difficult to keep the exciting light constant over long periods of time, all fluorescent methods require that a standard be run along with each set of samples.

The range of fluorescence is much smaller than colorimetry in that many more compounds are colored than are fluorescent. But fluorescent methods can be used to measure concentrations lower than for colorimetric methods by a factor of from 10-100. Accordingly, fluorometric methods are desirable for the measurement of small quantities of materials. Fluorometers are usually more expensive than the simpler photoelectric colorimeters, and fewer clinical methods have been adapted for them; consequently they are less commonly found in the typical clinical laboratory. They are essential for some important clinical procedures and are coming into more general use.

CHROMATOGRAPHY[8]

Chromatography is a technique used for the separation of small amounts of closely related substances. A solution of these substances in a suitable solvent is moved past a stationary phase which has a tendency to absorb the substances to some extent. The stationary phase absorbs the different substances in varying degrees. As the solution moves past the stationary phase, the rate of flow of the more strongly absorbed substances will be retarded the most. Substances that are not absorbed at all will move directly with the solvent flow. If the action of the stationary phase depends solely on the absorbing power of the solid, the process is termed **absorption chromatography.** If the stationary phase is an inert solid covered with a thin layer of absorbed liquid so that the process depends upon the partition coefficient of the substances being separated between the solvent and the absorbed immiscible liquid, the process is termed **partition chromatography.** Many actual chromatographic methods are combinations of the two.

Chromatography may be more concretely illustrated by citing the original experiments made 60 yr. ago by the botanist Tswett. He found that pigments appeared as separate colored zones along the column when a mixture of plant pigments (chlorophylls and xanthophylls) in petroleum ether was poured onto the top of a column of finely powdered calcium carbonate in a narrow glass tube and allowed to drain down the column while fresh solvent was added. These zones became more widely separated as more solvent was poured through the column. The various pigments were absorbed by the calcium carbonate in slightly different degrees. The less strongly absorbed pigments moved down the column the most rapidly, so that when sufficient solvent was poured through, the pigments could be almost completely separated. Tswett called his process chromatography because of the colored bands formed in the column. This method of column chromatography is still used today. Many types of substances can be separated depending upon the solvent and type of column used. Usually the method is not quite as simple as Tswett's original procedure since the substances separated may not be as intensely colored as the chlorophylls. Often one must analyze the successive small portions of the solution coming from the column to determine where the desired material is eluted. In the more complex instruments this analysis may be made automatically.

A simpler method, though not as accurate, is **paper chromatography.** In this method the stationary phase is a strip of absorbent paper. A small amount of solution containing the substances to be separated is applied near one end of the paper strip and the solvent is evaporated. If the paper strip is suspended so that the end nearest the point of application of the substances is dipped into a suitable solvent, the solvent will wet the paper and gradually rise through the strip by capillary attraction. The flow of this solvent through the paper will tend to carry substances along with it to varying degrees, depending upon how much they are absorbed by the paper. After the solvent has risen to the desired height in the paper, the strip is removed, the solvent is evaporated, and the strip is sprayed or dipped in a reagent that will give a color reaction with the substances one is seeking. If these are separated, there will be a series of distinct spots on the paper corresponding to the substances being sought. The size of the spot is roughly proportional to the amount of the particular substance present.

This is known as **ascending** paper chromatography because the solvent rises in the paper strip. In **descending** chromatography, one end of the strip dips into the liquid and the strip is then bent over the side of the container and hangs down so that the actual flow of solvent is downward. In both types the chromatography is carried out in an enclosed jar or other chamber that contains solvent. This prevents evaporation from the paper, which would seriously distort the results. A large number of substances have been determined by paper chromatographic methods. The methods must always be standardized with known substances since the actual rate of migration will vary with many conditions. The relative rates of migration are fairly constant and are usually tabulated in terms of R_f values. This is the ratio of the rate of migration of the substances in question to that of the solvent front. As the solvent rises in the paper strip, it carries along the applied substances at slower rates. If, in a given experiment, it was found that the solvent had wet the paper to a height of 20 cm. from the starting level and the spot for a particular substance was 10 cm. from the starting point, then this substance would have a R_f value of $10/20 = 0.50$ for these particular conditions.

For the separation of a large number of similar substances such as the amino acids in blood filtrates or urine, a method known as two-dimensional paper chromatography may be used. When a small amount of solution containing the substances to be separated (i.e., amino acids) is applied near one corner of a large square of filter paper and this is subjected to ascending chromatography with a particular solvent, the amino acids will be distributed on one edge of the paper. If the paper is then dried and the edge is dipped into a different solvent for further chromatography, the final result will be that the spots for the amino acids will be distributed over the entire sheet as the two solvents are chosen so that the amino acids have different R_f values.

Another variation is known as **thin-layer chromatography (TLC).**[9] In this method, substances often used in column chromatography (such as alumina, silica gel, or cellulose) are finely powdered and applied as a thin layer to glass plates. These are then used in a manner similar to paper sheets. The layer of material applied is commonly 0.2-0.5 mm. in thickness. Minute amounts of substances can be used in thin-layer chromatography and it is also a much more rapid technique than paper chromatography.

A recent development is **gas-liquid chromatography,** often simply termed gas chromatography.[10, 11] In this method the substances being analyzed or separated are gases, and they must be volatilized. The vapors are carried through the column by streams of an inert gas, commonly helium or nitrogen. The columns contain an inert material such as crushed firebrick on which is placed a thin layer of liquid having a very low vapor pressure. The columns are usually of small diameter and are many feet in length (coiled to conserve space). The temperature must be well above room temperature. The effluent gas from the column is automatically analyzed and the result is recorded on a strip chart. With the use of different column packing a wide variety of biologic materials can be analyzed Substances that are not sufficiently volatile can often be determined by converting them into chemical compounds that are more readily volatilized. The simpler forms are satisfactory for the determination of blood gases (oxygen, carbon dioxide, carbon monoxide) and relatively volatile compounds such as the lower al-cohols. Refinements are needed for the determination of more complex substances such as steroids and lipids.

MICROANALYSIS[12, 13]

In many instances, particularly in pediatrics, only very small samples of blood may be available for analyses. In such circumstances microanalytic methods may be helpful. Just what constitutes a micromethod is not always clear. In general, for most blood determinations, those requiring more than 0.5 ml. of the sample (whole blood, plasma, serum) may be considered to be macromethods (ordinary). Those requiring 0.05-0.2 ml. of the sample are usually classed as micromethods and those requiring 0.01-0.025 ml. are termed ultramicromethods. Many of the macromethods can be scaled down by using 1/5-1/10 the amount of the sample and all reagents. A number of precautions must be taken. Pipetting of small volumes requires extreme care. Pipettes can be obtained that have sufficient accuracy (0.05%) but which are somewhat less expensive than the regular micropipettes.* As with most micropipettes, these are usually "to contain" types and must be rinsed out. In working with small volumes, filtration is usually impracticable and centrifugation must be used. Often the limiting factor is the colorimeter, as the usual cuvettes may require 3-4 ml. of solution. Most instruments have adapters for obtaining a 10 mm. light path with only 1 ml. or so of solution. Due to the much larger ratio of surface to volume in the micromethods, one may encounter more evaporation of solvent, creeping of fluids on wettable surfaces, and absorption onto the glass of diluted ions. Although the micromethods require smaller quantities of blood and reagents, they are often more time-consuming and less precise.

Two manufacturers† have introduced complete ultramicro systems with all the apparatus required for the ultramicro determination of many blood constituents.

---

*Accupett, Precision Scientific, Chicago, Ill.
†Coleman Instruments, Inc., Maywood, Ill.; Beckman Instruments, Inc., Fullerton, Calif.

Use of disposable plastic containers eliminates the difficulties in cleaning small fragile glassware. These systems also use polyethylene or glass automatic pipettes for measuring the sample and reagents, special colorimeters or adapters, centrifuges, and other items. Usually all of the major items must be purchased in order to carry out any of the tests. Studies have shown that the systems are capable of good precision; to attain this requires considerable experience in manipulation of pipettes and other items. In order to maintain accuracy the technician must use the system components daily for many tests and not merely for an occasional test for which insufficient blood is available for ordinary methods. Some technicians find it very difficult to attain proper precision with the system components.

Micromethods are suggested for a number of procedures given in this book. In some instances mention is made of the fact that the method can be scaled down by using small volumes. In others, separate, different methods are suggested. This may also be helpful in another respect, as occasionally it is advantageous to determine the constituent in a sample by two different methods to find out whether the method or the sample is causing an unexpected result.

If micromethods that employ capillary blood rather than venous blood are used, it must be remembered that the values for all blood constituents are not the same for the two types of samples. Practically all tabulated normal values are for venous blood. It would appear that results for BUN, iron, phosphate, and Bromsulphalein are quite comparable for capillary and venous blood. The results for bilirubin and total protein are close enough for most clinical purposes, but the values for the electrolytes—sodium, potassium, chloride, and calcium—may be somewhat different and venous blood should be used for these.

AUTOMATION IN THE CLINICAL LABORATORY

With the development of many new tests and the greater use of older ones, many laboratories have had large increases in the work load in recent years. In an attempt to increase the number of tests that can be performed without great increases in personnel and space, consideration must be given to the many automatic and semiautomatic devices that have been developed to save both time and effort. Many of these devices are relatively simple and can be adapted to any laboratory, whereas others are more complicated and expensive. The latter may require a certain work load to justify their use. Mention will be made of a number of techniques and types of apparatus that may be of value in increasing automation in the clinical laboratory.

Although not directly concerned with the performance of the tests themselves, the washing of glassware is an essential part of the laboratory work load. Many of the automatic techniques mentioned will greatly reduce the amount of glassware used. However, the use of automatic washing machines will often prove helpful. Most laboratory personnel are familiar with the pipette washing machines based on the siphon principle, which automatically cycle wash or rinse water through the pipettes. If the work load is large, consideration should be given to the use of an automatic glassware washing machine.

The newer analytic balances offer a degree of semiautomatic operation. The weights are added or subtracted by turning appropriate knobs, which also indicate the value of the weight on a mechanical scale. The smaller milligram weights are usually read from an optical scale and the correct weight is easily determined. There is no question that these balances enable rapid and accurate weighings to be performed by semiskilled persons. If many weighings are to be done, this advantage may outweigh the greater cost of these instruments.

In pipetting, particularly when adding the same quantity of reagent to a number of tubes, use may be made of a variety of automatic or semiautomatic pipettes. The hand-operated type (Fig. 6-1) is very simple to operate and may be obtained in a number of different sizes. These may be obtained in a more rigid form attached

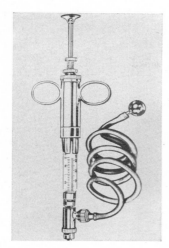

Fig. 6-1. Syringe pipette. (Courtesy Aloe Scientific Division, Brunswick Corp., St. Louis, Mo.)

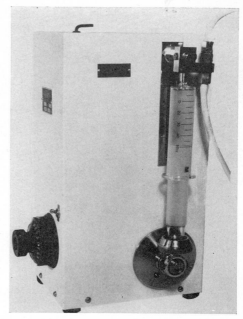

Fig. 6-2. Automatic pipetting machine. (Courtesy Aloe Scientific Division, Brunswick Corp., St. Louis, Mo.)

directly to the reagent bottle and of all-glass construction. They are more accurate and corrosion-free, but are more expensive and subject to breakage. With careful operation these pipettes will deliver a definite volume to within 1%. Some types may be difficult to set to deliver a definite volume such as 5 ml. However, for the addition of reagents, if the same amount is added to all tubes, samples, standards, and blanks, it usually makes little difference whether the amount delivered is 4.9 or 5 ml. For delivery of a larger number of samples one can obtain motor-driven syringe automatic pipetting machines such as were originally developed for bacteriologic use (Fig. 6-2).

For the dilution of samples and the preparation of protein-free filtrates the **Thomas-Seligson pipette** may be useful (Fig. 6-3). The sample is drawn up into the calibrated tip by gentle suction. The stopcock is then turned 90 degrees and the sample is rinsed into a tube by a definite amount of diluent from a burette. This is a relatively inexpensive device for the dilution of the sample. Saifer et al.[14] have described a system of analysis using this pipette and a syringe pipette which results in a considerable saving of time and glassware. The exact measurement of the diluent from a burette cannot be done

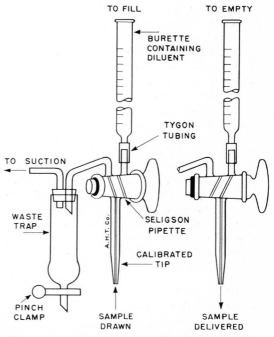

Fig. 6-3. Thomas-Seligson pipette. (Courtesy Arthur H. Thomas Co., Philadelphia, Pa.)

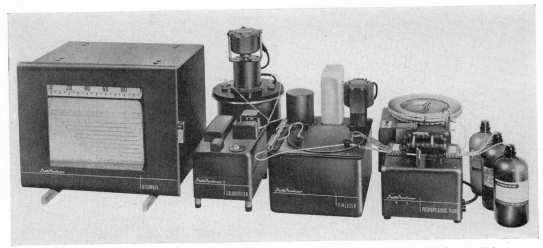

Fig. 6-4. Complete AutoAnalyzer. (Courtesy Technicon Instruments Corp., Ardsley, N. Y.)

too rapidly and is subject to errors. Measurement of the sample and the addition of one or two reagents can be done more rapidly and accurately by machines operating on the same principle but using motor-driven syringes for the measurement of the volumes. These are available from a number of manufacturers and are quite convenient for making dilutions. When standards and samples are diluted similarly in the machine, errors due to inaccuracies in the calibration of the syringe are greatly reduced.

In the colorimetric measurement of samples, recording spectrophotometers as well as recording attachments for spectrophotometers are available. These devices are also available for some of the smaller instruments so that readings may be made quite rapidly without the necessity of writing each one down. The results are automatically recorded on a strip chart. This may be conveniently used with another adaptation of the photometer. This is a cuvette, more or less permanently in place in the photometer, that can be rapidly emptied either by suction or gravity flow so that successive additions and readings on solutions can be made quite rapidly.

The most extensive application of automated methods in clinical chemistry has been the introduction of almost completely automatic systems such as the

AutoAnalyzer* (Fig. 6-4). The essential parts of the machine consist of a sample turntable from which the samples are taken from the sample containers; a proportioning pump by which the sample and the various reagents are added in varying proportions through the use of rollers over tubings of different internal diameters; a dialyzer used when necessary to separate diffusible material (such as glucose, chloride, urea, etc.) from the protein; a water bath for use when the reaction requires elevated temperatures; and a recording photometer in which the successive readings are recorded on a strip chart. The apparatus has been adapted for the determination of a large number of substances, including glucose, urea nitrogen, chloride, carbon dioxide, bilirubin, acid and alkaline phosphatase, glutamic oxalacetic transaminase, uric acid, calcium, total protein, albumin, inorganic phosphate, cholesterol, and serum iron. A flame photometer attachment is available for the determination of sodium and potassium. A digestion unit for the determination of protein-bound iodine and Kjeldahl nitrogen and a fluorometer for fluorometric measurements are also available.

Newer modifications allow the simultaneous determination of two substances

---

*Technicon Instruments Corp., Ardsley, N. Y.

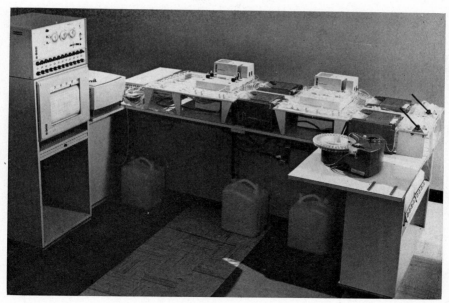

Fig. 6-5. Complete SMA-12 AutoAnalyzer. (Courtesy Technicon Instruments Corp., Ardsley, N. Y.)

on a single sample, such as glucose and urea nitrogen, total protein and albumin, calcium and inorganic phosphate, etc. For electrolyte studies the instrument can be set up with the addition of the flame photometer to determine sodium, potassium, chloride, and carbon dioxide on a single sample. The apparatus has proved to be as accurate as the manual methods and provides a great saving in time and effort. Since a certain amount of effort is involved in changing the setup to prepare for each different analysis, some laboratories may be inclined to reserve the use of the instrument for tests run in the largest volume, such as glucose and urea nitrogen. This enables technicians to use their time for analyses that are done in smaller numbers. However, with experience, the instrument will be found to save time, even when used with as few as 15 samples. A rather complete description of the instrument and methods is found in the review by Marsh.[15] Complete details concerning the instrument are available from the manufacturer.

In spite of the relatively high cost of the instrument, it has proved very valuable in laboratories having a sufficient volume of samples. The 12-channel SMA-12 AutoAnalyzer has been introduced recently (Fig. 6-5). This instrument will analyze and print on calibrated paper the results of 12 blood constituents from a single serum specimen, i.e., glucose, urea nitrogen, uric acid, total bilirubin, cholesterol, alkaline phosphatase, lactic dehydrogenase, total protein, albumin, glutamic oxalacetic transaminase, calcium, and inorganic phosphate. Such a machine has important applications in clinical chemistry. It can perform all of these tests at a cost similar to that of three or four tests carried out by the older manual methods. It has been noted that unsuspected abnormal results have been found in about 25% of cases when such a battery of tests is performed on all patients admitted to a hospital rather than just those ordered by the admitting physician. Some of these results might have been found in later tests ordered by the physician, but their early detection was an advantage to the patient. The increased use of automation will make it possible for many more tests to be performed at no great increase in cost and with a marked increase in the quality of diagnosis and medical care.[16, 17]

PROTEIN-FREE FILTRATES

For the determination of many blood constituents it is necessary to remove the plasma or serum proteins (and erythrocytes as well if whole blood is used). A number of methods for preparing **protein-free filtrates** have been introduced. Some methods are for specific determinations, whereas others are more widely applicable. In these methods some substance is added which combines with and precipitates the protein, leaving the desired constituents in solution. The most commonly used precipitants are tungstic acid, zinc hydroxide, and trichloroacetic acid. In the preparation of the filtrates the blood or serum is diluted in a definite ratio and this factor must be taken into account in the calculations. Most commonly the dilution is 1:10, i.e., to each 1 ml. of blood is added 9 ml. of other solutions to give a final volume of 10 ml. The solution is then filtered or centrifuged to separate the precipitate containing the protein. Filtration is often more convenient than centrifuging, but if only a relatively small volume of blood is available, a greater quantity of filtrate can be obtained by centrifugation. If a few particles of precipitate remain in the supernatant, it can be filtered through a small filter paper.

Folin-Wu filtrate[18]: This is probably the oldest method of blood deproteinization that is still in common use. The filtrate may be used for nonprotein nitrogen, chloride, creatinine, and some other tests. It has been used for glucose determinations, but it has been shown that this filtrate contains some nonsugar substances and gives a glucose value some 20-30 mg.% higher than a Somogyi filtrate. The latter gives a more accurate determination of true blood glucose, especially when used with a copper reduction method.

Reagents:
1. Sodium tungstate (10%). Dissolve 100 gm. reagent grade sodium tungstate in distilled water to make 1000 ml.

2. Sulfuric acid (2/3N). Mix together exactly 1000 ml. 1N sulfuric acid and exactly 500 ml. water. (See p. 432 for the preparation of standard acids.)

Method: Lake 1 vol. blood (measure with a "to contain" pipette and rinse well with the solution) with 7 vol. distilled water. Add 1 vol. 10% sodium tungstate solution and mix. Add 1 vol. 2/3N sulfuric acid and mix well, preferably by stoppering the container and shaking. Allow to stand until it turns a chocolate color. If after 10 min. a pink color still persists, cautiously add a small drop more of acid and shake again. Filter or centrifuge.

Haden's modification[19]: Lake 1 vol. blood with 8 parts 1/12N sulfuric acid (8.3 ml. 1N sulfuric acid diluted to 100 ml.), add 1 vol. 10% sodium tungstate solution, and mix by shaking. Centrifuge or filter.

Serum and cerebrospinal fluid: Serum and plasma contain less protein than whole blood and require only about one half as much protein-precipitating reagent. Mix 1 vol. serum or plasma with 8 vol. water and add 0.5 vol. 10% sodium tungstate solution. Mix and add 0.5 vol. 2/3N sulfuric acid. Mix, let stand 10 min., and centrifuge or filter.

Cerebrospinal fluid contains even less protein than serum. Mix 1 ml. spinal fluid with 8.5 ml. water, add 0.25 ml. sodium tungstate solution, and mix. Then add 0.25 ml. sulfuric acid. Mix, let stand 10 min., and centrifuge or filter.

Somogyi filtrate[20]: This may be used for blood sugar and urea nitrogen determinations.

Reagents:
1. Zinc sulfate solution (5%). Dissolve 50 gm. reagent grade zinc sulfate ($ZnSO_4 \cdot 7H_2O$) in distilled water to make 1000 ml. Zinc sulfate crystals tend to lose water on standing if the container is not tightly stoppered. Do not use crystals covered with a white powder, indicating a loss of water, as the solution will then be too concentrated.

2. Barium hydroxide (0.3N). Dissolve 95 gm. barium hydroxide ($Ba(OH)_2 \cdot$

$8H_2O$) in distilled water and dilute to 2 L. It is preferable to use distilled water that has been recently boiled and cooled to free it from carbon dioxide and to use fresh crystals of barium hydroxide that have been exposed to air as little as possible. Avoid contact of the solution with air as much as possible. If cloudy, filter or preferably allow to stand several days and carefully decant off the clear solution.

The actual concentrations of the zinc sulfate and barium hydroxide solutions are not as important as the fact that they must exactly neutralize each other. To check this, add exactly 10 ml. zinc sulfate solution to a 250 ml. flask; add about 50 ml. distilled water and 4 drops phenolphthalein indicator (1% in ethyl alcohol). Slowly titrate with barium hydroxide, using continual agitation. Too rapid a titration will give a false end point. The titration is carried out until 1 drop of the barium hydroxide solution turns the solution a faint permanent pink. The results should be that 10 ml. zinc sulfate solution requires 10 ± 0.05 ml. barium hydroxide.

If one or the other of the solutions is too strong, add distilled water in appropriate quantities and repeat the titration. For example, if 10 ml. zinc sulfate solution requires 10.33 ml. barium hydroxide solution for the titration, the zinc sulfate solution is too strong, and $\dfrac{10.33 - 10.00}{10.00}$ × 1000 or 33 ml. distilled water must be added to each liter of zinc sulfate solution. If 10 ml. zinc sulfate solution requires 9.68 ml. barium hydroxide solution, the hydroxide solution is too strong, and $\dfrac{10.00 - 9.68}{9.68}$ × 1000 or 33 ml. distilled water must be added to each liter of barium hydroxide solution. The solution may be stored in aspirator bottles. The bottle containing the barium hydroxide must be protected from air with a soda lime tube in the stopper. If it is desired to dispense the barium hydroxide solution from a burette, the top of the burette must be protected with a soda lime tube, and a burette with a Teflon plug in the stopcock must be used. The solution should be tested in advance by preparing a trial filtrate from blood. Filtration should proceed rapidly to give a clear filtrate that has little tendency to foam.

Method: Add 1 vol. blood (measured with a well-rinsed "to contain" pipette) to 5 vol. water. Add 2 vol. barium hydroxide and mix. Add 2 vol. zinc sulfate solution and mix. Filter or centrifuge. Note that in contrast to the Folin-Wu filtrate this precipitate will remain reddish in color and will not be a chocolate color.

Trichloroacetic acid filtrate[21]: This is used for the determination of phosphorus and may also be used for other tests requiring an acid filtrate.

Reagent:

1. Trichloroacetic acid (5%). Dissolve 50 gm. reagent grade trichloroacetic acid in distilled water to make 1000 ml. CAUTION! Trichloroacetic crystals are very, very corrosive to the skin. If spilled on the hands, wash immediately.

GLUCOSE

More methods have probably been used for glucose than for any other commonly determined blood constituent. Two similar methods are given here, one for use with Folin-Wu filtrate and one for use with Somogyi filtrate. Often it is desired to determine the blood glucose and nonprotein nitrogen or urea nitrogen on the same filtrate. **Nonprotein nitrogen** is best determined on **Folin-Wu filtrate** and **urea nitrogen** is best determined on **Somogyi filtrate**. Accordingly, the two methods for glucose are given here. As mentioned earlier, the Folin-Wu filtrate yields apparent glucose values 20-30 mg.% higher than the Somogyi filtrate. This may not be a serious disadvantage as long as the physician is aware of which method is being used and takes this into account in evaluating the analytic results.

Both methods are based on the principle that when glucose or other sugars are heated with an alkaline solution of cupric ions the copper is reduced to cuprous oxide. The extent of this reaction depends markedly upon the conditions of temperature, duration of heating, degree of alkalinity of the copper solution, etc. Hence the specified conditions must be followed closely in all determinations, and standards should always be run along with each set of samples. After heating, the cuprous oxide formed is estimated by allowing it to react with phosphomolybdic or arsenomolybdic acid to form a complex molybdenum blue, which is determined colorimetrically.

Somogyi method[20, 22, 23]:

Reagents:

1. Alkaline copper tartrate. Dissolve 24 gm. anhydrous sodium carbonate and 12 gm. sodium potassium tartrate in 200 ml. distilled water. Add, while stirring, 40 ml. 10% copper sulfate solution. When this has dissolved, add 16 gm. sodium bicarbonate and stir until dissolved. Dissolve 180 gm. anhydrous sodium sulfate in 600 ml. water. Heat to boiling, cool, and add to the copper solution. Transfer the mixture to a 1000 ml. volumetric flask and dilute to volume.

2. Arsenomolybdate solution. Dissolve 50 gm. ammonium molybdate in 900 ml. distilled water. Add 42 ml. concentrated sulfuric acid and mix. Add 6 gm. disodium orthoarsenate (Na_2-$HASO_4 \cdot 7H_2O$) dissolved in 50 ml. water. Mix and place in an incubator at 37° C. for 48 hr. This solution is stable indefinitely when stored in a glass-stoppered brown bottle.

3. Standards:

   A. Stock standard. Dissolve exactly 1 gm. reagent grade glucose in 0.2% benzoic acid solution and dilute to 100 ml. in a volumetric flask. This solution contains 10 mg. glucose/ml.

   B. Working standard. Prepare standard solutions containing 0.1 and 0.2 mg. glucose/ml. by diluting stock standard 1:100 and 2:100 with 0.2% benzoic acid. Prepare standards fresh weekly.

Procedure: Add 1 ml. 1:10 Somogyi filtrate to a Folin-Wu sugar tube. To three other tubes add 1 ml. water (blank) to the first, 1 ml. standard containing 0.1 mg. glucose to the second, and 1 ml. standard containing 0.2 mg. glucose to the third. Add 1 ml. alkaline copper tartrate to each tube. Mix and heat in a vigorously boiling water bath for 15 min. Cool, add 1 ml. arsenomolybdate solution, mix, dilute to 25 ml. with distilled water, and mix by inversion.

Read in a photometer at 500 nm., setting to zero with the blank. Since 1 ml. of a 1:10 filtrate is treated the same as 1 ml. standard containing 0.1 mg./ml. (10 mg.%) or 0.2 mg./ml. (20 mg.%), the calculation is:

$$\frac{OD\ sample}{OD\ standard} \times 10 \times 10\ (or\ 20) = Mg.\%$$

glucose in sample

Folin-Wu method[24]:

Reagents:

1. Alkaline copper tartrate. Dissolve 40 gm. anhydrous sodium carbonate in about 400 ml. distilled water and transfer to a 1000 ml. volumetric flask. Then add 7.5 gm. tartaric acid and 4.5 gm. crystalline copper sulfate ($CuSO_4 \cdot 5H_2O$). Mix and dilute to 1 L. With reagent grade chemicals this solution may be used immediately and is stable indefinitely. Should a small amount of cuprous oxide form, filter it off before use.

2. Phosphomolybdic acid. To 70 gm. molybdic acid (85%) and 10 gm. sodium tungstate add 400 ml. 10% sodium hydroxide and 400 ml. water. Boil for 20-40 min. to remove ammonia (the compound sold as molybdic acid [85%] is actually chiefly ammonium paramolybdate). Cool, add 250 ml. concentrated (85%) phosphoric acid, and dilute to 1 L.

3. Benzoic acid solution (0.2%). Add 4 gm. benzoic acid to 2 L. water. Heat (but do not boil) to dissolve. Benzoic acid acts as a preservative for the glucose standard solutions.

4. Standards:

   A. Stock standard. The same standard is used as in the Somogyi method.

   B. Working standard. Working standards containing 0.2 and 0.4 mg.

glucose/2 ml. are prepared fresh weekly by diluting the stock standard 1:100 and 2:100 with benzoic acid solution.

Procedure: Add 2 ml. 1:10 Folin-Wu filtrate (p. 298) to a Folin-Wu sugar tube. To three similar tubes add 2 ml. water (blank) and 2 ml. standard solutions containing 0.2 and 0.4 mg. glucose, respectively. To each tube add 2 ml. alkaline copper tartrate solution and mix. Immerse the tubes in at least 4 in. briskly boiling water and heat for exactly 8 min. Remove from water and, without cooling, add 2 ml. phosphomolybdic acid reagent and mix. Return to the boiling water bath for 3 min. more and then cool to room temperature. Dilute to 25 ml. with distilled water and mix well by inversion.

Read in a photometer at 420 nm. or with a filter having a maximum transmittance near this wavelength, setting the instrument to 0 OD or to 100% transmittance with the blank. Calculate the K as explained on p. 288. Then:

$$\text{Mg.\% glucose} = K \times \text{OD sample} \times \frac{\text{Dilution filtrate}}{\text{Ml. filtrate taken}} \times 100$$

which for the aliquot used reduces to:

$$\text{Mg.\% glucose} = K \times \text{OD} \times 500$$

This can also be calculated the same as for the Somogyi method since equal volumes of filtrate and standards are used.

Micromethod: Reagents are the same as for the Somogyi or Folin-Wu methods. When only a small quantity of blood is available, either of the methods can be adapted to a smaller scale. Use 0.2 ml. blood and proportionate amounts of the reagents in preparing the filtrate. For the Folin-Wu method use 0.2 ml. blood, 1.4 ml. water, 0.2 ml. sodium tungstate, and 0.2 ml. sulfuric acid. For the Somogyi filtrate use 0.2 ml. blood, 1.6 ml. zinc sulfate solution, and 0.2 ml. sodium hydroxide solution. By carrying out the precipitation in a small test tube and centrifuging strongly, a sufficient quantity of protein-free solution can be pipetted from the supernatant. Use one half the quantity of filtrate, standards, copper reagent, and molybdate. Use Folin-Wu tubes that are graduated at 12.5 ml. as well as at 25 ml. and dilute to the former mark. The calculations are the same as for previous methods and the results will be directly comparable with them.

Normal values and interpretation[25, 26]: The fasting venous blood sugar in normal adults is usually 80-125 mg.% when measured by the Folin-Wu method and is 65-95 mg.% when measured by the Somogyi method. It should be noted that the range of normal values for serum or plasma is somewhat higher. For the Folin-Wu method it is approximately 95-140 mg.% and for the Somogyi method it is approximately 80-115 mg.%. Capillary blood closely approximates arterial blood and contains about 25 mg.% more glucose. High blood sugar values are found in diabetes mellitus (up to 500 mg.% or more, according to the severity of the condition). Except in diabetes the fasting blood sugar rarely exceeds 120 mg.%. Small increases may be found in hyperactivity of the thyroid, pituitary, and adrenal glands (including in the latter condition that due to emotional stress).

In pancreatitis and pancreatic carcinoma there may be some increase in blood sugar, but it does not exceed 150 mg.% except in advanced cases. Moderate increases in blood sugar may be also found in infectious diseases and in some intracranial diseases such as meningitis, encephalitis, tumors, and hemorrhage. Anesthesia will also cause an increase in the blood sugar. Depending upon the duration and degree, a considerable rise may occur, sometimes exceeding 200 mg.%.

Hypoglycemia (lowered blood sugar) occurs most frequently as a result of insulin overdose in the treatment of diabetes. The fasting blood sugar may also be reduced in hypothyroidism (myxedema and cretinism), hypopituitarism (Simmonds' disease), and hypoadrenalism (Addison's disease), with values as low as 20 mg.% in severe cases of the last two conditions. Low blood sugar may also be found in glycogen storage disease.

GLUCOSE TOLERANCE TESTS

In studies on carbohydrate metabolism, particularly in the diagnosis of diabetes mellitus, a glucose tolerance test is done. This usually gives more information than can be secured from a fasting blood sugar level alone. If at all possible, the test should be made after the patient has been on a regular mixed diet for several days in order to obtain a true response to the test. Preceding carbohydrate starvation will cause an abnormal increase in blood sugar and a delayed decrease, suggesting a diabetic curve. A preceding high carbohydrate diet will cause a low blood sugar curve (Fig. 6-6).

Many of the earlier studies on glucose tolerance were done using the Folin-Wu or similar methods for the determination of glucose. Later work has shown that some of the methods used determined not only the "true" glucose of the blood but also other reducing substances as well. While these nonsugar reducing substances might not change markedly dur-

ing the tolerance test, the use of newer, more precise methods of glucose determination requires reevaluation of criteria for abnormal glucose tolerance curves. Various investigators have stated that the older methods in which a Folin-Wu filtrate was used gave blood sugar values from 15-25 mg.% higher than when a Somogyi filtrate was used, and that the Somogyi-Nelson method yields values close to the "true" glucose values as determined by enzymatic methods. The normal values for whole blood may be taken as 80-125 mg.% by the Folin-Wu method and as 65-95 mg.% by the Somogyi-Nelson method. However, Manger and Farese[27] have shown that even with the Somogyi-Nelson method the values for **whole blood** varied 5% or more, depending upon the exact procedure used in preparing the filtrate, as presumably much of the interfering material is in the red cells. When a filtrate was prepared using

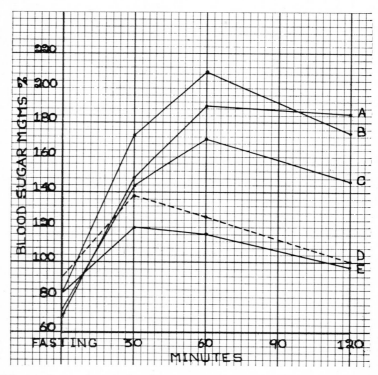

Fig. 6-6. Effects of preceding 48 hr. diets on glucose tolerance tests. **A**, Starvation diet; **B**, fat diet; **C**, protein diet; **D**, mixed (normal) diet; **E**, carbohydrate diet. Original chart has been modified by addition of curve after a mixed diet. (Modified from Sweeney: Arch. Intern. Med. [Chicago] **40:**818, 1927.)

plasma, the glucose concentration obtained was independent of the method of preparing the filtrate and the results compared well with those obtained by two different enzymatic methods. With the increasing use of automation it is often very desirable to be able to run several different determinations from the same sample. This usually requires that the sample be serum or plasma rather than whole blood. This is another reason for determining glucose on such samples rather than whole blood. Mainly because of the difference of water concentration of the cells and plasma, the concentration of glucose is not the same in plasma as in whole blood. The results obtained with plasma are consistently higher than those obtained with whole blood. Using the AutoAnalyzer, McDonald et al.[28] found a linear relationship that may be expressed as

$$P = 6.6 + 1.15\ W$$

and

$$W = -5.7 + 0.87\ P$$

where P is the glucose concentration in plasma and W is that in whole blood. These investigators gave somewhat more precise equations, but the ones cited are suitable for most purposes. These formulas can be used for the conversion of values from plasma to whole blood or vice versa. For example, if the blood sugar values for whole blood (Folin-Wu method) cited in Table 6-2 were converted to "true" glucose (Somogyi method), concentrations for fasting, ½, 1, 2, and 3 hr. specimens of approximately 65, 135, 145, 60, and 65 mg.%, respectively, would be obtained. With the use of the previous formula for conversion to plasma glucose, corresponding results of 82, 161, 173, 76, and 82 mg.%, respectively, would be obtained. This leads to the interesting result, which may be helpful to the physician, that the whole blood levels of glucose as determined by the older Folin-Wu method are approximately equal to the levels in plasma as determined by the more recent "true" glucose methods.

One-dose test: The test is usually performed in the morning after an overnight fast. Blood and urine specimens are obtained, and the patient is then given orally the glucose dissolved in water, with the juice of one lemon added to increase palatability. The amount of glucose recommended by many authorities is 0.9 gm./kg. body weight (0.4 gm./lb. body weight), with a maximum of 50 gm. Since this would be equivalent to nearly 50 gm. for most adults, it may be more convenient to give 50 ml. glucose dissolved in 250 ml. water in all cases since the solution can then be prepared beforehand. The exact volume of the solution is not critical; however, a concentrated solution may be more likely to cause some nausea on ingestion and a dilute solution may result in too large a volume to be conveniently ingested at one time.

Blood specimens are drawn at ½, 1, 2, and 3 hr. after ingestion of the glucose. Urine specimens are also obtained at these times. The blood specimens are analyzed for glucose, and the urine specimens are tested for glucose by one of the semiquantitative methods for urinary reducing sugars given in Chapter 2. Inclusion of 4 hr. specimens (blood and urine) is valuable in detecting hypoglycemia.

Normal values and interpretation: A typical normal response to a glucose tolerance test is given in Table 6-2 (Folin-Wu method).

The fasting blood sugar is within normal limits; the maximum blood sugar is usually between 140 and 180 mg.% and is reached in ½-1 hr. after ingestion of the glucose. The blood sugar then falls rapidly to normal limits, usually reaching this within 2 hr. There is sometimes a slight dip in the blood sugar toward the end of the test, as shown in Table 6-2. A similar example is shown by curve 4 in Fig. 6-7.

Table 6-2. Normal response to glucose tolerance test

	Fasting (mg. %)	½ hr. (mg. %)	1 hr. (mg. %)	2 hr. (mg. %)	3 hr. (mg. %)
Blood sugar	80	155	165	75	80
Urine	0	0	0	0	0

In normal individuals, as long as the blood sugar is below 160-190 mg.%, glucose in amounts detectable by most routine tests is not excreted by the kidneys. This level of blood sugar has been termed the renal threshold for glucose. Thus in the glucose tolerance of normal individuals there is usually no detectable sugar in the urine. The threshold varies with the individual and may occasionally be as low as 140 mg.% or less. Such an individual would show some urinary sugar with a normal tolerance curve. Little diagnostic significance can be attached to the occasional presence of small amounts of urinary sugar under these circumstances (Fig. 6-7, curve 5).

The effect of diet has been previously mentioned (Fig. 6-6). Both the average fasting level and the maximum to which the level rises tend to increase with age. In older people the maximum may reach 200 mg.%. A diminished glucose tolerance, i.e., an increase in the blood level after glucose ingestion, most commonly occurs in diabetes mellitus. Hyperactivity of the pituitary, adrenal, or thyroid glands may also lead to some degree of impairment. Fig. 6-7 indicates some of the conditions in which the blood sugar level may be above or below normal after the ingestion of glucose. Any condition in which there is impaired absorption from the intestinal tract may lead to a flat type of tolerance curve with only a slight rise in blood sugar. In a study of these cases an intravenous tolerance test may be used (see p. 305).

One-hour two-dose tolerance test: Exton and Rose[29] described a 1 hr. two-dose tolerance test based on Allen's paradoxical law. In normal individuals the more sugar given, the more is used, but in diabetic individuals the opposite is true.

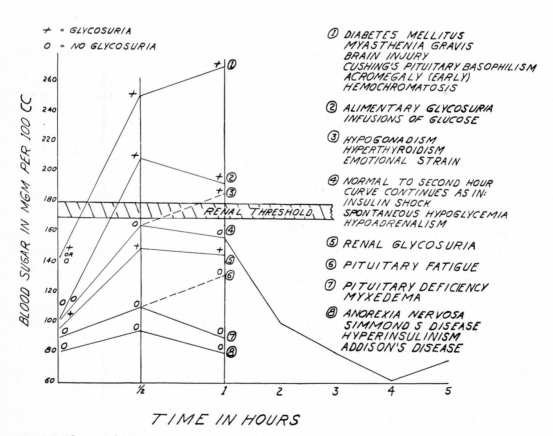

Fig. 6-7. Glucose tolerance curves.

The patient should be on a normal mixed diet for a day or two before the test. A low carbohydrate diet may cause a rise in the blood sugar of the 1 hr. specimen of as much as 25-35 mg./100 ml., suggesting diabetes.

Dissolve 100 gm. glucose in about 500 ml. water and flavor with lemon. Divide into two approximately equal portions. After an overnight fast, collect specimens of blood and urine and then give one portion of the glucose meal (50 gm.), allowing 1 or 2 min. for ingestion. At the end of 30 min. collect a specimen of blood and give a second portion of glucose, allowing 1 or 2 min. for ingestion. Again, 30 min. after the second dose, collect specimens of blood and urine. Determine the amount of sugar in the blood and urine specimens. Have the patient empty the bladder for each specimen.

Normally the fasting blood sugar is within the usual limits. The 30 min. sample shows the usual rise of not more than 75 mg.; the 1 hr. sample usually shows a decrease, but may show practically the same as the 30 min. sample (not more than 5 mg. increase). None of the urine specimens will show sugar. In diabetes mellitus the fasting blood sugar may be normal or above, the 30 min. sample will show a marked increase, and the 60 min. sample will show a further increase (not less than 10 mg.). The fasting urine may show sugar and the other specimens will show amounts which depend on the severity of the disease. In renal glycosuria and in alimentary glycosuria the blood sugar will follow the normal curve, but in the former (renal diabetes) the level is usually lower than normal. In both conditions the glycosuria, usually mild, is not in proportion to the carbohydrate intake. In renal glycosuria the fasting specimen of urine characteristically shows sugar (often only very small amounts), whereas in alimentary glycosuria the urine is sugar-free.

Postprandial blood glucose test: Sindoni[30] and other investigators have shown that the determination of **postprandial glucose concentration** is a reliable method for the detection of diabetes. They have demonstrated that the glucose concentration in blood specimens drawn 2 hr. after a meal is rarely elevated in normal individuals, while it is significantly increased in diabetic patients. This test has correlated well with other standard tests and is useful as a screening test. It has the advantage of requiring only one blood specimen.

Procedure: For best results the patient should be placed on a high carbohydrate diet for 2-3 days prior to the test.

Have the patient eat a breakfast of orange juice, cereal with sugar, toast, and milk. Two hours after this, draw a blood specimen and determine the glucose.

Interpretation: A normal response is a glucose level less than 140 mg.%. An abnormal response is a glucose level greater than 140 mg.%.

Intravenous glucose tolerance test[31]: The **intravenous method** should be used in sprue; in celiac disease; in hypothyroidism in which absorption is slow, thus giving low, flat curves; and in thyrotoxicosis in which absorption is accelerated, thus giving hyperglycemic curves.

Obtain specimens of blood and urine during the fasting state. Give intravenously 0.5 gm. glucose/kg. body weight, using a sterile 50% glucose solution and adjusting the rate of flow to require 5 min. for its administration.

Obtain specimens of blood and urine immediately after administration of the glucose is completed and thereafter at the end of 30, 60, 90, and 150 min.

Determine the amount of glucose in each specimen.

Significance: Normally the blood sugar will be increased immediately after glucose infusion is completed, perhaps reaching a maximum of about 250 mg./100 ml. The urine may contain glucose. In the 30 min. specimen there will be a marked drop in glucose and in the 60 min. specimen the amount will return to the fasting level ($\pm$10 mg./100 ml.).

In diabetes mellitus the glucose level is still elevated 60 min. after the glucose administration has been completed and remains elevated for 3 hr. or more. In no specimen of blood does the amount of glucose fall below the fasting level.

In liver insufficiency the return to a

normal level may be somewhat delayed—between 1 and 2 hr.

Insulin tolerance test[32]: Insulin administered to a normal person in the postabsorptive state causes a prompt decrease of the blood sugar and then a gradual return to the original level or above.

The response to insulin may be used to determine a patient's sensitivity to insulin (ability to store glycogen) and ability to recover after the induced hypoglycemia.

Take a fasting blood specimen for determination of glucose; then inject intravenously 0.1 unit regular insulin/kg. body weight. Take other blood specimens for glucose determinations at 30 min. and at 2 hr. CAUTION! Be prepared to administer glucose promptly if early clinical signs and symptoms of hypoglycemia occur (hunger, sweating, nervousness, tremulousness). Give carbohydrates after the test.

If marked symptoms are anticipated, use a smaller dose of insulin.

Normally the blood sugar falls to about 50% of the fasting level in 30 min. and returns to the original level or above in 2 hr. The duration of hypoglycemia is more important than the degree.

Abnormally there may be only a slight or a delayed fall in blood sugar (insulin resistance) or a delayed rise in blood sugar following the hypoglycemia (hypoglycemia unresponsiveness).

Insulin resistance may occur in hyperfunction of the adrenal cortex, in hyperfunction of the anterior pituitary, and sometimes in diabetes mellitus.

Hypoglycemia unresponsiveness occurs in hyperinsulinism, Addison's disease, hypofunction of the anterior pituitary (Simmonds' disease, pituitary myxedema, pituitary dwarfism), in some cases of hypothyroidism, and in some cases of glycogen storage disease (von Gierke's disease).

Epinephrine tolerance test[33]: Epinephrine accelerates glycogenolysis and promptly increases the blood sugar. This increase of blood sugar following administration of epinephrine is an index of the quantity and availability of liver glycogen for maintaining normal blood sugar.

Take a blood specimen for estimating the fasting blood sugar and then inject intramuscularly 10 minims of 1:1000 solution of epinephrine hydrochloride. Take another blood specimen for glucose at 30 min. Normally the blood sugar will increase over 30 mg./100 ml. in 30 min. (over 35 mg./100 ml. in 45-60 min.), returning to the fasting level in about 2 hr.

A diminished response occurs when the glycogen store is depleted (hepatocellular damage, including fatty liver and cirrhosis), in glycogen storage disease (von Gierke's disease) in which the glycogen is not readily available, and in hypoglycemia that does not respond normally to the insulin tolerance test (Addison's disease, pituitary cachexia, hyperinsulinism).

Tolbutamide diagnostic test for detection of diabetes mellitus[34-36]: This test is based on the difference in response of normal subjects and diabetic individuals to intravenous administration of a test dose of **tolbutamide (Orinase)**.

Reagents:
1. Orinase Diagnostic.* Available in sterile vials containing 1.081 gm. sodium tolbutamide, equivalent to 1 gm. tolbutamide, together with an ampule containing 20 ml. sterile water. Using a sterile syringe, transfer the water to the vial containing the tolbutamide. The material is dissolved and used at once.
2. Reagents for the determination of blood glucose by the Somogyi method (or other method yielding true glucose values).

Procedure: The precautions regarding previous dietary intake mentioned in the discussion of glucose tolerance apply here also. Severe hypoglycemic symptoms may develop in patients who have had previously fasting blood sugars in the hypoglycemic range. With such patients the test should be performed cautiously and should be terminated by the intravenous injection of 12.5-25 gm. glucose in 25 or 50% solution if severe hypoglycemic symptoms occur.

On the morning of the test after an

---

*The Upjohn Co., Kalamazoo, Mich.

overnight fast, obtain a blood specimen; then inject 20 ml. Orinase solution at a constant rate over a 2-3 min. period. Obtain blood specimens exactly 20 and 30 min. later, timing from the midpoint of the injection. Determine the blood sugar in the three specimens. The test is terminated after the last blood sample by feeding a high carbohydrate breakfast.

Interpretation: If the blood glucose value of the 20 min. specimen is 90% or more of the fasting level, the patient is definitely diabetic. If the 20 min. specimen is in the range of 85-89% of the fasting level, diabetes is probable; the range of 75-84% represents borderline cases and under 75% represents normal. The 30 min. specimen is of value in confirming the diagnosis. If it is more than 76% of the fasting level, diabetes is almost certain, but lower values have less negative significance (Fig. 6-8).

In patients suspected of having functioning adenomas of the pancreatic islet cells, the Orinase test may be helpful in differential diagnosis of spontaneous hypoglycemia. For this modification, after the injection of Orinase take blood samples at 15 min. intervals for the first hour and at 30 min. intervals for the next 2 hr. In normal patients there is a fall in blood sugar for 30-45 min., followed by a rise during the ensuing 90-180 min. to normal levels. In patients with insulomas the fall in blood sugar is somewhat greater, but more significantly, the hypoglycemia persists for several hours. It is this persistent lowering of blood sugar rather than the magnitude of the fall that is the significant criterion. The blood level at 90-180 min. is 40-65% of the fasting level as compared with a level of 78-100% in normal individuals.

NONGLUCOSE SUGARS[37]

The following method is suitable for determining nonglucose sugars such as galactose or levulose in the presence of

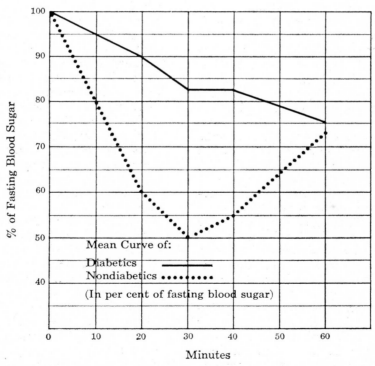

Fig. 6-8. Orinase diagnostic response curves in nondiabetic and diabetic subjects. The blood glucose responses are typical of nondiabetics and of mild diabetics. (Adapted from Unger and Madison: J. Clin. Invest. **37**:627, 1958.)

glucose, as in the galactose or levulose tolerance tests. In this method the glucose is eliminated by oxidation with glucose oxidase; the nonglucose sugar, which is not affected by the enzyme, is determined by the Somogyi-Nelson method.

Reagents:

1. Potassium phosphate (3.5%). Dissolve 3.5 gm. anhydrous monobasic potassium phosphate (KH_2PO_4) in water and dilute to 100 ml.
2. Glucose oxidase (1 mg./ml.). Weigh out several portions of 10 mg. glucose oxidase into separate 10 ml. graduated cylinders. Stopper and store in the refrigerator. Add 3.5% phosphate solution to 10 ml. when needed to make fresh glucose oxidase solutions. This solution is stable for only a day or two even when refrigerated.
3. Standards:
   A. Stock standard. Dissolve 1 gm. pure dried nonglucose sugar in 0.2% benzoic acid solution and dilute to 100 ml. This solution contains 10 mg./ml.
   B. Working standard. Dilute 1 ml. stock standard to 200 ml. with benzoic acid solution. This contains 5 mg.% of the sugar, but since a 1:20 dilution is made of the blood, it will be equivalent to 100 mg.% when used corresponding to the blood filtrate.
4. The following reagents are the same as those used in the Somogyi-Nelson method for glucose (p. 300): barium hydroxide (0.3N), zinc sulfate (5%), alkaline copper tartrate, and arsenomolybdate color reagent.

Procedure: To 0.8 ml. water in a plastic centrifuge tube add 0.1 ml. blood. Mix and allow to stand 2-3 min. to hemolyze. Add 0.2 ml. glucose oxidase solution, mix, stopper lightly, and incubate at 37° C. for 90 min. Every 20-30 min. mix well with the stopper removed. After incubation, add 0.5 ml. 0.3N barium hydroxide and mix. Add 0.4 ml. 5% zinc sulfate solution and mix. Centrifuge at high speed for 10 min. Decant supernatant and, if necessary, centrifuge supernatant again to obtain a clear solution. Pipette 1 ml. of the supernatant to a sugar tube. Also set up in separate tubes 1 ml. of working standard and 1 ml. of water as a blank. Add 2 ml. alkaline copper tartrate to each tube. Mix and heat in boiling water bath for 20 min. Cool, add 2 ml. of arsenomolybdate solution, mix, and dilute to 25 ml. Read standard and samples against blank in a photometer at 535 nm.

Calculation:

$$\frac{\text{OD sample}}{\text{OD standard}} \times 100 = \text{Mg.\% nonglucose sugar}$$

BLOOD UREA NITROGEN (BUN)

Urea may be determined colorimetrically by its reaction with **diacetylmonoxime** or by the use of **urease**. The latter converts urea to ammonia, which is then determined colorimetrically. The former method is fairly specific for urea; the latter method is very specific for urea except that any preformed ammonia in the sample will also be determined. Both methods are presented here. The oxime method is a modification of former methods; it has the advantage of producing a color that follows Beer's law much closer and it requires no strong acid solution. The determination is carried out on an aliquot of a protein-free filtrate. In the urease method the ammonia formed by the action of the enzyme on urea is determined by the Berthelot reaction with phenol and hypochlorite to produce an intense blue color. This may be used as a micromethod, requiring only 0.02 ml. of serum.

Oxime method[38]:

Reagents:

1. Oxime solution. Dissolve 1 gm. diacetylmonoxime* (also sold under the name of 2,3-butanedione monoxime), 0.2 gm. thiosemicarbazone, and 9 gm. sodium chloride in water and dilute to 1 L.
2. Acid solution. Cautiously add 60 ml. concentrated sulfuric acid and 10 ml. 85% phosphoric acid to about 800 ml. water. Add 0.1 gm. ferric chloride and dilute to 1 L.

---

*No. 86, Eastman Kodak Co., Rochester, N. Y.

3. Standards:
    A. Stock standard. Dissolve 2 gm. sodium benzoate in 1 L. water. Add 0.8 ml. concentrated sulfuric acid and mix. Use this solution for preparing and diluting the standard solutions. For the stock solution dissolve 322 mg. urea in some of the above solution and dilute to 500 ml. This solution contains 30 mg.% urea nitrogen.
    B. Working standard. Dilute 10 ml. stock solution to 100 ml. This solution contains 3 mg.% urea nitrogen and is equivalent to 30 mg.% when equal amounts of the standard and a 1:10 blood filtrate are used.

Procedure: Prepare a 1:10 Somogyi or Folin-Wu filtrate from blood. In separate test tubes place 1 ml. filtrate, 1 ml. diluted standard, and 1 ml. water as a blank.

To each tube add 3 ml. oxime solution and 3 ml. acid solution. Mix and heat in a boiling water bath for 15 min. Cool and read samples and standards against blank in photometer at 520 nm. If the color is too intense, the solutions may be diluted somewhat before reading. This is conveniently done if one carries out the reaction in tubes graduated at 10 or 15 ml.

Calculation: Since the standard and filtrate are treated similarly:

$$\frac{\text{OD sample}}{\text{OD standard}} \times 30 = \text{Mg.\% urea nitrogen}$$

Urease method[39, 40]: Since the final color reaction is very sensitive, ammonia-free water must be used for all reagents and dilutions. It is best to purify the distilled water by passage through a column of ion exchange resins such as Amberlite MB-3.

Reagents:
1. Alkaline hypochlorite. Dissolve 12.5 gm. sodium hydroxide in about 400 ml. water. Cool, add 20 ml. sodium hypochlorite solution (any commercial bleach solution containing 5.25% available chlorine), and dilute to 500 ml. Store in a polyethylene bottle in the refrigerator.
2. Phenol reagent. Dissolve 25 gm.

phenol and 0.13 gm. sodium nitroprusside in water to make 500 ml. Store in a brown bottle in the refrigerator. This remains stable for several months.
3. Buffer. Dissolve 5 gm. disodium salt of ethylenediaminetetraacetic acid in 200 ml. glycerin and 250 ml. water. Adjust to a pH of 6.5 with 4% sodium hydroxide (about 10 ml. required) and dilute to 500 ml.
4. Buffered urease. Dissolve 30 mg. urease type III* in 100 ml. buffer. This remains stable for several weeks when stored in the refrigerator.
5. Standard. Use the stock standard (not diluted) of the oxime method.

Procedure: To 0.5 ml. buffered urease add 0.02 ml. serum or standard with a "to contain" micropipette, rinsing well. (With a slight sacrifice of accuracy, Sahli pipettes may be used.) Incubate all tubes for 15 min. at 37° C. Also incubate a blank of 0.5 ml. buffered urease alone. After incubation, add to each tube 1 ml. phenol reagent and mix well; then add 1 ml. alkaline hypochlorite and mix again. Incubate for 15 min. at 37° C. Then add 10 ml. water and read samples and standard against blank at 620 nm. Conveniently, the 30 mg.% standard should give a reading of around 50% transmission. If the color is too intense, dilute the solutions further or use a shorter wavelength, e.g., 580 nm.

Calculation: Since standard and sample are treated similarly:

$$\frac{\text{OD sample}}{\text{OD standard}} \times 30 = \text{Mg.\% urea nitrogen}$$

Procedure for urine: The **oxime method** can be applied directly to diluted urine. Usually the urine is diluted 1:50 or 1:100. This dilution is then treated exactly like blood filtrate.

Calculation: Since the diluted standard actually contains 3 mg.% urea nitrogen, then

$$\frac{\text{OD sample}}{\text{OD standard}} \times 3 \times \frac{\text{B}}{\text{A}} = \text{Mg.\% urea nitrogen}$$

---

*Sigma Chemical Co., St. Louis, Mo.

where "A" ml. urine is diluted to a total volume of "B" ml.

Since urine contains some preformed ammonia, a slight modification of the **urease method** is required. This method uses serum directly; therefore the urine is diluted only 1:5 or 1:10. Determine the preformed ammonia by adding 0.02 ml. diluted urine to 0.5 ml. water; then add the color reagents and incubate for 15 min. along with a water blank. The sample is then read against the blank. Another aliquot of the dilute urine is treated with urease the same as the procedure for serum, along with a urease blank and standard.

Calculations:

For preformed ammonia:

$$\frac{OD\ sample}{OD\ standard} \times 30 \times \frac{B}{A} = Mg.\%\ ammonia\ nitrogen$$

For total nitrogen:

$$\frac{OD\ sample \times 30 \times B}{OD\ standard \times A} = Mg.\%\ total\ nitrogen$$

Total nitrogen – Ammonia nitrogen = Urea nitrogen

The OD values are the same for the respective samples, the same standard (run with urease) is used for both, and A and B refer to the dilution of urine.

Van Slyke et al.[41] stated that for urea clearance it is more correct to include the preformed ammonia along with the urea in the urine analysis. If this view is adapted, the analysis is simplified because only the total nitrogen is required.

Normal values and interpretation: The normal range of blood urea nitrogen is 10-18 mg.% (22-40 mg.% urea). The most common cause of increased blood urea nitrogen is inadequate excretion, usually due to kidney disease or urinary obstruction. Increased blood urea nitrogen in acute nephritis may vary from 25-160 mg.%. Urea retention occurs with extensive parenchymatous destruction of kidney tissue, as in pyelonephritis, advanced nephrosclerosis, renal tuberculosis, renal cortical necrosis, malignancy, suppuration, and chronic gout. (See also discussion of nonprotein nitrogen.)

The level of urea nitrogen in serum or plasma differs by only a few percent from that in whole blood, at least in the fasting state. Although serum contains more water than the erythrocytes, apparently the concentration of urea is higher in the erythrocyte water, so that the overall difference in urea concentration between the cells and plasma is slight. The values can thus be used interchangeably without serious error. Again, in regard to urea clearance it seems more logical to determine the concentration in plasma rather than in whole blood since it is the former that is filtered by the kidneys.

NONPROTEIN NITROGEN (NPN)

Nonprotein nitrogen is determined by digesting an aliquot of Folin-Wu blood filtrate with sulfuric and phosphoric acids, with a trace of copper as an added catalyst. The digestion converts all nitrogen compounds to ammonia, which is then determined by the reaction with **Nessler solution** (alkaline potassium mercuric iodide). For most clinical purposes a determination of the urea nitrogen is much simpler and gives as much information[26]; this determination has replaced the NPN in many laboratories.

Reagents[18, 42]:

1. Acid digestion mixture. Mix 300 ml. 85% phosphoric acid with 50 ml. 5% copper sulfate solution. Carefully add 100 ml. concentrated sulfuric acid. Dilute this mixture with an equal volume of water before use.

2. Nessler solution. Dissolve 45 gm. mercuric iodide and 37.5 gm. potassium iodide in about 200 ml. water and dilute to 500 ml. To 700 ml. 10% sodium hydroxide in a flask add 150 ml. double iodide as prepared previously and 150 ml. water. Allow to stand for a few days and decant from any precipitate formed. The 10% sodium hydroxide used should be fairly accurately standardized at 2.5N (see p. 432). It is advisable to check the alkalinity of the final solution by adding 1 ml. diluted digestion mixture to about 50 ml. water and titrating with the Nessler solution, using a phenolphthalein indicator. From 9-9.3 ml.

Nessler solution should be required to neutralize the acid.

3. Sodium citrate (15%). Dissolve 15 gm. trisodium citrate in water to make 100 ml.

4. Ammonium sulfate standard. Dissolve 0.472 gm. reagent grade ammonium sulfate (previously dried at 100° C.) in water, add a few drops concentrated sulfuric acid, and dilute to 1 L. This solution contains 0.1 mg. nitrogen/ml.

Procedure: Place 5 ml. Folin-Wu filtrate in a large, dry Pyrex digestion tube (25 × 200 mm.) graduated at 50 ml. Add 1 ml. diluted digestion mixture and two small glass beads. Support the tube vertically and boil the contents vigorously with a microburner to evaporate the water. Boil until heavy white fumes of sulfur trioxide begin to fill the tube. Begin heating rather cautiously as there may be some bumping before rapid boiling begins. Also there may be some initial foaming, but this will disappear as the solution concentrates. Remove the flame, cover the tube with a large glass marble or small watch glass, and continue to heat for 2 min., letting the acid mixture boil gently. Care should be taken to prevent appreciable loss of sulfur trioxide fumes. Oxidation is almost always complete by 2 min., as indicated by a clear, pale blue solution; but if this is not the case, further heating is required. Avoid prolonged or excessive heating.

Allow the tubes to cool somewhat, and then add about 30 ml. water and 2 ml. sodium citrate solution. Allow to cool completely to room temperature. During this period prepare a blank and two standards. Add to the blank tube 1 ml. diluted digestion mixture, water, and 2 ml. sodium citrate solution. To the standard tubes add in addition 1 ml. and 2 ml. ammonium sulfate standard, respectively. Dilute all tubes to 50 ml. If the digested samples are cloudy at this point, they may be poured into centrifuge tubes and centrifuged strongly.

Transfer 5 ml. aliquots from each tube to test tubes, add rapidly to each 1.5 ml. Nessler solution, and mix at once. After 10 min., read standards and samples

against blank in a photometer at 460 nm. If for a given instrument the lower standard gives too much absorbance, a somewhat longer wavelength (480 or 500 nm.) may be used or all solutions may be diluted somewhat.

If some samples give too high readings for good comparison with the standards, a smaller aliquot may be taken for color development. But to keep the acidity constant, the sample should be diluted with some of the blank solution instead of water (i.e., take 2.5 ml. of sample plus 2.5 ml. of blank). The color is not too stable and turbidity tends to develop on standing. When high samples must be diluted before color development, other aliquots of the standards and blank should be treated with Nessler solution at the same time.

Calculation: The two standards contain 0.1 and 0.2 mg. nitrogen and are treated exactly like 5 ml. of a 1:10 filtrate, which is equivalent to 0.5 ml. blood. Thus:

$$\frac{OD \text{ sample}}{OD \text{ standard}} \times \frac{0.1 \text{ (or } 0.2) \times 100}{0.5} =$$

$$\frac{OD \text{ sample}}{OD \text{ standard}} \times 20 \text{ (or } 40) = Mg.\% \text{ NPN}$$

Two standards are run since the color does not follow Beer's law too closely and the standard with the absorbance closest to a given sample should be used for the calculation of that sample. Also samples of over 60 mg.% will require further dilution in the manner previously mentioned. This dilution must be taken into account in the calculation.

An **alternative procedure** is to use the **Berthelot reaction** (as in the urease method for BUN) instead of the Nessler solution.[43] Most catalysts used in the digestion interfere with the color reaction, but by using a sufficiently small sample the digestion can be made with sulfuric acid alone. The following is suitable as a **micromethod for NPN** and might be simpler when only an occasional test is done.

Reagents: Ammonia-free water must be used as in the urease method.

1. Phenol reagent and hypochlorite reagent. These are the same reagents

used for the urease method for BUN.

2. Sulfuric acid (2/3N) and sodium tungstate (10%). Use for the preparation of Folin-Wu filtrate.

3. Standard. Dilute the previous NPN standard 1:5 to give a standard containing 0.02 mg./ml. or 2 mg.% nitrogen.

4. Sulfuric acid (30%). Cautiously add 30 ml. concentrated sulfuric acid to about 50 ml. water, cool, and dilute to 100 ml.

5. Sodium hydroxide (1N). Dissolve 4 gm. sodium hydroxide in water to make 100 ml.

Procedure: Prepare a 1:20 Folin-Wu filtrate by adding 0.1 ml. blood to 1.7 ml. water. Then add 0.1 ml. 2/3N sulfuric acid, mix, add 0.1 ml. 10% sodium tungstate, mix, and centrifuge.

Place 0.6 ml. water (blank), 0.1 ml. sample filtrate plus 0.5 ml. water (sample), and 0.1 ml. diluted standard solution for standard in three small Pyrex test tubes. Use "to contain" pipettes for standard and sample, rinsing well with water.

To each tube add 0.1 ml. 30% sulfuric acid and one small glass bead.

Digest carefully over a microburner until the water is driven off and dense white fumes fill the tube. Do not allow the ring of sulfuric acid condensate to go above half the length of the tube. The digest should be water clear; if not, digest further.

Cool, add 1 ml. phenol reagent to each tube, and mix. Then add 1 ml. 1N sodium hydroxide and mix. Immediately add 1 ml. alkaline hypochlorite solution and mix again. Incubate for 15 min. at 37° C.

Add 2 ml. water to each tube, mix, and read in a colorimeter at 600 nm. Read standard and samples against blank. As with the urease method, further dilution or reading at a shorter wavelength may be required to bring the readings of the standard in the desired range (about 50% transmission).

Calculation: Since 0.1 ml. standard containing 2 mg.% nitrogen is treated the same as 0.1 ml. of a 1:20 dilution of the

sample, the standard would be equivalent to $2 \times 20 = 40$ mg.%.

$$\frac{OD \text{ sample}}{OD \text{ standard}} \times 40 = Mg.\% \text{ NPN}$$

Normal values and interpretation[44]: The normal range of NPN values for blood is from 25-45 mg.%. A little more than one half of the nonprotein nitrogen is derived from urea, uric acid, creatinine, ammonia, and amino acids at normal levels. The remainder is made up of the nitrogen of glutathione, purine, pyrimidine compounds, and unknown constituents. Decreased kidney function is the chief cause of increased nonprotein nitrogen. In assessing the course of uremia some workers have considered it more valuable to determine blood urea than nonprotein nitrogen. Sometimes in the early stages of nephritis the variations in urea nitrogen are more readily apparent than changes in the NPN value since the other constituents change less than urea. In eclampsia, hepatic failure, or some other liver diseases there may be a disproportionate rise in NPN as compared to urea; in such instances a NPN determination may be of more value. In the assessment of kidney function the urea level is as satisfactory as the NPN and is technically somewhat simpler.

The concentration of nonprotein nitrogen (and, similarly, urea) in the blood is chiefly determined by the balance between urinary output of nitrogen and the protein catabolism since the kidneys are the main channel for nitrogen excretion. If, for example, in dehydration the amount of fluid available in the body for urine formation is small, the kidneys may not be able to excrete all the nitrogen metabolites and the NPN will rise. If the concentrating powers of the kidneys become impaired, more than the usual volume of urine will be required to sweep out a given amount of nitrogenous metabolites. Diuresis will, up to a certain limit, tend to increase the excretion of nitrogen and lower the NPN, but only to a limit of about 3 L./day. Beyond this, further diuresis does not greatly increase nitrogen excretion. The nonprotein nitrogen (or urea nitrogen) of the blood will not be a good criterion of kidney function unless the urine volume and protein catabolism are taken into account.

URIC ACID[45]

Uric acid is usually determined by its reducing action upon a phosphotungstic acid solution, producing a blue color that is measured in the photometer. Many variations have been introduced in the procedures to reduce interference by other reducing substances present. Since many of these interfering substances are found chiefly in the erythrocytes, better results are obtained by using serum or plasma rather than whole blood. In the method presented the mixture is allowed to stand at an alkaline pH before the addition of the phosphotungstic acid to eliminate some of the interfering substances by oxidation.

Uric acid has also been determined by the use of the enzyme **uricase;** this requires measurement of the absorbance in ultraviolet light, or one can measure the color produced with phosphotungstic acid before and after the oxidation of uric acid by uricase. This method is theoretically more specific, but the simpler methods are sufficiently accurate for most clinical purposes.

Reagents:
1. Phosphotungstic acid (Folin and Denis). Dissolve 50 gm. sodium tungstate in 400 ml. water, add 40 ml. 85% phosphoric acid, and reflux for 2 hr. in an all-glass apparatus. Cool and dilute to 500 ml. This solution is stable indefinitely when stored in a brown bottle and protected from contact with organic matter. For use, dilute a portion 1:10 with water. The diluted solution is stable for about 1 yr. when kept in the refrigerator.
2. Sodium carbonate (10%). Dissolve 100 gm. anhydrous sodium carbonate in water to make 1 L. Filter if cloudy and store in a polyethylene bottle.
3. Tungstic acid. To 800 ml. water add 50 ml. 10% sodium tungstate, 50 ml. 2/3N sulfuric acid (the reagents for Folin-Wu precipitation), and 0.05

ml. 85% phosphoric acid. Dilute to 1000 ml.
4. Uric acid standards:
   A. Stock standard. Dissolve 0.5 gm. lithium carbonate in 150 ml. hot water. Add 1 gm. pure uric acid and swirl to dissolve. When all the acid has dissolved, transfer quantitatively to a 1 L. volumetric flask, using about 300 ml. water. Then add 25 ml. 40% formalin and 3 ml. glacial acetic acid. Dilute with water to 1 L. This solution is stable for 1 yr. if protected from light. It contains 1 mg. uric acid/ml.
   B. Working standard. Dilute 1 ml. stock standard to 200 ml. with water. Store in refrigerator and make up fresh at least every 2 wk. This solution contains 0.5 mg.%/100 ml. and is equivalent to 5 mg.% when equal amounts of the standard and a 1:10 filtrate are used.

Procedure: Mix 9 ml. tungstic acid and 1 ml. serum. Allow to stand for 5 min.; then centrifuge or filter through a retentive paper. Since filtration is rather slow, rapid centrifugation may be preferable. To 5 ml. supernatant or filtrate add 1 ml. 10% sodium carbonate solution, mix, and allow to stand for 10 min. Then add 1 ml. diluted phosphotungstic acid and allow to stand for 30 min. Similarly, treat 5 ml. diluted standard and 5 ml. water as a blank. Read samples and standards against blank at 700 nm. (Since the absorption peak is quite broad, any wavelength between 660 and 720 nm. is satisfactory.)

Calculation: Since 5 ml. standard containing 0.5 mg.% uric acid is treated similarly to 5 ml. of a 1:10 dilution of serum:

$$\frac{\text{OD sample}}{\text{OD standard}} \times 5 = \text{Mg.\% uric acid}$$

Normal values and interpretation: The normal range of uric acid in plasma or serum is 2.5-8.0 mg.%. Some observers have stated that the values are slightly higher in men than in women.[46] Serum or plasma contains about twice as much uric acid as whole blood. Although the older values in the literature were for whole blood, the whole blood level is dependent upon the distribution between the cells and plasma and upon the hematocrit. Since the cells also contain much more of the interfering substances, it is more satisfactory to determine uric acid in plasma or serum.[47]

Increased levels of uric acid are associated with nitrogen retention and the increase in urea, creatinine, and the other nonprotein nitrogenous constituents of the blood. This must often be interpreted as another indication of decreased kidney function. Uric acid is formed from the breakdown of the cell nucleic acids and is often increased in the blood in conditions in which excessive cell breakdown and catabolism of nucleic acids occur. Increases in the blood level have been reported in the acute stages of infectious diseases, excessive exposure to roentgen rays, multiple myeloma, and leukemia. Increased levels of blood uric acid have been found in gout, but the increase may be slight in the early stages of the disease and the amount of the increase in level is not directly related to the severity of the disease.

Procedure for urine: If the urine is cloudy, warm to 60° C. to dissolve any precipitated urates. Dilute 1 ml. urine to 100 ml. with water. Treat 5 ml. of this dilution similarly to the serum filtrate. Note that the urine has been diluted 10 times more than blood (1:100 instead of 1:10) so that in the calculation given the figure 5 is replaced by 50. Depending upon the urine concentration, other dilutions may be necessary to bring the readings to a suitable range.

Normal values and interpretation: The amount of uric acid excreted in the urine depends in part upon the diet. With a diet that is low in purines the amount excreted is usually in the range of 0.3-0.5 gm./day. With an ordinary diet the normal amount excreted may vary more, i.e., from 0.4-0.8 gm./day. Increased excretion is sometimes found in conditions such as leukemia, which also leads to increased blood levels. The excretion of uric acid is usually increased during an attack of gout.

CREATININE AND CREATINE[48-50]

Creatinine is usually determined by quantitating the reddish color formed when an **alkaline picrate solution** is added to a creatinine solution (**Jaffé reaction**). Creatine is not estimated directly, but is usually determined after conversion to creatinine by heating with acid. In a mixture of the two substances the preformed creatinine is first determined in one aliquot, a second aliquot is heated with acid to convert any creatine present to creatinine, and the total creatinine is determined in this sample. The creatine is then determined by the difference.

In earlier methods the creatinine was often determined in whole blood. However, it has been shown by enzymatic methods that, although almost all of the material in plasma that gave a color with the Jaffé reaction was creatinine, less than 50% of such material in erythrocytes was actually creatinine. Since creatinine is apparently evenly distributed between the water of the cells and plasma, it seems more logical to determine the creatinine in plasma or serum. The creatine of the blood is chiefly in the cells; since the heating with acid necessary to convert the creatine to creatinine may further increase the noncreatinine chromogens, the measurement of creatine in whole blood is of little value. The creatine content of serum or plasma is very low, especially in adults, and there is some question as to whether the substance measured is actually creatine.

For most clinical purposes, creatinine may be determined directly in a Folin-Wu filtrate or in diluted urine with sufficient accuracy. It has been suggested, however, that for the measurement of creatinine clearance (where a slight overestimation of the creatinine concentration would be of more significance) the creatinine determination in plasma or serum should include the additional purification step of absorption of **Lloyd reagent.** This method is given as an alternative.

Reagents:
1. Sulfuric acid (2/3N) and sodium tungstate (10%). These are the

same reagents used in the regular Folin-Wu precipitation.

2. Picric acid (0.04M). The picric acid as purchased usually contains 10-12% water. Dissolve 10.5 gm. in water to make 1 L. If a good quality of reagent grade chemical is used, recrystallization is not required.

3. Sodium hydroxide (0.75N). Dissolve 30 gm. sodium hydroxide in water to make 1 L. Store in a polyethylene or alkali-resistant bottle.

4. Creatinine standards:
   A. Stock standard. Dissolve 150 mg. pure creatinine and 1 ml. concentrated hydrochloric acid in water to make 100 ml. This solution contains 1.5 mg./ml. and is stable when kept in the refrigerator.
   B. Working standard. Dilute 1 ml. stock standard with water to 100 ml. This solution contains 0.015 mg. creatinine/ml. It is not stable and should be prepared as needed.

Procedure for serum creatinine: To 2 ml. serum in a test tube add 3 ml. water and 1 ml. 10% sodium tungstate and mix. Then add 2 ml. 2/3N sulfuric acid, stopper, and mix well by inversion. Centrifuge at 2000 rpm for 5 min. Add 3 ml. centrifugate to a test tube. In another tube place 3 ml. water as a blank. Also set up tubes containing 1, 2, and 3 ml. working standard diluted to 3 ml. with water (when necessary). To each tube add 1 ml. picric acid and 1 ml. sodium hydroxide solution. Mix and, after standing at room temperature for 20 min., read in a photometer. Read samples and standards against the blank at 520 nm.

Calculation:

$$\text{Mg.\% creatinine} =$$

$$\frac{\text{OD sample}}{\text{OD standard}} \times \frac{8 \times 100}{2 \times 3} \times S =$$

$$\frac{\text{OD sample}}{\text{OD standard}} \times 133 \times (S)$$

In this calculation 2 ml. serum is diluted to 8 ml. in preparing the filtrate and 3 ml. of this is used in the color reaction; S is the actual amount of creatinine added to the standard tube, i.e., 0.015, 0.030, or 0.045 mg., when 1, 2, or 3 ml. of the working standard is used. Since Beer's law is not followed for this reaction, it is advisable to run several standards and use the standard giving a reading closest to that of a given sample for the calculation of that sample. Unless there is reason to believe the serum creatinine may be elevated, the lowest standard is usually sufficient. If the result is more than 8 mg.%, the determination should be repeated, using instead of 3 ml. supernatant, 1 ml. supernatant and 2 ml. water and multiplying the result by 3.

Procedure for serum creatine: The serum preformed creatinine must first be determined by the previous procedure. To determine the creatine, set up in graduated centrifuge tubes a blank containing 6 ml. water, a standard containing 1 ml. of the working standard used before plus 5 ml. water, and a sample tube containing 3 ml. water and 3 ml. of the same protein-free centrifugate as obtained previously. To each tube add 1 ml. picric acid solution and heat the tubes in a boiling water bath for about 2 hr. until the volume is reduced to below 4 ml. Remove from the bath, cool, and dilute to 4 ml. with water. Add to each tube 1 ml. 0.75N sodium hydroxide, mix, and read after 20 min. as for serum creatinine. The calculations are the same. It may be convenient to determine the serum creatinine first and then use the closest standard only for the total creatinine, or all three standards may be carried through the procedure.

$$\text{(Total creatinine - Preformed creatinine)} \times 1.16 = \text{Creatine}$$

Where 1.16 is the ratio of the molecular weight of creatine to creatinine.

Procedure for urine: The urine is diluted 1:100 and 3 ml. diluted urine is carried through the same procedure as for the serum centrifugate. Since the urine is diluted 1:100 instead of 1:4, the equations given must be multiplied by an additional factor of 25. Because of the greater variation in urine creatinine, it is usually advisable to run all three standards, and one may require another dilution of urine as well. It may be well to check the pH of the urine; if it is strongly acid or alkaline, add a few drops of acid or base during the dilution so that the diluted sample is approximately neutral.

Procedure with Lloyd reagent:

Additional reagents:

1. Lloyd reagent.*
2. Oxalic acid (saturated solution). Add about 18 gm. oxalic acid to 100 ml. water and shake until saturated.

Serum creatinine: Prepare a tungstic acid filtrate (as previously described). Set up tubes containing 5 ml. water as a blank, 3 ml. centrifugate plus 2 ml. water for sample, and 1, 2, or 3 ml. working standard made up to 5 ml. with water as a standard. To each tube add 0.5 ml. saturated oxalic acid and approximately 100 mg. Lloyd reagent. Stopper and shake at intervals during 15 min. Centrifuge the tubes strongly, decant off the supernatant, and drain. To each tube add 3 ml. water, 1 ml. picric acid solution, and 1 ml. 0.75N sodium hydroxide solution. Stopper and shake intermittently during 15 min. Centrifuge strongly, pour off the supernatant into cuvettes, and read in a photometer at 520 nm., reading samples and standards against the blank.

Calculation: The calculation is exactly the same as for the previous method.

Serum creatine: Prepare the protein-free centrifugate and heat in the boiling water bath exactly as in the previous method for creatine. After heating, dilute to about 5 ml. with water and add 0.5 ml. saturated oxalic acid and 100 mg. Lloyd reagent. Stopper and shake at intervals during 15 min. Centrifuge and decant. Treat the precipitate with 3 ml. water, 1 ml. picric acid, and 1 ml. sodium hydroxide. Shake, centrifuge, decant, and read exactly as for creatinine.

Calculation: The calculation is exactly the same as for the previous method.

Urine creatinine and creatine: Prepare a 1:100 dilution of urine and carry through the procedure the same as for serum centrifugates. Take into account the additional dilution in the calculation.

Normal values and interpretation: The normal values of creatinine in serum are from 0.6-1.2 mg.%. In chronic nephritis, when the blood urea nitrogen is above 50 mg.%, the creatinine rise is roughly proportional and values of over 5 mg.% are considered of grave diagnostic importance. In obstruction of the urinary tract and in acute nephritis the creatinine may be relatively higher than the urea and high values (10-15 mg.%) are not so unfavorable. Low values have been found in muscular dystrophy.

Creatine is found chiefly in the erythrocytes. The amount in serum is about 0.5-0.9 mg.%, but not all of this may actually be creatine.

BLOOD AMMONIA[51-53]

Blood ammonia is determined by laking the blood with water and absorbing the ammonia on an ion exchange resin. After the resin is washed, the ammonia is eluted and determined by the Berthelot phenol-hypochlorite reaction used in the determination of urea by urease. The blood may be collected with **potassium oxalate** or **heparin** as an anticoagulant, but it has been claimed that some brands of heparin will cause high results. Obviously the ammonium salt of heparin should not be used. Apparently the amount of ammonia in the blood increases quite rapidly after the blood is drawn, so analysis must be carried out as rapidly as possible. Immediately after collection of the sample, the blood should be cooled in ice. If determination cannot be performed within an hour or so, the specimen may be preserved by rapidly freezing in a mixture of dry ice and alcohol and storing in a freezer until ready for analysis.

Reagents: Ammonia-free deionized water must be used throughout.

1. Sodium chloride (4N). Dissolve 23.4 gm. sodium chloride in water and dilute to 100 ml.
2. Phenol reagent and alkaline hypochlorite. The same reagents are used as in the urease method for urea.
3. Ion exchange resin. Permutit Q,* so-

---

*A purified fuller's earth available from pharmaceutical supply houses.

*Permutit Co., New York, N. Y.; Ionac Chemical Co., Birmingham, N. J.

dium form (60-80 mesh size). The resin in the sodium form must be converted to hydrogen form and freed of ammonia. Digest 1 vol. resin with 5 vol. 1% sodium hydroxide for 1 hr. at 60° C. and wash with ammonia-free water until free of base. Then add 30 vol. 2% acetic acid/vol. resin. Stir the mixture well and allow the resin to settle. Wash resin with water by decantation five times and store moist in an airtight container.

4. Ammonia standard. Dissolve 70.7 mg. ammonium sulfate in water containing a few drops of sulfuric acid and dilute to 100 ml. This solution contains 15 mg.% ammonia nitrogen or 18.2 mg.% ammonia. For use, dilute 0.1 ml. standard and 0.3 ml. 4N NaCl with water to 10 ml. This standard contains 150 μg% ammonia nitrogen. (The standard used for the NPN procedure which contains 5 mg.% nitrogen can be used, taking 0.3 ml. and diluting to 10 ml.) This diluted standard should be made up fresh daily as required.

Procedure: Add 1 ml. blood to 2 ml. water and mix. Also set up a standard tube containing 1 ml. standard plus 2 ml. water and a blank tube containing 3 ml. water. To each tube add about 0.4 gm. wet resin and stopper. Mix well with gentle agitation for 5 min. Then add 10 ml. water to each tube and mix. Allow resin to settle and decant off water without loss of resin. Wash resin with two more 10 ml. portions of water. After second washing, add 1 ml. phenol reagent. Allow to stand for 3 min., occasionally mixing gently. Add 1 ml. alkaline hypochlorite and mix well. Incubate at 37° C. for 15 min. Add 3 ml. more water and read standard and sample against blank at 630 nm. If readings are too high, dilute sample or use a shorter wavelength. (See discussion of urease method.)

Calculation: If a 150 μg% standard has been used:

$$\frac{\text{OD sample}}{\text{OD standard}} \times 150 =$$

μg% blood ammonia nitrogen

Ammonia nitrogen × 1.22 = Ammonia

NOTE: If only an occasional ammonia determination is made, it may be more convenient to use the Ammonia Test Kit.* This contains all the reagents for the test, together with some additional resin for use in preparing ammonia-free water.

Normal values and interpretation: There is still some uncertainty as to the normal range of levels in whole blood. The older diffusion methods undoubtedly gave too high results due to the use of strong alkali that released additional ammonia from proteins or amino acids. Also, when comparing the results in the literature, one must note that some investigators report the results in terms of ammonia and others in terms of ammonia nitrogen. Using the previous method, the normal range may be from 35-100 μg% ammonia nitrogen. Since ammonia is removed from the blood chiefly by the liver with the formation of urea, the ammonia level rises in severe liver disease. Some of the toxic symptoms of hepatic coma are believed to be due to high blood concentrations of ammonia. Levels of over 150 μg% are usually indicative of severe liver damage.

AMINO ACID NITROGEN[54, 55]

Most amino acids react with ninhydrin to form a blue color when heated at a pH of over 3. The reaction is almost exclusively with the alpha amino acid nitrogen. Not all of the amino acid will give the color. Different amino acids give slightly different amounts of color on a molar basis, but the method is satisfactory for most clinical purposes. Some other nitrogen compounds also give a color with the reagent. In the method presented the use of a non-aqueous solvent greatly reduces the interference of urea, and ammonia is eliminated from urine by a preliminary treatment.

Reagents:
1. Carbonate buffer. Dissolve 14.3 gm. anhydrous sodium carbonate and 2.66 gm. sodium bicarbonate in water and dilute to 1 L.
2. Ethylenediaminetetraacetic   a c i d

*Hyland Laboratories, Los Angeles, Calif.

(EDTA) buffer. Dissolve 50 gm. disodium EDTA in about 900 ml. water and add 18.7 ml. glacial acetic acid and 10 ml. 1N sodium hydroxide. Dilute to 1 L. Check the pH and adjust to 3.7 if necessary.

3. Ninhydrin reagent. Dissolve 200 mg. ninhydrin in 100 ml. ethylene glycol. The material may dissolve rather slowly. The solution is stable for a few weeks when kept in the refrigerator.

4. Sodium tungstate and sulfuric acid. The same solutions are used as for preparation of a Folin-Wu filtrate.

5. Amino acid nitrogen standards:
   A. Stock standard. Dissolve 0.268 gm. glycine, 0.525 gm. glutamic acid, and 1 gm. sodium benzoate in about 400 ml. water. Add 4 ml. concentrated hydrochloric acid and dilute to 500 ml. This solution contains 20 mg.% alpha amino acid nitrogen and is quite stable.
   B. Working standard. Dilute 5 ml. stock standard and 0.5 ml. 1N sodium hydroxide to 100 ml. This solution contains 1 mg.% amino acid nitrogen. The pH of the diluted standard should be approximately neutral. The pH can be checked with narrow-range paper and the sodium hydroxide can be varied if necessary to bring the solution to near neutrality.

Procedure for plasma: Plasma (oxalated or heparinized) must be used since clotting causes an increase in the free amino acids. Prepare a 1:5 Folin-Wu filtrate using 1 ml. plasma, 3 ml. water, 0.5 ml. 2/3N sulfuric acid, and 0.5 ml. sodium tungstate. When this is centrifuged strongly, one can readily obtain 2 ml. clear supernatant. To 2 ml. supernatant add 0.5 ml. carbonate buffer and 2 ml. EDTA buffer. Similarly, set up 2 ml. diluted standard and 2 ml. water as a blank. Add 0.5 ml. of the mixture from each tube to separate tubes. To these add 6 ml. ninhydrin reagent and heat in a boiling water bath for 20 min. Cool and read samples and standards against blank at 570 nm.

Calculation: Since the diluted standard contains 1 mg.% amino acid nitrogen and is treated the same as a 1:5 dilution of plasma:

$$\frac{OD \text{ sample}}{OD \text{ standard}} \times 5 =$$

Mg.% alpha amino acid nitrogen

Procedure for urine: Urine requires a preliminary treatment to remove most of the ammonia that reacts to some extent with the reagent. The relative amount of ammonia present in plasma is negligible. The urine must be diluted with water. Unless abnormal values are expected, it is convenient to dilute the urine on the basis of the 24 hr. urine volume. If the volume is over 2 L., dilute the urine 5 ml. to 25 ml. For volumes between 1 and 2 L., dilute 5 ml. to 50 ml.; for lower urine volumes, dilute 5 ml. to 100 ml. In making the dilution, check the pH and add a few drops of acid or base as required before diluting to the mark so that the final dilution is approximately neutral. Pipette 2 ml. diluted urine to a 25 ml. Erlenmeyer flask, add 0.5 ml. carbonate buffer, and mix well. In the lower end of a one-hole rubber stopper that will fit the flask, insert a rolled up square of filter paper until it projects about 15 mm. from the bottom of the stopper. Moisten the filter paper with a drop or two of 1:10 sulfuric acid and insert stopper into flask, taking care that the paper does not touch the sides of the flask. Allow to stand at room temperature for 2-3 hr.; then remove stopper and discard paper. Add to the flask 2 ml. EDTA buffer and mix well. Also mix together 2 ml. diluted standard, 0.5 ml. carbonate buffer, and 2 ml. EDTA buffer. Prepare a blank by repeating the procedure, using water instead of the standard solution. Place 0.5 ml. of the mixtures from samples, standard, and blank in test tubes. Add to each tube 6 ml. ninhydrin reagent, mix, and heat in boiling water bath for 20 min. Cool and read standards and samples against blank at 570 nm.

Calculation: Since 2 ml. diluted urine

and 2 ml. diluted standard containing 1 mg.% amino acid nitrogen are treated similarly:

$$\frac{\text{OD sample}}{\text{OD standard}} \times 1 \times \frac{B}{A} =$$

Mg.% amino acid nitrogen

and

$$\text{Mg.\%} \times \frac{\text{Total volume in ml.}}{100} =$$

Total amino acid nitrogen excreted

where "A" ml. urine is diluted to a total volume of "B" ml.

Normal values and interpretation: Somewhat different values have been reported for plasma amino acid nitrogen, depending upon the method used. The usual range is 3.5-7 mg.%. Deamination of amino acids occurs in the liver, but this is impaired when there is severe liver damage. In acute yellow atrophy, values up to 20 mg.% have been noted. In acute infectious and toxic hepatitis and in chronic hepatitis the values are generally normal. Slight increases have been noted in advanced renal failure when the other nonprotein nitrogen constituents are also elevated.

In urine the amino acid nitrogen excretion is usually in the range of 50-200 mg./24 hr. It varies somewhat with the protein intake. It is higher with an increased intake. In those conditions in which the blood level of amino acids is increased without impaired kidney function, there may be some increase in the amount excreted. Very high levels have been found in Wilson's disease (hepatolenticular degeneration), with levels of over 1000 mg./day.

TOTAL NITROGEN BY MICRO-KJELDAHL METHOD[56-58]

The micro-Kjeldahl method may be used for the determination of total protein in blood serum as a check on the serum used for a standard in the biuret reaction for protein or for the determination of the total amount of protein or other nitrogenous compounds in other samples. Nitrogen is converted to ammonia by digestion with sulfuric acid and sodium sulfate, with the addition of selenium as a catalyst. The ammonia is distilled from an alkaline solution into a boric acid indicator solution and is titrated with standard acid.

Reagents:
1. Digestion mixture. Dissolve 15 gm. reagent grade sodium sulfate in 100 ml. water. Add slowly, with agitation and cooling, 100 ml. reagent grade sulfuric acid.
2. Selenized granules.*
3. Mixed indicator solution. Dissolve 0.1 gm. methyl red indicator in 100 ml. 95% ethyl alcohol. Dissolve 0.1 gm. bromcresol green indicator in 100 ml. 95% ethyl alcohol. Mix 1 part methyl red solution with 5 parts bromcresol green solution.
4. Boric acid indicator solution. Dissolve 20 gm. reagent grade boric acid in 1000 ml. distilled water, warming if necessary to aid solution. Cool and add 15 ml. mixed indicator solution. It may be helpful to vary the proportion of indicator somewhat to get the sharpest end point. To test this, add 15 ml. boric acid solution to a 125 ml. Erlenmeyer flask and then add 15 ml. distilled water and a drop or two of concentrated ammonia. Titrate with the 0.02N acid. The color change should be from green to almost colorless (end point) to pink.
5. Sodium hydroxide (50%). Dissolve 50 gm. sodium hydroxide in distilled water to make 100 ml. Keep in a polyethylene bottle.
6. Sulfuric acid (0.02N). Dilute 20 ml. 1N sulfuric acid (accurately standardized) to 1000 ml. with distilled water.

Special apparatus: A nitrogen still (Fig. 6-9) is connected to the 100 ml. Kjeldahl flask with a tight-fitting rubber stopper.

A fume hood or other device is necessary for removal of sulfuric acid fumes. If only a few digestions are made, a funnel connected to a water aspirator (made

---

*No. 132, Henger Co., Philadelphia, Pa., or may be obtained from most laboratory supply houses.

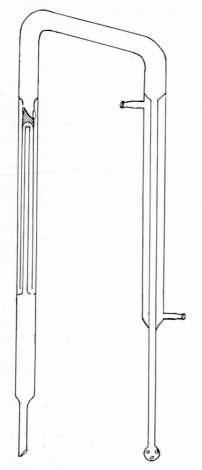

Fig. 6-9. Nitrogen still.

neath the other solution in the flask. Carefully withdraw the tube and, without mixing, connect the flask to the distillation apparatus prepared to collect the distillate in a 125 ml. Erlenmeyer flask containing 15 ml. boric acid indicator solution and sufficient distilled water to cover the end of the delivery tube (ammonia absorption tube) by at least 2 cm. Mix the contents of the flask by swirling and distill for 10 min. Then lower the receiving flask so that the liquid level is below the end of the delivery tube and continue the distillation for 3 min. more. Rinse the delivery tube with water. Titrate the distillate with 0.02N acid to the end point. Run a blank on the reagents by carrying through the digestion, distillation, and titration, using 5 ml. distilled water instead of the sample. The blank need be determined only when new reagents are used.

Calculations:

$$\begin{aligned}(\text{Ml. titration of sample} - \text{Ml. titration of blank}) \\ \times\ 0.28\ =\ \text{Mg. nitrogen in sample aliquot}\end{aligned}$$

$$\text{Nitrogen} \times 6.50 = \text{Protein}$$

For the total protein of serum the calculation would be:

$$\frac{(\text{Sample titration} - \text{Blank titration}) \times 0.28 \times 6.50}{\text{Ml. serum used} \times 1000}$$
$$\times\ 100\ =\ \text{Gm. protein/100 ml.}$$

Five milliliters of a 1:25 dilution is equivalent to 0.2 ml. serum. Hence:

$$\begin{aligned}\text{Gm.\% protein} = (\text{Sample titration} - \text{Blank} \\ \text{titration}) \times 0.910\end{aligned}$$

For accurate results on the total protein a correction must be made for the nonprotein nitrogen, as determined separately. The correction is mg.% NPN × 0.0650, which is subtracted from the total protein as previously determined. For normal sera the correction is small, and one may assume the NPN to be 25 mg. %, giving a correction of 0.16 gm. protein/100 ml. without serious error.

TOTAL PROTEIN, ALBUMIN, AND GLOBULIN[59-62]

Proteins are determined by reaction with an alkaline copper solution that

of glass or polyethylene) placed over the mouth of the digestion flask may be satisfactory.

Procedure: Pipette a sample containing 2-3 mg. nitrogen (for serum, 5 ml. of a 1:25 dilution with 0.9% sodium chloride or 0.2 ml. accurately measured) to a 100 ml. Kjeldahl flask. Add 5 ml. digestion mixture and a selenized granule. Heat over a microburner. Digest carefully at first to avoid foaming and then heat more strongly. Heat until clear; then heat for 2 hr. longer. Cool, add 30 ml. distilled water, and cool again. Connect a funnel to a length of glass tubing so that it will reach the bottom of the Kjeldahl flask and carefully add 12 ml. 50% sodium hydroxide so that it forms a layer be-

forms a dark blue-violet color (**biuret reaction**). The proteins are separated by precipitating the globulin by the addition of a concentrated sulfate-sulfite solution, determining the albumin in the remaining solution, and calculating the globulin by the difference.

Reagents:

1. Sodium hydroxide ([a] 0.2N and [b] 0.2N with 0.5% potassium iodide). (See p. 432 for preparation of standard acids and bases.) Add 5 gm. potassium iodide/L. to 0.2N sodium hydroxide to get solution b.

2. Stock biuret solution. Dissolve 45 gm. sodium potassium tartrate (Rochelle salt) in approximately 400 ml. 0.2N sodium hydroxide solution. Add, while stirring, 15 gm. copper sulfate ($CuSO_4 \cdot 5H_2O$) as fine crystals and continue to stir until the copper salt is completely dissolved. Add 5 gm. potassium iodide and dilute to 1000 ml. with 0.2N sodium hydroxide solution.

3. Dilute biuret solution. Dilute 200 ml. stock biuret solution to 1000 ml. with 0.2N sodium hydroxide solution containing 5 gm. potassium iodide/L.

4. Tartrate-iodide solution. Dissolve 9 gm. Rochelle salt in 0.2N sodium hydroxide containing 0.5% potassium iodide and dilute to 1 L. with this solution.

5. Ether (ethyl). Reagent grade is preferable but not absolutely necessary. The alcohol content must not be too great.

6. Standard serum. This method requires a standard serum. There is available commercially a number of satisfactory control sera, or pooled serum that has been accurately analyzed by the micro-Kjeldahl method may be used.

7. Sulfate-sulfite solution. Place 208 gm. anhydrous sodium sulfate and 70 gm. sodium sulfite in a 2 L. beaker. To 900 ml. distilled water in a separate container add 2 ml. concentrated sulfuric acid. Add the acidified water at once to the salts while stirring. When dissolved, transfer to a 1000 ml. volumetric flask and dilute to the mark. This solution should be stored at a temperature above 25° C. at all times.

Procedure for total protein only: Add 0.1 ml. serum (measured exactly with a calibrated Folin micropipette or other high-precision pipette calibrated "to contain") to 5 ml. biuret reagent, rinsing the pipette with the biuret reagent several times. Add 0.1 ml. water to 5 ml. biuret reagent as a blank. Also set up a serum blank by measuring 5 ml. tartrate-iodide solution and adding 0.1 ml. serum. The serum blank is essential only when opalescent or highly pigmented sera are used, but accuracy is improved by using it routinely. Set up a standard using 0.1 ml. serum of known protein content (or commercial protein standard) added to 5 ml. biuret reagent; also include a serum blank for the standard.

Place the cuvette in a water bath at 30°-32° C. for 10 min. (a pan of water adjusted to this temperature is satisfactory).

Read the samples and standards at 555 nm., using the biuret blank for zero setting. Also read the serum blanks at this wavelength, using the tartrate-iodide solution for zero setting.

Calculation for total protein only: Calculate K for the standard, using the OD of the standard serum biuret solution minus the OD of the standard serum blank. Then for the sample:

$$\%\text{Protein} = K \times (\text{OD sample biuret solution} - \text{OD samples serum blank})$$

Procedure for total protein, albumin, and globulin: Since the sulfate-sulfite solution tends to crystallize below approximately 25° C., all solutions and glassware must be kept above this temperature.

Measure 7.5 ml. sulfate-sulfite solution into an 18 × 120 mm. test tube. Add slowly, with continuous mixing, 0.5 ml. serum. Stopper and mix by inversion. Immediately pipette 2 ml. for total protein determination, adding it to 5 ml. biuret reagent. To the remainder of the protein suspension add 3 ml. ether, stopper, and shake exactly 40 times in 20 sec. This is a critical part of the procedure. Violent shaking should be avoided; an excursion of the arm about 15 in., 40 times in 20 sec., is optimal. Centrifuge the tubes for 10 min. at 2000 rpm. Tilt the tube to permit insertion of a 2 ml. pipette into the clear solution below the layer of globulin and, without disturbing the precipitate, remove 2 ml. solution and add it to 5 ml. biuret reagent; this is the albumin sample.

A standard should also be run. Since one does carry through the entire fractionation, a smaller quantity of standard can be used in the same proportion; i.e., add 0.2 ml. standard protein solution (accurately measured) to 3 ml. sulfate-sulfite, mix, and pipette 2 ml. of this solution into 5 ml. biuret reagent. If the serum is opalescent or highly pigmented, it may be advisable to run a serum blank. For highest accuracy a serum blank should always be run. Since the blank is relatively small, it can be measured with sufficient accuracy by adding 0.13 ml. serum (with a serologic pipette or a pipette graduated in 0.01 ml.) to a mixture of 5 ml. tartrate-iodide solution and 1.9 ml. sulfate-sulfite solution.

Place the biuret solutions containing standard and samples in a water bath at 30° C. for 10 min. Remove, cool to room temperature, and read in photometer at 555 nm., setting to zero with a blank of a mixture of 5 ml. biuret solution and 2 ml. sulfate-sulfite solution. Also read the serum blanks run at the same wavelength, setting the photometer to zero with tartrate-iodide solution.

Calculation for total protein, albumin, and globulin: The calculation is similar to that given previously for determining total protein alone. For each sample or standard, subtract the OD reading for the serum blank from that for the biuret reaction. With the corrected OD for the standard, calculate K using the given concentration of the standard in gm.% directly. Then when the aliquots recommended are used:

$$K \times (\text{Corr. OD}) =$$
$$\%\,\text{Total protein or albumin}$$
$$\text{Globulin} =$$
$$\text{Total protein} - \text{Albumin}$$

If after a number of standards have been run it is found that the K for the standards is quite constant, it may be sufficiently accurate to use this K without actually determining it every time a sample is run, but it must be checked each time a new batch of biuret reagent is used.

Normal values and interpretation: The normal range for total protein is 6-8 gm. %; for albumin, 4-5.5 gm.%; and for globulin, 1.5-3 gm.%. The albumin-globulin (A/G) ratio is usually between 1.5:1 and 2.5:1.

An increase in total protein is found in hemoconcentration due to dehydration from loss of fluid (vomiting, diarrhea, etc.). In such cases both the albumin and globulins increase in the same proportion so that the A/G ratio remains practically unchanged. This is the only instance in which an increase in albumin is found. In instances of increased total protein the albumin is unchanged or slightly decreased, whereas the globulin increases; as a result the A/G ratio falls markedly. Increases in globulins are found in severe liver disease, some infectious diseases, and multiple myeloma. The changes in liver disease will be discussed further in the section on liver function tests. The increases in infectious diseases may be due to increases in gamma globulins, which are the protein fractions concerned with antibody formation. The increases in multiple myeloma may be striking, with globulin concentrations up to 6% or more.

Low total protein levels are usually associated with low albumin levels, which are usually accompanied by a lesser change in globulins, so that the A/G ratio again is low. A low albumin level may be due to increased loss of albumin in the urine, decreased formation in the liver, or insufficient protein intake. Low serum protein levels may also be found in conditions in which there is severe hemorrhage since the plasma volume after hemorrhage is restored more rapidly than the protein level.

A low albumin level, if continued for any length of time, is one of the causes of edema since the oncotic pressure is such that water is able to pass from the serum into the tissue space and edema results. Agammaglobulinemia is a relatively rare condition, often due to a genetic metabolic defect, in which the gamma globulins are very low or nearly absent. The other blood fractions are relatively normal.

Protein in cerebrospinal fluid and urine: The biuret color reaction is not sensitive enough for analysis of protein in cerebrospinal fluid and urine. The **turbidimetric method** of Henry et al.[63] is chosen for these analyses.

Principle: The fluid is treated with trichloroacetic acid to precipitate the proteins as a fine suspension. The resulting turbidity is measured photometrically and is compared with protein standards similarly treated.

Reagents:

1. Trichloroacetic acid (TCA) (12.5%). Dissolve 12.5 gm. trichloroacetic acid in water and dilute to 100 ml.
2. Sodium chloride (0.85%). Dissolve 0.85 gm. sodium chloride in water and dilute to 100 ml.
3. Protein standard. Any clear normal serum of known protein concentration or commercially available control serum may be used. It should be diluted with 0.85% NaCl to a final protein concentration of 25 mg./ml. This dilution should be prepared on the day of use.

Procedure for cerebrospinal fluid: Set up two test tubes labeled standard and sample. Add 4 ml. diluted standard to standard tube; add 1 ml. clear spinal fluid (centrifuge if cloudy) and 3 ml. 0.85 NaCl to sample tube. To each tube add 1 ml. 12.5% TCA and mix immediately. Let stand between 5 and 10 min. and read OD in photometer at 420 nm. against a water blank. Tubes must be mixed before reading and care must be taken to avoid entrapment of air bubbles in the suspension.

Calculation:

$$\text{Mg.\% protein} = \frac{\text{OD unknown}}{\text{OD standard}} \times 100$$

Since 4 ml. standard containing 1 mg. protein is compared with 1 ml. spinal fluid, the factor of 100 is used to convert to mg./100 ml.

NOTE: If OD for the unknown is above the range following Beer's law, the sample must be repeated using a smaller amount and proper adjustment must be made in the calculation.

Procedure for urine: Set up three test tubes labeled standard, sample, and blank. To the standard tube add 4 ml. diluted protein standard; to the sample tube add 4 ml. clear urine (centrifuge if turbid); and to the blank tube add 4 ml. clear urine plus 1 ml. water. Add 1 ml. TCA to standard and sample tubes and mix immediately. Let stand between 5 and 10 min. and read OD in a photometer at 420 nm. Read the standard tube against water and the sample tube against urine blank. Before reading, tubes must be thoroughly mixed and entrapment of air bubbles in the suspension must be avoided.

NOTE: If OD for the unknown is above the range of Beer's law, the sample must be repeated using a smaller amount and proper adjustment must be made in the calculation.

Calculation:

$$\text{Mg.\% protein} = \frac{\text{OD of unknown}}{\text{OD of standard}}$$
$$\times 1 \times \frac{100}{4}$$

For 24 hr. urine protein the mg.% is multiplied by the total volume in liters to obtain the protein per day.

NOTES: Although Beer's law is usually obeyed up to an absorbance of about 0.8-1, the limitations of the photometer used should always be checked.

Analyses of xanthochromic spinal fluids may be inaccurate and it is suggested that a blank similar to that used for urine be run for color correction.

When certain drugs are excreted in the urine, the urine blank shows a different color than the urine to which acid has been added. In this case the method should not be used.

Normal values and interpretation[64]: The protein content of normal lumbar spinal fluid ranges between 15 and 45 mg.% and contains mostly albumin. Cisternal fluid has, on the average, a slightly lower level—about 20 mg.%. Ventricular fluids have appreciably lower levels—about 10 mg.%.

The most common abnormality found in spinal fluid is an increase in protein. In many conditions this increase is small, rarely exceeding 100 mg.%. In different types of meningitis, polyneuritis, and tumors, increases up to 400 mg.% may be found.

The normal protein content of urine ranges between 25 and 70 mg.%/24 hr. urine output. Normal newborn infants may have significant proteinuria during the first 5 days of life.

Significant increases in urine protein are found in nephrosis, where several gm.% may be found. Variable amounts of protein are found in the urine in various destructive lesions of the kidneys, but these amounts never approach the quantity found in nephrosis.

Electrophoresis: Fractionation of serum proteins by electrophoresis (Tiselius) is based on their rate of movement in an electric field. At constant field strength the rate for the different protein molecules will depend on their size (weight) and net electric charge. Since the latter will vary with the pH, electrophoresis is usually carried out in a buffered solution. Of the principal fractions of serum or plasma, albumin (the smallest molecule) generally moves the most rapidly; then, in order, alpha globulins, beta globulins, fibrinogen (in plasma), and gamma globulins.

Separation of the different protein fractions is relatively simple; the problem is how to estimate the fractions after separation. In the classic method devised by Tiselius,[65] electrophoresis was carried out in solution and the amount of different fractions present was determined by refined optical methods based on refractive index gradients. This method resulted in patterns similar to those shown in Fig. 6-10, where the amount of each fraction is proportional to the area under the respective peaks. Other methods give similar patterns, except that serum is generally used instead of plasma, so that the fibrinogen peak is absent. The Tiselius

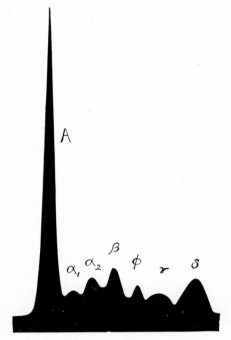

Fig. 6-10. Electrophoretic pattern of normal human plasma, ascending pattern. **A,** Albumin; α_1 and α_2, alpha globulins; β, beta globulin; ϕ, fibrinogen; γ, gamma globulin; δ, salt effect. (Courtesy Dr. H. R. Pearsall.)

method is regarded as the most accurate, but it is rather tedious and requires expensive apparatus. For clinical purposes the simpler methods are more commonly used.

Paper electrophoresis[66-68]: In paper electrophoresis the separation of proteins is carried out on paper strips moistened with a buffer solution. When a small amount of serum is applied near one end of the strip and an electric potential is applied along the strip that is kept moistened with buffer, the proteins will migrate along the strip at different rates. After a suitable period the strip is removed and dried. The proteins are fixed with acetic acid and then stained with a dye (bromphenol blue is now generally used). A series of colored bands will appear along the strip, corresponding to the different separated proteins; the albumin will migrate the greatest distance from the starting point. The amount of color in each band is proportional to

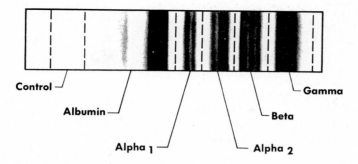

Fig. 6-11. For the elution technique, cut fractions at dotted lines.

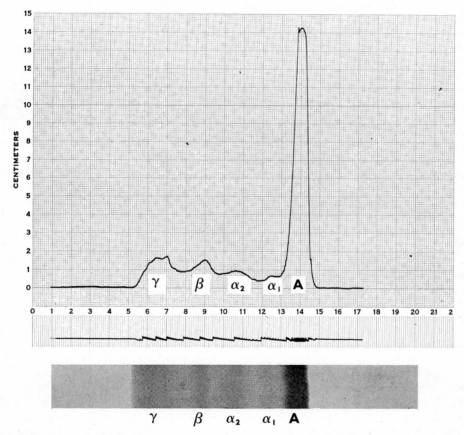

Fig. 6-12. Paper electrophoretic pattern of normal human serum. **A**, Albumin; α_1 and α_2, alpha globulins; β, beta globulins; and γ, gamma globulins.

the amount of protein present. The paper strip may be cut crosswise into a number of smaller pieces, each corresponding to one of the bands (Fig. 6-11). The dye can be eluted from the pieces with a definite amount of sodium hydroxide solution and the intensity of the resulting color is measured in a photometer at 590 nm. The optical density will be proportional to the amount of protein in that particular band. From these results the relative percentages of the individual protein fractions can be calculated. If the total protein is determined in another aliquot by the usual chemical methods, then the absolute amount of protein in each fraction can be calculated.

Instead of eluting the dye the color can be measured directly on the paper strip with a recording densitometer, obtaining a curve similar to that in Fig. 6-12, and from this, the proportion of proteins can be calculated. A number of manufacturers make types of apparatus for paper electrophoresis of serum proteins. The paper electrophoretic method is relatively simple, but it requires about 16 hr. to complete the electrophoresis, and the inevitable homogeneities in the paper cause some errors.

Cellulose acetate electrophoresis[69]: Recent methods have been devised in which the paper is replaced by a special material that is essentially cellulose acetate. With this material the electrophoresis can be completed in 1 hr. or less, depending upon the apparatus used. The strip is then fixed in dilute acetic acid and the proteins are dyed with Ponceau Red S. The dye may then be eluted from cut sections of the strip and the protein fractions quantitated as in paper electrophoresis (Fig. 6-11).

The strip may be further treated with methyl alcohol so that it is transparent when dried. This aids in quantitation of the dye with a densitometer. Since the cellulose acetate strips use much less protein, the amount of dye bound is also small; in the elution method, unless microcuvettes are available, the optical density readings are low, resulting in some error. The densitometer procedure is more rapid and accurate, but requires a relatively expensive apparatus.

Protein electrophoresis has been done with other media as well, such as **starch gel** and **polyacrylamide gel.** This latter media separates the serum proteins into as many as 15 different fractions, but the clinical significance of these fractions has not yet been established. Most of the data correlating electrophoretic patterns with disease are from results of paper electrophoresis, although cellulose acetate electrophoresis yields similar results (Tables 6-3 and 6-4).

Normal values and interpretation[70, 71]: Two conditions that give very characteristic electrophoretic patterns are hypogammaglobulinemia and analbuminemia. In hypogammaglobulinemia the gamma globulin fraction is very low, with the rest of the pattern not differing too much from normal. The gamma globulins average about 3% of the total protein or 0.2 gm., compared with a normal value of about 20% or 1.5 gm. In the rare condition of analbuminemia the albumin may amount to not more than 3% of the total protein, which is usually below 5 gm.

Various other conditions also give abnormal electrophoretic patterns, though not as striking. Table 6-5 shows the changes in protein fractions with other diseases. Elevated levels of beta globulins are frequently associated with hyperlipemia and hypercholesterolemia and thus may be found in such diseases as the nephrotic syndrome, idiopathic hyperlipemia, uncontrolled diabetes, and obstructive jaundice. The gamma globulins contain most of the immune bodies. Low values of gamma globulins are normally found in infants. At birth the gamma

Table 6-3. Normal range by paper electrophoresis

Fraction	Gm./100 ml.	% of total
Albumin	3.7-5.5	54-70
Globulin		
Alpha₁	0.1-0.3	2-5
Alpha₂	0.4-1.0	7-11
Beta	0.5-1.1	8-14
Gamma	0.5-1.2	10-20
Total protein	6.2-8.1	100

Table 6-4. Normal range by cellulose acetate electrophoresis

Fraction	Gm./100 ml.	% of total
Albumin	3.7-5.7	54-74
Globulin		
Alpha₁	0.1-0.3	1.1-4.2
Alpha₂	0.4-1.0	4.6-13.0
Beta	0.5-1.0	7.3-13.5
Gamma	0.5-1.5	8.1-19.9
Total protein	6.5-8.2	100

Table 6-5. Changes in electrophoretic protein fractions associated with disease*

	Total protein	Albumin	Alpha₁ globulin	Alpha₂ globulin	Beta globulin	Gamma globulin
Acute infection		D		I		
Asthma and other allergies with poor response to therapy		D		I		D
Carcinomatosis		D	I	I		
Chronic infection		D				I
Cryoglobulinemia						I
Diabetes mellitus		D	I	I		
Glomerulonephritis	D	D	I			
Hepatic cirrhosis	D	D				I
Hepatitis, viral		D	D	D	I	I
Hodgkin's disease	D	D		I		I
Leukemia, myelogenous		D				I
Lupus erythematosus		D		I		I
Lymphoma and lymphocytic leukemia	D	D				D
Macroglobulinemia	I	D			I	I
Myeloma	I	D				I
Myasthenia		D				I
Myxedema		D		I		I
Nephrosis (highest A₂ elevation)	D	D		I		D
Rheumatic fever		D		I		
Rheumatoid arthritis		D		I		I
Sarcoidosis	I	D		I	I	I
Scleroderma	D	D	D	D	D	D
Ulcerative colitis and other exudative enteropathies	D	D	I	I	D	D

*I = increase; D = decrease.

globulin level is characteristically about the same as in the maternal blood (0.9-1.6 gm.%), but it falls sharply during the first few months of life to a low value of 0.3-0.8 gm.% at the age of 3-4 mo. It then rises slowly, reaching a level of about 0.5-1.2 gm.% at 1 yr. and obtaining normal adult levels only after 5-10 yr. In multiple myeloma, although the total globulin is markedly increased, the increase is not always chiefly in the gamma globulin fraction. The so-called M globulins of this disease do not always migrate with the gamma globulins, and the increase may sometimes be found in the alpha or beta globulins.

Macroglobulins[72]: A number of pathologic conditions will cause abnormally high globulin fractions on electrophoresis. One of these conditions is **macroglobulinemia**. The following test is based on the fact that serum or plasma containing macroglobulin will form a white precipitate when diluted with water.

Procedure: Place 5 ml. water in a test tube. By means of a pipette brought close to the water meniscus, drop 0.2 ml. serum or plasma (oxalated, citrated, or heparinized plasma may be used) into the water. Observe the behavior of the drop of serum or plasma sinking in the water and the changes in the color of the medium.

Interpretation: If macroglobulins are present (1) the drop will sink, leaving a smoky trace, and (2) the entire solution will promptly assume a whitish color due to the condensation of transparent, slimy masses forming a precipitate that quickly sinks to the bottom. After centrifugation the separated precipitate will quickly dissolve in normal saline solution.

Normal serum, when tested by this method, shows no cloudiness or precipitate. A negative test does not exclude the possibility of the presence of macroglobulins.

Cryoglobulins[72]: The presence of this

type of globulin will also often give abnormal electrophoretic patterns. The following test may aid in its identification. When serum or plasma containing cryoglobulin is incubated at 4° C., it will undergo significant changes that are not observed at 37° C.

Procedure: Serum or plasma (oxalated, citrated, or heparinized) may be used. Transfer 2 ml. aliquots of serum or plasma to two test tubes. Incubate one tube at 4° C. (refrigerator) and the other at 37° C. (water bath) for 4 hr. Compare the serum incubated at 37° C. with that incubated at 4° C.

Interpretation: If cryoglobulins are present, no changes will be observed in the specimen incubated at 37° C. In the test tube incubated at 4° C. the following changes may be observed: the serum or plasma may appear to be wholly clotted or the plasma or serum may appear to be divided into two layers, the upper layer containing normal plasma or serum, the lower one containing the cryoglobulin (whitish in color) which has precipitated to the bottom of the tube. When this tube is warmed to 37° C. for a short time, the serum or plasma reverts to normal.

Normal plasma or serum does not show any precipitate or cloudiness when incubated at 4° C. The temperature at which cryoglobulin precipitates varies with other factors in the serum such as pH and the concentration of the other proteins. Precipitation has been observed at temperatures as high as 32° C. in severe cases.

Fibrinogen[73]: Fibrinogen is the blood protein specially concerned with clotting; its determination is often useful in conditions such as myocardial infarction, rheumatic fever, and liver disorders. The fibrinogen in oxalated blood is clotted by means of thrombin. The clot is separated and the amount of protein present is determined with biuret reagent.

Reagents:

1. Double oxalate. This is the same dried double oxalate used in hematology for the collection of blood counts (p. 98).
2. Sodium chloride (0.9%). Dissolve 9 gm. sodium chloride in water and dilute to 1 L.
3. Thrombin. Topical thrombin is used. This is generally obtained in vials containing 5000 NIH units. This is diluted to 100 units/ml. It is convenient to dilute the entire contents of a vial up to 50 ml. with saline solution and place 0.2 ml. aliquots in 15 × 125 mm. test tubes. These are then stoppered and kept frozen until use.
4. Sodium hydroxide (1%). Dissolve 10 gm. sodium hydroxide in water and dilute to 1 L.
5. Biuret reagent. This is the stock biuret solution used in the total protein determination (p. 321). Be certain that the **stock solution** is used directly in this procedure and not the diluted biuret solution that is used for total protein determination.
6. Protein standard. Use the same protein standard as in the total protein determination (fibrinogen gives the same amount of color as albumin with the reagent), but dilute to about 2 mg./ml. Using an accurate pipette, add 0.5 ml. protein standard to exactly 15 ml. 1% sodium hydroxide. This is a 1:31 dilution. If the original protein solution contained 6.3% protein, which is equivalent to 63 mg./ml., then a 1:31 dilution would contain 2.03 mg./ml. The exact concentration of the diluted standard will, of course, depend upon the concentration of the original standard.

Procedure: Draw 5 ml. blood and put into tube containing 0.5 ml. dried double oxalate. (Always keep blood and oxalate in this same proportion.) Mix well to prevent formation of clots. Centrifuge and separate plasma from the cells. Allow plasma to stand at room temperature for 2 hr. (This minimizes the fibrinolysis which may cause an error, but if a rapid result is needed, it can be omitted.) Add 5 ml. saline solution to each of the thrombin tubes and mix. Add 1 ml. plasma to tube and mix well. Clotting should begin within a few minutes. Allow this to stand for 30 min.

Loosen the clot from the walls of the tube by shaking the tilted tube. Rim with a fine-pointed glass rod if necessary. Usually the clot can be removed completely in one piece. Transfer the clot from the tube to the middle of a pile of three or four sheets of hard filter paper that have been placed on top of several sheets of coarse filter paper. Cover with several sheets of hard paper and place some coarse paper on top. Remove water by gently placing a flask of water weighing about 250 gm. on top of the pile. In about 10 min. all of the fluid should be absorbed by the filter paper, leaving a glistening membrane in the middle of the sheet. Loosen the clot carefully with a needle or fine-pointed glass rod. It should be easily removed in one piece. Rinse the clot with saline solution and drop into a graduated centrifuge tube. Add 5 ml. 1% sodium hydroxide and place in boiling water bath for about 15 min. until clot dissolves. Hasten hydrolysis by breaking up the clot with a small stirring rod. Cool, remove the glass rod, check the volume, and add more water if necessary to bring the volume to 5 ml. Also set up a blank with 5 ml. 1% sodium hydroxide and two standards of 1 and 2 ml. diluted protein standard made up to 5 ml. with sodium hydroxide solution. To each, add 1 ml. stock biuret solution (the concentrated stock solution, not the diluted solution used for protein analysis), mix, and allow to stand at room temperature for 30 min. Read samples and standards against the blank at 555 nm.

Calculation: Since the fibrin from 1 ml. serum is used for the determination:

$$\frac{\text{OD sample}}{\text{OD standard}} \times A \times 100 = \text{Mg.\% fibrinogen}$$

where A is the actual amount of protein in 1 (or 2) ml. diluted standard. (See preparation of standard for details.)

Normal values and interpretation[74, 75]: The normal range of fibrinogen in plasma is 200-400 mg.%. Fibrinogen is the component of plasma that most affects the erythrocyte sedimentation rate and is thus increased in rheumatic fever and other diseases in which there is an increased sedimentation rate (see discussion of sedimentation rate, Chapter 4). In patients in whom hypofibrinogenemia may be the cause of bleeding, such as obstetric patients after parturition, serial determinations of fibrinogen may be of value in the management of the patient. Serial determinations may also be of value in various other conditions such as acute myocardial infarction and hepatic disorders.

CALCIUM[76-78]

Calcium may be titrated with **ethylenediaminetetraacetic acid** (EDTA). A number of different indicators have been used for this titration. All are colored organic compounds that form a complex with calcium ions with a different color than the unreacted dye. In the presence of calcium ions the calcium dye color is formed. When enough EDTA has been added to react with all the calcium, the color changes to that of the unreacted dye. Unfortunately the color changes are seldom very sharp and some experience is required to distinguish the end point correctly. A number of other metallic elements also react with EDTA, but the only one likely to interfere in serum titration is **magnesium.** By using the proper indicator and a high pH (around 12), calcium alone can be titrated.

Reagents:
1. Standard EDTA solution. Dissolve 9.25 gm. EDTA reagent in water and dilute to 1 L. Keep in a polyethylene bottle.
2. Indicator. Calver II* is added as a powder to the solution as it is titrated.
3. Potassium hydroxide (8N). Dissolve 50 gm. potassium hydroxide in water to make 100 ml. Keep in well-stoppered plastic bottle.
4. Standards:
   A. Stock standard. Dissolve 2.497 gm. oven-dried reagent grade calcium carbonate (Iceland spar for standardization is also satisfactory) in a minimal amount of diluted hydrochloric acid (equal

---

*Hach Chemical Co., Ames, Iowa.

volumes of concentrated acid and water) in a beaker and evaporate almost to dryness in a water bath to remove most of the excess acid. Dissolve the resulting calcium chloride in water, transfer quantitatively to a volumetric flask, and dilute to 100 ml. This solution contains 10 mg. calcium/ml. (500 mEq./L.).

B. Working standard. Dilute 1 ml. stock standard to 100 ml. This solution contains 10 mg.% or 5 mEq./L. calcium.

Procedure: Pipette 1 ml. serum to a 50 ml. Erlenmeyer flask and add 10 ml. water and 3 drops of 8N potassium hydroxide. Add a small amount of indicator powder. (It may require some experimentation to determine the optimum amount of indicator that gives the sharpest end point.) Titrate with the EDTA solution, using a 5 ml. burette calibrated in 0.02 ml. The end point is reached when the last trace of red color disappears, leaving a pure blue color. (With serum there may be a greenish tinge due to yellow color from the serum.) Similarly, titrate 1 ml. standard.

Calculation: Since 1 ml. serum and 1 ml. calcium standard containing 10 mg.% calcium are titrated similarly:

$$\frac{\text{Titration of sample}}{\text{Titration of standard}} \times 10 = \text{Mg.\% calcium}$$

$$\frac{\text{Mg.\% calcium}}{2} = \text{MEq./L.}$$

Normal values and interpretation: The normal range of calcium in serum is 8.5-10.5 mg.% (4.25-5.25 mEq./L.). About one half of the calcium is combined with proteins in the serum and the other half is in diffusible form; this is the part that is physiologically active. There is, however, no simple method for the determination of ionized calcium alone. Increases in serum calcium are relatively uncommon. The highest values are found in **hyperparathyroidism,** when values up to 20 mg.% may be reached, although in this condition the level is often not over 15 mg.%. Excessive dosage of vitamin D may also raise the serum level of calcium,

at times up to 15 mg.%. This level may also be reached in some cases of multiple myeloma.

Low values are found in hypoparathyroidism, in which the level may be as low as 6 mg.%. Values do not fall this low in diseases involving impaired calcium absorption. In rickets the phosphorus level is depressed, but the calcium level may be normal or only slightly lowered to 8-9 mg.%. A low serum calcium value is found in adults with rickets and osteomalacia. In steatorrhea the serum calcium is normal or only slightly lowered. In advanced renal failure the high level of inorganic phosphorus is accompanied by a decrease in the calcium level, which may be as low as 6 mg.%. In diseases in which the plasma proteins are greatly reduced the calcium level may be lowered, but this reduction is chiefly in the calcium combined with proteins. Because this form is physiologically inactive the decrease has no clinical significance.

Urinary calcium: Direct titration of calcium in urine by EDTA is not satisfactory, possibly due to the high concentration of phosphate in urine. Satisfactory results are obtained if the calcium is first precipitated as the oxalate.

Additional reagents:

1. Ammonium oxalate (10%). Dissolve 10 gm. ammonium oxalate in water and dilute to 100 ml.
2. Sodium citrate (0.05M). Dissolve 14.7 gm. sodium citrate dihydrate in water to make 1 L.

Procedure: Mix the urine thoroughly and withdraw an aliquot of about 10 ml. Acidify with a few drops of concentrated hydrochloric acid to a pH of about 1 (wide-range paper). Warm the acidified mixture to 60° C. for 15 min., mixing occasionally. Pipette 1 ml. of this mixture to a conical centrifuge tube, add 0.2 ml. 10% ammonium oxalate, and mix. Add 1 drop methyl red indicator (0.1% in alcohol). Gradually add 5% ammonium hydroxide (concentrated ammonia diluted 1:6) to obtain an orange color. Place in boiling water bath for 20 min., then cool to room temperature and centrifuge. Decant the supernatant fluid, invert, and drain the centrifuge tube. Dissolve the precipitate in 0.5 ml. 1N hydrochloric acid and 0.5 ml. sodium citrate solution. Transfer quantitatively to a 50 ml. Erlenmeyer flask, using about 10 ml. water. Add 5 drops potassium hydroxide and indicator, and titrate as for serum. A standard may also be titrated directly without the precipitation.

Calculation: Since 1 ml. urine is used, the calculation is the same as for serum.

$$\text{Mg.\% calcium} \times \frac{\text{24 hr. urine vol. (ml.)}}{100} =$$
$$\text{Mg. calcium excreted/day}$$

The urine calcium concentration depends on the calcium intake. The normal range may be from 50-400 mg./day.

NOTE: A special problem sometimes encountered is the determination of calcium in the serum of patients who have been treated with EDTA. Under these conditions a direct titration cannot be used. The calcium may be precipitated from 1 ml. of serum with oxalate similar to the procedure for urine, except that the pH is adjusted to a slightly more acid state. After the addition of ammonium oxalate, add a few drops of ammonia and then add bromcresol green indicator (2 drops of a 0.1% solution). Add 10% acetic acid dropwise until the color just turns yellow. At this pH the calcium will be precipitated as the oxalate even in the presence of EDTA. After precipitation, proceed as for urine assay.

INORGANIC PHOSPHORUS[79, 80]

Although most of the phosphorus in the blood exists as **phosphates** or **phosphate esters** because of the diversity of compounds, it is usually reported as phosphorus (P) but often spoken of as phosphates. The phosphorus in the blood exists in a number of different types of compounds which include (1) inorganic phosphorus, the phosphates of alkalies, and alkaline earths; (2) **lipid phosphorus** and phosphorus in such lipid substances as lecithin, cephalin, and sphingomyelin; and (3) organic or **ester phosphorus,** including glycerophosphate, hexosephosphate, nucleotide phosphate, and others. Ester phosphates are chiefly in the cells,

while the other two compounds are present in somewhat similar concentrations in the cells and plasma. Usually determinations are made only of inorganic phosphorus and of lipid phosphorus; proteins are precipitated with trichloroacetic acid and phosphate is determined in the filtrate. In an acid solution, phosphate together with molybdate (or tungstate) will produce a blue color in the presence of a reducing agent. Many of the phosphate methods differ mainly in the use of different molybdate and acid concentrations and different compounds as the reducing agent.

Reagents:

1. Trichloroacetic acid (5%). Dissolve 50 gm. trichloroacetic acid in water and dilute to 1 L.
2. Acid molybdate solution. Dissolve 5 gm. sodium molybdate ($Na_2MoO_4 \cdot 2H_2O$) in about 600 ml. water, add 14 ml. concentrated sulfuric acid, and dilute to 1 L.
3. Reducing solution. Dissolve 1 gm. Elon* (*p*-methylaminophenol sulfate) in 100 ml. 3% sodium bisulfite solution. This solution should be filtered before use and made up fresh about once a month.
4. Standard solutions:
   A. Stock standard. Dissolve 0.4394 gm. anhydrous potassium dihydrogen phosphate (KH_2PO_4) in water and dilute to 1 L. This solution contains 0.1 mg. phosphorus/ml.
   B. Working standard. Dilute 4 ml. stock standard to 50 ml. with 5% trichloroacetic acid. This solution contains 0.008 mg. phosphorus/ml.

Procedure: To 1 ml. serum in a test tube add 9 ml. 5% trichloroacetic acid solution, mix thoroughly, and filter after 5 min. Pipette 2 ml. filtrate to a test tube. In another tube add 2 ml. 5% trichloroacetic acid as a blank and also set up two standards. To one tube add 1 ml. working standard (0.008 mg. P) and 1 ml. trichloroacetic acid; to the other tube add 2 ml. working standard (0.016 mg.

---

*No. 615-P, Eastman Kodak Co., Rochester, N. Y.

P). To each tube add 5 ml. acid molybdate and mix. Then add 0.25 ml. reducing solution to each tube, mix, and allow to stand for 45 min. Read the standards and samples against the blank in a photometer at 650-700 nm.

Calculation: Two ml. of a 1:10 filtrate of serum is equivalent to 0.2 ml. serum. If this is treated similar to a standard containing 0.008 (or 0.016) mg. P, then this is equivalent to $0.008 \times \dfrac{100}{0.2}$ or 4 mg.% P for the lower standard and 8 mg.% P for the higher standard. Usually for serum the 4 mg.% standard may be used. Hence:

$$\frac{\text{OD sample}}{\text{OD standard}} \times 4 = \text{Mg.\% P}$$

Urinary phosphates[81]: This method can also be used for urine. Treat the urine exactly like the serum. Precipitation with trichloroacetic acid may not always be necessary, but it removes traces of material that will cause turbidity and the urine must be diluted in any event. Since the phosphate concentration in urine varies much more than in serum, a different dilution may be needed to bring the final color in the range of accurate reading. If this is done, appropriate correction must be made in the calculation.

Organic phosphates, which are susceptible to hydrolysis, are found chiefly in erythrocytes, and the inorganic phosphate content of whole blood can increase markedly on standing at room temperature. Hence the serum should be separated from the cells as soon as possible. After separation, the inorganic phosphate content of serum or plasma is stable for several days in the refrigerator.[82] Acidified urine is quite stable for phosphate when kept in the refrigerator. To determine phosphate in urine the specimen must be acidified before sampling to dissolve any precipitated calcium or magnesium phosphates.

Normal values and interpretation: The normal range of inorganic phosphate in adults is 2.5-5 mg.%, with an average of 3.7 mg.%. The level is 1-2 mg.% higher in children. In severe nephritis the inorganic phosphate level may rise as high as 15 mg.%. In rickets the level may be lowered to 2 mg.% or less. There is also a decreased level in hyperparathyroidism to about 2 mg.%, but this fall is not so marked from the normal adult level as is the fall that occurs in children with rickets. In hyperparathyroidism there is a moderate increase in the level. The product of the concentrations of calcium and phosphate in serum seems generally to be more constant than the level of either, so that a fall in the level of one of the two elements usually means an increase in the level of the other. There is also a decrease to below 3 mg.% in increased carbohydrate metabolism and after the injection of insulin. The very low levels that may occur in the treatment of diabetic coma arise from this cause since phosphate esters such as hexosephosphates play an important role in the metabolism of glucose.

Inorganic phosphorus is sometimes expressed in terms of mEq./L. instead of mg.%. At the pH of blood (7.4), approximately 80% of the phosphate is present as HPO_4^{--} and about 20% is present as $H_2PO_4^-$. Hence each atom of phosphorus represents not 2 equivalents (as it would if it were all HPO_4^{--}), but only about 1.8. Therefore the equivalent weight of phosphorus for this purpose may only be taken as 31/1.8 or 17.2, and mg.%/1.72 = mEq./L., but it is probably better to express the P as mg.%. The phosphate in urine depends mainly on the amount of phosphorus in the diet. The daily excretion is about 1 gm. (as phosphorus). Phosphate clearance is increased in hyperparathyroidism and is decreased in hypoparathyroidism. Some tests have been suggested on this basis for the diagnosis of these diseases, but they have proved to be of limited value. They are based on the ratio of creatinine clearance to phosphate clearance.

$$R = \frac{\text{Phosphate clearance}}{\text{Creatinine clearance}} = \frac{P_c U_p}{P_p U_c}$$

P and U refer to plasma and urine concentrations and the subscripts c and p refer to creatinine and phosphate. One index that has been used is the **tubular reabsorbed phosphate** (TRP).

$$TRP = (1 - R) \times 100$$

The normal values are given as 84-95%. Reduced values occur in hyperparathyroidism.

Another index is the **phosphate excretion index** (PEI).

$$PEI = R - (0.055 \times Serum\ P - 0.07)$$

Normal values are from −0.09 to +0.09. Higher values occur in hyperparathyroidism.

MAGNESIUM[83, 84]

In alkaline solutions magnesium forms a colored compound (lake) with the dye **titan yellow**. The amount of color formed is proportional to the amount of magnesium present. Since the colored product is actually colloidal in nature and is not a true solution, polyvinyl alcohol is added to stabilize the color. The final solution is rather highly colored even in the absence of any magnesium. If too much dye is present, the blank will be high enough to increase the error in the readings. If too little dye is present, the magnesium color will not develop properly. It may be necessary to experiment with different lots of dye to find the best concentration. In the method presented, proteins are first removed by precipitation with trichloroacetic acid.

Reagents:

1. Sodium hydroxide (2.5N). Dissolve 100 gm. sodium hydroxide in water to make 1 L. Check the normality by titration and adjust to 2.5 ± 0.05N.
2. Polyvinyl alcohol (0.1%). Suspend 1 gm. polyvinyl alcohol* in about 40 ml. ethyl alcohol and pour into about 500 ml. water while swirling; then warm to dissolve and dilute to 1 L.
3. Titan yellow solutions:
   A. Stock solution. Dissolve 75 mg. titan yellow† in 100 ml. 0.1%

*Elvanol 70-05, E. I. du Pont de Nemours & Co., Inc., Niagara Falls, N. Y.
†Titan yellow, Eastman No. P4454, is the same as Clayton yellow, Eastman No. 1770.

polyvinyl alcohol. Store in a brown bottle.
   B. Working solution. Dilute stock solution 1:10 with the polyvinyl alcohol solution as needed.
4. Trichloroacetic acid (5%). Dissolve 50 gm. trichloroacetic acid in water and dilute to 1 L.
5. Magnesium standards:
   A. Stock standard. Dissolve 2.465 gm. uneffloresced crystals of reagent grade magnesium sulfate in water to make 1 L. This solution contains 20 mEq./L. magnesium.
   B. Working standard. Dilute stock standard 1:10 as required.

Procedure: To 5 ml. 5% trichloroacetic acid in a test tube add 1 ml. serum and mix. Allow to stand for 10 min. and centrifuge strongly. Pipette 3 ml. supernatant for the tests. Also set up a blank with 0.5 ml. water and 2.5 ml. 5% trichloroacetic acid and a standard with 0.5 ml. diluted standard plus 2.5 ml. 5% trichloroacetic acid. To each tube add 2 ml. titan yellow working solution, mix, and add 1 ml. 2.5N sodium hydroxide. Read standard and samples against the blank at 540 nm. It is preferable to read within 10-15 min. after the addition of alkali.

Calculation: Since 1 ml. serum is diluted with 5 ml. trichloroacetic acid to 6 ml., then 3 ml. supernatant is equivalent to 0.5 ml. serum. In the color development, 0.5 ml. serum is treated the same as 0.5 ml. standard containing 2 mEq./L. Hence:

$$\frac{OD\ sample}{OD\ standard} \times 2 = MEq./L.\ magnesium$$

The magnesium in cells is about three times that in the plasma or serum; hence hemolysis should be avoided.

Normal values and interpretation: The normal values in the serum of adults is 1.6-2.1 mEq./L. (mEq./L. × 1.2 = mg.%; hence the normal range is 1.9-2.5 mg.%).

Although in recent years there has been more interest in serum magnesium in diseased states, the findings are still few. Increases in serum magnesium occur in both acute and chronic renal disease, especially if there is reduced urine output, although it may be low in advanced renal disease. It may be raised in liver disease and diabetic coma. Low values have been found in the malabsorption syndrome, in diarrhea, and at times in pancreatitis. Low values have also been found in chronic alcoholism. It has also been stated that prolonged salicylate therapy will cause a substantial elevation in the serum magnesium level.

Urine magnesium: Very little is known about the relationship between excretion of magnesium in the urine and various diseased states. The titan yellow method could probably be adapted to urine, but even the best aliquot to use has not been accurately determined.

IRON AND IRON-BINDING CAPACITY[85-87]

Iron is transported in serum from the point of absorption in the intestines to the point of use in the erythropoietic system in combination with a fraction of the beta globulins known as **transferrin** or **siderophilin.** This is the iron available for the formation of hemoglobin and is measured in the serum iron determination. Usually the transferrin is not saturated with iron; i.e., it could absorb and transport much more iron than is actually in the serum. The amount of iron that the protein could absorb to be fully saturated is the latent or unsaturated iron-binding capacity.

In the determination of serum iron the metal is liberated from the protein complex by treatment with dilute hydrochloric acid and a reducing agent. The latter is used since ferrous iron is much more readily split off than ferric iron. The proteins are then precipitated with trichloroacetic acid and the iron is determined in the filtrate with a color reagent, sulfonated bathophenanthroline, that produces a red color with ferrous iron.

In the determination of serum iron-binding capacity the serum is treated with an excess of iron to saturate the transferrin. The excess iron over that required to saturate the protein is then removed by means of an ion exchange resin, and the iron in the fully saturated serum is measured by a modification of the method for serum iron. This gives the total iron-binding capacity of the serum. The total iron-binding capacity minus the serum iron is the latent or unsaturated iron-binding capacity.

Because iron is a very common contaminant in many reagents and since very small amounts of iron are being measured, care must be taken to avoid all contamination. Double-distilled or deionized water must be used for all reagents and for the final rinsing of all glassware, which must be thoroughly cleaned in dilute nitric acid, rinsed with ordinary distilled water, and then rinsed again with deionized water. When drying glassware, avoid all contact with metals. Pipettes and other glassware should be kept specially for this purpose to avoid contamination. However, much of the time involved in special washings can be avoided by using disposable plastic tubes, pipettes, and syringes. Hemolysis must be strictly avoided in the collection of samples since erythrocytes have a very high iron content. Although hemoglobin iron is not split off as easily as serum iron, it is best to avoid all hemolysis and discard any samples containing a visible amount of hemoglobin.

Procedure for serum iron:
Reagents:
1. Trichloroacetic acid (30%). Dissolve 150 gm. reagent grade trichloroacetic acid in deionized water and dilute to 500 ml. Trichloroacetic acid is one of the more frequent sources of contamination and the commercially prepared solutions have often been found to give very high blanks.
2. Thioglycollic acid (mercaptoacetic acid)* in water. Use as purchased. Store in a refrigerator.
3. Hydrochloric acid (0.2N). Dilute 17 ml. concentrated hydrochloric acid to 1 L. with deionized water.
4. Sodium acetate (35%). A saturated solution of the salt in water is satisfactory.
5. Color reagent. Dissolve 0.1 gm. sulfonated bathophenanthroline† in 50 ml. water. Store in a refrigerator.

---

*Matheson, Coleman & Bell, Norwood, Ohio.
†No. 274, G. Frederick Smith Chemical Co., Columbus, Ohio.

6. Iron standards:
   A. Stock standard. Dissolve 1.756 gm. AR ferrous ammonium sulfate (Mohr's salt), 25 mg. ascorbic acid, and 1.5 ml. concentrated hydrochloric acid in water and dilute to 500 ml. Store in a refrigerator. This solution contains 0.5 mg. Fe/ml.
   B. Working standard. Dilute 1 ml. stock standard to 250 ml. with water. This solution is not stable and should be prepared fresh as needed. It contains 2 μg/ml. Fe or 200 μg%.

Procedure: To 2 ml. plasma or serum add 3 ml. 0.2N hydrochloric acid and 1 drop thioglycollic acid and mix by swirling. Allow to stand at room temperature for 30 min. Also treat similarly 2 ml. working standard and 2 ml. water as the blank.

After the tubes have been left standing for the specific time, add 1 ml. 30% trichloroacetic acid. Mix well with a small, footed rod and allow to stand for 20 min. Remove the rod and centrifuge strongly (standards and blank need not be centrifuged). Carefully remove 4 ml. supernatant from each tube and add to labeled tube. Also pipette into separate tubes 4 ml. standard mixture and 4 ml. blank mixture. To each tube add 0.5 ml. sodium acetate solution and 0.5 ml. color reagent. Mix and allow to stand for 20 min. Read standards and samples against the blank at 540 nm. Ordinarily when the blank is read against water it should not have a color equivalent to more than 15-20 mg.% iron. If it is higher, there is some source of contamination.

Calculation: Since 2 ml. standard containing 200 μg% Fe is treated the same as 2 ml. serum:

$$\frac{\text{OD sample}}{\text{OD standard}} \times 200 = \mu g\% \text{ Fe}$$

Procedure for iron-binding capacity:
Reagents (in addition to those used for serum iron):
1. Ferric ammonium citrate. Dissolve 65 mg. ferric chloride in about 20 ml. water in a 50 ml. centrifuge tube. Make alkaline with about 10 drops concentrated ammonia to precipitate the iron. Centrifuge and decant off the supernatant. Add about 10 ml. water to the precipitate and dissolve with the aid of about 75 mg. citric acid, warming to about 60° C. When dissolved, cool, add a few drops of bromthymol blue indicator, and adjust with dilute ammonium hydroxide (1:10) to a lime green color. Transfer to a volumetric flask and dilute to 250 ml. This solution is stable in the refrigerator for about 6 mo.
2. Concentrated hydrochloric acid.
3. Barbital buffer. Dissolve 6.4 gm. sodium chloride, 6 gm. diethylbarbituric acid, and 2.3 gm. sodium diethylbarbiturate in water to make 1 L. The free barbituric acid is difficult to solubilize and it is usually necessary to make up to about 950 ml. and warm for some time to obtain solution. After the salts are dissolved, cool and dilute to 1 L. Store at room temperature.
4. Amberlite IRA-410.* Suspend the resin in two to three times its volume of approximately 3N hydrochoric acid (concentrated acid diluted 1:4) overnight. Wash well with water by decantation. Suspend the resin in some of the barbital buffer, bring to a pH of 7.5 with the aid of a little sodium hydroxide solution if necessary, filter, and dry at 95° C.

Procedure: Pipette 1 ml. serum or heparinized plasma (oxalate or citrate will interfere) to a centrifuge tube. Add 0.1 ml. ferric ammonium citrate solution and allow to stand at room temperature for 10 min. Add about 0.4 ml. resin (conveniently measured by volume) and stir occasionally for 5-10 min.; then add 5 ml. buffer and stir occasionally for 10 min. more. Centrifuge briefly, and carefully remove 5 ml. supernatant with a pipette without disturbing the resin. Place 5 ml. supernatant in a test tube, add 1 drop concentrated hydrochloric acid and 1 drop thioglycollic acid, mix, and allow to stand for 30 min. Add 1 ml. 30% trichloroacetic acid, and proceed as de-

---

*Mallinckrodt Chemical Co., St. Louis, Mo.

scribed for serum iron. It may be advisable to carry through a blank using 1 ml. water instead of 1 ml. serum, treating with resin as described for serum. The same standard is used as for the serum iron.

Calculation: The 5 ml. supernatant from the resin treatment corresponds to 5.0/6.1 ml. serum. This is treated exactly like 2 ml. serum plus 3 ml. diluted hydrochloric acid (total volume 5 ml.) in the serum iron determination. When the same standard is used as for serum iron, the result must be multiplied by $\dfrac{2}{(5.0/6.1)}$.

Hence:

$$\frac{OD \text{ sample}}{OD \text{ standard}} \times \frac{200 \times 2 \times 6.1}{5} = \frac{OD \text{ sample}}{OD \text{ standard}}$$
$$\times 488 = \mu g\% \text{ total iron-binding capacity}$$

This gives the total iron-binding capacity (TIBC).

TIBC – Serum iron = Unsaturated (or latent) iron-binding capacity (UIBC or LIBC)

(Serum iron/TIBC $\times$ 100 = %Saturation)

Normal values and interpretation: The normal range of serum iron is 70-150 $\mu g\%$ in men (average 125) and 60-135 $\mu g\%$ (average 90) in women. Low values are found in hypochromic types of anemias and often in individuals suffering from various infectious diseases. High values have been found in those anemias characterized by decreased hemoglobin formation not due to iron deficiency, such as pernicious anemia.

At birth the serum iron is somewhat high, in the range of 150-200 $\mu g\%$, but it rapidly falls to below 100 $\mu g\%$ and does not regain adult values for several years. There is a diurnal variation in the serum iron of as much as 20%. It is highest in the morning and falls during the day. There appears to be other random fluctuations in the serum iron levels and a single specimen taken at an unspecified time of day is not always satisfactory.

The total iron-binding capacity averages about 300 $\mu g\%$ in normal subjects, with about 40% saturation in men and 35% in women. Rather wide ranges of total iron-binding capacity have been given by different investigators, so that values of 200-400 $\mu g\%$ would not be considered abnormal.

In iron-deficiency anemia the total iron-binding capacity is normal or even elevated, but the serum iron is low, giving an increased unsaturated iron-binding capacity. The unsaturated iron-binding capacity is usually over 300 $\mu g\%$ in iron-deficiency anemia and is under 150 $\mu g\%$ in pernicious anemia. In hemochromatosis the serum iron is markedly elevated (200 $\mu g\%$) and the unsaturated iron-binding capacity is very low.

COPPER[88-90]

Although the exact role of copper in the body metabolism has not been completely explained, copper determinations in serum or urine are made in connection with certain diseases. Most of the serum copper is combined with a protein known as **ceruloplasmin.** This protein acts as an oxidase enzyme, and its determination on that basis is discussed in the section on enzymes. As with iron, the contamination of glassware and reagents with traces of the metal is often a problem. Redistilled or deionized water should be used for all solutions and reagents. The other suggestions mentioned in the determination of iron may also be used here.

Serum copper: In the method given here the copper is split off from the protein with hydrochloric acid and the protein is then precipitated with trichloroacetic acid. An aliquot of centrifugate is treated with oxalyl dihydrazide and acetaldehyde to yield a pink color with copper. Since a slight turbidity sometimes forms, this is corrected for by using a blank containing EDTA, which prevents the formation of any color with the reagents.

Reagents:
1. Hydrochloric acid (2N) with oxalyl dihydrazide. Dilute 84 ml. concentrated hydrochloric acid to 500 ml. In this, dissolve 0.5 gm. oxalyl dihydrazide.* This solution is stable for about 2 mo. Since copper determinations are usually done infrequently, it may be best to store the 2N hy-

---

*No. 7175, Eastman Kodak Co., Rochester, N. Y.

drochloric acid and dissolve 50 mg. in 50 ml. acid as required.

2. Trichloroacetic acid (20%). Dissolve 100 gm. trichloroacetic acid in water to make 500 ml. Store in a refrigerator.

3. Concentrated ammonium hydroxide (90%). Use as purchased.

4. Acetaldehyde solution (50% [v/v]). Mix well 1 vol. cold acetaldehyde with 1 vol. cold water. Store in refrigerator.

5. Ethylenediaminetetraacetic acid, disodium salt.

6. Citric acid crystals.

7. Copper standards:

   A. Stock standard. Dissolve 0.393 gm. uneffloresced crystals of reagent grade copper sulfate in water containing a few drops of concentrated sulfuric acid and dilute to 100 ml. This solution is stable and contains 1 mg. copper/ml.

   B. Working standard. Dilute 1 ml. stock standard to 500 ml. with water. This solution contains 200 μg% copper. It is not stable and should be made fresh as required.

Procedure: In a test tube place 1 ml. serum or heparinized plasma and 1 ml. hydrochloric acid with dihydrazide and mix well. Similarly, treat two water blanks (1 ml. water each) and a standard of 1 ml. diluted standard, adding hydrochloric acid to each. Allow to stand for 10 min. Add to each tube 1 ml. 20% trichloroacetic acid and mix well with a small, footed stirring rod. Cover with Parafilm and allow to stand for 5 min. Centrifuge the tubes rapidly for 15 min. Into tubes containing a pinch of citric acid crystals, pipette 2 ml. supernatant from samples, standard, and blanks. To only one of the two blanks add a pinch of disodium EDTA. To each tube add 0.5 ml. ammonium hydroxide and mix well. Then add to each tube 0.5 ml. acetaldehyde solution and mix. Allow to stand for 30 min. at room temperature. Read all tubes against the blank containing EDTA at 542 nm. Subtract the OD of the blank without EDTA from the OD of the standards and samples. If the colorimeter re-

quires more than 3 ml. volume for reading, the procedure can be carried using twice the quantities of all solutions.

Calculation: Since equal volumes of serum and standard containing 200 μg% copper are treated similarly:

$$\frac{\text{Corrected OD sample}}{\text{Corrected OD standard}} \times 200 = \mu\text{g\% copper}$$

This method is not satisfactory for urine without preliminary wet digestion with hydrochloric acid and nitric acid. This is time-consuming and introduces more chance of contamination from reagents. The following extraction method is suggested.

Copper in urine:
Reagents:

1. Zinc dibenzyldithiocarbamate (DBDC).* Dissolve 75 mg. reagent in 500 ml. reagent grade carbon tetrachloride.

2. Standards. The same standards are used as for serum copper.

Procedure: Pipette two 10 ml. aliquots of urine to separate tubes. Add 1 ml. concentrated hydrochloric acid to each tube and heat in a water bath just below boiling (95° C.) for 15 min. Cool and transfer to 125 ml. separatory funnels. To one funnel add 5 ml. DBDC reagent (urine sample) and to the other add 5 ml. carbon tetrachloride (urine blank). Shake vigorously for 1 min. Extract with DBDC reagent 10 ml. water plus 1 ml. hydrochloric acid (reagent blank) and 9 ml. water plus 1 ml. diluted standard and 1 ml. hydrochloric acid (standard). Shake each funnel vigorously for 1 min. After allowing phases to separate, draw off lower carbon tetrachloride layers into separate tubes. Centrifuge to clarify. Read all tubes at 436 nm., reading urine samples against urine blank and standard against reagent blank.

Calculation: Since the standard contains 2 μg/ml. copper and is compared with the extract from 10 ml. urine:

$$\frac{\text{OD sample}}{\text{OD standard}} \times \frac{2 \times 1000}{10} = \mu\text{g copper/L.}$$

Normal values and interpretation: Pub-

---

*Dibenzyldithiocarbamate may be obtained from Naugatuck Chemical Co., Naugatuck, Conn., as Arazate.

lished reports on normal serum copper levels vary somewhat, but an average range may be assumed to be 70-150 $\mu g\%$ in men and 80-160 $\mu g\%$ in women. The range is somewhat lower in children, having been reported as 15-65 $\mu g\%$ in newborn infants and 30-150 $\mu g\%$ in young children. Increased levels are found in pregnancy or in any condition in which there is an increased level of estrogen in the blood. Hypercupremia has also been reported in myocardial infarction, cirrhosis, rheumatoid arthritis, and many acute and chronic infections. Hypocupremia is associated with certain nutritional disorders, nephrosis, and Wilson's disease. This last-named condition is one in which there is the most interest in connection with serum copper levels. Values in the range of 40-60 $\mu g\%$ are common.

The urinary excretion of copper also shows considerable variation, but normal limits may be as much as 40 $\mu g\%$/day. It will tend to be higher when there is proteinuria or aminoaciduria because these substances tend to carry copper along with them. The urinary excretion of copper is very markedly increased in Wilson's disease; amounts of 500-1000 $\mu g\%$/day are not uncommon.

SODIUM[91, 92]

Sodium is usually determined by the use of the **flame photometer.** A general discussion of this instrument has been given. In the chemical method given here, sodium is precipitated as the triple salt of sodium zinc (or magnesium) uranyl acetate. The precipitate is dissolved in water and determined photometrically.

Reagents:
1. Trichloroacetic acid (10%). Dissolve 10 gm. trichloroacetic acid in water and dilute to 100 ml.
2. Uranyl zinc acetate. Add 14 ml. glacial acetic acid to 750 ml. water. Bring almost to boiling; then add 77 gm. uranyl acetate and dissolve. Add 231 gm. zinc acetate in divided portions while stirring; then add 7 ml. more acetic acid. Cool and make up to 1 L. Add 200 ml. 95% ethyl alcohol, place in refrigerator overnight, and filter.

3. Wash reagent. Add about 40 gm. magnesium acetate to 200 ml. absolute ethyl alcohol. Shake well at intervals during the next few hours and allow to stand overnight. Filter a portion as required just before use.
4. Sodium salicylate (1%). Dissolve 1 gm. sodium salicylate in water to make 100 ml.
5. Uranyl acetate (0.2%). Dissolve 0.2 gm. uranyl acetate in water to make 100 ml.
6. Sodium standards:
   A. Stock standard (90 mEq./L.). Dissolve 5.26 gm. dried reagent grade sodium chloride in water and dilute to 1 L.
   B. Working standard. Dilute stock standard 1:10 to make a solution containing 9 mEq./L.

Procedure: Add 0.3 ml. serum dropwise to 4.7 ml. 10% trichloroacetic acid while swirling. Shake well and centrifuge. Pipette 0.5 ml. supernatant ($=0.03$ ml. serum) to a conical centrifuge tube. Also set up a standard with 0.5 ml. working standard. To each tube add 3 ml. uranyl zinc acetate solution. Mix by rotation and allow to stand for 1 hr., swirling occasionally. Centrifuge strongly, decant off the supernatant, and then allow the tubes to drain while inverted on filter paper for 1 min. Wash down the sides of the tubes with 5 ml. wash solution. Mix the precipitate with the wash solution by "spanking" the tube; then centrifuge, decant the supernatant, and drain. Dissolve the precipitate in 5 ml. water, add 5 ml. 1% sodium salicylate, and mix. Read tubes at 460 nm. against a blank of 0.2% uranyl zinc acetate.

Calculation: Since the working standard contains 9 mEq./L. and 0.5 ml. of this is treated the same as 0.03 ml. serum, the factor is as follows:

$$\frac{9 \times 0.5}{0.03} = 150$$

Hence:

$$\frac{\text{OD sample}}{\text{OD standard}} \times 150 = \text{MEq./L. sodium}$$

While this method can also be applied to urine, the concentration of **sodium in**

urine varies so greatly, depending upon diet, urine output, etc., that it is difficult to choose a proper aliquot. This is not a serious problem with flame photometric methods since the only treatment required is a simple dilution; but with the chemical method, much time and effort would be lost with an improper aliquot. It is suggested that 0.5 ml. aliquots of two different dilutions of urine be set up. The aliquots of diluted urine are treated exactly like the aliquot of supernatant from the serum precipitation. Usually dilutions of 1:5 and 1:15 will bring at least one of the samples within the proper range. The calculation is then:

$$\frac{\text{OD sample}}{\text{OD standard}} \times 9 \times D = \text{MEq./L.}$$

where D is the dilution of urine, e.g., D = 5 for a 1:5 dilution.

NOTE: After separation from the cells, samples of serum for sodium determination are stable for at least 1 wk. in the refrigerator. Although the erythrocytes contain only about 1/10 of the sodium in the serum, small amounts of hemolysis do not dilute the serum sufficiently to cause an appreciable error.

Normal values and interpretation: Normal levels of sodium in serum are 135-145 mEq./L. Sodium is the chief base of the plasma and its function appears to be chiefly physicochemical in connection with the maintenance of osmotic pressure and acid-base balance. The body has a strong tendency to maintain a total base content, and only slight changes are found even under pathologic conditions. Significant decreases in sodium content of serum have been noted in pregnancy, in pyloric obstruction, in severe nephritis, and in Addison's disease. Since the loss of sodium is often accompanied by an equivalent loss of chloride, reference may be made to the discussion of chloride level, particularly in regard to Addison's disease.

The normal output of sodium in the urine is quite variable, depending upon the diet, kidney function, and other factors. With a normal diet the output is usually in the range of 40-220 mEq./ day (2.3-12.8 gm. as sodium chloride).

POTASSIUM[93-95]

Potassium is usually determined by flame photometry, which is the method of choice. A chemical method is presented which, like the chemical method for sodium, involves formation of a precipitate and requires considerable manipulation. Potassium is precipitated from serum as insoluble potassium sodium cobaltinitrite. After the precipitate has been washed to eliminate interfering substances, it is dissolved in water and potassium is determined indirectly by the colorimetric reaction of cobalt.

Reagents:
1. Sodium cobaltinitrite solutions:
   A. Solution A. Dissolve 25 gm. cobalt nitrate in 50 ml. water and add 12.5 ml. glacial acetic acid.
   B. Solution B. Dissolve 120 gm. sodium nitrite in 180 ml. water (about 220 ml. solution will be obtained).

   Mix 210 ml. solution B with all of solution A. Draw air through the solution until all brown fumes of nitrous oxide are driven off. Filter and store in a refrigerator. This is stable for about 1 mo.
2. Ethyl alcohol (35%). Mix 37 ml. 95% alcohol with water to make 100 ml.
3. Choline chloride (1%). Dissolve 1 gm. choline chloride in water to make 100 ml.
4. Potassium ferrocyanide (2%). Dissolve 2 gm. potassium ferrocyanide in water to make 100 ml.
5. Standards:
   A. Stock standard. Dissolve 3.728 gm. dried reagent grade potassium chloride in water and dilute to 1 L. This solution contains 50 mEq./L.
   B. Working standard. Dilute 10 ml. stock standard to 100 ml. to give a solution containing 5 mEq./L.

Procedure: Pipette 1 ml. serum into a 15 ml. graduated centrifuge tube. Also set up a tube containing 1 ml. diluted standard. To each tube add 3 ml. cobaltinitrite solution and mix by rotating the tube between the palms of the hands. Let stand at room temperature for 2 hr. and centrifuge at 2500 rpm for 10 min. Decant the supernatant. Wash the sides of the tube and the precipitate with 4 ml. 35% alcohol and mix with the precipitate, using a fine glass rod. Centrifuge again and decant. Repeat the washing twice. Add 3 ml. water to the final precipitate and heat in a boiling water bath until dissolved. Cool, add 1 ml. choline chloride and 1 ml. potassium ferrocyanide solution, make up to 6 ml., and mix. Read standard and sample against a blank of 4 ml. water, 1 ml. choline chloride solution, and 1 ml. potassium ferrocyanide at 630 nm.

Calculation: Since 1 ml. serum and 1 ml. standard containing 5 mEq./L. are treated similarly:

$$\frac{OD\ sample}{OD\ standard} \times 5 = MEq./L.\ potassium$$

Normal values and interpretation: The normal range of serum potassium is 4-5.6 mEq./L. (16-22 mg.%). An increase in serum potassium is often found in severe cases of Addison's disease (adrenal cortical insufficiency), particularly in the crisis of that disease. Values of up to 8 mEq./L. have often been found and levels of over 10 mEq./L. have been reported. Some increases in serum potassium have been reported in uremic coma and acute intestinal obstruction.

A decrease in serum potassium may be produced by severe diarrhea and vomiting and has been reported in Cushing's syndrome. In patients with familial periodic paralysis, a rare disease with intermittent attacks of paralysis of the somatic muscles, the serum potassium is lowered during the attacks, usually to about 2.5 mEq./L., but it is normal in the intervals between attacks.

Since the potassium content of erythrocytes is about 20 times that of plasma, any hemolysis during collection of the sample will give erroneously high results. It has been calculated that a just barely visible hemolysis will increase the potassium level of serum by about 0.2 mEq./L. Hence samples containing a readily noticeable hemolysis should not be used. Even without visible hemolysis there may be a shift of potassium from the cells to the serum when the latter stands in contact with the clot for a long time. Therefore the serum should be separated from the cells as soon as possible. After separation, the serum is stable for a week or more, even at room temperature.

It has been reported that opening and closing the fist 10 times with a tourniquet in place results in an increase in the potassium level of the sample by 10-20%, that this increase is due to forearm exercise, and that restricted blood flow persists for about 2 min. Hence either the blood sample should be taken without a tourniquet or the tourniquet should be released after the needle has entered the vein and 2 min. allowed to elapse before the sample is taken.

CHLORIDE[96-99]

Chloride ions may be determined by titration with **mercuric nitrate**. The mercuric chloride formed is so slightly ionized that it does not react with the indicator, **diphenylcarbazone**. When an excess of mercuric ions has been added, they react to give a violet-blue color with the indicator.

Reagents:

1. Mercuric nitrate solution. Dissolve 3 gm. reagent grade mercuric nitrate and 2.6 ml. concentrated nitric acid in 200 ml. water; then dilute to 1 L. This solution is quite stable.

2. Indicator solution. Dissolve 100 mg. s-diphenylcarbazone* in 100 ml. 95% ethyl alcohol. Store in a brown bottle in the refrigerator. This solution slowly deteriorates, especially on exposure to light, and should be prepared fresh monthly.

3. Sodium tungstate and sulfuric acid. These are the same as used for the preparation of Folin-Wu filtrate (p. 298).

4. Chloride standard. Dry reagent grade sodium chloride at 120° C. for several hours. Weigh out exactly 584.5 mg. of the salt and dissolve in water to make 1 L. This solution contains 10 mEq./L. chloride.

---

*No. 4459, Eastman Kodak Co., Rochester, N. Y.

Procedure: Pipette 2 ml. 1:10 Folin-Wu filtrate (=0.2 ml. serum) into a 25 ml. Erlenmeyer flask and add 2-3 drops indicator. Titrate with mercuric nitrate solution from a burette calibrated in 0.01 ml. intervals. (Some burettes have small hypodermic needles as tips; these have proved unsatisfactory as mercuric nitrate solution tends to react with the metal, thereby causing errors.) The burette should have a fine glass tip that delivers about 100 drops/ml. The clear solution becomes an intense violet on the addition of the first drop of excess mercuric nitrate (end point). To standardize the mercuric nitrate solution, similarly titrate 2 ml. standard chloride solution. Although the mercuric nitrate solution is stable, standardizations should be run frequently as a check.

Calculation: Since 2 ml. of a 1:10 dilution and 2 ml. of a 10 mEq./L. standard are titrated, this is equivalent to titrating 2 ml. serum and 2 ml. of a 100 mEq./L. standard. Hence:

$$\frac{\text{Ml. titration of filtrate}}{\text{Ml. titration of standard}} \times 100 =$$
$$\text{MEq./L. chloride}$$

The chloride concentration is sometimes expressed in terms of mg.% NaCl:

$$\text{MEq./L. chloride} \times 5.85 = \text{Mg.\%}$$
$$\text{(as sodium chloride)}$$

The serum may also be titrated directly. Add 0.2 ml. serum to 1.8 ml. water in a flask, add indicator, and titrate. When the first drops of mercuric nitrate are added, the solution will turn blue. As the titration is continued the blue color will disappear to a pale pink, with the blue color appearing again at the end point. The end point may not be quite so sharp as with the titration of the filtrate. For this quantity of serum the calculation is the same as previously given. Cerebrospinal fluid may be titrated without deproteinization, similar to serum.

Urine chloride: Titrate 2 ml. diluted urine (1:10 is usually satisfactory) as described for the filtrate of serum. If the chloride concentration is very low, the titration may be repeated using a different dilution of urine. The urine sample must not be alkaline at the start of the titration (test with paper). If the diluted urine is alkaline, add a few drops of diluted nitric acid (1:20) to a 2 ml. aliquot to bring the pH to approximately 4. If the acidity is too high, the indicator loses sensitivity. It may be convenient to add the acid dropwise to an aliquot of the diluted urine and count the drops required to bring the pH to 4. Then add the same number of drops to the aliquot to be titrated.

This method sometimes gives slightly high results in urine specimens that have been standing for several days, even if refrigerated. Hence only fresh specimens should be used.

Calculation: When 2 ml. standard and 2 ml. of a 1:10 dilution of urine are titrated, the calculation is the same as for serum. If another dilution of urine is used and 2 ml. standard is titrated, then:

$$\frac{\text{Titration of sample}}{\text{Titration of standard}} \times 10 \times \frac{\text{B}}{\text{A}} =$$
$$\text{MEq./L. chloride}$$

where "A" ml. urine is diluted up to a volume of "B" ml. Usually the total excretion per day is required.

$$\text{MEq./L.} \times 24 \text{ hr. urine vol. (L.)} =$$
$$\text{Total mEq. excreted}$$

The excretion of chloride is often expressed in terms of grams of sodium chloride:

$$\text{MEq.} \times 0.0585 = \text{Gm. sodium chloride}$$

Normal values and interpretation: The normal values for serum are 98-110 mEq./L. (575-645 mg.%); for whole blood, 77-88 mEq./L. (450-515 mg.%); and for cerebrospinal fluid, 125-135 mEq./L. (730-790 mg.% as NaCl). The chloride content of urine varies with dietary intake and, to a lesser extent, with the urine volume. On an average diet a normal adult will excrete about 170-250 mEq. chloride/day (10-15 gm. as NaCl).

Because of the relatively high concentration of chloride in the gastric secretion, prolonged vomiting from whatever cause may lead to considerable chloride loss and lowered serum level. In pyloric obstruction the level may fall to as low as

50 mEq./L. When there is vomiting in gastric disease in which there is achlorhydria, the loss is less. Severe diarrhea may also cause loss of chloride, but to a lesser extent. In ulcerative colitis the serum level may fall as low as 70 mEq./L.

In the normal individual the urinary excretion of chloride falls to a very low level whenever the serum level is much below 100 mEq./L.

Although the reason is not clear, low plasma chloride levels have been observed in a number of acute infections. The blood chloride is rather variable in renal disease. It is sometimes increased in acute glomerulonephritis; in nephrosis it may be almost normal. When renal failure is present, it may be reduced. This is a common finding in the latter stages of chronic glomerulonephritis. Plasma chloride can be maintained for years near normal limits even when a considerable degree of renal failure is present. Hence chloride determinations are of limited value in renal disease.

The chlorides in cerebrospinal fluid are usually decreased in meningitis. The reduction is generally more marked in tuberculous than in meningococcal meningitis. In other diseases of the nervous system the chlorides are usually within normal limits. A marked reduction in plasma chlorides in diseases not involving the nervous system is accompanied by lower levels in the cerebrospinal fluid.

In some conditions the urinary excretion of chloride is appreciable even when the serum level is as low as 85 mEq./L. or less. The chief condition of interest in this regard is Addison's disease, in which there is a deficiency of the adrenal hormone that controls the excretion of sodium and chloride. The **Robinson-Power-Kepler test** is often used for diagnosis of Addison's disease. It is described here because it is in part based on the measurement of serum and urinary chloride. The test is based on the fact that patients with Addison's disease usually do not experience rapid diuresis after the intake of a considerable amount of water and require a much longer time to excrete the excess water. There is a tendency to excrete excessive amounts of chloride and to retain urea.

Robinson-Power-Kepler test[100, 101]: On the day preceding the test the patient eats a regular meal but does not take any extra salt. If adrenal extracts or synthetic products are being given, they must be discontinued 2 or 3 days before the beginning of the test. On the day the test begins no food or fluid is allowed after 6 P.M. At 10:30 P.M. the patient empties the bladder and the urine is discarded. The patient is kept in bed at rest until completion of the test. All the urine voided from 10:30 P.M. until 7:30 the following morning is collected, including the specimen obtained by emptying the bladder at this time. No breakfast is allowed. A specimen of blood for estimation of urea and chloride is taken between 8 and 8:30 A.M. At 8:30 the bladder is emptied again and this specimen is discarded. The patient is then given 20 ml. water/kg. body weight (9 ml./lb.), drinking the entire amount within the next 45 min. The patient then empties the bladder at 9:30, 10:30, 11:30, and 12:30 and is kept in bed at rest except when passing urine specimens. These urine specimens are kept separately and the volume of each is measured. The volume of the largest specimen is noted.

The first part of the test is based on the urine volumes and is considered negative if the volume of the largest hourly morning specimen is greater than the volume of the night urine. If the volume of the largest morning specimen is less than that of the night specimen, Addison's disease may be present and the second part of the test is carried out.

Urea and chloride determinations are made on the night urine and on the plasma from the blood specimen collected as described. From these and the urine volumes a factor is calculated as follows:

$$A = \frac{\text{Urea N in urine (mg.\%)}}{\text{Urea N in plasma (mg.\%)}}$$

$$\times \frac{\text{Chloride in plasma (mEq./L.)}}{\text{Chloride in urine (mEq./L.)}}$$

$$\times \frac{\text{Vol. largest hourly morning specimen}}{\text{Vol. night urine specimen}}$$

If A is larger than 30, the patient probably does not have Addison's disease. If A is less than 25, the patient probably has Addison's disease, provided that nephritis, diabetes insipidus, and dehydration with fever have been ruled out.

Chloride determination by coulometric titration[102, 103]: Another method for the determination of chloride that is rather widely used is coulometric titration with silver ions, using the instrument devised by Cotlove. In this device silver ions are formed in the solution at a constant rate. These ions combine with any chloride ions present to form silver chloride when an excess of silver ions is present. This is detected electronically and the titration is stopped automatically. One merely compares the time required to titrate the sample with that required for the standard. The titration is carried out automatically, and when one has corrected the times by subtraction of the blank titration, then:

$$\frac{\text{Corr. time for sample}}{\text{Corr. time for standard}} \times \text{Conc. of standard} = \text{Conc. of sample}$$

Instruments are now available that have a direct readout reporting in milliequivalents per liter. The instrument can be used for direct titration of serum, plasma, spinal fluid, or urine without any preliminary treatment of the sample. When a large number of samples must be titrated, the instrument is very convenient and eliminates all subjective errors in titration. It is equipped with three titration rates so that samples ranging from 0.25-50 μEq. can be titrated and can be used for microtitrations with 0.01 ml. serum. The instruments are made by several manufacturers* and are available from most laboratory supply houses.

GASOMETRIC ANALYSIS

Laboratory analyses may be made by measuring the amount of gas liberated in a chemical reaction. This is the most practical method of determining the oxygen and carbon dioxide contents of blood. For these analyses the gas is liberated

from the blood by an appropriate reagent and is extracted by shaking under a partial vacuum; the amount of gas liberated is then measured. In oxygen determinations, not only is the oxygen combined with the hemoglobin determined but the oxygen and nitrogen physically dissolved in the plasma and some carbon dioxide are also determined. Carbon dioxide is reabsorbed in sodium hydroxide solution and the oxygen plus nitrogen is then measured; a correction can be made for the amount of physically dissolved gases (which is relatively constant) or the oxygen can be absorbed and the decrease in gas volume noted. The former, although theoretically less accurate, is preferable for an occasional analysis since the oxygen-absorbing reagent is rather unstable. In carbon dioxide determination the CO_2 can be absorbed and the change in volume noted, or a correction can be made for the amount of physically dissolved oxygen and nitrogen that is liberated along with the CO_2.

In the methods to be described the gas is measured by compressing it into a definite known volume and measuring the absolute pressure exerted by the gas. Then, in accordance with the gas laws: $PV = nRT$, where P is the pressure of the gas; V, its volume; n, the number of moles of gas present; R, a constant depending upon the units of measurement used; and T, the absolute temperature. When P is measured in millimeters of mercury, as is customary, and V is expressed in milliliters, then the value of R, in theory, can be expressed as:

$$\text{mM. of gas} = \frac{PV}{62.37} \times T$$

Since in the apparatus the gas is measured at a known volume, one could readily calculate a table relating millimoles of gas present and the pressure, P, as measured. In practice, two corrections must be applied to the formula. A correction may be applied for the amount of pressure exerted by the water vapor in the chamber. If the measurement is made by determining the difference in pressure before and after the absorption of the gas (such as carbon dioxide), then the correction for water vapor will be slight

---

*American Instrument Co., Silver Springs, Md.; Buchler Instruments, Inc., Fort Lee, N. J.

and is further reduced by running a blank determination. If the gas is extracted from the liquid under reduced pressure and the pressure then increased for the measurement, a slight amount of the gas may redissolve in the liquid. The solubility is slight for oxygen and nitrogen, but is greater for carbon dioxide. Corrections for the solubility of the gas have been determined empirically and are included in all tables of factors for the gasometric methods.

Van Slyke apparatus[104]: The conventional Van Slyke manometric apparatus is shown in Fig. 6-13. Some models have a magnetic stirrer instead of a shaker on the extraction chamber and are somewhat more convenient to use. The usual extraction chamber has calibrations at 0.5 and 2 ml., with a total volume of 50 ml.

A microchamber with calibrations at 0.1 and 0.2 ml. and with a total volume of 10 ml. is also available. This allows the use of smaller volumes of samples, but requires special micropipettes for the introduction of samples and a rather careful technique. For microsamples the Natelson apparatus, to be described later, is recommended.

A number of precautions must be taken in the use of the Van Slyke apparatus. The stopcocks must all be lubricated with a high-quality grease. The suppliers of the apparatus can usually furnish a grease made especially for the apparatus. Whenever a partial vacuum is to be formed in the extraction chamber, the capillaries in the stopcock at the top of the chamber must always be sealed with mercury. This is done by adding a little mercury through the cup every time a solution or gas is added to or removed from the chamber during the course of the analysis. It is convenient to have a source of suction (pump or water aspirator) to remove excess liquids rapidly from the cup, with a large bottle as a trap on the suction line to catch the liquid so that it will not enter the pump.

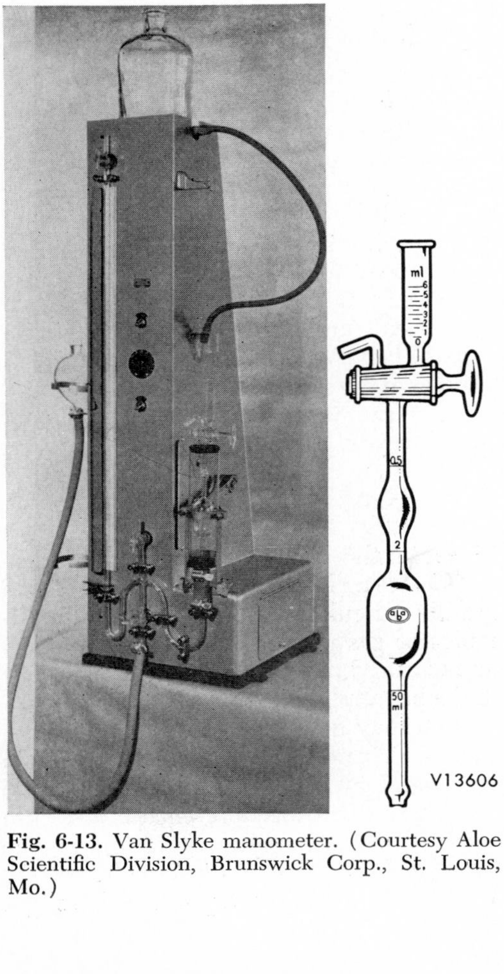

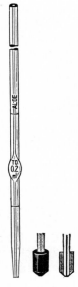

Fig. 6-13. Van Slyke manometer. (Courtesy Aloe Scientific Division, Brunswick Corp., St. Louis, Mo.)

Fig. 6-14. Van Slyke-Neill pipette. (Courtesy Aloe Scientific Division, Brunswick Corp., St. Louis, Mo.)

Care must be taken to keep metallic mercury from the drains because the mercury will amalgamate with and rapidly destroy brass or lead piping.

The best way to add a definite volume of a sample to the apparatus is by using the Van Slyke-Neill pipette that has a rubber delivery tip calibrated to deliver between two marks (Fig. 6-14). A small amount of mercury is placed in the cup (a reagent may be added above the mercury) and the pipette, filled to the upper mark, is placed in the cup with the rubber tip held firmly against the bottom. Then by carefully opening the chamber stopcock the sample will flow into the chamber. Some practice may be required to avoid going below the lower graduation. Reagents are usually measured by difference in the cup. To add 5 ml. reagent, for example, allow the liquid to flow slowly into the chamber

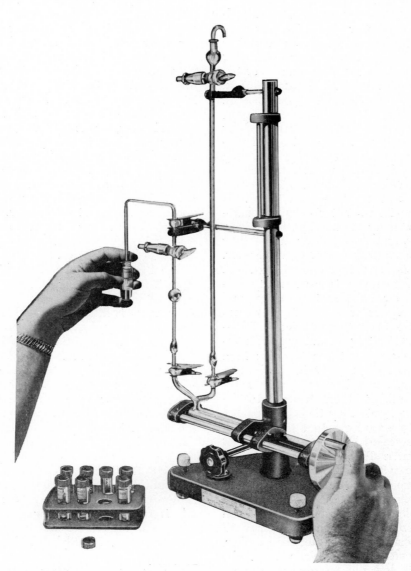

Fig. 6-15. Natelson Microgasometer, model 600. (Courtesy Scientific Industries, Inc., Springfield, Mass.)

until the level in the cup has been lowered from the 6 ml. mark to the 1 ml. mark; then after sealing the capillary with mercury, the excess reagent is removed from the cup by suction. In measuring the final pressure of a gas the fluid is slowly brought up to the meniscus. The flow is regulated by the lower stopcock on the apparatus. Care should be taken not to go past the calibration mark as this may cause some extra reabsorption of the gas, especially CO_2.

Natelson Microgasometer[105]: The Natelson Microgasometer (Fig. 6-15) is very convenient to use; it requires less time for operation and also uses a smaller sample than a conventional model of the Van Slyke apparatus. All samples and reagents are introduced through the tip, which is calibrated at 0.01, 0.02, 0.03, and 0.10 ml. The mercury is moved by means of a plunger attached to a handwheel, thus doing away with all leveling bulb manipulations. The extraction chamber has a volume of 3 ml. and the gas is measured at a volume of 0.12 ml. To operate the instrument the entire chamber and capillary are filled with mercury. In measuring a reagent or sample for introduction into the extraction chamber, the tip is inserted in the liquid, a small droplet of mercury is expelled to dislodge any air bubbles in the tip, and then the reagent or sample is drawn up into the tip to the appropriate calibration mark. The tube containing the sample is raised so that the tip dips in a small amount of mercury in the bottom of the tube, a small amount of mercury (0.01-0.02 ml.) is then drawn into the tip, and the liquid may then be removed and the tip wiped off. In this way each addition is sealed by mercury so that no air can enter. Before the next reagent is added a minute drop of this mercury is first expelled to eliminate any air bubbles clinging to the tip. When all the samples and reagents have been added, mercury is drawn in to carry all liquids over into the extraction chamber. The stopcock is then closed and the mercury is lowered to give a vacuum for the extraction. The gasometer may be shaken by hand or an automatic shaker can be supplied as an additional item. Models having a magnetic stirrer and a motor-driven handwheel for raising and lowering the mercury can also be obtained.

CARBON DIOXIDE CONTENT AND COMBINING POWER[106]

Carbon dioxide may be determined by acidifying plasma or serum with lactic acid and extracting the gas in the Van Slyke or Natelson gasometer. The pressure of CO_2 can be measured directly, with a correction for the other dissolved gases, or the CO_2 can be adsorbed by sodium hydroxide and the difference in pressure noted. Carbon dioxide has been determined as the CO_2 content, which is the actual content of the plasma or serum when collected and separated anaerobically, or as the CO_2-combining power, which is, in theory, the CO_2 content of the plasma after equilibration with a gas of a fixed carbon dioxide partial pressure of 40 mm. In practice, the technician's alveolar air is used to approximate the standard gas. The inadequacies of this technique are discussed in the section on interpretation and acid-base balance.

The best method for **anaerobic collection** is the use of heparinized Vacutainers.* When these are completely filled, there is little loss of carbon dioxide and they may be centrifuged without removal of the stopper. The blood may also be collected in a heparinized syringe (disposable plastic syringes are usually more airtight than glass syringes, even when the latter are oiled). In this case anaerobic separation of plasma is more difficult. It is usually recommended that the heparinized blood be transferred from the syringe to a tube containing a layer of mineral oil. But a careful interpretation of Van Slyke's original references shows that he concluded that mineral oil is not sufficient for preservation when the tube is to be centrifuged to obtain plasma. Van Slyke used tubes with

---

*No. 3204 AK, Becton, Dickinson & Co., East Rutherford, N. J.

a constricted neck and replaced the mineral oil with paraffin before centrifugation.

For carbon dioxide–combining power the plasma is collected without special precautions and is then equilibrated with alveolar air. Transfer about 3 ml. plasma to a separatory funnel and saturate it with alveolar air by blowing through a bottle of glass beads (to remove excess moisture from the breath) into the funnel. Without taking a deep breath, exhale normally and then blow through the funnel.

Close the funnel just before expiration is finished and rotate it in a horizontal position for 1 min. Repeat the blowing and rotation.

Reagents:
1. Lactic acid (1N). Add 90 ml. lactic acid (85%) to water and dilute to 1 L.
2. Sodium hydroxide (5N). Dissolve 100 gm. sodium hydroxide in water and dilute to 500 ml.

Procedure for Van Slyke apparatus: Introduce a small drop of capryl alcohol into the capillary of the stopcock. Then allow 0.5 ml. plasma to flow into the chamber from a Van Slyke-Neill pipette. Follow with 1.5 ml. lactic acid solution. Seal the stopcock with mercury and lower the mercury level in the chamber to near the 50 ml. mark. Shake for 2 min. Then carefully allow the liquid to rise to the 2 ml. mark. If the level is inadvertently allowed to rise above the mark, some carbon dioxide will be absorbed and the solution must be lowered and shaken again. With the meniscus at the 2 ml. mark, read the pressure and record as P_1. Allow the liquid to rise as far as possible in the chamber, add 0.5 ml. 5N sodium hydroxide, seal the stopcock with mercury, lower the level below the 2 ml. mark, and then bring the meniscus up to the mark. Read and record the pressure as P_2. Also note and record the temperature of the water jacket. Then:

$$P = P_1 - P_2 - C$$

where C is a blank obtained by carrying through the entire procedure with 2 ml.

lactic acid but no serum, then C is the difference between P_1 and P_2 for the blank. Calculate the vol.% carbon dioxide from the factor obtained in Table 6-6 as follows:

$$Vol.\% \ CO_2 = P \times Factor$$

If only a small amount of plasma is available, one can use 0.2 ml. plasma, add 1.8 ml. lactic acid, and make the readings at a volume of 0.5 ml. If it is desired to express the results in millimoles of carbon dioxide or milliequivalents of bicarbonate per liter, divide the vol.% by 2.24.

Carbon dioxide determination using the Natelson Microgasometer: Reagents are the same as used for the Van Slyke method.

Procedure: Add successively, measuring with the tip and sealing with mercury after each addition, 0.03 ml. sample, 0.03 ml. 1N lactic acid, and 0.01 ml. capryl

Table 6-6. Factors by which P is to be multiplied to obtain vol.% oxygen or carbon dioxide*

Temperature (° C.)	Oxygen (1 ml. sample; 2.5 ml. reagent) read at		Carbon dioxide lactic acid to 2 ml.	
	0.5 ml.	2 ml.	0.2 ml. sample read at 0.5 ml.	0.5 ml. sample read at 2 ml.
15	0.0623	0.2493	0.3370	0.5288
16	0.0621	0.2485	0.3354	0.5262
17	0.0619	0.2478	0.3338	0.5236
18	0.0617	0.2468	0.3322	0.5212
19	0.0615	0.2469	0.3307	0.5188
20	0.0613	0.2450	0.3294	0.5166
21	0.0610	0.2441	0.3278	0.5144
22	0.0608	0.2432	0.3263	0.5120
23	0.0606	0.2423	0.3248	0.5096
24	0.0604	0.2414	0.3234	0.5074
25	0.0602	0.2406	0.3220	0.5052
26	0.0600	0.2398	0.3206	0.5031
27	0.0598	0.2390	0.3193	0.5010
28	0.0596	0.2382	0.3179	0.4988
29	0.0593	0.2374	0.3166	0.4968
30	0.0592	0.2366	0.3153	0.4948
31	0.0590	0.2358	0.3140	0.4928
32	0.0588	0.2350	0.3128	0.4908
33	0.0586	0.2342	0.3115	0.4888
34	0.0583	0.2333	0.3103	0.4870

*From Van Slyke and Sendroy: J. Biol. Chem. 73:127, 1927.

alcohol. (The capryl alcohol is layered on top of the lactic acid so that both are measured from the same vial.) Then add 0.1 ml. water, followed by mercury to bring the liquids into the extraction chamber. Lower the mercury and shake the gasometer for 2 min. Raise the level in the chamber to the 0.12 ml. mark and read the pressure (P_1). Advance the mercury to release the pressure and add 0.02 ml. 5N sodium hydroxide, followed by mercury to bring the liquid into the extraction chamber. Lower the liquid to the 3 ml. mark, then raise to the 0.12 ml. mark, and read the pressure again (P_2).

As with the Van Slyke method:

$$P = P_1 - P_2 - C$$

where C is a blank correction found by carrying through the entire procedure without the addition of plasma. $C = P_1 - P_2$ is used for the blank determination. When recently boiled and cooled distilled water is used for making up the solutions and when they are protected from excessive contact with air, the blank should be only a few millimeters at the most. Then:

$$Vol.\% \ CO_2 = P \times Factor$$

where the factor is obtained from Table 6-6.

The normal values for plasma CO_2-combining power have been taken as 53-76 vol.% (24-34 mM./L.) for adults and as 40-55 vol.% (18-25 mM./L.) for infants. The CO_2 content in arterial plasma may be taken as 45-55 vol.% (20-25 mM./L.) and that of venous plasma as 50-60 vol.% (22-27 mM./L.). As will be mentioned in the discussion of acid-base balance, a determination of the CO_2 content or CO_2-combining power alone gives only incomplete information.

Gambino[107, 108] has suggested a method for preservation of plasma samples for carbon dioxide content analysis. This method was primarily intended for the AutoAnalyzer, but it can be used for other methods as well. It was found that when 1 drop 1N ammonium hydroxide was added to 1 ml. plasma, the carbon dioxide content did not change during 4 hr. of standing in AutoAnalyzer cups.

In the automated method the same amount of ammonia was added to the standards so that no dilution effect need be considered; but if the technique were to be applied to samples for gasometric analysis, this would have to be taken into account. However, it was found that when 1 drop ammonia from a disposable capillary pipette was added to 1 ml. plasma, the change in volume amounted to no more than 1-2%, so that a correction of 1.5% would reduce the dilution error to a negligible amount.

HYDROGEN ION CONCENTRATION (pH) IN BLOOD

The determination of the hydrogen ion concentration in blood is usually made by means of an electronic pH meter. This instrument is used to measure the electric potential across a thin membrane of special glass with a solution of known pH (usually 0.1N HCl) on one side and the unknown solution on the other side. The known solution is contained within the electrode and does not change. The other electrical connection to the unknown solution is usually made with a calomel electrode. Since the exact potentials will vary somewhat with the electrode setup, pH meters are always calibrated by the use of buffers of known pH. The manufacturers of the instruments furnish accurate buffers for standardization. The known solution is contained in the macroelectrodes in a small bulb of special glass, which is then dipped into the solution to be measured. These electrodes may require too great a volume for blood measurement, they do not protect the blood from exposure to air (which may change the pH), and they do not have water jackets (the blood pH should preferably be measured at 37° C.). Also, the simpler pH meters that are satisfactory for checking the pH of most buffers are not sufficiently accurate for blood pH determinations when readings must be made to within 0.005 pH unit or less.

There are on the market a number of accurate pH meters, together with thermostated microelectrodes, that are suitable for blood pH determinations. With these electrodes the solution to be measured (blood or plasma) is drawn up into a fine capillary made of the electrode glass and the known solution is in a small jacket around the capillary. This enables one to use small samples of blood and also protects the blood from exposure to air during measurement. These electrodes are also jacketed with a circulating water bath or heating device to keep them at a constant temperature. The operating details will vary somewhat from instrument to instrument, but the blood is usually drawn up into the capillary by gentle suction through a thin plastic tube attached to one end. This tube is then dipped into a saturated KCl solution for measurement. With care, reproducible measurements can be made to within 0.005 pH unit or better. Since the electrodes may not be quite linear, they are usually standardized with buffers of two different pH values.

As mentioned, the pH should be measured at 37° C. If the blood cannot be measured at body temperature, an approximate correction can be made. The pH of whole blood decreases about 0.015 pH unit for each degree C. rise in temperature. For example, at 27° C. blood will have a pH of 0.15 unit higher than at body temperature (37° C.). The difference for plasma is about –0.011 pH unit/degree C. The exact variation with temperature is different for different blood samples, particularly with changes in hematocrit, so that the correction can only be approximate. The pH of serum or heparinized plasma separated from blood at body temperature will be the same as that of the blood. However, if the cells are separated at a lower temperature and the pH of the plasma is then measured at 37° C., the pH will be too alkaline by 0.02-0.04 pH unit. Consequently, if plasma pH is to be determined, the blood should never be centrifuged while ice-cold. It should be warmed to room temperature or even to 30° C. before centrifuging.

The normal values for the pH of venous blood are 7.32-7.42; for arterial blood the values are about 0.03 unit higher. The significance of blood pH

changes will be discussed in relation to acid-base balance.

Acid-base balance[109]: An evaluation of the acid-base balance in blood requires a knowledge of the factors involved in the blood carbonic acid–bicarbonate buffer (a mixture of a weak acid and its salt) system. According to the Henderson-Hasselbalch equation, the general mathematical formulation for any buffer may be expressed as follows:

$$pH = pK + Log \frac{[Salt]}{[Acid]}$$

where the brackets denote concentrations.

The pK for carbonic acid is 6.1; then for the bicarbonate buffer this is:

$$pH = 6.1 + Log \frac{[HCO_3^-]}{[H_2CO_3]}$$

Normally the bicarbonate $[HCO_3^-]$ concentration is about 24 mEq./L. and the carbonic acid $[H_2CO_3]$ concentration is about 1.2. Then:

$$pH = 6.1 + Log \frac{24}{1.2} = 6.1 + Log\ 20 =$$
$$6.1 + 1.3 = 7.4$$

Table 6-7 illustrates the changes in blood pH and CO_2 content in various pathologic conditions. Note that in both respiratory acidosis and metabolic alkalosis the CO_2 content is high, so that a measurement of this would not assist in diagnosis as would the measurement of pH. In metabolic acidosis and respiratory acidosis the pH is low, so that this measurement would not distinguish between them, though a measurement of CO_2 content would. In compensated respiratory acidosis there would be a gradual retention of HCO_3^- to bring the pH to near normality. At this time a measurement of pH would not indicate the true condition of the patient, but a determination of CO_2 content would indicate a level even above that of the uncompensated condition. Other examples indicating that the single measurement of CO_2 content or pH alone is not sufficient to accurately assess the acid-base balance could also be given.

Gambino[110] has recently pointed out that many patients with severe intra-

Table 6-7. Acidosis and alkalosis—changes in blood pH and CO_2 content due to changes in bicarbonate buffer $\left(\dfrac{HCO_3^-}{H_2CO_3}\right)$

Clinical condition	Change in denominator H_2CO_3	Change in numerator HCO_3^-	Common causes
Respiratory acidosis (CO_2 content and P_{CO_2} high, pH low)	Increases due to pulmonary retention of CO_2*	May be increased late in compensation†	Impaired pulmonary function (asthma, emphysema, etc.)
Metabolic acidosis (CO_2 content and P_{CO_2} low, pH low)	May be decreased late in compensation‡	Decreases as result of loss of $NaHCO_3$* or displacement by other ions	Loss of base through diarrhea or impaired renal function in organic acids and in diabetes and starvation
Respiratory alkalosis (CO_2 content low, pH high)	Decreases due to hyperventilation*	May be decreased late in compensation†	Hyperventilation
Metabolic alkalosis (CO_2 content high, pH high)	May be increased in compensation‡	Increased as result of loss of Cl or ingestion of $NaHCO_3$*	Loss of HCl (vomiting), ingestion of alkali (peptic ulcer treatment)

*Primary changes that occur as the result of abnormal conditions.
†Changes made by the homeostatic mechanisms of the body to restore a normal pH and compensate for the abnormality. Changes in bicarbonate are chiefly mediated by an increase or decrease in the renal excretion of bicarbonate.
‡Changes in H_2CO_3 brought about by changes in respiratory function to accelerate or decrease elimination of CO_2.

abdominal or intracerebral diseases (peritonitis, liver coma, hypertensive encephalopathy) may have a normal CO_2 content of the serum (26-31 mEq./L.), but they have a high pH (over 7.5). Measurement of the CO_2 content alone would not indicate any serious disease process in such cases.

OXYGEN CONTENT AND OXYGEN CAPACITY

Procedure for Van Slyke apparatus: For determining oxygen content the blood must be collected and stored out of contact with air. If a glass syringe is used for collecting the blood, it is suggested that the inside of the syringe be lightly coated with mineral oil. Disposable plastic syringes have been found to be more airtight than glass syringes, especially those that have been used many times. **Heparin** is preferable as an **anticoagulant;** a few drops of the solution are placed in the syringe before drawing the blood. After drawing the blood, it is mixed with heparin by rotating the syringe horizontally between the palms of the hands. The blood is simply stored in the syringe by leaving the needle on and forcing the point of the needle into a small rubber stopper. If not analyzed at once, the blood for oxygen capacity should be stored in ice water. Another method of anaerobic collection is to use heparinized Vacutainers that are filled to capacity. These instruments may present some difficulty if arterial blood is desired, but it is quite possible to obtain such blood in these tubes. They should be kept stoppered until ready for analysis.

For determining oxygen capacity the blood is saturated with oxygen by adding about 5 ml. blood to a 250 ml. separatory funnel and rotating the funnel in a horizontal position to form a thin layer of blood over the interior. Preferably 100% oxygen from a tank should be passed into the funnel to aid in saturation. After about 5 min. of rotation, the funnel is turned upright and the blood is allowed to collect in the bottom. The actual chemical procedure is the same for both analyses. The oxygen content determination indicates the actual amount of oxygen present in the blood (principally combined with hemoglobin) and the oxygen capacity determination shows the amount of oxygen in the blood when fully saturated. Their ratio is the percent saturation.

Reagents:

1. Oxygen reagent. Add 1.6 gm. potassium ferricyanide, 0.3 ml. capryl alcohol, 0.4 ml. 85% lactic acid, and 0.6 gm. saponin to 100 ml. water. This solution is stable for several days in the refrigerator. Discard when it turns green.
2. Oxygen absorbent. (This is used only when the greatest accuracy is desired.) Add 5 gm. sodium hydrosulfite ($Na_2S_2O_4$) and 0.5 gm. sodium beta-anthraquinonesulfonate to 25 ml. 1N sodium hydroxide that has been boiled and rapidly cooled to room temperature without agitation. Overlay at once with a layer of mineral oil and stir gently to dissolve the salts. This is stable only 1 or 2 days in the refrigerator.
3. Sodium hydroxide (1N). Dissolve 20 gm. sodium hydroxide in water to make 500 ml. Deaerate a portion by boiling and cooling just before use.

Procedure: Mix the capryl alcohol in the oxygen reagent by vigorous rotation and add 7.5 ml. to the cup of the Van Slyke apparatus. Open the stopcock and allow the solution to flow into the chamber. Seal the upper stopcock with mercury. Lower leveling bulb and allow liquid in chamber to lower until the mercury meniscus is at the 50 ml. mark. Close lower stopcock and shake for 3 min. to deaerate solution. Slowly open the lower stopcock and allow fluid to rise in the chamber. Manipulate leveling bulb and stopcock so that 6 ml. liquid is expelled into the cup (leaving 1.5 ml. in the chamber).

Introduce 1 ml. well-mixed blood into the chamber from the pipette, followed by 1 ml. oxygen reagent. Seal capillary

with mercury and discard excess reagent. Lower mercury in chamber to 50 ml. mark and shake for 3 min. Allow liquid level to rise slowly to the 2 ml. mark and take the reading on the manometer (P_1). If the P_1 reading is less than 350, take this and all subsequent readings at the 0.5 ml. mark. The P_1 reading represents the combined pressure of carbon dioxide, oxygen, and nitrogen and is used only when the CO_2 content is desired. Lower liquid somewhat in chamber to give a gas volume of about 5 ml., add 1 ml. deaerated NaOH to the cup, and slowly add 0.5 ml. to the chamber. Seal capillary with mercury and discard excess NaOH. Bring meniscus up to 2 (or 0.5) ml. mark and read (P_2). When greatest accuracy is not desired and oxygen is not absorbed, raise leveling bulb and carefully eject all gas from the chamber without loss of liquid. Close upper stopcock, lower liquid level in chamber below 2 ml. mark, and carefully bring up to the mark and read (P_3).

The pressure due to the oxygen is then:

$$P = P_2 - P_3 - C$$

where C is a blank correction obtained by carrying through the procedure without blood, but using a total of 3.5 ml. deaerated reagent. The difference in the readings obtained is taken as C. This should be constant and need be determined only occasionally.

For highest accuracy the oxygen should be absorbed. After obtaining the P_2 reading as described, lower the liquid somewhat in the chamber so that the gas volume is about 5 ml. Add 2 ml. oxygen-absorbing reagent to the cup and allow 1 ml. to slowly enter the chamber over a period of 3 min. Close upper stopcock and slowly bring meniscus up to 2 (or 0.5) ml. mark and read (P_3). Again, $P = P_2 - P_3 - C$, where the blank C is determined for this procedure by carrying through all the steps including the absorption step.

The vol.% oxygen is then P × F, where F is obtained from Table 6-6. If it is desired to express the results in millimoles of oxygen per liter, divide the vol.% by

2.24. From the values thus obtained, there must be subtracted a correction factor for the physically dissolved gases. When the total oxygen is desired, a correction of 1 vol.% is subtracted as a correction for dissolved nitrogen when the method without oxygen absorption is used. When the oxygen is absorbed, the difference in pressure is due to oxygen alone. Usually in the determination of oxygen content one is interested only in the oxygen combined with the hemoglobin in the blood, and further correction must be made for the physically dissolved oxygen. This amounts to 0.1 vol.% for venous blood, 0.3 vol.% for arterial blood, and 0.6 vol.% for blood saturated with oxygen from air at 25° C.

The determination of percent oxygen saturation with the Van Slyke apparatus requires considerable experience since the results are based on two separate determinations of oxygen capacity. Since the oxygen is carried by the hemoglobin, it is obvious that an error will result if the hematocrit values for the blood specimen and the oxygenated specimen are not exactly the same. Apart from the difficulties in accurately sampling whole blood, it has been shown that when the blood is saturated with oxygen in the separatory funnel the sample withdrawn will not have the same hematocrit as that originally introduced. This is because of the different degrees to which the plasma and red cells will remain absorbed on the relatively large glass surface exposed.

However, this may be the only method available for many laboratories since the spectrophotometric methods require an accurate spectrophotometer with a narrow slit width. In these methods the hemolyzed blood is measured in a cell having a light path of 1 mm. or less at two different wavelengths. At one wavelength, hemoglobin and oxygen hemoglobin have different absorbances, while at the other wavelength they have the same absorbance (isobestic point). The ratio of the optical densities at the two wavelengths is a linear function of the percent of saturation. The measurements may be made at 650 and 805 nm. or at 560 and 522 nm. Since these methods depend on the ratio of the absorbances on the same sample of blood, they are independent of any errors in sampling. Details of these methods are given in the articles by Johnstone[111] and by Van Kampen and Zijlstra.[112]

Oxygen determination using the Natelson apparatus:

Reagents:

1. Saponin-ferricyanide. Prepare a solution of 1.2 gm. potassium ferricyanide in 100 ml. water. This is stable when stored in the refrigerator. Also dissolve 1 gm. reagent grade saponin in 100 ml. normal saline solution; this solution must be prepared weekly. On the day of use, mix together 1.5 ml. ferricyanide solution with 10 ml. saponin solution. Place in a small bottle, cover the solution with a layer of capryl alcohol, and deaerate as described below.

2. Sodium hydroxide (3N). Dissolve 12 gm. sodium hydroxide in water, cool, and make up to 100 ml. Store in polyethylene bottle. Transfer a portion to a 20 ml. vial, cover with mineral oil, and add mercury to a height of 2 cm., delivered to the bottom of the vial. This solution must also be deaerated.

3. Potassium hydroxide (1N). Dissolve 6 gm. potassium hydroxide in water and make up to 100 ml. Store in a polyethylene bottle.

4. Sodium hydrosulfite solution. Place 1 gm. sodium hydrosulfite in a 20 ml. vial and cover with mineral oil. Add 5 ml. 1N KOH and 2 ml. mercury. The hydrosulfite will dissolve as the solution is being deaerated.

Since the solutions cannot be deaerated in the apparatus, this must be done beforehand. One method is to place the vials, with the liquid covered with light mineral oil or capryl alcohol, in a vacuum desiccator and evacuate to a pressure of 25-35 mm. The pressure should not be so low that the liquids will tend to boil over. If a desiccator is not available, the individual vials may be connected to a vacuum source through small, one-hole rubber stoppers and a glass manifold. Deaeration should be continued for 25-30 min.

Procedure: Rinse the chamber with water and expel. Draw up 0.1 ml. 1N lactic acid into the bottom of the lower bulb. Shake for a few seconds and expel. Close the stopcock, move the piston back until the mercury is in the lower bulb, and then expel any trapped gases. Draw up 0.01 ml. capryl alcohol, then 0.1 ml. saponin-ferricyanide mixture, and 0.01 ml. capryl alcohol as a seal. Now draw up 0.03 ml. well-mixed blood, then 0.01 ml. capryl alcohol, followed by 0.1 ml. saponin-ferricyanide and 0.01 ml. capryl alcohol. This is followed by mercury to reach the 0.12 ml. mark. The stopcock is closed and the liquid brought down about halfway in the reaction chamber. Run piston back and forth several times to ensure complete mixing. Shake the gasometer for 3 min. to release the oxygen. Raise the capryl alcohol meniscus to the 0.12 ml. mark and take the pressure reading (P_1). Lower the liquid and repeat the shaking; then take another reading to ensure complete extraction of the oxygen.

The pressure is released by advancing the piston. Add 0.03 ml. 3N sodium hydroxide, followed by mercury to reach the 0.11 ml. mark. Lower the mercury to the 3 ml. mark and shake the gasometer for 3 min. Raise the capryl alcohol meniscus to the 0.12 ml. mark and take a reading (P_2).

Next, the oxygen is absorbed by introducing 0.03 ml. hydrosulfite solution, followed by mercury. Lower the mercury in the extraction chamber and shake the gasometer for 3 min. Raise the alcohol meniscus again to the 0.12 ml. mark and take a reading (P_3). As with the Van Slyke apparatus, a blank is run using all the reagents and steps but no blood. The $P_2 - P_3$ value for the blank is the correction C. Then the corrected pressure is:

$$P_2 - P_3 - C = P$$

and

$$P \times F = \text{Vol.\% } O_2$$

The factor for oxygen at various temperatures is given in Table 6-8.

The same correction for dissolved oxygen must be made as for the Van Slyke method if the hemoglobin oxygen deter-

Table 6-8. Factors for calculating O_2 and CO_2 concentration in vol.% using Natelson Microgasometer

Temperature (°C.)	Factor	
	Vol.% O_2	Vol.% CO_2
18	0.494	0.533
19	0.492	0.529
20	0.490	0.526
21	0.488	0.524
22	0.486	0.522
23	0.485	0.518
24	0.483	0.516
25	0.481	0.513
26	0.480	0.510
27	0.478	0.508
28	0.476	0.506
29	0.475	0.504
30	0.473	0.502
31	0.472	0.500
32	0.470	0.497

mination is desired. Normal venous blood may give a $P_2 - P_3$ value of only 40 mm.; the reading may be doubled by using 0.06 ml. blood. This is done by sampling the blood twice to the 0.03 ml. mark with a mercury plug in between. All reagents are doubled except the saponin-ferricyanide mixture. The factors are then divided by 2.

Normal values and interpretation: The oxygen capacity of blood is 1.34 ml./ gm. hemoglobin. In the absence of significant amounts of carboxyhemoglobin or methemoglobin, the oxygen capacity can be estimated quite well from an accurate hemoglobin determination and, conversely, oxygen capacity measurements have been used to calibrate hemoglobin methods. The oxygen capacity is normally about 20.7 vol.% (15.4 gm. Hb) for men and 19 vol.% (14.2 gm. Hb) for women. It is increased in polycythemia and in anhydremia and is decreased in anemia. As determined by gasometric methods, the oxygen saturation of arterial blood in normal individuals has been considered as 95%. Somewhat higher values, approaching 98%, are obtained by spectrophotometric methods. This is partially due to the hematocrit error in the saturation of the blood, as previously mentioned. The oxygen saturation of venous blood is 60-85%.

OSMOLALITY OF SERUM AND OTHER BIOLOGIC FLUIDS[113-116]

Osmotic pressure is one of the main factors regulating the homeostatic equilibrium between cytoplasm and extracellular fluid in living cells. It is a measurement of all particles in a solution, regardless of size, shape, or charge, and it can be measured by direct or indirect methods.

Direct measurement involves the use of a semipermeable membrane that allows water to pass through freely but restricts the movement of all solids, including electrolytes. This method is not practical because of the difficulty of finding membranes with sufficiently small pores.

The indirect methods involve measurements of freezing point, boiling point, or vapor pressure of the fluid. The most commonly used clinical method is the freezing point determination (a measurement of a solution's concentration). This requires a special apparatus known as an osmometer, which is rather expensive. With this instrument the osmolality of serum (or other biologic fluid) is determined by comparing its freezing point with that of a sodium chloride solution of known osmolality (osmotic pressure). Details for the operation of the various instruments available are furnished by the manufacturers.

Osmolality has been defined as the molality of an ideal substance dissolved in water in amounts sufficient to produce the same osmotic pressure and freezing point depression as the specimen. This ideal substance is assumed to be a nonelectrolyte, neither disassociating nor associating and not interacting with water. The amount of dissolved material equivalent in effect to 1 mole of the ideal substance is called 1 osmole.

Fresh serum, free of all particles, should be used for this determination. Serum that cannot be analyzed immediately should be stoppered securely and refrigerated or frozen.

Urine is collected without preservatives in sterile, clean, dry glassware and capped to avoid evaporation. Osmolality is determined in the freshly voided urine before and after centrifugation to avoid errors from changes in composition caused by chemical or bacterial action.

The normal range for serum osmolality has been reported to be 289 ± 8 mOsm./L. The same range applies to spinal, pleural, and peritoneal fluids when drawn at the same time.

Serum osmolality studies have been used in the evaluation of hypernatremia and hyponatremia, renal solute retention in acute renal failure, and hydration status. These studies are also used in detecting "undetermined solute" in cases of poisoning and for estimating the requirement for and effectiveness of dialysis. Most important, they are used to estimate serum water since water concentration determines the osmotic pressure.

The ratio of urine osmolality to serum osmolality has been used for the calculation of free-water and osmolar clearances in the differential diagnosis of polyuria and in the evaluation of renal solute excretion in certain hormonal and renal diseases.

The normal range of urine osmolality has been reported to be 855-1335 mOsm./L. Values will fall outside this range in cases of advanced renal disease or extrarenal disease affecting urine concentration. If osmolality is high, there is an increase in concentration; if low, there is a decrease.

LIVER FUNCTION TESTS

The liver is the largest organ in the human body and possesses a large and varied array of biochemical activities that are essential to proper function of the body. The liver plays a central role in the metabolism of carbohydrates and in the formation of proteins and other aspects of protein metabolism. It is concerned with detoxification of drugs and other harmful substances and with the metabolism of steroid hormones. It plays an important role in the production of some of the substances necessary for the coagulation of blood and in the metabolism of iron and the formation and breakdown of hemoglobin. It is also concerned in the production of bile, which aids in the digestion of fats and the absorption of fat-soluble vitamins. The liver has a great reserve capacity; nearly four fifths of the liver can be removed without seriously affecting its function. On the other hand, only a slight diffuse lesion (affecting the whole organ) is necessary to alter the results of liver function tests. In severe liver damage all of the functions will be decreased to some extent. This depends upon the type of disease; some functions may be affected more than others.

Liver function tests may be classified on the basis of the principal metabolic process or type of function with which they are concerned, on the basis of their sensitivity in detecting liver damage, or on the basis of the clinical conditions in which they are most useful. All three methods would have some validity for the purposes of this volume, but we have adapted a classification based mainly on the first—the specific function or metabolic process involved.

TESTS BASED ON BILE PIGMENTS

Bilirubin is formed by the breakdown of hemoglobin by the cells of the reticulo-endothelial system (spleen, bone marrow, Kupffer cells of the liver) and it circulates in the blood in low concentrations. A small amount is excreted by the kidneys into the urine. Bilirubin is excreted by the liver cells into the bile and passes with the bile into the intestines, where

Table 6-9. Early laboratory findings in jaundice (frequently used tests)

	Hemolytic	*Hepatogenous*	*Obstructive*
Bile pigments			
Urine			
Urobilinogen and urobilin	Markedly increased	Slight to moderate increase	Not increased; may be absent
Bilirubin	Negative	Positive	Positive
Blood			
Icterus index	Usually low increase	Increase variable	Greatly increased
Direct van den Bergh (1 min.)	Negative	Positive; increased	Positive; varies with degree of obstruction
Indirect van den Bergh (total)	Positive; moderate increase	Positive; moderate to marked increase	Positive; marked increase
Feces			
Urobilinogen compounds	Markedly increased	Normal or variable	Low or negative (alcoholic)
Blood			
Cholesterol (serum)	Normal	Decreased	Markedly increased
Alkaline phosphatase (serum)	Under 10 units	Normal or slightly increased; usually under 10 units	Markedly increased; over 10 units
Thymol or Hanger	Negative	Strongly positive	Negative
Prothrombin time	Normal	Increased	Normal, later increased
Response to vitamin K	Normal	Decreased or none	Normal
Albumin (serum)	Normal	Slightly decreased	Normal
Globulin (serum)	Normal	Increased	Normal
A/G ratio	Normal	May be reversed	Normal
Bromsulphalein retention	Usually negative	Usually positive	Positive

it is reduced by bacterial action to **uro-bilinogen.** The major portion of the uro-bilinogen is excreted in the feces. Some is reabsorbed into the blood and reex-creted by the liver as bilirubin or uro-bilinogen. A portion of the absorbed uro-bilinogen is also excreted by the kidneys into the urine.

An increase in bilirubin concentration in the bloodstream results in the clinical condition of jaundice (Table 6-9). This increase may be due to a number of causes. Because of increased hemoglobin destruction, the liver may not be able to properly excrete the greater load of pig-ment present and the bilirubin level in the blood will rise. This is the condition known as **hemolytic jaundice;** the liver function may be relatively normal but is simply unable to cope with the pigments from the marked increase in erythrocyte destruction. The second type of jaundice is due to damage to the liver parenchyma, which may be of toxic, infectious, or me-chanical nature. Excretion of bile is greatly decreased and the concentration of bilirubin in the blood rises. In the third type of jaundice the liver cells may have a normal or nearly normal ability to excrete bilirubin, but because of obstruc-tion in the biliary tract, the proper flow of bile is inhibited and the bile capillaries are dilated and even disrupted by the back-pressure. The bile flows into the peri-lobar lymphatics and hence into the blood-stream. This condition has been desig-nated as obstructive jaundice.

Icterus index[117]: Bilirubin is yellow in color. It has an absorption maximum (in the presence of protein) at around 460 nm. A simple method of estimating the approximate amount of bilirubin in the serum is to measure the yellow color. The color is compared with a standard solution of potassium dichromate and the results are reported in terms of units of icterus index. The method is only approx-imate as there are other compounds in the blood, chiefly carotenes, that will also give a yellow color, but it may be a sim-ple way of following the clinical state of the patient. In earlier methods the color of the serum was compared directly with the standard, but in the method presented the color is extracted with acetone and is therefore somewhat less subject to inter-ferences.

Reagents:
1. Acetone solution (78%). Place 78 ml. reagent grade acetone in a 100 ml. flask and dilute to the mark with water. Store in a refrigerator so that the solution will be cold when used.
2. Standards:
    A. Stock standard. Dissolve 0.61 gm. pure, dried potassium di-chromate ($K_2Cr_2O_7$) in water containing a few drops of con-centrated sulfuric acid and dilute to 100 ml. This solution is stable if protected from contact with organic matter.
    B. Working standard. Dilute 1 ml. stock standard to 100 ml. with water containing a drop or two of concentrated sulfuric acid. This corresponds to an icterus in-dex of 10 units.

Procedure: Place 1 ml. serum in a test tube. Add 9 ml. cold acetone solution, mix, and filter. Keep the top of the fun-nel covered with a watch glass to prevent evaporation. Read in a photometer at 450 nm. against a blank of 1 ml. water plus 9 ml. acetone solution. Also read the di-luted standard against water in the pho-tometer at the same wavelength.

Calculation:

$$\frac{\text{OD sample}}{\text{OD standard}} \times 10 = \text{Icterus index (units)}$$

Normal values and interpretation: The normal range of the icterus index is 2-6 units. In latent jaundice the index is 7-15 units. When the index is over 15, clini-cally obvious jaundice is usually present. An increase in the icterus index usually parallels the increase in bilirubin. Inges-tion of large amounts of food rich in caro-tene (carrots, tomatoes, spinach, etc.) may lead to carotinemia. This will in-crease the icterus index but not the bili-rubin level.

BILIRUBIN

Principle: Bilirubin reacts with diazo-tized sulfanilic acid to give a color that is red-violet in acid solution and blue in alkaline solution. It has been known for many years that not all of the bilirubin present in serum reacts at once with the diazo reagent in an aqueous solution. To obtain a complete reaction the addition of a fairly high concentration of alcohol (ethyl or methyl) or some other solubilizing agent is necessary. It is now generally believed that bilirubin exists in the serum in two forms—a "free" form (probably absorbed on protein) and a conjugated form (chiefly as glucuronates). The so-called **direct-reacting bilirubin** is the **conjugated form** that is more soluble in water and reacts relatively rapidly in aqueous solution. The free bilirubin is much less soluble in water and does not react (or reacts very slowly) in simple aqueous solution. The addition of methyl alcohol to a concentration of 40-50% will dissolve the bilirubin sufficiently to react with diazo reagent. This is the basis for the commonly used Malloy-Evelyn method. A solution containing a relatively high concentration of caffeine and sodium benzoate will also dissolve the free bilirubin for reaction. This is used in the method of Jendrassik and Grof.

Although widely used, the method of Malloy and Evelyn has several disadvantages that are not always kept in mind. The diazo color is slightly different in hue and intensity when the test is run on diluted serum than when it is run on a chloroform standard containing no serum or protein, as is often done with this method. Although convenient, a chloroform standard may introduce a slight error. Furthermore, unreacted bilirubin has some absorption at the wavelength used, so that in the standardization the blank should contain the same amount of bilirubin as the diazotized standard. The diazotized bilirubin is actually an indicator in which the color changes with the pH. As ordinarily run, the final solution is only slightly buffered so that changes in pH can occur, particularly if the serum used is one in which the pH has changed on standing. The high concentration of alcohol in the reaction for total bilirubin often causes some turbidity that is not always the same in the diazotized sample as in the serum blank. The presence of more than traces of hemoglobin will also interfere with the color reaction.

The method of Jendrassik and Grof suffers less from these disadvantages. The final color is read in a highly buffered alkaline medium in which changes in pH are negligible. This reduces the effects of varying protein content and the effects of hemolysis are also markedly reduced. Since the method of Malloy and Evelyn is still widely used, both methods will be presented.

It should also be mentioned that bilirubin is markedly **sensitive to light.** This applies to all methods; samples for bilirubin determination should not be exposed to strong light at any time. When serum samples that are not to be analyzed immediately are stored in the refrigerator, the effect of light is no problem; however, exposure to ordinary light in the laboratory for several hours could reduce the bilirubin content by 10% or more.

Bilirubin(Jendrassik-Grof method)[118, 119]: *Reagents:*

1. Caffeine solution. Dissolve 50 gm. caffeine, 75 gm. sodium benzoate, and 125 gm. crystalline sodium acetate (trihydrate) in warm water. Cool and dilute to 1 L. This solution is stable for at least 6 mo.
2. Diazo I. Dissolve 0.5 gm. sulfanilic acid and 15 ml. concentrated hydrochloric acid in water to make 1 L.
3. Diazo II. Dissolve 0.5 gm. sodium nitrite in 100 ml. water. This solution is stable for about 2 wk. when kept in the refrigerator. It may be convenient to weigh out 0.1 gm. portions of sodium nitrite into small stoppered vials or bottles to which 20 ml. water can be added as needed.
4. Diazo mixture. Mix 10 ml. diazo I and 0.25 ml. diazo II. Use within 30 min. after mixing.
5. Hydrochloric acid (0.05N). Dilute 4.5 ml. concentrated hydrochloric acid to 1 L.
6. Ascorbic acid (4%). Dissolve 200 mg. ascorbic acid in 5 ml. water. This should be freshly prepared. A convenient method for obtaining the

ascorbic acid solution is to use sterile ampules of ascorbic acid for parental injection. One ampule is then opened, diluted with water if necessary, and then used.

7. Alkaline tartrate. Dissolve 100 gm. sodium hydroxide and 350 gm. potassium sodium tartrate in water and dilute to 1 L. Store in polyethylene bottle.

Procedure for macromethod (total bilirubin): For each serum sample set up two tubes, sample and serum blank. Also set up one reagent blank, using water instead of diluted serum. Dilute 1 ml. serum with 4 ml. saline solution; this will give sufficient diluted serum for both direct and total bilirubin. For **total bilirubin** place 1 ml. diluted serum and 2.1 ml. caffeine mixture in test tubes and mix. To serum sample and reagent blank add 0.5 ml. diazo mixture; to serum blank add 0.5 ml. diazo I. Allow mixture to stand for exactly 10 min. To each tube add 1.5 ml. alkaline tartrate. Read the serum and serum blank against the reagent blank at 600 nm. 5-10 min. after the addition of the tartrate. Note that although the diazotized bilirubin is blue in alkali, the solutions appear green due to the yellow color from the reaction of the diazo reagent and the caffeine mixture. This yellow color has negligible absorbance at 600 nm. Subtract the OD of the serum blank from that of the serum for calculation. Experience will show that, except for noticeably hemolyzed sera, the blank reading is fairly constant and that a constant blank may be used without great error with unhemolyzed sera.

For hemolyzed samples the effect of hemoglobin may be reduced by using 2 ml. caffeine solution and then adding 0.1 ml. ascorbic acid solution just before the caffeine solution, as in the direct bilirubin method.

Procedure for direct bilirubin: The setup is similar to that for total bilirubin, using 1 ml. diluted serum, 2 ml. 0.05N hydrochloric acid, and 0.5 ml. diazo mixture. After exactly 10 min., add 0.1 ml. ascorbic acid solution, mix, and then add at once 1.5 ml. alkaline tartrate. Also set up a serum blank and reagent blank as

before, adding diazo I instead of the diazo mixture to the serum blank. Read as for total bilirubin.

Procedure for micromethod: To 0.25 ml. water and 1 ml. caffeine mixture add 0.05 ml. serum from a micropipette. Add 0.25 ml. diazo mixture and let stand exactly 10 min.; then add 0.75 ml. alkaline tartrate and read against blank as for macromethod. A serum blank and reagent blank should also be set up as in the macromethod. The solution is sufficient for reading in cuvettes such as the 12 mm. Coleman cuvettes.

Direct bilirubin can also be run by the micromethod, using 1 ml. 0.05N hydrochloric acid, 0.2 ml. water, 0.05 ml. serum, 0.25 ml. diazo mixture, 0.5 ml. ascorbic acid, and finally, 0.75 ml. alkaline tartrate.

Calculation: Bilirubin values are usually read from a calibration chart. The preparation of a chart will be discussed in the section on standardization. If a standard of a serum of known bilirubin content is used, then:

$$\frac{OD\ sample}{OD\ standard} \times Mg.\%\ standard = Mg.\%\ sample$$

where the OD of the standard and sample have been corrected, if necessary, for any blank readings.

All standards are calibrated in terms of total bilirubin only and are used to calibrate both the direct bilirubin and total bilirubin in the sample.

Total bilirubin − Direct bilirubin = Indirect bilirubin

Bilirubin (Malloy-Evelyn method)[120, 121]:
Reagents:
1. Diazo mixture. Prepare the same as for the previous method.
2. Hydrochloric acid (1.5%). Dilute 15 ml. concentrated hydrochloric acid to 1 L.
3. Methyl alcohol.

Procedure: Add 2 ml. serum to 18 ml. normal saline solution and mix. For **direct bilirubin** pipette 4 ml. diluted serum to each of two tubes, A and B. To tube A add 1 ml. diazo mixture and mix immediately. To tube B add 1 ml. 1.5% hydrochloric acid and mix. Read tube A against tube B in a photometer at 540 nm. at the required time interval. Some prefer to read exactly 5 min. after the addition of diazo mixture and record as direct bilirubin. Others read at 1 min. and again at 15 min. and report as 1 min. bilirubin and direct bilirubin, but it is probable that the 1 min. reading has little clinical significance.

For **total bilirubin** proceed as for direct bilirubin, but after the addition of diazo reagent add 5 ml. methyl alcohol, mix, and allow to stand for 30 min. before reading. Read tube A against tube B as for direct bilirubin.

Calculation: Note that in this procedure the final volume for total bilirubin is twice the final volume for direct bilirubin. Hence, if a known serum is used as a standard for total bilirubin, then:

Direct bilirubin:

$$\frac{OD\ sample}{OD\ standard} \times \frac{Mg.\%\ standard}{2} = Mg.\%\ sample$$

Total bilirubin:

$$\frac{OD\ sample}{OD\ standard} \times Mg.\%\ standard = Mg.\%\ sample$$

Total bilirubin − Direct bilirubin =
Indirect bilirubin

Bilirubin standardization[122]: Many commercial bilirubin preparations are by no means pure and all bilirubin solutions are subject to deterioration on storage. Consequently the standardization of a bilirubin curve is not simple. Chloroform solutions of bilirubin are relatively stable and have been used as standards, but they are not applicable to all methods. It has also been shown that absorption of diazo-bilirubin is different in the presence of protein (as in a serum sample) and in the absence of protein (as in a chloroform standard). It has been stated that this difference depends somewhat on the type of photoelectric colorimeter used (spectrophotometer or filter instrument). The best method seems to be the preparation of a standard curve using dilutions of a commercial lyophilized control serum. The serum should be used for bilirubin determination within 2 hr. after reconstitution and should not be exposed to bright light at any time.

Table 6-10

Tube No.	1	2	3	4	5	6
Serum A (ml.)	1.0	0.8	0.6	0.4	0.2	0.0
Serum B (ml.)	0.0	0.2	0.4	0.6	0.8	1.0
Equivalent mg.%	0.60	1.68	2.76	3.84	4.92	6.00

If the method used is sensitive to protein concentration (as is the Malloy-Evelyn method), it is preferable to use not merely dilutions of a high bilirubin serum with saline solution but mixtures of a low bilirubin serum and a high bilirubin serum to keep the protein content approximately constant. For example, if the one control serum contained 0.6 mg.% bilirubin (serum A) and the other serum contained 6 mg.% bilirubin (serum B) and the method required that 1 ml. serum be diluted with 9 ml. saline solution, then setting up the tubes as given in Table 6-10 would give a series of standards.

It is desirable to have an independent check on the bilirubin curve and we have found the "Harleco" Dripak bilirubin standard* very satisfactory for this purpose. The material is quite stable in the dry form. Standardization using this material is rather tedious and hence is most suitable as an occasional check on the calibration curve.

The "Harleco" bilirubin is supplied in plastic containers that hold exactly 40 mg. pure bilirubin each. The entire packet is dropped into exactly 40 ml. 0.1M sodium carbonate and swirled until dissolved. The bilirubin should form a clear solution within a few minutes. The entire standardization procedure should be carried through as rapidly as possible and in as dim a light as practicable.

In each of two test tubes place a dilution of a clear serum of low bilirubin content. Use the same volume of solution and the same dilution of serum as in the regular bilirubin procedure. To one tube add 0.05 ml. bilirubin solution, using an accurate "to contain" micropipette that has been rinsed well. To the other tube add 0.05 ml. sodium carbonate. The

---

*Hartman-Leddon Co. ("Harleco"), Philadelphia, Pa.

regular procedure for total bilirubin is then carried out for both tubes. The difference in optical density for the readings of the two tubes is the diazo color due to 0.05 mg. bilirubin (the bilirubin solution contains 1 mg./ml.). If the method under calibration regularly uses 0.4 ml. serum, then the color would be equivalent to that from a serum containing $\dfrac{0.05 \times 100}{0.4}$ or 12.5 mg.%. One could carry out a calibration curve by this method with different pipettes and dilutions of the strong bilirubin solution, but ordinarily this is used to check one or two points on the curve.

Normal values and interpretation: The normal values for the bilirubin fractions are direct bilirubin, 0.1-0.4 mg.%; indirect bilirubin, 0.2-0.8 mg.%; and total bilirubin, 0.3-1.3 mg.%.

In hemolytic jaundice the increase in indirect bilirubin is greatest, whereas in obstructive jaundice the increase in direct bilirubin is more pronounced. This may be explained by the fact that bilirubin is produced in the reticuloendothelial cells by the breakdown of hemoglobin and is transported in the blood in the form of free or indirect-reacting bilirubin to the liver, where it is conjugated to form the more soluble direct-reacting bilirubin. Thus in jaundice caused by increased destruction of red cells there will be more indirect bilirubin in the serum, whereas if the jaundice is caused by the fact that the bilirubin already conjugated by the liver cannot be properly excreted, the amount of direct-reacting bilirubin will rise. In jaundice due to liver parenchymal damage, both fractions may be greatly elevated. The ratio of direct to indirect bilirubin is still only of limited value in the differential diagnosis of jaundice. In infectious hepatitis the serum bilirubin rises to a peak and then steadily returns to normal when recovery ensues.

Other tests based on bile pigments are the determination of urinary **bilirubin** and urinary and fecal **urobilinogen**. Bilirubin is found in urine in obstructive jaundice, but is usually not present in hemolytic jaundice since the kidneys apparently excrete the more soluble direct-reacting bilirubin more readily. Urinary bilirubin is usually tested for only qualitatively, but a semiquantitative test for urinary and fecal urobilinogen is included here.

UROBILINOGEN IN URINE AND FECES[123, 124]

Principle: Urobilinogens found in urine and feces will give a red color with **Ehrlich reagent.** For a quantitative determination any urobilin present is reduced to urobilinogen by the use of alkaline ferrous sulfate. In urine the pigments are first extracted with petroleum ether to concentrate them, but this is not necessary for feces. Although there is no actual urobilinogen standard available and the material designated as urobilinogen may be more than one definite chemical compound, it has been found that the color produced with Ehrlich reagent approximates that produced by phenolsulfonphthalein (PSP) in alkaline solution; therefore this reagent has been used as an artificial standard. In alkaline solution 0.20 mg.% PSP will give the same color as 0.35 mg. urobilinogen when treated with Ehrlich reagent under the prescribed conditions.

Reagents:

1. Modified Ehrlich reagent (Watson). Dissolve 0.7 gm. *p*-dimethylaminobenzaldehyde in 150 ml. concentrated hydrochloric acid. Add 100 ml. water.
2. Ferrous sulfate (20%). Add 5 gm. ferrous sulfate to 23 ml. water to dissolve. This solution must be made up fresh as needed.
3. Sodium hydroxide (10%). Dissolve 50 gm. sodium hydroxide in water and dilute to 500 ml.
4. Sodium acetate (saturated solution). Add about 60 ml. water to 100 gm. crystalline sodium acetate, warm to dissolve, and then allow to cool. Some excess sodium acetate should crystallize out.
5. Petroleum ether.
6. Glacial acetic acid.
7. Artificial standard. Dissolve 20 mg. phenolsulfonphthalein in 100 ml. 0.05% sodium hydroxide. For the

colorimetric standard required, pipette 1 ml. of this solution to a 100 ml. volumetric flask and dilute with 0.05% NaOH. As mentioned, this solution containing 0.20 mg.% PSP gives the same color in alkaline solution as 0.35 mg. urobilinogen treated with Ehrlich reagent and made up to the same volume.

Procedure for urine: Collect a 24 hr. specimen in a brown bottle containing about 5 gm. sodium carbonate and 50 ml. petroleum ether. Measure the total volume and record. Transfer a 50 ml. aliquot to a 250 ml. flask. To this, add 25 ml. 20% ferrous sulfate and mix. Then add 25 ml. 10% sodium hydroxide and mix again. Stopper and allow to stand at room temperature in the dark for 1 hr.

Filter the solution through paper and transfer 50 ml. of the filtrate to a separatory funnel. Acidify with about 5 ml. glacial acetic acid and extract with three 30 ml. portions of petroleum ether, shaking well. Combine the ether extracts and wash with about 25 ml. water.

To the combined ether extracts in the separatory funnel add 2 ml. Ehrlich reagent and shake well. Add 4 ml. saturated sodium acetate solution and shake again. Allow the layers to separate and drain the lower aqueous layer into a test tube. Repeat the extraction of the petroleum ether with 2 ml. more Ehrlich reagent and 4 ml. sodium acetate solution. Combine the two aqueous extracts, mix, and read in a colorimeter at 540 nm. against a blank of a mixture of 2 ml. Ehrlich reagent and 4 ml. saturated sodium acetate. Also read the diluted PSP standard at this wavelength against a water blank.

Calculation:

$$\text{Mg.\% urobilinogen} = \frac{\text{OD sample}}{\text{OD standard}} \times \frac{100}{50} \times \frac{12}{50} \times 0.35$$

Since 50 ml. urine was taken and made up to a volume of 100 ml., and since 50 ml. of the filtrate was used, the final volume of the colored solution is 12 ml. and the standard is equivalent to 0.35 mg.% urobilinogen. This equation reduces to:

$$\frac{\text{OD sample}}{\text{OD standard}} \times 0.17 = \text{Mg.\% urobilinogen}$$

$$\text{Mg.\%} \times \frac{\text{Total urine vol. (ml.)}}{100} =$$

Total urobilinogen excreted

Normal values and interpretation: The normal range of urobilinogen excreted is given as 0.4-1 mg./day. Urinary urobilinogen is increased in hemolytic jaundice, and values up to 10 mg./day have been found. In obstructive jaundice the level is normal or low, often less than 0.3 mg./day. In infectious hepatitis the amount excreted may be normal or somewhat increased.

Procedure for feces: Use either a portion of a single stool specimen or, for a more accurate interpretation, an aliquot of a homogenized 24 or 48 hr. specimen.

Weigh out to within 10 mg. about 1.5 gm. stool. Transfer to a small flask with 9 ml. water and mix. Add 10 ml. 20% ferrous sulfate solution and mix. Add 10 ml. 10% sodium hydroxide and mix. Stopper and allow to stand at room temperature in the dark for 2 hr. Filter and pipette 2 ml. of the filtrate to a test tube. Add 2 ml. Ehrlich reagent and allow to stand for 10 min. Add 6 ml. saturated sodium acetate solution and mix. Read in a photometer at 540 nm. against a blank prepared from 2 ml. water, 2 ml. Ehrlich reagent, and 6 ml. sodium acetate solution. Also read the diluted standard against water as for the urine determination.

Calculation:

$$\frac{\text{OD sample}}{\text{OD standard}} \times \frac{30 \times 0.35 \times 10}{W \times 2} =$$

$$\frac{\text{OD sample}}{\text{OD standard}} \times \frac{52.5}{W} =$$

Mg. urobilinogen/100 gm. stool

W is the weight of the sample taken; this is made up to 30 ml., with 2 ml. of the filtrate taken and read in a final volume of 10 ml., and the standard is the same as used for urine:

$$\text{Mg. urobilinogen/100 gm. stool} \times$$
$$\frac{\text{Total weight (gm.)}}{100} =$$

Total urobilinogen in stool sample

Normal values and interpretation: The normal range is given as 30-220 mg./100 mg. stool or from 40-280 mg./day. Fecal urobilinogen is increased in those conditions in which there is an increased breakdown of hemoglobin, such as hemolytic jaundice. Values of 400-1400 mg. have been found in such conditions. Fecal urobilinogen is reduced when there is any obstruction to the flow of bile into the intestines. In obstructive jaundice, values as low as 5 mg./day have been found. In conditions such as infectious hepatitis the fecal levels may be low, but not as low as in obstructive jaundice. In cirrhosis of the liver the levels are low but may be in the normal range.

TESTS BASED ON CHANGES IN PLASMA PROTEINS

The liver plays an important role in the production of plasma proteins. The procedure for the determination of total protein, albumin, and globulin is given elsewhere in this chapter. Their determination often gives useful information in cases of chronic liver disease. In advanced stages of the disease, albumin is decreased and globulin is increased, so that the A/G ratio may be reversed. Albumin may fall to 2-3% and globulin may increase to 4-5%, a level which is said to indicate a poor prognosis. In acute hepatitis the protein levels are grossly normal in the early stages.

FIBRINOGEN

The procedure for the determination of fibrinogen has also been given. This protein is produced exclusively by the liver. Except in very severe forms of liver disease such as acute yellow atrophy, poisoning from phosphorus or carbon tetrachloride, and advanced stages of liver cirrhosis, the fibrinogen content of the blood is not altered greatly from normal values.

AMINO ACIDS

Along with changes in plasma proteins, changes in the plasma amino acids have been reported in liver disease. Any marked increase is found only in severe liver damage. The increased plasma levels also lead to increased urinary excretion. In severe liver disease the increase in amino acid excretion in the urine may be sufficient to cause the formation of leucine and tyrosine crystals in urinary sediment. There is a marked increase in urinary amino acid excretion in Wilson's disease (hepatolenticular degeneration).

There are a number of **flocculation tests** that depend upon alterations in the type or proportion of the proteins present in the plasma, usually involving one of the globulin fractions. The exact mechanism of these tests has not been completely explained, but they have proved to be of considerable value in the diagnosis of liver disease. An extensive review of the basis for these tests has been given by Reinhold.[125] He pointed out that the correlation between the results of the different tests is not always too great and seems to depend upon the clinical condition involved. The use of several different tests appears to improve the overall dependability. In his experience the three most useful tests are those presented here—the **cephalin-cholesterol flocculation** test, the **thymol turbidity and flocculation** test, and the **zinc sulfate turbidity** test.

CEPHALIN-CHOLESTEROL FLOCCULATION TEST[126, 127]

Normal blood serum does not produce flocculation with the cephalin-cholesterol reagent due to the inhibitory action of the albumin on the gamma globulin. When the albumin is decreased or the globulin is increased, there may be flocculation.

Reagent: The cephalin-cholesterol mixture for the preparation of the reagent is available commercially.* Dissolve the material from 1 unit in 5 ml. of ether. If a slight turbidity persists, add a small drop of water to obtain a clear solution. This solution is stable for some time when kept refrigerated and tightly stoppered to prevent loss of ether. To prepare the working reagent add 35 ml. water to a 50 ml. beaker marked at 30 ml.,

---

*Difco Laboratories, Detroit, Mich.

warm to 65-70° C., and add slowly 1 ml. ether solution while stirring. Heat slowly to boiling and let simmer until the volume is reduced to 30 ml. Cool to room temperature and store in the refrigerator. This solution is stable for about 1 wk.

Procedure: Dilute 0.2 ml. serum with 4 ml. 0.9% saline solution and add 1 ml. cephalin-cholesterol emulsion. Mix well, stopper with cotton, and allow to stand at room temperature in the dark. Also set up a control tube using 0.2 ml. water instead of serum. The reaction is sensitive to light and to large temperature variations. Observe the appearance at 24 and 48 hr., noting the amount of flocculation and precipitation. Normal sera will show no change in the state of flocculation and the test is described as negative. Positive reactions are graded from 1-4, based on the amount of flocculation; 4+ indicates complete precipitation with a clear supernatant fluid; 1+, 2+, and 3+ indicate intermediate degrees of flocculation. If possible, the reaction should be tested with known negative and 4+ sera, which can be kept for at least a month when frozen.

Flocculation is affected by light; hence the tubes are kept in the dark. It is also affected by temperature, so the room temperature should be kept relatively constant between 22° and 28° C. Serum samples may be stable for 1 day when kept in the refrigerator, but occasionally samples will deteriorate much more rapidly for unknown reasons. Traces of heavy metals or acids on the glassware will also cause false positive results; hence it is necessary to use care in obtaining chemically clean glassware.

Normal values and interpretation: Normal sera show no flocculation or, at most, only a very slight amount more than the control. The test will be positive in the early stages of infectious hepatitis before jaundice develops. In comparison with the thymol turbidity test, it was found that the cephalin-cholesterol test becomes positive earlier in hepatitis than does the thymol turbidity test, but the latter test may remain positive for a longer time. The test is usually negative in un- complicated obstructive jaundice. It may be regarded as an empirical test to detect early liver damage.

THYMOL TURBIDITY AND FLOCCULATION TEST

The thymol turbidity and flocculation test measures the degree of turbidity produced by blood serum when mixed with a buffered thymol solution having a pH of 7.55. Though normal sera produce little or no turbidity, sera from patients with liver disease can cause pronounced turbidity and precipitation on standing. The factors that control this reaction are mainly the presence of gamma globulins and phospholipids. The original procedure called for the use of a barbiturate buffer which was not too stable. The substitution of Tris buffer— Tris(hydroxymethyl)aminomethane—improved the stability and ease of preparation without changing the results of the test.[128]

Reagent:
1. Thymol buffer. Heat 1000 ml. deionized water to boiling in a 2 L. flask. Allow to cool to 80°-90° C. In another flask place 6 gm. thymol and 1.21 gm. Tris, add the hot water, and mix. When this has cooled at about 25° C., add some thymol crystals and shake vigorously. Filter and add exactly 7.3 ml. 1N hydrochloric acid to the filtrate. Check the pH, which should be 7.55 ± 0.03 at 25° C. (If measured at another temperature in the range of 18°-30° C., the pH should be 0.03 unit less for each degree above 25° C. and 0.03 unit more for each degree below 25° C.) If the pH is not at the required point, add more HCl or Tris as required.

Procedure: Place 6 ml. buffered thymol reagent in a test tube, add 0.1 ml. serum, and mix well. Allow to stand at room temperature for 30 min. Set up a blank by adding 0.1 ml. water to 6 ml. thymol buffer. Read sample against blank in a photometer at 650 nm. Allow to stand at room temperature for 18 hr. in the dark; then record the flocculation on the basis of 0-4+.

As originally devised by Maclagan,[129] the method called for a visual comparison against the Kingsbury turbidity standards for urinary protein.[130] The protein standard of 100 mg.% was taken as 10 thymol turbidity units. Thymol turbidity and albumin turbidity standards are available commercially in permanent form in sealed tubes. If the photometer can be adapted to accept tubes of the size used for these standards, and if the unknown samples are read in tubes of the same size, a satisfactory determination can be made (see following discussion as to units):

$$\frac{\text{OD sample}}{\text{OD standard}} \times \text{Units of standard} = \text{Sample units}$$

Standards can be prepared by the method of Shank and Hoagland.[131] Unfortunately there was an error in the original publication so that the 20-unit standard described by these authors actually corresponded to 10 Maclagan units. Thus, 1 Maclagan unit equals 2 Shank-Hoagland units. When using a commercial thymol turbidity standard, one must make certain of the units involved.

The following procedure gives the standard in terms of Shank-Hoagland units because they are more commonly applied in this country.

Dissolve 1.17 gm. barium chloride ($BaCl_2 \cdot 2H_2O$) in water and make up to 100 ml. in a volumetric flask. Dilute 6 ml. concentrated sulfuric acid to 1 L. Standardize against standard alkali and adjust to 0.2N. Pipette 0.7 ml. and 1.35 ml. barium chloride solution into two 100 ml. volumetric flasks. Dilute nearly to the mark with 0.2N sulfuric acid that has been cooled to 10° C. Warm to room temperature and dilute to the mark. Mix well and read in a photometer at 650 nm., using the 0.2N sulfuric acid as a blank. Mix the solution well just before adding to the cuvette and mix again in the cuvette just before reading. The OD obtained corresponds to 5 and 10 units.

The stability of serum for this test is also apparently quite variable, but usually it is stable for several days when kept in the refrigerator. Marked variations in room temperature may cause some change (up to 10%); if the room temperature is subject to wide variations, it is preferable to place the tubes in a pan of water at 25° C. for the incubation period. Lipemia will cause marked errors and lipemic sera should not be used.

Normal values and interpretation: The normal range is 0-5 units. After 18 hr. the flocculation should be very slight in normal samples. In infectious hepatitis the thymol turbidity is usually highest soon after onset of the disease, but may remain elevated for several weeks or more, even after the serum bilirubin has returned to normal.

The test is valuable in following the course of liver disease. In patients with stable liver disease there is usually a relatively constant thymol turbidity. The test is also high in other liver diseases such as cirrhosis that involve actual liver damage, but it is usually not elevated in obstructive jaundice. Other conditions such as Hodgkin's disease, coccidioidomycosis, disseminated tuberculosis, lobar pneumonia, and bacterial endocarditis may also be associated with increased thymol turbidity. The flocculation test sometimes proves to be positive in some cases in which turbidity is negative. It has been claimed that the sensitivity of the test is increased by this additional observation.

ZINC SULFATE TURBIDITY TEST[132]

The previously described flocculation and turbidity tests depend upon alterations in the gamma globulins plus other factors. The zinc sulfate turbidity test depends entirely on the amount of gamma globulins present. Serum is mixed with a buffered solution of zinc sulfate and the turbidity produced is read the same way as for the thymol turbidity test.

Reagent:
1. Buffered zinc sulfate solution. Dissolve 24 mg. zinc sulfate ($ZnSO_4 \cdot 7H_2O$), using only clear unefflo-resced crystals, 280 mg. barbital, and 210 mg. sodium barbital in distilled water to make 1 L.

Procedure: Add 0.1 ml. serum to 6 ml.

zinc sulfate solution, mix well, and allow to stand for 30 min. Then read in a photometer at 650 nm., using the zinc sulfate solution as a blank. The same standard is used as for the thymol turbidity test and the calculations are the same.

Normal values and interpretation: The normal range is 2-8 units. It has been found to be positive in all cases of cirrhosis, with an increase of up to 80 units in severe disease. Since the test is dependent on the increase of gamma globulins, it is not so specific for liver disease and gives a positive result in other conditions in which the gamma globulins are increased, such as multiple myeloma. The test has also been used to follow changes in gamma globulins in scarlet fever and rheumatic fever.

TESTS BASED ON CARBOHYDRATE METABOLISM

The liver plays an important role in carbohydrate metabolism, especially in the formation of **glycogen** from glucose. When the liver function is impaired in this respect, more of the ingested sugar absorbed from the intestines into the portal circulation passes into the peripheral circulation. The administration of glucose cannot be used as a test for this function because it is difficult to separate the part played by the liver from other factors (insulin, etc.) in glucose metabolism. Other sugars are used instead, principally galactose and levulose. **Galactose** is rapidly converted by the liver into glucose, and much of the latter is changed to glycogen. In a normal individual very little galactose appears in the blood after a test dose. **Levulose (fructose)** is also converted into glucose, chiefly in the liver.

Galactose may be determined in the blood by fermenting with yeast to remove glucose and determining the galactose remaining by use of the regular sugar reagents. Levulose cannot be determined directly by this method since it is also fermented by yeast. Although there are chemical methods for the determination of levulose, a simple and fairly satisfactory method is to determine the total blood sugar after the oral ad-

ministration of levulose since the rise in glucose after this procedure is generally small and any increase may be attributed to levulose.

ORAL GALACTOSE TOLERANCE TEST[133, 134]

With the patient in the fasting state, take a blood sample in the morning for a blank; then give 40 gm. galactose dissolved in 250 ml. water. Take blood samples at ½, 1, 1½, and 2 hr. after ingestion of galactose and determine the blood level of galactose in each specimen.

Determination of blood galactose[135]:
Reagents:
1. Sulfuric acid (2/3N) and sodium tungstate (10%). These are the same as used for the Folin-Wu precipitation.
2. Alkaline copper tartrate and arsenomolybdate. These are the same as used for glucose determinations (p. 300).
3. Yeast suspension. Suspend a quantity of bakers' yeast in 10 vol. water. Centrifuge and decant and discard the supernatant. Repeat washing procedure until supernatant is clear after centrifugation. Then make a 20% suspension in water. This may be used for about 1 wk. if kept in the refrigerator.
4. Galactose standard. Dissolve 100 mg. galactose in water to make 100 ml.

Procedure: Add 6 ml. well-mixed yeast suspension to a number of tubes. To separate tubes of yeast suspension add 1 ml. water and 1 ml. of various blood samples, including the blood sample taken before the ingestion of galactose. To a final tube add 1 ml. galactose standard and also 1 ml. of the blood sample taken before galactose ingestion. Mix well and incubate all samples at 37° C. for 20 min. To each tube add 1 ml. 2/3N sulfuric acid and mix; then add 1 ml. 10% sodium tungstate and mix well. Filter or centrifuge. Analyze aliquots of the filtrate for sugar by either the Somogyi or Folin-Wu method. Note that in these filtrates the blank (from blood obtained before galactose ingestion) and the standard (same blood plus standard) are automatically included. Increase the boiling times to 20 min. for the Somogyi method and to 10 min. for the Folin-Wu method.

Read all samples in the colorimeter, using appropriate wavelengths for the method chosen. Either read the samples against the blank or filtrate from blood taken before galactose ingestion or read all samples against the reagent blank as in the regular method for sugar; then substract the OD reading of the sample containing the blood taken prior to galactose ingestion from all the other samples and standard readings.

Calculation: Since the standard contains 100 mg. galactose and 1 ml. of this is treated similarly to 1 ml. blood:

$$\frac{\text{OD sample}}{\text{OD standard}} \times 100 = \text{Mg.\% galactose}$$

Normal values and interpretation: Values for the maximum level of galactose in the blood after oral ingestion have been given as 40-80 mg.% by different investigators. Maclagan uses an index that is the sum of the galactose levels for the blood samples. In normal individuals this should not exceed 160 mg.%. Increased values may be found in liver disease. In infectious and toxic hepatitis, values up to 500 mg.% may be found, decreasing slowly with improvement in the clinical condition. In cirrhosis the values may be 300 or 400 mg.% or more.

Intravenous galactose tolerance test[136]: An intravenous tolerance test has also been used in which the blood galactose is estimated at 5 min., ½, 1, 1½, and 2 hr. after intravenous administration of 0.5 gm. galactose/kg. body weight given as a sterile 50% solution. In this procedure a normal individual should have a curve beginning at about 200 mg.% and falling steeply, reaching 10 mg.% or lower at the end of 2 hr. In most cases of obstructive jaundice a normal curve is obtained, whereas with liver damage the curve falls more slowly. Although this test may avoid errors due to malabsorption, it has no other advantage over the oral test.

LEVULOSE TOLERANCE TEST

The procedure for the glucose tolerance test is followed, but the patient receives 50 gm. levulose (fructose) instead of glucose. Blood samples are taken as in the glucose tolerance test. Urine specimens are not taken. The blood sugar is determined by the usual method. This includes both glucose and levulose, but after levulose ingestion there is usually very little increase in the blood glucose so that the increase, if any, is due to levulose. In normal individuals the apparent rise in blood sugar is not more than 26-30 mg.% above the fasting level. In liver disease the rise is greater; the maximum levels may be 60-90 mg.% above the fasting level, but the differences are never striking.

TESTS BASED ON DETOXICATING FUNCTIONS

One of the important functions of the liver is its role in the **detoxification** of injurious substances. One of the mechanisms by which it performs this function is by chemical reactions to form substances that are less toxic or more readily excreted by the kidneys through conjugation with glucuronic acid, glycine, or other compounds. This is the basis of the hippuric acid test in which a dose of sodium benzoate is given and the amount of hippuric acid formed by the reaction of benzoic acid and glycine is determined. Since the test is based on the amount of hippuric acid formed as measured by the amount excreted in the urine, inaccurate results will be obtained if renal function is greatly impaired.

HIPPURIC ACID SYNTHESIS TESTS—ORAL AND INTRAVENOUS[137-140]

Benzoate may be given either orally or intravenously. For the oral test the patient ingests 6 gm. sodium benzoate dissolved in about 250 ml. water. All the urine passed during the next 4 hr. is saved, together with the urine obtained by emptying the bladder at the end of the period.

Because impaired absorption and nausea may occur when sodium benzoate is given orally, an intravenous test may be used. Sodium benzoate is available in sterile ampules containing 1.77 gm. sodium benzoate (equivalent to 1.5 gm. benzoic acid) in 20 ml. water. Have the patient empty the bladder and drink a glass of water. Inject the sodium benzoate, taking at least 5 min. for the injection. The bladder is emptied after 1 hr. and this urine is taken for analysis.

In the analysis for hippuric acid the urine is saturated with sodium chloride, acidified with sulfuric acid, and cooled to precipitate out the hippuric acid that is only slightly soluble. The precipitated hippuric acid is centrifuged, washed, and titrated with alkali. A correction is made for the slight solubility of the acid.

Reagents:

1. Sodium chloride (30%). Dissolve 30 gm. sodium chloride in water to make 100 ml. Since this solution should be cold when used, it is convenient to store it in the refrigerator. A slight crystallization is of no importance.
2. Sodium hydroxide (0.1N). Accurately standardize as given on p. 432.
3. Concentrated sulfuric acid.
4. Sodium chloride crystals.

Procedure: Measure the total volume of the urine obtained and take an aliquot amounting to 1/10 of the total volume for the oral test or 1/5 the volume for the intravenous test. It may be simpler to take a definite volume such as 10 or 20 ml. which is approximately the desired aliquot ratio. Transfer the aliquot to a suitably sized centrifuge tube. Add 3 gm. sodium chloride for each 10 ml. aliquot. Dissolve completely and warm slightly if necessary. Add 0.1 ml. concentrated sulfuric acid for each 10 ml. aliquot, mix well, and place in the refrigerator for at least ½ hr. If precipitation of hippuric acid has not occurred at the end of this time, scratch the inside of the tube below the surface of the liquid with a glass stirring rod and return to the refrigerator for another 30 min. or longer. If convenient, it may be left overnight in the refrigerator. Centrifuge at high speed and carefully pour off and discard the supernatant. Wash the pre-

cipitate by adding 10 ml. cold 30% sodium chloride solution and rinse down the sides of the tube. Mix the contents of the tube and recentrifuge. Pour off supernatant and repeat the washing. Dissolve the final precipitate in about 10 ml. boiling water, transfer to a small flask, and titrate with 0.1N sodium hydroxide, using phenolphthalein as an indicator. Some of the hippuric acid may precipitate out and redissolve slowly; therefore one must be certain that the final end point of the titration has been reached.

Calculation: Since 1 ml. 1N alkali is equal to 0.179 gm. hippuric acid:

$$\text{Gm. hippuric acid} = 0.179 \times (\text{Ml. alkali}) \times (\text{Normality of alkali}) \times \frac{\text{Total volume of urine}}{\text{Volume of aliquot taken}}$$

Add 0.12 gm. to the calculated amount for each 100 ml. of total volume of urine sample.

Normal values and interpretation: For the intravenous test 0.7-1.6 gm. should be excreted in the 1 hr. period. For the oral test at least 3-3.5 gm. hippuric acid should be excreted in the 4 hr. period. Amounts excreted above the limits have no significance. Excretion is normal in hemolytic jaundice and in uncomplicated gallbladder disease and obstructive jaundice. It is decreased in hepatitis, tumors, cirrhosis, and obstructive jaundice with liver impairment.

BROMSULPHALEIN TEST (BSP)[141-144]

The Bromsulphalein test is based on the ability of the liver to remove the injected dye, **Bromsulphalein,** from the blood. A definite amount of the dye is injected and the amount remaining in the blood after definite times is measured. Originally the amount injected was 2 mg./kg. body weight. Later, workers used 5 mg./kg., which is the amount suggested here because it is the most commonly used. Various time intervals have also been used. The times suggested here of 30 and 45 min. after injection of the dye are the most frequently used. The samples can be drawn at other intervals if requested by the physician. The injected dye is an indicator that is red in alkaline solution and colorless in acid solution. It may be estimated by measuring absorbance in alkaline solution and again after the color due to the dye has been eliminated by acidifying. The difference is a measure of the amount of dye present, with some correction for serum color or turbidity. Marked hemolysis or lipemia will interfere. The effect of proteins on the color of the dye is greatly diminished by the addition of sodium paratoluene sulfonate to the reagent.

Reagents:
1. Alkaline buffer. Dissolve 6.46 gm. anhydrous disodium phosphate, 0.76 gm. anhydrous trisodium phosphate, and 3.2 gm. sodium paratoluene sulfonate in water to make 500 ml. The pH of the solution should be between 10.6 and 10.7.
2. Acid buffer. Dissolve 27.6 gm. $NaH_2PO_4 \cdot H_2O$ (or 25.8 gm. anhydrous salt) in water to make 100 ml.
3. Bromsulphalein standards:
   A. Stock standard. The dye used for the test, in ampules containing 50 mg./ml., is also used for the preparation of the standard. Dilute 5 ml. to 50 ml. with water to make a stock solution containing 5 mg./ml. This solution is fairly stable when kept in a dark bottle.
   B. Working standard. As required, prepare a working standard from the stock standard by diluting 1 ml. to 100. This standard solution contains 5 mg.%.

Procedure: The dye is furnished in ampules containing 50 mg./ml. An amount equivalent to 5 mg./kg. body weight (0.1 ml./kg.) is injected. The dye should be injected slowly, taking at least 1 min. Care must be taken so that all of the solution enters the vein since it is quite irritating to the tissue. Severe and even fatal reactions, possibly allergic, have been reported; hence the injection should be made only under the supervision of a physician. Exactly 30 and 45 min. after injection of the dye (or at other times if desired), blood specimens are taken from the other arm. Take care

to avoid hemolysis as much as possible.

To 1 ml. serum add 7 ml. alkaline buffer and mix. Read in a colorimeter at 580 nm. (any wavelength in the range 560-600 nm. is satisfactory) against a water blank (A_1). Add 0.2 ml. acid buffer, mix, and read again (A_2). Treat 1 ml. working standard similarly, except that the reading need only be taken with the alkaline buffer (A_3).

Calculation:

$$\% \text{Retention} = \frac{A_1 - A_2}{A_3} \times 50$$

If 5 mg./kg. body weight of the dye is injected (as is usual) and it is assumed that the plasma volume is 50 ml./kg. body weight, then the initial concentration of the dye would be $\frac{5}{50} \times 100$ or 10 mg.%. Hence the 5 mg.% standard represents 50% retention. The assumption as to the ratio between plasma volume and body weight is only approximate and it has been suggested that a correction be applied. We find these corrections amount to only 1% retention except in persons weighing more than 200 lb. In this case a correction of 3% retention should be subtracted from the result.

The determination may be difficult when the serum is more than slightly hemolyzed or is highly lipemic. In these instances the following method may be used. For a reagent, mix 176 ml. acetone, 0.1 ml. glacial acetic acid, and water to make 200 ml. Add 2 ml. serum to 8 ml. reagent, stopper, and mix well. Centrifuge strongly and read the supernatant at 580 nm. against a blank of the reagent. Then add 2 drops 10% sodium hydroxide solution, mix, and read again. Treat an aliquot of the standard similarly. The difference between the reading in alkaline solution and that in the acid solution extract is proportional to the amount of dye present. Note that in this method the colorless form is read first and then the colored alkaline solution is read. If equal volumes of serum and working standard are used, the calculations are the same as for the other method.

Normal values and interpretation: In healthy adults not more than 15% of the dye should remain in the blood at the end of 30 min. and not more than 5% at the end of 45 min. Removal of the dye proceeds more slowly when liver function is impaired and in advanced cirrhosis; e.g., up to 40-50% of the dye may remain in the blood after 45 min. Since the dye is removed in the flow of bile, the test is accurate only when there is no obstruction to bile flow. It is most useful in liver cell damage without jaundice, in cirrhosis, and in acute hepatitis. In these chronic liver conditions it may be one of the most sensitive of liver function tests.

MISCELLANEOUS LIVER FUNCTION TESTS

A number of tests given elsewhere in this volume are also of value in the study of liver disease. Brief mention will be made of these tests, together with their application to liver function testing.

Cholesterol: The liver is concerned with the metabolism of lipids, especially cholesterol. Hypercholesterolemia is found in obstructive jaundice. The increase in cholesterol often parallels the increase in bilirubin during the course of the disease. In parenchymatous liver disease the findings are variable; the level is normal in many instances. Very high cholesterol levels are found in xanthomatous biliary cirrhosis. Changes in the ratio of free to esterified cholesterol are often found in liver disease. In infectious hepatitis and other conditions involving liver damage the amount of esters tends to fall relatively more than the total cholesterol, which may remain relatively constant. In severe acute liver necrosis the total serum cholesterol is usually low and may fall below 100 mg.%, with a marked reduction in the percentage of the esters.

Prothrombin time[145, 146]**:** Prothrombin time is used chiefly for the control of anticoagulant therapy; it has also been used in liver disease. Prothrombin is formed by the liver cells, which require vitamin K for the process. In liver disease the prothrombin formation may be reduced in two ways. In obstructive jaundice the absence of bile salts severely reduces the absorption of vitamin K from the intestines. In severe liver damage the liver is less able to form prothrombin, even in the presence of adequate amounts of the vitamin. These two conditions may be distinguished by the vitamin K tolerance test.

Vitamin K tolerance test: Determine the prothrombin time on several different days to find the range or level for the patient. Then give intravenously 76 mg. Sinkayvite* (2-methyl, 1,4-naphthohydroquinone diphosphate) for 4 consecutive days. The dose is equivalent to 60 mg. Hykinone.† Determine the prothrombin time daily just before the injection and on the day following the last injection.

In normal individuals there is a normal prothrombin time and no change occurs following administration of vitamin K. If an increased initial prothrombin time returns to normal (vitamin K deficiency) or the normal time is lowered following intake of the vitamin, the test for liver impairment is negative.

A positive test, indicating liver impairment, may show the following conditions after vitamin K has been administered: failure of an increased prothrombin time to return to normal, further increase in an abnormally high level, or a transient rise in a normal level.

Serum alkaline phosphatase[147]**:** Determination of serum alkaline phosphatase may be useful in differentiating obstructive jaundice from jaundice due to hepatocellular dysfunction; the level is usually elevated in the latter condition, but not in the former. The dividing line between the two conditions is approximately 8 Bessey-Lowry units. Frequently there is an increase in the serum alkaline phosphatase activity in patients with cancer of the liver or liver abscesses. Very high values are sometimes found in conditions such as xanthomatous biliary cirrhosis in which there is no extrahepatic obstruction. Determination of the serum alkaline phosphatase must be considered an em-

---

*Hoffman-LaRoche Co., Nutley, N. J.
†Abbott Laboratories, Chicago, Ill.

pirical test of liver function because it measures no known function and the source of the increased alkaline phosphatase has not been completely established.

Transaminases[148-150]: Determination of transaminase enzymes is of value in the diagnosis of liver disease as well as of myocardial infarction. The methods of determination and a more complete discussion are given on p. 406. In acute infectious hepatitis the serum glutamic pyruvic transaminase (SGPT) level may rise to around 600 Reitman-Frankel units and the glutamic oxalacetic transaminase (SGOT) to about 500 units in about 25 days after onset of the illness. The levels of both enzymes then usually decrease gradually, with a sharper downward slope for the SGOT. Both enzymes return to normal in 50-80 days after onset of the illness in uncomplicated cases.

In cirrhosis of the liver the SGPT level is usually normal or moderately elevated (up to 80 Reitman-Frankel units). The SGOT is always elevated (50-150 units). In cases of acute and subacute extrahepatic biliary obstruction the SGPT is usually greater than the SGOT.

Isocitric dehydrogenase (ICD)[151]: Preliminary work with this enzyme shows its usefulness in the differential diagnosis of jaundice. It has shown tremendous increases in acute viral hepatitis and in hepatitis with infectious mononucleosis, but no elevation occurs in cases of obstruction in most cases of cirrhosis. Normal values have been found in cases of myocardial infarction and in malignancies when there was no liver involvement.

Lactic dehydrogenase: Increases in the serum activity of this enzyme have been found in liver disease as well as in myocardial infarction. Usually in liver conditions the changes in lactic dehydrogenase are similar to but less marked than those in the transaminases. This is discussed further in the section on enzymes.

Cholinesterase: Since serum cholinesterase originates in the liver, its determination has been used in following the course of liver disease. The serum level decreases in compensated cirrhosis and to a greater extent in uncompensated

cirrhosis. Very low levels are considered a grave prognostic sign. The range of normal values widely overlaps the range of disease, but serial determinations may be helpful in following the course of the disease.

Ornithine carbamyl transferase (OCT)[152]: This enzyme catalyzes the formation of citrulline from ornithine and is found almost exclusively in the liver. The normal serum OCT activity is very low. Serum OCT activity is a sensitive, specific indicator of hepatocellular injury since any of the enzyme appearing in the serum almost certainly comes from liver tissue. The determination of OCT activity appears to have greater clinical value than the determination of GPT activity because of its greater specificity and sensitivity. The only proved cause of increased serum OCT activity is hepatocellular injury. Increased activity may occur secondary to cellular injury, with no histologic evidence of hepatocellular necrosis. Only recently have satisfactory chemical methods been developed that can be carried out in the average clinical laboratory. Reference to these methods will be found in the section on enzymes.

Guanase[153]: This enzyme catalyzes the deamination of guanine. In human beings it occurs principally in the liver, brain, and kidney, with little activity in other tissues. Serum guanase activity has been found to be increased in patients with viral hepatitis, but not in patients with cirrhosis or obstructive jaundice. In normal individuals the activity is very low, the range being up to 3 I.U. There is a rise to about 6 units in cirrhosis, and an increase of as much as twentyfold in the early stages of viral hepatitis. Guanase activity tends to parallel GOT activity. The lack of the enzyme in many other tissues makes it much more specific, and it should be helpful in deciding whether an increased LDH activity originates primarily in the liver. Only recently have chemical methods been developed that do not involve measurement in the ultraviolet range (245-290 nm.). Reference to the methods can be found in the section on enzymes.

Summary: The following tests can be

performed on a single specimen of serum, thus providing the maximum amount of information with a minimum of discomfort to the patient: bilirubin, albumin, globulin, A/G ratio, the three flocculation tests, alkaline phosphatase, and the transaminases. In addition to the study of specific conditions, the following extra tests may be performed. For the detection of liver damage in the absence of jaundice, urinary bilirubin, urobilinogen, and Bromsulphalein tests may be run. For detection of residual liver damage in the recovery stage of hepatitis and in chronic hepatitis, the BSP, prothrombin time, and serum cholinesterase tests may also be helpful. In following the course of jaundice in patients suffering from parenchymatous disease the prothrombin time is helpful; if the disease is severe, the cholesterol esters and cholinesterase tests may be used. In the differentiation of jaundice due to biliary disease from jaundice due to parenchymatous disease, the prothrombin time and the galactose tolerance tests may be useful.

Because of the many functions of the liver, and the fact that the various disease processes affect these functions differently, there is no single liver function test that can be said to be the best. Opinions differ as to which tests are most useful. In most cases the clinical symptoms suggest the tests that are most likely to be useful.

BLOOD LIPIDS

The term "lipid" is usually applied to a wide variety of substances that resemble fats in their solubility. Most lipids are concerned with the metabolism of the fatty acids. These substances constitute the principal and most efficient source of energy in the human body, not only because of their high caloric value but also because of their ability to be stored for use as needed. The determination of the various lipid constituents in blood is the subject of extensive literature which reveals a great deal of confusion and controversy. The lack of uniformity in the methods used and in the reporting of the results is responsible for some of this disagreement. This subject

is discussed in detail in a review by Peters and Van Slyke.[26]

The clinician may have one of several objectives in mind when requesting a determination of one or more of the blood lipid components. He may be interested in the malfunctioning of the digestion and absorption of fats that occurs in pancreatic disease or steatorrhea. The fasting levels of the blood lipids may be low in such conditions, but the determinations of such levels are of little value in assessing any of the malabsorption syndromes. A fat tolerance test, the measurement of the changes in the total blood fatty acids (or esterified fatty acids), or more simply the measurement of the changes in turbidity after a fat meal may be helpful. A fat balance test is often more satisfactory; this involves the determination of fat in the stool, which is not discussed in this section.

In recent years the role of lipids in the pathogenesis of atherosclerosis has received much attention. Determinations that have been emphasized in this connection are those of total cholesterol, cholesterol esters, phospholipids, triglycerides, and lipoproteins. In addition, the levels of cholesterol and cholesterol esters have been studied in a number of other conditions including diabetes, hypothyroidism and hyperthyroidism, and liver disease. The interpretation of the results in relation to these conditions will be discussed in connection with methods for the determination of these constituents.

This section will give simple methods in detail for those lipid constituents that can be readily determined in the average clinical laboratory. These are total lipids, cholesterol (total and esters), phospholipids, fatty acids (esterified and free), and triglycerides. Brief reference will be made to other constituents and their interpretation.

The total lipids include all the lipidlike substances found in blood serum, including cholesterol, phospholipids, free and esterified fatty acids, and other substances as well. Because of the heterogeneous nature of this material, no simple chemical reaction is available for its determination. Total lipids must still be determined by gravimetric methods after extraction from the serum with a lipid solvent. Modifications of the method of Sperry and Brand[154] are deemed to be the most accurate, but they are rather time-consuming. The simpler method presented here has been shown to be sufficiently accurate for clinical purposes. In this method the lipids are extracted from serum with a mixture of alcohol and ether. The extract is evaporated to dryness and the residue is reextracted with hot petroleum ether. This eliminates most of the interfering material. The petroleum extract is then evaporated and the residue is accurately weighed.

TOTAL LIPIDS (GRAVIMETRIC METHOD OF PERNOKIS, FREELAND, AND KRAUS)[155, 156]

Reagents:
1. Alcohol-ether mixture (3:1). Mix 3 vol. ethyl alcohol with 1 vol. ether.
2. Petroleum ether (boiling point, 30°-60° C.).

Procedure: Transfer about 60 ml. ethanol-ether solution to a 125 ml. Erlenmeyer flask and heat to boiling on a steam bath. Add slowly, while swirling, 2 ml. serum (use 1 ml. if lipemic). Cool and filter into clean 125 ml. Erlenmeyer flask. Add about 10 ml. alcohol-ether to extraction flask, heat to boiling, and pour through filter. Repeat the washing step twice. Evaporate filtrate just to dryness on steam bath. This can be hastened with the aid of a stream of nitrogen. Do not prolong heating of dried residue. Extract residue five times with 10 ml. portions of petroleum ether, bringing each to boil on the steam bath, and filter each into another 125 ml. Erlenmeyer flask. Evaporate solvent to about 10 ml. and transfer quantitatively to a preweighed weighing flask that has been stored in a desiccator prior to use. Rinse out the flask several times with small portions of petroleum ether and add these washes to weighing flasks. Evaporate solvent to dryness on steam bath. Transfer to vacuum desiccator over anhydrous $CaCl_2$ and dry overnight. Weigh to nearest 0.1 mg. Alternately, the residue in the weighing flask is dried in a vacuum oven at 65° C. for 2 hr., cooled to room temperature in a desiccator, and weighed.

Calculation: Subtract weight of flask alone from weight of flask plus lipid to obtain the weight of the lipid. Then:

$$\text{Mg. lipid/100 ml. serum} = \text{Mg. weight of lipid} \times \frac{100}{\text{Ml. serum used}}$$

Normal values and interpretation: The normal level of total lipids may be taken as 400-1000 mg.%. Published estimates of ranges vary rather widely. At birth the levels are usually in the range of 100-250 mg.% and increase to about twice this value within a few days, reaching the adult level after about 1 yr. The total lipids will be increased after a fat meal. They may be decreased in steatorrhea or other malabsorption syndromes, but a determination of some of the separate constituents (fatty acids, cholesterol, etc.) will give more valuable information. The reader is referred to the general discussion by Peters and Van Slyke.[26]

CHOLESTEROL

Cholesterol still remains the blood lipid constituent that is most often determined. In many of the methods the cholesterol is extracted from plasma or serum with an organic solvent. Some more recent methods use the direct addition of serum to the reagent. Although these methods are much simpler, they are also less accurate. Most methods still use some modification of the original **Liebermann-Burchard reaction,** with acetic anhydride and sulfuric acid for the development of the color. Free cholesterol is separated from the esters by precipitation with digitonin, which forms a precipitate with free cholesterol but not with esterified cholesterol. Since under most conditions the Liebermann-Burchard reaction may give slightly different amounts of color with equivalent amounts of free and esterified cholesterol, in many methods the esters are saponified (hydrolyzed) before color development.[157, 158] Because of their high degree of accuracy, these methods are used as the standard reference methods for cholesterol. While the direct methods are less accurate, their simplicity and time-saving procedures make them quite useful and the results obtained are adequate for most clinical purposes.

Total cholesterol and cholesterol esters (modified Bloor method)[159, 160]: In this method the cholesterol and other lipids are extracted from serum with an alcohol-ether mixture and the total cholesterol is determined in a portion of the extract by the reaction with acetic anhydride and sulfuric acid to give a blue-green color (Liebermann-Burchard reaction) that is determined colorimetrically. The esters are separated from free cholesterol by the addition of digitonin, which precipitates free cholesterol but not esterified cholesterol.

Reagents:
1. Acetic anhydride, reagent grade.
2. Chloroform, reagent grade.
3. Concentrated sulfuric acid, reagent grade.
4. Alcohol-ether (3:1). Mix 3 vol. ethyl alcohol with 1 vol. ethyl ether.
5. Color reagent. Cool a sufficient quantity of acetic anhydride in a glass-stoppered bottle or flask in ice. For every 20 ml. acetic anhydride, add slowly 1 ml. concentrated sulfuric acid while swirling. Cool for 10 min. more; then use at once.
6. Standards:
   A. Stock standard. Dissolve 100 mg. cholesterol in chloroform to make 100 ml. in a volumetric flask. This solution contains 1 mg. cholesterol/ml.
   B. Working standard. Dilute 20 ml. stock standard to 100 ml. with chloroform. This solution contains 0.2 mg. cholesterol/ml.

Procedure: Place about 35 ml. alcohol-ether mixture in a 50 ml. glass-stoppered volumetric flask; add 1 ml. serum while swirling. Warm to boiling in a water bath, with constant agitation to avoid bumping. Allow to stand without further heating for about ½ hr. When cool, dilute to 50 ml. with alcohol-ether mixture, stopper, and mix well. Filter into a large test tube, keeping the funnel covered with a watch glass to prevent excessive evaporation of the solvent.

Pipette 10 ml. filtrate to a 50 ml. beaker and evaporate to dryness in a water bath or on a hot plate at low heat. Place dried beakers in oven at 100° C. for 5 min. To the dried residue in the beaker add about 3 ml. chloroform and bring to a boil on a hot plate, evaporating about one half of the solvent. Carefully decant the remaining solvent into a 10 ml. graduated glass-stoppered cylinder. Repeat the extraction several times until the total volume of chloroform extract in the cylinder is exactly 5 ml. Carry out this extraction with adequate ventilation to avoid inhalation of chloroform vapors.

To one cylinder add 5 ml. chloroform as a blank. To three other cylinders add 1, 2, and 3 ml. cholesterol working standard (equal to 0.2, 0.4, and 0.6 mg. cholesterol, respectively) and dilute to 5 ml. with chloroform. Place all cylinders containing samples, standards, and blank in a water bath maintained at 25° C. A large pan of water with a thermometer and rack is satisfactory.

Add 5 ml. color reagent to each tube in order and mix. Time the addition so that each tube is read exactly 20 min. after addition of the reagent. Read in the photometer at 625 nm., setting to zero with the blank.

Calculation: Calculate the K as described, then:

$$\text{Mg.\% cholesterol} = K \times OD \times \frac{\text{Vol. extract}}{\text{Aliquot extract}} \times \frac{100}{\text{Ml. serum used}}$$

or for the recommended proportions:

$$\text{Mg.\% cholesterol} = K \times OD \times \frac{50}{5} \times \frac{100}{1}$$

$$= K \times OD \times 500$$

NOTE: Avoid contamination of the color reagent or solutions by water (from water bath, etc.) at every stage since this will give low results. During the color development the cylinders should not be placed near a strong light, although moderate illumination (away from windows) is not harmful.

Esterified and free cholesterol:
Additional reagents:
1. Digitonin solution (0.5%). Dissolve 500 mg. digitonin in 50% ethyl alcohol to make 100 ml.

2. Petroleum ether (boiling point, 30°-60° C.).

Procedure: Pipette 10 ml. alcohol-ether extracts as used for the total cholesterol method to a 50 ml. beaker. Add 2 ml. 0.5% digitonin. Evaporate to dryness, extract with several 10 ml. portions of petroleum ether, and evaporate to dryness. Then continue exactly as for total cholesterol. In this modification the free cholesterol is precipitated by the digitonin and is not extracted by chloroform; hence only the esterified cholesterol is determined. The calculations are exactly the same as for total cholesterol.

The free cholesterol is the difference between the total cholesterol and the esterified cholesterol.

Total cholesterol (direct method of Ferro and Ham)[161]: In this method the color is developed directly without extraction of the lipids. It is a very convenient and simple method, though possibly not as accurate as the longer extraction methods.

Reagents:
1. Acetic anhydride, reagent grade.
2. Glacial acetic acid, reagent grade.
3. Concentrated sulfuric acid, reagent grade.
4. Color reagent. Mix 30 vol. acetic anhydride and 20 vol. glacial acetic acid. Add 5 vol. concentrated sulfuric acid and cool to room temperature. Prepare the same day it is to be used.
5. Cholesterol standard. Dissolve 250 mg. pure cholesterol in glacial acetic acid to make 100 ml. in a volumetric flask.

Procedure: Dilute 0.5 ml. serum with 0.5 ml. distilled water. Add 0.2 ml. diluted serum to a 16 × 100 mm. test tube. Place the tip of a 10 ml. serologic pipette filled with the color reagent about ½ in. inside the test tube and allow 6 ml. reagent to run in rapidly, letting it fall directly into the serum in the test tube (not down the side). No further mixing is needed. Read the peak absorption (maximum color), which occurs in 90 ± 30 sec. and is maintained for about 1 min. more, at 640 nm., setting to zero with a blank of 0.2 ml. water plus 6 ml. reagent. For a standard place 0.1 ml. standard solution in a test tube and add 0.2 ml. water and then 5.9 ml. color reagent.

Calculation:

$$\frac{\text{OD serum sample}}{\text{OD standard}} \times 250 = \text{Mg.\% cholesterol}$$

Normal values and interpretation: The range of normal values for healthy young adults is 150-270 mg.%. It may be lower in children. The level increases somewhat with age until about 60 yr. Healthy individuals over 70 yr. of age may have cholesterol levels approaching those of young adults or even lower. The proportion of total cholesterol present as esters is usually between 68 and 74%.

Cholesterol, along with other lipids, is markedly increased in uncontrolled diabetes, but the level does not appear to be related to the severity of the disease. Cholesterol as well as other lipids may reach extremely high levels in the nephrotic syndrome, but the mechanism of this increase is not well understood. Little if any disturbance of the cholesterol level occurs in other renal diseases. Total cholesterol values in diseases of the liver may be increased or decreased, depending upon the nature and duration of the condition. Marked deviations from the normal ratio of free to esterified cholesterol occur in diseases of the liver and biliary tract, infectious diseases, and extreme hypercholesterolemia. A further discussion of the relation to liver diseases can be found in the section on liver function tests.

The cholesterol level tends to vary inversely with the basal metabolic rate, and its estimation has been used in the study of thyroid function. The level may be increased in hypothyroidism and decreased in hyperthyroidism, but because of the wide range of normal values, serum cholesterol can only be considered a secondary aid in the diagnosis of thyroid dysfunction. Changes in the levels may be of more value in following the course of the disease.

Marked increases in cholesterol levels are found in most cases of lipoidosis and xanthomatosis as well as in instances of familial or idiopathic hypercholesterolemia.

Cholesterol levels are not greatly affected by ordinary dietary changes, but they may be low in wasting diseases such as tuberculosis and terminal cancer.

In recent years much attention has been focused on the possible role of hypercholesterolemia in the pathogenesis of atherosclerosis. There is some evidence that populations consuming a smaller amount of their total calories as fats and ingesting vegetable rather than animal fats have a lower cholesterol level and a lower incidence of atherosclerosis and coronary artery disease than do populations with a higher fat intake. The exact role of hypercholesterolemia in the development of atherosclerosis is still the subject of some controversy. About all that can be definitely stated is that an individual with an elevated cholesterol level is, other things being equal, more likely to suffer from coronary artery disease than one with a normal level, but there are many other factors involved.

PHOSPHOLIPIDS (PHOSPHATIDES AND LIPID PHOSPHORUS)[162]

In the determination of phospholipids the organic portion of the phospholipids is oxidized by heating with a strong oxidizing agent (perchloric acid) and the phosphorus is converted to phosphate. Phosphate is determined by a reaction in which it is converted into a blue phosphomolybdate by a reducing agent. Phospholipid may either be precipitated with the protein or extracted with alcohol ether. If only the lipid phosphorus is to be determined or if it is to be determined along with the acid-soluble (inorganic) phosphorus, the trichloroacetic precipitation may be used. If other lipids such as cholesterol or fatty acids are to be determined as well, it may be more convenient to use the alcohol-ether extraction since the other lipids can be determined on further aliquots of the same extract. Other methods for inorganic phosphate may be used for the final colorimetric determination, provided the acidity of the standards and blank is kept the same as in the digested samples.

Use Pyrex test tubes calibrated to contain 10 ml. and a sand bath heated on a hot plate to 150° C.

Reagents:

1. Trichloroacetic acid (10%). Dissolve 100 gm. trichloroacetic acid in distilled water to make 1000 ml.
2. Perchloric acid (70%), reagent grade.
3. Concentrated sulfuric acid, reagent grade.
4. Ammonium molybdate (4%). Dissolve 4 gm. ammonium molybdate in distilled water to make 100 ml. This solution keeps several weeks in the refrigerator.
5. 1-Amino-2-naphthol-4-sulfonic acid (ANSA) stock solution. Mix 30 gm. sodium bisulfite, 6 gm. sodium sulfite, and 0.5 gm. 1-amino-2-naphthol-4-sulfonic acid and make to 250 ml. with distilled water. After 2-3 hr., remove any undissolved material by filtration and store in a dark bottle in the refrigerator. This solution will keep for 1 mo. or longer. For each series of determinations dilute 10 ml. stock solution to 25 ml. with distilled water.
6. Standard phosphate solutions:
   A. Stock standard. Dissolve 4.394 gm. potassium dihydrogen phosphate (KH_2PO_4) in distilled water to make 1 L. Add 1 drop chloroform as a preservative and store in a refrigerator. This stock solution contains 1 mg. phosphorus/ml.
   B. Working standard. Dilute 1 ml. stock standard to 100 with distilled water. This solution contains 0.01 mg. phosphorus/ml.

Procedure: Deliver accurately 0.2 ml. serum or plasma into a digestion tube containing 3 ml. water. Add 3 ml. 10% trichloroacetic acid, the first 1.5 ml. dropwise while swirling, the remainder more rapidly. Allow the tubes to stand for several minutes; then centrifuge until the precipitate is tightly packed.

Decant the supernatant and drain the tubes in an inverted position for 10 min. or until practically all the liquid has been removed. Add 0.5 ml. concentrated sulfuric acid and heat in the sand bath until fumes of sulfur trioxide appear. Remove from the bath, cool somewhat, add 0.5 ml. perchloric acid, and continue the digestion until clear.

It may be convenient to keep the two acid solutions in glass-stoppered dropping bottles and measure the acid by drops after checking the number of drops required to deliver approximately 0.5 ml. During the digestion, set up duplicate standards using 2 ml. working standard and a reagent blank. Add only 0.4 ml. of each acid to the standards and blank. After digestion, cool the tubes and add about 6 ml. distilled water to each. Dilute standards and blank to about 6 ml. with distilled water. Add 1 ml. ammonium molybdate to each tube. Then add 1 ml. ANSA reagent, dilute to 10 ml., and mix well. Add the ANSA reagent to the tubes in serial order, timing the addition so that each tube is read in the colorimeter approximately 20 min. after addition of the reagent. Read samples and standards against the blank at 660 nm.

Calculation:

$$\frac{\text{OD sample}}{\text{OD standard}} \times \frac{\text{Mg. P in standard}}{\text{Ml. serum used}} \times 100 =$$

$$\text{Mg.\% lipid phosphorus}$$

Or using the proportions mentioned:

$$\frac{\text{OD sample}}{\text{OD standard}} \times 10 = \text{Mg.\% lipid phosphorus}$$

Lipid phosphorus is conventionally converted to phospholipid by multiplying by the factor 25.

Alcohol-ether extraction: Prepare an alcohol-ether extract of 1 ml. serum in 50 ml. alcohol-ether as in the Bloor cholesterol method.

Evaporate 10 ml. of the filtrate to dryness in a digestion tube on a water bath with the aid of a stream of air. When the solvent has been completely removed, add the acids and digest, proceeding as in the previous directions. Complete the procedure as outlined for the previous method. Since here the equivalent of 0.2 ml. serum is used (10 ml. of a 1:50 extract), the calculations will be the same.

The use of calibrated tubes may be avoided by adding exactly the same amount of water to each tube. Add exactly 7 ml. water to each tube after digestion and also to the reagent blank. Add 5 ml. water plus 2 ml. standard to the standard tube before adding the other reagents. If one proceeds in this way, it may be more convenient to evaporate the alcohol-ether extract in a 30 ml. Kjeldahl flask, digest, and develop the color in the flask.

Many detergents used for cleaning glassware contain phosphates; accordingly, all glassware must be thoroughly rinsed with distilled water before using. It may be advisable to avoid the use of detergents entirely and to clean the tubes with sulfuric acid–chromic acid cleaning solution alone.

Normal values and interpretation: The normal serum level of lipid phosphorus in adults has been found to range from 6-14 mg.%, with an average of 9.2 mg.%. This corresponds to a range of 150-350 mg.% phospholipid, with an average of 230 mg.%. The phospholipid concentration in the serum parallels the cholesterol level in most instances. For lower lipid levels the cholesterol-phospholipid ratio is approximately 0.8 and approaches unity at higher levels. An increase in this ratio has been held by some investigators to be a more reliable index of a tendency toward atherosclerosis than the cholesterol level alone.

FATTY ACID ESTERS[163]

Since all but 2-5% of the fatty acids in serum are esterified (as cholesterol esters, phospholipids, or triglycerides), the simple colorimetric procedure given here to determine the esterified fatty acids is often satisfactory as a measure of the total fatty acids of the serum. It is based on the formation of hydroxamates from the reaction of the esters with hydroxylamine in alkaline solution and the formation of a colored complex on the addition of ferric chloride.

Reagents:
1. Alcohol-ether mixture (3:1). This mixture is the same as used in the Bloor cholesterol method.

2. Sodium hydroxide (3.5N). Dilute 115 ml. 50% (w/w) sodium hydroxide to about 500 ml. with distilled water. Titrate with standard acid and dilute to 3.5N.
3. Hydrochloric acid (4.2N). Dilute 200 ml. concentrated hydrochloric acid to 500 ml. with distilled water. Titrate against standard base and dilute to 4.2N.
4. Ferric chloride (10%). Dissolve 10 gm. ferric chloride ($FeCl_3 \cdot 6H_2O$) and 1 ml. concentrated hydrochloric acid in distilled water to make 100 ml.
5. Hydroxylamine hydrochloride (2M). Dissolve 14 gm. hydroxylamine hydrochloride in distilled water to make 100 ml. Store in refrigerator.
6. Standards:
   A. Stock standard. Dissolve 146 mg. triacetin or 428 mg. cholesteryl acetate in alcohol-ether mixture (3:1) to make 100 ml. This stock solution contains 20 μEq./ml.
   B. Working standard. Dilute 2 ml. stock standard to 100 ml. with alcohol-ether mixture. This contains 0.4 μEq./ml.

Procedure: Prepare an alcohol-ether extract using 1 ml. serum and 50 ml. alcohol-ether mixture exactly as described for the Bloor cholesterol method. Pipette 3 ml. extract to a test tube. Add 3 ml. alcohol-ether mixture to another tube as a blank. Prepare a series of standards by adding 1, 2, and 3 ml. working standard to separate test tubes and adding alcohol-ether mixture to make 3 ml. These standards contain 0.4, 0.8, and 1.2 μEq. fatty acid.

Add 0.5 ml. hydroxylamine solution to each tube, mix, then add 0.5 ml. sodium hydroxide solution, mix, stopper tightly, and allow to stand at room temperature for 30 min. Add 0.5 ml. hydrochloric acid solution, mix, and then add 0.5 ml. ferric chloride solution. Mix and read in a photometer at 520 nm., setting to zero with the blank.

Calculations: Calculate the K value for each standard as previously described. Then:

$$MEq./L. \text{ fatty acid esters} = K \times \frac{OD \text{ sample} \times Total \text{ vol. extract}}{Ml. \text{ serum used} \times Aliquot \text{ extract}}$$

For the proportions used in the procedure this reduces to:

$$MEq./L. = OD \times K \times \frac{50}{3}$$

since 1 μEq./ml. is the same as 1 mEq./L.

Normal values and interpretation: The normal range of fatty acids is 7-14 mEq./L. Since a considerable portion of the fatty acids are esterified with cholesterol and phospholipids, the total fatty acids will be high when the levels for these substances are elevated. The remainder of the fatty acids are chiefly triglycerides. Their significance will be discussed in the next section.

FREE (UNESTERIFIED) FATTY ACIDS[164]

The nomenclature of this lipid fraction is still somewhat controversial. The term "unesterified" is not strictly correct since some of the fatty acids in the sphingomyelins are not in an ester linkage. Some investigators have objected to the use of the term "free" since a greater part of these acids are bound to protein. Nonetheless they are free in the sense of being bound to covalent linkages. The same objection could be applied to the term "free cholesterol," which has the sanction of long usage. Free fatty acids are present in relatively small amounts (of the order of magnitude of 1 mEq./L.) and are determined by titration with alkali after direct extraction with a nonpolar solvent.

Reagents:
1. Isopropyl alcohol, reagent grade, redistilled.
2. Hexane, reagent grade, redistilled.
3. Sulfuric acid (1N). Dilute 28 ml. concentrated sulfuric acid to 1 L. with distilled water.
4. Extraction mixture. Mix together 40 vol. isopropyl alcohol, 10 vol. hexane, and 1 vol. 1N sulfuric acid.
5. Titration mixture. Mix together 1 vol. 0.1% aqueous solution thymol blue and 9 vol. redistilled ethyl al-

cohol. The titratable acidity of ethanol increases slowly over a period of several days but is easily reduced to a minimum value by the addition of alkali from the burette. A minimum of about 0.002 ml. 0.018N sodium hydroxide/ml. titration mixture is required to expel carbon dioxide from the system during titration.

6. Sodium hydroxide solution (approximately 0.018N). This is prepared fresh daily by 1/1000 dilution of 50% sodium hydroxide solution in freshly boiled and cooled distilled water. It is standardized against pure palmitic acid as described in the procedure.

7. Palmitic acid standards:
   A. Stock standard. Recrystallized palmitic acid* (obtainable in 99% purity) is used. Dissolve 256.4 mg. palmitic acid in hexane in a 100 ml. glass-stoppered volumetric flask. This stock solution contains 10 mEq./L.
   B. Working standard. Dilute 10 ml. to 100 ml. with hexane.

Procedure: As soon as possible after the separation of plasma, add 5 ml. extraction mixture to 1 ml. plasma in a glass-stoppered tube and shake vigorously for a moment.

Allow to stand 10 min. or longer; then divide the system into two phases by mixing into it an additional 2 ml. hexane and 3 ml. water. The phases should separate rapidly without centrifugation and form a sharp interface.

Transfer a 3 ml. aliquot of the upper phase to a 15 ml. conical centrifuge tube containing 1 ml. titration mixture. Nitrogen gas, delivered to the bottom of the tube with a fine glass capillary, expels the carbon dioxide from the sample and keeps the two phases mixed during titration. Titrate with the sodium hydroxide solution. As the yellow-green end point is approached, interrupt the gas stream from time to time to examine the indicator color in the alcoholic phase.

*Nutritional Biochemicals Corp., Cleveland, Ohio.

Run a blank using 1 ml. water instead of 1 ml. plasma and carry through the same procedure. Run a standard by adding to a glass-stoppered tube 1 ml. working standard, 4 ml. isopropyl alcohol, 0.1 ml. 1N sulfuric acid, and 1 ml. water. Shake the mixture and allow to stand for 10 min. Separate the phases by adding 2 ml. hexane and 3 ml. water as in the sample procedure. Titrate a 3 ml. aliquot of the hexane layer.

Calculation: Since the working standard contains 1 mEq./L. of palmitic acid and since 1 ml. each of standard and plasma is used, then:

$$\text{MEq./L. free fatty acids} = \frac{A - B}{C - B}$$

where A is the milliliters of sodium hydroxide required for titration of the sample; C, that required for the standard; and B, that required for the blank.

NOTE: The extraction must be carried out as soon as possible after drawing the blood to prevent any lipolysis on standing that might increase the free fatty acid concentration. Since heparinized plasma can be separated much more rapidly than serum from clotted blood, its use is preferable. If serum must be used or the extraction cannot be carried out immediately, the tubes containing the blood should be stored in an ice bath.

Normal values and interpretation: The normal range of free fatty acids in plasma is 0.35-1.2 mEq./L. The level is decreased somewhat after an ordinary meal, but shows some increase after a fat meal or the injection of epinephrine.

Unusually high levels are found in diabetes mellitus. These levels return to normal with treatment, and it has been shown that the response of the free fatty acids to treatment occurs more rapidly than do the responses of blood sugar, plasma CO_2, or excretion of urinary ketones.[165, 166]

SERUM TRIGLYCERIDES (MICROMETHOD OF VAN HANDEL AND ZILVERSMIT)[167]

This method is based on the quantitative removal of phospholipids from the sample by absorption with zeolite (silicic acid) and the subsequent determination of the glycerol hydrolyzed from the glycerides.

Glass-stoppered test tubes, 28 × 130 mm. (Corning* No. 8424 centrifuge tubes with stoppers are satisfactory), or screw-capped glass tubes, 16 × 125 mm. (Corning* No. 9825 culture tubes), may be used.

Reagents:

1. Chloroform. A redistilled technical grade is satisfactory. Store in a dark bottle.
2. Doucil.† Activate by heating for 4 hr. at 125° C. Store in a tightly stoppered bottle.
3. Alcoholic postassium hydroxide (0.4 %). Dissolve 2 gm. reagent grade potassium hydroxide in redistilled 95% ethyl alcohol and dilute to 100 ml. Dilute 10 ml. stock KOH solution to 50 ml. with 95% ethyl alcohol on the day of use.
4. Sulfuric acid (0.2N). Dilute 3 ml. concentrated sulfuric acid to 500 ml. with distilled water.
5. Sodium arsenite (0.5M). Dissolve 2.25 gm. sodium hydroxide and 5 gm. reagent grade arsenic trioxide in distilled water and dilute to 100 ml.
6. Sodium metaperiodate (0.05M). Dissolve 1.07 gm. sodium metaperiodate ($NaIO_4$) in 100 ml. distilled water.
7. Chromotropic acid (0.2%). Dissolve 2 gm. chromotropic acid or 2.24 gm. sodium salt‡ in 200 ml. distilled water. Add separately 600 ml. concentrated sulfuric acid to 300 ml. distilled water cooled in ice. When cool, add diluted sulfuric acid to the chromotropic acid solution.
8. Triglyceride standards:
    A. Stock standard (5 mg./ml.). Dissolve 0.5 gm. commercial corn oil in chloroform to make 100 ml., using a glass-stoppered volumetric flask. It is advisable to occasionally check the concentration of the standard solution gravimetrically to guard against increase due to evaporation of the solvent.
    B. Working standard. Dilute stock standard 1:100 with chloroform. This solution contains 0.05 mg. triglyceride/ml.

Procedure: Place 4 gm. Doucil in a glass-stoppered tube, add 2 ml. chloroform, and shake. Place 1 ml. plasma or serum on top of Doucil, mix thoroughly, and add 18 ml. chloroform. Stopper tube and shake intermittently but vigorously for about 10 min. Filter through fat-free paper and pipette 1 ml. portions of the filtrate to each of three screw-capped tubes. (If the triglyceride content is expected to be low, a larger aliquot of 2 or 3 ml. may be used.)

Similarly, pipette 1 ml. portions of the working standard to each of three tubes. Evaporate the solvent from all tubes by placing in a water bath at 60°-70° C.

To two of the three tubes in each set, standards and unknowns, add 0.5 ml. alcoholic potassium hydroxide (saponified sample); then add 0.5 ml. alcohol to the third tube (unsaponified sample).

Keep all tubes at 60°-70° C. for 15 min. Add 0.5 ml. 0.2N sulfuric acid to each tube and place in gently boiling water bath for about 15 min. to remove alcohol. It is advisable to keep the water level of the bath only slightly above the surface of the reaction mixture to avoid evaporation of water from the tubes.

Cool to room temperature. Add 0.1 ml. sodium periodate solution to each tube with a graduated pipette. After 10 min. add 0.1 ml. sodium arsenite solution to each tube. A yellow color of iodine appears and vanishes in a few minutes. Add 5 ml. chromotropic acid solution to each tube and mix. Cap tubes tightly and heat in boiling water bath for 30 min. in the absence of excessive light. After cooling, determine OD of all tubes at 570 nm. against water blank. The color remains stable for several hours.

---

*Corning Glass Works, Corning, N. Y.
†Doucil is a zeolite obtainable from W. A. Taylor Co., Baltimore, Md.
‡Obtainable as 4,5-dihydroxy-2,7-naphthalenedisulfonic acid, disodium salt, No. P-230, Eastman Kodak Co., Rochester, N. Y.

Calculation:

$$\frac{\text{OD saponified unknown} - \text{OD unsaponified}}{\text{OD saponified standard} - \text{OD unsaponified}}$$

$$\frac{\text{unknown}}{\text{standard}} \times 0.05 \times \frac{2000}{\text{Ml. chloroform extract}} =$$

$$\text{Mg.\% triglyceride}$$

To convert to mEq./L. multiply by 0.0342.

Normal values and interpretation: Normal values found by this method range from 40-145 mg.%, with an average of 79 mg.%, or from 1.4-4.9 mEq./L., with an average of 2.7 mEq./L. Values below the normal range are of no significance. It has been found that serum triglycerides are often elevated in atherosclerosis and coronary artery disease.[168, 169]

NOTE: Triglycerides can be estimated by calculating the difference between the total esterified fatty acids and those present as cholesterol esters and phospholipid esters. One formula is as follows:

$$\text{MEq./L. triglyceride fatty acids} =$$
$$\text{MEq./L. total fatty acids esters} - (0.0186 \text{ C} + 0.0232 \text{ P})$$

where C is mg.% cholesterol and P is the mg.% phospholipid. The derivation of this formula is given by Albrink. The normal range of triglycerides is 0-5 mEq./L.

POLYUNSATURATED FATTY ACIDS

There is some evidence that diets containing unsaturated fats (liquid fats) are less atherogenic than those containing an equivalent amount of saturated (solid) fats. In studies on atherosclerosis, one may wish to determine the percentage of fatty acids in the blood serum that is polyunsaturated (i.e., contains more than one double bond). The method requires the use of a spectrophotometer capable of making measurements in the ultraviolet range (234 nm.) and will only be mentioned here. The details are given in a paper by MacGee.[170]

LIPOPROTEINS

In their physiologic state in blood the lipids are largely associated with proteins as lipoproteins (except for the chy-lomicrons). In recent years more emphasis has been placed on the lipoproteins than on the simple lipid constituents in the pathogenesis of atherosclerosis. Lipoproteins have been estimated in a wide variety of ways, including ultracentrifugation, electrophoresis, low-temperature fractionation, direct precipitation, and immunochemical studies. These methods involve many different physical and chemical techniques, and as a consequence, the results obtained by the different methods are not always directly comparable.

The ultracentrifuge method involves centrifugation at very high speeds (up to 50,000 rpm) and gives results that are expressed in terms of S_f units, which is actually a flotation rate since lipoproteins tend to rise to the surface during centrifugation because they are less dense than the media used to dilute the serum. The actual methods are beyond the scope of this book. A discussion of the principles and techniques is found in the article by DeLalla and Gofman[171] and interpretation of the results is available in the review by Gofman and associates.[172] The S_f values have been used in the study of atherosclerosis, and an increase in certain ranges of S_f values has been stated to be indicative of a tendency toward atherosclerosis.

Other simpler methods have been devised for the approximate estimation of lipoproteins, either by precipitation upon the addition of certain high molecular weight compounds such as dextran sulfate, sulfonated amylopectin, or heparin[173, 174] or by an immunologic reaction with a specific antiserum.[175] These methods have not as yet come into general use, although they may serve as simple screening tests to select subjects for further study.

Lipoproteins have also been determined by electrophoresis, either on paper or by the starch zone method. Paper electrophoresis is similar to that used for proteins except that the paper is stained with an oil-soluble dye to distinguish the lipids. The paper electrophoretic method distinguishes between two classes of lipoproteins—the alpha and beta lipoproteins, which correspond roughly to the alpha and beta globulins. In normal individuals the alpha liproproteins comprise 30-50% of the total lipoproteins and the beta fraction comprises the remaining 50-70%. In individuals with atherosclerosis or coronary heart disease the proportion of beta lipoproteins increases to 75-85% of the total. Many investigators feel that an increase in the ratio of the beta or alpha lipoproteins above the normal value of 1-2 is a better index of the tendency toward coronary artery disease than is an increase in the level of any one of the lipid constituents such as cholesterol.

The starch zone method of electrophoresis, such as we used following the earlier work of Kunkel and Slater,[176] is a more elegant method for studying the lipoproteins. By this method the lipoproteins, measured in terms of their cholesterol content, are divided into three fractions, an alpha$_1$ fraction (25-35% in normal young adults), an alpha$_2$ fraction (8-12% in normal young adults), and a beta fraction (55-65% in normal young adults). In persons over 60 yr. of age the proportion in the alpha$_1$ fraction is somewhat lower (20-30%) and the beta fraction is higher (60-70%), with the alpha$_2$ fraction remaining unchanged. In patients with moderate to advanced atherosclerosis the percentage in the beta fraction is further increased—up to 80% or higher. It was also shown that in individuals with a history of previous myocardial infarction the alpha$_2$ fraction is increased.[177, 178] This fraction is also increased in nephrosis or extreme hyperlipemia; but in a large number of persons in whom these conditions could be excluded, 90% of the subjects having an alpha$_2$ proportion over 20% had a history of previous myocardial infarction, whereas in the subjects with an alpha$_2$ proportion of less than 16%, only slightly over 1% had any history of previous myocardial infarction, indicating a very striking relationship.

Fat tolerance test

The fat tolerance test has been used by many investigators in detecting derangement of lipid metabolism. The results are used as a criterion for assessing susceptibility to atherosclerosis and coronary heart disease.[179, 180]

A simple method for the study of fat tolerance is as follows. The subjects fast overnight. A fasting blood specimen is drawn and a standard fat meal consisting of 100 ml. of cream (approximately 40 gm. of fat), with cocoa and sugar for taste, is given. Succeeding blood specimens are drawn at intervals of 60, 120, 150, 180, and 210 min. The total esterified fatty acids (method of Stern and Shapiro) and visible lipemia are determined on each specimen. The visible lipemia is determined turbidimetrically by diluting serum 2½ times its volume with a 20% urea solution and reading the OD at 650 nm. Maximum fatty acid concentration and turbidity appear at about 180 min. in all subjects. The healthy individual will show an increase to about 17.5 mEq./L. In the atherosclerotic group, fatty acid will increase to about 23 mEq./L. and will show a slower return to the fasting level.

Atherogenic index (AI)[171, 181]

By using the ultracentrifuge, methods have been developed for characterization and quantitation of essentially all the serum lipoproteins. These various lipoproteins are conveniently classified by the rate of flotation under defined conditions in an intense centrifugal field. The unit of flotation rate is designated as the S_f unit (Svedberg unit of flotation). Thus, for example, a single lipoprotein may be referred to by its flotation rate as S_f4-10. For clinical purposes it has been more convenient to lump together the sum of all concentrations of lipoproteins between arbitrary flotation rate limits. Therefore one will note in the more recent reports reference to two major lipoprotein classes—standard S_f0-12 and standard S_f12-400. Both of these classes are significantly elevated in frank coronary heart disease. The determination of the index of coronary atherogenicity requires assessment of the relative importance of each group for coronary disease. This measurement permits preselection of individuals who may carry

$$AI = \frac{Mg\% \text{ standard } S_f 0\text{-}12 + 1.75 \times (Mg\% \text{ standard } S_f 12\text{-}400)}{10}$$

an abnormal risk of future overt coronary heart disease.

Numerous tests have indicated that intrinsically each mg.% of standard S_f12-400 lipoprotein is 1.75 times as important for atherogenesis as each mg.% of standard S_f0-12 lipoprotein. This information is converted into an atherogenic index as shown at the top of the page.

The denominator of 10 is used arbitrarily to provide a convenient scale of values. The AI is considered normal when it falls below 50 units, borderline when between 50 and 75 units, and elevated when above 75 units. Increased average AI values have been reported in patients with increased systolic blood pressure, increased diastolic blood pressure, increased weight, diabetes, and xanthomatosis.

ENZYMES

Enzymes are complex, naturally occurring compounds that catalyze many biologic reactions; i.e., they speed up reactions that might otherwise proceed very slowly. Most enzymes are very specific in their action in that they will catalyze only a definite type of chemical reaction or act on a particular compound (substrate). Many enzymes are named for the type of substrate on which they act: urease hydrolyzes urea, lipase hydrolyzes fats (lipids), phosphatases act on organic phosphates, etc. Recently a more systematic nomenclature was adopted by the International Union of Biochemistry. These names, while more accurate, are also more cumbersome; and although they may be useful in biochemical research, they are not likely to be adopted for clinical use in the near future.

The general reaction involving an enzyme may be written as follows:

$$E + S \rightleftarrows ES \rightarrow E + S^1$$

where E represents the enzyme; S, the substrate on which the enzyme acts; ES, the postulated enzyme-substrate complex; and S^1, the reacted substrate that may represent a changed molecular species for S or the splitting of S into two or more different molecules. The enzyme thus represents a true catalyst in that it is not changed in the reaction. The speed with which this reaction takes place depends, as in all chemical reactions, on the concentration of the reacting substances, E and S. If the concentration of the substrate, S, is sufficiently high in comparison with that of the enzyme so that it remains relatively constant, then the rate will be proportional to the concentration of the enzyme and the amount of product, S^1, formed in a given period of time will be proportional to the amount of active enzyme present.

This is the basis for most determinations of enzymes. The actual concentration of the enzymes is usually so low that it would be impracticable to determine their concentration in the same sense that one might determine the concentration of other blood constituents. The concentrations of the enzymes are usually expressed in **units**. The units are defined differently for each enzyme and are usually expressed in terms of micrograms or micromoles of substrate "acted upon" per unit time for a given amount of serum.

The actual units used in reporting enzyme concentrations are still in a state of flux. In all of the older procedures, arbitrary units were employed, and different units were used for the same enzyme in various procedures. For example, in the determination of the enzyme alkaline phosphatase, one method (Bodansky) uses a substrate of beta-glycerophosphate and defines the unit as 1 mg. phosphate phosphorus liberated from the substrate by 100 ml. serum during 1 hr. of incubation. Another method (original King-Armstrong method) uses a substrate of phenylphosphate and defines the unit as 1 mg. phenol liberated from the substrate by 100 ml. serum in 30 min. of incubation. A third method (Bessey-Lowry-Brock) uses *p*-nitrophenylphosphate as a substrate and defines the unit as millimoles of *p*-nitrophenol formed per hour per 1000 ml. serum. One could not expect these units to be directly comparable. It is best to run the same serum by the different methods and compare the results. For a rough correlation one can look up the range of normal values given for two methods and compare them. One compilation gives the range of normal values for the King-Armstrong method as 3.7-13.1 units and for the Bessey-Lowry-Brock method as 0.8-2.9 units. The ratios for the lower and upper limits are 3.7/0.8 = 4.6 and 13.1/2.9 = 4.5, so that one can say that approximately 4.5 K-A units equals 1 B-L-B unit.

Recently it has been proposed that all enzyme concentrations be expressed in terms of **international units** (I.U.). One unit is defined as 1 μM. of substrate used per minute per liter of serum under specified conditions of pH and temperature. These units have not come into general use in clinical chemistry because the older units are firmly established. In some instances the use of the international unit would make for better comparison between methods. For example, the normal ranges for three alkaline phosphatase methods (Shinowara-Jones-Reinhart, King-Armstrong, and Bessey-Lowry-Brock) are given as 2.2-8.6, 3.7-13.1, and 0.8-2.9 units, respectively. These all seem quite different, but when converted into international units, the ranges are essentially the same: 12.0-46.7, 13.0-46.0, and 13.3-48.3.

The rate of reactions involving enzymes is markedly influenced by temperature, pH, concentration of substrate, and a number of other factors. Accordingly, all the details of a given procedure must be followed exactly in order to give accurate results. The time as well as the temperature of incubation must be closely controlled. With some enzymatic procedures the reaction rate is not constant with time, so one cannot assume that incubation for 60 min. will utilize exactly twice the amount of substrate as will incubation for 30 min. One cannot always compensate for increased activity by halving the incubation time and then

multiplying the number of units found by 2. This may be true for some enzyme reactions, but not all. It cannot be assumed to be true unless specifically stated in the procedure.

There are a number of enzyme systems that involve the conversion of **nicotinamide adenine dinucleotide** (NAD) to its reduced form (NADH), or vice versa. The reduced form, NADH, has a much greater absorption at 340 nm. than does the oxidized form, and consequently the reactions may be followed by measuring the change in absorption at this wavelength. In addition, many other enzyme reactions that do not involve the NAD-NADH change directly can be coupled with another reaction involving NAD so that the change in NAD becomes a measure of the enzyme reaction. Thus a number of enzyme reactions can be determined by measurements at a wavelength of 340 nm. This wavelength is in the near ultraviolet range and most clinical photoelectric colorimeters do not operate at this wavelength. Good spectrophotometers that will operate in the ultraviolet range are rather expensive. However, there are instruments on the market that are relatively inexpensive and are specifically designed to read only at wavelength 340 nm.* This allows considerable simplification because these instruments can give accurate OD readings at this wavelength.

Most enzymes in biologic fluids are stable at refrigerator temperature for 24 hr. and at room temperature for a shorter time. When storing for longer periods, serum or plasma should usually be frozen. Exactness in pipetting, incubation time, and temperature must always be observed, and extreme cleanliness of the glassware must be ensured.

Because no primary standards are available, it is of extreme importance that all conditions for enzyme assays be maintained exactly the same each time they are run and that a quality control serum of a known value be included.

---

*Calbiometer, Calbiochem, Los Angeles, Calif.; Coenzometer, Macalaster-Bicknell Co., New Haven, Conn.

Throughout this section, reference to coenzymes **nicotinamide adenine dinucleotide** (NAD) and **nicotinamide adenine dinucleotide phosphate** (NADP) will be made. These compounds are also known as **diphosphopyridine nucleotide** (DPN) and **triphosphopyridine nucleotide** (TPN), respectively, and may be used interchangeably.

Only enzymes recognized as having clinical significance will be described in this section. Others will be mentioned briefly.

ALDOLASE[182-184]

Aldolase is the enzyme that takes part in the intermediary breakdown of glucose at the level of fructose-1,6-diphosphate and converts it into dihydroxyacetone phosphate and glyceraldehyde-3-phosphate.

$$\text{Fructose-1,6-diphosphate} \xrightarrow{\text{Aldolase}} \text{Dihydroxy-}$$

acetone phosphate + Glyceraldehyde-3-phosphate

In this method, hydrazine is added to the reaction mixture to combine with the products of the forward reaction, the triose phosphates, and prevents their disappearance due to other enzymes in the system. After the reaction has been stopped by precipitation of the proteins with trichloroacetic acid, the triose phosphates are hydrolyzed by alkali at room temperature to the corresponding trioses. The trioses are then reacted with 2,4-dinitrophenylhydrazine to form osazones, which give a characteristic color in alkaline solution. The intensity of the color produced is proportional to the amount of trioses. This is related to the aldolase activity.

Reagents:
1. Fructose-1,6-diphosphate (0.05M). Dissolve 250 mg. fructose-1,6-diphosphate sodium salt* in 10 ml. water. This is stable for approximately 2 wk. at 0°-5° C.
2. Hydrazine solution (0.56M, pH 7.4). Dissolve 7.28 gm. hydrazine sulfate in 50 ml. water. Adjust pH to 7.4

with 1N NaOH and dilute to 100 ml. with water.
3. γ-Collidine buffer (0.1M, pH 7.4). Dissolve 1.21 gm. γ-collidine in 50 ml. water. Adjust pH to 7.4 with 1N HCl and dilute to 100 ml. with water.
4. Iodoacetate (0.002M, pH 7.4). Dissolve 1.35 gm. iodoacetic acid (iodoethanoic acid) in about 80 ml. water. Adjust pH to 7.4 with 1N NaOH and dilute to 100 ml. This is a 0.2M solution and must be diluted 1:100 for the test.
5. 2,4-Dinitrophenylhydrazine (0.1% in HCl). Dissolve 100 mg. 2,4-dinitrophenylhydrazine in 100 ml. 2N HCl. Filter and store in the dark.
6. Sodium hydroxide (0.75N). Dissolve 30 gm. reagent grade sodium hydroxide in water and dilute to 1 L.
7. Trichloroacetic acid (TCA) (10%). Dissolve 20 gm. TCA in water and dilute to 200 ml.
8. Aldolase calibration solution (0.2% dihydroxyacetone). Dissolve 200 mg. dihydroxyacetone* in water and dilute to 100 ml. in a volumetric flask. This solution is kept in the refrigerator for 48-72 hr. before using to complete depolymerization.

Procedure: Label two test tubes "test" and "blank." Pipette into each tube 1 ml. γ-collidine buffer, 1 ml. serum, 0.25 ml. hydrazine, and 0.25 ml. iodoacetate. Place in water bath at 37° C. for a few minutes. To the "test" tube add 0.25 ml. fructose-1,6-diphosphate substrate and incubate for 60 min. Add 5 ml. TCA to both tubes; then add 0.25 ml. fructose-1,6-diphosphate substrate to the "blank" tube. Shake tubes well and filter or centrifuge. Add 1 ml. 0.75N NaOH to 1 ml. filtrate, mix, and let stand at room temperature for 10 min. Then add 1 ml. 2,4-dinitrophenylhydrazine, mix, and incubate at 37° C. for 1 hr. Add 7 ml. 0.75N NaOH, mix well, and let stand 5 min. Read in a spectrophotometer at 540 nm. against the "blank" tube. Obtain "dihydroxyacetone units" from the calibration curve. For values greater than 120 units, repeat as-

---

*Sigma Chemical Co., St. Louis, Mo.

*Mann Research Laboratories, New York, N. Y.

Table 6-11

Tube No.	Standard (ml.)	H₂O (ml.)	Dihydroxyacetone (mg.)	Dihydroxyacetone units
1	0	1.0	0	0
2	0.1	0.9	0.2	20
3	0.2	0.8	0.4	40
4	0.3	0.7	0.6	60
5	0.4	0.6	0.8	80
6	0.5	0.5	1.0	100
7	0.6	0.4	1.2	120

say using a fivefold dilution of the serum (1 part serum and 4 parts water) and multiply the results from the calibration chart by 5 to obtain the correct answer.

Calibration curve: Number a series of seven test tubes and pipette standard dihydroxyacetone solution and water in the proportions shown in Table 6-11.

The method is followed exactly as described. The 1 ml. portion of diluted dihydroxyacetone standard solution takes the place of the serum. Other reagents and steps are identical.

Plot OD (or %T) against corresponding dihydroxyacetone units. The curve will not necessarily be a straight line.

The dihydroxyacetone unit is defined as the amount of color developed by 0.01 mg. dihydroxyacetone under the conditions of this procedure. One dihydroxyacetone unit equals approximately 0.4 Sibley-Lehninger (S-L) unit.

Normal values and interpretation: The normal aldolase level according to this method is 6.1-21.3 dihydroxyacetone units. Significant elevations are found in acute infectious hepatitis, usually up to 20 times the average normal. Normal results are usually obtained in portal cirrhosis and obstructive jaundice.

A significant increase is also found in progressive muscular dystrophy (primary myopathy).[185] No elevation is found in muscular dystrophy secondary to alterations of the nerves or nerve centers.

Increases in aldolase activity have been reported after myocardial infarction,[186] advanced prostatic carcinoma, hepatoma, large pulmonary infarcts, hemorrhagic pericarditis, erythroblastosis fetalis, acute pancreatitis, and hemolytic anemia.[187, 188]

ALPHA-HYDROXYBUTYRATE DEHYDROGENASE (HBD)[189-192]

In the presence of reduced nicotinamide adenine dinucleotide (NADH) this enzyme catalyzes the reversible reduction of alpha-ketobutyrate to alpha-hydroxybutyrate. It is found in greatest concentration in the heart muscle, kidney, brain, and erythrocytes.

$$\text{Alpha-ketobutyrate + NADH} \underset{}{\overset{\text{HBD}}{\rightleftharpoons}}$$

Alpha-hydroxybutyrate + NAD

Serum is incubated with alpha-ketobutyrate substrate and reduced NADH. The reaction is stopped by the addition of 2,4-dinitrophenylhydrazine, which reacts with the unchanged alpha-ketobutyrate to form 2,4-dinitrophenylhydrazone. In the presence of excess sodium hydroxide this gives a brown color, which is determined colorimetrically. The intensity of this color is inversely proportional to the enzyme activity. The less color produced, the greater the enzyme activity. This reflects the decreased concentration of the substrate.

Reagents:

1. Sorensen phosphate buffer (0.067M, pH 7.4). Dissolve 7.61 gm. anhydrous disodium phosphate (Na₂HPO₄) and 1.78 gm. potassium phosphate dibasic (KH₂PO₄) in water and dilute to 1 L. Check pH and adjust to 7.4 if necessary.
2. Alpha-ketobutyrate stock solution (0.1M). Dissolve 1.02 gm. alpha-ketobutyric acid in phosphate buffer, adjust pH to 7.4 if necessary, and dilute to 100 ml. This is stable for 1 mo. at −18° C.

3. Alpha-ketobutyrate substrate. Dilute stock solution so that approximate OD differences shown in Table 6-13 are obtained when the calibration curve is prepared. Usually a dilution of 1:100 suffices. The substrate should be stored in 20 ml. glass bottles at −18° C. This is stable for 1 mo.

4. Reduced nicotinamide adenine dinucleotide solution (NADH). Dissolve 10 mg./ml. in phosphate buffer. Prepare on the day the test is run.

5. 2,4-Dinitrophenylhydrazine (0.04%). Dissolve 400 mg. reagent grade 2,4-dinitrophenylhydrazine in 85 ml. concentrated hydrochloric acid and dilute to 1 L. with water. This reagent is stable indefinitely.

6. Sodium hydroxide (0.4N). Dissolve 16 gm. reagent grade sodium hydroxide pellets in water and dilute to 1 L.

NOTE: All glassware must be chemically clean. Washing with chromic acid, followed by thorough rinsing in distilled water, is recommended. Clear serum, free from hemolysis, should be used since red cells contain more than 100 times the serum enzyme activity.

Procedure: A test and a blank are required for each serum tested. For each batch of tests a substrate blank and substrate NADH blank should be set up in duplicate. Set up a series of 10 × 175 mm. test tubes, label, and add reagents as described in Table 6-12.

Place all tubes in a water bath at 37° C. for about 5 min. Add 0.1 ml. NADH to the serum test and incubate all the tubes for exactly 60 min. at 37° C. Stop the reaction by adding 1 ml. dinitrophenylhydrazine reagent to each tube and mix thoroughly by gentle shaking. Remove tube from the water bath and allow to stand at room temperature for 20 min. Add to all tubes 10 ml. 0.4N sodium hydroxide and mix by inversion for 20 min. Allow to stand at room temperature no less than 10 min. or more than 30 min. and read OD in a photometer at 490 nm. against water.

Calculation: Subtract serum test OD from OD of serum blank. Subtract OD of blank substrate from OD of substrate NADH blank and add this difference to the OD obtained for the serum. This value is converted into international units of HBD per liter of serum by the calibration curve. If the activity of serum exceeds 310 units/L., the test should be re-

Table 6-12

Reagent	Serum test (ml.)	Serum blank (ml.)	Substrate blank (ml.)	Substrate NADH blank (ml.)
Alpha-ketobutyrate substrate	1.0	1.0	1.0	1.0
Serum	0.1	0.1	—	—
Phosphate buffer	—	0.1	0.2	0.1
NADH	—	—	—	0.1

Table 6-13

Tube No.	Substrate (ml.)	Phosphate buffer (ml.)	HBD activity (I.U./L. serum)	Net decrease in OD compared with tube No. 1
1	1.0	0.2	0	0
2	0.8	0.4	53	0.090
3	0.6	0.6	114	0.180
4	0.4	0.8	183	0.270
5	0.2	1.0	310	0.395

peated using 1 vol. serum diluted with 4 vol. phosphate buffer and multiplying the results from Table 6-13 by 5.

Calibration curve: Set up five test tubes and add reagents as shown in Table 6-13.

To all tubes add 1 ml. dinitrophenyl-hydrazine reagent, mix thoroughly, and let stand for 20 min. Add 10 ml. 0.4N NaOH to all tubes and mix well by inversion. Allow to stand at room temperature no less than 10 min. and no more than 30 min. Read OD in a photometer at 490 nm. against water. Plot OD vs. corresponding units of HBD, starting with the highest OD reading in tube No. 1 vs. 0 units, etc.

Normal values and interpretation: The normal range of HBD by this method is 56-125 I.U./L. serum. No significant changes occur with age after 10 yr., but slightly higher values have been obtained in children. Serum HBD is increased in myocardial infarction and in acute and chronic liver disease. In terms of duration and absolute value, elevation in HBD is considered superior to SGOT, total LDH, and CPK analyses for the confirmation of myocardial infarction.

AMYLASE (DIASTASE)

Methods for the determination of amylase involve measurement of the amount of **starch** hydrolyzed by the enzyme or the amount of reducing sugars formed in hydrolysis when definite amounts of starch and serum are incubated for an exact period of time. The following methods are those introduced by Somogyi and include recent modifications in the preparation of reagents. In one method the amount of reducing sugars formed are determined with the Somogyi high alkalinity sugar reagent. In the other method the disappearance of the starch is measured with the starch-iodine color reaction.

Method I (based on saccharogenic activity)[193, 194]:

Reagents:
1. Buffer solution. Dissolve 2.25 gm. anhydrous monobasic potassium phosphate (KH_2PO_4), 2.4 gm. anhydrous disodium phosphate (Na_2-HPO_4), 2.5 gm. sodium chloride, 2 gm. sodium fluoride, and 0.3 gm. propyl *p*-hydroxybenzoate* in distilled water and dilute to 1 L.
2. Starch solution. Best results are obtained with a starch purified as follows. Dissolve 4.5 gm. sodium hydroxide in about 1000 ml. water in a 2000 ml. beaker. Heat to 50°-55° C. Discontinue heating and introduce about 200 gm. cornstarch while agitating with a mechanical stirrer. Continue agitation for 1-2 hr.; allow starch to settle overnight. Decant the yellow liquid, suspend the starch in about 1800 ml. distilled water, and stir the mixture well before allowing it to settle again overnight. After the water is decanted, wash the starch twice more with water in a similar manner. After final removal of the water, allow the starch to dry in the air. For the preparation of the starch solution, suspend 15 gm. purified starch in 100 ml. buffer solution; heat 900 ml. buffer solution to boiling and add to the starch suspension with vigorous agitation. Further heating is unnecessary.
3. Barium hydroxide (0.3N) and zinc sulfate (5%). These are the same as used for the preparation of the Somogyi blood filtrate (p. 299).
4. Somogyi high alkalinity copper reagent. Dissolve 28 gm. disodium phosphate and 40 gm. potassium sodium tartrate in 700 ml. water. Add 100 ml. 1N NaOH and 80 ml. 10% copper sulfate and dilute to 1 L.

Procedure: Warm 5 ml. starch solution to 37° C. in a water bath, add 1 ml. serum, and incubate the mixture for 30 min. Then add 2 ml. 0.3N barium hydroxide and, after mixing, 2 ml. 5% zinc sulfate. Mix well and allow to stand for 30 min. Filter and determine the sugar in the filtrate using the Somogyi method, except that the high alkalinity copper solution is used and the samples are boiled for 20 min. rather than 15 min.

---

*No. 2992, Eastman Kodak Co., Rochester, N. Y.

Since the solution of the serum is 1:10, the calculations are exactly the same as for the blood sugar method. Also determine the blood sugar in the serum by the regular Somogyi method. Subtract the blood sugar value (in mg.%) found for the original serum from that found for the serum after incubation with starch (also expressed as mg.%). The result is the diastase activity of the serum in Somogyi units. If the value found is over 500 units, the incubation should be repeated using a 1 ml. aliquot of serum diluted with 0.5% sodium chloride (dilute 1:2 or 1:4 as required), and the results are multiplied by the appropriate dilution factor.

Method II (based on amyloclastic activity)[195]: This method is based on the measurement of the disapearance of the starch-iodine color.

Reagents:

1. Starch solution. This method requires a starch solution containing 75 mg. starch/100 ml. Five milliliters of the solution used in method I can be diluted to 100 ml. with the buffer solution. It is also available from a number of laboratory supply houses. The following method is best for preparing a satisfactory substrate for this test. Suspend 40 gm. purified cornstarch (see method I) in 200 ml. phosphate buffer and warm to about 55° C. Add with vigorous stirring 1800 ml. buffer solution that has been heated to boiling. Continue stirring for about 1 min. more. Transfer to an Erlenmeyer flask and allow to stand for several days until the starch solution breaks into a gelatinous sediment with a limpid, slightly opalescent supernatant layer. The supernatant layer is then siphoned off and used after proper dilution for the test. To determine the proper dilution pipette 5 ml. solution to a 25 × 200 mm. test tube, add 5 ml. 1N hydrochloric acid, and heat the tube in a boiling water bath for 2½ hr. After cooling, neutralize the acid hydrolysate with 1N sodium hydroxide, using 1 drop phenolphthalein solution for indicator,

and transfer the solution to a 50 ml. volumetric flask and dilute to the mark. Using 1 ml. diluted hydrolysate, determine the sugar content by the regular Somogyi method for blood sugar. (Since the original solution is diluted 1:10, the calculation will be the same as for a blood filtrate.) The mg.% sugar obtained multiplied by 0.9 will give the concentration of starch. Then dilute the starch solution to 75 mg.% with the phosphate buffer. For example, if the concentration was found to be 325 mg.%, pipette 75 ml. solution into a 500 ml. graduated cylinder and add buffer to the 325 ml. mark.

2. Iodine standards:
   A. Stock standard (0.1N). Dissolve 13 gm. iodine and 30 gm. potassium iodide in distilled water and dilute to 1 L. Store in a brown bottle in the refrigerator.
   B. Working standard (0.002N). Dilute 10 ml. stock standard and 1 gm. potassium iodide to 500 ml. with distilled water. Prepare fresh as needed.

Procedure: In a series of 13 mm. test tubes place 0.5 ml. diluted iodine solution. In another test tube place 4 ml. starch solution and warm in a water bath to 37° C. Then add 1 ml. serum (or other solution to be assayed), blowing it in from a "to contain" pipette (which is rinsed once with the reaction mixture) and simultaneously starting a stopwatch. After incubation for about 6 min., pipette 0.5 ml. into one of the test tubes containing the iodine solution and observe the color by transmitted light. Repeat the operation at intervals until the color of the iodine complex reaches the end point, when the time of incubation is read on the stopwatch. As the reaction progresses, the color of the starch-iodine complex changes from blue to purplish blue, purplish red, reddish brown, brown, and yellow. The transition is gradual, but a rather sharp line of demarcation is discernible when the purplish blue disappears, yielding the reddish brown color of erythrodextrin which is taken as the end point.

A little experience is necessary to estimate the time intervals after the first reading so that the final readings can be readily taken with the amount of solution available. If the reading at 6 min. is past the end point, the determination is repeated using serum diluted 1:5 or more with 0.5% saline solution.

Calculation:

$$\text{Amylase unit} = \frac{1800}{t \times D}$$

Here, t is the time in minutes for the end point, D is the dilution of the serum (e.g., 1 for undiluted serum, 5 for serum diluted 1:5), and 1800 is the K factor.

Normal values and interpretation: The normal range of amylase by either of the Somogyi methods is 60-200 units. Blood amylase is greatly increased in acute nonhemorrhagic pancreatitis early in the course of the disease. Increased levels are rarely found in chronic nephritis. Low values may be found after the elevation in acute pancreatitis and in hepatitis and liver cirrhosis.

Urinary amylase: The same method just described may be used merely by substituting urine for serum. A clean-voided, accurately timed specimen ranging from 1-24 hr. is required.

Normal values: Normal values range from 35-260 units/hr.

CERULOPLASMIN (COPPER OXIDASE)[196-203]

Ceruloplasmin is a blue copper protein found in serum associated with alpha$_2$ globulin. Although variations in its concentration are found in various pathologic conditions, its exact metabolic role is unknown; in vitro it catalyzes the oxidation of aromatic diamines. It is measured by its catalysis of the oxidation of p-phenylenediamine to form purple-blue compounds. The principal oxidation product is believed to be a compound known as Bandrowski base. This pure compound is used to standardize the enzyme activity.

Reagents:

1. Acetate buffer (ionic strength 1.2, pH 5.2 ± 0.05). Dissolve 163 gm. crystalline sodium acetate trihydrate and 20 ml. glacial acetic acid in water and dilute to 1 L. Store in the refrigerator.
2. Sodium azide (0.02%). Dissolve 10 mg. sodium azide in water and dilute to 50 ml. Prepare fresh daily as required.
3. Buffered p-phenylenediamine (PPD) (0.1%). Dissolve 10 mg. recrystallized p-phenylenediamine dihydrochloride* in 10 ml. acetate buffer. Prepare fresh daily.

Procedure: Serum or heparinized plasma may be used. Do not use ACD or EDTA plasma. Serum or plasma should be separated from the cells as soon as possible and frozen if the test is not done the same day.

Place 1 ml. freshly prepared buffered PPD in each of three test tubes (15 × 125 mm.) labeled blank, test 1, and test 2 (duplicate analysis) and incubate in water bath at 37° C. for about 5 min. Add 0.1 ml. serum to each tube; then immediately add 5 ml. sodium azide solution to the blank tube. Mix by inversion and incubate in water bath at 37° C. for 15 min. Make sure that the level of the reaction mixture in the test tubes is below the water level in the bath. After incubation, add 5 ml. sodium azide solution to the "test" tubes (not to the blank) to stop the reaction. Measure OD of test tubes 1 and 2 against the blank in a photometer at 540 nm. Dilutions should be made for specimens having very high activity.

Calibration using Bandrowski base†: Bandrowski base is a pure crystalline compound formed from the oxidation of p-phenylenediamine (PPD) in aqueous ammoniacal solution by hydrogen peroxide. This compound has been shown to have a spectral absorption curve identical to the pigment formed by the oxidase

---

*No. 207, Eastman Kodak Co., Rochester, N. Y. PPD is dissolved in a minimum amount of hot distilled water, decolorized with charcoal, filtered while hot, and recrystallized from the clear filtrate. The white crystals of PPD are dried and stored in a vacuum over calcium chloride.

†Nutritional Biochemicals Corp., Cleveland, Ohio.

activity of ceruloplasmin on *p*-phenylene-diamine. Measurements of absorbance at 540 nm. adhere strictly to Beer's law up to concentrations of 50 μg/ml. standard solution.

Weigh accurately 5 mg. Bandrowski base, transfer to a 100 ml. volumetric flask, add about 75 ml. acetate buffer, and agitate in a mechanical shaker for 2 hr. Dilute to 100 ml. with acetate buffer. This solution contains 50 μg/ml. base. It should be used for standardization within 1 hr. after preparation. Prepare six test tubes (15 × 125 mm.) and label as shown in Table 6-14.

Use any clear unhemolyzed serum. Mix all tubes and measure OD of standard tubes at 540 nm. against blank.

Calculation: One international unit is defined as the formation of 1 μM. Bandrowski base/min./L. serum. Since in our procedure 0.1 ml. serum is used and the incubation period is 15 min., the formation of 1 μg of base under these conditions would correspond to:

$$\frac{1}{318.4} \times \frac{1000}{0.1} \times \frac{1}{15} = 2.1 \text{ I.U.}$$

where 318.4 is the molecular weight converting micrograms to micromoles, 1000 converts to liters of serum, and 1/15 converts to the amount formed per minute. Accordingly, tubes 1-5 correspond to 10.5, 21, 42, 63, and 105 I.U. One can obtain a calibration curve by plotting the OD against the I.U.

Normal values and interpretation: The normal range of ceruloplasmin is 35-65 I.U. or 15-35 mg.%. Concentrations below the lower limit have been reported only in patients with Wilson's disease, in the neonatal period, in the nephrotic syndrome, and occasionally in unaffected relatives of patients with Wilson's disease. There may be a deficiency of ceruloplasmin in patients with kwashiorkor, tropical sprue, and in certain infants with a syndrome of anemia and hypoproteinemia.

Increased concentrations of ceruloplasmin have been noted in pregnancy, subacute or chronic infection, myocardial infarction, hepatic cirrhosis, hyperthyroidism, aplastic or refractory anemia, Hodgkin's disease, acute leukemia, and in patients receiving estrogen therapy. The ceruloplasmin activity generally parallels the copper content of the serum.

CHOLINESTERASE[204]

Cholinesterase is an enzyme that hydrolyzes **acetylcholine** to form choline and acetic acid.

$$\text{Acetylcholine} + H_2O \xrightarrow[\text{Acetic acid}]{\text{Cholinesterase}} \text{Choline} +$$

In the following method the change in pH due to the liberation of acetic acid is measured using metanitrophenol as indicator. The indicator is yellow in alkaline solution and colorless in acid; hence the amount of yellow color decreases as acetic acid is liberated. This decrease in color is a measure of the acetic acid formed and hence of the enzyme activity.

Reagents:
1. Buffered nitrophenol. Dissolve 6.65 gm. anhydrous disodium phosphate (Na_2HPO_4) and 0.43 gm. potassium dihydrogen phosphate (KH_2PO_4) in about 200 ml. distilled water. Dis-

Table 6-14

Tube No.	Sodium azide (ml.)	Serum (ml.)	Bandrowski base solution (ml.)	Acetate buffer (ml.)	Concentration (μg)	I.U.
Blank	5	0.1	0	1.0	0	0
1	5	0.1	0.1	0.9	5	10.5
2	5	0.1	0.2	0.8	10	21.0
3	5	0.1	0.4	0.6	20	42.0
4	5	0.1	0.6	0.4	30	63.0
5	5	0.1	1.0	0.0	50	105.0

solve 0.30 gm. metanitrophenol* in about 200 ml. distilled water (with the aid of slight heating if necessary). Mix the two solutions and adjust to pH 7.8 with 0.1N sodium hydroxide solution; then dilute to 1 L.

2. Acetylcholine solution (15%). Dissolve 15 gm. acetylcholine in water to make 100 ml. Store in the refrigerator.

3. Sodium chloride solution (0.9%). Dissolve 9 gm. sodium chloride in water and make up to 1 L.

Procedure: To each of two tubes add 0.1 ml. 0.9% sodium chloride solution and 0.1 ml. serum. Heat one tube to 60° C. in a water bath for 3 min. This is the blank tube; the heating inactivates the enzyme. The other tube is the sample tube. To each tube add 2.5 ml. buffered nitrophenol and 0.1 ml. acetylcholine solution. Mix and incubate at 25° C. for 30 min. Then read both tubes in a photometer at 420 nm., setting to zero with water. Read sample exactly 30 min. after addition of acetylcholine. Subtract the OD of the sample tube from the OD for the blank.

Calibration curve: Dilute 58 ml. glacial acetic acid to 1 L. with distilled water. Titrate against standard alkali solution with phenolphthalein indicator and adjust to exactly 1N. Dilute 1, 2, 3, 4, and 5 ml. of the 1N acid to 50 ml. in volumetric flasks. These solutions will correspond to 20, 40, 60, 80, and 100 units, respectively. Pipette 2.5 ml. buffered nitrophenol and 0.1 ml. pooled inactivated serum (heated to 60° C. for 3 min.) to each of six tubes. Do not use hemolyzed, icteric, or turbid serum. To one tube add 0.1 ml. distilled water; this is the blank. To the other tubes add 0.1 ml. diluted acetic acid solutions made up to correspond to 20, 40, 60, 80, and 100 units. Mix and read in a photometer at 420 nm., setting to zero OD with water. Subtract the reading of each standard tube from that for the blank. Plot the values obtained against the units of standard. The unknown sam-

ples are read from this curve. A new standard curve must be made up for every new batch of reagents. For values higher than 120 units, dilute the serum with an equal volume of sodium chloride solution and repeat the test, taking 0.1 ml. diluted serum and multiplying the result obtained by 2.

Normal values and interpretation: The normal values by this method are 40-80 units. Low values have been found in anemia, tuberculosis, hypoproteinemia, carcinoma, uremia, and shock. Increased values have been found in hyperthyroidism and diabetes. Serum cholinesterase activity is also reduced in poisoning by organophosphorus compounds such as those used in insecticides. Cholinesterase may be deficient in certain individuals who demonstrate a prolonged response to certain types of anesthetics, i.e., succinylcholine. The importance of this test in liver disease is explained in the discussion of liver function tests.

CREATINE PHOSPHOKINASE (CPK)[205-213]

Creatine phosphokinase is an enzyme that catalyzes the following reaction in the presence of magnesium ions:

$$\text{ATP} + \text{Creatine} \underset{Mg^{++}}{\overset{CPK}{\rightleftharpoons}} \text{ADP} + \text{Phosphocreatine}$$

$$\text{Phosphocreatine} \xrightarrow{\text{Hydrolysis}} \text{Creatine} + \text{Inorganic P}$$

The inorganic phosphorus present is then determined by the colorimetric method of King. A control and a test solution are analyzed concurrently; the difference between the two solutions in concentration of inorganic phosphate is used as a measure of creatine phosphate formation.

Reagents:
1. Creatine* (0.08M). Dissolve 104.9 mg. creatine in 10 ml. 0.001M Tris buffer at pH 9.0. It may be necessary to warm in order to dissolve. This solution must be prepared fresh each time determinations are run.

---

*No. 1340, Eastman Kodak Co., Rochester, N. Y.

*Pabst Laboratories, Milwaukee, Wis.

2. Adenosine triphosphate (ATP) (0.01M). Dissolve 0.605 gm. disodium salt of adenosine 5-triphosphate* in 10 ml. 0.001M Tris at pH 9.0. This solution is diluted 1:10 with distilled water just before using. The 0.1M stock solution can be stored from 1-2 wk. at refrigerator temperature (4° C.).

3. Magnesium sulfate (0.01M). Dissolve 1.204 gm. reagent grade magnesium sulfate in water and dilute to 100 ml. This stock solution is diluted 1:10 with water just before using.

4. Tris buffers:
   A. (0.4M, pH 9.0). Dissolve 48.5 gm. crystalline Tris(hydroxymethyl)aminomethane in about 900 ml. water, adjust pH to 9.0 with concentrated HCl, and dilute to 1 L. This is stable in the refrigerator for several months.
   B. (0.001M, pH 9.0). Dilute 5 ml. 0.4M buffer to 2 L. with water and adjust pH to 9.0 with 0.1N NaOH. This solution is stable for only a few days since it does not retain a pH of 9.0.

5. Aminonaphtholsulfonic acid (ANSA). Dissolve 1.54 gm. aminonaphtholsulfonic acid in 10 ml. warm distilled water. Allow to cool and filter into glass-stoppered brown bottle. This is stable at room temperature for about 2 wk.

6. Ammonium molybdate reagent. Dissolve 25 gm. ammonium heptomolybdate crystals in 200 ml. water, transfer quantitatively to a 1 L. volumetric flask containing 500 ml. 10N H_2SO_4, and dilute to volume. Stored in the refrigerator. This is stable for 2-3 mo.

7. Trichloroacetic acid (20%). Dissolve 200 gm. reagent grade trichloroacetic acid in water and dilute to 1 L. Store in the refrigerator (4° C.).

8. Phosphorus standards:
   A. Stock standard (1 mg. P/ml.). Dissolve 439.4 mg. monopotassium dihydrogen phosphate

(KH_2PO_4) in water and dilute to 100 ml. Store in the refrigerator (4° C.).
   B. Working standard (10 μg P/ml.). Dilute 1 ml. stock standard to 100 ml. with water. This solution is prepared fresh before analyses.

Procedure: It is of utmost importance that all glassware be scrupulously cleaned with chromic acid. Use of detergents should be avoided because they contain phosphates. Dilute serum with an equal volume of 0.001M Tris (i.e., 1.5 ml. serum + 1.5 ml. 0.001M Tris). Set up 15 ml. test tubes or centrifuge tubes for duplicate determinations as in Table 6-15.

Incubate all tubes at 37° C. for 10-15 min. Also incubate the 0.01M ATP solution. Add 1 ml. warm ATP to each tube at 30 sec. intervals, mixing thoroughly, and incubate for exactly 30 min. Following the same sequence, add 4.1 ml. cold TCA to each tube at 30 sec. intervals, agitating the tubes vigorously. This stops the reaction. Centrifuge tubes at 3000 rpm for 10 min. Transfer 5 ml. supernatant from each tube into correspondingly labeled (1 and 2) cuvettes or test tubes.

Add to all tubes 1 ml. ammonium molybdate and 4 ml. water; mix well. Prepare reagent blank containing 1 ml. ammonium molybdate, 6.5 ml. water, and 2.5 ml. TCA; mix well. Add 0.4 ml. aminonaptholsulfonic acid to each tube and mix thoroughly after each addition. Allow 15-20 min. for the color to develop and read OD or %T in a photometer at a wavelength of 660 nm. against reagent blank.

Calculation: Determine from the standard curve the micrograms of phosphorus in each reaction tube and multiply by

*Nutritional Biochemicals Corp., Cleveland, Ohio.

Table 6-15

Reagent	Tube 1 (control) (ml.)	Tube 2 (test) (ml.)
Creatine	0	1.5
Tris (0.001M)	1.5	0
Magnesium sulfate	0.3	0.3
Tris (0.4M)	1.2	1.2
Serum (diluted)	1.0	1.0

1.82 (the dilution factor for the color reaction tube with respect to the supernatant of the initial reaction tube). Then subtract the micrograms of phosphorus in tube 1 from that in tube 2 to obtain the amount transferred during the reaction. This value is multiplied by 2 (factor for the reaction time is 30 min. when the final units are expressed per hour) and divided by the actual amount of serum present in the initial reaction (0.5 ml.).

$$\mu g \text{ phosphorus transferred} =$$
$$1.82 \ (P_2 - P_1) \times \frac{2}{0.5} = 1.82 \ (P_2 - P_1) \times 4$$

$P_2 = \mu g$ of phosphorus in unknown tube from calibration curve; $P_1 = \mu g$ of phosphorus in control tube from calibration curve.

Calibration curve: Set up in test tubes or cuvettes the solutions given in Table 6-16 in duplicate.

Thoroughly mix all tubes, add 0.4 ml. aminonaphtholsulfonic acid, and mix after each addition. Let stand at room temperature for 15-20 min. and read in a photometer at 660 nm., using the blank as a reference.

Plot the phosphorus calibration curve on graph paper with the OD (or %T) values vs. corresponding micrograms of phosphorus.

Normal values and interpretation: Normally there is little or no creatine phosphokinase in serum or red blood cells; most all activity is found in striated muscle and in the brain. Due to errors in the procedure, low positive and slightly negative values are often obtained. The normal level by this method is 0-5 μg/hr./ml. Elevated CPK values have been reported after onset of myocardial infarction; elevations occur about 6 hr. after the onset of symptoms and reach peak levels in about 36 hr. There is usually a rapid return to normal levels by the fourth day. Extremely elevated values have been reported in Duchenne's muscular dystrophy; somewhat lower values have been reported in muscular dystrophy affecting the limbs and girdle. Following strenuous exercise, elevations of up to three times the normal CPK values have been observed. These elevations disappear within 24-48 hr. Significant elevations of CPK have been reported in cases of hypothyroidism.

NOTE: Recent literature indicates that the use of sulfhydryl groups increases the sensitivity of CPK procedures and prevents loss of activity even after several days of storage.

The method described in Sigma Technical Bulletin No. 661 includes such modifications and has given very satisfactory results in our laboratory.

ISOCITRIC DEHYDROGENASE (ICD)[214-216]

Isocitric dehydrogenase is an enzyme that catalyzes the conversion of isocitric acid to alpha-ketoglutaric acid (KGA) and carbon dioxide in the presence of coenzyme triphosphopyridine nucleotide (TPN) and manganese ions.

$$\text{Isocitrate} + \text{TPN} \underset{Mn^{++}}{\overset{ICD}{\rightleftarrows}} \text{TPNH} +$$
$$\text{Ketoglutarate} + CO_2$$

This conversion is assumed to take place through the enzymatic dehydrogenation to oxalosuccinic acid, followed by the spontaneous decarboxylation of oxalosuccinic acid to alpha-ketoglutaric acid

Table 6-16

	Working standard (ml.)	*TCA (ml.)*	*H_2O (ml.)*	*Molybdenum (ml.)*
Blank	0	2.5	6.5	1
Standard, 10 μg	1	2.5	5.5	1
Standard, 20 μg	2	2.5	4.5	1
Standard, 30 μg	3	2.5	3.5	1
Standard, 40 μg	4	2.5	2.5	1
Standard, 50 μg	5	2.5	1.5	1

and carbon dioxide. The amount of alpha-ketoglutaric acid formed is proportional to the amount of isocitric dehydrogenase activity present. The alpha-ketoglutaric acid reacts with 2,4-dinitrophenylhydrazine to form a hydrazone that is highly colored in alkaline solution.

It is essential to include a serum blank with each determination because the amount of color contributed by the serum itself is quite significant and variable from serum to serum, due partly to its bilirubin content. Since this enzyme is very sensitive to metals, all reagents should be made up with deionized water.

Reagents:

1. Sodium chloride (0.15M). Dissolve 8.55 gm. sodium chloride in distilled water and dilute to 1 L.
2. Manganese chloride (0.1M in 0.15-M NaCl). Dissolve 200 mg. manganese chloride ($MnCl_2 \cdot 4H_2O$) in 100 ml. 0.15M NaCl.
3. Tris buffer (0.1M, pH 7.5). Dissolve 12.1 gm. Tris(hydroxymethyl)aminomethane in 850 ml. water in a 1 L. volumetric flask. Adjust pH to 7.5 with 1N HCl (about 80 ml. will be required) and dilute to volume.
4. *d*-1-Isocitrate (0.1M in 0.15M NaCl). Dissolve 260 mg. trisodium isocitrate* in 10 ml. 0.15M NaCl.
5. Triphosphopyridine nucleotide (TPN*) (0.004M in 0.15M NaCl). Dissolve 30 mg. TPN in 10 ml. 0.15M NaCl. Store frozen. Be sure to melt completely and mix thoroughly before use.
6. Ethylenediaminetetraacetic acid (EDTA) (5% w/v). Dissolve 5 gm. EDTA (disodium) in 100 ml. water.
7. 2,4-Dinitrophenylhydrazine (DNPH) (0.001M in 1N HCl). Dissolve 19.8 mg. DNPH in 100 ml. 1N HCl. Stable for 1 mo. at room temperature.
8. Alpha-ketoglutaric acid (KGA) (0.001M for standardization). Dissolve 150 mg. alpha-ketoglutaric acid* (97.5% pure) in 1 L. water.

9. Sodium hydroxide (0.4N). Dissolve 16 gm. sodium hydroxide pellets in 1 L. water.
10. Hydrochloric acid (1N). Add 83 ml. concentrated HCl (AR) to a 1 L. volumetric flask containing about 500 ml. water. Mix, allow to cool to room temperature, and dilute to volume.

Procedure: It is essential that serum specimens have no trace of hemolysis since ICD is known to occur at very high concentrations in red blood cells. The serum should be stored frozen when analysis cannot be completed on the day blood is drawn.

Pipette 0.5 ml. serum into each of two test tubes labeled sample and blank. To both tubes add 0.4 ml. $MnCl_2$, 0.5 ml. Tris buffer, and 0.2 ml. isocitrate. Place tubes in water bath at 37° C. for a few minutes. Add 0.4 ml. TPN solution to the sample tube and 0.4 ml. NaCl solution to the blank tube. Incubate both tubes at 37° C. for 1 hr. Then add 1 ml. DNPH solution to each tube, followed by 0.2 ml. EDTA solution, and let stand at room temperature for a minimum of 25 min. (up to 1 hr.). Add 10 ml. NaOH solution and mix well. After standing 5-10 min., read in a photometer at a wavelength of 410 nm., setting the instrument to 100% T or 0 OD with the blank.

Calibration curve: A standard curve for the hydrazone of KGA is prepared as described in the procedure, except that no ICD or TPN is required and incubation is omitted. Any serum may be used to set up the calibration curve.

Prepare a series of test tubes as described in Table 6-17.

To each tube add 1 ml. DNPH solution and mix. Add immediately 0.2 ml. EDTA solution to all tubes, mix, and allow to stand at room temperature for a minimum of 25 min. Add 10 ml. NaOH to all tubes. Mix well, and after standing 5-10 min., read at 410 nm., setting to 100% T or 0 OD with the blank. Plot %T or OD vs. corresponding mμM. KGA/ml. serum. When using a Beckman DU spectrophotometer at 410 nm., the curve is linear up to 400 mμM. KGA.

---

*Sigma Chemical Co., St. Louis, Mo.

Table 6-17

Tube No.	Serum (ml.)	MnCl₂ (ml.)	Tris buffer (ml.)	0.001M KGA (ml.)	NaCl (ml.)	mμM. KGA
Blank	0.5	0.4	0.5	0	0.6	0
1	0.5	0.4	0.5	0.1	0.5	100
2	0.5	0.4	0.5	0.2	0.4	200
3	0.5	0.4	0.5	0.3	0.3	300
4	0.5	0.4	0.5	0.4	0.2	400
5	0.5	0.4	0.5	0.5	0.1	500
6	0.5	0.4	0.5	0.6	0	600

Units of activity are defined as the milli-micromoles of KGA formed by the enzyme in 1 ml. serum at 37° C. in 1 hr.

Calculation:

ICD activity in mμM./ml. serum =
mμM. KGA read from curve

$$\times \frac{1}{\text{Ml. serum used}} \times \frac{60}{\text{Incubation time (min.)}}$$

For values exceeding 600 mμM., either a smaller aliquot of serum may be used or samples can be incubated for a shorter time. This must be taken into consideration in the final calculation.

Normal values and interpretation: The normal values by this method are 238-686 KGA units/ml., with an average of 420 ± 138. Significant elevated values have been reported in viral hepatitis and in about 50% of patients with metastatic carcinoma involving the liver. Dawkins et al.[217] suggested that in the absence of liver disease an increase in serum ICD may indicate active placental degeneration (within 48 hr.) during pregnancy. The determination of ICD has been suggested for the differential diagnosis of intrahepatic vs. extrahepatic obstructive jaundice and as a screening test for blood donors.

LACTIC DEHYDROGENASE (LDH)[218-223]

Lactic dehydrogenase is an enzyme that reversibly catalyzes the following reaction:

$$\text{Lactate} + \text{DPN} \underset{}{\overset{\text{LDH}}{\rightleftharpoons}} \text{Pyruvate} + \text{DPNH} + \text{H}^+$$

The rate of catalysis is measured in either direction by the change in concentration

of DPNH as a function of time and is reflected by the change in absorbance of DPNH measured at a wavelength of 340 nm.

The spectrophotometric method of measuring the rate of reduction of DPN in the presence of lactate (the "forward" method) is simple, reproducible, and differentiates with certainty between normal and elevated serum LDH activities. The method may also be used to measure LDH activity in effusions, cerebrospinal fluid, and urine.

Reagents:

1. Diphosphopyridine nucleotide (DPN).*
2. DL-Lactic acid (AR).†
3. Sodium pyrophosphate (AR).‡
4. Buffered substrate coenzyme solution. Dissolve 6.2 gm. sodium pyrophosphate and 2 ml. lactic acid in 150 ml. hot distilled water, cool, add 1.1 gm. DPN, and dissolve. Adjust pH to 8.8 with 1N NaOH and dilute to 280 ml. Aliquots of 2.8 ml. stored in capped tubes at –20° C. are stable for 6 mo.§ This solution contains 50 mM. buffer, 77.5 mM. lactic acid, and 5.25 mM. DPN/L.

Procedure: Place tubes containing buffered substrate in a 25° C. constant temperature water bath and allow to come to bath temperature. Add 0.2 ml. serum to each tube and mix by gentle triple

---

*Pabst Laboratories, Milwaukee, Wis.
†Merck & Co., Inc., Rahway, N. J.
‡Baker Chemical Co., Phillipsburg, N. J.
§Lyophilized reagent tubes prepared by this procedure are available as LDH Determatubes from Worthington Biochemical Corp., Freehold, N. J.

inversion. Immediately transfer solution to a cuvette of 1 cm. light path and measure the increase in absorbance at 340 nm. every 30 sec. for 2 min. A buffered substrate tube to which 0.2 ml. water has been added serves as the reference solution. All reactions are measured at 25° C. with a spectrophotometer equipped with a thermospacer connected to a constant-temperature water bath or Macalaster Coenzometer.*

Calculation: One unit of LDH activity is defined as an increase in absorbance (OD) of 0.001/min./ml. serum under specified conditions. The formula used to calculate activity is:

$$\text{LDH activity} =$$
$$\text{Change in absorbance } (\Delta OD) \times \frac{5000}{\text{Min.}}$$

Sample calculation:

$$\text{Activity} =$$
$$(0.18 - 0.05) \times \frac{5000}{2} = 325 \text{ LDH units}$$

NOTES: LDH activities assayed by this method have zero-order kinetics; the activity is proportional to the amount of serum assayed and has a precision of 1.3%. Serum contains no inhibitors or interfering substances. The buffered substrate solution can be stored frozen for 6 mo. and in the lyophilized state indefinitely.

Serum with visible hemolysis (hemoglobin concentration above 0.1 gm.%) should not be used as this produces spurious elevations of LDH activity. Serum activity is stable for 48 hr. at 25° C. or for 1 mo. at –20° C.

Cerebrospinal fluid is collected in a sterile, chemically clean test tube without anticoagulant and should be processed within 4 hr. Activity is stable for 4 hr. at 25° C. or for 2 wk. at 4° C.

Serous effusions are allowed to clot and the clot is removed by centrifugation. Activity is stable for 3 wk. at –20° C.

Normal values and interpretation: The normal serum LDH activity by this method is 41-98 units. Increased values have been reported following myocardial

infarction. This increase often reaches 10 times the normal in 24-72 hr. after injury and somewhat parallels the extent of cardiac damage.

Elevations have been reported in leukemia, pulmonary infarction, sickle cell anemia, malignant lymphoma, trauma of striated muscle, and liver disease.

Because LDH activity is elevated in pulmonary infarction and the SGOT remains normal, these tests may be used for the differential diagnosis of these conditions.

LDH in urine: The procedure used for serum may also be used for the determination of LDH in urine by substituting 1 ml. dialyzed clear urine for serum and by using 2 ml. buffered substrate coenzyme solution. It is not desirable to store the urine for more than 6 hr. after collection because enzyme activity may decrease significantly.

Reagent:
1. Buffered substrate coenzyme solution. This is prepared exactly as described for serum LDH, except that the final volume is brought to 200 ml. Aliquots of 2 ml. stored in capped tubes at –20° C. are stable for 6 mo.

Equipment: Dialysis tubing (¼ in. diameter).* Wash tubing for 2 hr. in three changes of distilled water heated to about 90° C. Rinse with distilled water and store in distilled water at 4° C.

Procedure: Dialysis of urine prior to the determination of LDH is required to eliminate substances that inhibit LDH activity. Obtain an accurately timed, clean-voided 8 hr. overnight urine specimen (no preservatives needed). Measure and record the volume in milliliters and centrifuge about 10 ml. at 2000 rpm for 15 min. Transfer 6 ml. of the centrifuged urine sample to a dialysis sack as follows. Squeeze excess water from the dialysis sack and tie a knot at one end. Add 6 ml. urine to the sack by using a pipette or small graduated cylinder. With a squeezing action of the fingers, expel the air from the sack above the urine and tie a secure knot in the sack about 3 in.

---

*Macalaster Scientific Corp., Waltham, Mass.

*No. 8, Visking Co., Chicago, Ill.

above the level of urine. Weigh on trip balance to nearest 0.1 gm. and place the sack into a 250 ml. Erlenmeyer flask. Fasten length of soft rubber tubing to a cold water tap; adjust flow to at least 50 ml./min. Insert the rubber tube into flask so that the end is at the bottom. Set the flask so that the overflow runs down the drain and allow to dialyze for 2 hr. Remove the sack from the flask and reweigh. Centrifuge if there is any precipitate. The dialyzed urine and buffered substrate solution are brought to 25° C. in a water bath.

Proceed with the assay using the method described for serum. Simply substitute 1 ml. dialyzed, clear urine for serum and use 2 ml. substrate. Complete the determination as described.

Calculation: One unit of activity is defined as an increase in absorbance of 0.001/ml. urine/min. Then:

Total urinary LDH activity/8 hr. = Units/ml.

$$\times \text{ 8 hr. urine vol. } \times \frac{\text{Wt. after dialysis}}{\text{Wt. before dialysis}}$$

Normal values and interpretation: The normal urinary LDH activity by this method is 550-2050 units in 8 hr. specimens. Considerably elevated values have been reported by Wacker and Dorfman[224], [225] in cases involving carcinoma of the kidney or bladder. Significant elevations have also been reported in several other diseases involving the urinary system, including malignant hypertension, glomerulonephritis, lupus nephritis, acute tubular necrosis, and possibly pyelonephritis. However, these diseases are readily differentiated from malignant lesions. Urinary LDH increases as much as 5000% in carcinoma of the kidneys or bladder.

Spurious elevations may result from urologic instrumentation, hemolysis, and menstrual contamination. Low activities may result from incomplete urine collection or the use of unclean glassware.

Isozymes in LDH[226]: Because of the wide distribution of LDH throughout the various tissues in the body, an elevated serum LDH is of limited value in establishing the specific site of tissue damage. Several studies of LDH have shown that serum LDH is actually composed of at least five fractions (isozymes) that can be separated by electrophoresis or other methods. All of the five isozymes catalyze the same reaction and are generally referred to as LD_1, LD_2, LD_3, LD_4, and LD_5. The subscripts indicate increasing electrophoretic mobility at pH 8.6.

It has also been shown that all tissues contain these isozymes in amounts characteristic for that tissue. For example, liver contains a large proportion of LD_1 and very little of the other isozymes. Cardiac muscle, on the other hand, has a high content of LD_4 and LD_5 and is practically free of the other three isozymes. When a particular tissue is damaged, the isozymes characteristic of that tissue will increase in the serum. For example, when the liver is damaged, an elevation of LD_1 is observed, while after myocardial infarction, serum LD_4 and LD_5 are increased. This may serve as a means of differential diagnosis for these two conditions.

It has also been shown that LDH isozymes have different thermostability properties. Using these properties, it is possible to obtain an approximation of LD_1, LD_4, and LD_5 levels by a relatively simple heating technique. LD_1 is heat labile and is inactivated by incubation of the sample at 65° C. for 30 min., while LD_4 and LD_5 are relatively heat stable and most of their activity survives incubation at this temperature. LD_2 and LD_3 have heat stabilities intermediate between LD_1 and LD_5.

Procedure: Incubate approximately 0.5 ml. serum at 65° C. for 30 min. in a water bath. Transfer immediately to an ice bath for a few seconds and then to a 25° C. water bath. Determine the LDH by following the procedure exactly as described for serum. Determine also total LDH activity of the serum. Then:

$$\frac{\text{LDH activity after incubation}}{\text{Total LDH activity}} \times 100 =$$

%Heat-stable LDH

Interpretation: The heat-stable fractions (LD_4 and LD_5) are elevated in cardiac damage. The normal levels have not been clearly defined. Wroblewski and Gregory state that normal serum contains between 20 and 40% LD_4 and LD_5. In acute myocardial infarction, when the total serum LDH activity is elevated, the percentage of heat-stable fractions is always above 40% and may be as high as 90% of the total activity.

LDH isozymes by electrophoresis[227-232]: The LDH isozymes can be more accurately differentiated by electrophoresis. The electrophoresis has been carried out on agar gel, starch gel, polyacrylamide gel, and cellulose acetate strips. The serum is applied to the medium and electrophoresis is allowed to proceed for the required time. After electrophoresis, the isozymes are located on the strip by a special staining process. The strip is overlayed with a solution containing lactate, DPN, phenazine methosulfate, and a tetrazolium compound such as nitroblue tetrazolium (NBT). The reaction is:

$$Lactate + DPN \xrightarrow{\text{LDH}} Pyruvate + DPNH$$

In the presence of phenazine methosulfate the DPNH reduces the NBT to an intensely colored compound. Thus the strip will be stained blue, the amount of stain depending upon the concentration of LDH enzyme at that point. Five bands corresponding to the five isozymes (LD_1-LD_5) are usually obtained. One can estimate the relative proportion of the different isozymes either visually or quantitatively by using a densitometer as in paper electrophoresis. The method of choice will depend upon the equipment available. A sample kit may be obtained that has agar gel plates already prepared and that allows visual estimation of the isozymes.* If the apparatus for cellulose acetate protein electrophoresis is available, it can readily be adapted to LDH isozyme electrophoresis.

LDH using tetrazolium salt[218, 233, 234]: Lactic dehydrogenase catalyzes the reaction:

$$Lactic + NAD \xrightarrow{\text{LDH}} Pyruvate + NADH$$

where NAD and NADH are the oxidized

and reduced forms of the coenzyme nicotinamide adenine dinucleotide. In this method, lactate with NAD added is used as substrate. The amount of lactate changed is measured in terms of the amount of NADH produced and the latter is estimated by its action in reducing a tetrazolium salt to an intensely colored form. The reduction of tetrazolium salt by NADH requires the presence of an intermediate electron carrier and for this the compound phenazine methosulfate (PMS) is added. The result of the complex series of reactions is that for every molecule of lactate changed to pyruvate an equivalent amount of tetrazolium salt is reduced to a colored form, so that the final color produced is proportional to the enzyme action.

Reagents:

1. Buffer. Dissolve 1 gm. Lipal* (ethoxylated oleyl alcohol) in 10 ml. water by heating to 90° C. Dilute to about 50 ml. with water and add 12.1 gm. Tris(hydroxymethyl)aminomethane. Adjust to pH 8.2 with 3N hydrochloric acid (27 ml. concentrated acid diluted to 100 ml.) and dilute to 100 ml. Store under refrigeration and discard if any visible growth occurs. Lipal may be omitted if only serum is to be assayed.

2. L(+)-Lactic acid substrate (0.1M, pH 5.5). Add 5 ml. L(+)-lactic acid, 20% solution,† to about 50 ml. water. Adjust to pH 5.5 with 1N NaOH and dilute to 120 ml. with water. Saturate with a few drops of chloroform and store in the refrigerator.

3. Control reagent. Dissolve 0.2 gm. potassium oxalate and 0.2 gm. ethylenediaminetetraacetic acid disodium salt in 100 ml. water.

4. Color reagent. Dissolve 50 mg. 2-*p*-iodophenyl-3-*p*-nitrophenyl-5-phenyl tetrazolium chloride (INT)‡ in about 15 ml. water. Prolonged agitation

---

*Hyland Laboratories, Los Angeles, Calif.

*Lipal 10-OA, Drew Chemical Co., Boonton, N. J.
†Miles Chemical Co., Clifton, N. J.
‡May be secured from a number of supplies. Babson and Phillips[233] recommend Dajac Laboratories, Philadelphia, Pa.

with a magnetic stirrer or crushing with a stirring rod may be necessary to obtain complete solution. Add and dissolve 125 mg. nicotinamide adenine dinucleotide (NAD)*; then add 12.5 mg. phenazine methosulfate.* Transfer with washings immediately to a low-actinic 25 ml. volumetric flask and dilute to the mark with water. This reagent is very sensitive to light and must be protected from light at all times. It is stable for several weeks under refrigeration.

Procedure: Pipette 0.1 ml. serum and 0.2 ml. buffer to each of two tubes. Add 0.5 ml. substrate to one tube and 0.5 ml. control reagent to the other tube. Mix and warm to 37° C. At precisely timed intervals add 0.2 ml. color reagent, mix immediately, and return to the bath. Exactly 5 min. after the addition of color reagent, add 5 ml. 0.1N HCl and mix. The amount of HCl can be varied to suit the colorimeter, but a minimum of 2 ml. must be used to completely stop the enzyme reaction.

The difference in absorbance between the control and sample is measured at 520 nm. within 20 min. The color is linear with enzyme concentrations. With the use of an elevated control serum, dilutions with saline solution can be made and a calibration curve can readily be made by carrying the standards through the same procedure.

Normal values: The normal range as estimated by this procedure is 27-77 I.U.

LEUCINE AMINOPEPTIDASE (LAP)[235-240]

Leucine aminopeptidase is a proteolytic enzyme normally present in serum, urine, and bile. Its exact metabolic function in the body is unknown. In vitro it catalyzes the following reaction:

$$\text{L-Leucyl-beta-naphthylamide} + H_2O \xrightarrow{\text{LAP}}$$
$$\text{Leucine} + \text{Beta-naphthylamine}$$

The amount of beta-naphthylamine produced is proportional to the amount of LAP activity. Since beta-naphthylamine

*Sigma Chemical Co., St. Louis, Mo.

is colorless, it is diazotized with nitrous acid and then reacted with a dye base, *N*-(1-naphthyl)-ethylenediamine dihydrochloride, to form a purplish colored complex azo dye that is proportional to the amount of beta-naphthylamine formed and hence to the amount of LAP activity.

Reagents:*
1. Phosphate buffer (0.2M, pH 7.0).
    A. Dissolve 28.4 gm. anhydrous disodium phosphate (Na_2HPO_4) in water and dilute to 1 L.
    B. Dissolve 27.2 gm. anhydrous potassium dihydrogen phosphate (KH_2PO_4) in water and dilute to 1 L.
    C. Mix 7 parts solution A and 3 parts solution B. Check and adjust pH if necessary.
2. L-Leucyl-beta-naphthylamine hydrochloride (0.0012M, pH 7.1). Dissolve 400 mg. in water with gentle warming and dilute to 1 L.
3. Buffered substrate solution (0.1M, pH 7.0). Mix equal volumes of reagents 1C and 2. Make fresh every month.
4. Trichloroacetic acid (40%). Dissolve 40 gm. trichloroacetic acid in water and dilute to 100 ml.
5. Ammonium sulfamate (0.5%). Dissolve 0.5 gm. ammonium sulfamate in water and dilute to 100 ml.
6. Sodium nitrite (0.1%). Dissolve 100 mg. in water and dilute to 100 ml. in a volumetric flask. Make fresh daily.
7. *N*-(1-Naphthyl)-ethylenediamine dihydrochloride (0.05%). Dissolve 50 mg. in 95% ethyl alcohol and dilute to 100 ml. with the alcohol. This solution is stable for 30 days.

Procedure for serum: Dilute serum 1:50 (2%) with distilled water in a 50 ml. volumetric flask. Label three tubes 1, 2, and 3 for reagent blank, sample, and sample blank, respectively. Add 1 ml. water to tube 1 and 1 ml. diluted serum to tubes 2 and 3. Then add 1 ml. buff-

*All reagents and complete procedures may be obtained from Sigma Chemical Co., St. Louis, Mo. Reagents 2 and 7 are available from Dajac Laboratories, Philadelphia, Pa.

ered substrate to tubes 1 and 2 and 1 ml. phosphate buffer to tube 3. Mix well and incubate for 2 hr. at 37° C. Terminate hydrolysis by adding 1 ml. trichloroacetic acid to all tubes. Mix well and allow to stand about 5 min. for complete precipitation of the protein. Centrifuge and transfer 1 ml. supernatant from each tube to correspondingly marked tubes. Add 1 ml. sodium nitrite to all tubes, mix well, and let stand 3 min. Add 1 ml. ammonium sulfamate, mix well, and let stand 2 min. Add 2 ml. N-(1-naphthyl)-ethylenediamine dihydrochloride to all tubes, mix well, and let stand 10 min. Read all tubes against water in a photometer at a wavelength of 560 nm. Subtract OD of tubes 1 and 3 from tube 2. Convert corrected OD to micrograms of beta-naphthylamine from calibration curve. Calculate units as follows:

$$\text{Units} = \mu\text{g beta-naphthylamine} \times 3$$

where the factor 3 corrects for the 1 ml. aliquots diluted to 3 ml. To convert these units to those described by the original authors (Klett units) one must multiply by the factor 12. If the activity is too high to read, repeat the test with a more dilute sample. Units of serum LAP are defined as the micrograms of beta-naphthylamine liberated by 1 ml. 2% serum after 2 hr. of incubation.

Calibration curve: Use stock standard solution. Dissolve exactly 22.6 mg. beta-naphthylamine dihydrochloride in water and dilute to 500 ml. in a volumetric flask. This is equivalent to 0.036 mg./ml. free base $\left(\dfrac{22.6 \times 0.797}{500}\right)$. The factor 0.797 is for conversion of beta-naphthyl-

amine dihydrochloride to the free base. Prepare series of test tubes with standard solution as shown in Table 6-18.

Mix thoroughly all tubes containing working standard and pipette 1 ml. from each into correspondingly labeled test tubes. Add 1 ml. phosphate buffer and 1 ml. trichloroacetic acid to all tubes. Mix thoroughly, withdraw 1 ml. aliquot from each tube, and put into correspondingly labeled tubes or cuvettes. Proceed with color development as for the serum LAP assay. Read OD of all tubes against reagent blank (tube 8) in a photometer at a wavelength of 560 nm. Plot OD against micrograms of beta-naphthylamine as given in Table 6-18.

Procedure for urine: Collect 24 hr. urine specimen without preservative and refrigerate (4° C.). Measure and record total volume in milliliters. Because of the occasional presence of chromogens in the urine, it is necessary to dialyze a portion of the specimen before proceeding with the assay.

Dialyze a 50 ml. aliquot of urine overnight against running tap water (same procedure as for LDH). After urine is dialyzed, it may be stored, if necessary, at 4° C. for 7 days without significant loss of LAP activity.

Dilute 1 ml. dialyzed urine with 9 ml. water (1:10). Use 1 ml. of this dilution and follow procedure for serum LAP.

Calculation:

$$\text{Units} = \mu\text{g beta-naphthylamine (from curve)} \times$$
$$3 \times 10 \times \frac{1}{1000} \times \text{Vol. (ml.)} =$$
$$\mu\text{g beta-naphthylamine} \times 30 \times \text{Vol. (L.)}$$

The factor 3 corrects for the 1 ml. aliquots

Table 6-18

Tube No.	Stock standard solution (ml.)	Water (ml.)	Working standard (µg/ml.)	Beta-naphthylamine (µg) in aliquot used
1	6.0	0	36	12
2	5.0	1.0	30	10
3	4.0	2.0	24	8
4	3.0	3.0	18	6
5	2.0	4.0	12	4
6	1.0	5.0	6	2
7	0.5	5.5	3	1
8	0	6.0	0	0

diluted to 3 ml.; the factor 10 corrects for the 10% dilution of urine; and the factor 1000 converts micrograms to milligrams.

Units of urinary LAP are defined as the milligrams of β-naphthylamine liberated by a 24 hr. urine specimen under specified conditions of assay after 2 hr. of incubation.

Normal values and interpretation: The normal levels of serum LAP by this method are 5-20 units in adults and 5-24 units in infants. The values for urine are 2-18 units/24 hr. Serum LAP activity is increased in diseases of the liver (viral hepatitis, infectious mononucleosis, neoplasm, obstructive jaundice) and in carcinoma of the pancreas, where the increase is significant. There is a temporary elevation of LAP in acute pancreatitis. Patients with elevated serum LAP always show elevated urine levels; however, elevated urine LAP levels may be found with normal serum levels in diseases such as carcinoma of the colon and rectum, lymphomas, and leukemias.

LIPASE[241-244]

Lipase is an enzyme that hydrolyzes **fats** into fatty acid and glycerol. In this method an aliquot of serum is incubated with a stabilized olive oil emulsion and a buffer of pH 8.0 for 6 hr. The fatty acids liberated in the reaction are titrated with 0.05N sodium hydroxide, using thymolphthalein as indicator. The amount of 0.05N sodium hydroxide used to neutralize the fatty acids liberated (end point) is equivalent to the lipase units per milliliter of specimen.

Reagents:
1. Olive oil emulsion. To 100 ml. distilled water add 200 mg. sodium benzoate and 7 gm. gum arabic (acacia). Mix in a blender at low speed until dissolved. With the blender at low speed, slowly add 100 ml. pure olive oil. Mix for an additional 10 min. at high speed. This reagent should be kept at refrigerator temperature. Freezing or exposure to excessive heat will destroy the emulsion. A creamy layer on top of the emulsion may form during storage; shake the reagent thoroughly before using. Discard the reagent if excessive separation occurs after mixing. Olive oil should be purified as follows. To 300 ml. pure olive oil add 60 gm. aluminum oxide while stirring. Stir at 10 min. intervals for 1 hr. Let the aluminum oxide settle and filter through Whatman No. 1 filter paper. The olive oil may be checked by mixing 5 ml. purified oil with 5 ml. ether and 5 ml. 95% ethanol and titrating with thymolphthalein as indicator. If the titration requires more than 0.5 ml. 0.05N sodium hydroxide, repeat the purification.

2. Buffer:
   A. Stock solution. In a 500 ml. volumetric flask dissolve 48.55 gm. Tris(hydroxymethyl)aminomethane and dilute to volume.
   B. Working solution. Dilute 50 ml. stock buffer and 21.5 ml. 1N HCl with distilled water to 200 ml. in a volumetric flask. Adjust the pH to 8.0 using 1N HCl and refrigerate.

3. Sodium hydroxide (0.05N). In a 100 ml. volumetric flask dilute 5 ml. standardized 1N sodium hydroxide to volume with water.

4. Thymolphthalein indicator. Dissolve 1 gm. thymolphthalein in 95% ethanol and dilute to 100 ml.

5. Ethanol (95%).

Procedure: Into each of two test tubes labeled blank and test pipette 2.5 ml. water, 3 ml. olive oil emulsion, and 1 ml. working buffer solution. Add 1 ml. serum to the tube labeled test and stopper both tubes. Shake vigorously for a few seconds. Place both tubes in a water bath at 37° C. and incubate for 6 hr. Immediately after this, pipette 1 ml. "test" serum into a 50 ml. Erlenmeyer flask, label it blank, and store it in the refrigerator. At the end of the incubation period pour the contents of the "blank" tube into the cold "blank" flask containing "test" serum and pour the contents of the "test" tube into a clean Erlenmeyer flask labeled test. Rinse both tubes with 3 ml. ethanol. Add washings to the respective flasks. Mix the contents of the flasks by rotation and add 4 drops thymolphthalein. With the use of an accurate burette, titrate both flasks with 0.05N sodium hydroxide to a light, but distinct blue color (the test and blank must be titrated to the same color intensity). Icteric sera and some lighting conditions may cause the end point color of titration to be grayish green rather than blue.

Calculation: Subtract the milliliters of 0.05N sodium hydroxide taken by the blank from that taken by the unknown. The difference will be the units of lipase per milliliter of serum.

Example:

"Test" required 5 ml. sodium hydroxide
"Blank" required 4 ml. sodium hydroxide

Then:

$$5 - 4 = 1 \text{ unit/ml.}$$

Normal values and interpretation: Normal values found by this method range from 0-1 unit. Elevated serum lipase values are found in acute pancreatic disease. In this condition the elevation of the lipase may not parallel that of amylase. The latter may show an elevation earlier in the disease, but the elevation of the lipase may persist for a longer period. In chronic pancreatitis the lipase level may be normal. Moderate increases are found in some cases of pancreatic carcinoma. Occasionally elevated values are found in kidney diseases, intestinal obstruction, and duodenal ulcers.

PHOSPHATASES[245, 248]

Phosphatases are enzymes that catalyze the splitting off of phosphoric acid from certain phosphate esters, a reaction of considerable importance in several body processes. Two different phosphatases are commonly determined in blood serum. **Acid phosphatase** has an optimum activity at a pH of approximately 5 and is present in a number of tissues such as bone, kidney, spleen, and prostate glands. In clinical diagnosis it is used chiefly in connection with pathologic conditions of the prostate gland. **Alkaline phosphatase** has an optimum activity at a pH of approximately 10. It is found in a number of tissues but is used in clinical diagnosis chiefly in connection with bone and liver diseases.

Phosphatases are usually determined by measuring the amount of phosphatase ester split by the enzyme under specified conditions. A number of different substrates have been employed. Glycerophosphate was used in earlier methods (Bodansky). Disodium phenylphosphate has been widely employed (King-Armstrong). The methods given here use a substrate (*p*-nitrophenylphosphate) that has a colored reaction product (nitrophenol) so that it can be determined directly in the solution.

$$\text{\textit{p}-Nitrophenylphosphate} + H_2O \xrightarrow{\text{Phosphatase}}$$
(colorless in acid and alkali)

$$\text{\textit{p}-Nitrophenol} + H_3PO_4$$
(yellow in alkali)

Acid phosphatase:
Reagents:
1. Acid buffer solution. In a 1 L. volumetric flask dissolve 8.91 gm. citric acid in 180 ml. 1N sodium hydroxide. Add 100 ml. 0.1N hydrochloric acid, dilute to volume with distilled water, and mix. The pH of this solution should be 4.8.
2. Stock substrate solution. Dissolve 0.4 gm. disodium *p*-nitrophenylphosphate in 0.001N hydrochloric acid to make 100 ml. (100 ml. distilled water plus 0.1 ml. 1N hydrochloric acid).
3. Acid buffered substrate. Mix equal parts of acid buffer solution and stock substrate solution. This solution is not stable and should be kept frozen if possible. A convenient method is to pipette 1 ml. portions to test tubes that are then tightly stoppered (culture tubes with screw caps are excellent) and kept frozen. The number of tubes required are then thawed just before use.
4. Sodium hydroxide (0.1N). Dissolve 4 gm. sodium hydroxide in distilled water to make 1 L.

Procedure: Place two tubes containing 1 ml. buffered substrate in a 37° C. water bath for 5 min. to warm to this temperature (a slightly longer time may be required if the tubes are initially frozen).

Pipette exactly 0.2 ml. serum to one tube and start timing. Add 0.2 ml. water to the other tube as a reagent blank. Exactly 30 min. after the addition of serum add 4 ml. 0.1N sodium hydroxide to each tube. Read sample tube in a photometer at 410 nm., setting to zero with the reagent blank, and record the OD. To correct for any color contributed by serum add 0.2 ml. serum to 5 ml. 0.1N sodium hydroxide and read in a photometer, setting to 0 OD with 0.1N sodium hydroxide. Subtract the OD obtained from that for the sample determination. This is the corrected OD. Read units of activity from the calibration curve using the corrected OD.

Calibration curve: Prepare a solution of 139.1 mg. *p*-nitrophenol in distilled water and make to volume in a 100 ml. volumetric flask. This solution contains 10 mM./L. This stock solution is also used in preparing a curve for the alkaline phosphatase. Dilute 1, 2, 4, 6, 8, and 10 ml. stock nitrophenol solution, respectively, to 100 ml. in separate volumetric flasks with distilled water. To 0.2 ml. of each of the dilutions add 5 ml. 0.1N sodium hydroxide and read in a photometer against a reference tube containing water. Record the OD. The dilutions correspond to 0.2, 0.4, 0.8, 1.2, 1.6, and 2.0 Bessey-Lowry units. Plot the OD against the units to obtain the calibration curve.

Normal values and interpretation: The normal values range from 0.13-0.63 unit (Bessey-Lowry) for men and from 0.01-0.56 unit for women. In correlation with other units, B-L units × 1.8 = Bodansky units (approximate). The determination of acid phosphatase is usually carried out in connection with malignant disease of the prostate gland. Small increases are found in conditions such as Paget's disease in which there are very high levels of alkaline phosphatase. Very high values are often found in metastasizing carcinoma of the prostate.

Alkaline phosphatase:
Reagents:
1. Alkaline buffer solution. Dissolve 7.5 gm. glycine and 0.095 gm. magnesium chloride in about 750 ml. distilled water. Add 85 ml. 0.1N sodium hydroxide solution and dilute to 1 L. with distilled water. The pH of the solution should be 10.5.
2. Stock substrate solution. This is the same as used for acid phosphatase.
3. Alkaline buffered substrate. Mix equal volumes of alkaline buffer solution and stock substrate solution. This should be kept frozen.
4. Sodium hydroxide (0.02N). Mix 200 ml. 0.1N sodium hydroxide with 800 ml. distilled water.

Procedure: Place two tubes containing 1 ml. alkaline buffered substrate in a 37° C. water bath and warm to this temperature. Pipette 0.1 ml. serum to one tube and start timing. Add 0.1 ml. water to the other tube as a blank. Exactly 30 min. after the addition of serum add 10 ml. 0.02N sodium hydroxide to each tube. Mix by inversion and read the sample tube in a photometer at 410 nm., setting to zero with the blank tube, and record the OD. To each tube add 2 drops concentrated hydrochloric acid and mix. Read the sample tube again, using the blank tube as a reference. Subtract the OD obtained from the earlier reading on the sample. This is the corrected OD. Obtain units from the calibration curve.

Calibration curve: Using the same stock standard as for acid phosphatase, dilute 0.5, 1, 2, 3, and 5 ml. stock standard to 100 ml. with distilled water in separate volumetric flasks. To 1 ml. of each dilution add 0.1 ml. water and 10 ml. 0.02N sodium hydroxide solution. Read in a photometer with water as a reference. The dilutions correspond to 1, 2, 4, 6, 8, and 10 units (Bessey-Lowry). Plot the OD against units for the calibration curve.

Normal values and interpretation: The normal range for adults is 0.8-2.3 units (Bessey-Lowry) and for children it is 2.8-6.7 units. As stated, B-L units × 1.8 = Bodansky units (approximate).

Alkaline phosphatase may be elevated in liver disease (see discussion of liver function tests). In bone disease the alkaline phosphatase is increased in those conditions in which bone regeneration is taking place. It is not found when there is bone destruction unless there is simultaneous formation of new bone or osteoid tissue. In rickets the increase is very marked, the increases roughly paralleling the severity of the disease. Values from 20-60 units may be found. In osteomalacia (adult rickets) there is some increase, but not as marked as in children. In Paget's disease, values over 30 units are not unusual. In hyperparathyroidism the increase may be present, but it is less marked (15 units). In bone tumors the findings are variable. Serum alkaline phosphatase is usually normal in multiple myeloma, with never more than a very slight increase.

Prostatic acid phosphatase[249, 250]: Serum prostatic acid phosphatase activity is inhibited by the presence of **tartrate**, while acid phosphatase from other sources is not affected. By assaying for total acid phosphatase activity in the presence and absence of tartrate, one can determine by difference the activity due to prostatic secretion.

Reagents:
1. Acid buffered substrate and sodium hydroxide (0.1N). These are the same as used for acid phosphatase.
2. Tartrate (0.2M). Dissolve 3.002 gm. tartaric acid in about 50 ml. water in a 100 ml. volumetric flask. Add 35 ml. 1N sodium hydroxide. Adjust pH to 4.9 and dilute to the mark with water.

Procedure: Prepare four test tubes as shown in Table 6-19.

Pipette substrate, water, and tartrate in tubes 1, 2, and 3 and place in water bath at 37° C. for 5 min.

Add 0.2 ml. serum to tubes 2 and 3 and start timer. Incubate for exactly 30 min. While tubes 2 and 3 are incubating, prepare tube 4. At the end of the incubation period add sodium hydroxide to tubes 1, 2, and 3. Read tubes 2 and 3 against tube 1 and read tube 4 against water at a wavelength of 410 nm. Subtract OD of tube 4 from that of tubes 2 and 3 and convert to units by using the calibration curve from acid phosphatase. Subtract units in tube 3 from tube 2 and obtain units of tartrate-inhibited acid phosphatase.

NOTE: Prostatic acid phosphatase is very unstable. Blood should be refrigerated immediately after drawing. Centrifuge after standing 1 hr. and separate serum. Do not use if hemolyzed. Keep serum at 0°-5° C. at all times or add 0.02 ml. 20% acetic acid to each 2 ml. of serum to stabilize the enzyme.

Normal values and interpretation: The normal value may range up to 0.15 unit. Prostatic acid phosphatase assay is most valuable in cases of prostatic carcinoma, where it is found to be elevated even when the total acid phosphatase may be normal.

Alkaline phosphatase using phenolphthalein monophosphate[251]:

$$\text{Phenolphthalein monophosphate} + \underset{\text{Phosphatase}}{} $$
$$\text{H}_2\text{O} \xrightarrow{\hspace{1cm}} \underset{\text{(red in alkali)}}{\text{Phenolphthalein} + \text{H}_3\text{PO}_4}$$

The phenolphthalein formed is determined colorimetrically by its red color in an alkaline solution. It has an advantage over *p*-nitrophenylphosphate because the absorption peak of phenolphthalein is much farther from that of bilirubin and hemoglobin. Hence the interference from these compounds is reduced. Also, for a given enzyme concentration, much more color (greater OD) is produced by phenolphthalein. This increases the sensitivity of the method.

Reagents:
1. Stock substrate solution. Dissolve 0.39 gm. monohydrated dicyclohexylamine salt of phenolphthalein monophosphate* in a mixture of 73.2 gm. 2-amino-2-methyl-1-propanol and 21.9 ml. concentrated hy-

Table 6-19

	1	2	3	4
Step 1				
Substrate (ml.)	1.0	1.0	1.0	0
Water (ml.)	0.4	0.2	0	0.2
Tartrate (ml.)	0	0	0.2	0
Step 2				
Serum (ml.)	0	0.2	0.2	0.2
Step 3				
NaOH (ml.)	3.8	3.8	3.8	4.8

---

*At present phenolphthalein monophosphate is available as Phosphastrate Alkaline only from Warner-Chilcott Laboratories Division, Warner-Lambert Pharmaceutical Co., Morris Plains, N. J.

drochloric acid. This solution is 0.065M in phenolphthalein monophosphate and 7.8M in the buffer. The pH is 10.15. It is stable indefinitely when stored in the refrigerator and should be warmed to room temperature before use. This stock solution is diluted 1:26 before use (see procedure).

2. Color stabilizer (phosphate buffer, 0.1M, pH 11.2). Dissolve 9.3 gm. $Na_3PO_4 \cdot 12H_2O$ and 20.3 gm. $Na_2HPO_4 \cdot 7H_2O$ (or 10.8 gm. anhydrous salt) in water and dilute to 1 L. with water. The solution is stable at room temperature.

Procedure: Dilute 1 drop (0.04 ml.) stock substrate solution with 1 ml. water and warm to 37° C. Add 0.1 ml. serum and mix. After exactly 20 min., add 5 ml. color stabilizer and read absorbance at 550 nm. against a reagent blank without serum. The absorbance due to the serum has been found to be negligible.

Calibration curve: Dissolve 79.6 mg. phenolphthalein in 50 ml. alcohol in a 100 ml. volumetric flask and dilute to 100 with water. This stock solution is stable. Dilute 1 ml. stock solution to 50 ml. with water in a volumetric flask. This working standard contains 15.9 μg or 0.05 μM. phenolphthalein/ml. To 1, 2, 3, and 4 ml. working standard add, respectively, 5.14, 4.14, 3.14, and 2.14 ml. color stabilizer. This brings the volume of each standard up to that of the test samples (i.e., 1 ml. water, 0.04 ml. buffer concentrate, 0.1 ml. serum, and 5 ml. color stabilizer). Read these against a blank at 550 nm. If 1 I.U. is defined as the amount of enzyme that will liberate 1 μM. of product in 1 min. for each liter of serum, then the 0.05 μM. standard corresponds to:

$$\frac{0.05 \times 100}{0.1 \times 20} = 25 \text{ I.U.}$$

where the factor 1000 converts to liters, 0.1 ml. serum is used, and the incubation period is 20 min.

Thus the previous standards correspond to 25, 50, 75, and 100 I.U. and the OD may be plotted against the units to obtain a calibration curve. There may be some deviation from linearity with a filter

photometer because of the narrow absorption peak of phenolphthalein.

Normal values and interpretation: The normal range given for this method is 9-35 I.U. It may be noted that the method of Bessey, Lowry, and Brock, in which *p*-nitrophenylphosphate is used, defines the unit as millimoles per hour. By multiplying their values by 1000 (to change to micromoles) and dividing by 60 (from per hour to per minute), one obtains the range for this method of approximately 13-48 I.U. This does not differ greatly from the phenolphthalein monophosphate method.

Acid phosphatase using alpha-naphthylphosphate[252-255]: The alpha-naphthol liberated by enzymatic hydrolysis is measured by coupling with diazotized 5-nitro-*o*-anisidine.

Alpha-naphthylphosphate has been shown to be the substrate of choice for prostatic acid phosphatase; therefore this method is highly specific for its determination.

Reagents*:

1. Alpha-naphthylphosphate substrate (2.7 mM. in 0.07M citrate buffer at pH 5.2).
   A. Dissolve 5.30 gm. citric acid monohydrate and 13.18 gm. sodium citrate dihydrate in water and dilute to 1 L. Check and adjust pH to 5.2 if necessary.
   B. Dissolve 30 mg. alpha-naphthylphosphate in 50 ml. citrate buffer. This solution is stable for 1 wk. under refrigeration.
2. Diazonium salt. Dissolve 20 mg. diazotized 5-nitro-*o*-anisidine (Fast Red Salt B) in 100 ml. 0.1N HCl. Stable for 1 wk. under refrigeration.
3. Standards. Dissolve 86.5 mg. alpha-naphthol in 10 ml. ethanol and dilute to 100 ml. with water. Dilute 1 ml. of this solution to 10 ml. with pooled serum. Pipette 0, 1, 2, 3, and 4 ml. of this solution into correspondingly labeled test tubes and add 4, 3, 2, 1, and 0 ml. pooled serum. These mixtures are equivalent to 0, 5, 10, 15, and 20 I.U. acid phosphatase, re-

---

*Reagents are available from Warner-Chilcott Laboratories Division, Warner-Lambert Pharmaceutical Co., Morris Plains, N. J.

spectively, and are stable for several days under refrigeration. Alternately, mixtures of quality control sera of known activities may be used as standards. The latter has the further advantage of standardizing the enzymatic reaction in addition to the color reaction.

4. Sodium hydroxide (0.1N). Dilute 1N NaOH 1:10 in a volumetric flask.

Procedure: To 1 ml. substrate warmed to 37° C. add 0.2 ml. serum, mix, and return immediately to water bath. Exactly 30 min. later, remove from water bath and add 1 ml. diazonium salt, mix, and immediately add 5 ml. 0.1N NaOH. Mixing is accomplished by blowing the NaOH forcibly through a 5 ml. serologic pipette.

Read OD at 590 nm. against a water blank. The control is run the same way, except the substrate is not warmed to 37° C. and the diazonium salt is added immediately after the serum. Enzyme standards are treated exactly the same as unknowns and alpha-naphthol standards are treated the same as the controls.

Calculation: The optical densities of the alpha-naphthol standards minus the zero unit standard or of the enzyme standards minus controls are plotted against the known units. The activity of the unknowns can be read directly from the curve after subtracting the control reading.

The international unit is defined as the amount of acid phosphatase in 1 L. serum that will liberate 1 μM. alpha-naphthol in 1 min. under the conditions of assay.

Normal values: The normal serum level for men and women by this method is 1-1.9 I.U./L. The only interfering substance encountered was bilirubin, which forms a chromogen with the diazonium salt. The resulting increase in control color is equivalent to about 0.3 unit/ mg.% bilirubin.

TRANSAMINASES[256-259]

The transaminases are enzymes that catalyze the intraconversion of keto acids and amino acids, in the process of which the amino group is transferred from one molecule to the other. This results in the disappearance of one amino acid and the formation of a new one. **Serum glutamic oxalacetic transaminase** (SGOT) catalyzes the reaction:

$$\text{Aspartic acid} + \text{Alpha-ketoglutaric acid} \xrightarrow{\text{GOT}} \text{Glutamic acid} + \text{Oxalacetic acid}$$

Serum glutamic pyruvic transaminase (SGPT) catalyzes the reaction:

$$\text{Alanine} + \text{Alpha-ketoglutaric acid} \xrightarrow{\text{GPT}} \text{Glutamic acid} + \text{Pyruvic acid}$$

These enzymes are normally present in the blood in relatively low concentrations. They are present in much larger quantities in tissue, particularly heart muscle and liver. In instances of tissue destruction in these organs (myocardial infarction, liver necrosis, etc.) the enzymes are liberated into the bloodstream by the tissue and will be present in high concentrations.

The enzymes are determined by the reactions just given. The blood serum is added to a buffered solution of alpha-ketoglutaric acid and aspartic acid or alanine and the resulting oxalacetic or pyruvic acid formed after incubation is measured colorimetrically by reaction with dinitrophenylhydrazine.

Reagents:

1. Phosphate buffer. Mix 420 ml. 0.1M disodium phosphate (26.81 gm. $Na_2HPO_4 \cdot 7H_2O/L$.) and 80 ml. 0.1M potassium dihydrogen phosphate (13.61 gm. KH_2PO_4/L). The pH should be 7.4.

2. Pyruvate solution (2 mM./L.). Dissolve 22 mg. sodium pyruvate in 100 ml. phosphate buffer. This solution is used for the preparation of the standard curve.

3. Alpha-ketoglutarate-aspartate for substrate GOT. Place 29.2 mg. alpha-ketoglutaric acid and 2.66 gm. aspartic acid in a small beaker. Add 1N sodium hydroxide until solution is complete. Adjust to a pH of 7.4 with sodium hydroxide, transfer quantitatively to a 100 ml. volu-

metric flask with phosphate buffer, and dilute to the mark with the buffer.

4. Alpha-ketoglutarate-alanine substrate for GPT. Place 29.2 mg. alpha-ketoglutaric acid and 1.78 gm. alanine in a small beaker. Add 1N sodium hydroxide until solution is complete. Adjust to a pH of 7.4 with sodium hydroxide, transfer quantitatively to a 100 ml. volumetric flask with phosphate buffer, and dilute to the mark with the buffer.

5. 2,4-Dinitrophenylhydrazine solution. Dissolve 19.8 mg. 2,4-dinitrophenylhydrazine in 100 ml. 1N hydrochloric acid (90 ml. concentrated acid diluted to 1000 with distilled water).

6. Sodium hydroxide solution (0.4N). Dissolve 16 gm. sodium hydroxide in distilled water to make 1 L.

The concentrations of the substrate solutions and the dinitrophenylhydrazine solution are very critical. Under usual circumstances it is advisable not to attempt to make up the reagents (except the sodium hydroxide solution). It is advisable to obtain commercial preparations.*

Standard curve: Since the reaction does not yield a linear result, it is necessary to set up an empirical standard curve to calculate the results. Set up a number of tubes as shown in Table 6-20 and add the amounts of pyruvate solution, substrate, and water as indicated. Add 1 ml. dinitrophenylhydrazine solution to each tube. Mix and allow to stand for 20 min. Then add 10 ml. 0.4N sodium hydroxide

---

*Sigma Chemical Co., St. Louis, Mo.

Table 6-20

Tube No.	Pyruvate* (ml.)	Substrate† (ml.)	H₂O (ml.)	GOT	GPT
1	0	1.0	0.2	0	0
2	0.1	0.9	0.2	24	28
3	0.2	0.8	0.2	61	57
4	0.3	0.7	0.2	114	97
5	0.4	0.6	0.2	190	–

*Pyruvate solution for standard curve.
†Ketoglutarate-aspartate substrate for GOT.

solution to each tube. Mix and after 10 min. read in a photometer at 505 nm. (500-520 nm.). Set to zero with a blank and record OD reading for each tube. Plot the results against the corresponding units for GOT and GPT. Connect the points by a smooth curve.

Procedure for SGOT and SGPT. Pipette 1 ml. of the desired substrate into a test tube and place in 37° C. water bath for 5 min. Prepare one extra tube for blank. Pipette 0.2 ml. serum into tube, mix by swirling, and begin timing. Incubate exactly 60 min. for SGOT and 30 min. for SGPT. At the end of this time add 1 ml. dinitrophenylhydrazine solution, mix, and remove from bath. Allow to stand 20 min. at room temperature (a longer time is not harmful). Then add 10 ml. 0.4N sodium hydroxide, mix by inversion, and allow to stand for 10 min. Read as for standards, subtracting reading of blank from that of sample and reading units of enzyme from the prepared standard curve. If activities are too high to read on the curve, repeat with a 1:10 dilution of serum.

Normal values and interpretation: The normal values are 8-30 units for SGOT and 5-25 units for SGPT. Elevations in transaminase activity occur in myocardial infarction, infectious mononucleosis, and infectious hepatitis. Other conditions that often show some elevation are cirrhosis with active hepatic necrosis, biliary obstruction, acute interstitial pancreatitis, metastatic carcinoma of the liver, extensive traumatic injuries, and prolonged shock. Although the SGOT level is always increased in acute myocardial infarctions, the SGPT level does not always increase proportionately.

Glutamic oxalacetic transaminase using diazonium salt[260-262]: This enzyme catalyzes the following reaction:

Aspartic acid +

$$\text{Alpha-ketoglutaric acid} \xrightarrow{\text{GOT}} \text{Glutamic acid +}$$

Oxalacetic acid

In this method the oxalacetic acid formed is determined by reaction with a stabilized diazonium salt to form a red dye that is measured photometrically.

Reagents*:

1. Substrate buffer. Dissolve 0.731 gm. alpha-ketoglutaric acid, 2.66 gm. L-aspartic acid, 33.5 gm. K_2HPO_4, 1 gm. KH_2PO_4, 10 gm. polyvinylpyrrolidone† ,1 gm. sodium salt of ethylenediaminetetraacetic acid, and 5 ml. 1N NaOH in water and dilute to 1000 ml. Check pH and adjust to 7.4 if necessary. Store in the refrigerator.

2. Control buffer. Dissolve 28.6 gm. K_2HPO_4, 4.9 gm. KH_2PO_4, 10 gm. polyvinylpyrrolidone, 1 gm. disodium ethylenediaminetetraacetic acid, and 5 ml. 1N NaOH in water to make 1 L. Check pH and adjust to 7.4 if necessary. Store in the refrigerator.

3. Color reagent. Dissolve 0.2 gm. 6-benzamido-4-methoxy-meta-toluidine diazonium chloride‡ in 100 ml. 0.01N HCl (0.85 ml. concentrated HCl diluted to 1 L.). Store in the refrigerator. This is stable for only a few weeks. Discard when markedly colored or turbid.

4. Acid diluent. Dilute 1.7 ml. concentrated HCl and 5 ml. nonionic detergent such as Non-ionox,§ in water to make 1 L.

Procedure: Pipette 1 ml. aliquots of substrate buffer to test tubes, one tube for each sample plus one tube for the reagent blank. Place tubes in a 37° C. water bath to come to temperature. At timed intervals add 0.2 ml. serum to the respective tubes, except the blank, and replace in the water bath. After exactly 20 min. incubation and while still in water bath, add 1 ml. color reagent to each tube, including the blank, and incubate for another 10 min. Remove from

---

*Reagents may be obtained from Warner-Chilcott Laboratories Division, Warner-Lambert Pharmaceutical Co., Morris Plains, N. J., as "Transac."

†Polyvinylpyrrolidone, K-30, Oxford Laboratory, San Mateo, Calif., or through local laboratory supply houses.

‡Obtainable as Azoene Fast Violet B from Alliance Color and Chemical Co., Newark, N. J., and other suppliers.

§Aloe Scientific Division, Brunswick Corp., St. Louis, Mo.

bath and add 10 ml. acid diluent. Mix tubes thoroughly and read samples against reagent blank at 540 nm. Also set up a similar series of tubes, using the control buffer instead of the substrate buffer. Carry through the same procedure and read tubes against control reagent blank. For each serum sample subtract OD reading obtained with control buffer from that obtained with substrate buffer before converting to enzyme units.

Calculation: The method is best standardized by using dilutions of a control serum (such as Versatol E) with a high enzyme assay. For example, if the control serum contained 350 Karmen units, dilutions are made as follows:

Control serum (ml.)						
0.1	0.2	0.3	0.4	0.5	0.7	1
Saline solution (ml.)						
0.9	0.8	0.7	0.6	0.5	0.3	0
Units						
35	70	105	140	175	245	350

These mixtures are run exactly as in the previous procedure to obtain a calibration curve. A graph is constructed relating SGOT units to OD. A new curve should be constructed with each new lot of diazonium salt. Sera with enzyme activity greater than 350 units should be accurately diluted with saline solution (i.e., 1:5) and the analysis repeated. Final results from the calibration chart are multiplied by 5.

Normal values and interpretation: They are the same as for the previous method.

ERYTHROCYTE ENZYME DEFICIENCIES IN INBORN METABOLIC ERRORS

A number of enzymes are found in the red cells. Their measurements may be used to study certain inborn metabolic errors. These enzymes are all controlled by **autosomal recessive genes.** Usually an individual who is homozygous for the defective gene will have very low levels of the particular enzyme involved. A heterozygous individual will have values intermediate between those of homozygous and normal individuals. Usually a heterozygous individual shows no clinical signs of the enzyme deficiency. The determinations may be of value in the diagnosis of the particular enzyme deficiency involved and in the detection of heterozygous carriers for the purposes of genetic counseling. A screening method for these enzymes is discussed in the section on hematology. A further discussion of these enzymes can be found in a recent book by Hsia.[263]

Glucose-6-phosphate dehydrogenase[264]: This enzyme is concerned in one type of anaerobic glycolysis that is known as the direct oxidative pathway (hexose monophosphate shunt), which takes place to some extent as an alternative to the well-known citric acid aerobic cycle. This enzyme catalyzes the oxidation of glucose-6-phosphate to 6-phosphogluconic acid in the presence of nicotinamide adenine dinucleotide phosphate (NADP), which is changed to the reduced form (NADPH). The quantitative method for this enzyme involves this reaction, measuring the change in absorbance at 340 nm. as the NADP is reduced to NADPH.

Individuals having low concentrations of this enzyme in the red cells may experience little difficulty under favorable conditions, but after the ingestion of fava beans or a number of drugs such as primaquine or acetylphenylhydrazine, an excessive hemolysis of the erythrocytes occurs. This condition is known as favism if due to the fava bean or as primaquine defect if due to drugs.[265, 266]

6-Phosphogluconic dehydrogenase: This is another of the enzymes found in the erythrocyte that are concerned with the glucose metabolic pathway previously mentioned. The enzyme catalyzes the oxidation of 6-phosphogluconic acid to 3-deoxyphosphogluconic acid in the presence of NADP, which is changed to the reduced form (NADPH). An inborn metabolic error involving this enzyme occurs in some forms of congenital nonspherocytic hemolytic anemia. The enzyme may be measured by incubating a lysate of the erythrocytes with 6-phosphogluconic acid and NADP and measuring the change in absorption at 340 nm. This indicates the change from NADP to

NADPH and hence of the amount of enzyme present.

Pyruvic kinase (PK)[267]: Low levels of this enzyme in the erythrocytes also result in a form of congenital nonspherocytic hemolytic anemia. The enzyme catalyzes the conversion of phosphoenolpyruvate to pyruvate in the presence of adenosine diphosphate (ADP). It may be determined by incubating a hemolysate of the red cells with ADP and phosphoenolpyruvate. The amount of pyruvate formed in the reaction is measured by the additional reaction:

$$\text{Pyruvate} + \text{NADH} \xrightarrow{\text{LDH}} \text{Lactate} + \text{NAD}$$

The reaction is followed by the change in absorbance at 340 nm. from the conversion of NADH to NAD.

With this enzyme, heterozygous individuals have activities about halfway between the values for normal individuals and the very low values for homozygous individuals.

Glutathione reductase: This enzyme is also implicated in some types of congenital nonspherocytic hemolytic anemia. It is not concerned directly with the glucolytic process as are the previously mentioned enzymes, but it is necessary for the functional integrity of the cell membrane. The enzyme maintains glutathione in the reduced state in the presence of NADPH. It may be determined by incubating a dialyzed hemolysate under aerobic conditions with the oxidized form of glutathione and NADPH. The reduced glutathione formed may be determined colorimetrically by reaction with sodium nitroprusside or by the change from NADPH to NADP, which is followed by measuring the changes in absorption at 340 nm.

Galactose-1-phosphate uridyl transferase[268]: This enzyme catalyzes the reaction:

Galactose-1-phosphate + Uridine diphosphate glucose → Glucose-1-phosphate + Uridine diphosphate galactose

This is an important step in the metabolism of galactose by which it is converted into glucose. A deficiency of this enzyme is believed to be the basis for an inborn error of metabolism with the inability to use galactose. The test for this enzyme has been used in the study of this genetic trait, particularly in the detection of heterozygous carriers in whom the level of the enzyme in the erythrocytes is about half that of normal individuals, although it is still much higher than that of homozygous galactosemic individuals.[269] The enzyme may be determined by incubating a hemolysate of the erythrocytes with galactose-1-phosphate and uridine diphosphate glucose so that the above reaction takes place. After reaction the unchanged uridyl diphosphate glucose (UDPG) is measured by means of the coupled reaction:

$$\text{UDPG} + \text{NAD} \xrightarrow{\text{UDPG dehydrogenase}}$$

NADH + Uridine diphosphate gluconate

and following this reaction, by means of the change in absorption at 340 nm. due to the change in the amount of NAD present.

Ornithine carbamyl transferase (OCT)[152]: This is an enzyme that catalyzes the transfer of a one-carbon group—the carbamyl group—from carbamyl phosphate to ornithine-forming citrulline. This reaction is one of the steps in the formation of urea. The enzyme is found almost exclusively in the liver. The activity of the enzyme may be determined by incubating the serum with carbamyl phosphate and ornithine and determining the citrulline formed by a colorimetric reaction. Since urea interferes, it is removed by the addition of urease. Serum ornithine carbamyl transferase is increased only in cases of hepatocellular injury. Increased activity may occur secondary to cellular injury with no histologic evidence of hepatocellular necrosis. The determination of OCT is more specific for hepatocellular injury than the GPT and it is also more sensitive. It will complement rather than replace such regular tests as bilirubin, BSP, alkaline phosphate, and protein electrophoresis.

The earlier work on OCT was done by a radioisotope method that is not suitable for the average clinical laboratory.

An improved chemical method recently developed by Kulhánek and co-workers[270, 271] appears to be quite satisfactory, but when the equipment is available, the automated method of Strandjord[272] is suggested. This method gives an upper limit of normal of 2.3 I.U. in men and 2.0 I.U. in women.

Guanase[153]: This enzyme catalyzes the deamination of guanine to xanthine, which is one step in the conversion of guanine to the final end product of purine metabolism—uric acid. It is found chiefly in the liver, brain, and kidney, with very little of the enzyme in other tissue such as the heart, pancreas, spleen, skeletal muscle, and erythrocytes. The absence of the enzyme in cardiac and skeletal muscle should make this enzyme determination of value in differentiating cardiac and hepatic disease in instances of elevated GOT and LDH. The absence of the enzyme in the erythrocytes increases the use of the assay since slight hemolysis cannot interfere.

Unfortunately the earlier methods for the determination of the enzyme involved the use of ultraviolet absorption, either measuring the decrease in guanine by noting the decrease in absorbance at 245 nm. or by the addition of xanthine oxidase to the system, whereby the xanthine formed was oxidized to uric acid and the uric acid was measured by its absorbance at 290 nm.[273] Recently a colorimetric method has been developed by Caraway[274] which measures the ammonia formed in the deamination of guanine by the Berthelot phenate-hypochlorite reaction. The normal range of values by this method agrees well with that obtained by the ultraviolet method and may be taken as up to 3 I.U. Marked increases in the serum activity have been found in viral hepatitis and other acute hepatocellular disease, with but very little increase in obstructive jaundice and cirrhosis. This enzyme assay should prove helpful in distinguishing liver disease from other conditions that also give increases in the GOT and LDH.

Diaphorase: This enzyme catalyzes the reconversion of methemoglobin to hemoglobin in the presence of NADH. In the congenital deficiency of this enzyme the reconversion rate is slower and methemoglobin accumulates in the erythrocytes. In cases of methemoglobinemia the concentration of this enzyme may be measured as an aid in diagnosis. Here also, the parents of affected individuals have about half the concentration of the enzyme in the erythrocytes as normal individuals.[275] The enzyme may be determined by converting the hemoglobin in a hemolyzed sample with sodium nitrate to methemoglobin. The hemolysate, which contains both the enzyme and the methemoglobin, is incubated with NADH and the dye 2,6-dichlorobenzenoneindophenol (DCBIP). The oxidation of the dye is followed spectrophotometrically at 600 nm. as a blue color is formed. The rate of formation of the color is a measure of the enzyme concentration.

THYROID FUNCTION TESTS

The thyroid gland has a trapping mechanism that selectively removes inorganic iodides from the circulation and enzymatically oxidizes the iodides into free iodine. The free iodine combines with tyrosine and thyroglobulin and is stored in the colloid of the gland. The colloid also contains monoiodotyrosine and diodotyrosine, thyroxine, and triiodothyronine. Under the influence of the thyroid-stimulating hormone (TSH) of the pituitary gland the thyroglobulin is hydrolyzed enzymatically, releasing free thyroxine and triiodothyronine into the bloodstream. Upon entering the blood, thyroxine is quickly bound to plasma proteins (thyroxine-binding globulins and thyroxine-binding prealbumin). A minute amount of thyroxine remains free in the circulation. The thyroxine is concentrated in the liver, conjugated with glucuronic acid, and excreted in the bile. There is some reabsorption of thyroxine from the intestinal tract and some excretion by the salivary glands.

Iodine in blood is present as both organic and inorganic forms. Under normal conditions the organically combined iodine exists chiefly as thyroxine and triiodothyronine. Although triiodothyronine is considerably more active than thyroxine, its concentration is very low and it contributes very little to the total serum iodine. Thyroxine contributes most of the iodine of the blood (about 75-90%). The concentration of inorganic iodine depends more on the balance between the intake, metabolism, and excretion of iodine; hence it is not directly associated with thyroid function.

The functional state of the thyroid gland is regulated by the thyrotropic hormone of the anterior part of the pituitary gland (TSH). This hormone promotes not only iodine uptake by the gland but also the synthesis of the organic compounds and the hydrolytic dissociation of thyroxine from thyroglobulin. The secretion of TSH is directly controlled by the blood thyroxine level. An increase in this level diminishes TSH secretion; a decrease stimulates it.

Laboratory tests for the evaluation of thyroid function are divided into four main categories based upon their role in thyroid physiology: (1) tests based on the ability of the thyroid to concentrate iodine, such as radioactive iodine uptake (RAI); (2) tests based on the thyroid hormone transport system, i.e., thyroid-binding index (TBI) and ET_3; (3) tests based on thyroid hormone concentrations (PBI, BEI, and thyroxine—T_4); and (4) tests based on metabolic response, such as basal metabolic rate (BMR) and serum cholesterol levels. The speed of contraction and relaxation of the muscle in the tendon reflex (Achilles tendon reflex) has also been used as a measurement of thyroid activity. Of these tests, those based on the measurement of circulating hormone levels in the blood are the most accurate and dependable. All these tests will be discussed in this section. They can furnish valuable diagnostic information, either individually or as part of a battery of tests.

Radioactive iodine uptake by the thyroid gland[276, 277]

Radioactive iodine (I^{131}) has been used extensively as an aid in the diagnosis of thyroid disorders. The isotope is provided as sodium iodide by the Atomic Energy Commission and is available to persons approved by this commission. Numerous studies have been conducted and many methods have been proposed to achieve maximum accuracy in appraising the level of thyroid gland function by the use of radioactive iodine. No single procedure or combination of procedures has proved 100% accurate in diagnosis.

The most widely used method is the percent uptake by the thyroid gland 24 hr. after administration of a tracer dose of radioactive iodine. Each clinic must set up its own values for each thyroid state. In general this has been a very good test of hyperthyroidism and there is little overlap with the euthyroid state, but it has been less reliable in separating hypothyroidism from euthyroidism.

The main difficulty in the use of radioactive iodine is that many factors interfere with the iodine-trapping mechanism of the thyroid, but they do not change the thyroid function. Diagnostic x-ray procedures using organic iodides are the main offenders in that the 24 hr. uptake will be depressed to hypothyroid levels. Other substances that will falsely depress the iodine uptake are desiccated thyroid, cortisone, ACTH, antithyroid drugs, and inorganic iodides.

Significance: The percent uptake (24 hr.) of radioactive iodine in euthyroidism is 10-40; in hypothyroidism, less than 10; and in hyperthyroidism, over 40.

The radioactive iodine uptake measures the ability of the gland to trap iodine, to concentrate it, to convert it to a hormonal form, and finally to release it.

Increased uptake occurs in hyperthyroidism and endemic goiter. Decreased uptake occurs in hypothyroidism, treatment with thyroxine, and hypopituitarism.

Erroneous results may be recorded in iodine administration (contrast media), thiouracil treatment, and renal and cardiac diseases (reduced iodine clearance).

Thyroid-binding index (TBI)[278-282]

Thyroid hormone in the serum is primarily bound to the alpha$_1$ and alpha$_2$ globulins, which are referred to as the **thyroxine-binding globulins** or TBG. The TBG will combine with thyroid hormones in vitro as well as in vivo. It combines with thyroxine preferentially to triiodothyronine. Any thyroxine added to plasma will replace triiodothyronine combined with TBG, but added triiodothyronine will not replace thyroxine already bound by TBG. There is a direct relationship between the amount of free circulating TBG and the thyroid status of an individual. In hyperthyroidism there is an excess amount of thyroxine and triiodothyronine secreted by the thyroid gland into the circulation. This increased amount of thyroid hormone "ties up" more TBG than usual, resulting in less than normal amounts of free TBG. Conversely, in hypothyroidism there is more than normal amounts of free circulating TBG since there is less of the hormones secreted by the thyroid gland to combine with the TBG present.

The thyroid-binding index is an in vitro test used for the indirect measurement of the amount of free TBG in the blood. In this method the blood serum is incubated with an ion exchange resin in which has been adsorbed a definite amount of triiodothyronine labeled with I^{131}. The labeled triiodothyronine is held strongly enough by the resin so that it will not be eluted by simple solution, but will be preferentially adsorbed from the resin by any free TBG present in the serum. Accordingly, the greater the amount of TBG present, the greater the amount of labeled triiodothyronine that will be transferred from the resin to the serum. After incubation, the resin is separated from the serum and the radioactivity of the serum is measured by a scintillation counter; this is an index of the amount of I^{131}-labeled triiodothyronine adsorbed by the serum and thus of the amount of free TBG originally present since the amount of added triiodothyronine is more than sufficient to saturate the serum.

The amount of labeled hormone adsorbed is dependent somewhat on the conditions of the test; these are closely standardized. The measurements of each series of tests are compared with the measurements using a standard serum of known thyroxine-binding capacity. The results are then expressed in terms of thyroid-binding index or TBI, the ratio between the amount adsorbed by the sample serum and that of the standard serum. Serum from hypothyroid individuals will show a high index (increased amounts of free TBG because of low endogenous thyroid hormones). Serum from hyperthyroid individuals will show a lowered index (decreased amounts of free TBG due to increased saturation of the globulins by larger concentrations of endogenous hormones).

Normal values and interpretation: The normal values for serum TBI in euthyroidism are 0.9-1.1; in hyperthyroidism, less than 0.9; and in hypothyroidism, greater than 1.1.

In pregnancy, even in euthyroid individuals, there is a marked increase in TBI (decreased index of thyroid activity) due to an increase in thyroxine-binding globulins caused by increased estrogen secretion. This change in TBI usually occurs around the fifth or sixth week of pregnancy and remains until delivery.

Various clinical conditions will also show changes in TBI findings. Apparent increases in thyroid activity (decreased TBI values) will be found in nephrosis, severe liver disease, anticoagulant therapy (Dicumarol, heparin), metastatic malignancies, pulmonary insufficiency, and hyperandrogenic states.

The TBI test follows the clinical state of the patient very closely. As the hyperthyroid patient improves clinically under iodine or propylthiouracil therapy, the TBI increases to more normal levels. A decrease in the TBI value is shown during administration of thyroid hormones. The administration of various iodine compounds, whether organic or inorganic, usually does not affect the TBI values significantly. This is a very important advantage since these compounds are known to cause spuriously high values in the PBI test and in many cases also in the BEI and T_4 determinations. Trypan blue, sometimes used for diagnostic studies, is known to interfere with the TBI by combining with the thyroxine-binding globulins, which causes false low TBI results.

Erythrocyte uptake of I^{131}-labeled triiodothyronine (ET_3)[283]

This is another in vitro test, similar to the TBI, for the indirect measurement of free circulating TBG. In this method a tracer amount of I^{131}-labeled triiodothyronine is added to a previously obtained sample of the patient's venous blood. The tagged cells are incubated for a given time and the amount of I^{131}-labeled T_3 bound to the washed red cells is determined as a percentage of the total radioactive content of the same aliquot of whole blood. The value is corrected to 100 vol.% hematocrit. Normal uptake after incubation for 2 hr. is from 11-17%. It is higher in hyperthyroidism and lower in hypothyroidism.

Thyroxine-binding globulin capacity[284]

This test measures the total thyroxine-binding globulin capacity and indicates the amounts of TBG in circulation. It involves the addition of a large excess of I^{131}-labeled thyroxine (T_4) to the patient's serum, allowing equilibration to take place. This is followed by reverse-flow electrophoretic separation of the proteins and separation of the TBG inter-alpha band. The paper strip is scanned radiometrically for the distribution of I^{131} and the amount of TBG present is calculated by relating the proportion of I^{131} in the TBG to the total thyroxine in the supplemented serum. Normal values are 12-20 μg thyroxine-binding capacity/100 ml. serum.

PROTEIN-BOUND IODINE (PBI)

Protein-bound iodine represents the organic fraction of blood iodine that precipitates with the serum proteins. In normal subjects it consists primarily of thyroxine and triiodothyronine. The level of PBI in the serum correlates well with the thyroid status and is considered the most valuable method for evaluation of thyroid function.

Numerous methods have been used for the determination of PBI. Fundamentally, all present-day methods employ the following steps: treatment of the serum for elimination of inorganic iodine, either by precipitation and washing of protein or by treatment of serum with ion exchange resin; the subsequent destruction of organic matter and conversion of thyroxine to inorganic iodide, either by wet- or dry-ashing; and quantitation of the inorganic iodide formed by its catalytic effect on the ceric-arsenious acid reaction. The methods differ primarily in the steps used for the elimination of inorganic iodine and in the treatment of the organic iodine to a suitable form for use in the ceric-arsenious acid system.

Two methods will be described in this section: the chloric acid oxidation method of Zak (wet-ashing) and the alkaline-ashing method of Barker (dry-ashing). Although these methods are technically difficult, they can be performed by skilled technicians if sufficient care and ideal laboratory conditions are maintained.

METHODS OF SEPARATING INORGANIC IODINE FROM PROTEIN-BOUND IODINE:

Anion exchange resin method[285-289]: In this method the serum is treated with the anion exchange resin Amberlite IRA-401, AR. This is our method of choice because it has proved to be a quick, thorough, and efficient way of separating inorganic iodine from protein-bound iodine and may be used with any PBI procedure. We have used it for several years and consider it far superior to protein precipitation and washing. Besides saving time, it eliminates sources of contamination and loss of sample.

Reagent:
1. Amberlite IRA-401, AR (Cl⁻).* Suspend 1 lb. anion exchange resin in redistilled water in a large plastic container and wash several times by decantation to make certain that all the floating particles are removed. Then filter the resin under suction in a large Buechner funnel. Continue suction for about 1 hr. for partial drying. Spread out resin on filter paper and allow to dry for about 25-30 min. Store in airtight bottles. It is necessary to dry the resin sufficiently to prevent hydration of the serum. We have been informed by several laboratories that

---

*Mallinckrodt Chemical Co., St. Louis, Mo.

they use the resin as supplied by the manufacturer (without washing).

Procedure: The resin is most conveniently used by measuring approximate volume. Treat about 2 ml. serum with 0.5 ml. vol. resin (0.3 gm.) in a 12×100 mm. test tube, stopper tightly, mix thoroughly, and let stand about 10 min. Centrifuge for about 5 min. to settle the resin and pipette 1 ml. aliquots of serum for PBI determinations.

After some experience with the method is gained, the resin tubes may be prepared in advance by tapping the resin into test tubes to an approximate volume of 0.5 ml. The addition of serum can also be done by visually comparing it to a tube with resin to which 2 ml. serum has been added.

Precipitation and washing: This method requires zinc sulfate and sodium hydroxide, the same as used in the dry-ash method of Barker.

Reagents:
1. Redistilled water. Use to prepare all reagents and for the final rinsing of all glassware used in the procedure.
2. Zinc sulfate solution (10%). Dissolve 100 gm. zinc sulfate ($ZnSO_4 \cdot 7H_2O$) in redistilled water and dilute to 1 L.
3. Sodium hydroxide solution (0.5N). Dissolve 21 gm. NaOH in redistilled water and dilute to 1 L. Titrate against the zinc sulfate solution as follows: dilute 10 ml. zinc sulfate solution with 50 ml. distilled water and titrate with sodium hydroxide solution, using phenolphthalein as indicator, until a faint, permanent pink color is obtained. Adjust the hydroxide solution so that 10 ml. zinc sulfate solution requires between 10.8 and 11.2 ml. hydroxide.

Procedure: Pipette duplicate aliquots of 1 ml. serum (or plasma) to 15×125 mm. Pyrex tubes. Add 7 ml. water and 1 ml. 10% zinc sulfate and mix with a footed stirring rod. Add 1 ml. 0.5N sodium hydroxide to each tube, mix with rod, and allow to stand for 10 min. Have a separate stirring rod available for each test tube and use the stirring rod for the respective tube throughout, taking care to avoid contamination of the rod. Remove the rod and centrifuge the tubes for 10 min. at 2000 rpm. Pour off the supernatant fluid, add 10 ml. redistilled water, and resuspend the protein by means of the same stirring rod originally used. Stirring should be vigorous enough to distribute the zinc proteinate uniformly throughout the solution, but if over-zealously carried out, the precipitate may be so finely divided that it cannot be easily centrifuged down again. Centrifuge and discard the supernatant fluid. Repeat the washing twice more, making a total of three washings in addition to the original precipitation.

Run a reagent blank by using 1 ml. water instead of serum and carry through all the steps of precipitation and washing.

Perchloric acid method: This method requires perchloric acid, the same as used in the wet-ash method of Zak.

Reagent:

1. Perchloric acid (10%). Dilute 100 ml. 70% perchloric acid to 1 L. with redistilled water.

Procedure: Measure 1 ml. serum or plasma into a 15 × 125 mm. test tube. Add slowly, with agitation, 10 ml. 10% perchloric acid. This is conveniently added from a dispensing burette. Allow to stand 10 min., then centrifuge 15 min. at 2000 rpm, and decant the supernatant fluid completely. Again, add 10 ml. perchloric acid solution and resuspend the precipitated protein with the aid of a clean stirring rod. After use the rod may be rinsed with a small quantity of the perchloric acid solution. Recentrifuge at 2000 rpm for 15 min. Decant the supernatant fluid and allow the tubes to drain in an inverted position for 15 min. The precipitated protein may be stored in the freezing compartment of a refrigerator if one does not desire to proceed immediately with the analysis.

Method of Barker[290-292]: This is the **alkaline incineration** method of Barker et al., as modified by Foss et al. In this method the PBI is precipitated and washed by the zinc hydroxide technique; the washed precipitate is made alkaline by the addition of sodium carbonate and

dried in an oven. After complete drying, the protein is incinerated in a muffle furnace to convert iodine to iodide. The ash is dissolved and the iodide present is quantitated by the use of the ceric-arsenious acid reaction.

Equipment: The method requires a muffle furnace with a control to hold the temperature between 600° and 625° C. The precipitation and incineration is carried out in 15 × 125 mm. Pyrex test tubes. These are etched badly by the alkali and should not be used more than twice.

Reagents:

1. Redistilled water. All water used must be redistilled. It may be obtained from an all-glass still or by passing distilled water through an ion exchange column.

2. Sodium carbonate (4N) and potassium chlorate solution (2%). Dissolve 212 gm. anhydrous sodium carbonate and 20 gm. potassium chlorate in redistilled water and dilute to 1 L.

3. Antifoam solution. Dissolve 70 gm. Dow Corning Antifoam AF Emulsion* in redistilled water and dilute to 1 L.

4. Ceric ammonium sulfate solution (0.032N). Dissolve 20 gm. ceric ammonium sulfate† in 70 ml. redistilled water containing 49 ml. concentrated sulfuric acid. Cool and dilute to 1 L. Store in a dark bottle.

5. Arsenious acid reagent. Dissolve 0.986 gm. arsenic trioxide in 10 ml. 0.5N sodium hydroxide with the aid of heat. Add this solution to approximately 850 ml. redistilled water in a 1 L. volumetric flask. While mixing, cautiously add 20 ml. concentrated HCl and 39.6 ml. concentrated H_2SO_4. Cool to room temperature and dilute to 1 L.

6. Standard iodide solution. Dissolve 118.1 mg. sodium iodide or 130.8 potassium iodide in redistilled water to make 1 L. Use only highest purity salts that have been thoroughly

---

*Dow Corning Corp., Midland, Mich.
†G. Frederick Smith Chemical Co., Columbus, Ohio.

dried. This solution contains 100 μg iodine/ml.

A. Stock standard. Dilute 4 ml. standard iodide solution to 100 ml. with redistilled water. This contains 4 μg/ml. iodine.

B. Working standard. Add 0, 0.5, 1, 2, 3, and 4 ml. aliquots of stock standard to 100 ml. volumetric flasks containing 50 ml. 4N sodium carbonate and dilute to the 100 ml. mark. This solution contains 0, 0.02, 0.04, 0.08, 0.12, and 0.16 μg/ml., respectively. For the standard curve measure duplicate 1 ml. aliquots from each standard into 15 × 125 mm. Pyrex test tubes and dry in the oven at 110° C. for 2 hr. Dissolve residues in 10 ml. arsenious acid reagent, allow to leach for 15 min., mix, and centrifuge for 20 min. at 2000 rpm. From this point they are treated the same way as the incinerated samples.

Procedure: Add 0.5 ml. carbonate-chlorate solution and 1 drop Antifoam solution to washed precipitate (or alternately, to 1 ml. ion exchange resin–treated serum) and to the reagent blank. Do not mix. Place the tubes in a rack in an oven and dry for 2 hr. at approximately 110° C. Continue the incineration as follows. Place tubes containing the dry precipitates in a metal rack capable of withstanding a temperature of 620° C. Open the door of the muffle furnace, which has been heated to 620° C., and allow to cool to about 400° C. Place the rack inside and close the door. When temperature reaches 610° C., time for 30 min. At the end of this period remove the tubes and cool to room temperature. The incineration is the critical point of this method. The directions should be followed exactly. The muffle must have a tight-fitting door; if there is a vent in the rear of the furnace, it should be closed. Accurate control of temperature is also necessary.

Dissolve the ash in 10 ml. arsenious acid reagent, allow to leach for 15 min., mix, and centrifuge for 20 min. at 2000 rpm. Transfer 5 ml. aliquots of the clear supernatant to photometer cuvettes. Also set up standards and blank and place tubes in a water bath at 37° C.

Warm a quantity of the ceric sulfate solution to the bath temperature. Add 1 ml. ceric sulfate solution to a series of tubes at exactly 30 sec. intervals and immediately mix well by inversion, using a piece of Parafilm or Saran Wrap over the top of the tube. Exactly 20 min. after the addition of ceric sulfate, read each tube in the photometer at 420 nm., setting to zero with a water blank. The ceric sulfate must be measured very accurately and the timing must be the same for all tubes.

The readings in percent transmission (not optical density) for the standards are then plotted against the amount of iodine in the standards (0-0.16 μg) and a smooth curve is drawn through the points (the curve may not be exactly a straight line). The micrograms of iodine in the sample aliquots and reagent blank are then read directly from the curve. Subtract μg iodine found in reagent blank from all samples. For the aliquots used, the standards will be equivalent to 0, 2, 4, 8, 12, and 16 μg%.

NOTES: A number of special precautions must be taken in the use of these methods. Since minute quantities of iodine are being determined, great care must be taken to avoid contamination. It is best to carry out the determinations in a separate room devoted solely to this purpose. Solutions containing iodine (e.g., gram stain or Nessler reagent) should not be used in the same room with PBI determinations. All glassware must be scrupulously cleaned and rinsed well; redistilled water is used for the final washing.

Some lots of reagent grade chemicals may contain sufficient iodine to give excessively high blanks. Those manufactured by Mallinckrodt Chemical Co. have been found to be generally satisfactory. Before attempting to run any actual samples, a number of standards and reagent blanks should be run. As a final step before proceeding with the analysis of unknown samples, one of the commercially available lyophilized control serum should be run.

It has been found satisfactory to purify the water by passage through a commercially obtainable ion exchange demineralizing cartridge. If ordinary distilled water is passed through the cartridge, it should last for several months since the amount of material removed is very small.

The tubes used for the incineration are etched badly by the alkali, and it is recommended that they be used only once and certainly not more than twice.

If the incineration is carefully carried out, there should be no carbon particles left. They are difficult to remove by centrifugation and will interfere with the determination. If such particles persist, cool test tubes, add 1 drop distilled water to the tube containing the ash, redry the contents in the oven, and repeat incineration process for about 5 min.

The exact shape of the standard curve and the deviation from linearity will depend somewhat on the spectrophotometer used. If the decolorization proceeds too rapidly, the temperature of the water bath may be lowered somewhat.

Since standards are neither precipitated nor incinerated in this method, several quality control sera of various PBI concentrations should be run with each set to determine if iodine losses or contamination occurs during the analyses.

The use of some type of screening of unknown samples is of great importance in order to avoid contamination of the samples in the incinerator. A simple method is described below.

Rapid screening method (Ackerman-Meyers)[293]: Occasionally sera containing large amounts of iodine (over 40 μg%) may cause some cross contamination even with the present modification. The rapid screening method given by Ackerman and Meyers to eliminate those samples is as follows.

Procedure: To 0.1 ml. 4N sodium carbonate (21 gm. anhydrous salt/100 ml.) add 0.1 ml. serum and place in a boiling water bath for 3 min. Remove from the bath, cool, and add 1 ml. distilled water, followed by 1 ml. 2N hydrochloric acid (20 ml. concentrated acid diluted to 100 ml.). Shake the tube gently for 2-3 min., but not so hard as to break up the protein clot. Remove the protein clot with a stirring rod; any small remaining particles will not interfere. To the HCl solution add 0.5 ml. 0.1N sodium arsenite, followed by 0.25 ml. (0.032N) ceric sulfate solution, and start timing. Any tubes that show complete decolorization in 10 min. should be eliminated as contaminators.

Method of Zak[294-296]: This is the chloric acid oxidation of Zak et al. as modified by O'Neal and Simms and by us. In this method the PBI is precipitated and washed by the perchloric acid technique and digested with chloric acid and chromate to convert iodine to iodate. Iodate in the digestion residue is reduced by arsenious acid and determined as iodide by its catalytic action on the reduction of ceric sulfate by arsenious acid.

Equipment: Wash all glassware once with nitric acid or sulfuric-chromic acid cleaning solution. Rinse three or four times with tap water, three or four times with distilled water, and once with redistilled water.

1. Electrolytic beakers (250 ml.) for digestion and oxidation
2. Fisher Speedyvap or similar watch glasses for covering the electrolytic beakers
3. Glass beads (5 mm.)

The digestion and oxidation are performed on a hot plate at 150° C. under a fume hood.

Reagents:

1. Redistilled water. Obtain from an all-glass still or use distilled water purified by passing through an anion exchange column.
2. Concentrated sulfuric acid, reagent grade.
3. Chloric acid reagent with chromate. Dissolve 500 gm. potassium chlorate ($KClO_3$) and 200 mg. sodium dichromate (Na_2CrO_4) in 1 L. redistilled water with the aid of heat. While hot, add 370 ml. perchloric acid (72%), stir, and cool under running water. Store in the freezer compartment overnight and filter while cold. Store in a dark place that is below 4° C.
4. Arsenious acid with sodium chloride. Dissolve 2.64 gm. arsenic trioxide and 1.9 gm. sodium hydroxide in about 100 ml. redistilled water. Dilute to approximately 400 ml. and

neutralize to phenolphthalein with concentrated sulfuric acid. Add 30 ml. more of concentrated sulfuric acid and 6.6 gm. sodium chloride and dilute to 1 L.

5. Ceric ammonium sulfate (0.028N). Dissolve 17.7 gm. ceric ammonium sulfate, $(NH_4)_4Ce(SO_4) \cdot 2H_2O$, and 103 ml. concentrated sulfuric acid in 700 ml. redistilled water. Let stand overnight; then dilute to 1 L. Filter if cloudy and store in an amber bottle.

6. Iodate standards:
   A. Stock standard. Dissolve 168.5 mg. potassium iodate (KIO_3) that has been dried in a vacuum desiccator in redistilled water to make 1 L. This stock solution contains 100 μg iodine/ml.
   B. Working standard. Dilute 1 ml. stock standard to 2 L. with redistilled water. This solution contains 0.05 μg iodine/ml. and should be made fresh every 2 wk.

Before actually making any determinations it is advisable to run a blank through the actual procedure (see discussion of procedure) to check for contamination of the reagents. With the use of 19 mm. cuvettes at 420 nm., the $\Delta T/t$ for the blank should be less than 1. If the blank is too high, the reagents should be replaced one at a time to find the source of contamination.

Procedure: With the aid of a total of 10 ml. chloric acid, transfer the protein precipitate to a 250 ml. electrolytic beaker containing 8-10 glass beads or, alternately, add to 1 ml. ion exchange resin–treated serum. This is conveniently done by adding the acid in portions from a 10 ml. pipette. First add about 5 ml. acid; then by gently tapping the test tube on the desk top the precipitated protein can usually be loosened from the tube and the major portion transferred to the beaker in one clump. The small amount of protein remaining is rinsed into the beaker with small portions of the rest of the chloric acid. Too vigorous tapping may break up the clump entirely, rendering complete transfer more difficult. Cover with a watch glass and heat on the hot

plate. After crackling caused by the decomposition of chloric acid ceases and white fumes appear, add 0.5 ml. more chloric acid.

Add a few drops of chloric acid from time to time to maintain the chromium in its orange hexavalent state.

CAUTION: Reduction of chromium to the green trivalent state for more than a few seconds is associated with loss of iodine.

When the volume has been reduced to about 5 ml. and dense white fumes have been present for about 5 min., the watch glasses may be removed. The rate of digestion should be such that about 45 min. is required to reach this point from the beginning of the digestion.

Evaporate to an estimated volume of 0.3-0.5 ml. Iodine may be lost if complete dryness is obtained. With practice, the visual estimate of the desired volume can be made with negligible error. The final volume should just wet the glass beads with little excess liquid. Set up several blanks containing 1 ml. water and 10 ml. chloric acid. Also run standards containing 0.5, 1.0, 1.5, 2.0, and 3.0 ml. working standard with 10 ml. chloric acid. Digest and treat the same as the unknowns.

Allow beakers to cool after digestion and add 6 ml. arsenious acid solution to each. Warm the beakers gently on the hot plate to effect solution and allow to cool to room temperature. Pipette 5 ml. aliquots from each sample into labeled cuvettes and place in a water bath at 30° C. for about 15-20 min. Also warm an amount of ceric sulfate solution in the water bath. Since the temperature markedly affects the rate of reaction, the water bath should have an accurate thermostatic control.

At timed intervals of 30 sec. add 0.5 ml. ceric sulfate to each of eight or ten cuvettes and mix well by inversion with a piece of Saran Wrap or Parafilm over the top.

At 30 sec. intervals read the percent transmission at 420 nm. against a water blank. Thus each tube is read every 4-5 min. Two people can handle as many as 20 tubes at 15 sec. intervals; one technician removes the tubes from the bath at the proper time and the other takes the reading or adds the ceric sulfate. This can be done easily with a little practice. Keep the tubes in the water bath between readings.

Read the tubes at accurately timed intervals, each tube being read at exactly 5, 10, 15, and 20 min., etc. after the addition of ceric sulfate solution. Take readings until the percent transmission is close to 60%.

Calculation and reading: Calculate the rate of reaction by subtracting the spectrophotometric reading closest to 35% from that closest to 60% transmission (ΔT) and dividing by the time interval in minutes (t). With the use of the blank for zero iodine and the five standards previously mentioned that correspond to 2.5, 5.0, 7.5, 10.0, and 15 $\mu g\%$ iodine, plot the $\Delta T/t$ for each standard against the iodine concentration. From the $\Delta T/t$ for the samples, read the $\mu g\%$ directly from the curve.

As the curve is nearly straight, it may be extrapolated somewhat, but if the sample reading corresponds to over 20 $\mu g\%$, the spectrophotometric determination may be repeated using 2.5 ml. solution from the digestion of a blank and 2.5 ml. aliquot from the digestion of the sample and multiplying the results obtained by 2. An immediate decolorization of the sample tube indicates contamination, and the result may be reported merely as over 30 $\mu g\%$ because in this case the exact value is of no significance.

It is necessary to digest a series of standards each time samples are run because there will be some variation from day to day. Also quality control sera of various known concentrations of PBI should be included with each set of determinations.

NOTES: The principal sources of difficulty are the reagents. Some brands of reagent grade chemicals were found unsatisfactory.*

---

*Mallinckrodt's reagent chemicals are excellent. Ceric ammonium sulfate may be purchased from G. Frederick Smith Chemical Co., Columbus, Ohio, by specifying their special grade for PBI determinations. Few reagent difficulties have appeared with the use of these chemicals.

The digestion temperature is fairly critical. The beakers should not be overheated or allowed to boil vigorously. It should take about 45 min. of digestion before the white fumes appear. Then the watch glasses may be removed and the temperature lowered somewhat.

It should be noted that if the serum iodine is high and a smaller aliquot is taken the dilution to 5 ml. is made with the solution from the digestion of a blank, not with redistilled water.

When protected from contamination by organic matter, the ceric sulfate solution should be stable indefinitely. The arsenious acid solution is stable for at least 2 mo. The chloric acid solution slowly deteriorates on standing and should not be used after 2 wk. even when kept in the freezer.

Occasional difficulties have been encountered using chloric acid prepared from an old bottle of perchloric acid that apparently deteriorated on standing. This can be avoided by using fresh acid.

An alternate method of reading and calculation, which is outlined in the dry-ash method, may also be used if desired.

Occasionally a slight turbidity may occur in the solution from the digestion. In this event the solution may be centrifuged for a few minutes and the aliquot taken from the clear supernatant fluid.

Although mercury does not affect PBI results in the dry-ash method, extremely low results (under 0.5 $\mu g\%$) may be encountered in this method as the result of contamination with mercury due to the recent administration of mercurial diuretics or other mercury compounds.

Normal values and interpretation: Normal serum PBI values range from 4-8 $\mu g/100$ ml. In hyperthyroidism, values ranging from 8-25 $\mu g\%$ are found; in hypothyroidism, levels of 0-4 $\mu g\%$ are found. Low values are sometimes found in nephrosis or other conditions with very low serum proteins. In pregnancy there may be a mild elevation of the PBI level. Due to the interference of mercury (wet-ash method), erroneously low results may be found for a few weeks after the administration of mercurial diuretics or other drugs containing mercury. Many x-ray contrast media (such as Priodax, Neo-Iopax, Skiodan, etc.) used in the diagnosis of gallbladder and kidney disorders contain iodine and are apparently absorbed on the serum proteins. They will cause erroneously high values of protein-bound iodine for 6 mo. or longer after their use. Accordingly, all patients should be checked for the prior administration of these compounds before determination of protein-bound iodine. Drugs containing inorganic iodine (e.g., Lugol solution) will cause false high values for a week or so after administration.

Protein-bound iodine by automation[297-299]: Technicon Instruments Corp.* has developed a fully automated procedure using an automated digestion apparatus and standard automated colorimetric equipment for PBI determinations. The method used is a modification of the Zak wet-ash method. The serum is treated manually with an ion exchange resin (Amberlite IRA-401) for removal of inorganic iodine before analysis. This system has been thoroughly evaluated by our laboratories as well as by many other workers in the field of clinical chemistry and has been found to be accurate and precise. Good correlation has been found in comparing the results obtained by automation with those using the dry-ash method of Barker and the wet-ash method of Zak. Although the automated system is designed to analyze samples at the rate of 20/hr. with a sampling-wash ratio of 2:1, our laboratories have increased this rate to 30 samples/hr. by changing the sample-wash ratio to 1:1. The results obtained at these rates agree very well with those obtained at the slower rate.

In fact, today the automated procedure is considered to be the method of choice when a large number of samples are measured. In addition, it has also proved the reliability of the use of ion exchange resin for removal of inorganic iodine, a method we strongly recommend as a substitute for precipitation and washing of proteins in the manual methods.

In addition, the AutoAnalyzer digestor system can be adapted to measure bu-

---

*Technicon Instruments Corp., Ardsley, N. Y.

tanol extractable iodine and thyroxine (T_4) from column eluates.

Butanol extractable iodine (BEI)[300-303]

This is a more specific method for measuring thyroxine because it is less subject to interference by drugs containing inorganic iodine. In this method, thyroxine and triiodothyronine are extracted from acidified serum by butanol. The butanol extract is washed with alkali to remove inorganic iodine and iodotyrosines and is then evaporated.

The subsequent steps in the oxidation and spectrophotometric determinations may be carried out by any of the methods for PBI given previously. Accordingly, only the extraction step will be given here in detail, with such modifications as required for the final steps from the procedures already outlined.

Equipment: In addition to the equipment used in the PBI method chosen, the present method will require 50 ml. separatory funnels.

Reagents:
1. Sulfuric acid (10%). Dilute 10 ml. concentrated sulfuric acid to 100 ml. with redistilled water.
2. Albumin solution. Dissolve 5 gm. bovine albumin in redistilled water to make 100 ml. It is extremely important that this solution be iodine-free. As a precaution, this solution should be treated with anion exchange resin (Amberlite IRA-401).
3. Blau reagent. Dissolve 160 gm. sodium hydroxide and 50 gm. anhydrous sodium carbonate in redistilled water to make 1 L.
4. Normal butanol, reagent grade.

Procedure: Transfer 1 ml. serum to a 15 × 125 mm. test tube. Add, while mixing, 0.1 ml. 10% sulfuric acid, followed by 3 ml. butanol.

Extract serum by mixing with a stirring rod (use a different rod for each sample) and keep the precipitated protein in the lower part of the tube. Mix intermittently over a 10 min. period; then remove the stirring rod. (Keep the same stirring rod for use with the same sample all through the extraction and precipitation procedure.)

Centrifuge to pack the precipitate. Decant the butanol into a small separatory funnel. Make two additional extractions in the same manner and decant into the same funnel.

To the combined butanol extracts add 5 ml. Blau reagent and shake. One-minute extractions are adequate. Discard the lower aqueous layer and repeat the washing twice more. After the third extraction, allow at least 1 hr. for the organic layer to become clear before complete removal of the alkaline extract.

From this point the procedure will vary slightly, depending upon which method of oxidation is used.

Method for chloric acid oxidation: Transfer the butanol extracts to the electrolytic beakers by pouring the liquid from the top of the funnel. Rinse the funnel with about 0.5 ml. butanol and add the latter to the beaker. Also extract 60 ml. butanol with 35 ml. Blau reagent in a 250 ml. separatory funnel. Allow to separate completely and add 9 ml. butanol layer to each of six beakers for use as standards and blank.

Evaporate the butanol on a water bath with the aid of a current of clean air. Add 1 ml. bovine albumin solution to each beaker. Reserve one of the six beakers to which the plain butanol extract was added as a blank, and to the other five beakers add the standards as given in the original chloric acid procedure. To all the beakers add the glass beads and 10 ml. chloric acid solution as given in the original procedure, and proceed with the digestion, dilution, spectrophotometric determination, and calculation exactly as outlined previously.

Method for incineration: Transfer the butanol extract to test tubes such as are used in the incineration procedure. Rinse the funnel with 0.3 ml. butanol and add to the tube. Evaporate the butanol from the tubes in a water bath at 100° C. with the aid of a stream of clean air. Include the butanol blank with the set.

After the butanol has been completely removed, add 1 ml. bovine albumin solution and 1 ml. sodium carbonate-chlorate solution to the tubes. Proceed with the drying, incineration, dilution, and spec-trophotometric determination exactly as outlined previously in the procedure.

Normal values and interpretation: In normal individuals the BEI is approximately 70-80% of the PBI, with a normal range of 3.2-6.4 μg%.

In most instances the PBI gives an acceptable measure of thyroid activity. But there are certain instances in which the serum PBI does not correlate well with the clinical impressions. In studies on medically treated hypothyroid patients a number of PBI values proved unexpectedly high in light of clinical impressions. In hypothyroidism the BEI differs from the PBI by no more than 1 μg%. However, in Lugol-treated patients this difference was observed to be from 4-7 μg%. It is believed that these differences cannot be ascribed merely to inclusion of inorganic iodine in the PBI, but that when inorganic iodine is ingested in therapeutic amounts, some iodine compounds other than thyroxine may be included in the PBI determinations. In some cases, during treatment of thyroid disease the BEI may then be more helpful in following the actual level of thyroid activity than the PBI.

The fever of acute infections or severe liver dysfunction may affect the BEI; thus after the acute phase, the test should be repeated to confirm an abnormal observation obtained during the acute illness. Thiouracil, Itrumil, and similar compounds will exclude the use of the BEI for up to 6 mo.

Roentgenographic contrast media containing organic iodine will interfere with the BEI as they do with the PBI, and similar precautions must be taken. All other precautions in regard to the collection of samples and purity of reagents are as applicable to the BEI as they are to the PBI determination.

Thyroxine (T_4) by column chromatography[304-307]

In this method thyroxine and other iodine compounds are quantitatively removed and absorbed from acidified serum by means of an anion exchange resin column. Protein, iodotyrosines, and certain organic iodine compounds are eluted from the column by dilute acetic acid (pH 2.2) and the remaining organic iodine compounds are then quantitatively eluted with 50% acetic acid (pH 1.4). Three fractions are obtained with this method, and the iodine in each fraction is determined by the ceric-arsenious acid reaction, either by dry- or wet-ashing of the dried aliquots or by the direct method.

Equipment: In addition to the equipment used in the PBI method chosen for final analysis, this method requires a glass column* with an overall length of 260 mm. that has a funnel top (28 mm. ID), a 10 mm. ID column which is 150 mm. in length, a stopcock, and a 2 mm. ID tip which is 20 mm. in length.

Reagents:

1. Acetic acid (0.2N). Dilute 11.6 ml. glacial acetic acid to 1 L. with redistilled water.
2. Sodium acetate (0.2M). Dissolve 27.2 gm. sodium acetate trihydrate in distilled water and dilute to 1 L.
3. Acetate buffer (pH 4.0). Mix 625 ml. 0.2M acetic acid with 150 ml. 0.2M sodium acetate. The pH of this solution should be adjusted to 4.0 ± 0.1.
4. Acetic acid solution (pH 2.2). Mix 100 ml. glacial acetic acid with 1150 ml. redistilled water. Adjust pH to 2.2 ± 0.2.
5. Acetic acid solution (pH 1.4). Mix equal volumes glacial acetic acid and redistilled water. Adjust pH to between 1.3 and 1.4.
6. Glycine solution (12%). Dissolve 12 gm. glycine in water and dilute to 100 ml.
7. Sodium carbonate (4N) and potassium chlorate solution (2%). Dissolve 212 gm. anhydrous sodium carbonate and 20 gm. potassium chlorate in redistilled water and dilute to 1 L.
8. Anion exchange resin. Dowex AGi-X2† (Cl⁻), 200-400 mesh size, is washed three times with pH 1.4 acetic acid solution by a settling and decantation procedure. Then with a pH of 4.0, add acetate buffer until the wash solution reaches pH 4.0 ± 0.1 unit. Pour a slurry of the resin into the special glass column (with glass wool plug placed in bottom) to a height of 4-5 cm. The level of liquid (acetate buffer) is kept above the resin surface before adding serum sample.

NOTE: Bio-Rad Laboratories has recently introduced an accelerated T₄ disposable column that reduces the number of eluates to two and requires a total elution time of 90 min. These columns have been in use in our laboratory and have proved to be excellent for the separation of T₄. The time saved in the preparation of the columns as well as in the elution more than compensates for the cost of the columns.

Procedure: Acidify 2 or 3 ml. serum to pH 3.8 by adding 0.5 ml. pH 2.2 acetic acid solution for each 1 ml. serum. Transfer quantitatively to a prepared resin column, using additional pH 4.0 buffer to aid in the transfer. For each group of samples, carry a column without sample through the entire procedure to be used as a blank. Partially open the stopcock from the column and allow the sample to flow slowly through the column; discard all effluent. When the liquid level falls just below resin surface, add an additional 25 ml. pH 4.0 acetate buffer and allow the level to fall below the resin surface. Successively add two 25 ml. portions of pH 2.2 acetic acid and allow to flow through the column. Allow the column to drain until no further effluent appears. Discard all effluents and close the stopcock. Add to the column exactly 10 ml. pH 1.4 acetic acid and place a 15 ml. graduated centrifuge tube below the column; open stopcock and collect eluate in centrifuge tube. Allow column to drain dry. Label tube fraction No. 1. Repeat last step twice (fraction Nos. 2 and 3), making a total of three 10 ml. fractions collected. Record exact volume of each fraction and mix well by inversion. Pipette duplicate 4 ml. aliquots from each fraction (including the blanks) into 15 × 125 mm. test tubes (if dry-ash method is

*SGA No. 576212 "with stopcock," Scientific Glass Apparatus Co., Bloomfield, N. J.
†Bio-Rad Laboratories, Richmond, Calif.

used) or 250 ml. electrolytic beakers (if wet-ash method is used). Place tubes or beakers in water bath and evaporate contents to dryness. From this point the procedure will vary slightly, depending upon the method of oxidation used.

Dry-ash method: To test tubes containing dried extract add 0.5 ml. 12% glycine solution and 0.5 ml. sodium carbonate–potassium chlorate solution and proceed with the drying, incineration, dilution, and spectrophotometric determination exactly as outlined previously in the procedure.

Calculation: Obtain the micrograms of iodine in a 5 ml. aliquot from the PBI standard curve. Then:

$$\mu\text{g iodine/fraction} =$$
$$\frac{\mu\text{g iodine/5 ml. aliquot} \times 2 \times \text{Vol. of fraction (ml.)}}{4}$$

Subtract the column blank from each fraction and add the corrected iodine contents of the three fractions:

$$\mu\text{g ``thyroxine iodine''/100 ml. serum} =$$
$$\frac{\mu\text{g iodine content of 3 fractions} \times 100}{\text{Ml. serum used in test}}$$

Wet-ash method: To electrolytic beakers containing dried extract add 0.5 ml. 12% glycine solution, 8-10 glass beads, and 10 ml. chloric acid. Proceed with the digestion, dilution, and spectrophotometric determination exactly as outlined previously.

Calculation: Obtain the micrograms of iodine from the PBI standard curve. Then:

$$\mu\text{g iodine/fraction} =$$
$$\frac{\mu\text{g iodine obtained from curve} \times \text{Vol. of fraction (ml.)}}{4}$$

Subtract column blank from each fraction and add the corrected iodine contents of the three fractions. Then:

$$\mu\text{g ``thyroxine iodine''/100 ml. serum} =$$
$$\frac{\mu\text{g iodine content of 3 fractions} \times 100}{\text{Ml. serum used in test}}$$

Direct method: Pileggi and Kessler[304a]

recently described a method for the determination of thyroxine iodine in the column eluates that does not require wet- or dry-ashing. This results in a considerable saving of time and effort. It is considered to be more specific than the ashing methods because it has the ability to determine thyroxine in the presence of many organic iodine contaminants, including x-ray contrast dyes (except for Priodax and Telepaque).

Procedure: Pipette 2 ml. aliquots of the separate column eluates, including the column blank, and 2 ml. aliquots of working standards, including a zero standard of 50% acetic acid, to separate colorimeter tubes. Add 1 drop (0.05 ml.) saturated bromine water to each tube. (Shake 10 ml. water with several drops of liquid bromine and use the yellow supernatant after excess bromine has settled out. CAUTION! Liquid bromine is very corrosive.) After mixing, allow the tubes to stand for 5 min. Add 5 ml. arsenious acid solution to each tube. (Dissolve 1.44 gm. As_2O_3 in 15 ml. 0.5N NaOH, add H_2O to 850 ml., mix, and add 28 ml. HCl and 57.8 ml. concentrated H_2SO_4. Cool and dilute to 1 L.) Mix thoroughly and place in water bath at 37° C. After temperature equilibrium, add 1 ml. ceric sulfate (0.032N) and proceed with the colorimetric determination in the usual manner.

The authors also suggest using a pure thyroxine standard for this procedure since they found that the catalytic activity of T_4 in relation to that of iodide was only 92%. To prepare a standard, dissolve 8.85 mg. pure thyroxine (L-thyroxine, sodium salt, containing 11% H_2O*) in a mixture of 99 vol. methanol and 1 vol. ammonium hydroxide and make up to 50 ml. This solution contains 100 μg/ml. thyroxine iodine (65.4% of T_4 is thyroxine iodine). A working stock solution is prepared by diluting 1 ml. of the standard to 100 ml. with 50% acetic acid to give a solution containing 100 μg% thyroxine iodine. Prepare working standards fresh as needed by diluting 0.25, 0.5, 1.0, 2.0, and 3.0 ml. of working stock solution to

*Calbiochem, Los Angeles, Calif.

100 ml. with 50% acetic acid. These standards contain 0.25, 0.5, 1.0, 2.0, and 3.0 μg% thyroxine iodine. The standard curve is prepared as outlined previously. The values for the various eluate aliquots are read from the curve. Then:

$$\mu\text{g\% T}_4 \text{ iodine/fraction} = \frac{\mu\text{g iodine} \times 10}{2}$$

where 10 is the total volume of the column eluate and 2 is the volume of serum applied to the column, provided the same volume (2 ml.) is added to the colorimeter tubes for standard and sample aliquots. Subtract the column blank from each fraction and add the corrected iodine contents of the three fractions to obtain μg T$_4$ iodine/100 ml. serum.

Normal values and interpretation: The normal range for this procedure is 3.2-6.4 μg%. Normally in the elution pattern almost all the thyroxine is found in the first two fractions, with approximately 70-90% of the total found in the first fraction. The third fraction should not contain any thyroxine. In exogenous organic iodine contamination, significant amounts of iodine are found in the third fraction or the iodine content of fraction two is found to contain more iodine than fraction one. This usually renders the results unacceptable. Contaminants that interfere include Hippuran, Itrumil, Miokon, Orabilex, Telepaque, and Teridax.

Basal metabolism tests

Basal metabolism refers to the metabolism (heat production) during complete mental and physical rest in the postabsorptive (interdigestive or fasting) state and is a measure of the vital processes. It is essentially an index of the activity of the thyroid gland.

Warm-blooded animals maintain their body temperatures at uniform levels; therefore the study of heat production can be considered the principal characteristic of metabolism.

When food and muscular activity are ruled out, the basal metabolism is proportional to the surface area of the body, which in turn is determined by the height and weight, but it varies somewhat with age and sex. The **basal metabolic rate**

(BMR) is the percentage variation from the normal found for an individual of the same height, weight, age, and sex.

DuBois (1915) devised a method of estimating the surface area and published normal standards. Boothby and Sandiford[308] showed that 92.1% of normal individuals have a BMR within ±10% of the DuBois standards (Table 6-21), and 99.3% are within ±15%.

Since metabolism testing involves measurements and comparisons of gas volumes and since gases change with pressure and temperature, the volumes must be corrected to standard conditions: 0° C., 760 mm. Hg, and dryness.

In most basal metabolism machines a premeasured volume of oxygen is admitted to the breathing circuit and the time required for its consumption is estimated. A thermally responsive calibrating needle indicates the pressure at which the oxygen contained in the chamber is equivalent to the predetermined volume at standard temperature and pressure.

Fig. 6-16 shows the principles involved in the measurement of basal metabolism in the so-called closed-circuit apparatus. During inhalation an increase in vol. G_1 causes a decrease of G_2 by an equal

Table 6-21. DuBois normal standards as modified by Boothby and Sandiford*

Age (yr.)	Males	Fe- males	Age (yr.)	Males	Fe- males
		Cal./m.²/hr.			
5	53.0	51.6	20-24	41.0	36.9
6	52.7	50.7	25-29	40.3	36.6
7	52.0	49.3			
8	51.2	48.1	30-34	39.8	36.2
9	50.4	46.9	35-39	39.2	35.8
10	49.5	45.8	40-44	38.3	35.3
11	48.6	44.6	45-49	37.8	35.0
12	47.8	43.4			
13	47.1	42.0	50-54	37.2	34.5
14	46.2	41.0	55-59	36.6	34.1
15	45.3	39.6	60-64	36.0	33.8
16	44.7	38.5	65-69	35.3	33.4
17	43.7	37.4			
18	42.9	37.3	70-74	34.8	32.8
19	42.1	37.2	75-79	34.2	32.3

*From the Mayo Clinic preliminary report: Amer. J. Physiol. **90:**291, 1929.

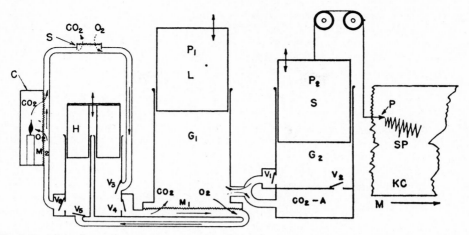

Fig. 6-16. Physiology of respiratory metabolism and measurement of closed-circuit spirometer type of metabolism apparatus. (From Glasser, editor: Medical physics, Chicago, 1951, Year Book Medical Publishers, Inc.)

amount. The opposite state of affairs holds true for exhalation. The spirometer movements are recorded by a kymograph. In addition to the volumetric exchanges between G_1 and G_2, there is a steady decrease in their combined volumes due to the diffusion of oxygen into the blood in response to metabolic requirements. The carbon dioxide that is released from the lungs is absorbed by lime in the metabolism apparatus at the same rate as it is produced, and therefore it does not volumetrically affect the system G_1 plus G_2. As oxygen diffuses from the lungs into the blood and tissues, there is a progressive decrease in the vol. G_1 plus G_2, and therefore a shift occurs in the level of the spirogram. Oxygen absorption within the lungs is thus a close measure of the rate of intracellular oxidation and heat production and thus of metabolism.

In recent years new machines have been developed commercially that either administer a standardized amount of oxygen and measure the consumption time or standardize the time and measure the amount of oxygen or air consumed. The Jones basal metabolism unit* supplies a standard liter oxygen. The Sanborn Me-

tabolator* standardizes the time that the patient breathes the oxygen-air mixture. The Jones air basal unit uses room air, and the volume of oxygen used by the patient can be read from a dial. The L-F basal meter† is a fully automatic, self-calculating, direct-reading machine.

Usual indications for metabolism tests: The indications include enlargement of the thyroid, exophthalmos, tachycardia, tremor, nervousness, marked loss or gain in weight, and sluggish mentality or vitality.

Preparation of patient: When the appointment for the test is made, explain to the patient that the test is very simple, that it measures the amount of oxygen consumed while the patient is comfortable and at rest, and that there is no reason for anxiety. The physician should not tell the patient that an operation may depend upon the result of the test.

Instruct the patient to eat a light dinner, to take no medicines, to go to bed by 10 P.M., to omit morning exercises, to take nothing whatsoever to eat or drink except water, and to report for the test with as little exertion as possible. The patient may smoke as usual. It is

---

*Jones Metabolism Equipment Co., Chicago, Ill.

*Sanborn Co., Waltham, Mass.
†The Liebel-Flarsheim Co., Cincinnati, Ohio.

not necessary to have the patient undress; this will afford the patient more comfort and require less exercise. However, tight clothing (collars, ties, shoes, corsets, girdles) should be loosened or removed.

Have the patient rest quietly in bed for 30 min. preceding the test. Ascertain whether the patient has carried out instructions. Take temperature, pulse, and respiration. Fill out record card completely.

Significance of basal metabolism: The BMR increases rapidly from birth to about 1½ yr. of age and then gradually declines (Table 6-22). The rate in men is about 7% greater than that in women. In Orientals the rate is 5-10% less than the DuBois standards.

Physiologically, in pregnancy there is an increase equal only to that of the fetus (10-25%) and a slight decrease occurs during sleep. Menstruation causes no significant change (lowest during the period and rising to a peak just before the next period), but when it is accompanied by marked pain or psychic changes, postpone the test.

Pathologically, the rate is increased by severe pain, fevers (about 7% for each degree F.), paralysis agitans, chorea, chills and convulsions, pernicious anemia (30%), leukemia (20-87%), dyspnea (50%), hyperpituitarism (up to 46%),

Table 6-22. Benedict-Talbot standards for children (Cal./hr.)*

Weight (kg.)	Boys	Girls	Weight (kg.)	Boys	Girls
3	6.3	6.3	18	33.5	31.7
4	8.8	9.2	19	34.6	32.5
5	11.3	11.9	20	35.8	33.5
6	13.8	14.6	21	36.9	34.6
7	16.3	16.9	22	37.9	35.6
8	18.5	19.2	23	39.2	36.7
9	20.6	20.8	24	40.2	37.5
10	22.7	22.5	25	41.3	38.8
11	24.6	24.2	26	42.5	39.6
12	26.0	25.4	27	43.5	40.6
13	27.5	26.7	28	44.6	41.7
14	29.0	27.7	29	45.4	42.5
15	30.2	28.8	30	46.5	43.5
16	31.5	29.6	31	47.5	44.6
17	32.5	30.6	32	48.3	45.4

*From Carnegie Institute of Washington, D. C., Publication No. 302.

adenoma of the thyroid with hyperthyroidism (10-40%), thyroiditis, carcinoma of the thyroid, and exophthalmic goiter (15-100%). The rate in hyperthyroidism tends to be higher when liver damage is present (hyperthyroid crisis). It is about normal in colloid goiter.

It is decreased in edema of heart failure or nephritis (20-30%), in nephrosis (15-20%), in hypopituitarism, in some cases of Addison's disease, in many cases of allergy and of chronic arthritis, in undernutrition, in obesity of endocrine origin (normal in other cases), and in hypothyroidism or myxedema (15-50%).

Drugs may affect the rate. Thyroxine increases the rate 2.8%/mg., with a maximum at 1 wk. and the effect lasting 6 wk. Atropine, caffeine, epinephrine, and Pituitrin increase the rate temporarily. Insulin should not be given within several hours before the test.

Morphine and barbituric acid derivatives decrease the rate (about 10%). Iodine decreases the rate in hyperthyroidism, with a maximum usually in 5-10 days, but it has no effect when the rate is normal. If the patient falls asleep, even after taking barbiturates, the slight decrease in the BMR, according to some authorities, only nullifies the increase due to tension from anxiety.

Smoking produces no significant constant change in rate.

Thiouracil given to patients showing hyperthyroidism reduces the BMR slowly, from a few weeks (2-3) to several months (sometimes as long as a year).[309] A rise in the BMR may occur during early treatment in those patients who have been treated with iodine due to loss of the iodine effect. Thiouracil may produce hypersensitiveness, resulting in a skin rash (maculopapular eruption), fever, leukopenia, or granulocytopenia.[310]

Propylthiouracil is less toxic but has been reported to give a severe febrile reaction. The therapeutic results appear similar in every respect to those following use of thiouracil.[311]

Treatment with these drugs is accompanied by an increase of blood cholesterol. A high blood level would indicate danger of myxedema.

Despite the newer thyroid function

tests, the determination of the basal metabolic rate is still a quick screening test of thyroid activity and a gauge of the response to therapy. It is essential for the diagnosis of such recently recognized conditions as euthyroid hypometabolism and hypermetabolism without hyperthyroidism.[312] The BMR measures the overall response of the tissues to the circulating thyroid hormone.

Modification of basal metabolism tests: Since determinations of BMR may be incorrect because of patient anxiety, lack of basal conditions, or youth of the patient, modifications such as the sleeping metabolic rate and the administration of sedatives prior to the test have been introduced.[313]

Achilles tendon reflex: Another test that has been used in the study of thyroid function is the measurement of the Achilles tendon reflex time. Duration of the reflex response upon tapping of the Achilles tendon with a percussion hammer has been found to be increased in hypothyroidism and decreased in hyperthyroidism as compared with that in normal subjects. There is a simple device available (Photomotograph*) for the photoelectric measurement of the reflex time using an electrocardiograph machine as a recorder. The test is very easy to perform and measurement of the time from the electrocardiograph record is relatively simple. With limits of under 290 msec. for hyperthyroid individuals, Squires and Langhorne[314] found the test to be slightly more reliable than the PBI and the radioiodine uptake. It is not subject to the interferences encountered in other methods. Although possibly not strictly a laboratory procedure, it is mentioned here as an additional method for testing thyroid function. For details, the papers by Chaney[315] and Gilson[316] may be consulted or information may be obtained from the manufacturer.

TSH suppression test[317]

The administration of thyroxine to euthyroid subjects will inhibit the secretion of endogenous thyroid hormone and will also suppress the secretion of the thyroid-stimulating hormone (TSH) of the pituitary gland, the level of which is controlled by the level of the circulating endogenous thyroid hormone (feedback mechanism). In hyperthyroidism the thyroid activity cannot be suppressed by the administration of exogenous thyroxine.

Thyroglobulin autoprecipitin test[318]

Circulating antithyroid autoantibodies have been demonstrated in cases of thyroiditis, Hashimoto's disease, and other thyroid diseases (myxedema, etc.). A commercially available latex thyroglobulin reagent (TA-test*) gives a reaction with sera containing precipitin antibodies to human thyroglobulins.

MISCELLANEOUS TESTS
VITAMIN A AND CAROTENE[319-322]

Carotenes are the precursors of vitamin A and are usually determined along with the vitamin. The proteins in the serum are precipitated with alcohol, and carotene and vitamin A are extracted with petroleum ether. The carotenes are measured directly by their absorbance at 450 nm. Vitamin A is determined by the reaction with antimony trichloride in chloroform solution, giving a transient blue color. Since carotenes also produce some color with antimony trichloride, a correction must be made.

Reagents:
1. Carr-Price reagent. Dissolve 25 gm. reagent grade antimony trichloride in chloroform to make 100 ml. Keep at room temperature in a glass-stoppered brown bottle and filter just before use if necessary.
2. Other reagents. Absolute alcohol, chloroform, acetic anhydride, and petroleum ether (boiling point, 30°-60° C.).
3. Standards:
   A. Carotene. Dissolve 50 mg. carotene† in 100 ml. petroleum ether. Keep in a tightly stoppered bottle in the refrigerator. This solution contains 50 mg.% carotene. As required, prepare a working standard by diluting 1 ml. stock

---

*Burdick Corp., Milton, Wis.

*Hyland Laboratories, Los Angeles, Calif.
†No. 3702, Eastman Kodak, Co., Rochester, N. Y.

standard to 50 ml. with petroleum ether to give a standard containing 1 mg.% or 10 μg/ml. Also needed is a standard containing 1 ml. stock standard diluted to 25 ml. with chloroform. This contains 2 mg.% carotene.

B. Vitamin A. Dissolve 40 mg. vitamin A alcohol* in chloroform to make 100 ml. Store in a tightly stoppered bottle in the refrigerator. As needed, prepare a working standard containing 0.4 mg. % or 4 μg/ml. by diluting 1 ml. stock standard to 100 ml. with chloroform.

Extraction procedure: Place 3 ml. plasma or serum in a screw-cap test tube and add dropwise, with agitation, 3 ml. absolute alcohol; then add 6 ml. petroleum ether. Stopper and shake vigorously for 10 min. Centrifuge at slow speed for about 1 min. Pipette off as much as possible of the upper petroleum ether layer, taking care not to remove any of the watery layer.

Carotene determination: Transfer a portion of this extract to a colorimeter cuvette and read at 450 nm. against a blank of petroleum ether. Also read a number of standards set up as follows: To a series of cuvettes add 0.5, 1, 2, and 3 ml. diluted carotene standard (1 mg.%). Then add sufficient petroleum ether to make a total volume of 10 ml. Since 6 ml. petroleum ether contains the carotenes from 3 ml. serum (a 1:2 dilution), the standards containing 5, 10, 20, and 30 μg in 10 ml. are equivalent to 100, 200, 400, and 600 μg% carotene.

Calculation:

$$\frac{\text{OD sample}}{\text{OD standard}} \times \text{Conc. of standard} =$$
$$\text{Conc. of sample } (\mu g\%)$$

One can use the standard with the OD closest to the sample or plot a calibration curve and read the results from the curve.

Vitamin A determination: Measure 4 ml. petroleum ether extract as obtained

---

in the carotene procedure into a colorimeter cuvette and evaporate in a water bath at 40°-50° C., preferably with the aid of a stream of nitrogen or carbon dioxide. Dissolve the residue in exactly 0.5 ml. chloroform and add 1 small drop acetic anhydride. Adjust the colorimeter to 100% T with a chloroform blank at 620 nm., quickly add 3 ml. Carr-Price reagent to the sample cuvette using a pipette with a wide tip, and immediately read in a colorimeter. The color develops rapidly, reaching a maximum in about 15-20 sec. and then fading. Record the maximum reading. Also make similar readings on a series of vitamin A standards by adding to a series of cuvettes 0.1, 0.2, 0.3, and 0.4 ml. diluted vitamin A standard and chloroform to make 0.5 ml. These standards are equivalent to 20, 40, 60, and 80 μg% vitamin A. A correction is made for the carotenes present, which give a small amount of color with the Carr-Price reagent. For this, treat 0.5 ml. chloroform solution of carotene (2 mg.%) with the Carr-Price reagent similar to the sample and vitamin A standards. This will give the color produced by 500 μg% carotene. From the previous standards the correction can be made.

Calculation:

$$\frac{\text{OD sample}}{\text{OD standard}} \times \text{Conc. of standard} =$$
$$\text{Vitamin A } (\mu g\%)$$

One may take the standard reading nearest to the sample or plot a calibration curve from the standard readings and obtain the sample concentration from the curve. In correcting for the amount of carotene, take:

$$\frac{\text{OD Carr-Price reaction of carotene 500 } \mu g\% \text{ standard}}{\text{OD Carr-Price reaction of vitamin A 80 } \mu g\% \text{ standard}}$$
$$\times \frac{80}{500} = \text{F} = \mu g\% \text{ vitamin A}$$

A correction is made per μg% carotene present; e.g., if F = 0.05 and if the carotene concentration is 150 μg%, a correction of 150 × 0.05 = 7.5 μg% must be subtracted from the measured vitamin A concentration.

Normal values and interpretation:
Carotene: The normal range for caro-

tene may be taken as 50-250 μg%. The level in the blood is influenced by the amount of carotene in the diet and may be high on a diet rich in vegetables such as carrots. Increased values have been reported in diabetes mellitus, myxedema, and chronic nephritis. Low values have been found in many patients with steatorrhea or malabsorption syndrome.

Vitamin A: The range of normal values reported in the literature varies considerably but may be taken as 25-75 μg% in adults and 15-60 μg% in infants. If the level is above 20 μg%, it may be assumed that there is no vitamin A deficiency. The absorption of vitamin A is decreased when there is decreased fat absorption, as in steatorrhea; a vitamin A tolerance test has been used in tests for this disease. The techniques vary somewhat, but in general, a dose of about 7500 I.U. vitamin A/kg. body weight is given orally and the blood levels are determined at several timed intervals after the ingestion. Usually, if the level rises to over 500 I.U. (150 μg)/ 100 ml. in 4 or 5 hr. after ingestion, steatorrhea may be excluded. Failure of the serum level to increase this much is not conclusive evidence of the disease. Vitamin A in dosage forms is usually given in terms of international units. One international unit is equivalent to 0.3 μg pure vitamin A alcohol, to 0.344 μg vitamin A acetate, or to 0.6 μg pure beta-carotene.

ASCORBIC ACID[323-325]

Ascorbic acid in plasma: A visual titration is used in this procedure. The proteins in the blood plasma are precipitated with trichloroacetic acid and the supernatant is used to titrate a standardized solution of **2,6-dichlorophenol-indophenol sodium.**

Reagents:
1. Trichloroacetic acid (10%). Dissolve 10 gm. TCA in water and dilute to 100 ml.
2. Acetic acid (10%). Dilute 100 ml. glacial acetic acid with water to 1 L. in a volumetric flask.
3. Ascorbic acid standard (0.02 mg./ ml.). Dissolve 40 mg. pure ascorbic

acid in 10% acetic acid and dilute to 100 ml. in a volumetric flask (0.4 mg./ml.). In a 100 ml. volumetric flask dilute 5 ml. of this solution to volume with 10% acetic acid (0.02 mg./ml.).
4. 2,6-Dichlorophenol-indophenol sodium solution.* Dissolve 40 mg. of the dye in 100 ml. distilled water. One milliliter of this solution is equivalent to 0.2 mg. ascorbic acid. This solution is unstable and should not be used for more than 1 wk.

Standardize against ascorbic acid as follows: Titrate 0.5 ml. dye solution with the diluted ascorbic acid standard solution. This should require 5 ml. to decolorize it. Then 1 ml. dye solution is equivalent to 0.2 mg. ascorbic acid.

Procedure: Mix 4 ml. plasma (separated immediately after withdrawing the blood) with 4 ml. TCA. Centrifuge or filter. Dilute 5 ml. dye solution to 25 ml. with water (equivalent to 0.04 mg. ascorbic acid). Pipette 0.2 ml. of the diluted dye into a test tube and titrate with the unknown filtrate until reddish color has disappeared (colorless).

Calculation: Since 0.2 ml. diluted dye is equivalent to 0.008 mg. ascorbic acid, then:

$$\text{Mg.\% ascorbic acid} = \frac{100}{\text{Ml. titration}} \times$$
$$2 \times 0.008 = \frac{1.6}{\text{Ml. titration}}$$

Normal values and interpretation: The normal range by this method is 0.5-2 mg.%. Plasma ascorbic acid levels are considered of limited value in diagnosing scurvy and subclinical conditions of vitamin C undernutrition. However, values below 0.4 mg.% suggest the possibility of ascorbic acid deficiency.

Ascorbic acid in urine: The same method as described for plasma is used to determine ascorbic acid in urine. The urine must be titrated within a few minutes after voiding or it must be preserved with glacial acetic acid in the proportions of 1 part acetic acid to 9

---

*No. 3963, Eastman Kodak Co., Rochester, N. Y.

parts urine. This will preserve the urine for several hours.

Procedure: Pipette 0.5 ml. standardized undiluted dye to a test tube and add 1 ml. glacial acetic acid. Titrate with urine until the red color disappears. Note the amount of urine required.

Calculation: Since 0.5 ml. dye is equivalent to 0.1 mg. ascorbic acid, then:

$$\text{Mg. ascorbic acid/100 ml. urine} =$$

$$\frac{0.1}{\text{Ml. urine required}} \times 100 = \frac{10}{\text{Ml. urine required}}$$

If the urine has been preserved with acetic acid as described, determine the volume required to decolorize 0.5 ml. dye. Then:

$$\text{Mg. ascorbic acid/100 ml. urine} =$$

$$\frac{11.1}{\text{Ml. urine required}}$$

Normal values and interpretation: The daily urinary output of ascorbic acid varies with the intake; it is approximately half of the intake. The average daily intake ranges from 30-80 mg., with an output of 20-30 mg./day. In vitamin C deficiency, urine ascorbic acid is significantly reduced and may disappear completely.

Ascorbic acid saturation tests: These tests are based on the assumption that previous intake of ascorbic acid has been insufficient; when large doses of the vitamin are administered, the tissues will take up most of the vitamin so that little or none is excreted in the urine. If the intake has been adequate, the individual will excrete appreciable amounts of the administered vitamin.

Ascorbic acid may be given orally or intravenously, and different times may be used for urine specimen collection. Normally, when 500 mg. ascorbic acid (in 5 ml. sterile distilled water) is given intravenously, at least 200 mg. should be excreted 4 hr. after injection.

Procedure: A dosage of 11 mg. ascorbic acid/kg. body weight is given orally. Only one urine specimen is needed for the period of 4-6 hr. after ingestion of the vitamin, which is the time when excretion is at its maximum.

The test is carried out as follows: At a designated time, 11 mg. ascorbic acid/kg. body weight dissolved in 4-6 oz. water is given orally. For an average individual weighing 70 kg. this will correspond to 770 mg. Empty the bladder completely 4 hr. later and discard the urine; then 2 hr. later empty the bladder completely and determine ascorbic acid content using the method previously described.

Repeat test daily until a normal response is obtained.

Normal values and interpretation: Normal individuals excrete approximately 0.8 mg./kg. or about 50 mg. In vitamin C deficiency the excretion may be below 10 mg.

CONGO RED TEST FOR AMYLOID DISEASE[326, 327]

The patient should be in the fasting state. Collect a specimen of urine. Inject intravenously 0.1 ml. Congo red solution containing 0.6% dye/lb. body weight, which is approximately equivalent to the 1% solution of the powdered material formerly used. Collect 15 ml. blood 2 min. later (let clot and retract) for a standard; 1 hr. after the injection collect another 15 ml. blood. Also collect another specimen of urine 1 hr. after the injection of dye.

Centrifuge blood after clotting to obtain clear serum. To 5 ml. of each serum specimen add 5 ml. acetone; mix and centrifuge. Transfer the clear supernatant to photometer cuvettes and read at 520 nm., setting to zero with a 1:1 mixture of distilled water and acetone. The 2 min. specimen is taken as 100% retention, and the amount retained after 1 hr. is calculated as follows:

$$\frac{\text{OD of 1 hr. specimen}}{\text{OD of 2 min. specimen}} \times 100 = \%\,\text{Retained}$$

$$100\% - \%\,\text{Retained} = \%\text{ that has disappeared}$$

Also test the specimen of urine for the dye by making it strongly acid with hydrochloric acid. A blue color is positive. The amount excreted may be calculated by comparing the color with that of a standard made up with urine of a similar color. Filter 5 ml. portions and add 10 drops gum ghatti and 2 drops concentrated hydrochloric acid to each and compare.

Normally less than 40% of the dye disappears from the plasma in 1 hr., and only traces are found in the urine. In nephrosis there is a rapid disappearance from the blood, usually 40-60% in 1 hr., but the dye is excreted in the urine adsorbed by the albumin. In amyloid disease, 30-100% (usually 90-100%) disappears in 1 hr., being adsorbed by the amyloid. When the plasma protein is decreased, even without albuminuria, the findings may suggest amyloid disease.

Congo red solution: A 0.6% solution of sterile dye for intravenous use may be obtained commercially.*

NOTE: The Congo red dye used should be known to be nontoxic to animals.

ANALYSIS OF BILIARY CALCULI

Grind up calculi in mortar. Extract 1 portion with ether (about 10 ml.) and filter. Test filtrate for cholesterol as follows:

1. Add equal parts of ether extract and alcohol, let evaporate, and examine microscopically for cholesterol crystals.
2. When dry, dissolve in about 2-3 ml. chloroform and add 1 ml. acetic anhydride and 2-3 drops concentrated sulfuric acid. Cholesterol gives a green color.

Test small portions of residue on microslides as follows:

1. For calcium. Dissolve in hydrochloric acid and add ammonium oxalate saturated solution, adjusting to a yellow color with methyl red and phenol red indicators, and examine microscopically for calcium oxalate crystals.
2. For phosphates. Dissolve in 1 drop concentrated nitric acid. Add a few drops of saturated ammonium molybdate solution and heat. A yellow precipitate indicates phosphates. Or dissolve in acetic acid and add ammonia. Phosphates give a white

precipitate which is crystalline if triple phosphates are present and amorphous if earthy phosphates are present.

3. For iron. Dissolve in 10% hydrochloric acid by heating to dryness. Add potassium ferrocyanide; ferric iron gives a blue color (precipitate). Add potassium ferricyanide; ferrous iron gives a blue color (precipitate). Or heat with a drop of nitric acid, evaporate to dryness, and add 1 drop potassium thiocyanate. A salmon-red color indicates iron.

Test another portion of the powder for bile as follows: Extract a portion with chloroform. Place a few drops on filter paper and add 1 drop Fouchet reagent. A green color indicates bile. Evaporate a portion and take up with water. Test with yellow nitric acid. A green color indicates bilirubin.

Extract again with hot alcohol and test with yellow nitric acid. A green color indicates biliverdin.

STANDARD SOLUTIONS AND BUFFERS
NORMAL SOLUTIONS

Standard acids and bases of known concentration are of great importance in analytic procedures. If only small amounts are used, they may be purchased already standardized. If larger amounts are used, it is often more convenient, besides being less expensive, to use standardized solutions made up in the laboratory. Since sulfuric acid solutions are probably the most stable and accurate solutions, this acid is the best for a secondary standard against which the other acids and bases can be standardized.

A normal solution contains 1 gm. replaceable hydrogen or its equivalent per liter; i.e., it contains 1 gm. equivalent weight (the molecular weight divided by the number of hydrogen atoms or hydroxyl radicals) per liter.

To make approximately 1N solutions of the common acids and bases the following amounts are required (for many purposes, such as reagents, exact normality is not required).

*George A. Breon & Co., Kansas City, Mo.

Acids: Dilute the following amounts of concentrated acids to 1 L. with distilled water:

1. Sulfuric acid, 28 ml.
2. Hydrochloric acid, 86 ml.
3. Nitric acid, 65 ml.
4. Glacial acetic acid, 58 ml.

Bases:

1. Ammonium hydroxide. Dilute 68 ml. concentrated solution to 1 L.
2. Sodium hydroxide. Dissolve 40 gm. in water to 1 L.
3. Potassium hydroxide, 60 gm. Dissolve in water to 1 L.

Preparation of standard acids and bases:

Sulfuric acid (1N). For most purposes requiring accurately known normality, acids stronger than 1N will not be required. Hence if a 1N solution is accurately prepared, lower normalities can be prepared by dilution, using volumetric pipettes and flasks. Add 60 ml. concentrated sulfuric acid to 2 L. distilled water (this solution will be slightly stronger than 1N). For standardization use Tris (hydroxymethyl)aminomethane. This compound is now available in a very pure form for use as a primary standard.* Accurately weigh out approximately 3 gm. Tris; any weight between 3 and 3.5 gm. is satisfactory, but the exact weight must be accurately known. Transfer quantitatively to a beaker with about 50 ml. distilled water and titrate with the sulfuric acid, using a few drops of ethyl orange as indicator† (0.2 gm. in 100 ml. 22% methyl alcohol). Calculate the exact normality of the sulfuric acid solution from the following formula:

$$\text{Normality} = \frac{\text{Wt. Tris}}{(\text{Ml. titration}) \times 0.12114}$$

Calculate the amount of distilled water necessary to dilute to exactly 1N by means of the following formula:

$$\frac{\text{Actual normality} - \text{Desired normality}}{\text{Desired normality}} \times \text{Vol.}$$

$$\text{solution to be diluted}$$

If, for example, the actual normality was

*Tham, Fisher Scientific Co., New York, N. Y.; Sigma 121, Sigma Chemical Co., St. Louis, Mo.
†No. A122, Eastman Kodak Co., Rochester, N. Y.

1.065 and it was desired to dilute 2 L. of this normality to exactly 1N, the required amount of water to be added would be as follows:

$$\frac{1.065 - 1.000}{1.000} \times 2000 = 130 \text{ ml. water to be}$$

added

Add slightly less than the calculated amount of distilled water to the sulfuric acid solution, mix well, repeat the standardization with another weighed sample of Tris, and calculate the new normality. If the normality is now between 1.005 and 1.000, repeat the standardization with two additional samples of Tris and calculate the normality from the average of the three values. Add the calculated amount of additional water to bring to exactly 1N and mix well. This solution is stable indefinitely if kept well stopped in a glass-stoppered bottle.

Sodium hydroxide standard solution: This is best prepared from 50% (w/w) solution that is available commercially and is practically carbonate-free. For a 1N solution dissolve 80 gm. solution in recently boiled and cooled distilled water to make 1 L. The concentrated solution should be weighed rapidly, avoiding excess contact with air, but need not be accurately weighed. Accurately pipette 25 ml. cooled sodium hydroxide solution to a beaker, add 50 ml. water, and titrate with the 1N sulfuric acid to the methyl red end point. Calculate the normality from the relationship.

$$\text{Normality of base} =$$
$$\frac{\text{Ml. acid} \times \text{Normality of acid}}{\text{Ml. base}}$$

Adjust to approximately 1N by the same method as used for the sulfuric acid, make several titrations, calculate the average normality, and adjust to exactly 1N. The sodium hydroxide solution should be kept in a well-stoppered polyethylene bottle. In preparing more dilute solutions of sodium hydroxide it is well to use distilled water that has been recently boiled and cooled.

Hydrochloric acid standard solution (1N). Dilute 86 ml. concentrated hydrochloric acid to 1 L. with water. Standardize either as for sulfuric acid or against the sodium hydroxide solution. Adjust to exact normality.

BUFFER SOLUTIONS[328-332]

The pH scale is a logarithmic scale for the expression of the acidity or alkalinity of a solution. It may be defined as the logarithm of the reciprocal of the hydrogen ion concentration. A 0.1N solution of a strong acid will have a pH of about 1, that of an exactly neutral solution (pure water) will have a pH of 7, and a 0.1N solution of a strong base, a pH of about 13. Many reactions, especially enzymatic reactions, will proceed only in a certain range of pH values; hence the solutions must be adjusted to the proper pH value. For rough measurements, indicator paper is used; e.g., Nitrazine paper, often used in testing the pH of urine, will indicate the pH in the approximate range of 4-8. There are available commercially a number of indicator papers covering any desired range of pH which enables one to estimate the value to about 0.5 unit or less. For a more accurate value such as is necessary in enzyme substrates, the use of a pH meter is necessary. Such instruments have been mentioned briefly in the discussion of blood pH. There are now on the market a number of line-operated, simple, and relatively inexpensive pH meters that are sufficient for most purposes except accurate blood pH. Such an instrument is a necessity for every laboratory that wishes to make up solutions requiring the control of pH.

Buffer solutions are solutions of a mixture of a weak acid (or base) and its salt which has a definite pH and tends to maintain this pH upon the addition of small quantities of acid or base. A number of buffer solutions have been used, some of them for specialized purposes. The following directions are for a few of the more common buffers which cover a wide range of pH. In the buffers given the pH is that measured at room temperature (about 25° C.); some of the buffers may have a slightly different pH at 37° C. The phthalate buffer will show no appreciable change with temperature, the acetate and phosphate buffers will have a pH of 0.03-0.05 unit less at body temperature, and the Tris and barbital buffers will have a pH of about 0.1 unit less at 37° C. The directions are given for preparing buffers with a definite concentration of salt and acid. The pH value will change somewhat on dilution of the buffer. A twofold dilution may change the pH value by 0.05 unit or more, depending upon the buffer. For many purposes these changes are unimportant, but they should be kept in mind when making up buffers of different concentrations. Unless great care is taken in weighing and using pure chemicals, the pH of the final solution may vary somewhat from the desired value. Hence it is best to check the buffers with a pH meter against known commercial pH standards unless only an approximate pH is desired. In Tables 6-23 to 6-27 the pH values are given in increments of 0.2 unit; interpolation may be readily made to obtain the amounts of solutions required for intermediate values.

Phthalate buffer (0.05M, pH 2.2-3.8): Weigh out 40.83 gm. reagent grade potassium acid phthalate that has been previously dried at 110° C. for several hours, dissolve in water, and dilute to 1 L. This solution is 0.2M in potassium acid phthalate. Also prepare a 0.2N solution of hydrochloric acid as directed in the section on the preparation of standard acids. To prepare the buffer solutions add 50 ml. phthalate solution to a 200 ml. volumetric flask. Add the amount of 0.2N HCl as given in Table 6-23 and dilute to the mark.

Acetate buffer (0.2M, pH 3.6-5.8): Prepare a 0.2M solution of sodium acetate

Table 6-23. Phthalate buffer

pH	0.2N HCl (ml.)	pH	0.2N HCl (ml.)
2.2	46.7	3.2	14.8
2.4	39.6	3.4	9.95
2.6	33.0	3.6	6.0
2.8	26.5	3.8	2.65
3.0	20.4		

Table 6-24. Acetate buffer

pH	0.2M sodium acetate (ml.)	0.2N acetic acid (ml.)	pH	0.2M sodium acetate (ml.)	0.2N acetic acid (ml.)
3.6	7.5	92.5	4.8	59	41
3.8	12.0	88.0	5.0	70	30
4.0	18.0	82.0	5.2	79	21
4.2	26.5	73.5	5.4	86	14
4.4	37.0	63.0	5.6	91	9
4.6	48.0	52.0	5.8	94	6

Table 6-25. Phosphate buffer

pH	M/15 Na_2HPO_4 (ml.)	M/15 KH_2PO_4 (ml.)	pH	M/15 Na_2HPO_4 (ml.)	M/15 KH_2PO_4 (ml.)
5.6	5.0	95.0	7.0	61.1	38.9
5.8	7.8	92.2	7.2	71.5	28.5
6.0	12.0	88.0	7.4	80.6	19.4
6.2	18.5	81.5	7.6	87.0	13.0
6.4	26.6	73.4	7.8	91.5	9.5
6.6	37.5	62.5	8.0	94.6	5.4
6.8	49.8	50.2	8.2	97.0	3.0

by dissolving 27.22 gm. crystalline sodium acetate in water to make 1 L. Prepare a solution of 0.2N acetic acid by diluting 11.5 ml. glacial acetic acid to 1 L. Standardize against sodium hydroxide as outlined in the section on preparation of standard acids, using phenolphthalein as indicator, and dilute to exactly 0.2N. To prepare the buffer solutions mix together the required amounts of the two solutions as given in Table 6-24.

Phosphate buffer (M/15, pH 5.4-8.2): Prepare a solution of M/15 disodium phosphate by dissolving 9.47 gm. reagent grade anhydrous Na_2HPO_4 in water to make 1 L. Prepare a M/15 solution of monopotassium phosphate by dissolving 9.08 gm. reagent grade KH_2PO_4 in water and diluting to 1 L. To prepare the buffer solutions mix together the amounts of the two solutions as given in Table 6-25.

Tris buffer (0.05M, pH 7.2-9.0): Prepare a 0.1M solution of Tris(hydroxymethyl)aminomethane by dissolving 12.11 gm. Tris in water and diluting to 1 L. Also prepare a 0.1N solution of HCl. To prepare the buffers add 50 ml. Tris solution to a 100 ml. volumetric flask, add the required amount of HCl as given in Table 6-26, and dilute to 100 ml.

Veronal buffer (0.1M, pH 6.8-9.4): Prepare a 0.1M solution of sodium diethylbarbiturate (sodium barbital) by dissolving 20.6 gm. salt in water and diluting to 1 L. Also prepare a 0.1N solution of hydrochloric acid. To prepare the buffers mix together the amounts of solutions given in Table 6-27.

ATOMIC WEIGHTS

In Table 6-28 are given the atomic weights of the elements which might be used in clinical chemistry or toxicology. They may be used to calculate the molecular weight of compounds not given in the text.

FORMULAS FOR CALCULATIONS

Gm./100 ml. $=$ sp. gr. $\times$ % by wt.
Approximate normality $=$

$$\frac{10 \, (\text{gm./100 ml.}) \, \surd}{\text{Mol. wt.}} =$$

$$\frac{10 \, (\text{sp. gr.} \times \text{\% by wt.}) \, \surd}{\text{Mol. wt.}}$$

where $\surd$ is the valence.

The number ml. required to make 1 L. approximately normal solution $=$

$$\frac{\text{Mol. wt.} \times 100}{\surd \, (\text{gm./100 ml.})} = \frac{\text{Mol. wt.} \times 100}{\surd \, (\text{sp. gr.} \times \text{\% by wt.})}$$

where $\surd$ is the valence.

The results of the calculations in Table

Table 6-26. Tris buffer

pH	0.1N HCL (ml.)	pH	0.1N HCl (ml.)
7.2	45.0	8.2	23.3
7.4	42.0	8.4	17.5
7.6	38.9	8.6	12.8
7.8	34.0	8.8	9.0
8.0	29.0	9.0	6.3

6-29 are approximately as follows (Table 6-30).

MILLIEQUIVALENTS

The results of the determinations of the electrolytes are sometimes expressed in milliequivalents per liter instead of milligrams per 100 ml.

Table 6-27. Veronal buffer

pH	0.1M Na barbital (ml.)	0.1N HCl (ml.)	pH	0.1M Na barbital (ml.)	0.1N HCl (ml.)
6.8	52.2	47.8	8.2	76.9	23.1
7.0	53.6	46.4	8.4	82.3	17.7
7.2	55.4	44.6	8.6	87.1	12.9
7.4	58.1	41.9	8.8	90.8	9.2
7.6	61.5	38.5	9.0	93.6	6.4
7.8	66.2	33.8	9.2	95.2	4.8
8.0	71.6	28.4	9.4	97.4	2.6

Table 6-28. International atomic weights (1961)

Element	Symbol	Atomic weight	Element	Symbol	Atomic weight
Aluminum	Al	26.9815	Magnesium	Mg	24.312
Antimony	Sb	121.75	Manganese	Mn	54.9380
Arsenic	As	74.9216	Mercury	Hg	200.59
Barium	Ba	137.34	Molybdenum	Mo	95.94
Bismuth	Bi	208.980	Nickel	Ni	58.71
Boron	B	10.811	Nitrogen	N	14.0067
Bromine	Br	79.909	Oxygen	O	15.9994
Calcium	Ca	40.08	Phosphorus	P	30.9738
Carbon	C	12.0111	Platinum	Pt	195.09
Cerium	Ce	140.12	Potassium	K	39.102
Chlorine	Cl	35.453	Selenium	Se	78.96
Chromium	Cr	51.996	Silicon	Si	28.086
Cobalt	Co	58.9332	Silver	Ag	107.870
Copper	Cu	63.54	Sodium	Na	22.9898
Fluorine	F	18.9984	Strontium	Sr	87.62
Gold	Au	196.967	Sulfur	S	32.064
Hydrogen	H	1.00797	Tin	Sn	118.69
Iodine	I	126.9044	Tungsten	W	183.85
Iron	Fe	55.847	Uranium	U	238.03
Lead	Pb	207.19	Vanadium	V	50.942
Lithium	Li	6.939	Zinc	Zn	65.37

Table 6-29

Grade CP		Molecular weight	Specific gravity	% by weight
Hydrochloric acid	HCl	36.5	1.19	37.0
Sulfuric acid	H_2SO_4	98.1	1.84	96.0
Nitric acid	HNO_3	63.0	1.42	70.0
Phosphoric acid (syrupy)	H_3PO_4	98.0	1.69	85.0
Acetic acid	CH_3COOH	60.0	1.06	99.5
Ammonium hydroxide	NH_4OH	35.0	0.90	28.0(NH_3) 57.6(NH_4OH)

The "equivalent" or the "equivalent weight" is the atomic weight divided by the valence.

The "milliequivalent weight" is one thousandth of the equivalent weight.

The weight in grams of any substance per liter divided by the milliequivalent weight (mEq. wt.) gives the number of milliequivalents per liter according to the following formula:

$$MEq. = \frac{Wt.\ in\ gm./L.}{MEq.\ wt.}$$

To convert milligrams per 100 ml. (mg.%) to milliequivalents per liter (mEq./L.) divide the amount in milligrams per liter (mg.% $\times$ 10) by the equivalent weight (Eq. wt.) of the substance.

$$MEq./L. = \frac{Mg.\% \times 10}{Eq.\ wt.\ substance}$$

For example, if serum sodium is 330 mg./100 ml., then there are 3300 mg./L. The equivalent weight of sodium is 23. Therefore:

$$MEq./L. = \frac{330 \times 10}{23} = 144$$

If the serum calcium is 10 mg./100 ml., then the mEq./L. would be:

$$\frac{10 \times 10}{40 \div 2}\ or\ \frac{10 \times 10 \times 2}{40} = 5$$

Table 6-30

	Normality (approximate)	Ml./L. to make 0.1N solution (approximate)
HCl	12.1	83.0
H$_2$SO$_4$	36.0	28.0
HNO$_3$	15.7	64.0
H$_3$PO$_4$	44.0	23.0
CH$_3$COOH	17.4	57.5
NH$_4$OH	14.8	67.5

Table 6-31. Table of equivalents

1 gr.	0.065	gm.	65	mg.
1 oz. (avoirdupois)	28.350	gm.	437.5	gr.
1 oz. (troy, apothecaries')	31.103	gm.	480.0	gr.
1 lb. (avoirdupois)	453.59	gm.		
1 lb. (troy, apothecaries')	373.2	gm.		
1 mg.	1/65	gr.	1000	μg
1 gm.	15.43	gr.	1000	mg.
1 kg.	2.2	lb. (avoirdupois)	1000	gm.
1 fl. oz.	29.573	ml.		
1 pt.	473.176	ml.		
1 qt.	0.946	L.		
1 gal.	3.785	L.	231.0	cu. in.
1 ml.	16	minims		
1 L.	1.0567	qt.	0.2642	gal.
1 cu. in.	16.387	ml.		
1 cu. ft.	28.3	liters	7.48	gal.
1 in.	25.4	mm.		
1 ft.	0.3048	m.		
1 yd.	0.9144	m.		
1 m.	39.37	in.	3.2808	ft.
1 mm.	1000	microns (μ)		
1 Ångström (Å or A)	0.1	mμ or nm.	0.0001	μ

Autoclave		
Pressure (lb.)	° C.	° F.
5	107.7	226
10	115.5	240
15	121.6	251
20	126.6	260

Temperatures
Degrees F. = (Degrees C. $\times$ 1.8) + 32
Degrees C. = (Degrees F. − 32) $\div$ 1.8

Since phosphorus in extracellular fluid is 20% univalent (BH_2PO_4) and 80% bivalent (B_2HPO_4), the valence is taken as 1.8.

The vol.% CO_2 is converted to mEq./L. by dividing by 2.22 or multiplying by 0.45.

The protein in gm./100 ml. is converted to mEq./L. by multiplying by the Van Slyke factor, 2.43.

NOTE: The mEq./L. may be calculated rapidly by multiplying the mg.% by the following factors: Ca × ½; Cl × 0.28; Cl from NaCl × 0.171; K × ¼; Na × 0.435; P × 0.58.

EQUIVALENTS

Equivalents are given in Table 6-31.

REFERENCES

1. Caraway, W. T.: Amer. J. Clin. Path. 37:445, 1962.
2. Sinton, S.: In Meites, S., editor: Standard methods of clinical chemistry, New York, 1965, Academic Press, Inc., vol. 5.
3. MacFate, R. P., Cohn, C., Eichelberger, L., and Cooper, J. A. D.: Amer. J. Clin. Path. 24:511, 1954.
4. Snell, F. D., and Snell, C. T.: Colorimetric methods of analysis, ed. 2, New York, 1937, D. Van Nostrand Co., Inc.
5. MacIntyre, H.: Advances Clin. Chem. 4:1, 1961.
6. Zettner, A.: Advances Clin. Chem. 7:1, 1963.
7. Udenfriend, S.: Fluorescence assay in biology and medicine, New York, 1962, Academic Press, Inc.
8. Block, R. J., Durrum, E. D., and Zweig, G.: Manual of paper chromatography and paper electrophoresis, ed. 2, New York, 1957, Academic Press, Inc.
9. Bobbitt, J. M.: Thin layer chromatography, New York, 1963, Reinhold Publishing Corp.
10. Littlewood, A. B.: Gas chromatography, New York, 1962, Academic Press, Inc.
11. Purnell, H.: Gas chromatography, New York, 1962, John Wiley & Sons, Inc.
12. Natelson, S.: Microtechniques of clinical chemistry, Springfield, Ill., 1957, Charles C Thomas, Publisher.
13. Knights, E. M., Jr., McDonald, R. D., and Ploompuu, J.: Ultramicro methods for clinical laboratories, ed. 2, New York, 1962, Grune & Stratton, Inc.
14. Saifer, A., Gerstenfeld, S., and Zymaris, M. C.: Clin. Chem. 4:127, 1958.
15. Marsh, W. H.: Advances Clin. Chem. 2:301, 1959.
16. Bruan, D. J., et al.: Clin. Chem. 12:137, 1966.
17. Skeggs, L. T., Jr.: In Meites, S., editor: Standard methods of clinical chemistry, New York, 1965, Academic Press, Inc., vol. 5.
18. Folin, O., and Wu, H.: J. Biol. Chem. 38:81, 1919.
19. Haden, R. L.: J. Biol. Chem. 56:469, 1923.
20. Somogyi, M.: J. Biol. Chem. 160:69, 1945.
21. Greenwald, T.: J. Biol. Chem. 34:97, 1918.
22. Somogyi, M.: J. Biol. Chem. 195:19, 1952.
23. Nelson, N.: J. Biol. Chem. 153:375, 1944.
24. Folin, O., and Wu, H.: J. Biol. Chem. 41:367, 1920.
25. Sunderman, W., and Fuller, J. B.: Amer. J. Clin. Path. (tech. section) 21:1077, 1951.
26. Peters, J. P., and Van Slyke, D. D.: Quantitative clinical chemistry, interpretations, ed. 2, Baltimore, 1946, The Williams & Wilkins Co., vol. 1.
27. Manger, M., and Farese, G.: Amer. J. Clin. Path. 44:104, 1965.
28. McDonald, G. W., Fisher, G. F., and Burnham, C. E.: Public Health Rep. 79:515, 1964.
29. Exton, W. G., and Rose, A. R.: Amer. J. Clin. Path. 4:381, 1934.
30. Sindoni, A., Jr.: Amer. J. Dig. Dis. 13:178, 1946.
31. Langer, P. H., and Fies, H. L.: Amer. J. Clin. Path. 11:41, 1941.
32. Thorn, G. W., et al.: J. Clin. Invest. 19:813, 1940.
33. Soskin, S.: J. Clin. Endocr. 4:75, 1944.
34. Unger, R. H., and Madison, L. L.: J. Clin. Invest. 37:627, 1958.
35. Unger, R. H., and Madison, L. L.: Diabetes 7:455, 1958.
36. Fajans, S. S., and Conn, J. W.: J. Lab. Clin. Med. 54:811, 1959.
37. Sondergaard, G.: Scand. J. Clin. Lab. Invest. 10:203, 1958.
38. Coulombe, J. J., and Favreau, L.: Clin. Chem. 9:102, 1963.
39. Fawcett, J. K., and Scott, J. E.: J. Clin. Path. 13:149, 1961.
40. Searcy, R. L., Gough, G. S., Korotzer, J. L., and Bergquist, L. M.: Amer. J. Med. Techn. 27:255, 1961.
41. Van Slyke, D. D., Page, I. H., Hiller, A., and Kirk, E.: J. Clin. Invest. 14:901, 1935.
42. Koch, F. C., and McMeekin, T. L.: J. Amer. Chem. Soc. 46:2066, 1924.
43. Chaney, A. L., and Marbach, E. P.: Clin. Chem. 8:131, 1962.
44. Mosenthal, H. O., and Bruger, M.: Arch Intern. Med. 55:411, 1935.
45. Caraway, W. T.: Amer. J. Clin. Path. 25:140, 1955.
46. Alper, C., and Seitchik, J.: Clin. Chem. 3:95, 1957.
47. Feichtmeir, T. V., and Wrenn, H. T.: Amer. J. Clin. Path. 25:833, 1955.
48. Bosnes, H. W., and Taussky, H. H.: J. Biol. Chem. 158:581, 1945.

49. Taussky, H. H.: J. Biol. Chem. **208**:853, 1954.
50. Brod, J., and Sirota, J. H.: J. Clin. Invest. **27**:645, 1945.
51. Hutchinson, J. H., and Labby, D. H.: J. Lab. Clin. Med. **60**:170, 1962.
52. Foreman, D. T.: Clin. Chem. **10**:497, 1964.
53. Miller, G. E., and Rice, J. D.: Amer. J. Clin. Path. **39**:97, 1963.
54. Khachadurian, A., Knox, W. E., and Cullen, A. M.: J. Lab. Clin. Med. **56**:321, 1960.
55. Siest, D., Siest, G., and Besson, S.: Bull. Soc. Pharm. (Nancy) **51**:19, 1961.
56. Scott, J. E., and West, E. S.: Industr. & Engin. Chem. **9**:50, 1937.
57. Sobel, A. E., Yuska, H., and Cohen, J.: J. Biol. Chem. **118**:443, 1937.
58. Kirk, P. L.: Advances Protein Chem. **3**:139, 1947.
59. Kinsley, G. R.: J. Biol. Chem. **131**:197, 1939.
60. Weichselbaum, T. E.: Amer. J. Clin. Path. **7**:40, 1946.
61. Gutman, A. B.: Advances Protein Chem. **4**:155, 1948.
62. Marrach, J. R., and Hoch, H.: J. Clin. Path. **2**:161, 1949.
63. Henry, R. J., Sobel, C., and Segalove, M.: Proc. Soc. Exp. Biol. Med. **92**:748, 1956.
64. Ellis, A. W.: Lancet, **1**:1, 1942.
65. Tiselius, A.: Biochem. J. **31**:313, 1937.
66. Armstrong, S. H., Jr., Budka, M. J. E., and Morrison, K. C.: J. Amer. Chem. Soc. **69**:416, 1947.
67. Dole, V. P.: J. Clin. Invest. **23**:708, 1944.
68. Jencks, W. P., Jetton, M. R., and Durrum, E. L.: Biochem. J. **60**:205, 1955.
69. Kaplan, A., and Savory, J.: Clin. Chem. **11**:937, 1965.
70. Sunderman, F. W., Jr.: Amer. J. Clin. Path. **42**:1, 1964.
71. Moore, D. H., et al.: Amer. J. Obstet. Gynec. **57**:312, 1949.
72. Stefanini, M., and Dameshek, W.: The hemorrhagic disorders, New York, 1955, Grune & Stratton, Inc.
73. Reiner, M., and Cheung, H. I.: Clin. Chem. **5**:414, 1959.
74. Losner, S., and Volk, B. W.: Amer. J. Med. Sci. **232**:276, 1956.
75. Jacobsson, K.: Scand. J. Clin. Lab. Invest. **14**:7, 1955.
76. Eliot, W. E.: J. Biol. Chem. **197**:641, 1952.
77. Kilbrick, A. C., Ross, M., and Rogers, H. E.: Proc. Soc. Exp. Biol. Med. **81**:353, 1952.
78. Bachra, B. N., Dauer, A., and Sobel, A. E.: Clin. Chem. **4**:107, 1958.
79. Gomori, G.: J. Lab. Clin. Med. **27**:955, 1942.
80. Maclay, E.: Amer. J. Med. Techn. **17**:265, 1951.
81. Hodgkinson, A.: Clin. Sci. **21**:125, 1961.
82. Nordin, B. E. C., and Frazer, R.: Lancet **1**:947, 1960.
83. Orange, M., and Rhein, H. C.: J. Biol. Chem. **189**:379, 1951.
84. Andreasen, K.: Scand. J. Clin. Lab. Invest. **9**:138, 1957.
85. Trinder, P.: J. Clin. Path. **9**:170, 1956.
86. Peters, T., et al.: J. Lab. Clin. Med. **48**:274, 1956.
87. Cartwright, G. E., and Wintrobe, M. M.: J. Clin. Invest. **28**:86, 1949.
88. Rice, E. W.: J. Lab. Clin. Med. **55**:325, 1960.
89. Giorgio, A. G., Cartwright, G. E., and Wintrobe, M. M.: Amer. J. Clin. Path. **41**:22, 1964.
90. Cartwright, G. E., and Wintrobe, M. M.: Amer. J. Clin. Nutr. **15**:94, 1964.
91. Stone, G. C. H., and Goldzieher, J. W.: J. Biol. Chem. **181**:511, 1949.
92. Butterworth, E. C.: J. Clin. Path. **4**:99, 1951.
93. Barry, J. M., and Rowland, S. J.: Biochem. J. **53**:213, 1953.
94. Jacobs, H. R. D., and Hofmann, W. S.: J. Biol. Chem. **93**:685, 1931.
95. Skinner, S. L.: Lancet **1**:498, 1961.
96. Shales, O., and Shales, S. S.: J. Biol. Chem. **140**:879, 1941.
97. Falconer, M. A., Osterberg, A. E., and Bargen, J. A.: Arch Surg. **38**:869, 1939.
98. Platt, R.: Clin. Sci. **9**:367, 1950.
99. Gamble, J. L.: Chemical anatomy, physiology and pathology of extracellular fluid, Cambridge, 1947, Harvard University Press.
100. Robinson, F. J., Power, M. H., and Kepler, E. J.: Proc. Staff Meet. Mayo Clin. **16**:577, 1941.
101. Kepler, E. J., Robinson, F. J., and Power, M. H.: J.A.M.A. **118**:1404, 1942.
102. Cotlove, E., Trautham, H. V., and Bowman, R. L.: J. Lab. Clin. Med. **51**:461, 1958.
103. Cotlove, E.: In Seligson, D., editor: Standard methods of clinical chemistry, New York, 1960, Academic Press, Inc., vol. 3.
104. Peters, J. P., and Van Slyke, D. D.: Quantitative clinical chemistry, methods, Baltimore, 1932, The Williams & Wilkins Co., vol. 2.
105. Natelson, S., and Manning, C. M.: Clin. Chem. **1**:165, 1955.
106. Holaday, D. A., and Verosky, M.: J. Lab. Clin. Med. **47**:634, 1956.
107. Gambino, S. R., and Scheiber, H.: Amer. J. Clin. Path. **45**:406, 1966.
108. Gambino, S. R.: In Meites, S., editor: Standard methods of clinical chemistry, New York, 1965, Academic Press, Inc., vol. 5, p. 169.
109. Weisberg, H. F.: Water and electrolyte balance, ed. 2, Baltimore, 1962, The Williams & Wilkins Co.
110. Gambino, S. R.: J.A.M.A. **198**:250, 1966.
111. Johnstone, J. W.: In Seligson, D., editor: Standard methods of clinical chemistry, New York, 1963, Academic Press, Inc., vol. 4, p. 183.

112. Van Kampen, E. J., and Zijlstra, W. G.: Advances Clin. Chem. **8**:167, 1965.
113. Johnson, R. B., Jr.: In Meites, S., editor: Standard methods of clinical chemistry, New York, 1965, Academic Press, Inc., vol. 5, p. 159.
114. Ehrmantraut, H. C.: In Sunderman, F. W., and Sunderman, F. W., Jr., editors: Clinical pathology of the serum electrolytes, Springfield, Ill., 1966, Charles C Thomas, Publisher.
115. Abele, J. E.: Amer. J. Med. Electronics **2**:32, 1963.
116. Hendry, E. B.: Clin. Chem. **8**:246, 1962.
117. Henry, R. J., Golub, O. J., Berkman, S., and Segalove, M.: Amer. J. Clin. Path. **23**:841, 1953.
118. Jendrassik, L., and Grof, P.: Biochem. Z. **297**:81, 1938.
119. Noslin, B.: Scand. J. Clin. Lab. Invest. **13**:1, 1960.
120. Malloy, H. T., and Evelyn, K. A.: J. Biol. Chem. **119**:481, 1937.
121. Malloy, H. T., and Evelyn, K. A.: J. Biol. Chem. **122**:597, 1938.
122. Henry, R. J., Jacobs, S. L., and Chaimori, N.: Clin. Chem. **6**:529, 1960.
123. Watson, C. J.: Amer. J. Clin. Path. **18**:84, 1936.
124. Maclaghan, N. F.: Brit. J. Exp. Path. **27**:190, 1946.
125. Reinhold, J. G.: Advances Clin. Chem. **3**:83, 1960.
126. Hanger, F. M.: J. Clin. Invest. **18**:261, 1939.
127. Hanger, F. M., and Patek, A. J.: Amer. J. Med. Sci. **202**:48, 1941.
128. Reinhold, J. G.: Clin. Chem. **8**:475, 1962.
129. Maclagan, N. F.: Brit. J. Exp. Path. **125**:234, 1944.
130. Kingsbury, F. P., Clark, C. P., Williams, G., and Post, A. L.: J. Lab. Clin. Med. **11**:981, 1926.
131. Shank, R. E., and Hoagland, C. L.: J. Biol. Chem. **162**:133, 1946.
132. Kunkel, H. G.: Proc. Soc. Exp. Biol. Med. **66**:217, 1947.
133. Maclagan, N. F.: Quart. J. Med. **9**:151, 1940.
134. Maclagan, N. F., and Rundel, F. F.: Quart. J. Med. **9**:215, 1940.
135. Meranse, D. R., Likoff, W. B., and Scheeberg, N. G.: Amer. J. Clin. Path. **12**:261, 1942.
136. King, E. J., and Aitken, R. S.: Lancet **2**:543, 1940.
137. Gaebler, O. H.: Amer. J. Clin. Path. **15**:452, 1945.
138. Lavers, G. D., et al.: J. Lab. Clin. Med. **34**:965, 1949.
139. Weichselbaum, T. E., and Probstein, J. G.: J. Lab. Clin. Med. **24**:636, 1939.
140. Mateer, J. G., et al.: Amer. J. Dig. Dis. **9**:13, 1942.
141. Seligson, D., Marino, J., and Dodson, E.: Clin. Chem. **3**:638, 1959.
142. Henry, R. J., Chiamori, M., and Ware, A. G.: Amer. J. Clin. Path. **32**:201, 1959.
143. Stewart, C. P., Scarborough, H., and Davidson, J. N.: Edinburgh Med. J. **44**:105, 1937.
144. Davidson, C. S., et al.: New Eng. J. Med. **234**:279, 1946.
145. Quick, A. J.: Amer. J. Dig. Dis. **6**:716, 1939.
146. Quick, A. J.: Arch. Intern. Med. **57**:544, 1936.
147. Knisely, M. H.: Transactions of tenth conference on liver injury, New York, 1951, The George Macy Companies, Inc.
148. Hsieh, K. M., and Blumenthal, H. T.: Proc. Soc. Exp. Biol. Med. **91**:626, 1956.
149. Wroblewski, F., and LaDue, J. S.: Proc. Soc. Exp. Biol. Med. **90**:210, 1955.
150. Bowers, G. N., Jr., Potter, J. P., Jr., and Norris, R. F.: Amer. J. Clin. Path. **34**:513, 1960.
151. Sterkel, R. L., et al.: J. Lab. Clin. Med. **52**:176, 1958.
152. Reichard, H., and Reichard, P.: J. Lab. Clin. Med. **52**:709, 1958.
153. Knights, E. M., Jr., et al.: J. Lab. Clin. Med. **65**:355, 1965.
154. Sperry, W. M., and Brand, F. C.: J. Biol. Chem. **213**:69, 1955.
155. Pernokis, E. W., Freeland, M. R., and Kraus, I.: J. Lab. Clin. Med. **26**:1978, 1941.
156. Jacobs, S. L., and Henry, R. J.: Clin. Chim. Acta **7**:270, 1962.
157. Schoenheimer, R., and Sperry, W. M.: J. Biol. Chem. **106**:745, 1934.
158. Abell, L., et al.: In Seligson, D., editor: Standard methods of clinical chemistry, New York, 1958, Academic Press, Inc., vol. 2.
159. Bloor, W. R., Pelkan, K. F., and Allen, D. M.: J. Biol. Chem. **52**:191, 1922.
160. Kelsey, H.: J. Biol. Chem. **127**:15, 1939.
161. Ferro, R. V., and Ham, A. B.: Amer. J. Clin. Path. **33**:545, 1960.
162. Zilversmit, D. B., and Davis, A. K.: J. Lab. Clin. Med. **35**:155, 1950.
163. Stern, I., and Shapiro, B.: J. Clin. Path. **6**:158, 1953.
164. Dole, V. P.: J. Clin. Invest. **35**:150, 1956.
165. Laurell, S.: J. Clin. Lab. Invest. **8**:81, 1956.
166. Bierman, E. L., Dole, V. P., and Roberts, T. N.: Diabetes **6**:475, 1957.
167. Van Handel, E., and Zilversmit, D. B.: J. Lab. Clin. Med. **88**:447, 1955.
168. Albrink, M. J.: J. Lipid Res. **1**:53, 1959.
169. Albrink, M. J., Man, E. B., and Peters, J. P.: J. Clin. Invest. **34**:147, 1955.
170. MacGee, J.: Anal. Chem. **31**:298, 1959.
171. DeLalla, O. F., and Gofman, J. W.: Meth. Biochem. Anal. **1**:459, 1954.
172. Gofman, J. W., et al.: Physiol. Rev. **34**:589, 1954.
173. Boyle, E., and Moore, R. V.: J. Lab. Clin. Med. **53**:272, 1959.

174. Burstein, M., and Samaille, J.: Clin. Chim. Acta **5**:609, 1960.
175. Kanabroki, E. L., et al.: Clin. Chem. **4**: 382, 1958.
176. Kunkel, H. G., and Slater, R. J.: J. Clin. Invest. **31**:677, 1952.
177. Ackermann, P. G., Toro, G., and Kountz, W. B.: J. Lab. Clin. Med. **44**:517, 1954.
178. Toro, G., Ackermann, P. G., and Kountz, W. B.: Proc. Soc. Exp. Biol. Med. **101**: 34, 1959.
179. Mann, E. B., and Gildea, E. F.: J. Biol. Chem. **99**:43, 1932.
180. Peters, J. P., and Mann, E. B.: J. Clin. Invest. **22**:707, 1943.
181. Gofman, J., et al.: J. Geront. **9**:4, 1954.
182. Friedman, M. M., and Lapan, B.: J. Lab. Clin. Med. **51**:745, 1958.
183. Sibley, J. A., and Lehninger, A. L.: J. Nat. Cancer Inst. **9**:303, 1948.
184. Sibley, J. A.: Ann. N. Y. Acad. Sci. **75**: 399, 1958.
185. Dreyfus, J. C., Schapira, G., and Schapira, F.: J. Clin. Invest. **33**:794, 1954.
186. Volk, B. W., et al.: Amer. J. Med. Sci. **232**:38, 1956.
187. Beck, W. S.: J. Biol. Chem. **212**:847, 1955.
188. Harris, M. L., Sr.: Amer. J. Med. Techn. **24**:99, 1958.
189. Wilkinson, J. H.: Workshop on clinical enzymology, technical manual, Chicago, 1964, American Society of Clinical Pathologists.
190. Rosalki, S. B.: J. Clin. Path. **15**:566, 1962.
191. Elliot, B. A., and Wilkinson, J. H.: Lancet **1**:698, 1961.
192. Knottinen, A., and Haolmen, P. I.: Amer. J. Cardiol. **101**:525, 1962.
193. Somogyi, M.: J. Biol. Chem. **134**:315, 1940.
194. Somogyi, M.: J. Biol. Chem. **142**:579, 1942.
195. Somogyi, M.: Clin. Chem. **6**:23, 1960.
196. Houchin, O. D.: Clin. Chem. **4**:519, 1958.
197. Ravin, H. A.: Lancet **2**:726, 1956.
198. Ravin, H. A.: J. Lab. Clin. Med. **58**:161, 1961.
199. Scheinberg, I. H., and Morrell, A. G.: J. Clin. Invest. **36**:1193, 1957.
200. Rice, E. W.: Anal. Biochem. **3**:452, 1962.
201. Wallace, J. W.: Workshop on clinical enzymology, technical manual, Chicago, 1964, American Society of Clinical Pathologists.
202. Scheinberg, I. H., et al.: Science **126**:925, 1957.
203. Morrell, A. G., and Scheinberg, I. H.: Science **127**:588, 1958.
204. Rappaport, F., Fischl, J., and Pinto, N.: Clin. Chim. Acta **4**:227, 1959.
205. Swaiman, K. E.: Workshop on clinical enzymology, technical manual, Chicago, 1964, American Society of Clinical Pathologists.
206. Sigma Technical Bulletin No. 661, St. Louis, 1965, Sigma Chemical Co.
207. DaCosta, W. A., and Friedberg, F.: J. Biol. Chem. **235**:3134, 1960.
208. Ebashi, S., et al.: J. Biol. Chem. **46**:103, 1959.
209. King, E. J.: Biochem. J. **26**:292, 1932.
210. Okinada, S., et al: Arch. Neurol. **4**:520, 1961.
211. Colombo, J. P., Richterich, R., and Rossi, E.: Klin. Wschr. **40**:37, 1962.
212. Craig, F. A., and Ross, G., Metabolism **12**:57, 1963.
213. Griffiths, P. D.: Lancet **1**:894, 1963.
214. Taylor, T. H., and Friedman, M. E.: Clin. Chem. **6**:209, 1960.
215. Bowers, G. N., Jr., and MacDuffee, R. C.: Clin. Chem. **5**:369, 1959.
216. Wolfson, S. K., and Williams-Ashman, H. G.: Proc. Soc. Exp. Biol. Med. **96**:231, 1957.
217. Dawkins, M. R., MacGregor, W. G., and McLean, A. E.: Lancet **2**:827, 1959.
218. Amador, E., Dorfman, L. E., and Wacker, W. E. C.: Clin. Chem. **9**:391, 1963.
219. Caboud, G. C., and Wroblewski, F.: Amer. J. Clin. Path. **30**:324, 1958.
220. Wroblewski, F.: Amer. J. Med. Sci. **234**: 301, 1957.
221. Snodgrass, J. J., et al.: New England. J. Med. **261**:1259, 1959.
222. MacDonald, R. P., Simpson, J. R., and Nossal, E.: J.A.M.A. **165**:35, 1957.
223. Berger, L., and Broida, D.: Sigma Technical Bulletin No. 500, St. Louis, 1963, Sigma Chemical Co.
224. Wacker, W. E. C., and Dorfman, L. E.: J.A.M.A. **181**:972, 1962.
225. Dorfman, L. E., Amador, E., and Wacker, W. E. C.: J.A.M.A. **184**:1, 1963.
226. Hill, B. R.: Ann. N. Y. Acad. Sci. **75**: 304, 1958.
227. Hill, B. R.: Cancer Res. **21**:271, 1961.
228. Blanchaer, M. C.: Clin. Chim. Acta **6**: 272, 1961.
229. Wroblewski, F., and Gregory, K.: Ann. N. Y. Acad. Sci. **94**:912, 1961.
230. Strandjord, P. E., Clayson, K. J., and Freier, E. L. F.: J.A.M.A. **182**:1099, 1962.
231. Synrniotis, F., et al.: Amer. J. Dig. Dis. **7**:712, 1962.
232. Markert, C. L.: Science **140**:1329, 1963.
233. Babson, A. L., and Phillips, G. E.: Clin. Chim. Acta. **12**:210, 1965.
234. Briere, R. O., Preston, J. A., and Batsakis, J. G.: Amer. J. Clin. Path. **45**:544, 1966.
235. Rutenburg, A. M., Goldbarg, J. A., and Pineda, E. P.: New Eng. J. Med. **259**: 469, 1958.
236. Goldbarg, J. A., and Rutenburg, A. M.: Cancer **11**:283, 1958.
237. Shay, H., Sun, D. C., and Siplet, H.: Amer. J. Dig. Dis. **5**:217, 1960.
238. Green, M. N., et al.: Arch. Biochem. **57**: 458, 1955.
239. Pineda, E. P., et al.: Gastroenterology **38**: 698, 1960.
240. Arst, H. E., Manning, R. T., and Delp, M. H.: Amer. J. Med. Sci. **238**:598, 1959.

241. Tietz, N. W., Borden, T., and Stapleton, J. D.: Amer. J. Clin. Path. **31**:148, 1959.
242. Cherry, I. S., and Crandall, L. A.: Amer. J. Physiol. **100**:266, 1932.
243. Overbeck, G. A.: Clin. Chim. Acta **2**:1, 1957.
244. Saifer, A., and Perle, G.: Clin. Chem. **7**: 178, 1960.
245. Bessey, O. A., Lowry, O. H., and Brock, M. J.: J. Biol. Chem. **164**:321, 1946.
246. Andersch, M. S., and Szcypinski, A. J.: Amer. J. Clin. Path. **17**:571, 1947.
247. Reinhold, J. G.: Clin. Chem. **1**:351, 1955.
248. Mendelsohn, M. L., and Bodansky, O.: Cancer **5**:1, 1952.
249. Fishman, W. H., and Lerner, F.: J. Biol. Chem. **200**:89, 1953.
250. Jacobsson, K.: Scand. J. Clin. Lab. Invest. **11**:358, 1960.
251. Babson, A. L., et al.: Clin. Chem. **12**:482, 1966.
252. Babson, A. L., and Phillips, G. E.: Clin. Chim. Acta **13**:264, 1966.
253. Babson, A. L., and Read, P. A.: Amer. J. Clin. Path. **32**:88, 1959.
254. Südhof, H., Meumann, G., and Oloffs, J.: Deutsch. Med. Wschr. **89**:217, 1964.
255. Van Gorkon, W. J.: Nederl. T. Geneesk. **106**:297, 1962.
256. Reitman, S., and Frankel, S.: Amer. J. Clin. Path. **28**:56, 1957.
257. Karmen, A.: J. Clin. Invest. **34**:131, 1955.
258. Annino, J. S.: Techn. Bull. Regist. Med. Techn. **36**:203, 1966.
259. Frankel, S.: Personal communication, 1967.
260. Babson, A. L., et al.: Clin. Chim. Acta **7**: 199, 1962.
261. Babson, A. L.: Clin. Chem. **6**:394, 1960.
262. Amador, E., and Wacker, W. E. C.: Clin. Chem. **8**:343, 1962.
263. Hsia, D. Y.: Inborn errors of metabolism, ed. 2, Chicago, 1966, Year Book Medical Publishers, Inc.
264. Marks, P. A.: Meth. Med. Res. **9**:26, 1961.
265. Brewer, G. J., and Dern, R. J.: Clin. Res. **12**:215, 1964.
266. Brewer, G. J., Tarlov, A. R., and Alving, A. S.: J.A.M.A. **180**:386, 1962.
267. Tanaka, K. R., Calenatine, W. N., and Minwa, S.: Blood **19**:276, 1962.
268. Carson, P., Brewer, G. J., and Ickes, C.: J. Lab. Clin. Med. **58**:804, 1961.
269. Walker, F. A., Hsia, D. Y., Slatis, H. M., and Steinberg, A. G.: Ann. Hum. Genet. **25**:287, 1962.
270. Kulhánek, V., et al.: Clin. Chim. Acta **8**:579, 1963.
271. Kulhánek, V., and Vojtíšková, V.: Clin. Chim. Acta **9**:95, 1964.
272. Strandjord, P. E., and Clayson, K. J.: J. Lab. Clin. Med. **67**:154, 1966.
273. Hue, A. C., and Free, A. H.: Clin. Chem. **11**:708, 1965.
274. Caraway, W. T.: Clin. Chem. **12**:187, 1966.
275. Scott, E. M.: J. Clin. Invest. **39**:1176, 1960.
276. Keating, F. R., Jr.: et al.: J. Clin. Invest. **28**:217, 1949.
277. McConahey, W., et al.: J. Clin. Endocr. **16**:724, 1956.
278. Scholer, J. F.: J. Nucl. Med. **3**:41, 1962.
279. Hamolsky, M. W., Stein, M., and Freedberg, A. S.: J. Clin. Endocr. **17**:33, 1957.
280. Dowling, J. T., Nicoloff, J., and Nicoloff, R.: Clin. Res. **7**:211, 1959.
281. Mitchell, M. L., and O'Rourke, M. E.: Clin. Res. **7**:241, 1959.
282. Cooper, T. J.: Personal communication, 1967.
283. Hamolsky, M. W., Golodegz, A., and Freedberg, A. S.: J. Clin. Endocr. **19**:103, 1959.
284. Sisson, J. C.: J. Nucl. Med. **6**:853, 1965.
285. Zieve, L., Vogel, W. C., and Schultz, A. L.: J. Lab. Clin. Med. **47**:663, 1956.
286. Farrell, P. L., and Richmond, H. M.: Clin. Chim. Acta **6**:620, 1961.
287. Toro, G., and Ackermann, P. G.: Personal communication, 1967.
288. White, W., and Erickson, M.: Personal communication, 1967.
289. Case, J., and Eibert, J.: Personal communication, 1967.
290. Barker, S. B.: J. Biol. Chem. **173**:715, 1948.
291. Barker, S. B., Humphrey, M. J., and Soley, M. H.: J. Clin. Invest. **30**:55, 1951.
292. Foss, O. P., Hankes, L. V., and Van Slyke, D. D.: Clin. Chim. Acta **5**:301, 1960.
293. Ackerman, J. A., and Meyers, J. T.: Clin. Chem. **5**:615, 1959.
294. Zak, B., Willard, H. H., Meyer, G. B., and Boyle, A. J.: Anal. Chem. **24**:1345, 1952.
295. O'Neal, L. W., and Simms, E. S.: Amer. J. Clin. Path. **23**:493, 1953.
296. Leffler, H. H.: Amer. J. Clin. Path. **24**: 483, 1954.
297. Austin, E., and Koepke, J. A.: Amer. J. Clin. Path. **45**:344, 1966.
298. Gambino, S. R., Schreiber, H., and Covolo, G.: Technicon international symposium, New York, 1965.
299. Strickler, H. S., Saier, E. L., and Grauer, R.: Technicon international symposium, New York, 1965.
300. Mann, E. B., Kydd, D. M., and Peters, J. P.: J. Clin. Invest. **30**:531, 1951.
301. Klein, D., and Chernaik, J. M.: Clin. Chem. **6**:476, 1960.
302. Kumaoka, S., and Toba, Y.: Acta. Med. Biol. **5**:20, 1957.
303. Chesky, V. E., et al.: Amer. J. Clin. Path. **23**:41, 1953.
304. Pileggi, V. J., et al.: J. Clin. Endocr. **21**: 1272, 1961.
304a. Pileggi, V. J., and Kessler, G.: Clin. Chem. **14**:339, 1968.
305. Ingbar, S. H., Bowling, J. T., and Greinkel, N.: Endocrinology **61**:321, 1957.
306. Wynn, J., Frabrikant, I., and Deiss, W. P.: Arch. Biochem. **84**:106, 1959.
307. Wynn, J.: Arch. Biochem. **87**:120, 1960.

308. Boothby, W. M., and Sandiford, I.: J. Biol. Chem. **54**:767, 1922.
309. Reveno, W. S.: J.A.M.A. **128**:419, 1945.
310. Moore, F. D.: J.A.M.A. **130**:315, 1946.
311. McGavock, T. H., Gerl, A. J., Vogel, M., and Schutzer, S.: Amer. J. Med. **2**:144, 1947.
312. Hamolsky, M. W., and Freedberg, A. S.: New Eng. J. Med. **262**:129, 1960.
313. Schwartz, J.: Triangle **3**:191, 1958.
314. Squires, R. B., and Langhorne, W. H.: Amer. J. Clin. Path. **46**:189, 1966.
315. Chaney, W. C.: J.A.M.A. **82**:2013, 1924.
316. Gilson, W. E.: New Eng. J. Med. **260**: 1027, 1959.
317. Werner, S. C., Goodwin, L. D., and Quimby, E. H.: J. Clin. Endocr. **9**:342, 1949.
318. Garrod, L. P.: Brit. Med. Bull. **16**:2, 1960.
319. Kimble, M. S.: J. Lab. Clin. Med. **24**: 1055, 1938.
320. Kaser, M., and Stekol, J. A.: J. Lab. Clin. Med. **28**:904, 1943.
321. Carr, F. H., and Price, E. A.: Biochem. J. **20**:497, 1926.
322. Paterson, J. C. S., and Wiggins, H. S.: J. Clin. Path. **7**:56, 1954.
323. Harris, L. J., and Ray, S. N.: Lancet **1**: 71, 1935.
324. Harris, L. J., and Abbasy, M. A.: Lancet **2**:1429, 1937.
325. Roe, J. H., and Kuethra, C. A.: J. Biol. Chem. **147**:399, 1943.
326. Lipstein, S.: Amer. J. Med. Sci. **195**:205, 1938.
327. Selikoff, I. J.: Amer. J. Med. Sci. **213**: 719, 1947.
328. Walpole, G. S.: J. Chem. Soc. **105**:2501, 1914.
329. Clark, W. M., and Lubs, H. A.: J. Biol. Chem. **25**:497, 1916.
330. Sorensen, S. P. L.: Biochem. Z. **21**:131, 1909.
331. Gomori, G.: Proc. Soc. Exp. Biol. Med.
332. Michaelis, L.: J. Biol. Chem. **87**:33, 1930. **62**:33, 1946.

Gastric, duodenal, and pancreatic juice analysis

Gastric secretion: Gastric secretion contains hydrochloric acid secreted by the parietal cells of the fundus and upper body of the stomach and an alkaline enzyme-mucoprotein complex secreted by the superficial mucosal cells (antral, pyloric, and fundal glands). The alkaline component contains enzymes such as pepsin, lipase, etc. and electrolytes such as sodium, potassium, calcium, chlorides, hydrogen, and phosphorus. The secretion is under central (vagal), chemical (intestinal), and hormonal (gastric) control.

GASTRIC ANALYSIS[1]

There are two laboratory methods for gastric analysis.

The tubeless technique investigates the ability of the stomach to produce acid.

The intubation technique allows measurement of gastric secretion under "basal" and "maximal" output conditions and lends itself to quantitative evaluation of gastric secretion.

Tubeless gastric analysis (Diagnex test*)[2, 3]

This test is a method for determination of the presence or absence of free gastric acidity without the use of intubation. The patient is asked to swallow an ion exchange resin that is coupled with a blue dye, azure A. In the presence of free gastric acid the blue of the resin is ex-

changed for the hydrogen ions of the acid. The dye that is thus split off is absorbed and excreted in the urine, usually coloring it blue. If no free acid is present in the stomach, the dye remains attached to the resin and does not appear in the urine within the prescribed period of 2 hr. The dye is administered in conjunction with caffeine sodium benzoate, which stimulates acid secretion.

The test is safe and allows the detection of the presence or absence of free gastric acidity, but it will not show quantitative changes of the free acid. The test does not function properly in the presence of pyloric obstruction, severe hepatic or renal disease, abnormalities of intestinal absorption, or urine retention.

Intubation method

MEASUREMENT OF GASTRIC ACID[4]: The most useful information is obtained by a single test that measures basal secretion as well as maximal (histamine-stimulated) secretion.

Intubation of patient: Place the stomach tube in ice water and slightly lubricate the tip with jelly. The patient is seated and is instructed to take deep breaths through his mouth while the tube is inserted into the floor of the nose and then slowly and gradually passed into the pharynx and esophagus. The tube has distance markers. The distance between the teeth and cardia of the stomach is about 45 cm., while the distance from a well-positioned tube tip to the teeth is about 60 cm. Fluoroscopic control is

---

*Diagnex blue, E. R. Squibb & Sons Division, Olin Mathieson Chemical Corp., New York, N. Y.

necessary to ensure proper tube placement. Aspirate the fasting basal juice and measure the amount. Histalog* is then administered.

Basal secretion: Basal secretion is the amount of gastric juice obtained in the absence of any stimuli. It may be obtained by continuous aspiration over a 12 hr. period overnight. It has been found that a 1 hr. morning collection of basal secretion is equivalent to a 12 hr. overnight collection.

Maximum secretion[5, 6]: Maximum secretion is measured after subcutaneous administration of an augmented dose of 0.05 mg./kg. histamine dihydrochloride or 2 mg./kg. Histalog. After the injection, the gastric secretion is collected for 60 min. in four 15 min. specimens by continuous aspiration.

Titration of acid with 0.1N NaOH, using Töpfer reagent and phenolphthalein: Filter contents of sample through two thicknesses of gauze, if necessary, to remove most of food residue and mucus. In a small graduated cylinder measure 10 ml. and transfer to a porcelain evaporating dish. Add 1 or 2 drops Töpfer reagent (dimethylaminoazobenzene, 0.5% alcoholic solution) and 1 or 2 drops phenolphthalein (1% alcoholic solution) and titrate with 0.1N sodium hydroxide from a burette until the last trace of red color disappears. Take this reading for free hydrochloric acid. Continue titration until the red color of phenolphthalein appears, titrating to the point at which further addition of alkali does not deepen the color. Take the burette reading for the total acidity, counting from the original reading.

The total acidity equals the hydrochloric acid plus the combined acidity. The latter is produced by organic acids (lactic, butyric, acetic, and carbonic), phosphates, and proteins.

Calculation: The number of milliliters from the beginning to the first reading × 10 = free HCl acidity percent.

The number of milliliters from the beginning to the last reading × 10 = total acidity percent.

Units of measurment: "Total acidity percent" is a clinical unit or degree of acidity and is equal to mEq./L. All of these units are the number of milliliters of 0.1N NaOH required to neutralize 100 ml. of gastric juice.

Normal values:
Basal secretion:
  Free HCl: usually none
  Total acidity: 20 mEq./L.
After stimulation:
  Free HCl: 15-55 mEq./L.
  Total acidity: 30-70 mEq./L.
Hypochlorhydria:
  Free HCl: below 15 mEq./L.
  Total acidity: below 30 mEq./L.

CONCENTRATION OF GASTRIC ACIDITY: The acidity (mEq./L.) of a specimen of gastric juice is not the same as the total amount of acid in the specimen secreted in a known period of time (volume in liters × acidity in mEq./L.).

$$\text{Concentration of acid (mEq.)} = \text{Vol. (L.)} \times \text{Acidity (mEq./L.)}$$

According to Segal,[4] titratable acid should be expressed in mEq. output per specific unit of time. He suggested titrating the gastric acid with sodium hydroxide to neutrality (pH 7.0-7.4) either electrometrically or colorimetrically with phenol red as indicator.

Values of gastric analysis expressed in concentrations[4]:
One-hour basal acid output:
  < 2 mEq.: normal, gastric ulcer, or gastric cancer
  2-5 mEq.: normal, gastric ulcer, or duodenal ulcer
  > 5 mEq.: duodenal ulcer
  >20 mEq.: Zollinger-Ellison syndrome
One-hour maximum acid output:
  0 mEq.: true achlorhydria, gastritis, or gastric cancer
  1-20 mEq.: normal, gastric ulcer, or gastric cancer
  20-35 mEq.: duodenal ulcer
  35-60 mEq.: duodenal ulcer, high normal secretion, or Zollinger-Ellison syndrome
  > 60 mEq.: Zollinger-Ellison syndrome

---

*Eli Lilly & Co., Indianapolis, Ind.

Ratio of basal acid output to maximum acid output:

20%: normal gastric ulcer, or gastric cancer

20-40%: gastric ulcer or duodenal ulcer

40-60%: duodenal ulcer or Zollinger-Ellison syndrome

> 60%: Zollinger-Ellison syndrome

Various other methods of measuring gastric acidity and of reporting the results have been suggested. Bock[7] suggested discontinuing the terms "free acid" and "total acid" and recording acidity obtained by titration to pH 7 with a glass electrode in milliequivalents of hydrochloric acid per liter. Baron[8] suggested the discontinuation of the titration of free acid to pH 3.5 with Töpfer reagent and of the titration of total acidity with phenolphthalein to pH 8-10. He replaced both titrations with measurement of the concentration of the acid, the titratable acidity (mEq./L.) obtained by titration with NaOH to neutrality (pH 7.0-7.4) electrometrically or colorimetrically with phenol red. Lubran[9] offered theoretic reasons and experimental data in favor of titrating gastric acid to a pH of 3.5 with Töpfer reagent or with a glass electrode.

Gross examination of gastric juice

Amount: The overnight secretion of gastric juice after 1 hr. of aspiration amounts to 50-80 ml. Over 80 ml. is pathologic. The fasting volume is increased in gastric hypomotility, pyloric obstruction, and Zollinger-Ellison syndrome. The volume is decreased, at times to almost zero, by gastric hypermotility.

Color: Normal gastric juice is almost colorless. Bile will stain it yellow-green and blood will produce a red to coffee-ground brown color.

Odor: Note fecal or rancid odor.

Character: Gastric juice usually separates into three layers: mucus is found in the top layer, opalescent fluid in the center, and sediment at the bottom. Mucus, which increases the viscosity of gastric juice, is increased in gastritis and pyloric obstruction.

Sediment: Note amount of undigested food.

pH: Add 2 drops Töpfer reagent. Free acid will produce a pink color.

Chemical investigation

Titration of hydrochloric acid

For titration of hydrochloric acid, see p. 444.

Lactic acid

Method: Add about 2 drops 10% ferric chloride solution to a test tube full of water and mix. The mixture should appear colorless when held before the light, but should present a faint yellow color when examined vertically over a white surface. Divide in two test tubes and to one add a small amount of gastric contents. Lactic acid gives a characteristic greenish-yellow (canary yellow) color. Compare with other test tube as control.

This method is neither specific nor accurate. Lactic acid associated with Boas-Oppler bacilli and with achlorhydria is seen in carcinoma of the stomach.

Blood

Hydrochloric acid transforms hemoglobin into brown acid hematin.

Method: Neutralize the gastric juice by adding 10% sodium bicarbonate to pH 7 (nitrazine paper) and shake with ether. Treat the aqueous extract just like urine when testing for blood.

Pepsin and pepsinogen[10]

Pepsin, an enzyme, is preformed as pepsinogen in the chief cells of the stomach mucosa and is activated by hydrochloric acid. About 1% of the predominantly exocrine secretion is discharged into the bloodstream (like a hormone) and excreted in the urine as uropepsinogen. The serum and urine pepsinogen levels reflect the rate of gastric pepsin production.

Pepsin test: Mix a portion of stomach contents with an equal amount of 0.1N hydrochloric acid. Divide this in three test tubes. To one add a small amount of pepsin for positive control; boil one tube in order to kill enzymes and cool for negative control. Place a small gelatin square into each test tube and incubate at 37° C. for 12 hr. Examine for evidence of digestion.

Insulin test[11]

The hypoglycemia produced by insulin causes increased gastric secretion by acting through the vagus nerves. Insulin is therefore used as a test to see whether vagotomy would be of value and to determine whether vagotomy has been complete.

Method: The stomach tube should be in place. Obtain fasting blood sugar specimen and fasting gastric juice. Inject 15 units of regular insulin intravenously. Obtain blood sugar specimens every 30 min. for 2 hr. and gastric aspirations every 15 min. for the same period.

Interpretation: Hypoglycemia associated with hyperacidity and an increased volume of gastric juice indicates intact vagal pathways.

MICROSCOPIC EXAMINATION

Mount 1 drop sediment, including any particles suspicious of food residue, on a slide and cover with a cover glass. Report all structures seen.

Add 1 drop gram iodine solution and 1 drop Sudan III or IV to the microscopic preparation in order to differentiate more easily between **fat, yeast,** and particles of **starch.** Fat will stain red, yeast yellow, and starch lilac-purple or blue-black.

Starch, yeast, mouth organisms, and a small amount of mucus are normally found.

Food taken previously, pus, blood, Boas-Oppler bacilli, sarcinae, fat droplets, increased mucus, protozoa or other parasites, and occasionally tissue fragments are abnormal findings.

Boas-Oppler bacilli are large nonmotile bacilli that are present in large numbers and in chains in gastric contents containing little or no free hydrochloric acid. They stain brown with gram iodine solution, which distinguishes them from mouth organisms that have been swallowed because the latter stain blue or black. They are lactic acid bacilli and indicate stasis with fermentation in the absence of free hydrochloric acid.

Sarcinae are large coccoid organisms that divide in three planes, forming packets that are often compared to bales of cotton. They stain brown with iodine. They are found in conditions associated with stasis and high acidity such as gastric ulcers.

Lugol's iodine stains **yeast** organisms slightly yellow. They are found in the same conditions as sarcinae.

Special methods must be utilized to obtain a satisfactory specimen for screening for **cancer cells.**

• • •

Duodenal secretion: Duodenal juice consists of (1) the duodenal excretion of Brunner's glands, (2) bile (of hepatic origin), and (3) pancreatic juice (trypsin, lipase, and diastase).

PANCREATIC JUICE ANALYSIS

Have the patient fast 12 hr. Introduce a stomach tube as for gastric analysis and aspirate the fasting stomach contents. Have patient lie on right side with knees flexed and hips elevated 6 or 8 in. on cushions and swallow the tube to about 75 cm. Usually within ½-1 hr. the tip will be in the duodenum, and the contents will siphon off.

The tip is in the duodenum when a colorless or yellow viscid alkaline fluid is obtained. The entire procedure must be fluoroscopically controlled.

To drain the biliary tract by the Meltzer-Lyon method, introduce 50-100 ml. 25% magnesium sulfate through the tube. Whereas originally three specimens were obtained separately, it is usually sufficient, after drainage is well started, to collect all in one bottle. Use a dark amber bottle and examine promptly (within 30 min.).

GROSS EXAMINATION OF PANCREATIC JUICE[12, 13]

Volume: 700-2000 ml./24 hr.
Character: clear and watery
Viscosity: varies from thin, watery secretion during periods of activity to a thick, more viscid secretion in the basal state

Specific gravity: 1.007-1.042
pH: 7.0-8.7

Pancreatic enzymes

Pancreatic enzymes are digestive enzymes. Trypsin hydrolyzes proteins, amylase hydrolyzes carbohydrates, and lipase hydrolyzes fats.

Trypsin:

Normal values: 100-200 units/L.

Screening test: Make duodenal contents slightly alkaline (faint pink with phenolphthalein) with 2% sodium carbonate and add 1 vol. 1:1000 sodium carbonate. Place a small amount in three tubes. Boil one tube and cool for negative control and add a small amount of trypsin to another tube for positive control. Place a small gelatin square into each tube and incubate overnight at 35° C.

Interpretation: Trypsin digests gelatin (see below).

Rough quantitative test: Make duodenal contents slightly alkaline (faint pink with phenolphthalein) with 2% sodium carbonate. The optimum pH is 8-9. Into six tubes put 1, 0.5, 0.25, 0.10, 0.05, and 0.01 ml. adjusted contents. Run a seventh tube without contents as control. To each tube add 2.5 ml. 0.1% casein in 1:1000 sodium carbonate (filtered) and mix. Incubate in water bath at 38° C. for 15 min. Add a little water to each tube, make acid with a few drops of 10% acetic acid, and mix.

Note the least amount of duodenal fluid producing complete digestion (giving a clear mixture with the acid) and report the number of milliliters of the casein solution digested by 1 ml. duodenal fluid.

Interpretation: Normal is 25-50 ml. Ten milliliters or less indicate pancreatic deficiency. In chronic cystic fibrosis of the pancreas there is an absence or only a trace of trypsin, and none of the tubes will be clear.

Amylase and diastase:

Normal values: 1000-2000 units/L.

Screening test: Prepare a 1:10 dilution of duodenal contents. Add 2 ml. of dilution to 2 ml. 1% starch solution and incubate at 37° C. for 30 min. Add 1 drop gram iodine solution.

Interpretation: A blue color indicates diastase deficiency.

Quantitative tests: For a discussion of quantitative tests, see the section on clinical chemistry.

Urinary amylase[14]*:* The urine often shows a prolonged elevation of amylase in patients with acute pancreatitis as compared to the short-lived serum peak. The 2 hr. amylase excretion in the urine is a more sensitive test than either the serum amylase or lipase test. (For technique, see clinical chemistry section.)

Normal values: 200 units/hr.

Lipase and steapsin:

Normal values: 30,000-60,000 units/L.

Screening test[15]*:* Place 1 ml. duodenal contents in two large test tubes, boil one tube to destroy the lipase, and cool. To each tube add 1 ml. ethyl butyrate, 10 ml. water, and 1 ml. toluol. Mix and incubate at 37° C. for 24 hr., shaking several times. Titrate each tube with 0.1N sodium hydroxide, using 2 drops phenolphthalein. Subtract the amount used to neutralize the boiled specimen (blank) from the amount used in the other. The difference represents the amount of digestion due to the lipase, expressed in terms of the number of milliliters of 0.1N sodium hydroxide required to neutralize the fatty acids formed in the unheated specimen as a result of lipase activity. Normal is 0.2-2 ml.

Serum enzyme measurements: Serum amylase and lipase are elevated in acute pancreatitis. (See clinical chemistry section.)

Secretin and pancreozymin stimulation test of pancreatic function[16]

Principle: Pancreatic secretion is measured after intravenous injection of secretin and pancreozymin. Serum amylase and lipase measurements are made at the same time since the levels may rise in the presence of pancreatic duct obstruction.

Technique: Give the patient a skin test with 0.1 ml. of an isotonic saline solution of secretin and pancreozymin containing 1 unit/ml. Under fluoroscopic observation insert a Dreiling double-lumen gastroduodenal tube and connect each tube to a suction pump, providing continuous aspiration. Samples are collected for 20 min. before stimulation and for 10 min. after pancreozymin administration (100 units intravenously), followed by 10, 10, 20, and 20 min. fractions after secretin administration (75 units).

Blood samples for serum diastase are taken before pancreozymin administration and at 1, 2, and 4 hr. after secretin stimulation.

The duodenal aspirate is examined for amount, color, pH, bicarbonate concentration, and amylase output.

Normal values of duodenal aspirate[17]:
Postpancreozymin (10 min. period):
Volume: 16-72 ml.
Bicarbonate concentration: 8-24 mEq./L.
Amylase: 19,720-164,200 mg. glucose
Postsecretin (60 min. period):
Volume: 99-377 ml.
Maximal bicarbonate concentration: 69-126 mEq./L.

Interpretation: A reduction in bicarbonate concentration is a reliable index of pancreatic dysfunction. A rise in serum enzymes above the normal limit is indicative of ductal obstruction. Bile staining should be intermittent. Absence of bile indicates obstruction of the duct.

Titration of bicarbonate in duodenal aspirate[18]

Principle: An excess of acid is added to liberate CO_2 from bicarbonate, and the equivalent amount of hydrogen is used for the formation of water.

Reagents:
1. HCl (0.05N). Prepare from 1N solution by 1:20 dilution (see p. 432).
2. NaOH (0.01N). Prepare fresh from 1N solution by 1:100 dilution (see p. 432).

Technique: Measure pH value as soon as specimen is obtained. Add 1 ml. duodenal aspirate to 1 ml. 0.05N acid and mix well. Add water so that the fluid level reaches the electrodes. Back-titrate with 0.01N NaOH to original pH value.

Calculation:

Bicarbonate (mEq./L.) = 50 – (ml. NaOH × 10)

Interpretation: Reduction in the bicarbonate level is indicative of pancreatic damage.

Tolerance tests in investigation of pancreatic function

Glucose tolerance test: Destruction of the islets by chronic pancreatitis or by a tumor produces a diabetic type of curve. (For technique, see clinical chemistry section.)

Starch tolerance test: This is similar to the glucose tolerance test, but the patient receives 100 gm. starch instead of 100 gm. glucose.

The test represents an attempt to measure the amylolytic activity of the pancreatic juice. It requires 2 days. On the first day a 3 hr. glucose tolerance test is performed (100 gm. glucose), and on the second day 100 gm. soluble starch is administered. The maximal rise in blood sugar after the glucose tolerance test is compared with that after ingestion of starch. The result is expressed in percent and ranges from –39 to +83%, with an average of +19%. It is calculated on the basis of the following formula:

$$\frac{(P^1 - F^1) - (P - F)}{P - F} \times 100 = \%$$

In the formula, P^1 is the peak and F^1 the fasting blood sugar levels of the glucose tolerance test; P and F are the peak and fasting blood sugar levels of the starch tolerance curve.

Leucine aminopeptidase (LAP)

This test was thought to be of value in the diagnosis of cancer of the pancreas and posthepatic obstruction. Extensive clinical trials have failed to bear this out. A commercial kit is available.*

Tests for malabsorption

Radioactive iodine (I^{131}) triolein test: Fecal fat studies are important in the investigation of fat metabolism in all forms of steatorrhea but they are time-consuming. I^{131} triolein is a fat consisting of oleic acid groups esterified with 1 mole of glyceryl. In the process of absorption of this fat there is no appreciable loss of iodine, and therefore the amount of I^{131} in the blood or feces can

---

*Sigma Chemical Co., St. Louis, Mo.

be accepted as evidence of absorption or lack of it. The maximal total blood level of 8-12% of the original dose should be reached rapidly in 3-4 hr. under normal circumstances. In steatorrhea the maximal absorption of 3-5% is reached only slowly. In the case of poor absorption it may be due to either absence of pancreatic enzymes or mucosal inadequacy. These two conditions can be distinguished by administration of I^{131} oleic acid, which requires no hydrolysis and is absorbed normally in the absence of enzymes, but not if there is a mucosal block. (See discussion of steatorrhea, p. 455.)

MICROSCOPIC EXAMINATION

Examine within 30 min. Mix specimen and centrifuge a portion for 15 min. at highest speed. Pour off supernatant fluid and mount sediment on slide under cover glass.

Record whatever is found, but note especially the presence or absence of bile-stained columnar epithelial cells, bile-stained pus cells (give approximate number per high-power field when present), increased cholesterin crystals, increased calcium bilirubinate crystals, other crystals, and parasites.

Bile-stained cells and increased numbers of crystals indicate stasis. An occasional cholesterin or calcium bilirubinate crystal is normal. Amebas, hookworms, *Ascaris*, flagellates, and *Strongyloides* have been reported.

Special double-lumen gastrointestinal tubes allow the aspiration of neoplastic cells from lesions of the duodenum, pancreas, and biliary tract following stimulation with secretin.

FIBROCYSTIC DISEASE OF THE PANCREAS (MUCOVISCIDIOSIS)

This disease is congenital, probably enzymatic, and clinically can be classified into three groups, depending on the age of onset. In newborn infants it is called meconium ileus. In children it is called fibrocystic disease and is characterized by repeated pneumonia, failure to gain weight, and large foul stools, producing a clinical picture similar to that of celiac disease. In adults it manifests itself as a tendency to repeated pulmonary infections.

LABORATORY DIAGNOSIS
Changes in exocrine secretions

Duodenal fluid: The outstanding feature is an increase in viscosity associated with a decrease in pancreatic enzymes. (See discussion of tests for fecal trypsin.) The increased viscosity, which is readily measured by the Ostwald viscosimeter, is in part due to changes in the mucopolysaccharide composition, such as low sialic acid and high fucose content.

Bronchial secretion: The secretion is unusually viscid and forms a good culture medium for coagulase-positive staphylococci *(Staphylococcus aureus)* and *Pseudomonas aeruginosa*.

Saliva: The sodium and chloride concentrations are increased.

Sweat: In sweat the concentration of sodium and chloride is two to five times the normal values. The rise in the concentration of these two electrolytes may not be equal.

There are a few other conditions in which chloride concentration in the sweat is elevated, e.g., in adrenal insufficiency and in some cases of nephrosis. Parents or siblings of patients with fibrocystic disease may also have increased concentrations.

Normal values: Chlorides vary from 4-60 mEq./L. and average 25 mEq./L. Sodium normally varies from 10-80 mEq./L. and averages 45 mEq./L.

Pathologic values in fibrocystic disease: Chlorides vary from 60-160 mEq./L. and average 106 mEq./L. Sodium varies from 80-190 mEq./L. and averages 133 mEq./L.

Screening tests for chloride in sweat:
Hand sweat test: The test is based on the quantitative precipitation of the chloride ion with silver nitrate on the surface of potassium chromate agar.

A finger, hand, or toe imprint is made on the surface of the agar plate 15 min. after the hands or feet are washed with plain water and dried. When there is little chloride on the skin surface, the imprint is barely detectable; however, if the chloride content is increased, a whitish-yellow discoloration occurs immediately. This discoloration can be graded 1+ to 3+ according to sodium chloride standards from 50-250 mEq./L., small amounts of which are applied to the agar surface as controls. The test is commercially available in the form of impregnated filter paper* and as silver chromate agar plates.†

Pilocarpine iontophoresis technique:

Principle: Sweating is induced by pilocarpine nitrate ions introduced into a small area of skin by an electric potential. The positive electrode is moistened with pilocarpine and placed on the skin. The negative electrode is moistened with sodium nitrate solution and placed opposite the positive electrode. Some time is allowed for the sweat to wash out of the sweat glands; it is then collected on a previously weighed filter paper disk placed exactly over the site of iontophoresis and covered by a plastic sheet to prevent evaporation. The current source is commercially available. After 30 min., the paper disk is removed, returned to the weighing bottle, and reweighed. The sweat is then eluted from the disk with 20 ml. distilled water and analyzed for chlorides in the Cotlove chloridometer.

As an alternate procedure, the sweat can be collected in small capillary tubes and the electrolyte concentration determined using the electrical conductivity method.

Technique using the chloridometer: Weigh filter paper pad in stoppered weighing bottle before and after absorption of sweat by pad. The difference in weight is the grams of sweat absorbed. Do not handle the pad with the fingers, only with forceps.

After the test, add 5 ml. deionized distilled water to the pad in the weighing bottle. (NOTE: All mention of water in this procedure refers to deionized distilled water.) Allow stoppered bottle to stand 15 min., occasionally swirling every

2 or 3 min. Transfer as much of the water as possible to a graduated **Pyrex** centrifuge tube with a pipette, press any remaining water from the pad with a **clean** flat surface (the bottom of one of the vials used with the chloridometer is satisfactory), and transfer any expressed water to the centrifuge tube.

Repeat extraction with two additional 3 ml. portions of water and allow to stand 10 min. each time, swirling occasionally. Transfer all extract to centrifuge tube and dilute to 12 ml. Stopper with Parafilm* and mix by inversion. Centrifuge to pack filter paper fibers in bottom of tube.

Chloride analysis: Use "low" setting on chloridometer. For blank use 1 ml. water and 1 ml. double-strength ($2\times$) chloride diluent. For sample use 1 ml. diluted extract and 1 ml. double-strength diluent. For standard use 0.75 ml. water, 0.75 ml. double-strength diluent, and 0.5 ml. "low" standard (2 mEq./L.). Run several blanks and standards to obtain consistent results before running sample in duplicate. Subtract the average seconds for blank titration from average seconds for sample and standard titrations to obtain net seconds for sample and standard titrations.

The actual chloride concentration in the diluted extract in mEq./L. is:

$$\frac{\text{Net seconds for sample}}{\text{Net seconds for standard}} \times$$
$$\frac{\text{Volume of standard used}}{\text{Aliquot of extract used}} \times$$
$$\text{Concentration of standard}$$

For the volumes and standard used as given, this reduces to:

$$\text{MEq./L. Cl in diluted extract} = \frac{\text{Net seconds for sample}}{\text{Net seconds for standard}}$$

And the chloride concentration in the sweat is:

$$\text{MEq./L. Cl in sweat} = \text{MEq./L. Cl in diluted extract} \times \frac{\text{Total vol. of extract}}{\text{Gm. sweat collected}}$$

---

*Fibron paper, Consolidated Laboratories, Inc., Chicago Heights, Ill.
†Hyland Laboratories, Los Angeles, Calif.

---

*American Can Co., Neenah, Wis.

Example:

Average seconds for blank	10.1
Average seconds for standard	71.2
Average seconds for sample	28.3
Volume of extract	12.0
Grams of sweat	0.15

$$\text{Cl in extract} = \frac{28.3 - 10.1}{71.2 - 10.1} = 0.3 \text{ mEq./L.}$$

$$\text{Cl in sweat} = 0.3 \times \frac{12}{0.15} = 54 \text{ mEq./L.}$$

Heated aluminum silver electrode sweat test[19]: This method is used for testing newborn infants for cystic fibrosis.

Procedure: A heated aluminum cylinder (48° C.) covered with Parafilm is applied to a washed skin area (interscapular) to stimulate sweating. The cylinder is removed after 5 min. and a modified silver chloride-coated, silver billet combination electrode is applied to the skin, which is moist with sweat. Within 10-15 sec. the concentration of chloride in the sweat is indicated on the pH meter and can be converted into milliequivalents per liter on the basis of a graph.

Examination of hair by atomic absorption analysis

The hair of an infant can be examined within a few hours after birth. In cystic fibrosis, sodium and potassium are increased and calcium and magnesium are decreased.[20]

Estimation of fecal fat and enzymes

In pancreatic fibrosis the pancreatic ferments in the stool are markedly depressed. Small amounts of lipase and amylase are sometimes present, but trypsin is never present in significant amounts. The stool is bulky, the fat content is very high, and most of the fat is unsplit (neutral fat), producing the so-called butter stool. (See discussion of fecal fat, p. 445.)

REFERENCES

1. Rovelstad, R. A.: Gastroenterology **45**:90, 1963.
2. Segal, H. L., Miller, L. L., and Morton, J. J.: Proc. Soc. Exp. Biol. Med. **74**:218, 1950.
3. Segal, H. L., Miller, L. L., and Plumb, E. J.: Gastroenterology **28**:402, 1955.
4. Segal, H. L.: J.A.M.A. **196**:655, 1966.
5. Laudano, O. M.: Gastroenterology **50**:653, 1966.
6. Zaterka, S., and Neves, D. P.: Gastroenterology **47**:3, 1964.
7. Bock, O. A.: Lancet **2**:1101, 1962.
8. Baron, J. H.: Gastroenterology **45**:1, 1963.
9. Lubran, M.: Lancet **2**:1070, 1966.
10. Seljffers, M. J., et al.: Gastroenterology **48**:122, 1965.
11. Ross, B., and Kay, A. W.: Gastroenterology **46**:379, 1964.
12. Rosenberg, I. R., and Janowitz, H. D.: Gastroenterology **48**:350, 1965.
13. Haverback, B. J.: J.A.M.A. **193**:279, 1965.
14. Kirshen, R., Gambill, E. E., and Mason, H. L.: Gastroenterology **46**:746, 1964.
15. Goldstein, N. P., and Roe, J. H.: J. Lab. Clin. Med. **28**:1334, 1942.
16. Fitzgerald, O., et al.: Gut **4**:193, 1963.
17. Sun, D. C.: Gastroenterology **44**:602, 1963.
18. Van Slyke, D. D., and Cullen, G. E.: J. Biol. Chem. **30**:289, 1917.
19. Warwick, W. J.: J.A.M.A. **198**:177, 1966.
20. Shwachman, H.: Lab. Manage. **3**:9, 1965.

Chapter 8

Stool analysis

ROUTINE PHYSICAL EXAMINATION

Odor: Putrid, inoffensive, rancid, sour.

Color: The normal color of stool is due to stercobilin, the oxidation product of stercobilinogen, which owes its existence to bilirubin-reducing bacteria.

Yellow to yellow-green: The stool of breast-fed infants who lack the normal intestinal flora contains bilirubin but no stercobilin. Severe diarrhea and sterilization of the bowel produce similar results.

Black: This color may be the result of bleeding into the upper gastrointestinal tract, or it may be due to drugs such as iron, charcoal, etc. Bleeding into the lower segments of the large bowel leads to blood-streaked stool.

Tan: Blockage of the common bile duct produces pale, greasy, acholic stool.

Consistency: Fluid, semisolid, formed, hard.

Macroscopic mucus: Strings, balls, casts, ribbons.

Macroscopic blood: In mucus, localized, diffuse, changed.

Concretions: Intestinal sand, enteroliths, coproliths (fecaliths).

Parasites: Adult roundworms, segments of tapeworms, flukes (trematodes).

Macroscopic pus: Note color, quantity, consistency.

Fat: A significant increase of fat is usually detected grossly. In obstruction of the common bile duct the fat gives a puttylike appearance to the stool (acholic stool). In sprue and celiac disease the appearance of the feces often suggests aluminum radiator paint due to the fatty acid crystals. In cystic fibrosis of the pancreas the increase of neutral fat gives the greasy "butter-stool" appearance.

CHEMICAL EXAMINATION
Tests for blood

Most of the methods for detecting blood in the stool employ phenolic compounds such as gum guaiac, benzidine, etc. They are oxidized to colored compounds by oxygen liberated from hydrogen peroxide by the peroxidases contained in the heme portion of the hemoglobin. Huntsman and Liddell[1] investigated these tests as well as the commercially available Hematest* and Occultest* and found them too sensitive (falsely positive), even after a meat-free diet, except for the guaiac test.

Guaiac test[2]:

Reagents:
1. Saturated guaiac solution. This solution is stable for 1 mo.
2. Guaiac crystals, 10 gm.
3. Ethyl alcohol (95%), 50 ml.
4. Hydrogen peroxide (3%). Keep in refrigerator.
5. Glacial acetic acid.

Technique: Smear a pea-sized fecal specimen on clean filter paper. Add 2 drops guaiac solution, 2 drops glacial acetic acid, and 2 drops 3% hydrogen peroxide.

Interpretation:

Immediate blue color	4+
Deep blue color in 30 sec.	2-3+
Blue color in 1-3 min.	1-2+
No blue color or a slowly developing faint blue	Negative

A negative result should be confirmed by repeating the test with 1 drop diluted blood to test the reagents.

---

*Ames Co., Inc., Elkhart, Ind.

According to Morgan and Roantree,[2a] a reaction of over 1+ is always indicative of blood.

As guaiac is difficult to obtain, two other filter paper methods are included. A modified guaiac test[2b] is available.*

Benzidine test:

Reagents:

1. Benzidine hydrochloride powder, 0.025 gm.
2. Barium peroxide powder, 0.2 gm.
3. Acetic acid (50%) in water, 5 ml.

Technique: Prepare stool specimen on filter paper as previously described. Add 2 drops reagent, examine after 15-30 sec., and grade the same as for the guaiac test. Disregard color change after 30 sec.

Interpretation: Same as for guaiac test.

Orthotoluidine test[3]:

Reagents:

1. Sodium perborate (2%) in water, equal parts
2. Orthotoluidine (2%) in glacial acetic acid, equal parts

Prepare fresh mixture before use. Individual reagents keep for 1 wk. at room temperature.

Technique: Make a thin smear of a pea-sized piece of stool on Whatman No. 1 filter paper and add 6 large drops reagent mixture.

Interpretation: A positive test is indicated if a blue color forms outside the area of the fecal smear within 2 min.

Orthotoluidine tablet tests: Occultest and Hematest tablets are commercially available.

INFLUENCE OF IRON ON OCCULT BLOOD TESTS[4]: Ferrous fumarate and ferrous carbonate may produce false positive results with the orthotoluidine test tablets and with the guaiac filter paper procedure. Other iron preparations do not interfere.

Test for ingested iron[5]:

Principle: Iron plus potassium ferricyanide produces ferrous ferricyanide (Turnbull's blue). The presence of blood does not interfere with the test.

Technique: Emulsify a small amount of stool in 2N hydrochloric acid with two orange sticks. Using the sticks again,

---

*Hemoccult Slides, Laboratory Diagnostic Co., Roselle, N. J.

transfer 1 drop of emulsion to Whatman No. 1 filter paper. The consistency of the specimen must be such that after 1 or 2 min. a 3-4 mm. halo of fluid surrounds the fecal drop. Place 1 drop 0.25% potassium ferricyanide close to the fecal specimen so that the two fluids meet. A positive result is evidenced by the immediate appearance of a blue color at the interface of the liquids.

Tests for bile pigments and derivatives

Gmelin test for bile: Make a thin smear on filter paper and test with 1 drop yellow nitric acid or Fouchet reagent as for urine or make an emulsion and perform a ring test with yellow nitric acid.

This test is used for the detection of bilirubin, which normally does not occur in the stool except under the conditions mentioned in the discussion of stool color.

Qualitative screening procedure for fecal urobilin and urobilinogen (Watson)[5]: Urobilin and urobilinogen are extracted with a saturated alcoholic (95% ethyl alcohol) solution of zinc acetate. Urobilin gives a green fluorescence, and after the addition of Ehrlich aldehyde reagent, urobilinogen imparts a pink color to the mixture.

Reagents:

1. Saturated solution of zinc acetate:

   Zinc acetate ($2H_2O$), 50 gm.
   95% ethyl alcohol, 1 L.

Heat in water bath to 50° C., stirring frequently. The cooled solution must show crystals at the bottom of the container.

2. Saturated solution of sodium acetate:

   Sodium acetate ($3H_2O$), 140 gm.
   Distilled water, 100 ml.

Heat to 60° C. and allow to cool. There must always be crystals at the bottom of the container.

3. Ehrlich aldehyde reagent:

   p-Dimethylaminobenzaldehyde (colorless), 0.7 gm.
   Concentrated hydrochloric acid, 150 ml.
   Distilled water, 100 ml.

Store in brown bottle with glass stopper.

Method: Emulsify about 2 gm. stool in 10 ml. saturated alcoholic solution of zinc acetate and filter. If urobilin is present, the solution will show green fluorescence. To 2.5 ml. filtrate add 2.5 ml. Ehrlich aldehyde (Watson modification) and after 15 sec. add 5 ml. saturated aqueous solution of sodium acetate. If urobilinogen is present, the solution will be pink.

Interpretation: A pink color indicates urobilinogen. Green fluorescence of the untreated zinc acetate filtrate in transmitted light is a rough quantitative measurement of urobilin in the filtrate. To determine urobilinogen the stool specimen must be fresh; however, any stool specimen can be used to test for urobilin. Urobilinogen may be present in normal amounts as compared to a normal control specimen, or it may be decreased, absent, or increased.

Semiquantitative estimation of fecal urobilinogen: See Chapter 6.

Summary: **Bilirubin** occurs physiologically in the stool of newborn infants and pathologically in severe diarrhea and following administration of antibiotics.

Stercobilin (urobilin) is normally present in stool and absent as a result of complete obstruction to bile flow.

Urobilinogen is normally present in stool although in somewhat decreased amounts in infants. It is increased in hemolytic anemia and decreased as the result of partial obstruction to the flow of bile, the administration of antibiotics, and diminished blood production (aplastic anemia).

Urobilinogen may be absent if all of it is converted to urobilin, the test for which should be positive. No urobilinogen and no urobilin are evidence of complete obstruction of the common bile duct.

Test for trypsin

The test for trypsin in feces of adults is not very satisfactory because of the presence of leukocytes and bacteria. Prepare a 1:10 suspension of feces in saline solution, allow to settle, and set up test with the supernatant fluid, using the amounts given previously for duodenal contents. Report the milliliters of casein solution that are completely digested. Normal is about 2.5-5 ml.

X-ray film method: As a screening test in infants, the x-ray film method[5a] for feces is of value in detecting cystic pancreatic fibrosis. Trypsin can be demonstrated in 95% or more of the stools of normal infants. Absence of trypsin is presumptive evidence of pancreatic deficiency and is usually accompanied by the absence of the other ferments, lipase and amylase.

Technique: Make a suspension of feces in distilled water in dilutions of 1:5, 1:10, 1:20, and 1:40. Place a large drop of each dilution on the surface of an unexposed, unfixed gelatin (x-ray) film and incubate at 37° C. for 1 hr. or at room temperature for 2 hr. The drops should be large enough to prevent drying or caking during the test. Wash in cold running water with gentle rubbing. Complete digestion (clearing) is read as 4+ and a slight clearing only at the periphery of the drop as 1+.

Run a control with the feces of a normal infant. Run the test on three separate fresh stools. Positive tests should be checked once or more at intervals of a week in order to rule out the possibility that the positive reaction might be due to the temporary bacterial flora of the intestines. For older children, test stools following a cathartic.

Malabsorption and steatorrhea

Steatorrhea (increased fat in stool) is evidence of malabsorption and is due to many conditions of varying etiology.

1. Genetic atrophy of intestinal mucosa: celiac disease, idiopathic steatorrhea, and tropical sprue
2. Failure of digestion of fat: obstructive jaundice, pancreatic disease (pancreatic cirrhosis, fibrocystic disease), and total gastrectomy
3. Abnormal intestinal flora: blind loops, fistulas, and resections
4. Blockage of intestinal lymphatics: Whipple's disease and scleroderma
5. Iatrogenic steatorrhea: irradiation and antibiotics
6. Miscellaneous: pneumatosis intestinalis

7. Failure of blood supply: mesenteric endarteritis

LABORATORY INVESTIGATION OF STEATOR-RHEA[6, 7]: Steatorrhea may be determined by gross examination of feces, microscopic examination for free fat, and measurement of total fat in feces.

To determine the cause of steatorrhea test for small bowel competence (D-xylose excretion test), pancreatic competence (secretin-pancreozymin test, p. 447), plasma protein leakage into the bowel (rate of degradation of injected I^{131}-labeled albumin), disaccharidase deficiency (lactose tolerance test), and small bowel morphology (transoral biopsy of intestinal mucosa).

Gross examination of feces: Typically the feces are foamy, greasy, soft, and foul-smelling.

Microscopic examination for free fat: Mix a drop of emulsion with 1 drop glacial acetic acid and 1 drop Sudan IV, apply a cover glass, and examine for fat.

Fat occurs as neutral fat, fatty acids, and soaps. Neutral fat appears as droplets that stain deep orange or red (or occasionally as yellowish flakes); fatty acids appear as fine needlelike crystals that do not stain (or as flakes like those of neutral fat); soaps, chiefly calcium soaps, appear as coarse unstained crystals or as yellowish opaque masses, round or irregular in shape.

Measurement of total fat in feces[8-11]:

Principle: Fecal fat may be determined by extracting the fat from the stool and either weighing the amount of extracted material or titrating the fatty acids extracted after hydrolysis. In the gravimetric methods any mineral oil or any other nonfat material soluble in ether or petroleum ether will be included in the weight of fat. In the titration methods one must assume an average molecular weight for the titrated fatty acids to calculate their actual amount. Although there will be some variation with the type of diet, the differences are rarely large enough to influence the clinical interpretation. The method chosen for presentation is a wet-extraction method, with titration of the extracted fatty acids.

Collection: Collection of the specimen presents some problems. The determination of fat on a random specimen is of little value. It is generally agreed that, if possible, all the stool excreted over a 3-5 day period should be collected for analysis. Also it is preferable that the patient be on a fairly constant diet, one in which the fat content is at least approximately known, for 2 or 3 days prior to and throughout the collection period. The samples should be preserved in the refrigerator until analyzed. If more than an occasional determination is made, it is helpful to collect the specimens in new preweighed 1 gal. metal paint cans. These have tight-fitting covers, and after the entire specimen has been collected it can be well mixed in the original can by adding some water if necessary and shaking on a paint-shaking machine. This usually gives a homogeneous sample. Subtract the weight of the can from the weight of the can plus contents to obtain the weight of the specimen. The addition of water makes no difference since one is determining the fat in an aliquot from an entire 3 day specimen. If the feces are collected in other containers, the entire specimen must be well mixed. This is best accomplished with a Waring blender or similar machine and with the addition of a small amount of water. The weight of the total homogenized specimen must then be obtained.

Reagents:
1. Ethyl alcohol containing 0.4% amyl alcohol. Add 0.4 ml. amyl alcohol to 100 ml. 95% ethyl alcohol.
2. Potassium hydroxide (33%). Dissolve 33 gm. potassium hydroxide in water, cool, and dilute to 100 ml.
3. Hydrochloric acid (25% w/v). Mix together 250 ml. concentrated hydrochloric acid and 125 ml. water.
4. Thymol blue indicator solution. Dissolve 0.2 gm. thymol blue in 100 ml. 50% alcohol.
5. Sodium hydroxide (0.1N), standardized, or dilute from standardized 1N solution (see p. 432).
6. Hydrochloric acid (2.5%) with 25% sodium chloride. Add 10 ml. 25% HCl and about 60 ml. water to a

flask. Add 25 gm. sodium chloride, dissolve, and dilute to 100 ml.

Technique: Weigh out to the nearest 10 mg. 5-7 gm. feces into an Erlenmeyer flask. Add 10 ml. 33% potassium hydroxide and 40 ml. ethyl alcohol containing 0.4% amyl alcohol. A simple way of determining the weight is to use small screw-capped vials of about 10 ml. capacity. These are first weighed, the stool is then added, and they are weighed again. The material is then rinsed into the flask with the KOH and alcohol solutions.

Boil the solution gently under a reflux condenser for 20 min. Cool, add 17 ml. 25% HCl, and cool again. Add exactly 50 ml. petroleum ether, stopper, and shake for 1 min. Allow the layers to separate. Since the petroleum ether is rather volatile, separation is best accomplished by allowing the flask to stand in a refrigerator to avoid loss of the petroleum ether.

Remove exactly 25 ml. of the petroleum ether layer, taking care not to include any of the aqueous layer. Transfer this to a flask and evaporate to dryness on a steam bath. (CAUTION: Flammable!) Add about 20 drops thymol blue indicator to 100 ml. ethyl alcohol. Then add 0.1N NaOH dropwise until the color changes to green; avoid any excess. Add 10 ml. of this neutralized alcohol to the flask containing the residue from the petroleum ether evaporation. Warm slightly to dissolve and titrate with 0.1N sodium hydroxide. The color change of the indicator is from yellow to blue, but the end point may not be pure blue in the yellow material usually extracted from the feces.

Calculation:

$$\text{Gm. fatty acids/100 gm. stool} = \frac{n \times 284 \times 1.04 \times 2 \times 100}{10{,}000 \ W} = \frac{5.91n}{W}$$

Where n is the milliliters of 0.1N NaOH required for the titration, W is the weight of stool taken, 284 is the average molecular weight of the fatty acids, and 1.04 is a factor to compensate for incomplete extraction.

This gives the total amount of fatty acids. If one wishes to determine the split fat, weigh another sample, add 22 ml. 2.5% HCl with NaCl, boil under a reflux condenser for exactly 1 min., cool well, and add 40 ml. ethyl alcohol containing 0.4% amyl alcohol and 50 ml. petroleum ether. Proceed with the extraction and titration as for total fat. The calculations are the same.

Normal values and interpretation: The amount of fat in the stool depends on the dietary intake. On the usual diet the normal excretion is 1-7 gm./day for adults, which is usually less than 10% of the intake. The normal value has been given as 1-9% of the intake. In steatorrhea the fat excretion is increased; in some cases as much as 40% of the ingested fat may be excreted. This increase in fat in the stool is indicative of malabsorption, but for accurate results one must at least know the approximate fat intake.

Formerly it was considered of value to determine the amount of fat in the split and unsplit form, the former being the fats hydrolyzed to fatty acids. Impaired absorption or pancreatic dysfunction would increase the amount of unsplit fat. It has been found that even at refrigerator temperature some fats will still be slowly hydrolyzed, and the value of the determination has been doubted on theoretic grounds. Usually one can consider that the ratio of split fat to unsplit fat is about 3:1, so that about 75% of the fat is in the split form.

Microanalysis of fecal fat[12]: This method measures total lipids in small quantities of stool dried on glass fiber paper and is useful for analyses in newborn infants.

I[131] **triolein adsorption test:** See p. 448.

D-Xylose excretion test[13-15]:

Principle: This test is used as an indirect measure of intestinal absorption. A definite amount of the pentose xylose which is not metabolized by the body is administered, and the amount excreted in the urine in the next 5 hr. is measured. In the absence of severely impaired kidney function the amount excreted is dependent upon the amount absorbed in the intestines.

Reagents:

1. *p*-Bromoaniline reagent. Prepare a saturated solution of thiourea in glacial acetic acid by shaking about 5 gm. of the material with 120 ml. of the acid. Allow crystals to settle and decant off solution. Dissolve 2 gm. of *p*-bromoaniline in 100 ml. of the acid. Prepare fresh weekly.

2. Xylose standards:

   A. Stock standard. Dissolve 200 mg. pure xylose in 100 ml. saturated benzoic acid. This stock standard contains 200 mg.% xylose.

   B. Working standard. Dilute 1 ml. stock solution with 9 ml. water on the day required. This working standard contains 20 mg.% xylose.

Technique: Have the patient ingest 5 gm. xylose dissolved in about 250 ml. water. Collect all the urine voided during the next 5 hr. Give additional water to drink during this period, if necessary, since a very low urine volume may lead to unreliable results.

Dilute the total urine excreted to 1 L. Then further dilute a portion 1:10. Add to separate tubes 1 ml. diluted urine, 1 ml. xylose working standard, and 1 ml. water as blank. To each tube add 5 ml. aniline reagent and heat in water bath at 70° C. for 10 min. Then allow to stand at room temperature in the dark for 90 min. Read standard and sample against blank at 545 mμ.

Calculation:

$$\frac{\text{OD sample}}{\text{OD standard}} \times 0.2 \times \frac{1000 \times 10}{1000} =$$
$$\text{Gm. xylose excreted}$$

Since each milliliter of the standard contains 0.2 mg. xylose, the urine is diluted to 1000 ml. and then diluted an additional 10 times. The denominator 1000 converts milligrams to grams.

The formula then reduces to:

$$\frac{\text{OD sample}}{\text{OD standard}} \times 2 = \text{Gm. xylose excreted}$$

Interpretation: Some workers have administered 25 gm. xylose instead of 5 gm., but this occasionally causes nausea or diarrhea which interferes with the test. Five grams is sufficient for good results. When 5 gm. xylose is given in the absence of impaired kidney function, an excretion of more than 1.2 gm. is indicative of satisfactory intestinal absorption. Excretion of 0.9-1.2 gm. would be a doubtful result but may indicate some degree of malabsorption. If less than 0.9 gm. is excreted, malabsorption is present if kidney function is near normal.

Lactose tolerance test[16, 17]:

Principle: Under normal conditions lactose is hydrolyzed to glucose and galactose by lactase, an enzyme found in the small bowel mucosa; therefore scarcely any lactose appears in the blood. The diagnosis of lactase deficiency is based, among other criteria, on a flat blood sugar curve associated with diarrhea following an oral test dose of lactose.

Technique: The patient, who has been fasting (12 hr.), is given 50 gm. lactose in 500 ml. water. Blood specimens for glucose determination are obtained in the fasting state and at 30, 60, 90, 120, and 150 min. after the test dose.

Interpretation: A flat blood sugar curve associated with diarrhea following the test dose is found in lactose intolerance, but it must be noted that it is also found in asymptomatic adults.

Lactosuria[18]: Following administration of the test dose, all urine may be collected for 5 hr. and tested for lactose excretion. Patients with lactose intolerance show increased lactosuria.

REFERENCES

1. Huntsman, R. G., and Liddell, I. J.: J. Clin. Path. **14**:436, 1961.
2. Moss, D. G.: J. Med. Lab. Techn. **13**:22, 1955.
2a. Morgan, T. E., and Roantree, R. J.: J.A.M.A. **164**:1664, 1957.
2b. Greegor, D.H.: J.A.M.A. **201**:943, 1967.
3. Wahba, N.: J. Clin. Path. **18**:687, 1965.
4. Illingworth, D. G.: J. Clin. Path. **18**:103, 1965.
5. Afifi, A. M., et al.: Brit. Med. J. **1**:1021, 1966.
5a. Shwachman, H., Patterson, P. R., and Laguna, J.: Pediatrics **4**:222, 1949.
6. Jeffries, G. H., Weser, E., and Sleisenger, M. H.: Gastroenterology **46**:434, 1964.
7. Kalser, M. H.: J.A.M.A. **188**:37, 1964.
8. van de Kamer, J. H., ten Bokkel Huinink, H., and Weyers, H. A.: J. Biol. Chem. **177**: 347, 1949.

9. Cooke, W. T., et al.: Quart. J. Med. **15:** 141, 1946.
10. van de Kamer, J. H.: In Seligson, D., editor: Standard methods of clinical chemistry, New York, 1958, Academic Press, Inc., vol. 2, p. 347.
11. Jover, A., and Gordon, R. S., Jr.: J. Lab. Clin. Med. **59:**878, 1962.
12. Searcy, R. L., Dunn, J. M., Simms, N. M., and Bergquist, L. M.: Amer. J. Clin. Path. **41:**477, 1964.
13. Roe, J. H., and Rice, E. W.: J. Biol. Chem. **173:**507, 1948.
14. Kerstell, J.: Scand. J. Clin. Lab. Invest. **13:**637, 1961.
15. Santini, R., Jr., Sheehy, T. W., and Martinez-De Jesus, J.: Gastroenterology **40:**772, 1961.
16. Friedland, N.: Arch. Intern. Med. (Chicago) **116:**886, 1965.
17. Peternel, W. W.: Gastroenterology **48:**299, 1965.
18. Weser, E., and Sleisenger, M. H.: Gastroenterology **48:**571, 1965.

Chapter 9

Methods in parasitology

The methods employed for investigation of parasitic infections depend on the biologic behavior of the parasite, the organ or organs it involves, and where and by what method it reproduces and is transmitted. In some cases the method involves search for the adult form; in others, examination for ova and larvae or examination of imprints of smears of blood or tissues.

The material examined includes stool, sputum, urine, blood, or tissue, depending on the nature of the parasite.

INTESTINAL PARASITES[1-5]
EXAMINATION OF FECES
Specimen collection

Use a clean container that allows ready access to and visualization of the specimen. The specimen must be adequately identified and should be examined as soon as possible. It should not be kept warm. If immediate examination is not possible, store the specimen in the refrigerator.

Macroscopic examination

Wire sieve method: Liquefy the specimen with water and strain through a wide-mesh sieve (10-20 mesh) that allows medium-sized worms to pass through but retains bulky fecal components. Then strain the sieved material through a finer sieve (40-50 mesh) to retain scolices and smaller worms.

Microscopic examination

Direct wet-film method:
Reagents:
1. Iodine solution for protozoa (D'Antoni):

Potassium iodide, 1 gm.
Iodine, 1 gm.
Distilled water to make 100 ml.
Grind the potassium iodide and the iodine together in a mortar with about 5 ml. water; then add the remaining portion of water. There will be a slight excess of iodine. Transfer (including the excess of iodine) to a dark glass-stoppered stock bottle. Filter before use.
2. Normal saline solution

Procedure: Use a 3 × 2 in. microscope slide. Place 1 drop saline solution on one end of the slide and 1 drop iodine solution on the other. Emulsify 1-2 mm.[3] of fecal material with an applicator stick, first in the saline solution and then in the iodine solution. Choose mucoid hemorrhagic particles if looking for amebas and *Schistosoma* eggs. Remove fibers and large particles and cover each emulsion with a 22 × 22 mm. cover glass. The emulsion should be just thin enough to allow reading of print.

Interpretation: In the saline preparation, trophozoites are characterized by their motility. When the objective is moved up and down for a short distance, cysts, which are somewhat refractile, can be recognized as glistening, round to ovoid objects that are usually about two to four times as large as red blood cells. In the iodine preparation, trophozoites and cysts stain light brown.

Concentration methods

Zinc sulfate centrifugal flotation:
Reagent:
Zinc sulfate solution (specific gravity 1.18):

1. Zinc sulfate, 331 gm.
2. Distilled water to make 1000 ml.

Check specific gravity frequently with hydrometer.

Procedure:

1. Take a small test tube, approximately 12 × 115 mm. with round bottom and without a lip, and add sufficient distilled or tap water to fill to a height of 1-1½ in.
2. With the aid of a wooden applicator, place a sufficiently large portion of the stool, about the size of a large red bean, in the water in the test tube. Emulsify the sample of stool thoroughly in the water with the aid of two wooden applicators. Add more water to the tube gradually and mix well each time until the fluid in the tube is within ½ in. of the top.
3. Centrifuge for 1 min. at 2500 rpm.
4. Pour off all of the supernatant fluid. Add a few milliliters of water. Resuspend the sediment and add sufficient water to refill the tube. Mix well during the addition of the water.
5. Centrifuge again for 1 min.
6. After the second centrifugation, the supernatant fluid should be poured out completely. The washed and packed sediment should be at least ¼ in. high in the tube if the proper amount of fecal material was employed initially.
7. Add zinc sulfate solution with a specific gravity of exactly 1.18. Mix well, preferably by striking the thumb against the bottom of the tightly held tube or with an applicator. Fill the tube to exactly 2-3 mm. of the top with additional zinc sulfate solution. Add the solution with a dropper and with sufficient force to mix the contents or mix with the applicator.
8. Centrifuge again for 1 min.
9. Place a small drop of iodine stain in the center of a clean slide.
10. Do not remove tube from centrifuge. With a wire loop remove 1 or 2 loopfuls of surface film and mix with iodine on slide. Apply cover slip and examine.

NOTE: The method is not suitable for fatty stools and does not concentrate the eggs of most trematodes.

Brine flotation method:

Procedure: Emulsify 0.5-1 gm. feces in 10-20 vol. saturated salt solution. Filter through two layers of gauze into a 25 ml. cylinder (without spout). With a pipette add more salt solution until a convex meniscus is formed; let stand 30-60 min. Remove a large drop by touching the meniscus with a cover glass or with a wire loop and mount it between the cover glass and a microslide.

NOTE: Larvae do not float and are not found by this method.

Formalin-ether sedimentation:

Procedure:

1. Comminute 2 ml. stool in 3 ml. saline solution in a 15 ml. conical centrifuge tube.
2. Add saline solution to mark 15.
3. Centrifuge at 1500-2000 rpm for 2 min. Decant the supernatant fluid.
4. Resuspend the sediment in fresh saline solution, centrifuge, and decant as before. This step may be repeated if a cleaner sediment is desired.
5. Add about 10 ml. 10% formalin to the sediment, mix thoroughly, and allow to stand for 5 min.
6. Add 3 ml. ether, stopper the tube, and shake vigorously; remove the stopper carefully.
7. Centrifuge at 1500 rpm for about 2 min. Four layers should result: a small amount of sediment containing most of the parasites, a layer of formalin, a plug of fecal debris on top of the formalin, and a topmost layer of ether.
8. Free the plug of fecal debris from the sides of the tube by ringing with an applicator stick and carefully decant the top three layers.
9. Mix the remaining sediment with the small amount of fluid that drains back from the sides of the tube. Prepare iodine and unstained mounts of the sediment in the usual manner for microscopic examination.

The formalin-ether sedimentation technique is excellent for the detection and identification of protozoa and ova of most intestinal parasites. The technique is also very useful for examining stools containing fatty substances that interfere with the performance of the zinc sulfate centrifugal flotation method.

Preservation of fecal specimens

Refrigeration: Refrigerate specimen at 3°-5° C.

Formalin: Add 5 parts 10% formalin to 1 part specimen.

PVA fixative: Add 5 parts fixative to 1 part specimen. Mix and stopper. The material is suitable for preparation of slides.

Reagents:
1. Mercuric chloride (saturated aqueous), 62.5 ml.
2. Ethyl alcohol (95%), 31 ml.
3. Glacial acetic acid, 5 ml.
4. Glycerol, 1.5 ml.
5. Polyvinyl alcohol (PVA) powder (Elvanol 90-26*), 5 gm.

Mix materials 1 to 4 at room temperature. Heat to 75° C. or higher until suspension clears.

Merthiolate-iodine-formalin stain (MIF): This preservative is useful for all types of parasites.

Reagents:
1. Lugol solution, 0.1 ml.
   Potassium iodide, 2 gm.
   Iodine, 1 gm.
   Distilled water, 100 ml.
2. Tincture of Merthiolate (No. 99, 1:1000†), 0.775 ml.
3. Formaldehyde solution (USP), 0.125 ml.

Procedure: The Lugol iodine solution must be freshly prepared. One milliliter of fixative is adequate for 25 fecal specimens. Place test tube containing 1 ml. stain and another test tube containing distilled water in a rack. Put a medicine dropper in each tube. Place a small drop of distilled water at one end of a glass slide and add an equal size drop of stain solution. To this mixture add a small amount of fecal sample. Mix thoroughly and apply cover slip.

---

*E. I. DuPont de Nemours & Co., Inc., Pharmaceuticals Div., Wilmington, Del.
†Eli Lilly & Co., Indianapolis, Ind.

Staining procedures

Iron hematoxylin stain[6]:
Reagents:
1. Schaudinn solution. Mix 2 parts saturated solution of mercuric chloride in distilled water (6.9 gm./100 ml. H_2O) and 1 part 95% alcohol. Add 10% glacial acetic acid just before use. Slides must be scrupulously clean or the film will not adhere. The preparation is best fixed if the slide is held film-side down against the fixative for 1 sec. before immersion.
2. Ferric ammonium sulfate. Use only violet crystals.
3. Hematoxylin crystals. Use only certified crystals. Dissolve 5 gm. hematoxylin in 100 ml. absolute alcohol. Add distilled water to 1000 ml. The hematoxylin solution should be allowed to stand at least 1 wk. before using. Stock solution will keep indefinitely. Pour about 150 ml. into a glass-stoppered bottle for use. Hematoxylin can be reused but should be tested each time by pouring a few drops into about 100 ml. tap water. If the solution becomes violet, the stain is satisfactory; but if it turns orange-brown, it should be discarded.

Film preparations must be thin, wet, and fresh and must not be allowed to dry during the procedure.

Procedure:
1. Fix smear in Schaudinn fluid—5 min.
2. Remove residual mercury in 70% alcohol (with iodine added to give a port-wine color)—1 min.
3. Remove residual iodine in 70% alcohol, two changes each—½ min.
4. Mordant in 4% aqueous ferric ammonium sulfate—3-5 min.
5. Wash in running tap water—1 min.
6. Stain in 0.5% aqueous hematoxylin —1 min.
7. Remove excess stain by dipping in water.
8. Differentiate in 2% phosphotungstic acid—2 min.
9. "Blue" the hematoxylin in tap water—1 min.

10. Dehydrate in 95% alcohol and then in absolute alcohol—1 min. each
11. Clear in xylol—1 min.
12. Mount in Piccolyte.*

NOTE: Fogging will result in steps 10 to 12 if dehydration is not complete. Use absolute alcohol and water-free xylol for the final steps.

The characteristics of nuclei stained with iron hematoxylin are shown in Table 9-2.

Kohn one-step rapid staining technique (modified) for intestinal protozoa:

Reagents:
1. Kohn stain (modified)†[7]
2. HSR†-xylene solution

Procedure: Prepare thin smears of fecal specimen on plain glass slide. Immerse immediately in stain and allow to stain for 2-3 hr. at 37° C. Wash 10-15 sec. in 95% alcohol. Immerse 5 min. in carbolxylol. Immerse 5 min. in xylene. Mount with HSR-xylene solution.

Appearance of specimen: In fresh specimens the organisms are gray-green to black. Occasionally *Entamoeba coli* will appear pink. Ingested red blood cells are pink to dark red. In unpreserved stools (2-3 days old) the protozoa are gray to black. Within the cells the nuclei, chromatoid bodies, karyosomes, and cell membranes are dark green to black.

EXAMINATION OF SPECIMENS OTHER THAN FECES

Urine: The sediment of the centrifuged specimen may contain *Schistosoma haematobium* eggs.

Duodenal contents: The centrifuged specimen may contain larvae of *Strongyloides* and *Giardia*.

Sputum: The sputum is digested in 5% sodium hydroxide (see methods for tubercle bacilli) and is then centrifuged and examined for *Paragonimus* ova.

Blood: Fresh preparations and fixed smears may be examined for microfilariae and malarial plasmodia.

---

*Turtox, General Biological Supply House, Inc., Chicago, Ill.
†Hartman-Ledden Co., Inc., Philadelphia, Pa.

PROTOZOA

LABORATORY DIAGNOSIS

A. **Stool examination**
  1. Three or more fresh stool specimens
     (a) Direct smear in saline solution and iodine for trophozoites and cysts
     (b) Zinc sulfate centrifugal flotation or formalin-ether sedimentation for cysts
  2. Fresh warm stool specimen obtained after saline purgative
     (a) Same as steps a and b above

B. **Sigmoidoscopic examination**
  1. Visual examination for lesions
  2. Aspiration of material for microscopic study
     (a) Employment of glass tube for aspiration in place of swab
     (b) Direct smear in saline solution for trophozoites

C. **Culture of stools and of aspirate on suitable medium**

D. **Serologic examination**

E. **Surgical biopsy** (e.g., of rectum)

Stool examination

Examination for protozoa should be made while the specimen is fresh because the active or vegetative forms of the organism soon disintegrate. If the examination cannot be made at once, keep the specimen at 3°-5° C. Urine, soap, water, and antiseptics kill protozoa quickly. Specimens collected after administration of oil, barium, and bismuth are not satisfactory. Body temperature destroys trophozoites.

Formed stools usually contain cysts; fluid stools contain the vegetative forms. The life cycle of the common pathogenic protozoa is simple and takes place entirely in the host's intestine. Encystment occurs only in the intestines, not after the stool is voided. Both encystment and excystment may occur in cultures.

Collection of specimen: Have patient void before collecting the specimen. Collect stool in a clean, dry container. (1) Normal stool is best for encysted forms. In dysenteric stools, examine blood-streaked mucus. (2) Stools after a mild

Table 9-1. Most important intestinal parasitic infections of man

Protozoa		
Class	*Name*	*Incidence (%)*
Amebas	*Entamoeba histolytica**	9
	Entamoeba coli	20
	Endolimax nana	
	Iodamoeba bütschlii	
	Dientamoeba fragilis	
Flagellates	*Giardia lamblia**	12
	*Trichomonas hominis**	3
	*Chilomastix mesnili**	4
Infusoria (ciliates)	*Balantidium coli**	
Sporozoa	*Isospora hominis**	

Helminths		
Scientific name	*Common name*	*Habitat*
Cestodes		
Diphyllobothrium latum	Fish tapeworm	Small intestine
Hymenolepis nana	Dwarf tapeworm	Small intestine
Taenia saginata	Beef tapeworm	Intestine
Taenia solium	Pork tapeworm	Intestine
Echinococcus granulosus	Hydatid cysts or echinococcus cysts	Liver and other organs
Nematodes		
Strongyloides stercoralis		Small intestine
Necator americanus	American hookworm	Small intestine
Ancylostoma duodenale	Old World hookworm	Small intestine
Trichinella spiralis	Trichina	Small intestine and muscles
Trichuris trichiura	Whipworm	Large intestine
Ascaris lumbricoides	Roundworm	Small intestine
Toxocara canis	Dog roundworm	Intestine
Enterobius vermicularis	Pinworm or seatworm	Large intestine, cecum, and appendix
Trematodes		
Fasciola hepatica	Sheep liver fluke (large liver fluke)	Liver
Fasciolopsis buski	Giant intestinal fluke	Small intestine
Clonorchis sinensis	Chinese liver fluke	Biliary capillaries
Opisthorchis felineus	Cat liver fluke	Biliary capillaries
Paragonimus westermani	Lung fluke	Lung
Schistosoma haematobium	Blood fluke	Venous plexuses of urinary bladder, uterus, prostate
Schistosoma mansoni	Blood fluke	Inferior and superior mesenteric veins and hemorrhoidal plexus
Schistosoma japonicum	Oriental blood fluke	Inferior and superior mesenteric veins and hemorrhoidal plexus

*Pathogenic.

laxative (Alophen pills*) are best for vegetative forms. (3) Saline enema may be given or a rectal tube passed, and the small amount of fecal matter or mucus recovered is examined. (4) Administration of bile salts may aid in the finding of amebas. (5) Material from proctoscopic examinations should be obtained by aspiration into glass tubing (slightly bent at one end, with flame-polished tip) and not by wiping with a cotton swab.

Since protozoa appear intermittently in the stool, more than one examination should be made. Three specimens (one every other day) are usually recommended.

*Parke, Davis & Co., Detroit, Mich.

There seems to be a more distinct periodicity in the appearance in the stools of *Entamoeba histolytica* than of *Entamoeba coli*. Amebas are found only on about one half to three fourths of the days on which examinations are made. One examination is successful in only two thirds of the cases; six examinations are successful in about 98% of the cases if some examinations follow a laxative or purge. One proctoscopic examination will detect about 30% of the positive cases.

MACROSCOPIC STOOL EXAMINATION: Look for blood, mucus, and pus.

MICROSCOPIC STOOL EXAMINATION: Use direct wet-film preparation (p. 459).

Emulsify a small amount of specimen in saline solution and in iodine solution. Trophozoites will move actively in saline solution but are killed and easily overstained by iodine.

Cysts are refractile in saline solution and stain brown with iodine.

Iodine staining: Iodine stains the cysts light brown, makes the nuclei prominent by staining the nuclear membrane and the karyosome, and deeply colors glycogen (brown). If stool has been fixed in formalin, the glycogen disappears, and only the vacuoles are seen. Addition of a drop of 50% acetic acid makes the nuclei of cysts even more distinct, but acid will immediately destroy the trophozoites of flagellates.

In the fresh preparation in saline solution, nuclear outlines of amebas or of their cysts can hardly be recognized. The addition of iodine allows the breakdown of amebas into two groups on the basis of nuclear characteristics: *E. histolytica* and *E. coli* trophozoites and their cysts show nuclei with nuclear membranes, while nonpathogenic trophozoites and their cysts usually show only chromosomal granules and not well-defined nuclear membranes.

Iron hematoxylin staining: Findings may be confirmed when necessary by

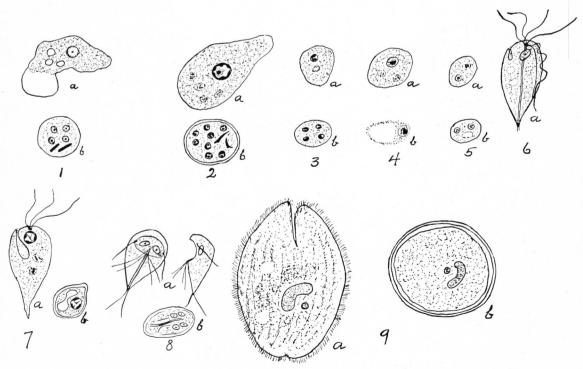

Fig. 9-1. Drawings illustrating protozoa as seen in stained preparations. a, Trophozoites and, b, cysts. **1,** *Entamoeba histolytica.* **2,** *Entamoeba coli.* **3,** *Endolimax nana.* **4,** *Iodamoeba bütschlii.* **5,** *Dientamoeba fragilis.* **6,** *Trichomonas hominis.* **7,** *Chilomastix mesnili.* **8,** *Giardia lamblia.* **9,** *Balantidium coli.* (**1** to **8,** ×1000; **9,** ×800.)

staining with iron hematoxylin (Fig. 9-1) or by culture.

Fluorescent microscopy[8]: Acridine orange in McIlvaine buffer at pH 3.0-5.0 has been used as a staining method to make identification of amebas easier.

Culture of protozoa

All the amebas and flagellates (except *Giardia lamblia*) grow in the initial culture, but only *E. histolytica* grows vigorously in subcultures.

Entamoeba **medium of Cleveland and Collier*** is commercially available for the cultivation of *E. histolytica*. The slants are covered with Bacto-Horse serum–saline solution (1:6 mixture), sterilized by filtration, and 1 loopful Bacto-Rice powder, sterilized in a dry-heat oven at 160° C. for 1 hr.

Procedure: Mix a pea-sized sample of feces with the medium or, if liquid, introduce 0.5 ml. of material with a pipette. Incubate at 35° C. and examine three wet preparations microscopically at 24-48 hr., pipetting from the bottom of the tube. Make transfers every 2-3 days.

Serologic diagnosis of amebiasis

Serologic methods are not very helpful in the diagnosis of amebic dysentery, but they do allow diagnosis of amebic liver abscess with some accuracy.

Amebic gel diffusion precipitation test[9]: This test, described by Powell and Maddison, appears to be more sensitive than the older complement-fixation test in detecting tissue invasion and involvement by amebas.

Indirect fluorescent antibody test[10]: By this method the level of antibody titer clearly distinguishes hepatic amebiasis (titers from 1:64-1:16,384) from nonspecific titers obtained in controls (1:8 or less, a few 1:16).

Hemagglutination technique[11]: The hemagglutination technique has been described by Kessel et al.

Complement-fixation test[12]: This test detects about 83% of all cases of amebic hepatitis. It is 100% positive in amebic liver abscess, while it is positive in only 15% of cases of intestinal amebiasis.

*Difco Laboratories, Detroit, Mich.

AMEBAS

Six species of amebas are found in the intestines of man, one of which is definitely pathogenic, i.e., *E. histolytica*.

Entamoeba histolytica:
Size:
1. Trophozoite: 20-30μ diam.
2. Cyst: 10-20μ diam.
3. Small and large races occur. The small race cyst is not larger than a red blood corpuscle. The large race trophozoite varies from 20-30μ.

Characteristics (Table 9-2 and Fig. 9-1):
Vegetative stage (Plate 8):
1. Explosive (sluglike) expulsion of pseudopodia.
2. Ingestion of red blood cells.
3. Nucleus contains a small amount of chromatin with central position of the karyosome.
4. In lesions the trophozoites reproduce by binary fission; in the lumen of the intestine they form cysts.

Cyst stage:
1. One to four nuclei, similar to trophozoite nucleus.
2. Inconspicuous glycogen vacuole.
3. Rodlike chromatoid bodies with rounded ends.

Entamoeba coli:
Size:
1. Trophozoite: 20-30μ diam.
2. Cyst: 10-30μ diam.

Characteristics (Table 9-2 and Fig. 9-1):
Vegetative stage:
1. Protrusion of pseudopodia not explosive.
2. Ingestion of bacteria, but not of red cells.
3. Nucleus contains considerable chromatin, with a distinct peripheral layer and an eccentric karyosome.

Cyst stage:
1. Eight or more nuclei, similar to trophozoite nucleus.
2. Distinct glycogen mass.
3. Usually no chromatoid bodies, but when present resemble splintered glass.

Dientamoeba fragilis:
Size:
1. Trophozoite: 8-10μ diam.
2. Cyst: Encysted stage has not been identified.

Table 9-2. Differential diagnosis of human intestinal amebas

	Entamoeba histolytica	*Entamoeba coli*	*Endolimax nana*	*Iodamoeba bütschlii*	*Dientamoeba fragilis*
Trophozoite					
Unstained					
Diameter	20-30μ	20-30μ	6-12μ	9-20μ	8-10μ
Motion	Active; explosive extension of pseudopodia	Slow; pseudopodia flow out slowly	Very slight; several blunt pseudopodia at one time	Like *E. coli*	Wavelike action of pseudopodia; leaflike indented edges
Nucleus	Faint or invisible	Clearly visible	Faint	May or may not be visible	Usually 2 (about 60%); indistinct
Food inclusions	Tissue fragments, leukocytes, RBC; no bacteria	Bacteria and debris; no RBC or tissue	Bacteria and debris; no RBC or tissue	Bacteria and debris; no RBC or tissue	Bacteria; no RBC
Cytoplasm	Ectoplasm sharply differentiated	Ectoplasm not sharply differentiated	Ectoplasm not sharply differentiated	Ectoplasm not sharply differentiated	Ectoplasm hyaline
Stained					
Nucleus	Small, central, 4-7μ; karyosome small, central	Large, eccentric, 4-8μ; karyosome large, eccentric	1-3μ; one or several large karyosomes connected by strands	2-3μ; large central karyosomes surrounded by refractile granules	1-2μ; 2 nuclei; several large central karyosomes
Nuclear peripheral chromatin	Thin; often beaded	Heavy, thick membrane	None; nuclear membrane dimly stained	None	None; delicate membrane
Cyst					
Unstained					
Diameter	5-20μ	10-30μ	7-10μ	8-12μ	Cyst stage is not known
Shape	Spheroidal	Spheroidal	Ellipsoidal	Irregularly spheroidal	
Nucleus	Faint or invisible	Distinct	Faint	Faint or invisible	
Stained with iodine (brown)					
Glycogen	Present in young cysts; absent in old	Well defined in young cysts	Sometimes present in young cysts	Large, distinct, and characteristic	
Number of nuclei	1-4	Usually 8	4 when mature	1	
Stained with iron hematoxylin					
Nucleus	Like trophozoite	Like trophozoite	Like trophozoite	Large karyosome on one side, with nuclear granules on opposite side	
Chromatoid bodies	Usually 1 or more; rodlike with rounded ends	Resembles fragments of splintered glass	None usually; sometimes small dots or minute rods, often in vacuoles	None	

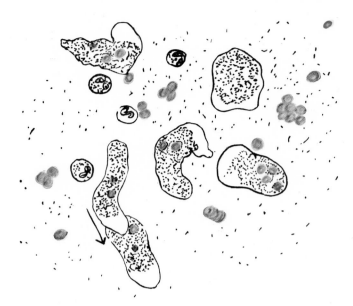

Plate 8. *Entamoeba histolytica.*

High-power field showing ameboid activity and phagocytosis of red blood cells.

Characteristics (Table 9-2 and Fig. 9-1):
Vegetative stage:
1. Trophozoite is characteristically bi-nucleated. With iron hematoxylin stain the delicate nuclear membrane is hardly visible and only the large lobulated central karyosome stands out. The karyosome is composed of groups of chromatin granules. The nuclei may be connected by a dark-staining thread. Nuclei cannot be seen in the fresh preparation.
2. Pseudopodia are clear and indented, producing a cloverleaf-like appearance.

Endolimax nana:
Size:
1. Trophozoite: 6-12μ diam.
2. Cyst: 7-10μ diam.
Characteristics (Table 9-2 and Fig. 9-1):
Vegetative stage:
1. Trophozoite is sluggish and shows only minimal locomotion.
2. Projects blunt hyaline pseudopodia.
3. The large karyosome is only seen well in the iodine preparation.
4. Nucleus is spheroidal; when stained with iron hematoxylin, it shows a thick nuclear membrane that lacks

chromatin beading. The karyosome is large, irregular, and lobulated.
Cyst stage:
1. It is thin-walled and oval or spherical.
2. Nucleus is similar to trophozoite nucleus.

Iodamoeba bütschlii:
Size:
1. Trophozoite: 9-20μ diam.
2. Cyst: 8-12μ diam.
Characteristics (Table 9-2 and Fig. 9-1):
Vegetative stage:
1. Trophozoite is rarely seen; it is a sluggish organism that produces broad hyaline pseudopodia.
2. Nucleus is not seen in the unstained preparation. In the stained preparation the nucleus is large, with an achromatic nuclear membrane and a large centrally placed karyosome.
Cyst stage:
1. It is thick-walled, irregular in shape, and characteristically contains a large round or oval glycogen mass.
2. Stained nucleus shows an unbeaded, thin membrane and a large, often eccentric karyosome in contact with the nuclear membrane.

3. The nucleus is not visible in the unstained preparation and the glycogen mass appears as vacuoles. In the stained preparation (iodine) the glycogen mass is well delineated and dark brown.

Free-living amebas in soil: Culbertson[13] identified *Acanthamoeba* or *Hartmanella* species as a cause of brain abscess.

FLAGELLATES

The most important are *Giardia lamblia*, *Trichomonas hominis*, and *Chilomastix mesnili*. The incidence varies greatly, but the distribution is cosmopolitan. Smaller flagellates, *Embadomonas intestinalis* and *Enteromonas hominis*, are less frequently found and may be confusing. Reproduction is by longitudinal division. Resistant forms (cysts) occur except in *Trichomonas* (Table 9-3).

The **diagnostic procedures** for flagellates are the same as for amebas and include the direct wet-film preparation with saline solution and iodine solution and the concentration procedures.

Chilomastix mesnili:
Habitat: Intestine, chiefly colon.
Size:
1. Trophozoite: 7-18μ in length.
2. Cyst: 6-9μ diam.
Characteristics:
Motile form:
1. Pear-shaped; rounded anteriorly and pointed posteriorly; characteristic oblique spiral groove across ventral surface.
2. Three flagella from anterior end and a fourth (not usually seen) within the large mouthlike cavity or cytostome.
3. Large oval nucleus near anterior end.

Table 9-3. Morphologic differentiation of intestinal flagellates

	Trichomonas hominis	*Chilomastix mesnili*	*Giardia lamblia*
Incidence	3%	5%	12%; high among children
Habitat	Cecum and colon	Cecum and colon	Duodenum and jejunum
Trophozoite Shape	Pear-shaped (variable); rapid tapering	Pear-shaped (not variable as *Trichomonas*); gradual tapering	Pear-shaped; bilaterally symmetric
Size	10-15μ	7-18μ	10-15μ
Anterior flagella	4 (3 and 5)	3	1 pair (plus posterior, ventral, and caudal pairs)
Undulating membrane	+	−	−
Cytostome	Very small	⅓-½ of body length	−
Axostyle	+ (beyond posterior end)	−(posterior spine present)	+ (1 pair)
Movement	Jerky	Jerky and twisted	Kitelike
Inclusion	Bacteria and other semi-digested material	Bacteria and food vacuoles	−
Sucking disc	−	−	+ (anterior and ventral)
Parabasal body	−	−	+
Cyst Size	No cyst stage	6-9μ	7-12μ
Shape	−	Oval or lemon-shaped	Oval
Other characteristics		Nucleus and cytostome	2-4 nuclei; axostyle fibrils

+ = present; − = absent.

Cyst form:
1. Pyriform or spherical (lemon-shaped).
2. A single nucleus.
3. Remains of cytostome extending across the cyst.

Diagnosis: The unstained organism is pear- or carrot-shaped and has a counter-clockwise twist of the body. The organism moves with a spiraling counter-clockwise rotation of the body.

Trichomonas hominis:

Habitat: Intestine, chiefly colon.

Size:
1. Trophozoite: 10-15μ in length.
2. Cyst: The encysted stage has not been identified.

Characteristics (Table 9-3 and Fig. 9-1):
Motile form:
1. Pear-shaped; rounded anteriorly and pointed posteriorly, with a central axostyle that projects beyond the posterior end.
2. Undulating membrane on one side terminating in a flagellum posteriorly.
3. Four flagella from anterior end; varies with the species.
4. Nucleus near anterior end.

Two other species of *Trichomonas* have been described, although many authorities consider them individual variants of *Trichomonas hominis: Trichomonas vaginalis* is found in the vagina in cases of trichomonas vaginitis and also in urine, prostatic fluid, and semen; *Trichomonas buccalis* is found as a nonpathogen in the mouth.

Diagnosis: The salient diagnostic feature of the unstained organism is the rapid, jerky, darting movements of a flagellate with an undulating membrane.

Giardia lamblia:

Habitat: Duodenum chiefly; gallbladder.

Size:
1. Trophozoite: 10 × 15μ in length.
2. Cyst: 7 × 12μ diam.

Characteristics (Table 9-3 and Fig. 9-1):
Motile form:
1. Pear-shaped.
2. Concavity on ventral side of blunt end for attachment to epithelial cells.
3. Two nuclei.

4. Four pairs of flagella.
Cyst form:
1. Oval and refractile.
2. Two or four nuclei, usually at one end.
3. Two curved longitudinal axostyles in center.

Diagnosis: The unstained organism is top-shaped, has a suction cup, and resembles the face of a tennis racquet. The organism has a spinning and flip-flop movement.

INFUSORA (CILIATES)

The **diagnostic procedures** are the same as for all protozoa (see p. 464).

Balantidium coli:

Distribution: Cosmopolitan.

Incidence: Rare in man; common in pigs.

Size:
1. Varies greatly.
2. Trophozoite: 65-100 × 40-70μ.
3. Cyst: 45-65μ diam.

Characteristics (Fig. 9-1):
Motile form:
1. Oval and covered with short cilia in parallel rows.
2. Anterior end somewhat pointed, presents a deep cytostome.
3. Food vacuoles and two contractile vacuoles usually present.
4. Ingests blood, tissue, and bacteria.
5. One large kidney-shaped nucleus (macronucleus) and a small micronucleus usually lying in the concavity of the macronucleus.
6. Reproduction by binary transverse division.
Cyst form:
1. Spheroidal; greenish or yellowish with doubly outlined cyst wall.
2. Macronucleus and micronucleus like the trophozoite.
3. In young cysts the cilia may be seen; in older cysts the outline of the organism is lost.

Diagnosis: The unstained organism is large, shows rapid motility, and has a rim of moving cilia.

STRUCTURES RESEMBLING INTESTINAL PROTOZOA

Blastocystis hominis: This yeast is often found in feces and is sometimes

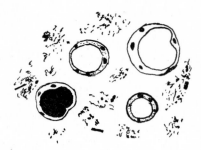

Fig. 9-2. *Blastocystis hominis* from human feces. (Oil-immersion lens.)

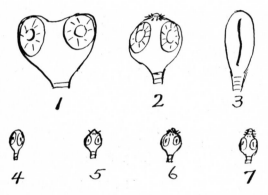

Fig. 9-3. Scolices of tapeworms. 1, *Taenia saginata*. 2, *Taenia solium*. 3, *Diphyllobothrium latum*. 4, *Hymenolepis diminuta*. 5, *Hymenolepis nana* (one row of hooklets). 6, *Echinococcus granulosus* (two rows of hooklets). 7, *Dipylidium caninum* (three or more rows of hooklets).

mistaken for a cyst of some intestinal parasite.

It is ovoid or spherical, 10-15µ diam., and surrounded by a cyst wall-like membrane (Fig. 9-2). The cytoplasm is hyaline and refractive. The outer layer of the cytoplasm contains refractile granules. One or more nuclei are often seen in unstained as well as in iodine-stained preparations. Entire cytoplasm stains brownish with iodine.

Macrophages: The cytoplasm is hyaline, uninucleate, vacuolated, and may contain red blood cells. Macrophages lack mobility, but they send out pseudopodia. They are usually accompanied by polymorphonuclear cells and the nucleus is more prominent than it would be in the unstained trophozoite.

HELMINTHS
Cestodes or Tapeworms[14]

These flat tapelike or ribbonlike worms consist of a series of segments (proglottids) which arise by a budding process from a specially modified smaller segment (the scolex) provided with sucking grooves or sucking discs, with or without hooklets for attachment to the mucosa (Fig. 9-3). The young segments are small, but as they are pushed distally by new ones, they increase in size and become sexually mature. The scolex is sometimes called the head and the most immature segments the neck of the tapeworm. The tapeform has no alimentary tract and, in fact, is a multiple parasite, like a chain of cocci or yeast cells. It derives its food by osmosis. Each mature segment is a complete individual with nerves, excretory canals, and a reproductive system that includes organs of both sexes. The mature proglottid consists chiefly of a uterus dilated with ova (Fig. 9-4). The segmented portion (strobila) varies in length in the different species, from 3-8 mm. (*Echinococcus granulosus*) to 10-12 m. (*Diphyllobothrium latum*).

The adults inhabit the intestinal tract of vertebrates, and the larvae inhabit the tissues of vertebrates and invertebrates. The vertebrate harboring the adult parasite is known as the **definitive host**; the host harboring the larval form is the **intermediate host**.

There are two orders of cestodes that are important medically. In the *Pseudophyllidea* the scolex has grooves (or bothria) for attachment to the intestinal mucosa; the uterine pore is on the flat surface of the proglottid; the uterus has a saccular or rosettelike appearance; the vitellaria are scattered; the ova are operculated, and the oncospheres, which have six hooklets, are usually ciliated. In the *Cyclophyllidea* the scolex has four cup-shaped suckers, with or without a rostellum and hooklets. There is no birth pore, but the ova are liberated when the gravid proglottid disintegrates; the vitellaria are concentrated; the ova do not have opercula, and the oncospheres, which have six hooklets, are not ciliated.

The **diagnosis of all tapeworms** (Figs.

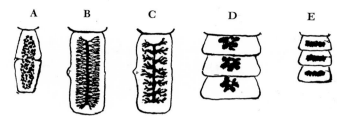

Fig. 9-4. Mature segments of tapeworms (schematic). **A,** *Dipylidium caninum.* **B,** *Taenia saginata.* **C,** *Taenia solium.* **D,** *Diphyllobothrium latum.* **E,** *Hymenolepis nana (Hymenolepis diminuta* is similar but larger).

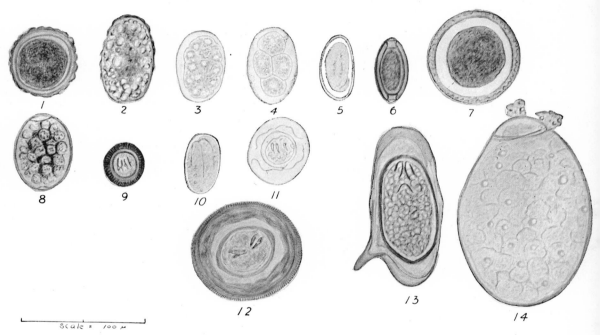

Scale = 100 μ

Plate 9. Ova of intestinal parasites.

1. *Ascaris lumbricoides* (fertilized egg)
2. *Ascaris lumbricoides* (unfertilized egg)
3. *Necator americanus* (late segmentation)
4. *Necator americanus* (four-cell stage)
5. *Enterobius vermicularis*
6. *Trichuris trichiura*
7. *Toxocara canis*

8. *Diphyllobothrium latum*
9. *Taenia saginata*
10. *Rhabditis hominis*
11. *Hymenolepis nana*
12. *Hymenolepis diminuta*
13. *Schistosoma mansoni*
14. *Fasciolopsis buski*

9-3 and 9-4 and Plate 9) rests on the recognition of *Taenia* eggs in the stool and also on the finding of gravid proglottids since specific identification cannot be made by the eggs alone. The macroscopic sieve method and the microscopic wet-film preparation with saline solution and iodine are used (see p. 159).

Visualization of uterine pattern: The uterus of the proglottids can be injected with diluted **India ink** to outline its branches. A 25-gauge needle fits the birth pore. The proglottid is squashed between two slides and the uterine branches can be counted with a hand lens or a low-power microscope.

Taenia saginata (beef tapeworm) (Fig. 9-5 and Plate 9):

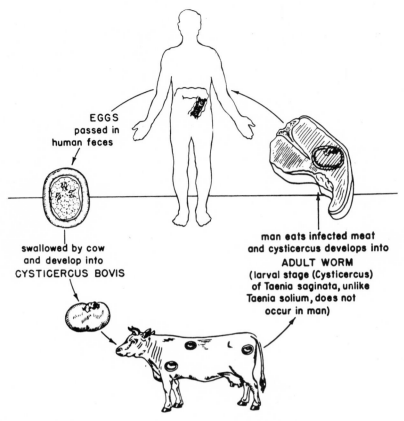

EGGS passed in human feces

swallowed by cow and develop into CYSTICERCUS BOVIS

man eats infected meat and cysticercus develops into ADULT WORM (larval stage (Cysticercus) of Taenia saginata, unlike Taenia solium, does not occur in man)

Fig. 9-5. *Taenia saginata.* (From Ash and Spitz: Pathology of tropical diseases: an atlas, Philadelphia, 1945, W. B. Saunders Co.)

Habitat: Upper part of small intestine.

Size: 9-13 ft. long and 5-7 mm. wide; scolex (head) is about the size of a pinhead, 1-2 mm. diam.

Ova: Spheroid, stained yellow or brown with bile, and about 30-40μ diam. They have a thick radially striated shell surrounding a thin clear space, which in turn surrounds the embryo (onchosphere) containing six characteristic hooklets.

Life history: The egg containing the embryo with the hooklets is swallowed by cattle, the shell is digested, and the embryo (hexacanth onchosphere) bores through the intestine, after which it loses its hooklets. It becomes encysted (*Cysticercus bovis*) in the muscles and organs of the animal, where it lies dormant. Meat so infected is recognized on inspection and is called "measly meat." When

this meat is eaten insufficiently cooked, the capsule is digested and the young parasite is set free in the intestine, where it develops in to the adult form in 2-3 mo.

Diagnosis: Ova and segments of the parasite may be found in the feces. After treatment, search should be made for the **scolex** (head) since the parasite will develop again unless this part is removed. The scolex is tetragonal, without hooklets, and has four cup-shaped suckers. **Segments**—uterus branches dichotomously, with 15-30 branches on each side. The genital pores are irregularly alternating. The segments are more actively motile than those of *Taenia solium* and are more long than broad.

The eggs have been found to contain some acid-fast material. They are deposited at times in the anal folds and

Table 9-4. Differential characteristics of important tapeworms in man

	Taenia saginata	*Taenia solium*	*Diphyllobothrium latum*
Length	4-8 m.	3-5 m.	4-10 m.
Scolex			
Shape	Quadrilateral	Globular	Almondlike
Size	1 × 1.5 mm.	1 × 1 mm.	3 × 1 mm.
Rostellum			
and hooklets	−	+	−
Suckers	4	4	2 (grooves)
Proglottids			
Number	2000	700-1000	3000-4000
Genital pore	Lateral border	Lateral border	Ventral surface
Uterine pore	−	−	+
Terminal segments (gravid)			
Size	19 × 7 mm.	11 × 5 mm.	3 × 11 mm.
Uterine branches	15-30 on each side	5-10 on each side	Rosette-shaped
Color	Milky white	Milky white	Red-brown
Appearance in feces	Usually appears singly	5 or 6 segments	Varies from a few inches to a few feet in length
Ova			
Shape	Oval	Oval	Oval, with operculum
Size	35 × 28μ	35 × 31μ	70 × 45μ
Color	Rusty brown	Rusty brown	Yellow-brown
Larvae	*Cysticercus bovis*	*Cysticercus cellulosae*	Plerocercoid (sparganum)
Size	5-9 mm.	5-10 mm.	2-15 mm.
Color	Milky white	Milky white	Chalky white

can be diagnosed by Scotch tape preparations.

Taenia solium (pork tapeworm) (Fig. 9-6 and Plate 9):

Habitat: Upper part of small intestine.

Size: 6-10 ft. long and 5-6 mm. wide; scolex (head) is about 0.5-1 mm. diam.

Ova: Similar to those of *Taenia saginata*.

Life history: Similar to *Taenia saginata*, except that the larval stage infects swine instead of cattle, and the scolex or head does not lose the hooklets. The larval form *(Cysticercus cellulosae)* is sometimes found in man, especially in the subcutaneous tissue and in the central nervous tissue (brain, eye).

Diagnosis: **Ova** and **segments** of the parasites may be found in the feces. After treatment, search should be made for the **scolex** because the parasite will develop again unless this part is removed. The scolex is globular, with two rows of hooklets and four cup-shaped suckers. **Seg-** ments—uterus branches dendritically, with 5-10 branches on each side. The genital pores are rather regularly alternating.

The gravid proglottid, though shorter, cannot be readily differentiated from the proglottid of *Taenia saginata*, except for the uterine pattern.

Diphyllobothrium latum (fish tapeworm) (Fig. 9-7 and Plate 9):

Habitat: Small intestine.

Size: 9-15 ft. long and 10-12 mm. wide. The segments are short, about 3 mm.

Characteristics: The **scolex** is almond-shaped, with one lateral groove on each side, and has no hooklets. **Segments**— uterus has a rosette shape and is centrally located. The gravid proglottid is more broad than long, creamy white, and motile.

Ova: About 45 × 70μ, ovoid, yellowish brown, and operculate (with a lid), so that pressure on the cover slip may open them. The ovum contains a globular

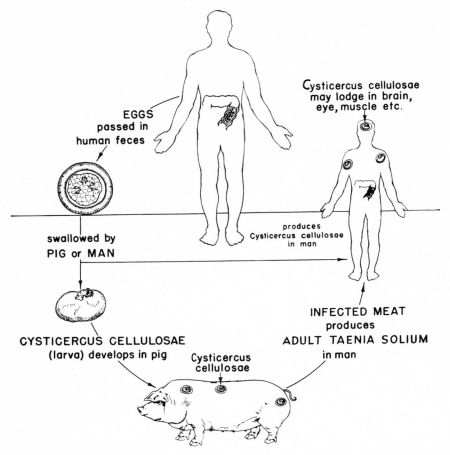

Fig. 9-6. *Taenia solium.* (From Ash and Spitz: Pathology of tropical diseases: an atlas, Philadelphia, 1945, W. B. Saunders Co.)

mass. *Diphyllobothrium latum* eggs must be differentiated from those of *Paragonimus westermani*, which are more ovoid, slender, and pointed at one end, while the operculum rests on a delicate ridge at the other end.

Life history: The ova passed in human stool find their way into some body of water and develop ciliated embryos (ciliated hexacanth onchospheres) which hatch out (coracidia), leaving the shells through the opercula. The embryo soon enters a crustacean (*Cyclops, Diaptomus*) as its first intermediate host and makes its way through the stomach wall into the body cavity, where it develops. The crustacean is eaten by some freshwater fish (pike, trout, etc.), the second intermediate host, in which the parasite migrates to the muscle tissue and lives without forming cysts. When the infected fish is eaten without being sufficiently cooked, the larval forms develop in the human intestine into the adult worms.

Diagnosis: The **ova** and sometimes **segments** of the parasite are found in the stool.

As mentioned in the discussion of macrocytic anemias, this tapeworm is responsible for a vitamin B_{12}-deficiency anemia. Investigations with Co^{60}-labeled vitamin B_{12} show that this parasite selectively takes up significant amounts of vitamin B_{12}.[15]

Echinococcus granulosus (hydatid cyst or echinococcus cyst) (Figs. 9-3 and 9-8):

Habitat: Adult worm is found in the intestine of the dog; larval stage(cyst)

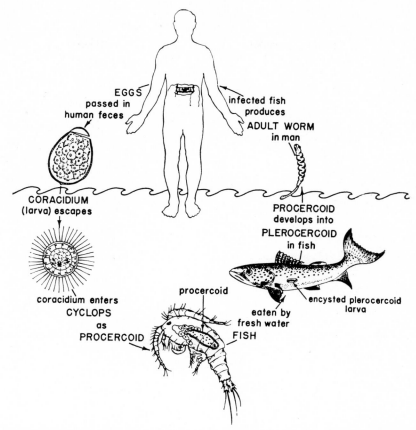

EGGS
passed in
human feces

infected fish
produces
ADULT WORM
in man

CORACIDIUM
(larva) escapes

PROCERCOID
develops into
PLEROCERCOID
in fish

coracidium enters
CYCLOPS
as
PROCERCOID

procercoid

eaten by
fresh water
FISH

encysted plerocercoid
larva

Fig. 9-7. *Diphyllobothrium latum.* (From Ash and Spitz: Pathology of tropical diseases: an atlas, Philadelphia, 1945, W. B. Saunders Co.)

is found in the tissues of sheep and man. The cysts are found chiefly in the liver and lungs; sometimes in the brain or eye.

Size: The adult worm is very small, 0.5 cm. long, and consists of only four segments.

Ova: Not found in human feces, but in feces of infected animals. Spheroidal, $30\text{-}50\mu$ diam., with thin radially striated shell containing embryo with six hooklets.

Life history: When the ova find their way into the digestive tract of man, the embryos are set free and make their way to the liver chiefly, but also to other organs, where they form cysts (Fig. 9-8). Smaller cysts, daughter cysts, may develop within the larger ones. The cysts are made up of two layers contributed by the parasite, an outer lamellated dense hyaline portion and an inner granular one, called the brood membrane, from which develop numerous larvae similar to the scolex, or head, of the parent worm. Should these reach the digestive tract of the dog or wolf, they develop into the adult form (scolex with a double row of hooklets; mature proglottid with a longitudinal uterus irregularly coiled). The cycle is completed in the wolf and other cannibalistic animals. Hydatid cysts are frequently found in sheep, cattle, and pigs.

Diagnosis: In man the disease (presence of cysts) must be suspected on clinical grounds. Serologic tests such as complement-fixation, hemagglutination precipitation, and skin tests are reliable.

Sometimes a positive skin reaction may be obtained with antigen made from a

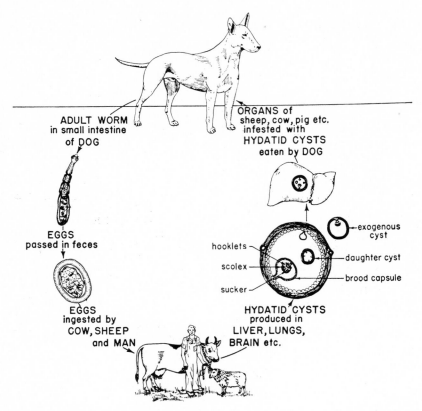

Fig. 9-8. *Echinococcus granulosus (Taenia echinococcus).* (From Ash and Spitz: Pathology of tropical diseases: an atlas, Philadelphia, 1945, W. B. Saunders Co.)

closely related species (group reaction). An antigen prepared from *Dipylidium caninum* is frequently used.

Microscopic examination of the cyst fluid shows scolices, free hooklets, cholesterin crystals, and granular debris from the degenerated scolices and cyst wall (Figs. 9-9 and 9-10). These may be found in the urine or sputum when a cyst ruptures into the urinary or respiratory tract. Since the fluid is infectious, it is dangerous to puncture the cyst to confirm a diagnosis.

In several papers Fischman[16, 17] describes a new serologic technique of diagnosing human hydatid disease employing polystyrene latex particles coated with hydatid cyst fluid and a modified technique using bentonite particles. Upon request the Communicable Disease Center (C.D.C.) of the United States Public Health Service, Chamblee, Georgia, will perform the complement-fixation test, the bentonite flocculation test, and the hemagglutination procedure.*

Hymenolepis nana (dwarf tapeworm) (Figs. 9-3, 9-4, and 9-11):

Size: From 1.5-2.5 cm. long and 0.5 mm. wide.

Characteristics: There are about 150-200 **segments**. The **scolex** bears four small suckers and a short rostellum with 20-30 hooklets arranged in a single ring.

Ova: Nearly spheroidal, colorless, and transparent; about 40μ diam. There are two distinct walls, between which is a gelatinous appearing substance. At each pole of the inner wall is a slight protuberance from which arise two hairlike processes. These processes may be so

---

*Specimens should be sent to the laboratory of the local state health department, where it will be transmitted to the C.D.C.

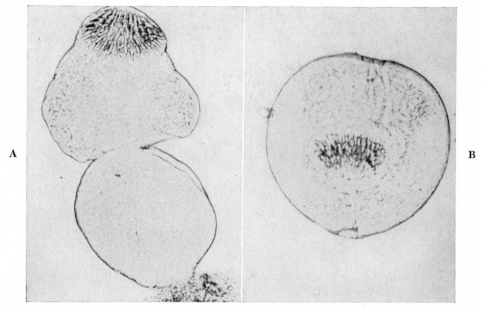

A   B

Fig. 9-9. Scolices of *Echinococcus granulosus.* **A,** Hooklets and suckers evaginated. **B,** Hooklets and suckers invaginated.

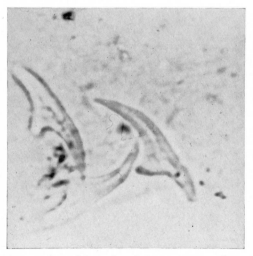

Fig. 9-10. Hooklets of *Echinococcus granulosus.*

placed that they simulate a third wall. Within the inner wall is a fully developed embryo with three pairs of hooklets.

Life history: There is no intermediate host. The eggs are passed in the feces and ingested by man or mice, where they hatch and develop into onchospheres in the intestinal tract. They penetrate the intestinal mucosa and develop into cysticercoids, the larval form from which the tapeworm develops. The worms penetrate the mucosa and escape into the lumen of the bowel, where they attach themselves to the small bowel wall, mature, and lay eggs (Fig. 9-11).

Diagnosis: The ova are found in the feces. (See description of diagnostic points, i.e., shape, size, shell, embryo, and filaments.)

Hymenolepis diminuta (rat tapeworm)[18]**:**

Habitat: Intestine of man.

Size: Up to 2.5 in. long.

Characteristics (Fig. 9-3): The **scolex** has four suckers and an unarmed retractile rostellum. The mature **proglottid** is more wide than long and carries a central ovary. It is seldom seen in stool. The organism may have up to 1000 proglottids.

Ova: Nearly spherical; $50 \times 70\mu$. The distinct outer yellowish membrane is thick and has an irregular inner border. It is separated by a gelatinous layer (space) from the delicate inner membrane that surrounds the six-hooked onchosphere. There are no polar filaments.

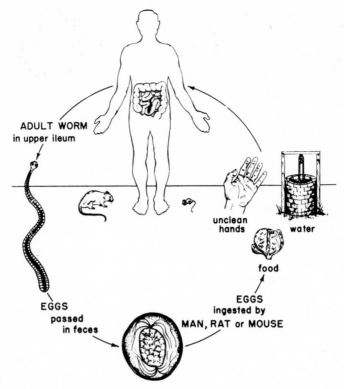

ADULT WORM
in upper ileum

unclean
hands

water

food

EGGS
passed
in feces

EGGS
ingested by
MAN, RAT or MOUSE

Fig. 9-11. *Hymenolepis nana.* (From Ash and Spitz: Pathology of tropical diseases: an atlas, Philadelphia, 1945, W. B. Saunders Co.)

Life history: Eggs are contained in the feces of the final host animals and are acquired by various insects such as roaches, fleas, and mealworms in which the larvae develop. The insects in turn are ingested by various animals that act as final hosts and reservoirs, e.g., dogs, mice, rats, etc. Man acquires infection through ingestion of parasitized insect hosts such as larvae in grains and cereals.

Diagnosis: Diagnosis depends on the characteristic eggs.

Dipylidium caninum (common tapeworm of dog):

Habitat: Small intestine.

Size: 10-50 cm.

Characteristics (Fig. 9-3): The **scolex** has three or four rows of hooklets; **segments** are shaped like cucumber seed. The gravid proglottid is pink because of the red-colored ova.

Ova: In groups of 8-15, surrounded by one embryonic membrane; measure 25 ×

40μ and are spherical. The ova resemble those of *Taenia saginata* but do not have striated shells. The outer shell is brick red. The ova are liberated by the disintegration of the segments and contain embryos with three pairs of hooklets.

Life history: Ova are ingested by fleas of dogs, cats, and man and by the dog louse, which serve as intermediate hosts. The infected fleas or lice are ingested by the dog, the final host.

Diagnosis: The ova or the segments are found in the feces.

NEMATODES OR ROUNDWORMS

These parasites have a complete intestinal tract and a body cavity (without epithelial lining) into which project four longitudinal chords. They have nervous, excretory, and reproductive systems, and the sexes are separate.

In cross section, as sometimes found in sections of the appendix, the type of mus-

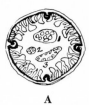 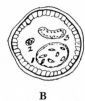 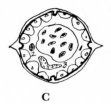

A   B   C

Fig. 9-12. Cross sections of female nematodes (schematic). **A,** Polymyarian type *(Ascaris* and *Toxocara). **B,** Holomyarian type *(Trichuris). **C,** Meromyarian type *(Enterobius, Ancylostoma,* and *Necator).* **1,** Uterus; **2,** ovary; **3,** digestive tract.

culature aids in distinguishing the species (Fig. 9-12).

There are two large groups of nematodes: intestinal nematodes and tissue-inhabiting nematodes.

Intestinal nematodes

Trichuris trichiura (whipworm):

Habitat: Large intestine, usually cecum or appendix.

Size: 3-5 cm. long.

Characteristics: Anterior three-fifths is slender and threadlike; posterior two-fifths is thicker, bulbous, and whiplike. The worm is white. The coiled posterior end of the male resembles a watch spring.

Ova: Ovoid; stained brown, yellow, or green with bile; measure about $50 \times 23\mu$ diam. There is a characteristic clear refractile plug at each end. They are barrel-shaped and have a thick double wall; the inner wall is lighter than the outer. The unsegmented immature embryo fills the entire egg (Plate 9).

Life history: The ova require from a few weeks to about 18 mo. in polluted soil to develop to the mature embryo stage, at which time they are infectious. When they reach the digestive tract of man after they become infectious, usually with contaminated food and water, they develop to the adult form.

Diagnosis: The characteristic ova are found in the feces.

Enterobius vermicularis or Oxyuris vermicularis (pinworm):

Habitat: Man is the only host; the organisms are found in the large intestine and appendix.

Size: Female measures $5\text{-}10 \times 0.5$ mm. diam. The male is almost microscopic in size and has a curved pointed tail.

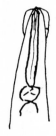

Fig. 9-13. Head of *Enterobius vermicularis* showing cuticular expansion.

Characteristics: The posterior end of the female is drawn out into a long pointed structure. The vulva opens at the junction of the anterior and middle third of the body. The anterior end has cuticular expansions resembling lips, but there is no true buccal cavity. The esophagus ends in a bulb (Fig. 9-13).

Ova: Asymmetrically ovoid, colorless, and about $50 \times 20\mu$ diam. One side is characteristically flattened. The shell is thick and double-contoured. The mature larva is coiled inside. (See Fig. 2-11, p. 51.)

Life history: The gravid female wanders out from the intestine to deposit the ova in the rugae about the anal margin. This produces itching and scratching so that some ova burst. The ova contain embryos which are infectious so that auto-infection is the rule. This also accounts for the extremely heavy infections. When the ova are taken into the digestive tract, they hatch, moult twice, mate in the small intestine, and migrate to the large intestine. The complete life cycle requires about 2 wk.

Diagnosis: Ova may be found in the

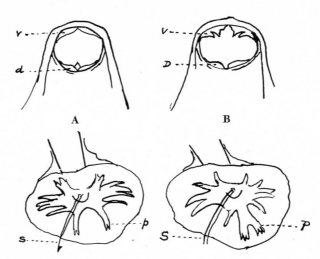

Fig. 9-14. Mouths and caudal bursae of hookworms. **A**, *Necator americanus:* **v**, ventral cutting plates; **d**, dorsal cutting plates and median tooth; **s**, pair of copulatory spicules, fused distally and ending in a barbed tip; **p**, characteristic posterior muscle ray. **B**, *Ancylostoma duodenale:* **V**, two pairs of ventral teeth; **D**, dorsal cutting plates; **S**, pair of copulatory spicules, not fused and without barbs; **P**, characteristic posterior muscle ray.

scrapings from the anal margin, especially in the morning before the patient has had a bath, and sometimes under the fingernails. Adult worms may be found after an enema given when the itching is worst, usually in the early evening.

Scotch tape preparation: Over one end of a tongue depressor curve a 3 in. long strip of ¾ in. wide Scotch tape, sticky side out. Spread the anal folds apart and firmly touch all four quadrants of the mucocutaneous junction with the sticky tape. Spread the sticky surface of the tape on a microscope slide and examine microscopically for *Enterobius* ova. If none are found, lift the tape off the slide, place 1 drop toluene on the slide, and replace the tape. The toluene will clear the extraneous matter on the slide but will not harm the ova.

Necator americanus (American hookworm):

Habitat: Small intestine.

Size: Female is 9-11 mm. long and 0.35 mm. diam. Male is 5-9 mm. long and 0.30 mm. diam.

Characteristics: The anterior end of the adult hookworm is curved sharply into a dorsal hook. The **mouth cavity** has one pair of broad semilunar chitinous plates

anteriorly, one pair of smaller ones posteriorly, and a prominent dorsal toothlike structure projecting into the cavity from the posterior wall (Fig. 9-14). The vulva of the female is anterior to the middle of the body.

The **male bursa**, a cuticular expansion over the caudal end, contains a number of muscular groups or rays, the two posterior ones of which are characteristic. They are small, and their tips are divided into two fingerlike portions. The two spicules (long bristlelike structures extending from the caudal end of the male parasite) are barbed, and their distal ends are frequently fused.

Ova (Plate 9): Ovoid, colorless, 40 × 60μ, and hyaline. The shell is thin and transparent. It contains an immature segmented embryo in the 2-8 cell stage. It is surrounded by a clear outer zone that separates it from the shell.

Life history (Fig. 9-15): The ova develop in warm moist soil, and the young worms, the **rhabditiform larvae,** hatch out in a few days. The larvae grow and moult twice, being transformed into the **filariform type** and becoming infectious in about 3-6 wk. The usual mode of infection is through the skin, though the larvae may

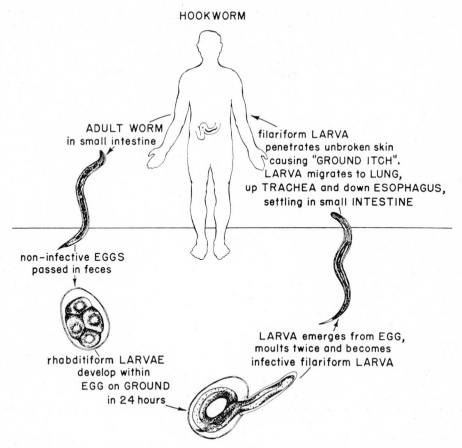

HOOKWORM

ADULT WORM
in small intestine

filariform LARVA
penetrates unbroken skin
causing "GROUND ITCH".
LARVA migrates to LUNG,
up TRACHEA and down ESOPHAGUS,
settling in small INTESTINE

non-infective EGGS
passed in feces

rhabditiform LARVAE
develop within
EGG on GROUND
in 24 hours

LARVA emerges from EGG,
moults twice and becomes
infective filariform LARVA

Fig. 9-15. *Necator americanus.* (From Ash and Spitz: Pathology of tropical diseases: an atlas, Philadelphia, 1945, W. B. Saunders Co.)

reach the digestive tract directly with food or water from polluted soil. When infected earth is placed upon the skin, the larvae are found to enter through the skin within 5 min. This produces dermatitis, the so-called **ground itch.** The larvae migrate by blood and lymph vessels to the lungs, enter the air sacs, make their way to the bronchi and pharynx, and are swallowed. They attach themselves to the mucosa of the small intestine by means of the buccal cavity and mature to adult forms. The ova are found in the feces in from 7-10 wk. after the infection.

Diagnosis: Ova are found in the feces and are diagnostic. When the larva first hatches (**rhabditiform larva**), the writhing snakelike motion and the long buc-

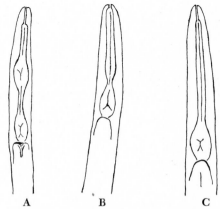

A   B   C

Fig. 9-16. Diagram showing the mouth and esophagus of rhabditiform larvae of the following. **A,** *Rhabditis hominis.* **B,** *Strongyloides.* **C,** *Necator americanus.*

cal cavity (about the diameter of the larva) distinguish it from the rhabditiform larva of *Strongyloides intestinalis,* which has a characteristic lashing motion (purposeless) and a very short buccal cavity (Fig. 9-16). The larva of the hookworm is not found in fresh feces but may be found in specimens that are a day old or more; the larva of *Strongyloides* is found in fresh specimens.

Ancylostoma duodenale (Old World hookworm):

Size: Female is 10-13 mm. long; male measures 8-11 mm. in length.

Characteristics: This parasite is very similar to *Necator americanus,* but it is very slightly larger, and the head does not curve so sharply in a dorsal hook as that of the American type. The ova are somewhat more ovoid. The chief differences, however, are in the mouthparts and in the male bursa (Fig. 9-14). The **buccal cavity** of *Ancylostoma duodenale* has two pairs of rather sharp curved teeth ventrally and one platelike pair posteriorly. The vulva of the female is posterior to the middle of the body. The posterior rays in the **male bursa** are fused proximally, and each tip is divided into three fingerlike portions. The two spicules are without barbs and are not fused.

Ancylostoma braziliense (dog and cat hookworms):

Size: Female is 9-11 mm. long; male measures 8-8.5 mm. in length.

Characteristics: This hookworm is the smallest one affecting man. It has two pairs of ventral teeth, the inner (medial) pair being much smaller than the outer pair (Fig. 9-17). It is frequently found in the intestine of cats and dogs, but rarely in the intestine of man.

Creeping eruption (cutaneous larva

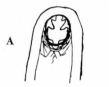 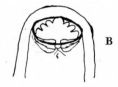

Fig. 9-17. Buccal cavities of the dog hookworms. **A,** *Ancylostoma braziliense.* **B,** *Ancylostoma caninum.*

migrans): The disease is due to infective filariform larvae of the dog and cat hookworms, which invade the unprotected human skin and wander about in the stratum germinativum, forming a serpiginous tunnel, the course of which is outlined by redness and elevation, followed by scaliness. Itching is intense, and secondary infection often follows scratching. The cutaneous lesion may progress from a few millimeters to several centimeters a day, the larva being in advance of the raised reddened portion of the tunnel. The larva (larva migrans) may continue the migration for weeks or months, apparently unable to penetrate through the skin in order to complete the life cycle. The skin lesion occurs along the coast of the United States during the swimming season wherever dogs and cats are permitted on beaches.

Ancylostoma caninum (dog hookworm):

Size: Female is 14 mm. long; male is 10 mm. long.

Characteristics: It is the most common hookworm of the dog. The filariform larva may cause mild dermatitis in man. The dog hookworm is characterized by three pairs of ventral teeth in a wide buccal cavity (Fig. 9-17).

Ascaris lumbricoides (large roundworm):

Habitat: Small intestine.

Size: Female is 20-35 cm. long (longer than the male) and 3-6 mm. diam. Male is 15-25 cm. long and 3-6 mm. diam.

Characteristics: The adult worm is white or pink and has fine striations of the cuticula. The anterior end has three lips. The posterior end of the male is curved.

Ova: The ova may be present in several different forms (Fig. 9-18).

1. Fertilized eggs: They are ovoid and measure $50\text{-}75 \times 40\text{-}60\mu$. They are yellow to brown. They have a thick shell with a mammillated outer covering and a thick transparent hyaline inner shell. There is a crescentic inner clear space at either pole of the egg.
2. Unfertilized eggs: When only females are present in the intestine, the ova are elongated, have thinner

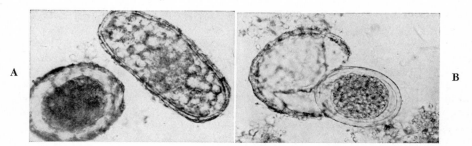

Fig. 9-18. Ova of *Ascaris lumbricoides.* **A,** Fertile and unfertile eggs. **B,** Fertile egg expressed from its ruptured outer mammillated membrane. (×400.)

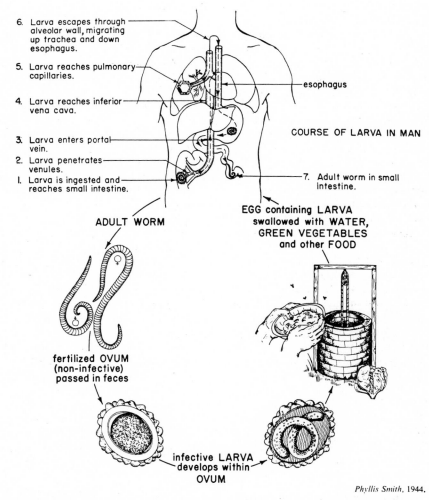

Fig. 9-19. *Ascaris lumbricoides.* (From Ash and Spitz: Pathology of tropical diseases: an atlas, Philadelphia, 1945, W. B. Saunders Co.)

shells, and are filled with a coarse granular or globular protoplasm. They are stained yellow or brown with bile. They lack the crescentic clear space and are often misshapen and distorted.

3. Decorticated eggs: The outer mammillated shell is at times absent, leaving only the inner thick hyaline membrane. The eggs may or may not be fertile.

One female worm may produce 200,000 ova per day and a total of 25 million.

Life history: In the feces the eggs are unsegmented. After 2-5 wk. in polluted soil, the eggs contain a wormlike embryo and are infectious. These eggs are very resistant and can withstand winter without injury. They are viable for 5-6 yr. at least. They can also withstand 5% formalin for long periods. When the infectious ova are taken into the digestive tract, the embryos leave the shell in about 15 hr., make their way through the intestines, and migrate through the liver to the lungs, chiefly through the blood vessels. During this migration they grow to a length of 2 mm. From the lungs they make their way into the bronchi and are coughed up and swallowed. They develop in the intestine to the familiar adult worm in about a month (Fig. 9-19).

Diagnosis: Diagnosis depends on finding the various types of eggs and all of the adult form in the stool. In severe infestations, *Ascaris* larvae may be found in the stool. All the previously described methods of direct wet-film preparation and concentration methods should be used.

Toxocara cati (roundworm of the cat): The adult is characterized by three lips (like *Ascaris*) and a pair of broad lateral cervical alae, giving its head an arrowhead appearance.

In other respects this parasite is similar to *Toxocara canis,* the head of which has narrow lateral cervical alae, the shape suggesting a bow (Fig. 9-20).

Toxocara canis (roundworm of the dog):

Habitat: Small intestine.

Size: Female is 6-12 cm. long; male is 4-6 cm. long.

Ova: Spheroidal, with thin shell; grayish (or very slightly bile stained after standing); thin albuminous envelope with alveolated surface.

Life history: Probably similar to that of *Ascaris lumbricoides.* Children are infected by playing with dogs.

Visceral larva migrans[19, 20]**:** This clinical syndrome is due to ingestion of eggs of nonhuman parasites, especially *Toxocara canis* and *Toxocara cati.* It occurs mainly in children, and gives rise to a pronounced eosinophilia in the peripheral blood, a granulomatous enlargement of the liver with eosinophilia, and bronchopneumonia with eosinophilia. Man is an abnormal host and the parasite does not mature in the human body.

Stoll egg-counting technique: This method is used to obtain a **quantitative estimation** of the number of worm eggs in a measured sample of feces.

Procedure:

1. Fill a special Stoll flask with 0.1N sodium hydroxide to the bottom mark etched on the neck of the flask (56 ml.).
2. Using two applicators, add sufficient feces to the fluid to raise the level to the upper mark etched on the neck (60 ml.).
3. Add 6-8 glass beads and firmly insert a rubber stopper.
4. If the feces is very hard, allow the preparation to soak for a while.
5. Shake vigorously with a straight up-and-down motion for 1 min. to secure a homogenous suspension. Some investigators recommend shaking the flask in an inverted

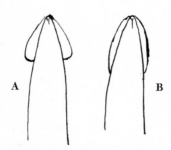

Fig. 9-20. Head showing cervical alae. **A,** *Toxocara cati.* **B,** *Toxocara canis.*

position. It is very important to avoid a circular motion since this may concentrate the ova in a small area.

6. It is the best routine to run the sample to this point in the afternoon and to set it aside until the next morning. Reshake (up and down) the contents of the flask the following day. Complete comminution of the feces is essential for an accurate result.

7. The ova and debris will begin to settle out immediately after shaking stops. Using a Stoll pipette calibrated to 0.15 ml. with rubber bulb attached, **quickly** withdraw 0.15 ml. sample. Insert the tip of the pipette in the center of the flask to decrease the error due to settling.

8. Expel the entire contents of the pipette onto a 3 × 1½ in. slide.

9. Cover the drop with a 22 × 40 mm. No. 2 cover slip.

10. Examine under low-power lens, moving the slide with a mechanical stage.

11. Count **all** the hookworm ova present in the preparation, including those not confined under the cover slip.

12. Multiply the number obtained by 100. This will yield the total number of ova per milliliter of formed feces. For mushy stools multiply this latter number by the correction factor 2; for diarrheic stools multiply by 4.

13. By multiplying the number per milliliter by the total weight of the 24 hr. fecal specimen, the daily output of eggs can be derived. With knowledge of the average number of eggs laid per day by a single female worm of the parasite, a reasonably accurate estimate of the female worm burden of an individual can be made. The following are estimates of the number of **eggs per female per day:**

Necator americanus: 9000
Ascaris lumbricoides: 70,000-250,000
Trichuris trichiura: 5000-7000

Since the number of male and female worms is usually about equal, the total number of worms may be computed roughly as twice the estimated number of female worms.

Keller and associates[20a] used the following classification for their surveys of hookworms:

Intensity grouping (eggs/ml. feces)	Clinical classification
100-699	Very light
700-2599	Light
2600-12,599	Moderate
12,600-25,099	Heavy
25,100 and over	Very heavy

Strongyloides stercoralis:

Size and morphology: The adult parasitic worm is microscopic, filariform, and measures about 2 mm. in length. The cylindric esophagus is one-third the length of the body. The parasitic male, which is seldom found, is rhabditiform like the free-living male and measures 0.7 mm. in length.

Ova: Ova are not found in feces except when active diarrhea exists because they hatch in the intestines. When found, they are similar to hookworm ova.

The larvae are found in feces (see diagnosis).

Life history: The parasitic female bores deeply into the mucosa, chiefly that of the duodenum, and deposits eggs that hatch in situ.

The parasite has three types of life cycle.

1. Indirect cycle. The actively motile **rhabditiform larvae** make their way into the lumen of the intestines and are voided with the feces. These larvae (Fig. 9-15) are rather short and thick; outside the body in the soil they develop into adult free-living male and female forms. These free-living forms resemble the filariform larvae of the hookworm but have a shorter mouth cavity, a longer esophagus, and a notch in the tail (Fig. 9-21). After fertilization the free-living female produces eggs that develop into rhabditiform larvae. These rhabditiform larvae become infective **filariform larvae** in a short period of time. They may repeat the free-

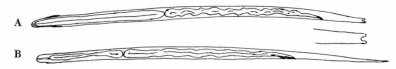

Fig. 9-21. Filariform larvae. **A,** *Strongyloides stercoralis* with notched tail (inset shows notch enlarged). **B,** *Necator americanus.*

living generation or they may enter new hosts.

2. Direct cycle: After 2 or 3 days the rhabditiform larvae transform into the slender infective filariform larvae that penetrate the skin of man and thus enter the venous circulation and are finally carried to the lungs. From the lungs the parasites ascend to the glottis and are swallowed and reach the intestines, where they develop into adult forms. The parasitic female then enters the mucosa of the small bowel, deposits eggs, and starts the new generation.

3. Autoinfection cycle: The rhabditiform larvae develop into filariform larvae within the intestines and penetrate the intestinal mucosa or the perianal skin to start a developmental cycle within the host.

Diagnosis: Rhabditiform larvae are found in the feces and are the diagnostic stage. They are microscopic, measuring 200-250μ in length. They exhibit a characteristic lashing, purposeless motion. The buccal or mouth cavity is short, the length being less than half the diameter of the body.

Differential diagnosis of rhabditiform larvae:

HOOKWORM LARVAE: The buccal cavity of the hookworm larva is longer than the buccal cavity of the *Strongyloides* larva. Its length is about the same as the diameter of the body. Otherwise the hookworm larva is very similar to the *Strongyloides* larva. Hookworm larvae are usually accompanied by hookworm eggs and will only be found in the stool specimen that has been left standing for some time. If only rhabditiform larvae are found in a fresh specimen, *Strongyloides* should be suspected.

RHABDITIS HOMINIS: This free-living parasite is harmless and resembles the rhabditiform larva of *Strongyloides.* *Rhabditis hominis* worms show variation in length and have a buccal cavity that is longer than that of *Strongyloides,* thus resembling the buccal cavity of the hookworm. The esophagus presents an anterior tubular portion followed by a bulb, then another tubular portion, and then the posterior bulb (see Fig. 9-14). Both adults and larvae are found in the feces.

Demonstration of rhabditiform larvae of Strongyloides: The zinc flotation and formalin-ether concentration methods are suitable for the demonstration of larvae. If no larvae are found after several attempts, duodenal aspiration is advisable.

DUODENAL ASPIRATION: Rhabditiform larvae and eggs may be found within mucus and bile-stained fragments. Duodenal aspirate may contain several parasites in addition to *Strongyloides,* such as the trophozoites of *Giardia lamblia* and the eggs of hookworms. *Strongyloides* rhabditiform larvae within their eggs will hatch at room temperature in 15-20 min.

Demonstration of filariform larvae:

PRINCIPLE: After 24-48 hr. of incubation, rhabditiform larvae transform into filariform larvae.

PROCEDURE: Moisten stool in a glass jar with several drops of water (not saline solution), cap the jar loosely, and allow to stand at room temperature. After 24-48 hr. of incubation, examine the sides of the glass jar with a hand lens for almost microscopic infective filariform larvae.

Additional laboratory findings in Strongyloides infestation: There is usually a marked eosinophilia of the peripheral blood.

Trichostrongylus:

Habitat: Intestine of man. This is one of the most common intestinal nematodes in some areas of Japan.

Morphology: Female measures 5-8 mm. in length. The head is unarmed, there is no buccal dilatation, and a notch indicates the excretory pore. Male is a small roundworm, measuring 4-6 mm. in length. It has a copulatory bursa with rays and spicules.

Ova: They resemble hookworm eggs, but are much larger, 85-115μ. They are elongate and oval and have a transparent hyaline shell that is separated by a clear space from the embryo in the morula stage.

Diagnosis: Diagnosis includes detection of adult worms in stool and finding the characteristic egg.

• • •

Gordiacea

Intestinal nematodes must be distinguished from a group of free-living roundworms, the Gordiacea.

This class of nemathelminthes differs from the nematodes in that the posterior part of the digestive tract in the adult is atrophied. The gonads are discontinuous with their ducts, and the body cavity is chiefly filled with germ cells. The body cavity is lined with a layer of muscle cells of the holomyarian type (see Fig. 9-12), but the cells are taller than those in *Trichuris,* and beneath the muscular layer is a characteristic hypodermal single layer of clear cuboidal cells (Fig. 9-22).

The adults are free-living roundworms found in fresh water or in the vegetation along the water's edge. The larvae are parasites of the insects found in such places. In the body cavity of these insects the larvae become threadlike worms and then emerge into the water, where they mature.

The long threadlike adult (10-50 cm. or 4-20 in. long) is frequently called a hairworm, hair snake, or cabbage worm. The worm is not pathogenic. It may be accidentally swallowed as a free-living form or as a form still within the insect host.

The anterior ends of the worms are bluntly rounded. The posterior ends may be rounded, bifurcated, or trifurcated, depending upon the species and the sex.

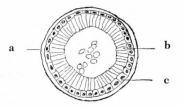

Fig. 9-22. Cross section of *Gordius* sp. (schematic). **a,** Cuticle; **b,** hypodermal cell layer; **c,** muscle layer.

Some species are tuberculated. These worms are passed in feces and urine and are sometimes found in vomitus.

• • •

Tissue-inhabiting nematodes

Nematodes that inhabit tissues include the filariae, *Dracunculus medinensis,* and *Trichinella spiralis.*

FILARIAE[21]:

Classification: The following nematodes belong to the filariae: *Wuchereria bancrofti, Wuchereria malayi, Onchocerca volvulus, Loa loa, Acanthocheilonema perstans,* and *Mansonella ozzardi.*

Morphology: The threadlike adult worms vary in length from 19-60 cm. The female is twice as long as the male. The parasites are white and are covered with a smooth or patterned cuticle.

Microfilariae: The larvae produced by the female are called microfilariae and measure from 177-300μ in length. Some retain their shells, or **sheath,** while others discard it and remain "unsheathed." The sheath closely surrounds the organisms but can be detected where it projects beyond the tail or head.

The embryos may migrate into the peripheral circulation, often periodically, or may be found in chylous urine, chylous exudate, or nodular swellings. Stained preparations of microfilariae show deeply colored columns of nuclei within the body.

Life history: The microfilariae are ingested by a blood-sucking insect vector (mosquito, fly, or midge), in which they develop to the infective stage and migrate to the proboscis of the insect. When the insect feeds on man, the parasites enter the body of the final host and migrate

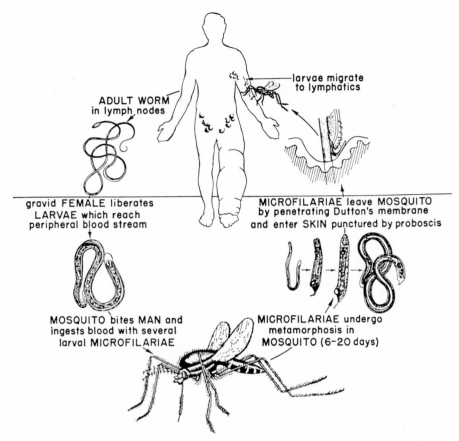

ADULT WORM
in lymph nodes

larvae migrate
to lymphatics

gravid FEMALE liberates
LARVAE which reach
peripheral blood stream

MICROFILARIAE leave MOSQUITO
by penetrating Dutton's membrane
and enter SKIN punctured by proboscis

MOSQUITO bites MAN and
ingests blood with several
larval MICROFILARIAE

MICROFILARIAE undergo
metamorphosis in
MOSQUITO (6–20 days)

Fig. 9-23. *Filaria (Wuchereria) bancrofti.* (From Ash and Spitz: Pathology of tropical diseases: an atlas, Philadelphia, 1945, W. B. Saunders Co.)

to their specific tissues, where they develop into the mature worm. After mating, the adult female gives birth to a new generation of microfilariae.

The adult threadlike worms, male and female, are found in pairs in lymph vessels, lymph nodes, body cavities, or subcutaneous tissue, where they often obstruct the lymph flow and cause elephantiasis, chyluria, chylous exudates, or nodular swelling (Fig. 9-23).

Diagnosis:

Examination of blood: In the case of *W. bancrofti* and *W. malayi*, more parasites are found in the blood if examined at night.

Unstained preparation: Mount 1 drop capillary blood under cover glass and examine for microfilariae.

Stained preparation: Stain thick and thin smears with hematoxylin-eosin, a method especially good for staining the details of the microfilariae and the sheaths. To prepare a thick smear, collect 2-3 drops of blood in one small area of the slide and mix. When dry, lake the smear in water, dry in air, fix in equal parts of ether and 95% alcohol for 10 min., dry in air, and stain with hematoxylin-eosin (see Chapter 16). Wright stain may be decolorized with acid alcohol and restained with hematoxylin-eosin. Prepare thin smear as for hematology.

Concentration by centrifugation: Obtain a larger amount of capillary blood (better than venous blood) by puncture of the finger and place in a centrifuge tube containing 2% acetic acid. When laked, centrifuge and examine sediment under cover glass.

DIFFERENTIAL DIAGNOSIS OF MICROFILARIAE: Identification of the species is based on the presence or absence of a sheath and the distribution of nuclei in the tail.

SHEATHED LARVAE: The larvae of the following species are enclosed in sheaths:

Wuchereria bancrofti (Filaria bancrofti):

General characteristics: The parasite is widely distributed in tropic and subtropic zones and has been found in the United States at Charleston, S. C. It produces elephantiasis of the lower extremities and scrotum, but many patients present no symptoms. The intermediate host is a mosquito *(Culex fatigans,* especially). The larvae vary greatly in size (150-500 × 7.5μ), are enclosed in a sheath (the egg capsule or shell), and show a nocturnal periodicity in the blood. They tend to collect in the capillaries of internal organs (especially the lungs) during the day. The granules of the body cells do not extend to the tip of the tail. The tail is pointed.

Very similar to this larva is the microfilaria of *Wuchereria malayi* (Dutch East Indies, New Guinea, and China), which is characterized by two nuclei in the tail, with enlargement at these levels.

Loa loa:

General characteristics: The filarial worm is common in Africa and lives in the subcutaneous tissues, where it causes fugitive swellings (Calabar swellings). The intermediate host is a fly *(Chrysops).* The larvae measure about 250-300 × 7μ, are enclosed in a sheath, and show a diurnal periodicity. The granules of the body cells extend to the tip of the tail, which is less sharply pointed.

UNSHEATHED LARVAE: The larvae of the following species are not enclosed within sheaths:

Acanthocheilonema perstans:

General characteristics: The worm is prevalent in tropical Africa, coastal South America, and the West Indies. The adults live in the mesentery and retroperitoneal tissue, usually without causing symptoms. The intermediate host is a midge, a kind of gnat *(Culicoides).* The larvae (microfilaria) are small, 200 × 5μ, do not occur in sheaths, and do not show any periodicity, but usually there are more in the peripheral blood at night. The granular body cells extend to the tip of the tail, which is blunt.

The microfilaria of *Mansonella ozzardi,* a very similar parasite, is distinguished by a rather blunt tail in which the granules of the body cells do not extend to the tip.

Onchocerca volvulus:

General characteristics: The parasite is widely distributed in Africa and is found also in Guatemala and southern Mexico. The adults live in the connective tissues, causing nodules, most commonly at the junction of long bones and under the scalp. The intermediate host is a black gnat *(Simulium damnosum).* The larvae measure about 250 × 7.5μ and are unsheathed, and the granules of the body cells do not extend to the tip of the pointed tail. These microfilariae are found in the nodules with the adults or in the adjacent lypmh vessels, rarely in the blood.

Examination of skin: *Onchocerca volvulus* is best diagnosed by the following method. Cleanse an area of skin, raise a fold and pinch slightly until it is blanched, and make several shallow punctures with a sterile lancet to obtain tissue fluid without blood. Mount fluid on a microslide and examine stained or unstained.

• • •

Dracunculus medinensis (guinea worm):

Distribution: The guinea worm is common in Asia, Africa, and Arabia and is less common in the West Indies and Brazil.

Size: The male is rarely found and is small, about 25-40 mm. The female measures about 80-120 cm. × 1.6 mm. and has been likened to a catgut thread.

Life history: The gravid female wanders through the subcutaneous tissues to the foot or the ankle and forms a nodule which ulcerates. The head of the parasite protrudes, and whenever the foot is in contact with fresh water, numerous larvae are discharged (through prolapse of uterus

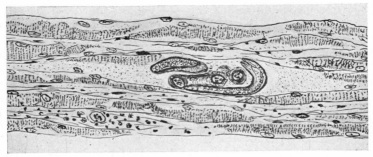

Fig. 9-24. Larva of *Trichinella spiralis* in striated muscle fiber at tendinous insertion. Low-power field showing myositis with infiltration of polymorphonuclear leukocytes and eosinophils. (Hematoxylin-eosin stain.)

through the esophagus or head portion), and the parasite dies. The unsheathed larvae are $600 \times 20\mu$. A crustacean (*Cyclops*) is the intermediate host, and the infection is spread by swallowing the *Cyclops* in the contaminated water. The parasite has been reported in North America in the fox, the raccoon, and the mink.

Diagnosis: It is based on finding the pregnant adult female worm immediately below the skin in an ulcerated area. Washings of the ulcer will produce microfilariae discharged by the worm.

Trichinella spiralis[22]:

Habitat: Small intestine and muscles.

Size: Very small. The male is about 1.5 mm. long, and the female is 3 or 4 mm. long. Larvae are about 100μ in length soon after birth (in feces, blood, and cerebrospinal fluid) but grow rapidly to about 1 mm. (encysted larvae).

Ova: None. The parasite is viviparous.

Life history: The infection is continuous in rats through cannibalism. Hogs are infected by eating scraps of infected slaughtered hogs and by feeding on infected rats. Man becomes infected by eating raw infected pork. In the intestine the encysted larvae within the animal skeletal muscle are freed and penetrate the duodenal mucosa, where they mature and mate. Live larvae are discharged by the pregnant female within the intestinal wall, from where they reach the bloodstream. While in the bloodstream, in heavy infections the larvae must be distinguished from the *Filarioidea*, from

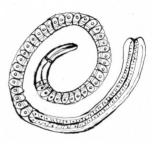

Fig. 9-25. Larva of *Trichinella spiralis* showing clear cell bodies around the esophagus.

which they morphologically differ. After reaching muscle in man they grow to about 1 mm. in size and become encysted. In man the cysts usually become calcified and the larvae die. In animal infestations a second host is required to liberate the encysted larvae.

The parasite is killed by thorough cooking or by freezing at $-30°$ C. for 24 hr.

Diagnosis: Diagnosis is based on demonstration of tissue parasites. The larvae may be found in a bit of muscle obtained from the gastrocnemius or at the insertion of the deltoid. The muscle should be teased out, pressed between slides, and examined under the low-power lens. It may be fixed, sectioned, stained with hematoxylin-eosin, and examined (Fig. 9-24). Or it may be digested with pepsin and hydrochloric acid (0.5N HCl containing about 0.25 gm. pepsin and 0.9 gm. sodium chloride/100 ml.), centrifuged, and examined. Young larvae (up to 15 days old) and adult intestinal forms are de-

Table 9-5. Flukes of man, excluding schistosomes

Parasite	Diagnostic stage	Egg
Fasciola hepatica (sheep liver fluke, mainly a disease of sheep)[23]	Eggs in stool and duodenal or bile drainage	$150 \times 80\mu$; yellow; flat; operculum
Fasciolopsis buski (intestinal fluke)	Eggs in stool; parasites after treatment	$135 \times 82\mu$; similar to *F. hepatica*
Clonorchis sinensis[24] (Chinese liver fluke)	Eggs in stool and duodenal or bile drainage; adult organisms in liver (autopsy)	$29 \times 16\mu$; small, deep-set operculum and prominent rim at narrow pole; yellow-brown, flask-shaped; knob opposite operculum; knob often hooklike; mature miracidium within egg (Fig. 9-28)
Paragonimus westermani (oriental lung fluke)	Eggs in stool and sputum; adult organism in lung (autopsy)	$120 \times 80\mu$; yellow-brown; operculum flattened (Fig. 9-29)
Opisthorchis felineus (cat liver fluke)	Eggs in stool; adult organism in liver (autopsy)	$30 \times 11\mu$; elongated; small and slender; operculum at narrow pole; buttonlike thickening at pole opposite operculum; mature miracidium within egg (Fig. 9-28)

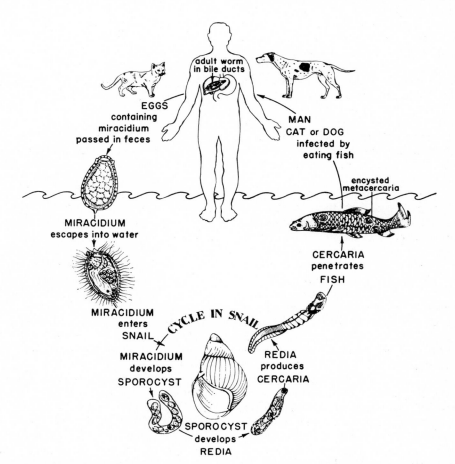

Fig. 9-26. *Clonorchis sinensis.* (From Ash and Spitz: Pathology of tropical diseases: an atlas, Philadelphia, 1945, W. B. Saunders Co.)

stroyed by the digestion technique. The large clear cell bodies around the esophagus are characteristic (Fig. 9-25).

During the period of migration the larvae may be found in the blood. The blood is obtained from a vein, laked in 2% acetic acid solution, and centrifuged; the sediment is examined under a cover glass with the low-power lens. During the period of migration the larvae may also be found in the spinal fluid.

Serology: The intracutaneous test with extract of the larvae is positive in most cases but not diagnostic because false positive tests occur (5%). The reaction is immediate rather than delayed. The complement-fixation, flocculation, and precipitin tests become positive from the second to the fifth week.

The United States Public Health Service (C.D.C.) performs the complement-fixation test and a newer bentonite flocculation test (send specimen to local state health department laboratory).

Eosinophilia: Except in the acute stage, the infection is accompanied by a marked increase in eosinophils.

TREMATODES OR FLUKES

There are two kinds of trematodes: **hermaphroditic** and **diecious** (blood flukes).

HERMAPHRODITIC TREMATODES

The trematodes that most commonly infect man are *Fasciola hepatica, Opisthorchis felineus, Fasciolopsis buski, Clonorchis sinensis,* and *Paragonimus westermani* (Table 9-5).

They are fleshy, flat, leaflike organisms that vary in length from 1-8 cm. and are provided with characteristic suckers, one of which is at the extreme anterior end. The eggs are operculated.

Life history: The life cycle of all trematodes is similar. The operculate eggs are deposited in feces or sputum. When the eggs reach shallow surface water, the ciliated mature larvae, the miracidia, escape through the operculum and swim about until they enter a mollusk (snail). Eggs of *Clonorchis* and *Opisthorchis* are ingested by the snail before hatching. In the snail the miracidium develops into

a sporocyst, which produces rediae (germ cells). Finally, they become free-living cercariae and emerge. They are like the adult trematode, but with a tail or rudder for swimming. They swim about until they encyst and become infective metacercariae attached to water vegetation or to a specific second host (Fig. 9-26). The metacercaria of *Fasciola hepatica* is found attached to water vegetation. The metacercaria of *Paragonimus* enters a second intermediate host, the crayfish or crab, and causes infection when the host is eaten raw or is insufficiently cooked. The cercaria of the small liver flukes (*Clonorchis sinensis* and *Opisthorchis felineus*) penetrates certain freshwater fish and becomes encysted. Man acquires the infection by eating the encysted metacercaria.

Diagnosis: Diagnosis is based on the recognition of ova in feces or sputum or of the adult worm at autopsy. All trematode eggs (except those of schistosomes) are spined or knobbed and possess a lid, or operculum. When found in the stool, the eggs usually contain only the fertilized yolk mass.

The methods of diagnosis include the direct wet-film method, concentration methods, and sieve methods. Complement-fixation tests are available.

Concentration methods for trematodes[25]
Acid-ether concentration:
1. Emulsify 1 gm. feces in 5 ml. 40% hydrochloric acid (40 ml. stock hydrochloric acid diluted to 100 ml.).
2. Filter through two layers of moist gauze into a 15 ml. centrifuge tube.
3. Add equal quantity of ether and shake vigorously.
4. Centrifuge at 1500 rpm for 1 min.
5. Loosen debris at the interface with wooden applicator.
6. Decant.
7. Examine sediment for eggs.

Efficiency is increased if 0.06 ml. Triton* NE is added with the ether.

Sedimentation:
1. Homogenize 10-100 gm. fecal specimen.

---

*Rohm & Haas Co., Philadelphia, Pa.

2. Suspend in 0.5% glycerin in 20 vol. tap water.
3. Strain through four layers of gauze into a tall cylinder.
4. Suspend sediment three times, decanting and resuspending in 20 vol. 0.5% glycerin water: first settling, 1-2 hr.; second settling, 45 min.; third settling, 30 min.
5. Examine sediment.

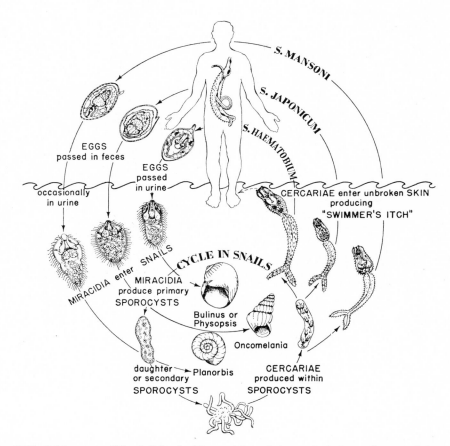

Fig. 9-27. *Schistosoma* (blood flukes). (From Ash and Spitz: Pathology of tropical diseases: an atlas, Philadelphia, 1945, W. B. Saunders Co.)

Table 9-6. Schistosomes

Parasite	*Adult*	*Diagnostic eggs*
Schistosoma mansoni (blood fluke)	Male: 6-10 mm., has gynecophoral canal in which female lies, integument has tubercles; female: 7-14 mm.	$140 \times 60\mu$; nonoperculate with lateral spine; contains miracidium (Plate 9); found in feces, rarely in urine
Schistosoma japonicum (oriental blood fluke)	Male: 12-20 mm. and has integument with minute spines, not tubercles; female: 26 mm.	$90 \times 70\mu$; broadly oval, no spine; some may have a small lateral spine or knob; no operculum (Fig. 9-30); found in feces only
Schistosoma haematobium (vesical blood fluke)	Male: 10-18 mm. and has integument covered with small tubercles; female: 20 mm.	$140 \times 50\mu$; stout terminal spine; nonoperculated, elongated, spindle-shaped (Fig. 9-30); found in urine

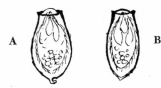

Fig. 9-28. Ova of small liver flukes. **A,** *Clonorchis sinensis.* **B,** *Opisthorchis felineus.* (×500.)

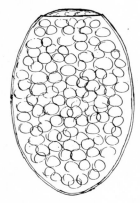

Fig. 9-29. Ovum of *Paragonimus westermani.* (×500.)

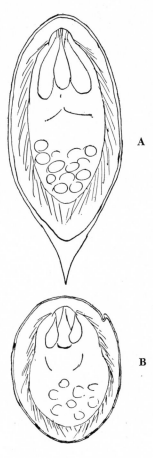

Fig. 9-30. **A,** Ovum of *Schistosoma haematobium.* **B,** Ovum of *Schistosoma japonicum.* (×500.)

SCHISTOSOMES OR BLOOD FLUKES

There are three main species: *Schistosoma haematobium, Schistosoma mansoni,* and *Schistosoma japonicum.*

Life history: The life cycles of all three schistosomes are similar. The eggs hatch as they reach water and liberate the miracidia which invade specific snails, where they develop into cercariae that swim to the water surface and search for a host. They penetrate the skin (**swimmers' itch**) and enter the venous circulation of the host. In the portal vein they mature and finally reach the venules of the intestines, in the case of *S. mansoni* and *S. japonicum,* or of the urinary bladder, in the case of *S. haematobium.* The lesions are produced primarily by the eggs, which penetrate the intestinal or bladder wall (Fig. 9-27).

Diagnosis: Blood flukes are identified by their eggs (*S. haematobium* in urine and *S. mansoni* and *S. japonicum* in feces) on direct smears of flecks of blood or mucus. Surgical biopsy of bladder or of rectum may be diagnostic.

RED BLOOD CELL PARASITES
MALARIAL PARASITES

The parasite of malaria has the characteristics of an ameba and is found in the red blood cells. Similar parasites are found in other animals (especially monkeys and birds).

Malaria induced therapeutically or accidentally (contaminated needles and syringes) differs from natural malaria in the absence of relapses (no tissue phase), in irregular brood formation, and in smaller numbers of gametocytes.

Species: In man there are four common species: *Plasmodium vivax* of tertian malaria, *Plasmodium malariae* of quartan malaria, and *Plasmodium falciparum* of estivoautumnal (or malignant tertian) malaria. A fourth species, *Plasmodium ovale*, resembles both *Plasmodium vivax* and *Plasmodium malariae* as follows. Like the latter, it is not actively ameboid, the host cell is not greatly enlarged, and the segmenting form contains 6-10 (usually 8) merozoites. Like the former, the pigment is fine and light brown, the host cells regularly show Schüffner's granules (even when containing the young ring forms, a finding which is rare in *Plasmodium vivax*), and the asexual cycle requires 48 hr. Perhaps the most striking characteristics are the oval shape of the infected corpuscles and the ragged appearance of their edges.

Life history: The life history includes the **asexual cycle in man** and the **sexual cycle in the female *Anopheles*** mosquito. The cycle in man is called **schizogony** and that in the mosquito **sporogony**. Man is the intermediate host, and the mosquito is the definitive host (Fig. 9-31).

Cycle in man:

Asexual cycle:

Exoerythrocytic schizogony (tissue phase): The form of the parasite introduced into the blood with the salivary secretion of the mosquito is elongated, narrow, and spindle-shaped and is called the **sporozoite.** The sporozoite enters the reticuloendothelial cells of the liver, where it develops and multiplies. After this stage in the fixed tissues, some parasites enter the red blood cells (erythrocytic stage). The forms of the exoerythrocytic cycle in man are nonpigmented and resemble *Toxoplasma* organisms.

Erythrocytic schizogony (peripheral blood phase): When the sporozoite enters a red blood cell, it assumes a spheroidal shape and is then called a **trophozoite.** Growth and development take place in the red cell, the hemoglobin of which is used by the parasite. Each parasite consists of a nuclear mass called chromatin, which stains red with Wright stain, and of cytoplasm, which stains blue. A few hours after the sporozoites enter the red cells, a ring of cytoplasm appears, indicating the young trophozoites. The parasite becomes actively ameboid, and in 8-10 hr. pigment granules representing

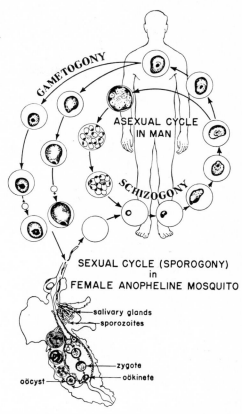

Fig. 9-31. Life cycle of malarial parasite. (From Ash and Spitz: Pathology of tropical diseases: an atlas, Philadelphia, 1945, W. B. Saunders Co.)

the product of catabolism are seen in the pseudopodia or in the periphery of the parasite. As the trophozoite enlarges, it grows more rapidly and becomes less active, and the chromatin divides into distinct masses, after which it is called a **schizont.**

Most of the parasites undergo internal change during the last 8-12 hr. of this cycle in preparation for sporulation. The chromatin is distributed in fine granules throughout the parasite and becomes invisible, the pigment begins to collect in masses that tend to assume a radial distribution, and the periphery tends to become scalloped or regularly notched (**presegmenters** or **immature schizonts**). Then the organism becomes divided into a definite number of spores (**merozoites**), each of which contains a small chromatin mass or dot, whereas the pigment between the merozoites becomes arranged in masses near the center. These forms are called **segmenters** or **mature schizonts.** Finally the infected red cell ruptures, and the merozoites, the future young trophozoites, and pigment are set free in the plasma. The parasites enter new red cells, and the pigment is taken up by phagocytic monocytes that transport it to the reticuloendothelial tissue. In plasma a number of the merozoites are destroyed, chiefly by leukocytes.

Sexual cycle: After the infection has become established, some of the merozoites, apparently due to an unfavorable environment developing in the body about 12 days after the infection, will not continue the asexual cycle but will differentiate into **sexual forms** called **gametocytes,** of which there are males (**microgametocytes**) and females (**macrogametocytes**). They develop slowly, requiring about twice as long for maturing as the asexual forms, and persist in the blood (free in the plasma after rupture of the red cell membrane) for a very long time or until taken by a mosquito in feeding. These resistant forms are responsible for the preservation of the species and go through a developmental cycle in the female *Anopheles* mosquito. The female mosquito requires blood for reproduction; the male mosquito does not bite.

All of the asexual and sexual forms described in the cycle in man appear in the peripheral blood, except in estivoautumnal infection *(Plasmodium falciparum),* where only ring forms and crescents (gametocytes) are found. The older asexual forms of this species remain in the capillaries of the internal organs, where sporulation occurs. The red blood cells infected with *Plasmodium falciparum* tend to adhere to the capillary walls and to block the vessels, giving rise to the special clinical forms of this type of malaria. To complete the cycles, *P. vivax* and *P. ovale* require 48 hr., *P. malariae* require 72 hr., and *P. falciparum,* from 24-48 hr.

The chill occurs at the time of sporulation and is considered to be due to the liberation of the pigment, which is a neurotoxin. It is estimated that at least 1 billion parasites in the body, or 200/ mm.^{3}, sporulating at the same time are necessary to produce a chill. This is about one parasite per 100 oil-immersion fields since there are about 250 cells per field in thin blood smears. After the infection is established, there is a tendency, except in estivoautumnal infection, for the parasites to become grouped into one or more broods so that all of the same brood will sporulate about the same time. When more than one brood is formed, the broods usually sporulate on different days, often producing a chill each day. This is called a **multiple infection,** e.g., double tertian. If more than one species is present, the condition is called a **mixed infection,** e.g., tertian and quartan or estivoautumnal and tertian.

The number of parasites in the peripheral blood is small during the incubation period but increases rapidly to a peak during the acute clinical stage. The number decreases very rapidly (suggesting a crisis) and then more slowly, with irregular variations, until none can be found in the thick-thin smear during the period of latent infection.

Cycle in the mosquito: In the stomach of the mosquito the **macrogametocyte** casts off the polar body (becoming a **macrogamete**) and the **microgametocyte** throws out four to six very motile threadlike filaments (**microgametes**).The macrogamete fertilized by a microgamete is called a **zygote** and, becoming actively motile (**ookinete**), penetrates the stomach mucosa and forms a cyst (**oocyst**).

The cyst enlarges as numerous minute, slender, spindle-shaped **sporozoites** are formed by multiple division of the parasite, and when mature, it ruptures into the body cavity. The sporozoites invade the body of the mosquito, including the salivary glands from which they are injected into the next host upon which the mosquito feeds.

This cycle requires about 12 days, after which the mosquito remains permanently infectious.

EXAMINATION FOR MALARIAL PARASITES (Plate 10):

Thin blood smear (Table 9-7): Make a blood smear and stain with Wright (or Giemsa) stain. Since the larger parasites

MALARIAL PARASITES

PLASMODIUM VIVAX (MALARIA TERTIANA)

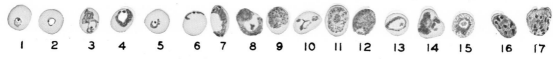

1 2 3 4 5 6 7 8 9 10 11 12 13 14 15 16 17

PLASMODIUM MALARIAE (MALARIA QUARTANA)

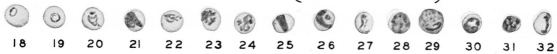

18 19 20 21 22 23 24 25 26 27 28 29 30 31 32

PLASMODIUM FALCIPARUM (MALARIA TROPICA)

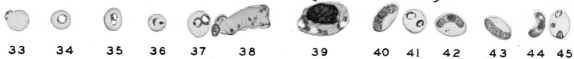

33 34 35 36 37 38 39 40 41 42 43 44 45

Plate 10. Malarial parasites. (From Gradwohl: Clinical laboratory methods and diagnosis, St. Louis, 1956, The C. V. Mosby Co.)

Plasmodium vivax (malaria tertiana)

1, 2. Ring forms
3, 4. Early ameboid forms
5. Double-ring form
6. Ring form
7-10. Ameboid forms
11. Microgametocyte
12. Macrogametocyte
13, 14. Ameboid forms
15. Ameboid form showing Schüffner's punctation
16, 17. Division forms

Plasmodium malariae (malaria quartana)

18, 19. Ring forms
20-27. Ameboid forms showing malaria pigment

28. Beginning division
29. Macrogametocyte
30. Ameboid form showing malaria pigment
31. Division form
32. Ameboid form showing malaria pigment

Plasmodium falciparum (malaria tropica)

33-36. Ring forms
37. Double-ring form
38. Section of brain capillary showing malaria pigment
39. Macrophage showing malaria pigment
40. Microgametocyte
41. Double-ring form
42. Macrogametocyte
43. Microgametocyte
44. Macrogametocyte
45. Multiple ring forms

are easiest to find, obtain the blood just before a chill occurs whenever possible. When only ring forms are present, repeat the examination 8 hr. or more later in order to identify the species. If only ring forms are present again, the species is estivoautumnal. When the parasites are scarce, as in carriers, make the usual smears and also a thick and thin preparation.

Thick blood smear (Table 9-8):

Principle: The blood cells in a thick drop are lysed, rendered transparent, and examined for parasites after staining. The method allows many more red cells to be examined than the thin smear method.

Stain:

Giemsa solution: Dilute Giemsa stain 1:50 with distilled water (pH 7.0-7.2).

Technique: Make a thick drop and incubate ½ hr. to dry completely. Put in Giemsa solution for ½ hr. Decolorize in

Table 9-7. Differential diagnosis of malaria in Wright-stained thin blood smears

	Plasmodium vivax	*Plasmodium malariae*	*Plasmodium falciparum*	*Plasmodium ovale*
Disease	Benign tertian malaria	Quartan malaria	Malignant tertian malaria (estivo-autumnal malaria)	
Length of asexual cycle (schizogony)	48 hr.	72 hr.	48 hr.	49 hr.
Infected red blood cells	Larger than normal; Schüffner's dots; pale	Normal size or sometimes slightly smaller; normal color	Normal size or sometimes smaller; pale	Larger than normal; oval; Schüffner's dots; irregular edge at times; similar to *P. vivax*
Multiple infections	Occasional	Rare	Common	Occasional
Pigment in parasite	Fine granules of yellowish brown pigment	Coarse granules of dark brown pigment	Coarse granules of black pigment	Pigment similar to *P. vivax*
Young trophozoite	Ring is one-third diameter of cell; cytoplasmic circle around vacuole; heavy chromatin dot	Ring similar to *P. vivax* and often smaller; heavy chromatin dots	Small signet rings; delicate with vacuole, delicate chromatin dots; 1 or often 2 organisms; sometimes at edge of red cell (appliqué) or filamentous, stretched out into "tenue" forms	Ring is smaller and thicker than *P. vivax* and at times filled in
Mature trophozoite	Irregular mass of cytoplasm filling cell; increased amounts of brown pigment; vacuole retained until late	Vacuole disappears early; elongated chromatin mass is dense; cytoplasm is compact, oval, band-shaped, or round, almost filling the cell; peripheral large pigment granules	Usually not seen in peripheral blood; growth takes place in internal organs	Compact; vacuoles soon disappear; very similar to *P. malariae;* pigment is lighter, similar to pigment of *P. vivax;* oval cell
Mature schizont	Larger than normal red cell; 12-24 merozoites arranged around central mass; schizont fills red cell	6-12 merozoites in rosettes or irregular clusters filling normal-sized cell and arranged around central mass	Rarely found in peripheral blood; if present, similar to but smaller than *P. malariae;* 8-24 small merozoites irregularly arranged around central pigment mass	Usually 8 merozoites in rosettes or irregular clusters; cell is enlarged and often oval; Schüffner's dots
Macrogametocyte	Rounded or oval homogeneous blue cytoplasm; diffuse delicate pigment nearly fills cell when grown; eccentric, compact chromatin	Similar to *P. vivax;* compact, abundant pigment; fills cell when grown	Sausage-shaped or crescentic; red chromatin mass near center; surrounded by pigment	Similar to *P. vivax,* though smaller; normal-sized red cell; Schüffner's dots

Table 9-7. Differential diagnosis of malaria in Wright-stained thin blood smears—cont'd

	Plasmodium vivax	*Plasmodium malariae*	*Plasmodium falciparum*	*Plasmodium ovale*
Remarks	Schüffner's dots not always present; several phases of growth often seen in one smear; gametocytes appear early	Band forms not always seen; gametocytes appear late; parasite appears intensely stained	Crescents not always seen; frequently numerous parasites; development following ring stage takes place in internal organs	Resembles aberrant *P. vivax* and *P. malariae*; most infrequent form of malaria
Main criteria	Red cell is large and pale; trophozoite is irregular; fine pigment; Schüffner's dots	Red cell is normal in size and color; trophozoites compact; coarse pigment; no stippling of red cell	Characteristic delicate ring; no other growing forms; gametocyte	Red cell is frequently oval and contains Schüffner's dots

Table 9-8. Differential diagnosis of malaria in Wright-stained thick blood smears

	Plasmodium vivax	*Plasmodium malariae*	*Plasmodium falciparum*	*Plasmodium ovale*
Young trophozoite	Ring forms with irregular cytoplasmic borders; fine pigment; older forms also present	Ring forms with prominent chromatin; often solid cytoplasm; older forms also present; rings may be infrequent	Many small delicate ring forms with small chromatin dots; no older stages seen; forms may resemble exclamation marks, commas, or swallows and may show open rings	Resembles *P. vivax* and *P. malariae* and cannot be differentiated on thick smears
Mature trophozoite	Irregular dark-staining mass of cytoplasm; 1 or 2 vacuoles; fine brown pigment	Dark, heavily pigmented mass; band forms may become rounded	Not seen in peripheral blood unless there is severe infection	See above
Mature schizont	10-16 merozoites clustered around central pigment	Rosette of 8 merozoites, each with large chromatin dots; compact or separated; central black pigment	Not seen in peripheral blood	See above
Mature gametocyte	Large parasite with diffuse, light pigment; dense cytoplasm; resembles mature trophozoite	Similar to *P. vivax*, but smaller and more compact; much pigment present; may resemble rounded *P. falciparum* gametocyte	Crescent or sausage-shaped forms with pigment near center; may become rounded	See above

distilled water until outer rim is pink and the center is blue.

The slides may be covered with Diaphane* after they are dry and before they are examined under oil. Oil can be removed with xylene. Diaphane is applied across the width of the slide and is then spread toward the opposite side with a glass rod. Diaphane solvent is used to remove any excess.

Saponin hemolysis technique[26]:

Technique: Obtain EDTA anticoagulated venous blood and add 1.5 ml. 1% solution of saponin in normal saline solution to 2 ml. blood. Lysis is complete in 30 sec. Centrifuge in Sero-Fuge for 1 min. at 3500 rpm. Save supernatant and prepare smears, using the bottom portion of the sediment.

Centrifuge the supernatant for 10 min. at 3500 rpm and smear sediment again. Stain both smears with Wright or Giemsa stain.

This method preserves the morphology of the parasites and allows a higher concentration of parasites than the thick smear method.

Species identification:

Stained preparations: In stained preparations the chromatin appears red, the cytoplasm blue, and the pigments brown or black.

Other laboratory findings in malaria[27]:

Immunofluorescent technique: It provides a sensitive tool for detecting specific malarial antibodies.

Hypo- or ahaptoglobinemia: The hemolytic component of malaria may account for the reduction in haptoglobin.

INTESTINAL SPOROZOA

Isospora hominis:

Incidence: Uncommon.

Habitat and life history: All developmental stages of the organism are not known. It probably matures in the mucosal cells of the small intestine. The trophozoites are found in the epithelial cells of intestine and bile ducts, where they enlarge (schizonts) and undergo multiple division (merozoites), rupturing the cells. Some of the merozoites formed

---

*Will Corporation, Rochester, N. Y.

enter other cells and repeat the cycle; some (gametocytes) form oocysts, probably in the lumen of the intestine, which appear in the feces.

Characteristics:

Oocysts:

1. Ovoid; $28 \times 15\mu$ diam.
2. Shell-like wall with a micropyle at the narrow end; colorless.
3. Protoplasm unsegmented in fresh specimen, but soon divides into two parts (sporoblasts) which become surrounded by a thin wall, forming sporocysts, within each of which develop four vermiform sporozoites (Fig. 9-32). When liberated in the intestine, the sporozoites invade the epithelial cells of the intestine and bile ducts, becoming trophozoites.

Diagnosis: Diagnosis is based on detection of the oocyst in the stool.

HEMOFLAGELLATES

Hemoflagellates are blood and tissue flagellates, two forms of which are of medical importance: *Leishmania* and *Trypanosoma*. Each has a vertebrate and an invertebrate host.

They produce six important diseases in man: Three are produced by *Leishmania* and three are produced by *Trypanosoma*.

Leishmania produces kala-azar, oriental sore, and mucocutaneous leishmaniasis.

Trypanosoma produces West African trypanosomiasis, East African trypanosomiasis, and Chagas' disease.

Morphologic forms of hemoflagellates

Each organism contains a nucleus with a karyosome, a cytoplasmic body, a kinetoplast consisting of a rodlike parabasal

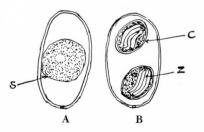

Fig. 9-32. Oocysts of *Isospora hominis* (schematic). **A,** Immature: **S,** sporoblast. **B,** Mature: **C,** sporocyst; **Z,** sporozoites.

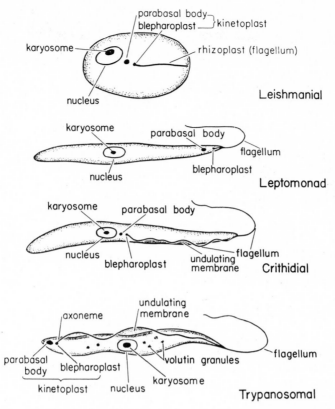

Fig. 9-33. Leishmanial, leptomonad, crithidial, and trypanosomal forms of ·*Trypanosoma*. (From Hunter et al.: Manual of tropical medicine, ed. 4, Philadelphia, 1966, W. B. Saunders Co.)

body and a dotlike blepharoplast, and a rhizoblast (flagellum). The latter extends from the blepharoplast beyond the anterior (flagellar) end as a free flagellum.

There are four morphologic forms of hemoflagellates: **leishmanial, leptomonad, crithidial,** and **trypanosomal** (Fig. 9-33).

Leishmanial form (Leishman-Donovan or L.D. bodies): The parasite is intracellular in the reticuloendothelial system (RES). It is ovoid, measures 1.5-5μ, and contains the previously mentioned structures but no undulating membrane or free flagellum (Fig. 9-34).

Leptomonad form: It is a slender, elongated, spindle-shaped organism (14-20 × 1.5-3.5μ) that exhibits the previously mentioned structures except for an undulating membrane. The kinetoplast is situated close to the anterior (flagellar) end and gives rise to a single flagellum.

Crithidial form: It is a spindle-shaped organism (10-20 × 1-3μ) that exhibits all structures mentioned, including an undulating membrane, a flagellum, and a kinetoplast close to the anterior end.

Trypanosomal form: It is a spindle-shaped organism exhibiting all structures mentioned, including a flagellum and an undulating membrane. The kinetoplast is posterior to the nucleus.

Not all species exhibit all four forms. *Leishmania* usually exists in leishmanial form in man and in leptomonad form in the insect host. *Trypanosoma* exists in trypanosomal form in man and in crithidial form in the insect host; *T. cruzi* and *T. rangeli* show all four forms.

Leishmania

Three species are found in man, but morphologically they are identical: *Leish-*

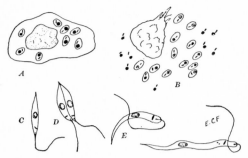

Fig. 9-34. *Leishmania donovani.* **A** and **B,** Leishmanial form from endothelial cells of spleen. **C** to **F,** Flagellate stage from culture. (×1000.) (From Faust: J. Lab. Clin. Med. **17:**654, 1932.)

mania donovani, the cause of visceral leishmaniasis, Dumdum fever, or kala-azar; *Leishmania tropica,* the cause of oriental sore; *Leishmania braziliensis,* the cause of mucocutaneous leishmaniasis.

The parasite occurs in the leishmanial and leptomonad forms only.

Leishmania donovani: The leishmanial form occurs in the reticuloendothelial system and the leptomonad form occurs in the insect vector (sandfly) and in culture (Fig. 9-34).

Leishmania tropica: The leishmanial form occurs in the reticuloendothelial cells of the skin and the leptomonad form occurs in the sandfly and in culture.

Leishmania braziliensis: The leishmanial form occurs in the reticuloendothelial cells of the skin and mucous membrane and the leptomonad form occurs in culture and in the sandfly.

Laboratory diagnosis:

Diagnosis of Leishmania donovani (kala-azar, visceral leishmaniasis): The intracellular leishmanial form (L.D. bodies) within the reticuloendothelial cells of the RES organs (e.g., liver, spleen, bone marrow) or within the mononuclear cells of the peripheral blood is diagnostic (Fig. 9-34). The L.D. bodies must be distinguished from *Histoplasma capsulatum,* which lacks the kinetoplast.

The leptomonad form appears in culture.

Smears: Bone marrow and splenic aspiration smears and imprints are stained with Giemsa stain and examined for re-

ticulum cells containing L.D. bodies. In blood smears, L.D. bodies may be present in large mononuclear cells stained with Giemsa stain. The blood smear is not a satisfactory method.

Liver biopsy: Examine tissue sections for L.D. bodies.

Animal inoculation: Hamsters, mice, and guinea pigs are susceptible to intraperitoneal injection of blood and splenic or lymph node material.

Culture: Leptomonad forms are produced in the condensation water of rabbit blood culture medium (NNN medium) or of its modification, NN medium without peptone.

NNN medium for Leishmania:

1. Bacto-agar,* 14 gm.
2. Sodium chloride, 6 gm.
3. Distilled water, 900 ml.

Neutralize boiling mixture with 0.1N NaOH. Sterilize medium and store in refrigerator.

Melt agar in 50°-55° C. water bath and, using sterile technique, add sterile defibrinated rabbit blood. Mix and distribute 5 ml. into tubes to produce slant.

Formol-gel test: To 1 ml. serum add 2 drops 40% formalin. If the test is positive, the serum will become opalescent and opaque within a few minutes and will finally solidify. This test is basically for increased gamma globulins and is therefore not diagnostic of leishmaniasis.

Trypanosomes[28]

There are three species: *Trypanosoma gambiense,* *Trypanosoma rhodesiense,* and *Trypanosoma cruzi.*

The first two are the cause of African sleeping sickness and are transmitted by the bite of the tsetse fly. *T. cruzi* is the cause of Chagas' disease in Central and South America and is transmitted by the reduviid bug.

The first two trypanosomes mentioned are similar in morphology; they produce similar diseases characterized by a febrile stage with enlargement of lymph nodes and spleen when the parasites can be demonstrated in the peripheral blood and in the fluid aspirated from lymph nodes,

---

*Difco Laboratories, Detroit, Mich.

and by a chronic sleeping stage when the parasites can be demonstrated in the cerebrospinal fluid, not in the blood. Both are transmitted by the bites of tsetse flies (*Glossina palpalis* and *Glossina morsitans*, respectively). The cycle in the tsetse fly is complicated and requires about 3 wk. After several reproductive and developmental stages the parasites reach the salivary glands, after which the fly is infective. In man these trypanosomes divide by binary longitudinal fission. *T. rhodesiense* produces a more acute and severe infection, death occurring usually within a year. *T. gambiense* produces a more chronic disease with a longer sleeping stage.

T. cruzi, on the other hand, is transmitted by the reduviid bug (*Panstrongylus megistus*), the feces of which, containing the infectious parasites, are rubbed into the bite. This trypanosome does not divide in the blood, but loses its flagellum and undulating membrane, invades endothelial or tissue cells (especially heart muscle), and divides by binary fission, producing numerous leishmanial forms within a cystlike cavity. The leishmanial forms develop into trypanosomes and are liberated into the blood (accompanied by fever) when the cystlike structure ruptures. The symptoms are varied and are due to degeneration of the infected tissue of the various organs.

FORMS OF TRYPANOSOMES FOUND IN MAN: The trypanosomal forms are found free in the bloodstream and the crithidial forms are found in the insect vector; the leishmanial forms are mostly intracellular.

T. gambiense and *T. rhodesiense* (Figs. 9-35 and 9-36) exhibit the trypanosomal forms in blood, spinal fluid, brain, and lymph nodes in man and also in the tsetse fly. The crithidial forms are seen in the insect host (tsetse fly).

T. cruzi exhibits all four forms in man: the leishmanial forms in the heart and lymph nodes, the leptomonad forms in the brain, and the trypanosomal forms in the blood. The crithidial forms are seen in human tissue and in the reduviid bug.

LABORATORY DIAGNOSIS: Diagnosis is

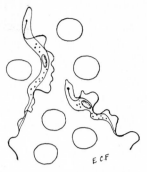

Fig. 9-35. *Trypanosoma gambiense* in blood. (×1000.) (From Faust: J. Lab. Clin. Med. **17**: 654, 1932.)

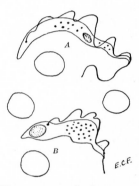

Fig. 9-36. *Trypanosoma rhodesiense* in blood. **A,** Usual form. **B,** Posterior nucleate type from rodent host. (×1000.) (From Faust: J. Lab. Clin. Med. **17**:654, 1932.)

based on the demonstration of trypanosomes.

Diagnosis of Trypanosoma gambiense and Trypanosoma rhodesiense:

Smears: During the febrile stage, examine the peripheral blood, unstained and stained with Wright or Giemsa stain. Thick blood smears (p. 497) may be helpful. During the sleeping stage, examine smears of cerebrospinal fluid. Smears may also be prepared from aspirates of enlarged lymph nodes.

Animal inoculation: Inoculate hamsters, mice, or guinea pigs and examine blood for trypanosomes. The material used for injection may be blood or macerated lymph nodes. When inoculated into mice, *T. rhodesiense* is rapidly fatal; smears of blood and organs may reveal posterior nucleated forms, the nucleus being behind the kinetoplast. *T. gambiense* produces a chronic infection, and posterior nucleated forms are scarce.

Culture: The organism will grow on NNN medium for *Leishmania.*

Diagnosis of Trypanosoma cruzi: Same as above. Trypanosomal forms are found in blood of man and animals after inoculation. In addition, the leishmanial stage can be seen in tissues obtained at biopsy or at autopsy from man or laboratory animal.

Xeno diagnosis: Uninfected laboratory-bred reduviid bugs are allowed to feed upon suspected patients. After about 2 wk. the crithidial forms may be found in the gut of the bugs.

Complement-fixation and slide agglutination tests are available.

PRESERVATION OF SPECIMENS

Preserve specimens of feces containing ova and larvae by emulsifying the feces in 10% formalin. Add about 5% glycerin to prevent loss by drying in case of a loose stopper.

Wash nematodes with water or physiologic saline solution and drop into hot 70% alcohol (heated to bubbling). Store in 70% alcohol, adding glycerin to make 5%.

Wash trematodes with water or saline solution and drop into hot 10% formalin (heated to bubbling). Store in 70% alcohol containing glycerin to make 5%.

Wash cestodes with water and leave in water until they are dead (a few hours for small specimens; overnight for large ones). Fix in 10% formalin. Store in 70% alcohol containing glycerin to make 5%.

Place spiders, ticks, mites, fleas, lice, or other arthropods in a mixture of 97 parts 20% alcohol and 3 parts ether (room temperature) until dead.[29] Store in 70% alcohol containing glycerin to make 5%.

Drop fly larvae or mosquito larvae into boiling water. Store in 70% alcohol containing glycerin to make 5%.

Small insects and parasites may be mounted directly without previous dehydration and clearing in Turtox* nonresinous mounting medium.

*Turtox, General Biological Supply House, Inc., Chicago, Ill.

TOXOPLASMA GONDII[30]

This protozoan parasite was first observed in the gondi (North African rodent) and in the rabbit (Brazil)[31-33] and is pathogenic to a large number of hosts (rabbit, guinea pig, mouse, rat, squirrel, dog, monkey, and pigeon). It is found in many parts of the world. It is crescentic, pyriform, oval, or round and is about 6-7μ long and 2-4μ wide. With Wright stain the cytoplasma is pale blue, and the large nucleus, which occupies the whole width of the posterior portion of the parasite, is deep purple (Fig. 9-37).

It is an obligate intracellular parasite found in tissue cells (brain, heart, muscle, and lung), leukocytes, and endothelial cells. When the infected cells rupture in the preparation of slides, the parasite is freed. In tissue cells the parasite appears in closely packed colonies from which it can be freed by the rupture of the involved cells. A second form in which the parasite appears is the **pseudocyst,** which is found in chronic infections; the parasites are not easily liberated even if the cell is ruptured.

Life history: Domestic animals and man are reservoirs of the organism. The exact mode of transmission has not been established.

Clinical classification:

Congenital toxoplasmosis: Congenital toxoplasmosis may lead to fetal death or, if a viable infant is born, it may lead to

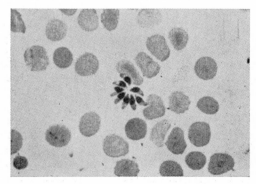

Fig. 9-37. *Toxoplasma* in Giemsa-stained smear from the omentum of a guinea pig. (From Pinkerton and Henderson: J.A.M.A. **116**:807, 1941.)

the development of the symptoms and signs of toxoplasmosis in childhood.

Acquired toxoplasmosis: Acquired toxoplasmosis is one of the causes of eye infection.

Latent toxoplasmosis: Latent toxoplasmosis is the most common form of the disease and is found in a large percentage of the population in which antibodies can be detected.

LABORATORY DIAGNOSIS

Laboratory diagnosis is based on isolation of the parasite and immunologic diagnosis.

Isolation of the parasite

Animal inoculation: After centrifugation (30 min. at 3000 rpm), inject cerebrospinal fluid intracerebrally and intraperitoneally into six laboratory-bred mice. If the mice remain well after 14 days, aseptically remove the brain and spleen in two, and effect passage to another group of six mice.

Animal inoculation with tissue digest: Tissue digest is prepared with pepsin solution, using 125 gm. tissue/100 ml. solution.

Pepsin solution:
1. Pepsin, 0.26 gm.
2. NaCl, 0.5 gm.
3. Concentrated HCl, 0.7 ml.
4. Distilled water to 100 ml.

Incubate tissue-pepsin mixture for 2 hr. at 35° C. Filter through cloth, centrifuge, and wash sediment twice with saline solution. Resuspend sediment in small amount of saline solution and inject mice as previously described. If the mice die, examine imprints and sections of brain, lungs, and liver. The imprints and smears of peritoneal fluid are stained with Giemsa stain. The tissue sections are stained with hematoxylin-eosin. The toxoplasma cysts are PAS positive (see tissue section). The cyst wall can also be demonstrated by Wilder silver stain.

Immunologic methods

Dye test of Sabin and Feldman:

Principle: Living *Toxoplasma* organisms killed by antibodies in the patient's serum plus a heat-labile serum factor (proper-din system) are not stained by alkaline methylene blue.

Results: Dye test titer of "normal" sera rarely exceeds 1:64. If the dye test titer is 1:256 or higher, a positive diagnosis can be made provided the patient is over 4 mo. old and the same or higher titer is obtained on a repeat test 4 mo. after the first test. A newborn infant may have a high titer due to passive transfer of antibodies from the mother and therefore a repeat test after 4 mo. is necessary as the passively transferred antibodies will have disappeared by then.

Hemagglutination test:

Principle: Tannic acid–treated sheep cells or human Rh-negative O cells are sensitized by an antigen prepared from water-lysed parasites. The sensitized cells are brought in contact with suitably diluted serum. The agglutination pattern is graded 0-4+.

Complement-fixation test: The antigen is peritoneal exudate of infected mice. The complement-fixing antibodies develop more slowly and disappear more rapidly than the dye test antibodies. In acute congenital toxoplasmosis the dye test may show a high titer in both mother and child, while the complement-fixation test titer will be high only in the mother.

PNEUMOCYSTIS CARINII[34, 35]

This parasite is thought to be a protozoan that occurs in two forms: the vegetative trophozoite and the encysted organism.

Morphology:
1. Trophozoite: It varies from 5-12μ diam. and has a central nucleus measuring 0.5μ that is surrounded by a clear zone.
2. Cyst: It is round, 5-8μ diam., and has a prominent cyst wall.

Life history: Adults are carriers of the organism and appear to be able to transmit it to infants and debilitated individuals. The common denominator appears to be a lack of resistance due to absence or diminution of immune globulins. The infants affected are usually 2-3 mo. old, a time when their antibodies are lowest. The transplacentally transmitted maternal antibodies have almost disappeared and their own are just beginning to appear. In affected adults the immune mechanisms are depressed by such diseases as plasma-lymphocytic proliferative disorders or by therapeutic procedures such as administration of antimetabolites and cortisone or radiation.

Disease production: The organism is an opportunistic invader able to produce interstitial plasma cell pneumonia in infants and hyaline membrane type of disease and pulmonary proteinosis-like conditions in adults. The organism is endemic in some areas in Europe.

Diagnosis: The organism is demonstrated in tissue sections (lung), in smears of sputum and bronchial aspirations, and in imprints of lung parenchyma by the PAS, trichrome, or hematoxylin-eosin stains if it is present in the vegetative form. The cysts are best demonstrated by the Gomori methenamine silver nitrate method, by Giemsa stain, or by the toluidine blue method.[36]

REFERENCES

1. Marsden, P. D., and Hoskins, D. W.: Gastroenterology **51**:701, 1966.
2. Harris, A. H., and Coleman, M. B., editors: Diagnostic procedures and reagents, ed. 4, New York, 1963, American Public Health Association, Inc.
3. Swartzwelder, J. C.: Parasitology, a diagnostic workshop for medical technologists, St. Louis, 1961, The Catholic Hospital Association of the United States and Canada.
4. Gould, S. E., Hinerman, D. L., Batsakis, J. G., and Beamer, P. R.: Amer. J. Clin. Path. **39**:626, 1963.
5. Gould, S. E., Hinerman, D. L., Batsakis, J. G., and Beamer, P. R.: Amer. J. Clin. Path. **39**:512, 1963.
6. Tompkins, V. N., and Miller, J. K.: Amer. J. Clin. Path. **17**:755, 1947.
7. Kohn, J.: Med. Quart. Israeli **19**:160, 1960.
8. Doxiades, T., and Candreviotis, N.: Brit. Med. J. **1**:1810, 1962.
9. Powell, S. J., and Maddison, S. E.: Lancet **1**:566, 1966.
10. Jeanes, A. L.: Brit. Med. J. **1**:1464, 1966.
11. Kessel, J. F., Lewis, W. P., Pasquel, C. M., and Turner, J. A.: Amer. J. Trop. Med. **14**:540, 1965.
12. Kasliwal, R. M., et al.: Brit. Med. J. **1**:837, 1966.
13. Culbertson, C. G.: Amer. J. Clin. Path. **35**:195, 1961.
14. Gould, S. E., Hinerman, D. L., Batsakis, J. G., and Beamer, P. R.: Amer. J. Clin. Path. **40**:83, 1963.
15. Scudamore, H. H., Thompson, J. H., and Owen, C. A.: J. Lab. Clin. Med. **57**:240, 1961.
16. Fischman, A.: J. Clin. Path. **13**:72, 1960.
17. Fischman, A.: New Zeal. Med. J. **59**:485, 1960.
18. Edelman, M. H., Spingarn, C. L., Nauenberg, W. G., and Gregory, C.: Amer. J. Med. **38**:951, 1965.
19. Hogan, M. J., Kimura, S. J., and Spencer, W. H.: J.A.M.A. **194**:1345, 1965.
20. Bisseru, B., Woodruff, A. W., and Hutchinson, R. I.: Brit. Med. J. **5503**:1583, 1966.
20a. Keller, A. E., Leathers, W. S., and Densen, P. M.: Amer. J. Trop. Med. **20**:493, 1940.
21. Harder, H. I., and Watson, D.: Amer. J. Clin. Path. **42**:333, 1964.
22. Gould, S. E., Hinerman, D. L., Batsakis, J. G., and Beamer, P. R.: Amer. J. Clin. Path. **40**:197, 1963.
23. Jones, I., and Smith, P.: Lancet **1**:1241, 1963.
24. Gibson, B. J., and Sun, T.: Int. Path. **6**:94, 1965.
25. Hood, M.: Amer. J. Clin. Path. **22**:396, 1952.
26. Keffer, J. H.: Techn. Bull. Regist. Med. Techn. **36**:153, 1966.
27. Kuvin, F. S., Beye, H. K., Stohlman, F., Contacos, P. G., and Coatney, G. R.: J.A.M.A. **184**:1018, 1963.
28. Leading Article: Brit. Med. J. **1**:939, 1965.
29. Boardman, E. T.: J. Parasit. **30**:57, 1944.
30. Eichenwald, H. F.: Ann. N. Y. Acad. Sci. **64**:207, 1956.
31. Nicolle, C., and Manceaux, L.: Compt. Rend. Acad. Sci. **147**:763, 1908.
32. Nicolle, C., and Manceaux, L.: Compt. Rend. Acad. Sci. **148**:369, 1909.
33. Splendore, A.: Bull. Soc. Path. Exot. **2**:462, 1909.
34. Callerame, M. L., and Nadel, M.: Amer. J. Clin. Path. **45**:258, 1966.
35. Esterly, J. A., and Warner, N. E.: Arch. Path. **80**:433, 1965.
36. Chalvardjian, A. M., and Grawe, L. A.: J. Clin. Path. **16**:383, 1963.

Chapter 10

Examination of biologic fluids (serous fluids, cerebrospinal fluid, synovial fluid, amniotic fluid, sputum, pus)

The liquid contained in the pleural, pericardial, and peritoneal cavities is called **serous fluid** because it somewhat resembles serum. All serous fluids have common characteristics. They are mainly watery ultrafiltrates of the plasma and are influenced by changes in osmotic and hydrostatic pressures, protein concentrations of the plasma, and permeability of the lining of the blood vessels and of the serosal cavities.

Joint fluid is produced by modified connective tissue (synovia) and is not the result of mesothelial activity or filtration.

Cerebrospinal fluid is a secretion of the choroid plexuses and therefore has a relatively constant chemical and cellular composition as well as volume. Diseases of the meninges are reflected in spinal fluid profile.

SEROUS FLUIDS

Collection of specimens: Collect about 50 ml. fluid in a sterile flask containing 10 ml. 4% sodium citrate. This is used for cell counts, smears, and animal inoculations. Also collect a small amount of fluid without citrate in order to observe clot formation.

LABORATORY INVESTIGATION

Color and transparency
Specific gravity
Protein
Glucose
Lactic acid dehydrogenase
Amylase
Gram stain
Acid-fast stain
Culture
Cell count and differential count
Papanicolaou smear

Characteristics of normal serous fluids:
Color and transparency: straw colored, clear
Specific gravity: less than 1.016
Total protein: less than 3 gm./100 ml.
Noncolloidal solutes: same level as in plasma
Coagulation: will not clot

The protein electrophoretic patterns of serous fluids show them to contain more albumin than plasma and little or no fibrinogen.

Physical examination

Amount: Measure.

Color: Note blood (fresh or changed) and bile.

Transparency and general appearance: Fluids may be serous, fibrinous, purulent, putrid, sanguineous, chylous, chyloid, or combinations of these.

Make alkaline with sodium hydroxide and shake with ether. Fat dissolves in ether, and fluid becomes clear. Chyloid or pseudochylous fluids contain only small amounts of fat, the milky appearance being due to lecithin. Gently warm a few milliliters with 5 vol. alcohol and filter. This precipitates albumin and dissolves lecithin. Evaporate filtrate to original volume. This precipitates lecithin. The turbidity is increased by adding water.

Reaction to litmus: The pH of inflammatory and noninflammatory fluids varies from 6.8-7.6.

Specific gravity: This reflects the protein content of the fluid; it is low in noninflammatory fluids and high in inflammatory fluids.

Clot formation: Record presence or absence and state whether clot formation is slight, weblike, or en masse.

Clot formation reflects fibrinogen content. Fibrinogen is a large molecular substance and does not escape unless there is considerable damage to the mesothelium.

Chemical examination

Total protein (Table 10-1): For clinical purposes, subtract 1.007 from the specific gravity and multiply by 343 to obtain the percent protein or use method as for urine. For more accurate methods, see plasma protein methods in the section

Table 10-1. Total protein in exudates and transudates

Specific gravity	Total protein* (gm./100 ml.)
1.035	9.60
1.034	9.25
1.033	8.92
1.032	8.58
1.031	8.22
1.030	7.87
1.029	7.53
1.028	7.18
1.027	6.84
1.026	6.51
1.025	6.16
1.024	5.81
1.023	5.47
1.022	5.12
1.021	4.78
1.020	4.44
1.019	4.10
1.018	3.77
1.017	3.43
1.016	3.08
1.015	2.74

*Data according to following formula: protein = 343 (specific gravity − 1.007).

on clinical chemistry. Refractometry (TS meter*) is an adequate method.

Globulin (Rivalta test): Add 1 drop glacial acetic acid to 100 ml. water in a graduated glass cylinder. Allow a drop of the fluid, free from cells, to fall into this solution. Normal body fluids give no cloud; transudates give only slight clouds; inflammatory exudates give heavy precipitates, often falling to the bottom with the drop of fluid.

Sugar: Use Clinistix† and perform the test for glucose as given in the section on clinical chemistry. The concentration is that of plasma glucose.

The blood sugar level should always be determined at the same time the sugar level of the serous fluid is measured. In bacterial infections, rheumatoid arthritis, and malignancies the sugar level is depressed.

Lactic acid dehydrogenase: The serum level must be determined simultaneously. In the pleural fluid the level is elevated in tumors metastatic to the pleura. The biochemical method is described in the section on clinical chemistry.

Microscopic examination

The following examinations are made:
1. White cell count unless fluid is purulent
2. Sediment
   (a) Unstained preparations
   (b) Stained preparations—gram, Wright, and acid-fast (when necessary) stains
   (c) Papanicolaou smear
   (d) Culture
   (e) Inoculation

The specimen may have to be anticoagulated for all these procedures.

White cell count: If fluid is not very cloudy or bloody, moisten a small pipette with glacial acetic acid, blowing out excess. Mix specimen thoroughly and draw 1-3 drops fluid into pipette. Mix by rotating pipette and transfer to a blood counting chamber. If cells are few in number, count 10 fields, 1 mm.^{2} each, and add. This gives the number of cells/mm.^{3}

*American Optical Co., Buffalo, N. Y.
†Ames Co., Inc., Elkhart, Ind.

When there are many cells, count the same as for leukocytes in blood (p. 116).

When the cell count is low, a chamber differential may be made, as described in the discussion of cerebrospinal fluid (p. 512), to determine the predominant type of leukocyte. Use the following stain (Greenthal): cresylecht violet, 0.07 gm.; methylene blue, 0.10 gm.; glacial acetic acid, 3 ml.; and distilled water, 100 ml. Filter before using.

NOTE: With synovial fluid use physiologic saline solution instead of acetic acid solution, which produces a precipitate.

Differential count: Centrifuge citrated specimen, pour off supernatant, make smear, and stain with Wright stain. Study the types of cells present in the Wright stain. Make a differential count or record the predominant type of cell. Predominance of polymorphonuclear cells suggests pyogenic infection; predominance of lymphocytes suggests a tuberculous infection, a chronic pyogenic infection, virus infection, or certain blood diseases. Predominance of mesothelial cells suggests a transudate or a malignant disease when these cells are in great numbers and many red blood cells are present. Frequent tappings often give a predominance of eosinophils, as do diseases due to hypersensitivity.

Culture: See section on bacteriology.

Malignant cells:

Papanicolaou smear technique: Prevent clotting by the addition of heparin or ADTA. Centrifuge specimen and prepare smears as soon as the fluid is delivered to the laboratory. If delay is unavoidable, add ⅓ vol. 50% ethyl alcohol, mix well, and store in refrigerator until the material can be centrifuged and smeared.

Prepare smears by evenly distributing the sediment over frosted slides* and immediately (before drying) fixing them in 95% ethyl alcohol. If only a small amount of sediment can be expected, augment it by the method described in the urine section (p. 50).

Tissue sections: Pack the sediment by centrifuging, carefully decant supernatant fluid, and fix by overlaying the sediment

---

*No longer commercially available.

with 10% formalin. With a fine capillary glass rod carefully loosen the sediment from the sides of the centrifuge tube and allow to harden. Use paraffin method as for tissue specimen.

Transudates and exudates

Transudates: Transudates are clear, serous, light yellow fluids. Their specific gravity is below 1.015, and they do not form clots. The protein content is less than 3 gm./100 ml., and the Rivalta test is negative. The sugar content is approximately the same as in blood, and there are few mesothelial and blood cells. Cultures are negative. Repeated tappings tend to cause an increase of neutrophils and sometimes of eosinophils. Transudates are noninflammatory in origin and are usually due to cardiac failure, to venous obstruction (portal vein), or to hypoproteinemia (nephrosis or nephritis).

Exudates: Exudates are inflammatory in origin, may be clear or cloudy, and are serous, fibrinous, purulent, hemorrhagic, chylous or chyloid, or combinations of these. Their specific gravity is above 1.018, and they clot spontaneously. The protein content is more than 3 gm./100 ml., and the Rivalta test is positive. The sugar content is decreased. Many cells are present (see discussion of cytodiagnosis), and bacteria may be present or absent. In pulmonary tuberculosis the pleural effusion is usually serofibrinous; in pyogenic infections it is usually purulent (pneumococcus and staphylococcus) or

Table 10-2. Differentiation of inflammatory (exudates) and noninflammatory (transudates) serous fluids

	Noninflammatory	Inflammatory
Specific gravity	Less than 1.016	1.016 or more
Protein	Less than 3 gm./100 ml.	More than 3 gm./100 ml.
Leukocytes	A few lymphocytes	Many white cells of all types
Coagulation	Does not clot	Often clots

serosanguinopurulent (streptococcus); in malignancy it is usually hemorrhagic.

True chylous fluid is usually due to trauma to lymphatic vessels or ducts or to obstruction of the lymph channels by tumor, filaria, or scarring.

CEREBROSPINAL FLUID

Cerebrospinal fluid is the product of the secretory activity of the choroid plexus. It circulates from the lateral ventricles through the third and fourth ventricles into the subarachnoid space. About four-fifths flows over the brain and one-fifth flows down around the spinal cord. It is absorbed through the arachnoid villi into the large sinuses and through the capillaries into the bloodstream.

Collection of specimens: Cerebrospinal fluid is usually obtained by lumbar or suboccipital puncture and occasionally directly from the ventricles of the brain. The specimen should be collected in three sterile, labeled, capped tubes that are numbered 1, 2, and 3 in the order in which they were obtained. Each one should contain 2-4 ml. of specimen. Tube No. 3 should be reserved for bacteriologic investigation.

If tuberculous meningitis is suspected, another portion is collected and left standing without being shaken in order to observe clot formation. The total amount withdrawn should not exceed about 6-10 ml. as a rule.

Cultures should be made whenever the spinal fluid is cloudy. If the fluid is very cloudy or highly colored, a portion should be collected in a tube containing citrate in order to prevent clotting until the cell count and sediment examination can be made.

Pressure: The pressure of the spinal fluid should always be recorded. This observation is made before any fluid is withdrawn.

The normal pressure in the horizontal position is from 100-200 mm. H_2O in adults and 50-100 mm. H_2O in infants. Small fluctuations are due to the heartbeat and to respiration; wider ones occur upon straining or coughing.

Fluid from different levels: As previously indicated, the composition varies with the level from which the specimen is obtained. The protein varies from about 10 mg. in the ventricles to about 45 mg. in the spinal region. The chlorides show no variation, and the reducing substances only slightly decrease from above downward.

LABORATORY INVESTIGATION

Examination of cerebrospinal fluid should be made at once. **Characteristics of normal spinal fluid:**
Color: colorless like water
Transparency: clear like water
Osmotic pressure: hypertonic to blood plasma
Specific gravity: 1.006-1.008
pH: 7.35-7.70
Glucose: 44-100 mg./100 ml.
Urea: 8-28 mg./100 ml.
Chlorides: 118-127 mEq./L.
Total protein: 14-45 mg./100 ml.
  Lumbar: 20-40 mg./100 ml.
  Cisternal: 15 mg./100 ml.
  Ventricular: 10 mg./100 ml.
Fibrinogen: none
Pressure (supine position): 100-200 mm. H_2O
Cells: 1-5 cells/mm.³

Physical examination

Color: Normally cerebrospinal fluid is colorless. Note color of blood and xanthochromia (yellow color).

Blood: If much blood is present grossly, omit chemical examination, cell count (unless corrected for the presence of blood), and colloidal gold test.

Traumatic blood due to the puncture is not evenly distributed in the different specimens collected, there being more in the first tube and little or none in the last one. The supernatant fluid is clear and colorless, and the specimen tends to clot.

In subarachnoid hemorrhage the blood is evenly mixed, the supernatant fluid becomes yellowish a few hours after the hemorrhage, and the fluid will not clot.

Clear spinal fluid, however, does not rule out intracranial hemorrhage.

Blood in the cerebrospinal fluid is accompanied by 1 leukocyte for each 700 red blood cells if the blood leukocyte and erythrocyte counts are normal. Blood contributes 1 mg. protein/100 ml. cerebrospinal fluid for each 700-750 RBC/mm.[3] cerebrospinal fluid if the blood is normal.

Xanthochromia: Xanthochromia is a yellow discoloration of the spinal fluid. It may be due to bilirubin, hemoglobin derivatives, or a lipidlike substance resulting from brain tissue destruction.[1]

A yellow cerebrospinal fluid containing a large amount of protein and tending to clot en masse (**Froin's syndrome**) indicates the formation of a cul-de-sac below some obstruction such as a tumor. The tests for blood (benzidine) and for bile (van den Bergh) are usually negative. In jaundice the cerebrospinal fluid is not yellow except in severe and chronic cases and in premature infants. A yellow color is more often due to the presence of blood that has disintegrated, as after subarachnoid hemorrhage or after hemorrhage caused by previous puncture. The benzidine test for blood will be positive unless the change in the blood pigment has progressed too far, and sometimes the test for bile (delayed direct van den Bergh test or oxidation with Obermayer reagent) is positive due to the presence of old blood pigment.

Xanthochromia occurs in the cerebrospinal fluid of normal premature infants and may persist for several weeks, depending upon the degree of jaundice. The indirect van den Bergh test is positive.

Transparency: Note whether the fluid is clear or cloudy. Record degree of cloudiness. Fewer than 200 WBC/mm.[3] does not give rise to macroscopic clouding of fluid.

Clot formation: Clot formation indicates the presence of fibrinogen. Record presence or absence of clot and also type of clot when present. Normally no clot forms. In paresis there are many small clots, in tuberculous meningitis a web-like clot, in purulent meningitis a large clot, and in blockage of spinal fluid circulation a tendency to clot en masse.

Test for increased fibrinogen: Add ⅓ vol. 10% NaOH, shake, and observe fine fibrin flocculation that ultimately condenses on the surface.

Chemical examination

Globulin:

Ross-Jones test; Nonne-Apelt test: In a test tube overlay 2 or 3 ml. saturated ammonium sulfate solution (or about 0.5 ml. in a small test tube) with the spinal fluid after centrifuging (supernatant fluid). Observe for gray ring at line of contact. Let stand 3 min. before recording the test as negative.

When blood is absent, this test is positive only with pathologic fluids.

Pandy test: To 1 ml. saturated aqueous solution of phenol crystals add 1 drop cerebrospinal fluid (clear). A bluish-white cloud indicates an increased amount of globulin. A very slight turbidity is normal. This is due to the fact that phenol precipitates albumin also.

Pandy reagent: Use saturated aqueous solution of phenol crystals. Add 10 gm. phenol crystals to 100 ml. distilled water. Leave in incubator for several days, shaking frequently. Use the clear supernatant fluid.

NOTE: When blood due to trauma is present, the serum accompanying a very few red blood cells (seen microscopically or grossly after settling) will not give a positive test for globulin. If the number is sufficient to cause haziness, however, the accompanying serum may give a positive reaction. When blood is mixed with spinal fluid, about 20,000 RBC/mm.[3] is sufficient to give a 1+ globulin reading.

Procaine (Novocain) gives a false positive Pandy test.

Total protein: For quantitative measurements, see section on clinical chemistry.

Normal values and interpretation: The usual normal range of total protein in the spinal fluid is between 14 and 45 mg./100 ml. The amount increases from above downward, being sometimes as little as 5 mg./100 ml. in ventricular fluid. Normally the protein is chiefly albumin (A/G ratio about 4:1). The protein is normal in meningismus. It is normal or slightly increased in multiple sclerosis, central nervous system syphilis, encephalitis, and anterior poliomyelitis; it is moderately to markedly increased in purulent meningitis, tuberculous meningitis, and subarachnoid block.

In inflammatory diseases (meningitis) the globulin is relatively increased; in arachnoid block, polyneuritis, and radiculomyelitis the albumin is relatively increased.

Chromatography: The normal spinal fluid contains 16 amino acids, the most important of which is glutamine (58 μg/ml.). The concentration of the others varies from 1-7 μg/ml. Changes in disease, with the exception of multiple sclerosis (normal pattern), have not been published to date.[2, 3]

Electrophoresis: Cerebrospinal fluid gamma globulin is increased in multiple sclerosis, encephalitis, central nervous system syphilis, and conditions accompanied by serum gamma globulin elevations. Microimmune electrophoretic methods are used to determine fibrinogen.[4] Use the concentration method described for urine, p. 21.

Cerebrospinal fluid enzymes[5]: The two enzymes that are most frequently tested for are glutamic oxalacetic transaminase and lactic acid dehydrogenase.

Transaminase is increased in cerebrovascular disease, head injury, convulsive disorders, and degenerative diseases of the central nervous system.

Lactic acid dehydrogenase is increased in head injury, convulsive disorders, and degenerative diseases.

Tryptophan test: Mix 2 or 3 ml. spinal fluid, 15-18 ml. concentrated hydrochloric acid, and 2 or 3 drops 5% formalin and let stand 5 min. Overlay with 1 or 2 ml. sodium nitrite solution (0.06%, fresh, i.e., 60 mg./100 ml.). Observe for 2 or 3 min.

A delicate violet is positive; no color or a brown color is negative. A purple ring is given by bloody, purulent, or xanthochromatic fluids.

The test is positive in a very large percentage of patients with tuberculous meningitis, but it is not diagnostic. It is usually negative in syphilitic meningitis, encephalitis, poliomyelitis, and brain tumor.

Reducing substances:

Glucose: Quantitative measurements are discussed in the section on clinical chemistry.

Normal values and interpretation: The spinal fluid sugar normally amounts to a little more than half of the blood sugar, the fluctuation of which it follows. The level of the spinal fluid glucose should always be measured together with a blood sugar specimen obtained immediately prior to the spinal puncture since this procedure itself may increase the cerebrospinal fluid glucose content. If possible the patient should be fasting, and there should be no delay in performing the determination.

Normal is about 60-90 mg./100 ml. Reducing substances are absent in acute pyogenic infections and decreased in tuberculous meningitis (20-40 mg./100 ml.). They may be increased in encephalitis lethargica and are usually normal or slightly reduced in poliomyelitis. Glucose is increased in diabetic coma (hyperglycemia) and reduced in hypoglycemia.

Chlorides: The method is the same as for blood.

Normal values and interpretation: The normal level is 118-127 mEq./L. There is no change in encephalitis, hydrocephalus, tumors, or syphilis. Chlorides are reduced in pyogenic meningitis and tuberculous meningitis. They are said to be normal or slightly decreased in poliomyelitis but are often found to vary greatly. Similar to glucose, cerebrospinal fluid chlorides also reflect plasma chloride changes.

Microscopic examination

WHITE CELL COUNT: Cells should be counted as soon as the specimen is received since they are only well preserved in a fresh specimen. The method of counting will vary with the number of cells expected.

Method for low white cell count: The spinal fluid appears completely clear.

Technique: Transfer 1 drop well-mixed undiluted fluid to a counting chamber and count all the cells in 9 large squares (see p. 112). Since this represents a volume of 9/10 mm.[3], the result is multiplied by 10/9 to obtain the number of cells/mm.[3]. For practical purposes the multiplication may be omitted.

Method for moderate white cell count: *Diluting fluid:*
1. Crystal violet, 0.2 gm.
2. Glacial acetic acid, 10 ml.

3. Distilled water, 100 ml.

Technique: Mix specimen thoroughly. If not very cloudy or bloody, draw diluting fluid to mark 1 in a white cell counting pipette and well-mixed spinal fluid to mark 11, producing a dilution of 1:10. The dilution procedure is the reverse of that for the low white cell count.

Mix, discard one-third, and place 1 drop on each side of the blood counting chamber as in the method for leukocyte counting. Count the cells in 5 squares, 1 mm.² each (4 corner squares and the central square), in each of the 2 drops, and add. Divide the sum by 10 to obtain the number per single large square. Multiply by 10 × 10 = 100 to obtain the number of cells in 1 mm.³. The first 10 converts the number found in 0.1 mm.³ to the number found in 1 mm.³, and the second 10 represents the dilution factor.

If the count is low, a rough estimate of the differential count can be obtained by classifying the cells seen in the counting chamber.

Method for high white cell count: The white cell count in purulent cerebrospinal fluid is made as outlined for white cells in the peripheral blood (see p. 116).

Method for counting mixture of white and red cells: To find the true white cell count when the cerebrospinal fluid is bloody, make red and white cell counts on the patient's blood as well as on the cerebrospinal fluid specimen. Multiply the ratio of the red cell count of the fluid to the red cell count of the blood by the blood leukocyte count and subtract this product from the white cell count of the spinal fluid.

Example: RBC of blood is 5,000,000 and of spinal fluid, 25,000; WBC of blood is 12,000 and of spinal fluid, 70.

$$\frac{25,000 \times 12,000}{5,000,000} = 60$$

$$70 - 60 = 10 \text{ WBC/mm.}^3$$

Normal blood will add 1 leukocyte for each 700 red cells.

Normal values and interpretation: The normal count is 0-5 cells (lymphocytes). The cell count is usually normal in multiple sclerosis, epilepsy, brain tumor, and meningismus as well as in cerebral arteriosclerosis. It is elevated in syphilis (20-100), viral meningitis, and in 50% of patients with encephalitis. It reaches its highest levels in pyogenic meningitis.

DIFFERENTIAL COUNT:

Estimating differential count in white cell counting chamber: When the total count is low, make a chamber differential count by identifying the cells in the counting chamber, using the high-power dry lens.

Stained smear: When the cells are numerous, make a smear of the sediment (after centrifuging) using the technique given for blood smears (p. 125).

Significance of count and differential count: The normal count is 0-5, chiefly lymphocytes. An increase of lymphocytes (and by usage of total leukocytes) is called pleocytosis. Infants up to a few weeks of age may have as many as 30. A great increase, chiefly polymorphonuclear cells, occurs in acute pyogenic meningitis. A slight to moderate increase of polymorphonuclear cells (total cell count usually less than 1000) occurs in the meningitis accompanying brain abscess and in the early stages of tuberculous meningitis, syphilitic meningitis, and poliomyelitis (first 24 hr.), after which the lymphocytes predominate.

A moderate increase of cells, lymphocytes chiefly, occurs in neurosyphilis, tuberculous meningitis, poliomyelitis, and lymphocytic choriomeningitis. Sometimes the increase is marked.

As many as 400 lymphocytes/mm.³ may not cause distinct clouding; the same number of polymorphonuclear cells will.

The cell count in the different tubes of fluid may vary markedly. The first tube will contain more cells in spinal disease, and the last tube will have more cells in disease of the brain only. The first tube shows more traumatic blood.

Sometimes the cell count and the protein are not increased together. The cells are increased without a corresponding increase in the protein in aseptic meningitis, and the protein is increased without an increase of cells in Guillain-Barré syndrome.

CYTOLOGY: The Papanicolaou technique, used in conjunction with the Millipore filter, has been applied to the examination of the cerebrospinal fluid for tumor cells. In primary tumors of the brain the results are disappointing, but they are somewhat improved in metastatic tumors with meningeal involvement.[6]

Serologic examination

Perform serologic test for syphilis and colloidal gold test.

Colloidal gold test:

Principle: Quantitative and qualitative changes in the spinal fluid protein level produce color changes and precipitation of a colloidal gold solution. The normal protein content of spinal fluid has no effect on the gold solution since the normal albumin content prevents the precipitation of the colloidal gold by globulin. As long as the albumin-globulin ratio remains the same, an increase of total protein has little effect on the colloidal gold curve; but should the ratio change, the colloidal curve will reflect the alteration (Fig. 10-1).

Reagent:

Colloidal gold solution: This reagent should be purchased.

Technique: Clean glassware with white soap (Ivory, etc.) and water and then with cleansing fluid; then rinse with running water and finally with distilled and double-distilled water. Sterilize in hot air.

Place 10 test tubes in a rack. Into the first tube place 1.8 ml. 0.4% sodium chloride solution and 1 ml. into each of the others. Centrifuge and add 0.2 ml. clear spinal fluid to the first tube and mix. Transfer 1 ml. to the second tube and mix. Continue in this manner, discarding 1 ml. from the tenth tube. Add to each tube 5 ml. colloidal gold solution and mix. Let stand overnight at room temperature.

Each time, carry the following controls in one rack as tubes 11 and 12. In tube 11 put 1.7 ml. 1% sodium chloride solution and in tube 12 put 0.5 ml. Add 5 ml. colloidal gold solution to each. Tube 11 should be colorless, and tube 12 should show no change.

NOTE: It is more economical to use half the quantities in the directions given.

Novocain is a contaminant that will give abnormal curves similar to those in cer-

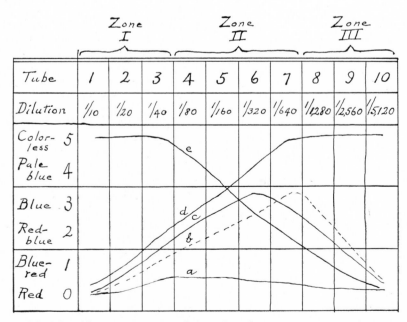

Fig. 10-1. Colloidal gold curves. **a,** Normal; **b,** tuberculous meningitis; **c,** tabes, meningovascular syphilis, and some virus infections; **d,** pyogenic meningitis and aseptic meningitis; **e,** paresis and multiple sclerosis (50%).

tain diseases. The change is most marked in zone II.[7]

Record results in each tube on a scale of 1-5 as follows:

        0 = no change
        1 = bluish red
        2 = reddish blue
        3 = blue
        4 = pale blue
        5 = colorless

Significance: Normally there is no change above 1 in any tube, e.g., 0001100000. A marked change in the first three tubes (zone I reaction) occurs in general paresis (with a reactive test for syphilis) and in active multiple sclerosis, e.g., 5554321000. The greatest change in the fourth and fifth tubes (zone II reaction) occurs in tabes and meningovascular syphilis and sometimes in multiple sclerosis, encephalitis lethargica, and poliomyelitis, e.g., 1124320000, the change being rarely above 3 or 4. The greatest change in the last three tubes (zone III reaction) occurs in pyogenic meningitis, e.g., 0012234553.

Many nonsyphilitic fluids with increased protein (old hemorrhage, tumors, etc.) give positive reactions. In tuberculous meningitis the greatest change is usually in tube 6 or 7 (zone II), e.g., 0000243000.

Culture

Cerebrospinal fluid should be cultured without delay. The sediment of the centrifuged specimen should be handled as outlined on p. 532.

Mix the sediment with dilute India ink and examine for *Cryptococcus neoformans.* If a virus disease is suspected, spinal fluid and serum should be frozen in a deep freeze in sterile containers and paired with a second specimen obtained 8-14 days later for virus identification or viral serology.

CHANGES IN CEREBROSPINAL FLUID IN DISEASE (Table 10-3)

Lymphocytic choriomeningitis[8]**:** The cell count varies from 500-1000 WBC/mm.[3], rarely reaching 2000 WBC/mm.[3]. While polymorphonuclear cells may predominate in the first few days, they are soon replaced by lymphocytes that continue to dominate the picture for several weeks. The protein is moderately elevated in the neighborhood of 250 mg./100 ml. and may give rise to clot formation. The lowered glucose level may suggest tuberculous meningitis as a differential diagnostic consideration.

Leukocytes of the blood are usually within the normal range and the differential count is also normal. Antibodies can be demonstrated in the serum from about the third week. Inoculation of serum into mice is usually fatal in about 7 days, although the animals may appear well as late as the sixth day. Mice show paralysis of the hind legs and tonic spasms as in tetanus. Intracerebral inoculation is most successful, although subcutaneous and intraperitoneal inoculation may be used.

St. Louis encephalitis: The spinal fluid is usually under slightly increased pressure and is clear; cells are usually slightly increased (0-250), occasionally over 1000, chiefly lymphocytes; globulin is slightly increased; and sugar and chlorides are within normal range. Mice inoculated intracerebrally are very susceptible, showing tremors, prostration, and death after 4-8 days.

Subarachnoid hemorrhage: Spinal fluid shows blood evenly mixed in all tubes, absence of clot, and xanthochromia. None of these are found in traumatic hemorrhage caused by the spinal tap. The blood shows moderate leukocytosis and the urine shows transient (1-10 days) massive albuminuria without renal lesions.

Ruptured nucleus pulposus: In about three fourths of the cases of herniation of the intervertebral cartilaginous disc, the cerebrospinal fluid protein is increased below the level of the lesion (75-100 mg./100 ml.). Often this is the only positive finding. The determination is usually made on the first 2 ml. specimen (blood-free) obtained, but sometimes the amount of protein is greater in the other portions.

Infectious mononucleosis: This disease may involve the central nervous system, producing symptoms of encephalitis, lymphocytic choriomeningitis, or poliomyelitis.[9] The spinal fluid findings are not characteristic, but the globulin and

Table 10-3. Cerebrospinal fluid in disease

Disease	Pressure (mm. H₂O)	Appearance	Clot	No. and type of cells	Protein (mg./100 ml.)	Sugar (mg./100 ml.)	Chlorides (mEq./L.)	Colloidal gold	Remarks
Normal	100-200	Clear; colorless	0	0-15 lymphocytes	20-40	60-90	118-127	0000000000	
Meningitis									
Pyogenic	3+	Cloudy	Large	3+ PMN	3+	D (0)	Slightly D	V	See Chapter 11
Tuberculous	3+	Clear or slightly turbid	Web	2+ lymphocytes	2+	20-40	D < 600	0002344100; tube 6 or 7 (zone II)	Tubercle bacilli (see Chapter 11)
Lymphocytic choriomeningitis	2+	Clear or opalescent	0	50-2000 lymphocytes	+	N	N	V; slight meningitic curve	See text
Cord tumor	N	Clear; deep yellow	En masse	N - + lymphocytes	3+	N	N	V	
Brain abscess	1+ - 3+	Clear or turbid	±	+ PMN	+ - 2+	N	N - slightly D	V	
Brain tumor	3+	Clear; yellow	±	N lymphocytes	± - 2+	N	N	V	
Poliomyelitis	N	Clear or opalescent	0	50-2000 PMN early; lymphocytes later	+	N	N - slightly D	N - 1123210000	Filtrable virus
Encephalitis	N - +	Clear; colorless	0	N - + lymphocytes	±	N	N	N - 1123210000	Filtrable virus (see text)
Subarachnoid hemorrhage	1+ - 2+	Bloody; yellow	0	Blood	3+	N	N	V; meningitic curve	See text
Neurosyphilis									
Meningovascular	+	Clear; colorless	Rare	20-100 PMN early; lymphocytes later	+ - 2+	N	N	0244321000; zone II	Serologic test for syphilis nearly always reactive
Tabes	+	Clear; colorless	Rare	25-75 lymphocytes	+	N	N	0244321000; zone II	Serologic test for syphilis 80% reactive
Paresis	+	Clear; colorless	Many; small	25-50 lymphocytes	+	N	N	5555441000; zone I	Serologic test for syphilis 100% reactive

N = normal; ± = normal to slight increase; + = slight increase; 2+ = moderate increase; 3+ = marked increase; D = decrease; V = variable.

total protein are usually increased. The cell count varies from normal to over 1000 cells, chiefly lymphocytes.

The blood picture and the heterophil reaction of the serum should help in the differential diagnosis, but symptoms of central nervous system involvement may appear as much as 2 wk. before lymphadenopathy. The cerebrospinal fluid does not give the heterophil reaction.[10]

Polyneuritis: In this disease (Guillain-Barré syndrome), which is accompanied by painful paralysis, the protein of the cerebrospinal fluid is markedly increased without any increase of cells.

Poliomyelitis[11]**:** Since an increase in the cerebrospinal fluid protein may be the only positive routine laboratory finding (though pleocytosis is the rule), the presence of over 45 mg./100 ml. in patients with signs (stiff neck, muscular tenderness or weakness, and central nervous system involvement) and symptoms (fever, headache, and upper respiratory infection) consistent with a diagnosis of poliomyelitis seems to justify a tentative diagnosis of the disease.

In laboratories especially equipped for virus studies a definite diagnosis of poliomyelitis can be made in 7-14 days by the use of tissue culture methods, employing monkey kidney epithelial cells in fluid medium. The cytopathogenic virus can be identified and typed by specific antiserum (monkey). Cultures from stools are most successful, but may be made from throat swabs, rectal swabs, or cerebrospinal fluid (least successful). Tests for specific antibodies, neutralizing and complement-fixing, are made on two serum samples, one from the early phase and the other from the convalescent phase.

SYNOVIAL FLUID[12]

Synovial fluid is a modified connective tissue fluid found in joints and tendon spaces. It is characterized by a high mucin content, which gives it its viscid nature. It is a product of the secretory activity of the synovial lining. Other components of the fluid are dialysates of the plasma such as glucose, electrolytes, and nonprotein nitrogen, showing the same concentration as in plasma. Analysis of the synovial fluid is of value in the study of arthritis.

LABORATORY INVESTIGATION

Characteristics of normal synovial fluid:
Transparency: clear
Color: straw
Viscosity: high
Total cell count: 200-600 WBC/mm.³, 25% segmented forms
Differential count:
    Polymorphonuclear cells: 0-25%
    Lymphocytes: 0-78%
    Monocytes: 0-71%
Wet preparation:
    No crystals
    No RA cells
    No cartilage fibers
    No bacteria
Total protein: 1.07-2.13 gm./100 ml.
    Albumin: 1.02 gm./100 ml.
    Globulin: 0.05 gm./100 ml.

Transparency: Normal fluid is clear and transparent. In inflammatory joint diseases it becomes cloudy to purulent. Cloudy fluid should always be cultured.

Color: Normal fluid is straw colored or lighter. After trauma it may be bloody or xanthochromatic. Blood-streaked fluid is due to the aspirational procedure; in pathologic conditions the blood is usually evenly distributed throughout the fluid.

Total cell count: The white blood cell counting technique is used, but isotonic saline solution is substituted for the usual acid white cell diluting fluid since the latter may clot synovial fluid. A 0.3% saline solution has the advantage of laking red cells in a bloody specimen and still preserving white cells.

Interpretation: The white cell count in inflammatory arthritis is high, varying from 5000-60,000 WBC/mm.³. In osteoarthritis it is only moderately elevated, the average value being 2000 WBC/mm.³.

Differential count: Prepare a smear of synovial fluid, allow to dry, and stain with Wright stain. In osteoarthritis the predominant cell is lymphocytic, while in rheumatoid arthritis and infective arthritis the polymorphonuclear cells predominate.

Mucin clot production (Ropes test): Add

1 ml. glacial acetic acid to 5 ml. synovial fluid and observe the ropy clot of mucoproteins that follows the heavy acid to the bottom of the tube. In osteoarthritis the clot is firm and the surrounding fluid remains clear even after agitation. In rheumatoid arthritis the clot is friable and the surrounding fluid is turbid. In acute rheumatic fever the clot is firm, and in lupus erythematosus the clot is firm, i.e., normal.

Crystals in wet preparation: Place 1 drop uncentrifuged fluid on a microscope slide, apply cover slip immediately and seal with fingernail polish. Examine the preparation by ordinary light microscopy under high magnification and also by polarized light and phase microscopy. In

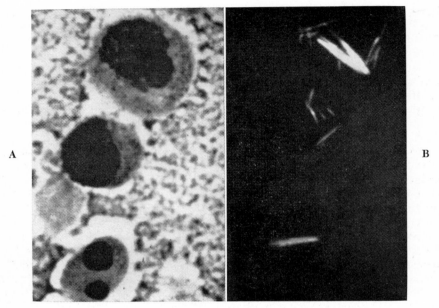

Fig. 10-2. Synovial fluid from knee involved with acute gout. **A,** Inflammatory cells viewed with ordinary light. **B,** Same cells viewed with polarized light show birefringent intracellular sodium urate crystals. (From Good and Frishette: J.A.M.A. **198:**80, 1966.)

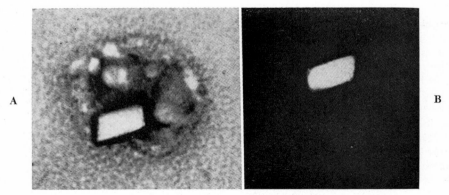

Fig. 10-3. Synovial fluid obtained from knee involved with acute pseudogout. **A,** Mononuclear leukocyte containing rhomboid-shaped calcium pyrophosphate crystals viewed with ordinary light. **B,** Same cell viewed with polarized light shows birefringence of crystals. (Wright stain; ×2000.) (From Good and Frishette: J.A.M.A. **198:**80, 1966.)

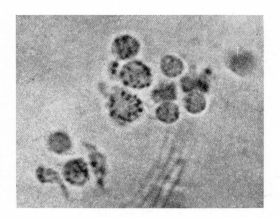

Fig. 10-4. Polymorphonuclear leukocytes containing typical cytoplasmic inclusions in wet preparation of synovial fluid from patient with rheumatoid arthritis. (Courtesy George B. Backer; from Hollander et al.: Med. Clin. N. Amer. **50:** 1281, 1966.)

about 90% of fluids from acutely inflamed joints, two kinds of **birefringent crystals** are found[13, 14]: **monosodium urate crystals** are found in gouty fluids and **calcium pyrophosphate crystals** are found in chondrocalcinosis. The urate crystals are needle shaped, doubly refractile under polarized light, and are found free as well as within neutrophils. The pyrophosphate crystals are only weakly birefringent. Also found within wet preparations are cartilage fibers, cholesterol crystals, and **RA cells** (Figs. 10-2 to 10-4).

Tests for rheumatoid factor

Rheumatoid factor[15]**:** The serum (and synovia) of 80-90% of patients suffering from rheumatoid arthritis contains a macroglobulin type of antibody called rheumatoid factor (RF), the agglutinating properties of which are the basis for many of the tests for rheumatoid arthritis. The RF differs from normal macroglobulin antibodies such as anti-A and anti-B isoagglutinins by its ability to bind gamma₂ globulins. The RF agglutinates latex particles coated with gamma globulin fraction II or sheep erythrocytes sensitized with rabbit antisheep antibody (modified Rose-Waaler sheep erythrocyte test).[16]

Gm groups and rheumatoid factor: Group O, Rh-positive erythrocytes coated with incomplete anti-Rh₀ antibody are agglutinated by most AB sera, Coombs sera, and sera containing RF. The addition of serum of some individuals inhibits the agglutination (Gm-Test) and the factor responsible for this inhibition is a genetically controlled serum gamma globulin called Gm factor. There is apparently some relationship between Gm groups and RF.

RA cell[15]**:** Under ordinary light microscopy wet preparations of synovial fluid from a patient with rheumatoid arthritis show dark, small, multiple nodular inclusions within polymorphonuclear cells and macrophages, which can be visualized even better by phase microscopy. These inclusions are of immune gamma globulin nature (Fig. 10-4).

Screening test for rheumatoid factor: The rheumatoid factor may be found in synovial fluid before it can be detected in serum. The fluid should be tested in the same way as serum.

The **RA-Test*** (rapid slide screening test) is useful. Latex globulin will agglutinate in the presence of suitably diluted serum or synovial fluid containing RF. If the screening test is positive, the **macroscopic tube test*** may be used to titrate the factor. Agglutination in a dilution of 1:80 or over is considered positive.

Biochemical tests

Glucose: The level usually reflects the plasma glucose level but is decreased in severe inflammatory arthritis.

Total protein: Total protein is elevated in osteoarthritis and in some cases of rheumatoid arthritis and lupus erythematosus, but it is still below 5 gm./100 ml. In severe infectious arthritis it is above the 5 gm. level.

Culture

Synovial fluid should be cultured if the total white count is 20,000 WBC/mm.³ or over. A tuberculous and gonorrheal etiology should be considered in septic arthritis. See gonorrheal antibody test, p. 558. For culture, see p. 557.

---

*Hyland Laboratories, Los Angeles, Calif.

Table 10-4. Synovianalysis in arthritis*

Disease	Appearance	Viscosity	Mucin clot	White cell count	Crystals	Cartilage debris	Special features
Normal	Straw; clear	High (normal)	Good	200-600; 25% PMN	0	0	0
Traumatic arthritis	Cloudy; bloody	Normal	Good	2000 ± (many RBC)	0	0 or +	0
Osteo-arthritis	Yellow; clear	Normal	Good	1000 ±; 20% PMN	0	Fragments; fibrils	0
Rheumatic fever	Yellow; slightly cloudy	Low	Fair	10,000 ±; 50% PMN	0	0	Few inclusion body cells
Systemic lupus erythematosus	Yellow; slightly cloudy	Normal	Good	3000 ±; 10% PMN	0	0	L.E. cells on smear
Gouty arthritis	Yellow; cloudy	Low	Poor	10,000 +; 75% PMN	Many (urate)	0	Crystals in cells or free negative birefringence
Pseudogout	Yellow; slightly cloudy	Normal or low	Good	6000 +; 75% PMN	Few to many (Ca pyrophosphate)	0 to many	Crystals in cells, free, or in cartilage fragments (weakly positive birefringence)
Rheumatoid arthritis and variants	Yellow to greenish; cloudy	Low	Poor	8000-40,000; 70% PMN	Rare (cholesterol)	0	5-95% of PMN show inclusions; latex positive
Tuberculous arthritis	Yellow; cloudy	Low	Poor	25,000 ±; 40-50% PMN	0	0	Glucose low; latex negative; acid-fast bacterial culture
Septic arthritis	Grayish to bloody; turbid	Low	Poor	80,000 ±; 90% PMN	0	0	Latex negative; culture positive; inclusion body cells negative for RF; decreased glucose

*From Hollander et al.: Med. Clin. N. Amer. **50**:1281, 1966.

AMNIOTIC FLUID[17]

The method of formation of amniotic fluid has not been established. Undoubtedly both fetus and mother take part in its formation. The fluid is partially ingested by the fetus.

Volume: The volume gradually increases until the last trimester, when it reaches a level of 850-1000 ml.

Color and transparency: It is a watery, clear, colorless fluid that is clouded by desquamated cells, blood, meconium, etc. It is composed of about 98% water and 2% solids.

Biochemistry: The total protein is much lower in amniotic fluid than in maternal serum. Urea, creatinine, and uric acid are higher in amniotic fluid; glucose is only slightly lower. The composition somewhat resembles that of the interstitial portion of extracellular fluid contaminated by the end products of fetal activity.

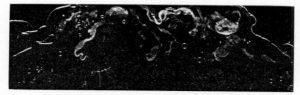

Fig. 10-5. Curschmann's spirals in sputum from patient with asthma. Specimen of sputum is pressed between slides over a black background. (Natural size.)

For discussion of bilirubin in amniotic fluid, see p. 276.

SPUTUM

Collection of specimen: Sputum should be obtained from the respiratory tract below the larynx. For routine examination it should be fresh, and for culture it should be obtained in a sterile petri dish or other sterile container after the teeth have been washed and the mouth rinsed thoroughly.

The early morning specimen or a 24 hr. specimen of sputum is usually the most satisfactory in searching for the tubercle bacillus.

Since infectious diseases may be spread by means of sputum, all specimens should be kept covered, handled with aseptic precautions, and afterward disinfected by chemicals, autoclaving, or burning.

Heated aerosol techniques have been developed (1) to produce sputum not mixed with other secretions and (2) to induce patients whose pulmonary lesion is not cough-producing to expectorate.

Laboratory investigation
Physical examination

Amount: Note whether the amount is small, moderate, or large. Large amounts are characteristic for bronchiectasis, abscesses, cavities with bronchial connections, and pulmonary adenomatosis.

Color: Sputum is normally gray or colorless. The color is influenced by such components as blood, pus, mucus, saliva, and jaundice. Pneumonia produces a rust-brown sputum, whereas tumors frequently lead to a raspberry-colored sputum. The blood of true hemoptysis is bright red and foamy, while vomited blood is brown, often likened to the color of coffee grounds (acid hematin).

Consistency: Sputum may be mucoid, purulent, sanguineous, serous, or combinations of these. On standing, the sputum of abscesses and bronchiectasis separates into two or three layers.

Odor: Note unusual odors such as fetid, rancid, etc. Enteric gram-negative bacteria impart a fecal odor.

Macroscopic structures:

Cheesy masses: These are fragments of necrotic tissue.

Dittrich's plugs: These are plugs from the bronchi or bronchioles and consist of cellular detritus, fat, and bacteria. Similar plugs are often found in the crypts of the tonsils.

Curschmann's spirals: These are spirally twisted mucoid strands (Fig. 10-5) enclosing epithelial cells and leukocytes, chiefly eosinophils, and sometimes Charcot-Leyden crystals.

Casts: Bronchial casts are molded in the bronchi and consist of fibrin and mucus. They are usually grayish white, but they may be reddish brown due to blood pigment. They are frequently so tangled that they cannot be recognized until they are floated in water over a black background. They are found in the sputum of patients with chronic fibrinous bronchitis, lobar pneumonia, tuberculosis, chronic heart disease (mitral valve), and diphtheria.

Concretions: These are usually formed by a deposit of calcium in exudate. Sometimes the core is a small foreign body or a fungus growth.

Foreign bodies and parasites: Foreign material may include concretions formed in the bronchi made of calcium carbonate and phosphate (bronchial calculi) and aspirated substances such as pollen, seeds, and dust.

In pneumoconiosis, asbestos bodies and silica particles as well as other foreign material may be found.

Only a limited number of parasites can be seen grossly; they are *Echinococcus granulosus* (hydatid sand in sputum), *Toxocara canis* (visceral larva migrans), and *Paragonimus westermani*.

Microscopic examination

Pick out cheesy masses, purulent particles, rusty portions, and suspicious structures and examine in both unstained and stained preparations.

Unstained preparations: Place on slide under cover glass. Examine for Curschmann's spirals, myelin globules, elastic tissue fibers, crystals, parasites, and phagocytic cells containing pigment, dust particles, mineral oil, or fat.

White and red blood cells: White blood cells form the majority of all cellular elements in sputum and are markedly increased when pus is present. The usual chemical tests for blood (guaiac and benzidine) cannot be used to confirm the presence of blood in sputum. The diagnosis of blood is therefore based on the finding of red blood cells or of derivatives of blood pigment (hemosiderin). Eosinophils are commonly seen in the sputum of allergic patients (asthma) and can be demonstrated by Wright stain.

Phagocytic cells (heart-failure cells): These are endothelial cells containing in their cytoplasm very fine particles of matter that they have engulfed as foreign bodies: carbon particles in normal sputum, especially marked in smokers who inhale; dust from coal, silica, iron, or marble in pneumoconiosis; blood pigment (hemosiderin) in heart failure; or mineral, animal, or vegetable oil in lipoid pneumonia.

Hemosiderin can be stained for iron with the Prussian blue reaction (see p. 138).

Myelin globules: These are round or irregularly shaped highly refractile bodies with a very slight greenish tinge and markings of concentric rings. They vary greatly in size and must be distinguished from fat droplets and yeastlike fungi. They apparently arise from degenerating mucus. They are found characteristically in normal mucoid sputum after it has stood for a long time, and they are notably absent (or scarce) in specimens containing inflammatory exudate.

Crystals: These consist of Charcot-Leyden, hematoidin, cholesterol, or fatty acid crystals.

Crystals indicate stasis and decomposition of the sputum in the body or in an old specimen that is often unsatisfactory.

Charcot-Leyden crystals are colorless hexagonal double pyramids with bases together and sharply pointed apexes. They arise from the disintegration of eosinophils and are usually abundant in the typical sputum of asthma. The crystals stain black with hematoxylin (as in feces stained for protozoa) and red with eosin.

Hematoidin crystals are usually rhombic and brownish red, although they may appear as yellow needles arranged in rosettes. These crystals result from the breaking down of old blood and are found in pulmonary infarcts, lung abscess, bronchiectasis, and perforating empyema.

Cholesterol crystals are colorless thin rhombic plates with a notched corner (reentrant angle). They indicate stasis with fatty degeneration of the exudate and are found often in lung abscess and in empyema.

Fatty acid crystals are long colorless needles, often arranged in sheaves. They indicate stasis and fatty degeneration and are found especially in bronchiectasis, abscess, and gangrene of the lung.

Parasites: They are *Paragonimus westermani*, *Toxocara canis*, *Ascaris lumbricoides*, *Endamoeba histolytica* (in abscess), *Taenia solium*, *Echinococcus granulosus*, *Schistosoma japonicum*, and *Schistosoma mansoni*.

Elastic tissue fibers: These indicate tissue destruction and are found in tuberculosis, lung abscess, bronchiectasis, infarction, and gangrene of the lung.

The presence of elastic tissue fibers may be due to the involvement of the lung, the bronchus, or a blood vessel.

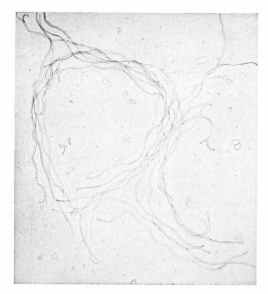

Fig. 10-6. High-power field showing elastic tissue fibers in sputum of patient with lung abscess. (Sodium hydroxide preparation.)

When the fibers appear in alveolar arrangement, however, the destructive process is in the lung.

To demonstrate elastic tissue fibers, select the most purulent portions and warm in 20% sodium hydroxide. Mount under cover glass. Elastic tissue fibers are highly refractive and curly, and the ends are often split (Fig. 10-6). Distinguish from cellulose structures, which are also not destroyed.

Stained preparations: Smears should be stained by the Gram method for general bacterial flora and by the acid-fast method for tubercle bacilli. A smear may also be stained by the Wright method for making differential counts in asthma, etc. and by the Giemsa method for demonstrating spirochetes, as in bronchial spirochetosis (organisms similar to Vincent's).

Culture: See Chapter 11 for a discussion of culture methods.

Fungi: The most common ones are *Blastomyces, Actinomyces, Monilia, Streptothrix, Torula, Coccidioides immitis, Aspergillus, Alternaria,* and *Mucor.* (See Chapter 12.)

When molds, yeasts, and *Actinomyces*

are suspected, mount the suspicious particles in 20% potassium or sodium hydroxide. This dissolves the cellular debris so that the fungi are more easily seen. This method is also useful for demonstrating elastic tissue fibers and asbestos bodies. Culture for fungi.

Malignant cells

Special methods of collection, preservation, and concentration are advised. The fresh early morning specimen is used for cytologic smears, or the patient is requested to inhale a heated (100° F.) aerosol of 20% propylene glycol solution in 10% sodium chloride to induce expectoration.[18] The sputum should be either smeared immediately or preserved in ethyl alcohol or polyvinyl alcohol fixative[19, 20] (PVA; Elvanol*), or it should be concentrated.

CONCENTRATION OF CELLS IN SPUTUM:
Aqueous dissolution technique:
1. Transfer specimen to 250 ml. Erlenmeyer flask. If specimen is in fixative (alcohol or formalin), centrifuge first and transfer sediment to flask.
2. Add sufficient absolute alcohol to cover specimen (usually about 20 ml.).
3. Allow to stand for 10 min., swirling several times. Add distilled water.
4. Stopper and shake vigorously by hand or in mechanical shakers until mucus is dissolved. Dissolution is indicated by a homogeneous, milky appearance with only finely suspended particles. Shaking time is usually from 5-20 min. If after 20 min. the mucus still persists, add more water and repeat shaking.
5. Transfer specimen to 50 ml. polyethylene round-bottom centrifuge tubes. Centrifuge at 2000 rpm for 10 min. in standard swinging tube head or 5 min. in an angle-head centrifuge.
6. Decant. Aspirate sediment with pipette and place on clean albuminized slides.

*E. I. DuPont de Nemours & Co., Inc., Wilmington, Del.

7. Spread evenly with wooden applicator stick or between two slides, using gentle pressure.
8. Place slides in ether-alcohol mixture and proceed with routine Papanicolaou technique, or stain with acridine orange for fluoroscence microscopic examination.

SPUTUM IN DISEASE

The type of sputum is not diagnostic of any disease but depends upon the type of **inflammation,** the severity of the infection, and the presence or absence of blood. The causative organism may often be found in sputum as a predominating type except in gangrene, abscess, or bronchiectasis, in which the flora is mixed. In mild infections (acute bronchitis) the sputum is scanty at first and mucoid, changing later to an abundant mucopurulent or purulent sputum. Microscopically, pus cells, a few red cells, and desquamated respiratory epithelial cells are found. Later on, degeneration of the pus cells and red blood cells may occur, especially when there is stasis (abscess or bronchiectasis), in which case the amount of sputum will vary periodically with posture. There may be phagocytic leukocytes often containing tissue debris or blood pigment, and crystals (cholesterol, fatty acid, or hematoidin) may be present. When there is tissue destruction, there will be elastic fibers. Characteristically in asthma there are Curschmann's spirals and eosinophils and often Charcot-Leyden crystals. In tuberculosis, sputum may vary from the small normal mucoid expectoration to a frankly bloody mucopurulent type. Tubercle bacilli may be present, but failure to find them does not rule out tuberculosis. In lobar pneumonia the sputum is rusty and gelatinous. Later, the sputum becomes frankly purulent and often yellowish or greenish in color.

Sulfonamides and antibiotics may produce pleomorphic change in various organisms.[21]

In **pneumoconiosis** there will be a large number of phagocytic leukocytes containing small particles of the inhaled dust, e.g., silicosis (silica or sand), anthracosis (coal), siderosis (iron), calicosis (marble or lime), and asbestosis (asbestos). The **asbestos bodies** are extracellular, highly refractile bodies with a central needlelike crystal (greenish tinge) around which is deposited a yellowish homogenous substance. The bodies often have clubbed ends and show segmentation. They give the Prussian blue reaction for iron.

In **bagassosis** the sputum is usually scant, mucoid, and often blood streaked. Bagassosis appears to be a hypersensitivity reaction caused by the inhalation of the dust of bagasse, the broken sugar cane from which the juice has been pressed. The fiber contains about 1% protein and about 5-7% silica. Saline extract of the dust of bagasse gives a positive intracutaneous reaction (immediate). Secondary bacterial infection probably accounts for the absence of eosinophils in the sputum and the blood smear. Slight leukocytosis is usually present.

In **lung abscess** the sputum is purulent, pus cells are degenerated, and the bacterial flora is mixed, showing cocci and bacilli of various types, especially influenza bacilli and diphtheroids. Elastic tissue fibers are present. In gangrene of the lung, fusospirochetal forms (Vincent's) also are present.

In **malignant disease,** blood is common, and sometimes clusters of malignant cells can be found.

Infarction in the lungs is characterized by a mucoid and bloody sputum without many leukocytes or bacteria. Other laboratory findings include leukocytosis, increased sedimentation rate, and frequently bilirubinemia.

Edema of the lung shows abundant frothy pink sputum which is serosanguineous in character. In decompensated heart disease the sputum is watery, yellowish, and characterized microscopically by masses of heart-failure cells, phagocytes containing hemosiderin.

In **lipid pneumonia**[22] macrophages containing liquid petrolatum or vegetable and animal oils can be demonstrated. Animal and vegetable oils stain both with Sudan IV (scarlet red) and osmic acid; mineral oil stains with Sudan IV, but not with osmic acid.

PUS

Pus is a yellow to yellow-green liquid that contains many polymorphonuclear cells in all stages of degeneration, much granular and fatty debris from disintegrated pus cells and tissue, and the causative organisms as well as secondary invaders at times. Some pus contains many eosinophils (gonorrheal pus, purulent pleuritic fluids, and asthmatic sputum). Pus from old abscesses may show numerous fatty acid and cholesterol crystals, and when there has been hemorrhage, hematoidin crystals are also present. In some liver abscesses, bilirubin crystals are found. Gram-negative enteric bacteria produce a fecal odor.

LABORATORY INVESTIGATION
Physical examination

Note amount, consistency, general character, color, odor, and presence (or absence) of sulfur granules.

Microscopic examination

Unstained preparations: For *Actinomyces* and other fungi and yeasts, mount suspicious granules in 20% potassium or sodium hydroxide.

For amebas, scrape material from abscess wall, mount in saline solution, and examine at once.

For crystals, mount drop on slide under cover glass in a small amount of saline solution if necessary.

Stained preparations:

Gram stain: Note types of organisms and of cells. In a mixed flora the offending organism is likely to be found in some of the polymorphonuclear cells.

Acid-fast stain: Prepare this stain when indicated, especially in pus from chronically inflamed joints, cold abscesses, etc.

Wright stain: This stain is prepared when indicated in order to study the types of cells.

NOTE: For stained preparations, make thin smears, preferably as for blood smears. When making smears from swabs, tissue, or platinum loop, do not cover the same area twice. Going over the areas more than once breaks up the cells and ruins the smear.

Culture

Plant on blood agar plates and on special media when indicated. For bacteriologic examination of pus from various sources, see Chapter 11.

REFERENCES

1. Crosby, R. M. N., and Weiland, G. L.: Arch. Neurol. & Psychiat. **69:**732, 1953.
2. Logothetis, J., and Bovis, M.: World Neurol. **2:**747, 1961.
3. Bronnestam, R., Dencker, S. J., and Swahn, B.: Arch. Neurol. **4:**288, 1961.
4. Ivers, R. R., McKenzie, B. F., McGuckin, W. F., and Goldstein, N. P.: J.A.M.A. **176:**515, 1961.
5. Fleisher, G. A., Wakin, G., and Goldstein, P.: Proc. Staff Meet. Mayo Clin. **32:**188, 1957.
6. McMenemey, W. H., and Cumings, J. N.: J. Clin. Path. **12:**400, 1959.
7. Kercher, G.: Amer. J. Clin. Path. (tech. sect.) **22:**812, 1952.
8. Dickens, P. F.: Southern. Med. J. **30:**728, 1937.
9. Landes, R., Reich, J. P., and Perlow, S.: J.A.M.A. **116:**2482, 1941.
10. Lyons, H. A., and Harrison, J. G.: Blood **4:**734, 1949.
11. Casey, A. E., Fishbein, W. I., and Bundensen, H. N.: J.A.M.A. **129:**1141, 1945.
12. Hollander, J. L., Reginato, A., and Torralba, T. P.: Med. Clin. N. Amer. **50:**1281, 1966.
13. Good, A. E., and Frishette, W. A.: J.A.M.A. **198:**80, 1966.
14. McCarty, D. J., Jr., Gatter, R. A., Brill, J. M., and Hogan, J. M.: J.A.M.A. **193:**129, 1965.
15. Hollander, J. L., McCarty, D. J., Astorga, G., and Castro-Murillo, E.: Ann. Intern. Med. **62:**271, 1965.
16. Ball, J.: Lancet **2:**520, 1950.
17. Fuchs, F., editor: Clin. Obstet. Gynec. **9:** (entire issue), 1966.
18. Barach, A. L., et al.: Canad. Med. Ass. J. **83:**211, 1960.
19. Pons, E. R.: Arch. Intern. Med. (Chicago) **106:**230, 1960.
20. Collins, D. N., Katz, S. S., and Harris, A. H.: Amer. J. Clin. Path. **36:**92, 1961.
21. Frisch, A. W.: Amer. J. Clin. Path. **12:**16, 1942.
22. Loughlen, G. F.: Amer. J. Path. **1:**407, 1925.

Chapter 11

Methods in microbiology, with reference to methods in virology

Microbiology includes the study of bacteria, rickettsiae, viruses, and fungi. The latter are discussed in Chapter 12.

BACTERIOLOGY*

INTRODUCTION TO CLINICAL BACTERIOLOGY

The clinical bacteriologist's main concern is the rapid and exact identification of pathogenic bacteria. To render this service the bacteriologist must know the origin of the submitted specimen and the nature of the investigation the clinician has in mind. The bacteriologist must be familiar with the normal flora and its physiologic changes to appreciate pathologic alterations. The routine bacteriologic methods must be rapid and accurate. For clinical purposes the identification of the genus of a microorganism should be sufficient in many instances so that treatment is not delayed. Rapid examination of a direct smear may allow a preliminary report within a few minutes or hours after the specimen has been received. The final identification of an organism must be based on all methods available: smears, cultures on routine and special media, biochemical tests, and serologic analysis. Accurate records must be kept that indicate not only the identity of the specimen but also the steps taken in the identification of the organism such as the media employed and the biochemical and serologic tests performed.

*See Cowan and Steel,[1] Harris and Coleman,[2] and Bailey and Scott.[3]

Bacteria are minute plantlike (no chlorophyll) microorganisms that vary in length from $0.2\text{-}10\mu$, with an average length of 1.5μ. The average diameter is less than 1μ. Clinical bacteriology is concerned with the parasitic bacteria (pathogens) that may injure the host, depending on such factors as host resistance and defense, bacterial toxicity, virulence, and invasive power.

The generally accepted classification of bacteria is based on morphologic, cultural, physiologic, serologic, and biochemical characters as contained in the seventh edition of *Bergey's Manual of Determinative Bacteriology.*

Morphologic classification of bacteria

Morphologically, bacteria are classified into the following types: cocci, which are oval or round; bacilli, which are rod shaped; and vibrios and spirochetes, which are curved or spiral shaped (Fig. 11-1 and Table 11-1).

Division of bacteria

Bacteria divide by binary fission, usually transversely, into equal parts. Cocci form characteristic groups, depending on the direction of splitting and the number of planes (diplococci, chains, clusters, etc.). The average rate of reproduction varies from every 16-20 min. (*Escherichia coli*) to once a day (*Mycobacterium tuberculosis*). Some species do not remain in a single form and are described as pleomorphic. This type of regularly encountered irregularity is one of the diagnostic

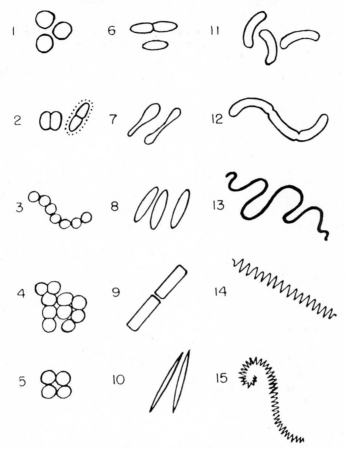

Fig. 11-1. Morphology of bacteria. **1**, Single cocci; **2**, cocci in pairs; **3**, cocci in chains; **4**, cocci in clusters; **5**, cocci in tetrads; **6**, coccobacilli; **7**, club-shaped bacilli; **8**, bacilli with rounded ends; **9**, bacilli with square ends; **10**, fusiform bacilli; **11**, vibrios; **12**, spirilla; **13**, *Borrelia;* **14**, *Treponema;* **15**, *Leptospira.* (From Smith and Conant: *Zinsser bacteriology,* New York, 1960, Appleton-Century-Crofts Co., Inc.)

Table 11-1. Examples of morphologic types

Cocci (spherical)	Bacilli (rod shaped)		Vibrios (comma shaped) and spirochetes (spiral shaped)
	Nonspore forming	Spore forming	
Staphylococci	*Escherichia coli*	Clostridia	*Treponema*
Streptococci	Corynebacteria	*Bacillus anthracis*	*Leptospira*
Gonococci	*Brucella*	*Bacillus subtilis*	*Borrelia*
Meningococci	*Shigella*		*Vibrio fetus*
			Spirillum minus

criteria of some bacteria, e.g., corynebacteria.

Structure of bacteria

Structurally, all bacteria possess a nucleoid structure containing DNA, cytoplasm containing RNA, a cell membrane, and a cell wall. Surrounding the cell wall is an outer slime layer that is called a capsule (Fig. 11-2). The motile bacteria possess appendages called cilia or flagella which are responsible for their motility and are antigenically different (with the exception of *Proteus*) from the somatic (body) antigen. The position and number of flagella can also be used to classify bacteria. The capsule, which consists of mucopolysaccharides, is related to the virulence of the organisms. In cultures the composition of the medium determines capsule production. Encapsulated forms produce smoother or more mucoid colonies than nonencapsulated cells.

Gram stain: Stains combine chemically with the bacterial protoplasm, the composition of which apparently determines one of the most important bacterial characteristics, their response to gram stain (Table 11-2). During the staining procedure, gram-positive cells retain the crystal violet–iodine complex, remaining blue, whereas gram-negative cells are completely decolorized by alcohol and take on the red color of the counterstain (safranin). Gram-positive bacteria contain less lipid than gram-negative bacteria.

Spores: Two genera, *Bacillus* and *Clostridium*, form spores, one cell giving life to only one spore, which may be located centrally, terminally, or subterminally according to the species. Spores represent resistant dormant bacterial forms that can survive extremely unfavorable conditions.

Pigments: Some bacteria produce pigments or fluorescing material. Some pigments are water soluble, e.g., that of *Pseudomonas;* others are not, e.g., that of *Staphylococcus aureus.*

Bacterial enzymes and toxins

Bacteria produce various enzymes that are able to split food elements and are responsible for the fermentation reactions of bacteria, i.e., the formation of acid and acid and gas as a result of carbohydrate metabolism, as well as for putrefaction and decay, resulting in production of hydrogen sulfide, amines, ammonia, and ptomaines. Some enzymes are characteristic of certain organisms, e.g., coagulase production of pathogenic staphylococci or streptokinase synthesis of streptococci. The energy for these metabolic activities

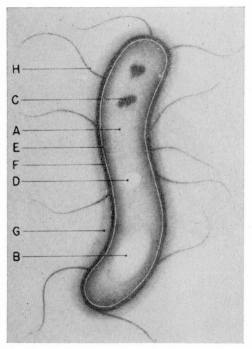

Fig. 11-2. Morphologic structure of a bacillus. **A,** Cytoplasm; **B,** nucleus; **C,** cytoplasmic granules; **D,** vacuole; **E,** cytoplasmic membrane; **F,** cell wall; **G,** slime layer or capsule; **H,** flagellum. (From Smith and Conant: Zinsser bacteriology, New York, 1960, Appleton-Century-Crofts Co., Inc.)

Table 11-2. Gram stain reaction of some important bacteria

Gram negative	Gram positive
Gonococci	Staphylococci
Meningococci	Streptococci
Coliform bacteria	Pneumococci
Proteus vulgaris	Clostridia
Pasteurella pestis	*Actinomyces*
	Diphtheria bacilli
	Bacillus subtilis

is derived from light (photosynthesis) or from oxidation of chemical substances (chemosynthesis).

Bacteria also produce toxins (exotoxins and endotoxins) which, if they are anti-erythrocytic, are called hemolysins. The endotoxins are closely linked to the bacterial cell body and are responsible for the occurrence of bacterial shock.

Hemolysis: The hemolytic activity of bacteria is tested on blood agar plates. **Beta hemolysis** consists of complete destruction of hemoglobin and red blood cell stroma so that the blood agar surrounding the bacteria becomes completely transparent and, on microscopic examination of the culture, fails to show red blood cells. In **alpha hemolysis** the red blood cell stroma remains, but the oxyhemoglobin is destroyed and converted into a greenish methemoglobin product. The agar around the colonies is not completely transparent, having a greenish tinge, and red cell ghosts can be seen on microscopic examination. In **gamma hemolysis**, no hemolysis is noted on blood agar plates, though in liquid blood-containing media, oxyhemoglobin leaves the cells, but is not degraded.

The chemical composition of bacteria varies according to the species and the media on which they are grown. The **growth** of bacteria in culture media is determined by environmental factors such as moisture, composition of air, pH, temperature, salt, availability of carbon and nitrogen, and growth factors such as thiamine. The gas requirements vary; **obligate aerobes** grow only in free oxygen and **obligate anaerobes** grow only in an oxygen-free atmosphere. There is a tendency to call aerobes and anaerobes that do not clearly belong to either group "facultative." Most bacteria grow better with the addition of carbon dioxide. The optimal pH is close to neutral or is slightly alkaline. The optimal temperature for most pathogens is 35° C., and the optimal salt concentration is below 1%. Media may produce temporary chemical and/or morphologic changes in bacteria called **adaptations,** or they may produce **transmissible** permanent changes called **mutations.**

Involution and L forms

The nongenetic adaptations produce the so-called involution forms which are related to changes in pH, culture media, salts, nutrients, etc. A mutation that may be of clinical significance is the L form (L for Lister Institute). Penicillin in the nutrient media can produce L forms from such organisms as *Salmonella, Shigella, Escherichia coli, Proteus,* and *Corynebacterium diphtheriae.* The L form possesses no rigid bacterial shape but is a mass of protoplasm lacking a rigid cell wall; it is surrounded by an electron-dense layer and can be maintained in pure culture. The L forms of certain bacteria have some characteristics in common with the PPLO—the pleuropneumonia-like organisms *(Mycoplasma)*—and with certain viruses.

Colonies

Groups of bacteria forming on solid media as a result of repeated division of one or a few organisms are called colonies; these colonies may vary in their characteristics according to the genus or species they represent.

Normal flora

Following is a list of flora normally present in human beings:
1. Skin: Yeast, *Staphylococcus epidermidis,* streptococci (gamma), sarcinae, *Bacillus subtilis,* diphtheroids, and *Escherichia coli* in some areas.
   NOTE: Resistant staphylococci on skin of hospital personnel.
2. Mouth: Lactobacilli, streptococci (gamma and alpha), sarcinae, micrococci, spirochetes, fusiform bacteria, yeast, *Neisseria catarrhalis,* pneumococci, and diphtheroids.
3. Conjunctiva: *Staphylococcus epidermidis* and sarcinae.
4. Vagina: Before puberty, occasional cocci; after puberty, *Lactobacillus doederleini.*
5. Intestinal tract: Stomach—sterile if acid, Boas-Oppler bacilli if achlorhydric; jejunum and ileum—lactobacilli; cecum and colon (feces)—*E. coli, Bacteroides,* and smaller numbers of *Proteus,* enterococci

(gamma streptococci), lactobacilli, *Pseudomonas,* clostridia, *Enterobacter,* and yeast. These bacteria appear gradually within the first 24-48 hr. after birth. If any one group predominates, a pathologic condition may be produced.

6. Sputum: Streptococci (alpha and gamma), *Neisseria catarrhalis,* diphtheroids, pneumococci, *Candida,* spirochetes, fusiform bacilli, *Haemophilus,* and *Staphylococcus.* Any of these organisms except the first three may cause disease when present in large numbers.

Collection and handling of specimens

Specimens for culture should be sent to the laboratory without delay.

Specimens should be cultured and smeared as soon as they are obtained because some bacteria are sensitive to air and standing at room temperature may change the relative number of bacteria by enhancing the growth of some and suppressing others.

Specimens should be labeled with the patient's name and age (e.g., important to note pathogenic *E. coli* in infants), the date, and the time of collection (if important as in blood cultures). Note delays in reaching the laboratory that may produce misleading culture results, as in quantitative urine cultures where delays allow bacteria to multiply.

Save material and cultures from which transfers are made until satisfactory growth is obtained.

Save blood cultures for 3 wk. before making a final report.

Make a direct smear from each material cultured if sufficient specimen is submitted and stain by the Gram method. This will often help in the choice of culture media, as does knowledge of the source of the material.

Specimens must be representative of a lesion and should not be contaminated by extraneous material.

All containers and cups must be sterile and suitable in size and shape so that the submitted material can be received without danger of contamination. All containers must be closed and labeled.

For scanty material use sterile cotton swabs (at least two) and return to the laboratory in sterile containers. To prevent drying of specimen and to retard differential growth of organisms, insert swabs into a holding medium such as Pre-Med.*

If the material is from a patient receiving antibiotic therapy, use neutralizing agents if available. Penicillinase, a penicillin antagonist, may be used. For amounts, see manufacturer's instructions. No antagonists to the newer antibiotics are known. Simple dilution of part of the specimen by inoculation into broths, e.g., thioglycollate, is effective in negating the effect of antibiotics. This is one of the reasons for using thioglycollate broth routinely.

Examine cultures daily; subculture to special media as indicated on the basis of cultural appearance and of gram-stained smear. Disinfect hands after handling cultures and infectious material. Disinfect and clean up if cultures and infectious material are spilled. Autoclave discarded cultures. Dispose of specimens in a safe manner, e.g., by autoclaving. Keep stock and reagent bottles clean, properly labeled, and in their proper places.

Sterilization

Dry heat: All glassware should be absolutely dry when placed in the sterilizer; if not, keep the flame low and leave the door ajar until drying is complete. Sterilize at 170° C. for 1½ hr. Dry heat is not an efficient method of sterilization. It is the method of choice for oils, however, as they are not wettable.

Moist heat (steam)—autoclaving: Sterilize at 15 lb. pressure (121.6° C.) for 15 min. after the temperature and pressure both reach the proper levels. Media and other material for sterilization must not be more than 5 cm. thick. Autoclave culture media, vaccine bottles, discarded blood cultures, and any dangerous or spore-forming organisms. Steaming under pressure is an effective method of sterilization.

Bacterial spore strips: The efficiency of

---

*Hyland Laboratories, Los Angeles, Calif.

the autoclave must be checked daily with commercially available dried strips impregnated with bacilli. After completion of the sterilization these strips are cultured in thioglycollate broth. Color indicators that change color if the time-temperature ratio is correct are also available.

Filtration: Filtration through special filters is useful for removing bacteria from materials which would be coagulated or broken down by heat, e.g., serum, ascitic fluid, and sugars. Several kinds of such filters are available. The Seitz filter made of asbestos is most commonly used. Other filters are made of cellulose. They are used in the Swinny adapter which is fitted with syringes and allows filtration of small amounts of liquid.

Chemical disinfection: A great number of chemical disinfectants are commercially available and fall in five main groups: quaternary ammonium ion agents, phenolics, alcohols, iodophors, and heavy metals. Their advantages and disadvantages have been extensively reviewed.[4]

Gaseous sterilization: Ethylene oxide[5] is an effective, safe agent for sterilization of objects that may be injured by steam sterilization. Another gas, beta-propiolactone, is being investigated as a sterilizing agent.

Ultraviolet radiation[6]**:** Bactericidal radiant energy acts primarily as an oxidizing agent.

Detergents: These are surface-active agents containing both a fat-soluble group and a water-soluble group. They insinuate themselves between the lipid-containing bacterial cell membrane and the surrounding aqueous medium. There are two types: anionic and cationic.

Handling of clinical material

The importance of prompt and correct culturing and staining of direct smears cannot be overemphasized.

For special procedures of identification, see discussion of the organism concerned. This section includes only general outlines for tentative identification. Definitive identification may require special media and procedures.

1. **Routine bacterial smears.** Stain smear with gram stain.

2. **Routine bacterial cultures.** Use blood and chocolate agar incubated at 35° C. aerobically, and also under increased carbon dioxide tension (CO_2 jar) if indicated, and thioglycollate broth incubated at 35° C.

3. **Routine fungus smear.** Use a wet preparation made with 10% sodium hydroxide.

4. **Routine fungus culture.** Use duplicate slants of Sabouraud agar with and without antibiotics incubated at 35° and 26° C. and duplicate blood agar plates incubated at 35° and 26° C. Omit 35° C. cultures on Sabouraud agar and 26° C. cultures on blood agar if material is scanty. Spreading material too thin may result in no growth because there are not enough organisms in any one medium to initiate growth.

5. **Acid-fast routine.** Use a direct smear for acid-fast bacilli stained by the Kinyoun method and a concentration method for preparation of a second smear stained by the same method. Culture on special media such as Lowenstein-Jensen or Petragnani media after concentration. Perform guinea pig inoculation if requested. The fluorescent method is very useful for screening of a large amount of material. The *N*-acetyl-L-cysteine digestion procedure and Middlebrook 7H 10 agar are discussed in the section on *Mycobacterium tuberculosis*.

6. **Anaerobic culture.** Insert streaked blood agar plates into sealed containers rendered anaerobic by various methods. Material is also cultured in thioglycollate broth.

Swabs and transport media[7]**:** The swab must not be allowed to dry. If delay is unavoidable, the swab should be inserted into a transport medium that may be stored in the refrigerator. At the time of culturing the swab is twirled in broth and then rubbed on the desired solid medium with a rotating motion. After inoculation the broth is rolled between the palms of both hands to distribute the material so that levels of subsequent growth may be meaningful (aerobic vs.

anaerobic bacteria). Because the amount of material on most swabs is small, smears are made last.

Blood and bone marrow: In the course of any bacterial infection there are transient phases of bacteremia. In some diseases the resulting bacteremia persists and becomes the dominant clinical feature. The primary focus may not be known, and the organism involved may not be generally accepted as a pathogen.

Blood culture: Blood cultures should be obtained before any treatment is instituted; take one every 2 hr. for 6-8 hr. or obtain all cultures at one time.

Media: Use trypticase soy agar, with added agar containing 0.1% L-cystine solidified on the side of the bottle and covered with trypticase soy broth under 10% carbon dioxide, and thioglycollate broth.[8] Ideally two bottles should be used —one containing trypticase soy broth and one containing thioglycollate broth.

When possible, take blood culture when the patient's temperature is rising. Aseptic technique is essential (sterile needle and syringe). Paint site, usually over median basilic vein, with tincture of iodine. The iodine may be removed from a small area directly over the vein with 95% alcohol. Place tourniquet over arm above elbow. Insert needle into vein and withdraw about 10 ml. blood into syringe. Remove tourniquet, withdraw needle, and place a sterile dry sponge over point of puncture. Transfer blood to appropriate media using sterile precautions. Label cultures and place at once in incubator. Use about 5 ml. blood for 50 ml. media, and incubate at 35° C. To reduce danger of contamination, transfer can also be accomplished by using sterile transparent tubing. If it is necessary to check donor's blood or blood bank bottles for sterility, use 10 ml. blood and 100 ml. liquid medium and incubate at 35° C., or preferably, duplicate specimens held at room temperature and at 35° C.

Isolation of *Salmonella* from blood is best accomplished in bile medium (5 ml. blood added to 15 ml. reconstituted ox bile.*

*Bacto-Oxgall, Difco Laboratories, Detroit, Mich. Dissolve 10 gm. in 100 ml. sterile water.

Blood culture bottles containing solid and liquid media are turned daily in the incubator so that the liquid medium covers the solid agar for 1 hr. The bottle must not be entered until growth is seen on the agar. This procedure will reduce contamination to a minimum.

Blood culture bottles are inspected grossly every day. If culture shows growth or becomes cloudy or discolored, prepare gram-stained smears and subculture to appropriate media. If smear shows organisms, set up a direct sensitivity test. A preliminary report should also be given to the physician. All blood cultures are kept 21 days, unless growth occurs earlier. After 7 days and after 21 days, make smears of the blood cultures, transfer to chocolate agar, and incubate at 35° C. under CO_2 for 2 days.

Organisms that grow only anaerobically and not aerobically are anaerobic streptococci, bacteroides, clostridia, and actinomycetes. The only organisms that at times do not grow in thioglycollate broth are *Pseudomonas, Neisseria, Haemophilus,* and aerobic diphtheroids. If only one bottle shows growth, it may be that the organism cannot adjust itself to the medium of the other bottle, or it may be a contaminant.

Bone marrow culture: Add 5 ml. of the marrow and blood mixture aspirated from the sternum (see p. 202) to 50 ml. trypticase soy broth. This method is superior to blood cultures in the isolation of *Brucella* species. For the diagnosis of generalized histoplasmosis, marrow may be cultured on blood agar and on Sabouraud agar at room temperature and at 30° C.

Bile: The specimen is usually obtained at the time of operation or through a T tube. The methods outlined for feces also apply to bile. Keep in mind the possibility of *Salmonella* infection.

Cerebrospinal fluid: If the fluid is submitted in two or three tubes, obtain culture from the second or third tube rather than from the first. Be sure to anchor stopper or cotton plug before centrifuging. Centrifuge specimen at 3000 rpm for 15 min., decant supernatant, and use sediment to inoculate thioglycollate broth and chocolate agar (CO_2) and also to make two smears, in this order. If there is a sufficient amount of sediment, it should also be cultured on blood agar and the remaining sediment and supernatant fluid should be saved in the incubator. Place the chocolate plate in a candle jar. Use the Gram and Kinyoun staining methods. Examination of the direct smear is very important, and any organism found should be reported to the physician immediately.

If tuberculous meningitis is suspected, look for pellicle formation and use pellicle or sediment to inoculate one Lowenstein-Jensen slant and one Petragnani slant, in addition to the media just mentioned. Incubate the slants at 35° C. for 8 wk.

Use India ink preparation for the demonstration of *Cryptococcus* if any sediment is left.

Feces: The patient should collect the stool in a clean container and avoid contamination with urine. With a sterile spatula, transfer a small portion into a disposable sterile plastic container with lid. Stool may also be collected on a swab moistened with thioglycollate broth, either by blind insertion into the rectum after cleaning of the anal area or under proctoscopic guidance, using commercially available protected swabs (recommended if *Shigella* infection is suspected). Select purulent, mucoid, or bloody portions and inoculate the following media: phenylethyl alcohol blood agar (staphylococci and yeast), MacConkey or Endo blood agar, *Salmonella-Shigella* (SS) medium, Mycosel agar* (fungi), and selenite-F broth. Inoculate these plates in the order given with increasing amounts of material. Bismuth sulfite medium should be included in cases of suspected typhoid fever. Incubate all media at 35° C. After 12-24 hr., examine for nonlactose-fermenting bacteria and other stool pathogens and plate selenite-F medium onto SS agar.

If *Salmonella* or *Shigella* infection is suspected, it is preferable to collect the stool specimen directly into a selective enrichment medium such as GN broth or into a preservative such as buffered glycerol-saline mixture.

Use ether concentration method for tubercle bacilli (see section on mycobacteria).

---

*Baltimore Biological Laboratory, Baltimore, Md.

Make a direct gram-stained smear for staphylococci, yeast, and vibrios.

Fluids from serous cavities (pleurae, pericardium, peritoneum, joints, etc.): Since most of these fluids are exudates and have a tendency to clot (fibrinogen contents), the laboratory should have large, graduated, screw-topped, sterile centrifuge tubes containing sterile mixed oxalate, heparin, or sodium citrate (1 ml. of 20%). Mix specimen well and centrifuge at speed of at least 3000 rpm for 15-30 min. Use the sediment to make routine and acid-fast smears and to inoculate routine culture media and media for acid-fast organisms.

Culture joint fluids on chocolate agar and incubate under CO_2 at 35° C.

Genital tract: Venereal infections require a special approach; other infections can be handled in the same way as infections of the urinary tract.

Gonorrhea:

Male patient: Milk urethra and collect material on cotton swab. Make a direct gram-stained smear. Material obtained by prostatic massage can also be used.

Female patient: Swab cervix, vagina, and urethra. Make three smears. For culture use chocolate agar medium or Thayer medium under CO_2 and incubate at 35° C.

Syphilis: For the primary chancre make a dark-field examination; for secondary lesions, a dark-field examination of moist patches; for tertiary lesions, a serologic investigation.

Dark-field examination[9]: With a gloved hand, clean surface of lesion with saline solution and squeeze and scrape base of the ulcer to produce serum. Touch slide to moist ulcer base, cover immediately with cover glass, and rim with petrolatum. Examine under dark-field microscope with the oil-immersion lens and oil on the condenser.

Chancroid: Stain smears by the Gram method and culture on blood agar medium (*Haemophilus ducreyi*).

Granuloma inguinale: The diagnosis is based on surgical tissue biopsy or tissue impressions that show the presence of Donovan bodies.

Pus and purulent exudates: If enough material is available, make a direct gram-stained smear. If organisms are seen on the smear, perform routine bacterial cultures. Investigate specimen for tubercle bacilli if no organisms are seen and hold blood agar plate and thiogycollate broth for 5 days before discarding as negative. If gonococci are suspected, inoculate a chocolate plate or Thayer medium[10] and incubate under CO_2 at 35° C. Clostridia will grow in thioglycollate broth.

Sputum: The material should be processed as soon as it is obtained so that it is suitable for the detection of predominant organisms. Sputum should be obtained in the early morning and should be expectorated into disposable sterile plastic containers with lids. The patient should be instructed as to the purpose of the test, and should brush his teeth and rinse his throat before the specimen is collected. Every attempt should be made to exclude saliva and nasal secretions.

Select hemorrhagic, purulent, or cheesy particles. Make routine bacterial and acid-fast smears and employ routine bacterial and acid-fast staining methods. Also employ routine smear and culture methods for fungi and tubercle bacilli. For the detection of certain fungi such as *Histoplasma capsulatum,* the blood agar plate should be kept for 3 wk. at room temperature and tightly closed with a wide rubber band.

Tissue (autopsy and surgical): If the tissue specimen is small in amount, mince with sterile forceps and scissors and use the entire material. If the specimen is medium in amount, grind with a sterile pestle in a sterile mortar containing sterile sand or alundum. If a large amount of tissue is available, remove several small representative portions from the desired areas with sterile instruments and transfer them to a sterile mortar for maceration. Store the remaining tissue in the deep freeze. On the basis of history, gross examination, or frozen section, choose routine culture methods or selective and inhibitory media as well as procedures for fungi and tubercle bacilli. Inoculate three sets of plates, one for incubation aerobically at 35° C., one under CO_2 at 35° C., and one at 26° C. (room tempera-

ture). The frozen specimen is suitable for virus investigation.

Throat, ears, eyes, nose, nasopharynx, and sinuses: These specimens are usually collected on sterile swabs (see previous discussion of swabs). Nasopharyngeal material is obtained by means of wire swabs protected from contamination enroute by glass or plastic tubing. Calcium alginate wool is suggested to take the place of absorbent cotton as it will dissolve in saline solution. The swabs should be moistened with sterile broth, or preferably, inserted into holding media. Throat swabs are plated on sheep blood agar plates and incubated anaerobically (see discussion of streptococci). If diphtheria is suspected, inoculate a Loeffler slant and a tellurite plate in addition to the routine culture media. Material from eyes and throat suspected of infection by *Neisseria, Haemophilus,* or microaerophiles should be cultured on chocolate agar or on Thayer medium under 10% CO_2. Cultures of material suspected of containing fungi should be kept for 3 wk. even though bacteria are found. Initial plating on MacConkey agar may be required for presumptive identification of enteric gram-negative organisms sometimes found in throat cultures from children.

Make two smears, one for gram stain and one for Loeffler methylene blue stain, which is helpful in the demonstration of *C. diphtheriae.*

Urine:

Male patient: Thoroughly clean glans penis and collect final portion of urinary stream in disposable, sterile plastic container with lid.

Female patient: Catheterization may be avoided by placing the patient in lithotomy position, cleaning the vulva from front to back, separating the labia, and collecting the urine specimen from midstream in sterile container.

• • •

Urine specimens for culture should not be allowed to stand at room temperature for more than 2 hr. Urine is an excellent culture medium so that rapid bacterial proliferation in the specimen will render a quantitative approach inaccurate. If the specimen cannot be handled immediately after receipt, it should be stored in the refrigerator. One of the quantitative or semiquantitative methods should be used when the urine specimen is plated on blood agar, Endo agar, or EMB agar. It is not necessary to use thioglycollate broth.

In most cases quantitative bacterial counts allow differentiation of true bacterial urinary tract infection from contamination of the urine by bacteria from the urethra and the external genitalia. A concentration of 100,000 or more bacteria/ml. urine is generally accepted as "significant bacteriuria."

Methods for estimating number of bacteria in urine[11]:

1. Screening tests: Griess nitrite test and TTC test
2. Semiquantitative test: standard loop method
3. Quantitative test: counting of colonies

Screening tests:

Griess nitrite test[12]:

Reagents: Dissolve 1.5 gm. sulfanilic acid in 450 ml. 10% acetic acid. Add this solution to 0.6 gm. alpha-naphthylamine in 60 ml. boiling distilled water. Filter through Whatman No. 1 filter paper (stable 2-4 wk.).

Test: Add 1 ml. Griess reagent to 1 ml. urine. A pink color develops in seconds if the urine *Escherichia coli* count is greater than 100,000/ml.

The reagent tests for the presence of nitrites that are produced by coliform bacteria from the ever-present urinary nitrates. This test gives only about 61% correlation with quantitative counting.

Triphenyl tetrazolium chloride (TTC) test (Uroscreen*): Living bacteria will reduce the colorless TTC within 4 hr. to a pink-red precipitate of triphenyl formazone when present in clinically significant numbers (10,000 organisms/ml. urine). This red precipitate may be so fine as to require a concave mirror held below the test tube to read the result of the test. In infections due to gram-negative bacteria

in the range of 100,000 organisms/ml. the test is about 98% accurate. In infections due to gram-positive and gram-negative bacteria in a concentration below 100,000 organisms/ml. the accuracy of the test falls to 87% and 70%, respectively.

Semiquantitative test:

Standard loop method: Mix the specimen thoroughly and inoculate each side of a divided blood agar and MacConkey agar plate with a standard loopful (3 mm. diameter equal to 0.01 ml.) of urine. Spread evenly over the whole area. Incubate at 37° C. Use gram strain on all colony types. Report number of colonies present per milliliter of urine (colony count × 100). The small amount of material used reduces the accuracy of this method.

Leigh and Williams[13] utilize a measured area of a sterile blotting paper to transfer a constant aliquot of urine onto the surface of the culture medium. The number of bacterial colonies in the inoculated area corresponds to the number of organisms in the urine.

Quantitative test:

Counting of colonies: Prepare a tenfold or a thousandfold dilution of urine in sterile distilled water (1 or 0.01 part urine plus 9 parts water) and spread 0.1 ml. diluted urine (sterile, 1 ml., 1-in-0.1 disposable serologic pipette) on a blood agar plate and 0.1 ml. on a MacConkey agar plate. Kass[13a] suggests a 1 ml. pour plate technique. Report colony counts per milliliter of urine (colony count × 100 or × 10,000).

Collection, handling, and shipment of bacteriologic specimens

The Department of Health, Education, and Welfare publishes detailed instructions on the collection, handling, and shipment of diagnostic specimens.*

Organisms most likely to be isolated from clinical material

Although the most common organisms are listed, it must be remembered that

---

*Chas. Pfizer & Co., Inc., New York, N. Y.

*Public Health Service Pub. No. 976, Washington, D. C., 1962, U. S. Government Printing Office.

any organism may be found in clinical material.

Blood cultures:
Staphylococci (pathogenic and saprophytic)
Coliform bacilli and related organisms
Alpha and beta hemolytic streptococci
Pneumococci
Enterococci
Clostridium perfringens
Proteus species
Bacteroides species and related anaerobes
Neisseria meningitidis
Salmonella species
Brucella species
Pasteurella tularensis
Listeria monocytogenes
Herellea species
Streptobacillus moniliformis
Vibrio fetus and related vibrios
Pathogenic yeasts and molds

Cerebrospinal fluid cultures:
Haemophilus influenzae, type b (infants and children)
Neisseria meningitidis
Pneumococci
Mycobacterium tuberculosis
Staphylococci and streptococci, including enterococci
Cryptococcus neoformans
Coliform bacilli, *Pseudomonas* and *Proteus* species
Bacteroides species
Listeria monocytogenes
Mima polymorpha
Leptospira species

Ear cultures:
Nonpathogens:
Coagulase-negative staphylococci
Diphtheroids
Gaffkya tetragena
Bacillus species
Pathogens:
Pseudomonas aeruginosa
Staphylococcus aureus
Proteus species
Alpha and beta hemolytic streptococci
Pneumonocci
Coliform bacilli
Aspergillus fumigatus

Eye cultures:
Staphylococcus aureus
Neisseria gonorrhoeae
Pneumonococci
Alpha and beta hemolytic streptococci
Moraxella lacunata
Haemophilus species
Herellea species
Diphtheroids, including *Corynebacterium xerosis*
Pseudomonas species and other enteric rods
Viruses and fungi

Gastrointestinal tract cultures (stool):
Coliform bacilli
Proteus species
Salmonella species
Shigella species
Enterococci
Clostridia
Bacteroides species
Various yeast forms, including *Candida albicans*
Vibrio species
Escherichia coli

Genital tract cultures:
Coliform bacilli, enterococci, and other intestinal commensals, including *Bacteroides* species
Lactobacilli
Haemophilus species (probably *Haemophilus vaginalis*)
Beta hemolytic streptococci of groups B and D
Nonpathogenic mycobacteria
Anaerobic streptococci (peptostreptococci)
Neisseria gonorrhoeae
Haemophilus ducreyi
Mycobacterium tuberculosis

Cultures from newborn infants:
Staphylococci
Vibrio fetus
Group E streptococci
Enteric rods

Sinus tract cultures:
Mycobacteria
Fungi
Bacteroides species
Proteus species
Streptococci
Staphylococci

Sputum cultures:
Pneumococci or *Diplococcus pneumoniae*
Klebsiella species
Haemophilus influenzae
Staphylococcus aureus
Streptococcus species
Mima polymorpha
Cryptococcus or other fungi
Pasteurella bronchoseptica

Throat cultures:
Nonpathogens:
Alpha hemolytic streptococci
Neisseria catarrhalis and other species, including pigmented forms
Coagulase-negative staphylococci and occasionally *Staphylococcus aureus*
Haemophilus haemolyticus and *influenzae*
Pneumococci
Nonhemolytic (gamma) streptococci
Diphtheroid bacilli
Coliform bacilli (particularly after penicillin therapy)
Yeasts, including *Candida albicans*
Beta hemolytic streptococci other than group A

Pathogens:
Beta hemolytic streptococci of group A and occasionally groups B, C, and G
Corynebacterium diphtheriae
Bordetella pertussis
Meningococci
Predominance of *Staphylococcus aureus*, coliform bacilli, pneumococci, *Haemophilus influenzae*, *Candida albicans*, etc.

Urinary tract cultures:
Nonpathogens:
Coagulase-negative *staphylococci*
Diphtheroids
Coliform bacilli
Enterococci
Proteus species
Alpha and beta hemolytic streptococci
Saprophytic yeasts
Bacillus species

Pathogens:
Coliform bacilli
Proteus species
Pseudomonas species
Enterococci

Staphylococci
Alcaligenes species
Herellea species
Haemophilus species
Candida albicans
Beta hemolytic streptococci, usually groups B and C
Gonococcus
Mycobacterium tuberculosis
Salmonella species

Wound cultures:
Staphylococcus aureus
Streptococcus pyogenes
Coliform bacilli
Proteus species
Pseudomonas species
Clostridium species
Anaerobic cocci (peptostreptococci)
Enterococci
Bacteroides species

METHODS OF EXAMINATION
EXAMINATION OF UNSTAINED MATERIAL
Motility

Hanging drop method: Prepare a saline suspension of young culture and place 1 drop in center of a cover glass which is inverted over the depression in a well slide. Examine for motility, as evidenced by the organisms moving away from each other. Motility is best seen at lower temperature, 15°–25° C. Brownian movement, which is not an expression of motility, is a constant to-and-from movement.

Semisolid medium technique: Motility is evidenced by growth away from the line of inoculation. Nonmotile organisms grow only along the line of inoculation (Fig. 11-3).

Wet preparation

Emulsify small segment of colony in loopful of water, saline solution, sodium hydroxide, or dilute iodine. Cover with cover glass and rim with petrolatum or nail polish.

Dark-field preparation

The wet preparation just described is used. Insert dark-field condenser, adjust light and plane mirror, and insert funnel stop into the lower half of the oil-immersion lens.

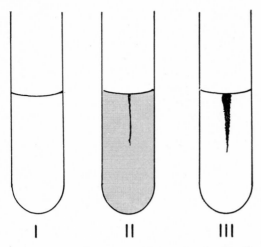

Fig. 11-3. Motility test. **I,** Uninoculated tube. **II,** Motile organism. **III,** Nonmotile organism.

STAINING METHODS

Smears: Prepare the smear as follows: With forceps, remove a clean slide that has been stored in 70% ethyl alcohol and flame. Identify the slide, and if several preparations need to be made, divide into sections with wax pencil. Then draw a key to the slide on a 3 × 4 in. card, indicating which cultures are in which spaces. Using a flame-sterilized loop, transfer a loopful of well-shaken liquid medium or emulsify segment of colony of solid medium in a loopful of sterile water. Spread over an area of about 1 cm. Make heavy smears of broth cultures and thin smears of emulsified colonies taken from solid media. Allow to air dry and fix by passing the slide quickly through the top of a Bunsen flame. Allow to cool and then stain. The stained preparation should be examined for size and shape, arrangement and grouping of bacteria (e.g., singly, in clusters, in pairs, etc.), and for special morphologic features such as spores and capsules.

Routinely employed stains

Albert stain: Albert stain is used for detection of diphtheria bacilli.
   Reagents:
   Solution I:
      Toluidine blue, 0.15 gm.
      Malachite green, 0.2 gm.

Glacial acetic acid, 1 ml.
      Ethyl alcohol (95%), 2 ml.
      Distilled water, 100 ml.
   Dissolve dyes in alcohol and then add water and acetic acid. Mix well, let stand for 24 hr., and filter.
   Solution II:
      Iodine crystals, 2 gm.
      Potassium iodide, 3 gm.
      Distilled water, 300 ml.
   Grind iodine crystals and potassium iodide in about 10 ml. water and then add the remaining portion of water. The usual gram iodine solution may be substituted for solution II.
   Technique: Allow smear to dry and fix with heat. Stain with solution I for 2 min. Rinse with water and blot dry. Apply solution II for 1 min. Rinse with water, blot dry, and examine.
   Result: The granules of diphtheria bacilli stain black; the cytoplasm stains light green.

Carbolfuchsin-Kinyoun stain for mycobacteria (acid-fast stain): This stain is used for the detection of mycobacteria, which are surrounded by a waxy envelope that is resistant to staining, but which, once stained, retains the stain, whereas other bacteria are decolorized by acid alcohol and accept the blue counterstain. Acid-fast bacilli are stained red.
   Reagents:
   1. Carbolfuchsin-Kinyoun:
      Basic fuchsin, 4 gm.
      Phenol crystals, 8 gm.
      Alcohol (95%), 20 ml.
      Water, 100 ml.
   Dissolve fuchsin in alcohol and add to phenol crystals that have been melted in a hot water bath; then add the water. To increase the rapidity of staining add a detergent (Tergitol No. 7 or Aerosol), 1 drop to each 30-40 ml. stain. Since the rapid staining property is lost after a few days, the detergent must be renewed accordingly.
   2. Acid alcohol:
      Ethyl alcohol (95%), 97 ml.
      Concentrated hydrochloric acid, 3 ml.
   Add the acid to the alcohol.
   Technique: Fix the dried smear with heat. Stain with carbolfuchsin for 5 min.

Wash and decolorize with acid alcohol. Wash well and counterstain 1 min. with 1% methylene blue or 1% malachite green.

Gram staining method: Cultures 24-48 hr. old are used in the differential staining method described by Gram. The gram staining property may not be characteristic in exudates, pus, or in very young, old, dead, or degenerating cultures. It is also not dependable when the organisms have been grown on sugar media. Acids in media or staining solutions interfere with the gram stain.

Reagents:

1. Hucker crystal violet:

   Solution A:

   Crystal violet, 2 gm.
   Ethyl alcohol (95%), 20 ml.

   Solution B:

   Ammonium oxalate, 0.8 gm.
   Distilled water, 80 ml.

Mix solutions A and B and allow to mature for 24 hr.

2. Burke iodine:

   Potassium iodide, 2 gm.
   Iodine crystals, 1 gm.
   Distilled water, 100 ml.

Grind iodine crystals and potassium iodide together in a mortar with a pestle, adding only a little water. The iodine is readily soluble in strong potassium iodide solution. As soon as the iodine is dissolved, add the balance of water and mix thoroughly.

3. Hucker counterstain:

   Solution A:

   Safranin O, 2.5 gm.
   Ethyl alcohol (95%), 100 ml.

   Solution B:

   Solution A, 10 ml.
   Distilled water, 100 ml.

Technique: Make thin smear, dry in air, and fix in flame. Apply 1.5% crystal violet for 1 min. Wash and apply gram iodine solution for about 1 min. Wash and decolorize with 95% alcohol or with acetone until no further violet washes off. Wash and counterstain with dilute safranin for about ½ min. Wash with water and dry by blotting.

Technique for feces: Fat interferes with the stain and must be removed. Make smear and let dry. Fix with methyl alcohol for 5 min. Wash with xylene and dry. Apply the gram stain as usual.

Results: Gram-positive organisms stain dark blue. They retain the violet stain, the iodine acting as mordant. Gram-negative organisms stain red. They are decolorized and restained by the red counterstain.

The stain is satisfactory if pus cell nuclei stain deeply with the counterstain and if control spots of gram-negative and gram-positive bacteria stain correctly. Use carbolfuchsin as counterstain when searching for small gram-negative organisms such as *Bordetella pertussis, Haemophilus influenzae,* Koch-Weeks bacilli, etc.

Loeffler methylene blue stain: This stain is used for the identification of diphtheria bacilli since its differentiates the deeply staining metachromatic granules from the pale blue-staining cytoplasm.

Reagents:

1. Methylene blue (certified), 0.3 gm.
2. Ethyl alcohol (95%), 30 ml.
3. Distilled water, 100 ml.

Dissolve stain completely before adding water.

Technique: Apply the stain for 1 min. to the heat-fixed smear. Wash and blot dry.

Fluorescent antibody technique: Fluorescein-labeled antibodies are potentially applicable to the detection of all bacteria. The fluorescent technique allows the detection and localization of organisms or substances because of their ability to fluoresce under certain conditions. Fluorescence is the property of converting invisible light rays of short wavelengths into visible rays of longer wavelengths. The fluorescence may be primary (natural) or secondary only after treatment with certain dyes. The light source is usually a high-pressure mercury arc lamp. The microscope is equipped with a dark-field condenser and with filters which determine the wavelengths and the color of the light. Between the lamp and the object is the primary or exciter filter, which allows only the fluorescence-exciting waves of the light source to reach the stained object. Between the object and the eye of the observer there is placed the secondary or excluding filter so that the eye is protected and only the light characteristic of the fluorescent dye in use is seen. Nonfluorescing oil is applied to the undersurface of the slide beneath the area of the specimen and also to the surface of the specimen.

The following fluorescent methods are given in detail in the appropriate sections: identification of group A streptococci, *Neisseria gonorrhoeae*, enteropathogenic *E. coli*, and rabies and the fluorescent treponemal antibody test.

CULTURE METHODS

Examine liquid media for turbidity, sediment, arrangement of colonies (floating, snowflake, chains, etc.), pellicle formation, color development, and gas and odor production.

Examine solid media for size, shape, color, outline and consistency of colonies, changes in the medium, and odor production.

Technique of inoculation of liquid media

Hold all tubes almost horizontally. Remove cap (or cotton plug) and hold between fingers to avoid contamination. Pass mouth of tube through flame. Sterilize loop by heating it until it is red hot; cool, obtain inoculum, and transfer into liquid. Mix by tapping on tube, reflame mouth of tube, and replace cap or cotton plug.

Technique of inoculation of solid media

Four techniques are used for solid media: (1) streak plate, (2) pour plate, (3) streak-pour plate, and (4) slants.

Streak plate (Fig. 11-4): The purpose of the streak plate is to isolate organisms in pure culture. Collect specimen in sterile (flamed) loop that is slightly bent so that it will glide smoothly over the surface of the medium. Deposit inoculum at one edge and streak back and forth over the area, progressing across the agar until one fourth of the plate surface is covered. Flame the loop, streak at right angles to the originally inoculated agar, and cover

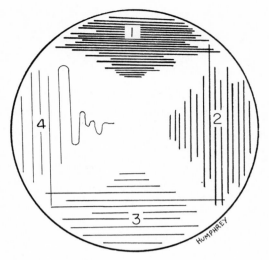

Fig. 11-4. Streaking of medium.

the second quarter of the plate. Flame loop again and repeat procedure until third and fourth quadrants are covered. Instead of flaming the loop, which is time-consuming, two loops may be used alternately or the loop may be used to cut deeply twice into the agar before progressing from one quadrant to the next. Whichever method is used, a small area of the agar should be undercut with the loop to streak the undersurface of the agar.

Pour plate: Melt a tube of agar in water bath, cool to 45° C., and inoculate tube. Pour inoculated agar into sterile petri dish. Distribute evenly by tilting plate and cool, leaving the top half of the petri dish partially open for a few minutes to allow water vapor to escape.

Streak-pour plate: Streak agar as for streak plate and cover streaked surface by melted blood agar. This is a good method to study hemolysis.

Storage of media: Except for thioglycollate broth, store most media in refrigerator. Plate media that are not to be used within a few days should be sealed with Parafilm.* Dried media is a most common cause of culture failure.

Stack cultures upside down in the in-

---

*American Can Co., Neenah, Wis.

cubator so that water from condensation does not drop on culture.

Slants: Slants are tubes containing media gelled in such a way that the upper surface is slanted.

Anaerobic cultures

Oxygen requirements of bacteria: Aerobes grow in the normal atmosphere. Microaerophiles require reduced oxygen tension. Anaerobes require relative or absolute absence of oxygen. Obligate anaerobes require complete absence of oxygen; facultative organisms grow either aerobically or anaerobically.

Reduced oxygen tension can be produced in three ways:

1. Production of carbon dioxide: candle jar (This method cannot be used for growth of obligate anaerobes; it is not a method of anaerobiasis.)
2. Exhaustion of oxygen: biologic methods, e.g., cooked meat media; chemical method; replacement method; and combustion methods
3. Absorption of oxygen: thioglycollate medium

Candle jar: Place the culture plates and tubes into a large-mouthed jar with a well-fitting ground-glass lid or any other well-fitted top. Pull one of the petri dishes close to the top of the stack about halfway out and place on it a medicine glass containing a short, thick candle. The candle should be in the upper half of the jar rather than on the bottom. Light candle. Close jar airtight, using Plasticine if necessary. The candle flame will die when the atmosphere contains 2-3% carbon dioxide, which accumulates at the bottom.

Biologic methods:

Streak plate: Plate *Bacillus subtilis* on first half of a plate and the anaerobic culture on the second half. Close airtight with Plasticine.

Cooked meat medium: To 1 part beef heart or lean beef (free from fat and minced fine) add 1 part water and cook slowly. Restore loss of water and add normal sodium hydroxide until slightly alkaline to litmus (about pH 8.5). Add 5 mg. *p*-aminobenzoic acid/100 ml. Distribute into tubes, add 1-2 ml. melted petrolatum, and autoclave. The cooked meat not only

contains many reducing substances but also provides substances for bacterial growth. The petrolatum button covering the surface of the medium is melted before inoculation; the medium is then inoculated and the button reforms on cooling.

Chemical method (alkaline pyrogallol method): The streaked plates are placed in a large, wide-mouthed glass jar with a screw cap or tight-fitting lid that is reinforced by Plasticine applied around its free edge. Inside the jar is placed an open test tube containing 1 gm. pyrogallic acid and 10 mg. 2.5N sodium hydroxide for each 100 ml. of jar capacity. The disadvantages of this method are the production of some carbon monoxide, which may be injurious to some bacteria, and the absorption of CO_2 formed by sodium hydroxide.

Replacement method: The Anaero-jar* is based on the principle that air is evacuated and then replaced by the desired gas such as 10% carbon dioxide in air or by a mixture† of 80% nitrogen, 10% carbon dioxide, and 10% hydrogen, which is supplied in cylinders. The jar is equipped with a gauge and requires an efficient vacuum pump.

Combustion methods:

Brewer jar: In this apparatus an electrically heated platinized asbestos is used to burn out oxygen which is replaced by a commercially available mixture† of 80% nitrogen, 10% carbon dioxide, and 10% hydrogen.

The BBL Gaspak,‡ which contains a special wick and zinc chloride and magnesium in balanced amounts so that the addition of 10 ml. water generates enough hydrogen to produce anaerobic conditions, can be used to great advantage in the Brewer jar.

Varney phosphorus jar: In this method a stick of yellow phosphorus is inserted into a jar with a tight-fitting lid. The phosphorus ignites spontaneously and remains burning until all the oxygen is used up. The petri dishes are inverted and held in a metal rack. The phosphorus

---

*Case Laboratories, Inc., Chicago, Ill.

†Matheson Co., Inc., Joliet, Ill.

‡Baltimore Biological Laboratory, Baltimore, Md.

should be contained in a small metal cup. The stock phosphorus should always be kept under water, handled with long metal forceps, and transferred to the jar as rapidly as possible.

NOTE: In all types of anaerobic jars it is necessary to include an **indicator of anaerobiasis.** Such an indicator is methylene blue, which is reduced to a colorless compound in an anaerobic environment (Anaerobic Indicator No. 06-115*).

Thioglycollate medium: This medium maintains the proper redox potential and utilizes methylene blue as the indicator of degree of oxidation. Screw caps should be tightened immediately after autoclaving. This liquid medium should be used routinely except for culturing feces and urine. It should not be refrigerated because it absorbs more oxygen at lower temperatures. The degree of oxidation of the medium can be judged by the depth of the color zone on the surface. If more than 20% of the medium shows the surface change, reheat the medium once only. Store at room temperature in screw-capped tubes in the dark.

Selection of media

Most media are available in dry powder form. For details, consult *Manual of Dehydrated Culture Media and Reagents for Microbiological and Clinical Laboratory Procedures†* and *Products for the Microbiological Laboratory.** They contain lists of many kinds of culture media for various purposes. No one laboratory ever employs all these media, but each laboratory has a few favorite combinations.

PRIMARY MEDIA:

Basic nutrient media: Basic nutrient media support the growth of most organisms. They include trypticase soy broth and agar, tryptose phosphate broth and agar, and thioglycollate broth.

Enriched media: Because of their enrichment with serum, ascitic fluid, blood, and carbohydrates, these media support the growth of most organisms. The following media fall into this group: blood agar, chocolate agar, and serum agar.

---

*Baltimore Biological Laboratory, Baltimore, Md.
†Difco Laboratories, Detroit, Mich.

Blood agar contains 5% sterile defibrinated rabbit or sheep blood. Human blood may be used but it is not recommended as it may contain inhibitory substances such as drugs, antibodies, etc. Blood agar plates are used for the study of hemolysis.

Hemolysis: Hemolysis at times develops best when the cultures are incubated anaerobically or kept at 4° C. Hemolysis is the result of the action of bacterial toxins or antibodies on the red blood cell membrane which allows release and denaturation of the hemoglobin. This leads to discoloration of the agar beneath and surrounding the colonies. (See discussion of streptococci for alpha, beta, and gamma hemolysis.)

Chocolate agar contains lysed blood that releases factors X and V, which are beneficial for some organisms.

SPECIAL MEDIA: Some organisms require special media, e.g., Lowenstein-Jensen medium for *Mycobacterium tuberculosis,* Fletcher medium for *Leptospira,* and W medium for *Brucella,* etc. Bordet-Gengou agar base enriched with 20% blood is recommended for the isolation of *Haemophilus pertussis.*

DIFFERENTIAL MEDIA: These media contain a carbohydrate and an indicator to distinguish carbohydrate fermenters from nonfermenters. They have, in addition to a basic medium, some substrate, e.g., a sugar or an amino acid with a color indicator of utilization added; they may contain inhibitors, e.g., KCN, active against only certain bacteria; or their composition may be such that only certain known organisms will grow on them, e.g., Simmons citrate or Cetrimide agar.

Some media test the biochemical behavior of organisms and can be used to identify **ferments** which may be characteristic for certain bacteria. Such enzymes include urease, fibrinolysis, decarboxylases, and carbohydrases.

SELECTIVE MEDIA: These media contain substances such as dyes, chemicals, etc. that inhibit the growth of certain organisms and permit the growth of others, e.g., phenylethyl alcohol agar and chloral hydrate agar; dyes such as crystal violet, brilliant green, and basic fuchsin; and substances such as sodium desoxycholate

Table 11-3. Indicators used in bacteriology

Dye	pH range	Change of color	
		Acid	Alkaline
Bromphenol blue	3.0–4.6	Yellow	Blue
Methyl red	4.2–6.3	Red	Yellow
Bromthymol blue	6.0–7.6	Yellow	Blue
Litmus	4.5–8.3	Red	Blue
Cresol red	7.2–8.8	Yellow	Purple
Phenol red	6.8–8.4	Yellow	Red

and potassium tellurite. Strains isolated on inhibitory media must be checked carefully for purity and should be transferred by touching the dome only, as the base may contain suppressed contaminants. A combination of both types of media is called a selective and differential medium.

SELECTIVE AND DIFFERENTIAL MEDIA: MacConkey medium contains sodium taurocholate, which inhibits many gram-positive organisms, and lactose, which, with neutral red as indicator, differentiates lactose-fermenting from nonlactose-fermenting organisms. The lactose-fermenting organisms produce acid and absorb the neutral red. The nonlactose-fermenting organisms produce an alkaline reaction, do not absorb neutral red, and produce colorless colonies.

Selenite-F broth at a neutral pH is an excellent selective enrichment medium for *Salmonella* because it suppresses *E. coli.* Tetrathionate broth is satisfactory for the same purpose.

ANTIBIOTIC SENSITIVITY[14, 15]

A number of microorganisms so consistently respond to adequate and well-chosen antibiotic therapy that sensitivity testing is hardly ever indicated. They are pneumococci, meningococci, gonococci, group A streptococci, *Haemophilus influenzae, Shigella, Salmonella typhosa,* and *Brucella.* On the other hand, **sensitivity testing is necessary** when (1) the culture reveals organisms that are known to be frequently resistant to antibiotics, e.g., *Proteus, Pseudomonas,* enterococci, and staphylococci; (2) the clinical picture warrants the use of a rapid bactericidal drug (not merely bacteriostatic), e.g., in

bacterial meningitis, endocarditis, osteo-myelitis, etc.; and (3) in the course of therapy the bacteria become resistant in varying degrees to certain drugs or to the dosage used.

Several methods[14] are available to ascertain the sensitivity of bacteria to antibiotics:

1. Diffusion tests, e.g., disk sensitivity test
2. Dilution tests, e.g., test tube dilution method

In vitro testing does not take into consideration the patient's own resistance, the concentration of the drug in the tissues, and most important, its concentration at the site of infection.

Disk sensitivity test: This is a rapid, economical, and easy to perform method that allows the testing of many antibiotics at the same time.

Procedure: Culture the organisms on trypticase soy agar enriched with sheep or rabbit blood or on special sensitivity test medium.* Spread the inoculum evenly and heavily with a cotton swab. Using aseptic precautions, place paper disks impregnated with antibiotics in maximal concentrations on the agar surface. Place one disk at a time 2 cm. or more apart and handle with flamed forceps or distribute with a disk dispenser. Make certain that disks are in contact with the agar surface. Gently press each disk onto the agar surface with flamed forceps, flaming the instrument each time. If direct sensitivities are desired, prepare three plates. Incubate one aerobically at 35° C., one anaerobically at 35° C., and one under 10% CO_2 at 35° C. Incubate plates

---

*Difco Laboratories, Detroit, Mich.

for no longer than 12-18 hr. since antibiotics are unstable at 35° C.

Interpretation: A clear zone around the disk will indicate that the antibiotic carried by the disk has diffused into the surrounding agar and that it inhibits the growth of the streaked organism.

Controls with known sensitive and resistant organisms should be included with the daily tests.

The disk method is clinically useful despite the fact that the formation of clear zones depends on many factors, e.g., composition of the agar, solubility and rate of diffusion of antibiotics, rate of growth of bacteria, and size of inoculum.

Direct sensitivity testing of mixed cultures[15-21]: This method allows speedy results at times but will depend on the adequacy of the initial inoculum and the rate of growth. Penicillinase produced by some bacteria (e.g., coliform bacteria) may interfere, but it diffuses rather poorly. Direct testing should be followed by sensitivity tests of the pure culture.

Errors in disk sensitivity testing: The most frequent errors in disk sensitivity testing are due to difficulties associated with (1) sulfonamide testing, (2) failure to recognize the difference in the appearance of the inhibition zones produced by penicillin-sensitive and penicillinase-producing staphylococci, and (3) *Proteus* sensitivity testing.

The technique of disk sensitivity testing must include built-in controls that also embrace commercially produced and tested products such as media, stains, etc. (See section on quality control in bacteriology.)

Selection of disks: The selection of suitable disks will somewhat depend on the preference expressed by the physician and on the development of more effective drugs. The following guidelines are suggested. Identification of certain uniformly drug-susceptible microorganisms eliminates the necessity for sensitivity testing of these organisms, e.g., alpha streptococci, pneumococci, etc. Only one member of each major class of drugs should be presented. The disk method does not differentiate bactericidal from bacteriostatic drugs. The difference between a bactericidal and a bacteriostatic agent is probably quantitative rather than qualitative. At a given concentration for a given period a drug may be bacteriostatic, but increasing the exposure time and the concentration may impart bactericidal properties.

Bactericidal antibiotics act on the cell wall of growing bacteria, e.g., penicillin, streptomycin, cephalothin, kanamycin, and vancomycin.

Bacteriostatic antibiotics interfere with protein synthesis, e.g., tetracycline, Chloromycetin, erythromycin, and lincomycin.

Sulfonamide disks are rarely indicated. Furadantin is only active in urine and not systemically. Mandelamine disks should not be used. Three sets of disks are suggested. For **gram-positive organisms** use penicillin V and penicillin G, phenethicillin, or methicillin. If the organisms are resistant to these, use erythromycin, novobiocin, methicillin, vancomycin, kanamycin, Keflin, Chloromycetin, or ristocetin. For **gram-negative organisms** use streptomycin, tetracycline, penicillin, kanamycin, Chloromycetin, Coly-mycin, or polymyxin B.

Test tube dilution method: This method determines the least amount of drug (mg./ml.) that will inhibit the organism in pure culture. This test is more accurate than the paper disk technique and is indicated in testing "resistant" organisms.

Selection of culture media: The liquid medium used must be the medium in which the best and most rapid growth of the recovered organisms can be obtained. Growth requirements of the organisms must be ascertained before the medium is selected.

1. Trypticase soy broth supports the growth of most organisms.
2. Fluid thioglycollate medium must be used for microaerophilic streptococci, anaerobic streptococci, clostridia, and *Bacteriodes*.
3. *Haemophilus* must be grown in medium with 1% blood added.

Concentration of inoculum: Usually an inoculum of 1:1000 dilution of an 18 hr. broth culture is used if the organisms are rapidly growing. If the organisms grow

Table 11-4

Tube No.	Broth (ml.)	Antibiotic stock solution	Final concentration of penicillin (units/ml.)	Final concentration of Aureomycin, Chloromycetin, streptomycin, or Terramycin (µg/ml.)
1	3.6	0.4 ml. stock solution	10	100
2	2	2 ml. from tube 1		
3	2	Continue with twofold serial dilutions until tube 9	5	50
4	2		2.5	25
5	2		1.25	12.5
6	2		0.625	6.25
7	2		0.313	3.13
8	2		0.156	1.56
9	2	Discard 2 ml.	0.078	0.78
10	2	No antibiotic	0.0	0.0

slowly, a concentration of 1:100 or even 1:10 of a 24 or 48 hr. broth culture may be used. If adequate growth cannot be obtained in 24 hr., the organism cannot be tested for antibiotic sensitivity since the antibiotics deteriorate at incubator temperature with prolonged time.

Antibiotic solutions: It is recommended that new, fresh stock solutions of antibiotics be prepared each day they are to be used.

The following concentrations for stock solutions are prepared: Aureomycin, Chloromycetin, streptomycin, and Terramycin, 1000 µg/ml.; penicillin, 100 units/ml.

Setup for test tube sensitivity: Use 10 sterile Kahn tubes, the tenth tube being the control without any antibiotic, prepared as shown in Table 11-4. Mix and incubate at 35° C. for 48 hr.

Reading and interpretation of test:

1. The first clear tube that indicates no growth is the end point.
2. This end point is the minimum concentration of the antibiotic necessary to inhibit the growth of the organism tested and indicates the sensitivity of that organism to the antibiotic.
3. If tube No. 8 is the first clear tube, then the organism is sensitive to the antibiotic in that concentration (0.156 unit/ml. if penicillin is the antibiotic used; 1.56 µg/ml. if other antibiotics are used).

Test tube testing of antibiotics in combination:

1. Double the concentration of each antibiotic since each antibiotic serves to dilute the other.
2. Set up protocols to include dilutions. Be prepared to repeat the procedure if the solutions are too strong (no growth) or too weak (no end point with growth in all tubes).

Sensitivity determination of anaerobes

Disk method: The technique is the same as described for aerobic organisms except for incubation under anaerobic conditions.

Disk-thioglycollate method: Dispense thioglycollate medium in 100 ml. amounts and autoclave. Transfer 2.5 ml. broth aseptically into 15 × 85 mm. sterile tubes and incubate for 24 hr. at 35° C. to test for sterility. If sterile, drop high-concentration disks into the fluid, refrigerate the tubes for 2 hr., and then use 2.5 ml. thioglycollate broth dilution of the organism for inoculum. Shake the tubes, incubate at 35° C. for 24 hr., and read for complete inhibition (dilution of culture—1:100 in broth of an 18-24 hr. broth culture of organism).

Sensitivity testing for Mycobacterium tuberculosis

These tests are described in the section on *Mycobacterium tuberculosis.*

Sulfonamide sensitivity tests

Sulfathiazole solutions of 1, 5, and 10 mg.% are incorporated in Mueller-Hinton medium, which contains a little *p*-aminobenzoic acid, but not enough to neutralize the action of the sulfonamide. Inoculate the surfaces of these plates with a 1:1000 dilution of the bacterial culture to be tested. The inoculum must be small since sulfonamides act only on a small number of bacteria. If growth occurs on the plates, the organisms are resistant. Include a known resistant (*Aerobacter*) and a known sensitive organism (meningococcus) as control.

BACTERIAL VACCINE

A vaccine is a suspension of killed (by heat or antiseptics) organisms that may stimulate production of active immunity when parenterally introduced in the body.

There are several types of bacterial vaccines: autogenous vaccine, containing the organism isolated from the patient; mixed vaccine, containing two or more organisms; and polyvalent vaccine, containing different strains of the same organism.

Technique of preparation[22]: The organism must be obtained in pure culture and is then planted on several blood agar plates. After 18 hr. of incubation at 35° C., 6 loopfuls of the growth (keep bacteria free of blood agar) are homogeneously suspended in 6 ml. sterile stock normal saline-formalin mixture. This mixture consists of 0.2 ml. 37% formalin in 140 ml. sterile normal saline solution. This suspension is referred to as the stock suspension. Incubate the stock suspension for 24 hr. at 35° C. and after this period test for sterility by inoculating several loopfuls of suspension into thioglycollate broth and onto blood agar plates. Incubate for an additional 3 days at 35° C. and check daily for sterility. Assuming that the suspension is sterile, proceed with the preparation of the following suspensions of the stock suspension.

Vial I: to 25 ml. stock saline-formalin mixture add 0.1 ml. bacterial stock suspension
Vial II: to 12 ml. stock saline-formalin mixture add 0.5 ml. bacterial stock suspension
Vial III: to 15 ml. stock saline-formalin mixture add 5 ml. bacterial stock suspension

All three vials are then incubated in a water bath at 60° C. for 45 min., after which time they are again checked for sterility. Inject subcutaneously 0.5 ml. of vial III into two young white mice; they should show no ill effects.

Administration (intramuscular injection):

1st day:	Vial I	0.5 ml.
2nd day:	Vial I	1.0 ml.
3rd day:	Vial I	2.0 ml.
4th day:	Vial II	0.5 ml.
5th day:	Vial II	1.0 ml.
6th day:	Vial II	2.0 ml.
7th day:	Vial III	0.5 ml.
8th day:	Vial III	0.75 ml.
9th day:	Vial III	1.0 ml.
10th day:	Vial III	1.75 ml.

Standardization of vaccine: Opacity tubes for standardization of bacterial vaccines are commercially available* and are based on standards issued by the National Institutes of Health.

GRAM-POSITIVE COCCI

Gram-positive cocci include the following: streptococci, staphylococci, *Gaffkya tetragena, Sarcina,* and pneumococci.

STREPTOCOCCUS

Streptococci are spherical or spheroid organisms that occur singly, in pairs, or in short or long chains. They divide at right angles to their long axis. They are gram positive, but some decolorize easily. Most species are aerobic, but many are anaerobic (or microaerophilic). They are typically nonmotile, are catalase negative, and ferment sugars.

LABORATORY DIAGNOSIS
MORPHOLOGY

The morphology of streptococci, like that of other bacteria, may be markedly changed by sulfonamides and antibiotics.

Microaerophilic strains may be found in deep or closed lesions.

Classification on morphologic grounds is not reliable; therefore other criteria are used for diagnosis[23, 24]:

1. Hemolysis in blood agar at 35° or 22° C.

---

*Burroughs Wellcome & Co., Inc., Tuckahoe, N. Y.; McFarland barium sulfate standards, Difco Laboratories, Detroit, Mich.

2. Serologic characteristics
3. Sensitivity to Optochin or bacitracin
4. Catalase activity
5. Fluorescent antibody identification
6. Behavior when brought in contact with bile salts, heat, and 6.5% sodium chloride (methylene blue)

HEMOLYSIS

Blood agar made of defibrinated sheep or rabbit blood is used to show the effect of streptococci on red blood cells. A pour plate is superior to a streak plate in bringing out hemolysis unless the latter is incubated anaerobically. The anaerobic substreak method can also be employed in place of anaerobic incubation, wherein the agar is cut with the loop and its undersurface is streaked. The blood agar pH should be 7.3-7.4. The blood, as previously stated, should be defibrinated because anticoagulants such as citrates and oxalates are at times toxic to streptococci. Sheep blood is preferred because human blood may contain antistreptolysins; sheep blood has the added advantage of inhibiting the hemolysis of *Haemophilus haemolyticus,* which macroscopically might be confused with streptococci. On the basis of presence (or absence) and type of hemolysis, the streptococci are divided into three groups designated by the Greek letters alpha, beta, and gamma. Schottmueller divides streptococci into (1) alpha hemolytic streptococci (viridans); (2) beta hemolytic streptococci (hemolytic); and (3) gamma hemolytic streptococci (anhemolytic).

Alpha hemolytic streptococci: There is greenish discoloration of the hemoglobin within the red blood cells beneath and around the streptococcal colonies. The red blood cells beneath remain intact. Macroscopically, there is a green or brown discoloration around the colonies, which may or may not be surrounded by a hazy zone of hemolysis that may be widened by refrigeration. Microscopically, there is a zone of intact cells, often better seen in the deeper layers around the colonies.

Beta hemolytic streptococci: There is clearing (disappearance) of the red blood cells beneath and around the streptococcal colonies. Macroscopic examination reveals a clear transparent zone around colonies; microscopically, no intact red blood cells are seen. Some beta hemolytic streptococci are oxygen labile, their streptolysin O enzyme being active only at reduced oxygen tension (necessitating pour plates, anaerobiosis, or streaking of the undersurface of the agar). Streptolysin S is stable and active in the presence of oxygen and can be appreciated on surface colonies. Some beta-type strains which contain hot-cold hemolysins produce a double zone of lysis when they are refrigerated after incubation at 35° C. (Lancefield group B).

Gamma hemolytic streptococci: There is complete absence of hemolysis of the red blood cells and of the blood agar below the streptococcal colonies. Macroscopic and microscopic (low-power objective) examination reveals no change in the medium.

APPEARANCE OF CULTURE

On solid medium the typical colony is small, discoid, and 1-2 mm. in diameter. The colonies may be matt or glossy. Matt colonies are more likely to be virulent. There may or may not be hemolysis. Streptococci from solid media often resemble staphylococci microscopically.

SEROLOGIC CHARACTERISTICS

On the basis of the capsular polysaccharide C, Lancefield grouped the streptococci into serologic groups from A to S (Table 11-5).

Lancefield group A streptococci (Streptococcus pyogenes)[25]

Eighty-five percent of all streptococcal infections are caused by group A beta hemolytic streptococci. Group A streptococci are characteristically sensitive to bacitracin, though 10% of groups B, C, and G may also be sensitive. Group C is usually resistant to bacitracin.

Lancefield grouping by the precipitin test

This method has two phases: (1) preparation of streptococcal extract by acid heat extraction of the C capsular antigen and (2) grouping by the precipitin test,

Table 11-5. Identification of beta hemolytic streptococci[*]

Characteristics	Group A	Group B	Group C human	Group D (enterococci)
On blood agar				
Surface colonies	White to gray, opaque, hard, dry; 2 mm. zones of hemolysis	Gray, translucent, soft; narrow hemolytic zone; a few RBC may be observed microscopically under colonies	Similar to group A	Gray, translucent, soft; zone of hemolysis wider than colony
Subsurface colonies	2-2.5 mm. zones of hemolysis, with sharply defined edges	0.5 mm. zone of hemolysis after 24 hr.; 1 mm. zone of hemolysis after 48 hr.; refrigeration produces double zones of hemolysis	Similar to group A	3-4 mm. zones of hemolysis
Bacitracin susceptibility	Susceptible	Resistant	Resistant	Resistant
Sodium hippurate	Not hydrolyzed	Hydrolyzed	Not hydrolyzed	Not hydrolyzed
Growth at 10° C.	−	−	−	+
Growth at 45° C.	−	−	−	+
SF medium	No growth	No growth	No growth	Growth, acid reaction
6.5% NaCl broth	No growth	No growth	No growth	Growth
Source	Throat, blood, wounds, rarely spinal fluid	Urine, peritoneum, rarely blood, occasionally human throat	Throat, nose, vagina, intestinal tract	Urine, peritoneum, feces; milk and milk products
Pathogenicity	Septicemia, tonsillitis, scarlet fever, puerperal sepsis, pneumonia, erysipelas	Rare cases of endocarditis and meningitis	Erysipelas, puerperal sepsis, throat infections; opportunist pathogen	Subacute bacterial endocarditis; urinary tract infections

[*]From Bailey and Scott: Diagnostic microbiology, St. Louis, 1966, The C. V. Mosby Co.

Note: Groups A, B, and C will not grow at pH 9.6 or in 0.1% methylene blue milk—two criteria which will distinguish them from group D (enterococci).

using commercially available group A streptococcus antiserum.

Preparation of streptococcal extract:

1. Transfer a pure culture of streptococci to 30 ml. Todd-Hewitt broth and incubate overnight at 37° C.
2. Centrifuge broth culture for 30 min. at 2000 rpm and discard supernatant into disinfectant.
3. Add to the sediment 1 drop 0.04% metacresol purple (200 mg. powder ground with 26.7 ml. 0.2N NaOH, diluted to 500 ml. with distilled water for working solution) and 0.3 ml. 0.2N HCl in physiologic saline solution. Mix with capillary pipette and transfer to small tube. The suspension should be pink (pH 2.0-2.4). If necessary, add another drop or two of 0.2N HCl.
4. Place suspension in a boiling water bath for 10 min. Shake several times.
5. Centrifuge for 30 min. at 2000 rpm.
6. Decant the supernatant, which is the extract, into the clean tube. Discard the sediment into disinfectant.
7. Neutralize extract by adding 0.2N NaOH carefully and slowly drop by

drop until the color is lavender (pH 7.4-7.8). Avoid too alkaline a reaction, as evidenced by a deep purple color. It may give rise to false positive tests.

8. Centrifuge for 10 min. at 2000 rpm.
9. Decant the supernatant, which represents the extract, into a small test tube. It can be stored in the refrigator in a small screw-capped vial.

Group precipitin test for group A streptococci: Rehydrate commercial group A streptococcus antiserum. Dip sterile capillary tube (supplied by manufacturer of antiserum) into group A streptococcus antiserum and allow a 1 cm. long column to rise in the tube by capillary attraction. Remove tube and keep finger on free end to prevent air from replacing serum. Wipe capillary, insert into the prepared extract, and allow an amount equal to the antiserum to enter the tube. Remove tube, keeping one finger on free end, and wipe outside. Allow fluid column to rise to midportion of the tube. There should be no air at the interface of extract and antiserum, but there should be an air column at either end of the tube. Invert capillary and insert gently into soft Plasticine block. After 10 min., examine tube against dark background for white ring at the center of the column. Examine at frequent intervals between 10 and 30 min. False positive results may appear after 30 min.

SENSITIVITY TESTING
Sensitivity to bacitracin

Place a bacitracin differentiation disk (not sensitivity disk) on heavily surface-streaked segment of agar plate. After 18-24 hr. of incubation a clear zone will be seen around the disk if the organisms are group A streptococci.

Sensitivity to Optochin

Streptococci are not sensitive to Optochin (Optochin differentiation disks) and can thus be differentiated from pneumococci, which are inhibited.

CATALASE TEST FOR STREPTOCOCCI

Technique: Add 1-2 ml. fresh 3% H_2O_2 to a plain agar slant or plain broth culture

of the organisms to be tested. Observe for bubbling or foaming of O_2, indicating the presence of catalase.

Interpretation: Streptococci are catalase negative, whereas other cocci and diphtheroids are catalase positive. Do not use media that contain body fluids because they are catalase positive. Always use a negative (streptococci) and a positive (staphylococci) control. The H_2O_2 should be kept in the refrigerator.

A modification of the catalase test can be used to detect significant bacteriuria.[26]

FLUORESCENT ANTIBODY (FA) IDENTIFICATION OF GROUP A STREPTOCOCCI[27]

Direct smear method: This method is similar to the one described below, but the culture phase is eliminated. It may be used if a duplicate gram-stained smear shows streptococci in chains. Troublesome FA reactions of groups C and G streptococci and *Staphylococcus aureus* may occur.

Method utilizing smears from cultured streptococci:
Phosphate buffered saline solution (pH 7.5):
1. NaCl, 8.77 gm.
2. Na_2HPO_4, 1.42 gm.
3. $NaH_2PO_4H_2O$, 1.38 gm.
4. Distilled water to 1 L.
Technique:
1. Transfer beta hemolytic colonies as seen on blood agar to 1 ml. Todd-Hewitt broth.
2. Incubate broth for 4 hr. at 37° C.
3. Centrifuge for 5 min. to pack the bacteria.
4. Pour off supernatant into disinfectant and resuspend bacteria in 1 ml. phosphate buffered saline solution, pH 7.2.
5. Prepare duplicate smears of suspended bacteria, spreading 1 loopful throughout each etched circle and both FA microscopic slides.*
6. Air dry over lighted microscope lamp.
7. Fix with Bunsen burner flame. These smears may be stored in the

---

*Fluoroslides, Aloe Scientific Division, Brunswick Corp., St. Louis, Mo.

deep freeze as future controls and reference.

8. Cover smear nearest to the etched end of the slide with a small drop of group A streptococcus antiserum labeled with fluorescein. Cover second smear on slide with mixture of labeled group A streptococcus antiserum (0.1 ml.), labeled group C streptococcus antiserum (0.15 ml.), and buffered saline solution (2.75 ml.). Spread conjugate over entire smear with applicator sticks held horizontally. Also stain previously prepared known positive and negative controls that have been stored in the deep freeze.

9. Cover slides with a large petri dish lid fitted with moist filter paper and allow to stand for 30 min. in darkness at room temperature.

10. Pour off excess conjugate and rinse in free-flowing buffered saline solution. Continue rinsing in a container filled with buffered saline solution for 10 min. in darkness. Rinse quickly in distilled water.

11. Blot slides very gently with new bibulous paper and cover with small drops of buffered glycerin-saline solution (1 part buffered saline solution and 9 parts glycerin) and cover with a No. 1 cover slip. The completed preparations may be stored in the refrigerator.

12. Examine smears with fluorescent microscope under oil immersion with dark-field condenser.

Interpretation: If group A streptococci are present, both smears on each slide will show fluorescing cocci in chains. The fluorescence should be of grade 3+ (bright yellow-green).

LANCEFIELD GROUP B STREPTOCOCCI (STREPTOCOCCUS AGALACTIAE)

Group B streptococci, together with groups C, G, and F, are found in normal flora but may be resistant to antibiotics after group A streptococci have been treated. Serologic typing is necessary for identification. They may be alpha or beta hemolytic. These organisms are the cause of mastitis in cattle, meningitis in infants, cervical infections in women, and occasionally, sore throat.

LANCEFIELD GROUP C STREPTOCOCCI (STREPTOCOCCUS DYSGALACTIAE)

Group C streptococci produce mastitis in cows but are also occasionally found in throat cultures and in puerperal sepsis. They may be alpha or beta hemolytic.

LANCEFIELD GROUP D STREPTOCOCCI— ENTEROCOCCUS GROUP (STREPTOCOCCUS FAECALIS)

The organism is found in genitourinary tract infection and in the throat after treatment with antibiotics. The organism is characterized by resistance to antibiotics and to physical insults; it grows in 6.5% NaCl broth and on 10% bile blood agar. It is a facultative anaerobe, able to grow at a pH of 9.6 and to resist heat, e.g., 70° C. for 15 min. Enterococcus on blood agar may resemble staphylococcus, which may also grow on 6.5% NaCl. The growth pattern in broth will distinguish the two, but the coagulase test will not because the enterococcus utilizes the citrate from citrated plasma, which will then clot. Most organisms show gamma hemolysis, but they may be alpha or beta hemolytic. These hemolysins are not water soluble, as can be proved with the soluble hemolysin test.

Soluble hemolysin test:

Technique: Mix 1 ml. of an 18 hr. broth culture with 1 ml. 4% washed horse red cells. Incubate at 35° C. for 1 hr. in a water bath. Lysis of the cells indicates a positive test. *Streptococcus faecalis* gives a negative test.

Heat-resistance test:

Technique: Plate a broth culture onto one half of a blood agar plate. Heat the culture for 15 min. at 35° C. and plate it onto the other half of the plate. If the organism has withstood the heating, equal growth will occur on both sides of the plate. *S. faecalis* resists heating.

ANAEROBIC STREPTOCOCCI (PEPTOSTREPTOCOCCUS)

Anaerobic streptococci may be found in pelvic material. Strict anaerobiasis is required.

Selective medium:

SF medium*: This medium contains sodium azide, which suppresses all streptococci except enterococci. Bromcresyl purple is added as indicator of fermentation (acid gives a yellow color). The organisms should initially be grown on phenylethyl alcohol medium.

Antibody reactions

Antibody reactions include the demonstration of neutralizing antibodies (**antistreptolysin O**) and of precipitating antibodies (**C-reactive protein** and **MG agglutinin**).

Antistreptolysin O titer[28]: The hemolysin liberated by group A streptococci is antigenic and results in the production of antistreptolysin O after infection with these organisms. Antistreptolysin O appears in the serum from 1 wk. to 1 mo. after the onset of a streptococcal infection.

Test: The reagents are commercially available† and are supplied with complete directions. Streptolysin O is capable of lysing human or rabbit erythrocytes and can be neutralized by its specific antibody—antistreptolysin O antibody. Various dilutions of the patient's serum are mixed with constant amounts of streptolysin O antigen and a 5% suspension of washed human or rabbit cells. After incubation, the end point is determined by noting the tube with the highest dilution of serum showing no hemolysis. The titer is expressed as the reciprocal of the serum dilution (**Todd units**).[29] Modifications of this test using latex particles are available.

Clinical significance: The ASO titer is useful in the diagnosis of rheumatic fever and glomerulonephritis and in the differential diagnosis of early rheumatoid arthritis. It is an aid in the diagnosis of hemolytic streptococcal infection.

Interpretation: Absence of infection with hemolytic streptococcus is indicated by the presence of 50 units or less; 500 units or more indicate the presence of infection with hemolytic streptococcus. Serial determinations with a rising titer

are more significant than a single determination.

C-reactive protein: This is a protein that is not present in normal sera and occurs in response to a variety of inflammatory stimuli. It appears early in the acute phase and declines during convalescence.

NOTE: C-reactive protein is destroyed if heated above 65° C.

C-reactive protein was first described by Tillett and Francis,[30] who obtained a precipitin reaction upon mixing somatic pneumococcal C polysaccharide with the serum of patients in the acute phase of pneumococcal pneumonia. C-reactive protein is not specific for any one disease but appears as a result of some inflammatory reaction, infectious or noninfectious in origin.

The protein has been isolated and injected into the rabbit to form a specific C-reactive protein antiserum[31, 32] (CRPA-Schieffelin, available commercially) which is now being used instead of the C polysaccharide as a more sensitive reagent for the precipitin test.

Test: Collect blood from patients who are in the fasting state. Let clot and centrifuge if necessary to obtain clear serum. The procedure is essentially that described by Anderson and McCarty.[33]

Draw into a capillary glass tube (0.7-1 mm. outside diameter or 0.4 mm. inside diameter) a column of C-reactive protein antiserum about 1.5 cm. long, controlling with the finger over the clean tip of the capillary tube, and wipe the used tip with cleansing tissue.

Before removing finger from the tip of the tube, insert the other tip into the patient's serum, avoiding any air bubbles between the two serums, and draw an equal amount of the patient's serum into the tube. Wipe tip again.

Move serum column near the middle of the tube, close tip with the finger, and mix sera by slowly inverting the tube about 10 times. Stand the tube vertically with the patient's serum on top in a special rack (obtainable commercially) or in modeling clay, making certain that the bottom of the serum column is well above the surface of the clay.

---

*Baltimore Biological Laboratory, Baltimore, Md.
†Difco Laboratories, Detroit, Mich.

A slide test (CR test) is available commercially.[*]

Significance: A positive or negative reaction indicates, respectively, the presence or absence of inflammation, but not the etiology of the process. The test is positive in rheumatic fever, rheumatoid arthritis, disseminated lupus erythematosus, and myocardial infarction. It has been found especially useful in following the progress of rheumatic fever under treatment, becoming negative and indicating that the inflammatory reaction has disappeared even when the sedimentation rate remains elevated.[34] The test is negative in chorea.

The test is helpful in the interpretation of the sedimentation rate, which is also elevated in the absence of inflammation; in anemia, due to a decreased number of red blood cells; in pregnancy, due to increased fibrinogen; in multiple myeloma and in other cases of hyperglobulinemia; and in nephrosis, due to loss of albumin and relative increase of globulin.

Serum from viral hepatitis gives a negative test with C polysaccharide, but in some cases (about 50%) the C-reactive protein is present in sufficient amount to be detected with the antiserum. The reaction is not strong and is not limited to the initial acute phase.[35] The results in poliomyelitis and in infectious mononucleosis have not been helpful.

AGGLUTININS FOR STREPTOCOCCUS MG

Streptococcus MG is a strain of anhemolytic streptococci. The agglutinins are present in 20-75% of the cases of primary atypical pneumonia, which is now considered to be caused by *Mycoplasma pneumoniae* infection. They may be demonstrated after the second week, reaching a peak in the fourth or fifth week. The agglutinins are found only in low titer (under 1-20) in normal individuals and in other conditions (acute respiratory diseases and streptococcal infection). A fourfold increase in titer in the course of the disease is significant. Absence of agglutinins does not rule out primary atypical pneumonia.

Streptococcus MG agglutination test: *Streptococcus MG* antigen is commercially available.[*]

Preparation of antigen: If the antigen is not obtained commercially, use 0.1 ml. of an 18 hr. stock culture of *Streptococcus MG* to inoculate about 400 ml. trypticase soy broth. Incubate for 18-24 hr. at 35° C. Centrifuge and wash sediment three times with saline solution. Suspend in saline solution to give a turbidity of about No. 5 McFarland standard. Kill by heating 30 min. at 56° C. Heating at 60° C. for 30 min. is said to destroy the agglutinogens.

Technique: Set up a twofold serial dilution of the serum, from 1:5-1:1280, with saline solution. The serum is not inactivated since heating decreases the titer. Add an equal amount of the streptococcus suspension (antigen). Final dilutions are 1:10-1:2560.

Set up 10 tubes and number from 1-10. To tube 1 add 0.8 ml. normal saline solution, and add 0.5 ml. to the remaining 9 tubes. To tube 1 add 0.2 ml. serum, mix, and transfer 0.5 ml. of tube 1 mixture to tube 2; mix and continue transfer, discarding 0.5 ml. from tube 9. Tube 10 is the saline solution control. The initial serum dilutions are 1:5, 1:10, 1:20, 1:40, 1:80, 1:320, 1:640, and 1:1280.

Add 0.5 ml. antigen to each tube, giving a final serum dilution of 1:10, 1:20, 1:40, 1:80, 1:160, 1:320, 1:640, 1:1280, and 1:2560.

Place in water bath at 35° C. for 2 hr. and then refrigerate (4° C.) for 18 hr.

Place again in water bath at 35° C. for 2 hr. to rule out nonspecific agglutination. Shake and read.

Interpretation: *Streptococcus MG* agglutinin titer is the highest dilution of the patient's serum that produces agglutination.

Capsular swelling with Streptococcus MG antiserum: The antigen used in the *Streptococcus MG* agglutination test gives a positive quellung reaction with the MG antiserum. The serum can also be used to test unknown organisms.

Technique: Mix 1 loopful of an 18 hr.

---

[*]Hyland Laboratories, Los Angeles, Calif.

[*]Difco Laboratories, Detroit, Mich.

broth culture of the organism with 1 loopful of 1% methylene blue solution on a slide. Add 1 loopful of *Streptococcus MG* antiserum. Mix the preparation, add a cover slip, and microscopically observe for capsular swelling.

STAPHYLOCOCCUS[36, 37]

Staphylococci are gram-positive spheres that characteristically appear in grapelike clusters, but also appear singly, in pairs, and occasionally in chains of three or four and are then difficult to distinguish from streptococci.

On the basis of cultural and chemical characteristics, two groups are distinguished: (1) *Staphylococcus aureus*, which is aerobic, coagulase positive, and mannitol positive, and (2) *Staphylococcus epidermidis*, which is aerobic, coagulase negative, and ferments dextrose but not mannitol. The latter species leads a saprophytic existence on normal skin and mucosa. The first species is responsible for skin infections (carbuncles, abscesses, and furuncles) and is also found in infections of bone and lung. If certain strains grow in food, their enterotoxins produce a severe form of food poisoning. The skin of hospital personnel may harbor epidemic strains of resistant *Staphylococcus aureus*.

LABORATORY DIAGNOSIS
Morphology

Smear: Smear from lesion or culture shows gram-positive cocci in clusters.

Culture: After 12-18 hr. on blood agar, large opaque colonies surrounded by zones of hemolysis appear. In some strains, hemolysis does not appear until later. **Pigment** production may not occur until several days later and is improved by exposure to sunlight and to room temperature. It appears earlier if the material is subcultured to special media such as Loeffler agar or Champman-Stone agar. If several colonies are scraped together on the agar surface, it is sometimes easier to appreciate pigment production. The color of the colonies (white, gold, lemon) bears little relationship to pathogenicity. The colonies are round and slightly convex and have a smooth edge.

Thioglycollate broth is a suitable liquid medium, in which they form small granules.

Differential media: **Blood agar with 5-7% sodium chloride** serves as a selective medium for isolation of staphylococci from a mixed culture. **Chloral hydrate** and **phenylethyl alcohol media** suppress gram-negative organisms, allowing identification of staphylococci and streptococci in autopsy material and in feces. The latter investigation is of importance in the diagnosis of diarrhea in postoperative patients receiving antibiotic therapy. Do not omit direct smear of the original specimen in cases of suspected pseudomembranous (staphylococcal) enterocolitis.[38]

Staphylococcus aureus
Laboratory methods to determine pathogenicity and virulence[39]

Pathogenic staphylococci tend to be coagulase positive, hemolytic, pigment producing, mannitol fermenting,[36] and gelatin liquefying.

CULTURE METHODS:

Mannitol salt agar: This medium is good for isolation from contaminated sources such as feces. Mannitol salt agar consists of 7.5% sodium chloride added to phenol red mannitol agar. Coagulase-positive staphylococci grow well and the colonies are surrounded by yellow zones, while nonpathogenic staphylococci grow poorly and their small colonies are surrounded by red or purple zones. Other bacteria are generally inhibited.

Enzymatic methods:

Coagulase test: In a small test tube mix a loopful of organisms or 2 drops of an 18 hr. broth culture with 0.5 ml. reconstituted commercial desiccated coagulase plasma. Let stand 3 hr. in the incubator and examine for clotting. Any clotting (firm clot, flocculi, or gelatinous globule) is positive. The earlier the clotting, the more coagulase is present. This test is critical for the diagnosis of pathogenic staphylococci.

Untested human or rabbit plasma may be unsatisfactory for the test; therefore pretested commercial plasma is preferable. Stock cultures of coagulase-positive staphylococci suitable for pretesting plasma may in time become coagulase negative. The plasma must contain adequate supplies of coagulase reacting factor (CRF) and fibrinogen and must lack inhibitors. Commercial plasma is not sterile and incubation for over 3 hr. is not recommended.

Slide test for clumping factor of staphylococci: The clumping factor, or bound coagulase, is different from free coagulase, and the slide test can only be used as a screening test.

Emulsify a single colony in 1 small drop of 0.85% NaCl on a slide. Add 1 small drop of coagulase plasma and mix. Read within 5 sec. Agglutinated strains are almost all coagulase positive. If there is no clumping, perform the coagulase test because many coagulase-positive staphylococci are negative with the slide test.

Other enzymes and toxins produced by pathogenic staphylococci can be investigated by tests for fibrinolysin, phosphatase, hyaluronidase, enterotoxin, leukocidin, alpha toxin, and deoxyribonuclease.

DNAse test agar*:* Deoxyribonuclease activity closely parallels coagulase activity.

Technique: After incubation, flood the streaked plate with 0.1% toluidine blue. A light pink zone will surround colonies of DNAse-producing bacteria.

Phage typing[40]: This method is based on the lysis of staphylococci by specific bacteriophages. The phage type is a stable genetic characteristic based on a surface antigen. This method, which identifies about 60% of all staphylococci, has no diagnostic value, but is important in the epidemiologic investigation of hospital infections, etc. The type most frequently identified is arbitrarily designated 80/81/KS6.

Reference is given only to the investigation of staphylococcal food poisoning.[41]

Sensitivity testing: The so-called community strains are usually sensitive to penicillin or tetracycline, but the so-called epidemic strains may be resistant and may require synthetic penicillinase-resistant drugs (see previous section on sensitivity testing).

Bacteriologic survey— staphylococcal infections in hospitals[42, 43]

The duty to investigate hospital cross-infections or potential sources of such an infection is usually that of the laboratory. The methods employed have already been described.[44]

There are three main problems in the investigation of actual or potential hospital infections: (1) to establish the source, (2) to discover the reservoir, and (3) to discover the spread.

The primary sources of infection are individuals with staphylococcal infections, and the reservoirs are people who are nasal and cutaneous carriers of staphylococci (patients, staff, visitors, etc.). Obtain culture material from the lesions of infected patients and prepare nasal cultures from all possible carriers. Investigation of the reservoirs and spread of infection includes culturing the air, patient's utensils, bedding, floors, and walls, surgical instruments and gloves, nursery utensils, and supplies and checking on the efficiency of the sterilizing processes (bacterial spore strip method). All findings should be recorded and reported to some central body (infections committee, etc.). Some of these investigations, such as the investigation of the obstetric division, nursery, operating rooms, autoclaves, etc., should be done routinely once a month.

A detailed outline of the hospital areas to be investigated has been prepared by Litsky.[45, 46]

The use of Rodac plates* is suggested for sanitary examination of surfaces. Trypticase soy agar is a suitable medium. Lecithin and polysorbate 80 (Tween 80*) are included in the medium to inactivate residual disinfectant cationic surface-active material from which the specimen is being collected.

---

*Baltimore Biological Laboratory, Baltimore, Md.

*Baltimore Biological Laboratory, Baltimore, Md.

Some of the counts one may expect are as follows:

Floor: After cleaning and mopping with disinfectant-detergent and before traffic has begun, 0-12 colonies/Rodac plate.

Hands: Provided that the hands are regularly exposed to surgical technique, 50 colonies/ml. test rinse water before scrubbing. Immediately after scrubbing the count should be close to 0-10 colonies/ml. test rinse water. Hands that are simply washed and not surgically scrubbed average 12,000-15,000 colonies/ml. test rinse water.

Lights: After cleaning, the overhead lights in surgical suites should have a count of 0-5 colonies/Rodac plate.

Staphylococcus epidermidis

Morphologically, tinctorially, and culturally, *Staphylococcus epidermidis* is similar to *Staphylococcus aureus* except that the colonies are usually white and the organism is coagulase and mannitol negative. It is a ubiquitous saprophytic organism which is nevertheless a potential pathogen.

GAFFKYA TETRAGENA (MICROCOCCUS TETRAGENUS)

These organisms are gram-positive cocci arranged in tetrads. Each coccus is surrounded by a mucoid capsule. There is no hemolysis on blood agar. The colonies are grayish white and mucoid.

These organisms are related to staphylococci and may thus be found in staphylococcal pus.

SARCINA

These organisms are large gram-positive cocci growing in cuboidal packages. On solid media they are pigmented, varying from pale yellow to yellow and orange. They can be cultivated from stomach contents and from the air.

PNEUMOCOCCUS (DIPLOCOCCUS PNEUMONIAE)

Pneumococci are encapsulated lance-shaped cocci that are gram positive, bile (and desoxycholate) soluble, and produce a green color on blood media.

LABORATORY DIAGNOSIS
Morphology

Smear: Smear of sputum and culture shows pairs and short chains of gram-positive lanceolate diplococci, with the long axis of the organisms in a line. The free ends of the cocci are pointed, while the opposite ends, which are facing each other, are round.

The strongly gram-positive staining reaction of the young colonies is quickly lost as the culture ages. After 6 hr. the organisms may become gram negative. Capsular stains can be used to prove the presence of a well-developed capsule.

Culture: Small, round, translucent, alpha hemolytic, glistening colonies are present on blood agar. They are dome shaped when young, but later develop central depressions (autolysis). Colonies of type 3 pneumococci are larger and have the appearance of drops of water. Subculture alpha hemolytic colonies to blood agar for Optochin disk test and to tryptose-phosphate broth for bile solubility test.

The organism grows diffusely in thioglycollate broth, forming a faint cloud.

Bile solubility test:

Reagent: Prepare 2% solution of sodium desoxycholate in water and add Merthiolate to make 1:50,000 dilution.

Technique: Set up two tubes. Add 0.5 ml. of 2% sodium desoxycholate to one tube and 0.5 ml. saline solution to the other.

To each tube add 0.5 ml. broth culture. Incubate at 35° C. Examine every 10 min. for 1 hr.

Interpretation: Lysis of organisms is evidenced by clearing of the medium. Pneumococci are readily soluble. Other bacteria, e.g., *Haemophilus*, are also bile soluble, but gram stain will help to differentiate.

Precautions: Desoxycholate is precipitated by sodium citrate and by acid (below pH 6.5). The optimum pH is about 7.6. Cultures to be tested should not contain citrate or sugars. Also remove red cells, which are laked by desoxycholate.

Neutralization of an acid broth culture with 2 or 3 drops 0.1N NaOH will prevent clouding produced by desoxycholate at a low pH.

Inhibition by Optochin:

Optochin disk (ethylhydrocupreine hydrochloride, 1:4000): Place disk on heavily streaked blood agar plate and incubate 17 hr. at 35° C. Pneumococci in the vicinity of the disk will be lysed, whereas alpha hemolytic streptococci (viridans) will be unaffected. Morphologically, alpha hemolytic streptococci may closely resemble pneumococci on blood agar. The Optochin disk test is superior to the bile solubility test.

Controls: Use known pneumococci and alpha hemolytic streptococci.

Pneumococcus typing—capsular swelling (quellung): Types 1-8 are responsible for most cases of pneumonia in adults, whereas type 14 is the most common in children.

Technique: Place 1 drop fresh sputum or 1 loopful of culture suspension or broth on a microscope slide. Add 1 drop antiserum pool* for which the organism is to be tested. Add 1 loopful of Loeffler methylene blue. Mix with applicator stick, add cover slip, and examine under oil-immersion lens.

A positive reaction should occur within 3-5 min. up to 1 hr. and is indicated by a definite increase in capsular size.

Prepare a control to which 0.85% saline solution is added instead of the antiserum pool. Examine this slide first to establish the normal size of the capsule.

Mouse method: Collect fresh sputum in a clean receptacle. Make gram stain to determine presence of pneumococci.

Wash a small portion of sputum the size of a fingertip with sterile broth or saline solution, selecting the bloody or characteristic portion. Emulsify in a sterile mortar, and inoculate mouse intraperitoneally. When mouse appears ill, usually after 6-8 hr., puncture peritoneal cavity with capillary tip of pipette and secure 1 drop of fluid for gram stain. If fluid shows 12 or more pneumococci per field, identify pneumococci by capsular swelling.

---

*Difco Laboratories, Detroit, Mich.

Antigenic structure: The capsular polysaccharide is specific for each type and is the basis of the capsular swelling test. M protein is characteristic for each type, whereas C protein is common to all pneumococci. C-reactive protein is the nonspecific substance appearing in the serum of patients with inflammatory lesions that precipitates pneumococcal C carbohydrate (see p. 551).

GRAM-NEGATIVE COCCI

Gram-negative cocci consist of *Neisseria* (*gonorrhoeae, meningitidis,* and *catarrhalis*).

NEISSERIA

These organisms are gram-negative diplococci; the individual coccus is kidney shaped, with adjacent flat or concave sides. The pathogenic forms autolyze quickly. They occur in single pairs or in groups of pairs. They vary in their O_2 requirements and in their pigment production. They are oxidase and catalase positive. Group I contains pathogens, while group II consists of bacteria that are usually classified as nonpathogens but which may be responsible for disease.

Group I: *Neisseria gonorrhoeae* and *meningitidis,* which grow only on special media without pigment production, preferably under CO_2 tension and strictly at 35° C.

Group II: *Neisseria catarrhalis, sicca,* etc., which grow without pigment production, and *N. flava,* etc., which grow with pigment production on blood agar. With the possible exception of *N. catarrhalis,* they form dry, wrinkled opaque colonies that can be differentiated macroscopically from the moist opaque colonies of group I.

Gonococcus (Neisseria gonorrhoeae)
LABORATORY DIAGNOSIS
Morphology

Smear: Obtain smear from lesions (genital, synovial, ophthalmic, etc.) or

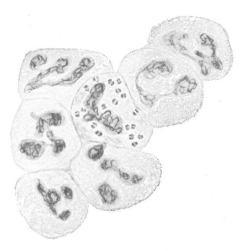

Plate 11. Gonococci in a cervical smear showing well-preserved pus cells and the characteristic clear spaces around the organisms.

from cultures. It shows intracellular gram-negative diplococci within pus cells, often in groups, and also some that are extracellular (Plate 11).

NOTE: It is not wise to make a diagnosis of gonococci without a culture since some gram-negative coccobacilli, e.g., *Mima* and *N. catarrhalis*, have forms suggesting *N. gonorrhoeae*.[47, 48] These organisms may be found in urine, blood, pleural exudate, cerebrospinal fluid, conjunctival exudate, and vaginal smears. The report of the smear should read "Intracellular gram-negative diplococci resembling gonococci were (were not) found." As the intracellular location is an important feature, if only extracellular organisms are seen after adequate search, a repeat specimen should be examined or the material should be cultured. A statement as to the number of pus cells should also be included, i.e., few, many, etc.

Culture: Immediate culture is necessary. Cultures should be made directly onto chocolate agar, or preferably onto Thayer-Martin medium, because drying kills the organism. If it is not possible to make the culture promptly, place the swab in a holding medium such as Stuart transport medium. The medium is unsuitable

if it turns bluish. The combination of transport medium and culture is superior to diagnosis by smear only. Streak chocolate agar and place in candle jar at 35° C., the atmosphere of which is kept moist by inserting wet filter paper into the screw top. The colonies are small (1-3 mm. in diameter), are slightly elevated to convex, and are grayish and buttery mucoid so that a portion of a colony cannot be easily separated. They are transparent and have undulate margins.

On the basis of their colony characteristics, gonococci can usually be differentiated from young colonies of diphtheroids and streptococci. Prepare gram-stained smear from selected colonies. Because of the rapid autolysis, many atypical forms may be seen.

Oxidase test: Colonies of *Neisseria* can be detected in mixed cultures by the oxidase test.

Technique: Drop on the suspicious colonies 1 drop freshly prepared 1% solution of the oxalate of *p*-aminodimethylaniline (which has stood about 15 min. or just long enough to become purple). In a positive reaction the colonies become pink, then red, and finally black. Colonies usually remain viable through the pink stage and may be subcultured, but they are killed by the reagent upon longer contact. The reagent does not interfere at any stage, however, with the gram stain. The test is based on the presence of the enzyme oxidase produced by *Neisseria*. Streptococci and diphtheroids, which by direct colony inspection may be confused with *Neisseria*, are oxidase negative. *Pseudomonas* are oxidase positive but differ culturally from *Neisseria*.

Fluorescent antibody identification of Neisseria gonorrhoeae[49]: This procedure may be performed as an immediate direct test or as a delayed test on an 18 hr. culture. The latter method will be described.

Delayed method—smears from growth on chocolate agar or Thayer-Martin medium:

1. Swabs from the cervix, urethra, and vagina of female patients and from the urethra of male patients are rolled on chocolate agar slants and left in the tubes. Place the tubes in

a CO_2 candle jar and incubate at 37° C. for 18 hr.

2. After 18 hr., smears are made from the cultures on FA slides and are air dried (do not heat).
3. Fix smears in 3% formalinized buffered saline solution (pH 7.2) for 10 min.
4. Rinse slides in distilled water and blot gently with bibulous paper.
5. Place 1 drop (approximately 1/30 ml.) fluorescein-labeled *N. gonorrhoeae* antiserum (previously absorbed with bone marrow) on each smear and spread with a smooth glass rod. (Use a clean rod for each smear; do not use wooden applicator sticks.)
6. Place the slides (do not drain conjugate) in a petri dish with a wet paper towel in the top and incubate for 1 hr. at 37° C.
7. Rinse off in buffered saline solution and allow to soak for 10 min.
8. Rinse slides in distilled water and blot gently between two layers of bibulous paper.
9. Add 1 drop glycerin-buffered saline mounting fluid and apply a cover slip. Allow to stand for 5 min. and examine.
10. Use a previously prepared frozen slide as a positive control and use a smear of *Aerobacter cloacae* as a negative control (can be purchased in desiccated form*).
11. Read the slides with a microscope that has a dark-field condenser and a fluorescent light source. Organisms that have typical morphology

(capsular staining) and stain with a 3+ or 4+ fluorescence are reported as positive.

NOTE: Stained slides keep in the refrigerator for 1 mo. Air-fixed slides keep in the deep freeze for several months (6 or more). For details of mounting fluids and saline buffer, see method of fluorescent antibody identification of group A streptococci, p. 549.

The fluorescent method is particularly useful for the identification of gonococci in chronic cases.

Carbohydrate fermentation: A semisolid medium such as cystine trypticase agar,* to which 1% solutions of carbohydrates have been added, is the preferred medium. The carbohydrates are glucose, maltose, and sucrose. After surface inoculation the cultures are incubated for 48 hr. at 35° C. The fermentation of glucose only differentiates *N. gonorrhoeae* from other *Neisseria* (Table 11-6).

Instead of cystine trypticase agar, a medium can be used that contains semisolid agar enriched with 20% sterile bile-free acetic fluid and 1% solutions of the various carbohydrates.

Serologic diagnosis: Recently Hess et al.[50] described a much-needed indirect immunofluorescent method using formalin-fixed smears of *N. gonorrhoeae* for the demonstration of antigonococcal antibodies in acute gonococcal arthritis.

Meningococcus
(Neisseria meningitidis)

Meningococci are gram-negative diplococci with flattened adjacent sides that ferment glucose and maltose and are

---

*Difco Laboratories, Detroit, Mich.

*Baltimore Biological Laboratory, Baltimore, Md.

Table 11-6. Differentiation of *Neisseria*

	Sugar fermentation			Oxidase reaction
	Glucose	*Maltose*	*Sucrose*	
N. meningitidis	+	+	−	+
N. gonorrhoeae	+	−	−	+
N. catarrhalis	−	−	−	+
N. sicca and *N. flava*	+	+	+	+

+ = acid (yellow); − = no reaction.

morphologically similar to *N. gonor-rhoeae.*

LABORATORY DIAGNOSIS
Morphology

Smear: Obtain smear from spinal fluid sediment or from cultures of spinal fluid, sputum, and material from throat. Prepare spinal fluid smear as soon as specimen is received. The organism is an intracellular and extracellular gram-negative diplococcus. The positive-appearing smear must be confirmed by culture. (*Haemophilus influenzae* may be very pleomorphic.) The physician should be informed as soon as meningococci are suspected.

Culture: Use chocolate agar in a candle jar. The colonies are smooth, moist, gray, and mucoid. A moist atmosphere must be maintained.

The spinal fluid itself is a good culture medium and should be incubated at 35° C.

Inoculation of the yolk sac of an embryonated egg is a rapid culture method.

Oxidase test: This test is performed the same way as for *N. gonorrhoeae.*

Carbohydrate fermentation: Table 11-6 shows differentiating fermentation reactions of gram-negative diplococci. Inoculate semisolid cystine trypticase agar (CTA) slants containing 1% solutions of glucose, maltose, and sucrose.

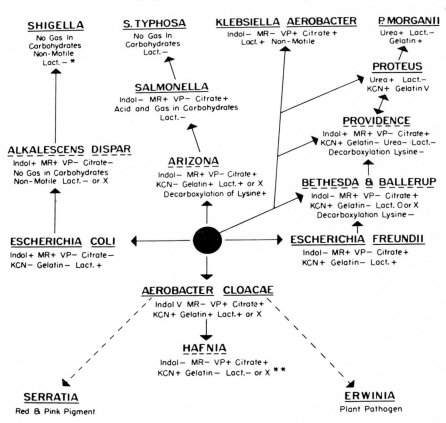

Fig. 11-5. Principal groups of Enterobacteriaceae. (From Smith and Conant: Zinsser bacteriology, New York, 1960, Appleton-Century-Crofts Co., Inc.)

Serologic tests: Polyvalent antisera* are available and should be used to confirm the diagnosis of meningococci by means of a slide test. If agglutination occurs in the polyvalent serum, repeat the test with antisera of meningococcal groups A to D. Slide agglutination sera may also be used for typing by capsular swelling. This procedure can be done directly on spinal fluid. There is some importance to the typing of meningococci because group A is usually associated with epidemics, while groups B and C are linked to sporadic cases.

GRAM-NEGATIVE AEROBIC NONSPORE-FORMING BACILLI

ENTERIC GRAM-NEGATIVE BACTERIA (ENTEROBACTERIACEAE)

The Enterobacteriaceae include (1) coliform organisms, e.g., *E. coli, Klebsiella-Enterobacter,* which are part of the normal flora of the intestinal tract; (2) pathogens, which include *Salmonella* and *Shigella*; and (3) some miscellaneous saprophytic to potentially pathogenic bacteria such as *Mimeae-Herellea, Hafnia, Citrobacter, Arizona,* and Bethesda-Ballerup groups (Fig. 11-5).

Coliform organisms are normally found in the intestinal tract; but outside the tract, in urine, blood, uterus, etc., they are pathogens. Certain forms are pathogenic if found in the intestinal tracts of infants.

Gram-negative bacteremia may rapidly lead to irreversible shock due to release of endotoxins (gram-negative bacteremic shock).[51, 52]

LABORATORY DIAGNOSIS

Collection of specimens: Collect fecal specimens in waxed boxes or preferably in GN broth or some other enrichment medium.

GN broth (Hajna) is a selective enrichment broth that accelerates the growth of *Shigella* and *Salmonella,* limits the growth of *Proteus* and coliform bacteria, and suppresses the growth of gram-positive bacteria.

Sachs buffered glycerol–sodium chloride

*Difco Laboratories, Detroit, Mich.

solution with added phenol red is an acceptable preservative for mailing stool specimens.

Sachs buffered glycerol–sodium chloride solution:

1. Sodium chloride, 4.2 gm.
2. Distilled water to make 700 ml.
3. Glycerol, 300 ml.
4. Dipotassium phosphate (anhydrous), 3.1 gm.
5. Monopotassium phosphate (anhydrous), 1 gm.

Technique: Dissolve sodium chloride in part of the water and make up to 700 ml. Add glycerol and phosphates. The phosphate concentration is about 0.025M. Determine the reaction, which should be pH 7.2. If necessary, adjust the pH with 0.1N HCl or 0.1N NaOH. Filter through paper and cotton. Dispense in 8-10 ml. amounts in the tubes or jars used in the outfits distributed for collection of fecal specimens. Cap loosely and autoclave for 40 min. After removing from the autoclave, allow jars or tubes to cool to 50°-60° C., fasten the caps or stoppers securely, and leave standing overnight in an inverted position. Discard leaky jars or tubes.

Prior to adding 1 gm. feces, add sufficient phenol red to give solution a pink color. Acid produced by coliform bacteria inhibits *Shigella*; therefore if indicator changes from pink to yellow during transport, the specimen is unsuitable for isolation of *Shigella*.

Direct smear: Prepare a gram stain from all liquid stools (hemorrhagic and mucoid particles) and from material submitted in preservative solution or in enrichment medium. Enteric bacteria are gram-negative, nonspore-forming, straight, plump, small rods. If the material is old, long filamentous forms may appear. Usually *E. coli* does not have a well-developed capsule. The appearance of the smear cannot be relied upon for distinction of enteric gram-negative rods, but the smear allows recognition of the normal flora and of the presence of staphylococci, yeast, and pus. The presence of much pus indicates shigellosis and contraindicates amebiasis (wet saline preparation). Candidiasis is suggested by budding yeast cells and pseudohyphae.

PRIMARY ISOLATION:

Fluid enrichment media: By inhibiting the growth of coliform bacteria, fluid enrichment media support the growth of *Salmonella* and *Shigella.* Suggested media are **GN broth (Hajna), tetrathionate broth,** or **selenite broth.** The latter, by means of buffers, maintains a neutral pH for 12-18 hr. after inoculation, at which pH it is toxic for enterococci but allows the growth of *Salmonella.* Emulsify 1 gm. feces (or 2-3 ml. liquid material) in 8-10 ml. broth. Mix and incubate at 35° C. for 18 hr. After incubation, streak a loopful on SS and Endo agar plates. Selenite broth is kept in the refrigerator and is discarded after 2 wk.

Plating media: Use at least three plates for each culture.

Blood agar: Blood agar serves for identification of **staphylococci** and **yeast.** Enteric gram-negative organisms grow aerobically and anaerobically on blood agar and produce shiny, convex, opaque colonies. *Pseudomonas* produces pigmented colonies and a fruity odor. Pigmentation is also characteristic of *Serratia* and *Flavobacterium.* **Blood agar with phenylethyl alcohol** suppresses gram-negative organisms, thus supporting the growth of staphylococci and streptococci.

SELECTIVE AND INHIBITORY MEDIA: Grouped on the basis of increasing inhibitory action, these are Endo agar, EMB agar, desoxycholate agar, MacConkey agar, and SS agar. They contain a red indicator dye and lactose to differentiate **lactose-fermenting from nonlactose-fermenting organisms.**

On Endo, MacConkey, EMB, and SS agar, almost all nonpathogenic enteric gram-negative organisms that ferment lactose produce red colonies, the color of which spreads into the surrounding medium. Almost all pathogenic enteric gram-negative rods are nonlactose-fermenting organisms and produce colorless colonies against a pink background.

On MacConkey agar, *E. coli* forms moist, smooth, flat, opaque colonies with a metallic sheen. *Klebsiella-Enterobacter* colonies are more mucoid, larger, are pink to red, and often have colorless borders. They sometimes string when touched with a straight wire. Young colonies of *Citrobacter* are usually colorless, but they may acquire color later. Colonies of *Shigella* and *Salmonella* are translucent, colorless, or delicate pink. *Proteus, Pseudomonas, Hafnia, Providencia, Mimeae-Herellea,* and *Alcaligenes faecalis* are also late or nonlactose fermenters, thus producing colorless colonies that may be mistaken for pathogens.

Endo agar: It slightly suppresses gram-positive organisms, but does not prevent *Proteus* from swarming.

MacConkey agar: It suppresses the swarming of *Proteus* and thus may be instrumental in the discovery of some colonies of *Shigella* which do not grow on SS agar and which may be lost in the swarming colonies of *Proteus* on Endo agar.

SS agar: This is a highly selective medium for *Shigella* and *Salmonella,* suppressing the growth of coliform bacteria and preventing *Proteus* from swarming by means of bile salts, citrates, and brilliant green. *Shigella* and *Salmonella* colonies are colorless and translucent, but *Salmonella* colonies may be black due to the production of H_2S and black sulfide salts. Lactose-fermenting organisms are colored red by the neutral red indicator. SS agar may suppress some strains of *Shigella.*

Bismuth sulfide agar: If typhoid fever is suspected on clinical grounds, bismuth sulfide agar should be included. Colonies of *S. typhosa* are flat, black (H_2S, black sulfide salt), and surrounded by a metallic halo.

Enrichment medium: After 18 hr. of incubation the enrichment broth should be plated lightly on the same media that are used for primary isolation, i.e., MacConkey (or EMB) agar and SS agar.

PRELIMINARY BIOCHEMICAL IDENTIFICATION:

Triple sugar iron agar slants (TSI): After 18 or 24 hr., only colorless or black colonies are transferred from MacConkey agar and SS agar to TSI agar. Touch the center of the colony with a straight wire (do not penetrate to the level of the agar, as only pure colonies must be transferred), streak the TSI slant, and stab the butt to a depth of 2 cm. Incubate at 35° C.

Table 11-7. Group differentiation of Enterobacteriaceae by biochemical tests (reactions of typical cultures)*

| | Salmonella-Arizona-Citrobacter | | | Shigella-Escherichia | | Klebsiella-Enterobacter-Serratia | | | | | Proteus-Providence | | | | |
	Salmonella group	Arizona group	Citrobacter group¹	Shigella group¹	Escherichia group	Klebsiella group	Enterobacter group	Hafnia group 37° C.	Hafnia group 22° C.	Serratia group	Proteus vulgaris	Proteus mirabilis	Proteus morganii	Proteus rettgeri	Providence group
Indole	-	-	-	d	+	-	-	-	-	-	+	-	+	+	+
Methyl red	+	+	+	+	+	-	-	+	-	-	+	+	+	+	+
Voges-Proskauer	-	-	-	-	-	+	+	d	+	+	-	d	-	-	-
Simmons citrate	+	+	+	-	-	+	+	d	+	+	d	d	-	+	+
H₂S (TSI agar)	+	+	+	-	-	-	-	(+)	-	- or (+)	+	+	-	-	-
Urease	-	-	-	-	-	(+)	d	-	-	-	+	+	+	+	-
KCN	-	-	+	-	-	+	+	+	+	+	+	+	+	+	+
Motility	+	+	+	-	+	-	+	d	+	+	+	+	+	+	+
Gelatin	-	(+)	-	-	-	-	d	-	-	+	+	+	-	-	-
Lysine decarboxylase	+	+	-	-	+	+	d	+	+	+	-	-	-	-	-
Phenylalanine deaminase	-	-	-	-	-	-	-	-	-	-	+	+	+	+	+
Gas from glucose	+	+	+	-†	+	+	+	d	+	d	+	+	+	d	d
Lactose	-	+ or ×	+ or ×	-†	+ or ×	+	+ or ×	×	×	- or ×	-	-	-	d	-
Sucrose	-	-	d	-†	d	+	+	×	×	+	+	×	d	d	d
Mannitol	+	+	+	d	+	+	+	+	+	+	-	-	-	+	d
Dulcitol	+²	-	d	d	d	d	-	-	-	-	-	-	-	-	-
Salicin	-	-	d	-	d	+	d	d	d	+	+	d	-	d	-
Adonitol	-	-	-	-	-	+	d	-	-	d	-	-	-	+	d
Inositol	d	-	- or ×	-	-	+	d	-	-	d	-	-	-	+	d

*Courtesy Dr. P. R. Edwards and Dr. W. H. Ewing, Communicable Disease Center, Atlanta, Ga.

¹Formerly *Escherichia freundii*.

²*Salmonella typhi, Salmonella pullorum, Salmonella paratyphi* A, *Salmonella choleraesuis*, and a few others do not ferment dulcitol promptly.

†Certain biotypes of *Shigella flexneri* 6 produce gas; *Shigella sonnei* cultures ferment lactose and sucrose slowly.

+ = positive; - = negative; × = late and irregularly positive; d = different biochemical types; (+) = gelatin liquefied slowly, urea hydrolyzed slowly, or hydrogen sulfide produced slowly and in small amounts.

and examine after 18-24 hr. The screw caps of the TSI tubes must allow air to enter so as to prevent erroneous results.[53]

TSI agar contains 1% lactose, 1% sucrose, 0.1% glucose, ferrous sulfate, and phenol red as indicator. All Enterobacteriaceae ferment glucose, but not all ferment lactose or sucrose, and some ferment lactose only gradually.

The combination of urea agar and TSI medium allows rapid identification of *Proteus* species in group 2 and 3 TSI reactions (Fig. 11-6). *Proteus* produces a pink color in the urea medium within 2-4 hr. by virtue of its urease (Table 11-8 and p. 568).

Reactions on TSI agar:
1. Fermentation of glucose only (by nonlactose- and nonsucrose-fermenting organisms) produces acid

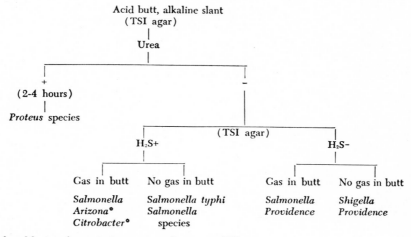

*Delayed lactose fermentation may not show up on TSI agar.

Fig. 11-6. Presumptive identification of group 2 and 3 TSI reactions on basis of combined use of urea and TSI media. (From Bailey and Scott: Diagnostic microbiology, St. Louis, 1966, The C. V. Mosby Co.)

Table 11-8. Presumptive identification of organisms on basis of 18-24 hr. culture on TSI agar

Reaction			Production of		Carbohydrates fermented			
Group	Slant	Butt	Gas (CO₂)	H₂S	Glucose	Lactose	Sucrose	Possible organisms
1	Acid	Acid	+	–	+	+	+	E. coli, Klebsiella-Aerobacter (Enterobacter), Proteus-Providence, Hafnia
2	Alkaline	Acid	+	+	+	–	–	Proteus, Salmonella, Arizona, Citrobacter
3	Alkaline	Acid	–	–	+	–	–	Shigella, S. typhosa,* Proteus-Providence, Salmonella, Alkalescans-Dispar
4	Acid	Acid	+	+	+	+	+	Arizona, Citrobacter
5	Alkaline	Alkaline	–	–	–	–	–	Alcaligenes, Pseudomonas, Mimeae-Herellae

*S. typhosa produces a small amount of H₂S, but no gas.

Table 11-9. Differentiation of principal divisions within Enterobacteriaceae by biochemical methods (reactions of typical cultures)[*]

Substrate or test	Shigella-Escherichia division	Salmonella-Arizona-Citrobacter division	Klebsiella-Aerobacter-Serratia division	Proteus-Providence division
Indole	d	–	–	d
Methyl red	+	+	–	+
Voges-Proskauer	–	–	+	–
Simmons citrate	–	+	+	d
Hydrogen sulfide (TSI)	–	+	– or (+)	d
Urease	–	–	– or (+)	+ or –
KCN	–	d	+	+
Phenylalanine deaminase	–	–	–	+

[*]From Ewing and Edwards: The principal divisions and groups of Enterobacteriaceae and their differentiation, Atlanta, 1962, U. S. Department of Health, Education, and Welfare, Public Health Service, Communicable Disease Center.

Note: *S. typhi, S. paratyphi A,* and some of the rare types are citrate negative. *S. paratyphi A* and other rare types are H_2S negative. *P. mirabilis* may be Voges-Proskauer positive.

+ = positive in 1 or 2 days; – = negative; (+) = delayed positive; d = different biochemical types.

throughout the medium (yellow) at first (12 hr.); but as soon as the small amount of glucose (0.1%) is used up, oxidation at the surface of the slant leads to neutralization of the acid so that the final results, after about 24 hr., is an acid butt (yellow) and alkaline slant (red).

2. Fermentation of lactose and sucrose produces enough acid throughout the medium to maintain butt and slant yellow. Some bacteria that ferment lactose slowly can nevertheless metabolize sucrose readily so that they still produce enough acid to maintain butt and slant yellow.

3. Fermentation of sucrose only does not produce enough acid to change the pH of the entire medium so that the butt turns yellow but the slant changes to red.

4. If none of the three sugars is fermented, the butt and slant become alkaline (red).

5. Gas-forming organisms produce gas bubbles in the butt which are evident on inspection if the butt has been carefully stabbed.

6. Hydrogen sulfide production leads to blackening of the butt.

TSI is a poor medium by which to judge H_2S production because the medium is deficient in sulfhydryl groups and contains ferrous sulfate as indicator, which is less sensitive than lead acetate paper.

DEFINITE IDENTIFICATION OF BACTERIA PREVIOUSLY GROUPED ON THE BASIS OF THEIR TSI REACTIONS: In general, bacteria should be identified by their biochemical and serologic pattern (Table 11-9). The serologic reactions should be strong and rapid to exclude weak and delayed nonspecific cross-reactions. If carbohydrate solutions are not obtained commercially, they should be sterilized by Seitz filtration.

ESCHERICHIA COLI

These organisms are gram-negative rods that ferment lactose with the production of acid and gas. Most strains are motile and the motility improves at lower temperatures. They are indole and methyl red positive and Voges-Proskauer and citrate negative. Sixty-two percent ferment salicin and 80% are lysine decarboxylase positive (Table 11-10). Most strains ferment lactose (acid and gas) promptly and must be differentiated from the *Klebsiella-Enterobacter* group by the use of malonate broth and the IMViC reaction. *E. coli* leaves malonate broth unchanged (green), while *Klebsiella-Enterobacter* turns it blue. If *E. coli* orga-

Table 11-10. *Shigella-Escherichia division**

Substrate or test	Shigella group	Escherichia group
Gas from glucose	−†	+ (−)
Lactose	−†	+ or ×
Salicin	−	d (approx. 62% +)
Motility	−	+ (−)
Lysine decarboxylase	−	+
Ornithine decarboxylase	−†	+ or −
Mucate	−	+ (−)
Christensen citrate	−	+ (−)
Sodium acetate agar	−	+

*From Ewing and Edwards: The principal divisions and groups of Enterobacteriaceae and their differentiation, Atlanta, 1962, U. S. Department of Health, Education, and Welfare, Public Health Service, Communicable Disease Center.

†Certain biotypes of *S. flexneri* 6 form gas. *S. sonnei* cultures ferment lactose slowly and decarboxylate ornithine.

Note: There is no difficulty in the differentiation of typical *E. coli* cultures and shigellae. However, the anaerogenic nonmotile varieties of *E. coli,* some of which are often referred to as *Alkalescens-Dispar* types, may require closer examination before they can be definitely classified as *E. coli.* In attempting to classify a particular strain as *E. coli* or as a member of the *Shigella* group, the biochemical reactivities of the culture should be considered as a whole. Shigellae are much less reactive than *E. coli* strains and a culture that produces acid promptly (i.e., within 24 hr.) from all or most of a wide variety of carbohydrates such as maltose, rhamnose, xylose, sorbitol, and dulcitol undoubtedly is not a member of the *Shigella* group.

+ = positive in 1 or 2 days; − = negative; + (−) = majority of strains positive but negative varieties occur; × = late and irregularly positive; d = different biochemical types.

nisms are slow lactose fermenters, they may produce an acid butt and alkaline slant on TSI and be confused with *Proteus* and *Shigella. Proteus* is urea and phenylalanine deaminase positive, while *E. coli* is negative. *Shigella* may be agglutinable with *Shigella* antiserum and will ferment salicin and decarboxylate lysine (Table 11-10). However, the anaerogenic nonmotile varieties of *E. coli,* referred to as *Alkalescens-Dispar,* may require more detailed examination and agglutination by antiserum to *Alkalescens-Dispar* O antigen.

IMViC reactions

When it is necessary to differentiate *Escherichia* from other coliform organisms, the use of four tests designated by the mnemonic formula IMViC (indole, methyl red, Voges-Proskauer, and citrate reactions) is indicated (Fig. 11-7). However, in practice the performance of only one test, e.g., the indole test, may be sufficient. Test tablets are commercially available for all these procedures.* The tablets are handled with sterile forceps, dissolved in sterile distilled water, and the solution of distilled water and dissolved tablets is then inoculated.

PRINCIPLES AND TECHNIQUES OF IMViC REACTIONS:

Indole production:

Principle: In the presence of oxygen some bacteria are able to split tryptophan into indole and alpha-aminopropri-

---

*Key Scientific Products Co., Los Angeles, Calif.

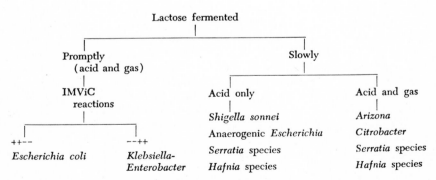

Fig. 11-7. Differentiation of lactose-fermenting Enterobacteriaceae. (From Bailey and Scott: Diagnostic microbiology, St. Louis, 1966, The C. V. Mosby Co.)

onic acid. The presence of indole can be proved by the addition of **Ehrlich** or **Kovac reagents** (*p*-dimethylaminobenzaldehyde), which produce a red color and are soluble in ether, chloroform, and alcohol.

Kovac reagent:
1. *p*-Dimethylaminobenzaldehyde, 5 gm.
2. Amyl alcohol, 75 ml.
3. Concentrated HCl, 25 ml.

Mix alcohol and aldehyde and heat in water bath at 50° or 60° C. until aldehyde is dissolved. Cool and slowly add the HCl. Store in stoppered brown bottle in the dark.

Technique: Add 0.5 ml. Kovac reagent to 3 ml. of a 2-day-old peptone water culture (must contain tryptophan). Use as controls an uninoculated broth tube, one inoculated with *E. coli,* and one inoculated with *Salmonella typhosa.* Red color, indole positive; no change, indole negative.

Salmonella and *Klebsiella* are indole negative, while *Proteus* and *E. coli* are indole positive.

Voges-Proskauer (acetoin) reaction and methyl red test:

Principle: One of the intermediary products of the anaerobic breakdown of glucose (Embden-Meyerhoff pathway) is the production of pyruvic acid. Some bacteria are able to condense pyruvic acid into acetoin (acetylmethylcarbinol), while other bacteria metabolize pyruvic acid to lactic and acetic acids, producing a strongly acid reaction of the medium. As both tests are based on glucose metabolism, the same 3-day-old peptone-dextrose-phosphate broth is used.

Voges-Proskauer reaction:

Principle: Acetoin is oxidized by the addition of alkali to diacetyl, which gives a pink color.

Technique: One half of a 3-day-old peptone-dextrose-phosphate culture is mixed well with equal amounts of 10% KOH. Let stand at room temperature for 1 hr. Pink color, positive; no change, negative.

Salmonella and *Shigella* are Voges-Proskauer negative; *Klebsiella-Enterobacter* and *Proteus* are Voges-Proskauer positive.

Methyl red test: This test depends on the strongly acid reaction of the medium.

Technique: To the other half of the peptone-dextrose-phosphate culture add 2 or 3 drops of methyl red (methyl red, 0.1 gm.; ethyl alcohol, 300 ml.; H_2O to 500 ml.). Red color, positive; yellow color, negative.

E. coli is methyl red positive; *Klebsiella-Enterobacter* is methyl red negative.

Citrate utilization:

Principle: Some organisms are able to use citrate as the only source of carbohydrates. These organisms quickly use up the citrate and metabolize the proteins in the medium, releasing NH_4 which changes the pH of the medium from acid to alkaline. In the case of slower acting bacteria the citrate is used up slowly and spares the protein so that no ammonia is released. *Klebsiella-Enterobacter* and some *Salmonella* are able to grow in this medium and to metabolize citrate and therefore are citrate positive. In Simmons citrate agar, citrate-positive bacteria produce an alkaline pH and a change from green to blue. *E. coli, Shigella, S. typhosa,* and *S. paratyphi* do not grow in citrate agar, and Simmons medium therefore remains unchanged (green).

Technique: Inoculate medium by stab and streak.

Serology

The coliform bacteria possess a somatic O, capsular K, and Vi antigen, and if motile, also an H flagellar antigen. The capsular K antigen occurs in three varieties—L, B, and A—and interferes with O agglutination.

The **antigen** O is not inactivated by heat (120° C. for 1 hr.). The **K antigen** is inactivated by heat and inhibits O agglutination of the living organism. Boiling at 100° C. for 1 hr. destroys the L and B antigens, while boiling at 121° C. for 2½ hr. is necessary to destroy the A antigen. The **H antigen** is inactivated by heating to 100° C. for 1 hr.

Enteropathogenic Escherichia coli (EPEC)[54]

Enterocolitis in newborn infants and in children under 2 yr. of age may be produced by a group of *E. coli* called enteropathogenic *E. coli* (EPEC). They may also be found in pregnant women.

LABORATORY DIAGNOSIS

Enteropathogenic *E. coli* cannot be differentiated from nonpathogenic *E. coli* biochemically, but they can be identified antigenically. They are nonhemolytic and ferment sorbitol. In infants they are usually present in pure culture, whereas only a small number is found in carriers and convalescents.

SEROLOGIC INVESTIGATION: EPEC can be typed by multivalent and specific antisera. The most common offenders fall into groups arbitrarily labeled 055:B5, 0111:B4, and 0127:B8. All enteropathogenic *E. coli* are of the B capsular type. They share O and B antigens with nonpathogenic *E. coli* types and both O and B antigens must be determined.

PRESUMPTIVE IDENTIFICATION:

Slide agglutination test for enteropathogenic E. coli: Suspend material from five colonies in 0.5 ml. normal saline solution.

On a slide mix 1 standard loopful (2.5 mm. in diameter) of suspension with an equal amount of polyvalent OB antisera A, B,* etc. Spread the mixture over 1 cm.² area.

Include phenolized saline solution* as a negative control.

The agglutination must be complete and rapid. Weak cross-reactions may be given by *Citrobacter, Salmonella, Providence,* and bile salts. Dextrose may also interfere with the agglutination. In case of agglutination, reexamine a single colony with the OB antiserum indicated.

FINAL IDENTIFICATION: Test colony with group-specific OB antisera.

Fluorescent antibody method for identification of enteropathogenic E. coli[55]: Initial screening is performed by using two pools of fluorescent antibody sera, e.g., Bacto-FTA *E. coli* Poly A and B.* Positive and negative controls are also included.

Technique: Rehydrate FTA *E. coli* Poly A and B with 5 ml. FTA buffer per vial

(for buffer, see p. 680). Prepare bacterial smears, air dry, and fix by passing through flame. Place drop of desired FTA *E. coli* globulins on slide. Distribute evenly with glass rod, place slide in a petri dish containing moistened absorbent paper in the top half, and allow to stand 3 min. at room temperature.

Rinse with FTA buffer and place in buffer-filled Coplin jar for 10 min. with two changes. Blot slides gently between layers of bibulous paper. Apply a drop of FTA mounting fluid (see p. 681) and add cover slip. Examine under fluorescent microscope with ultraviolet light for fluorescent *E. coli* cells.

CITROBACTER GROUP (ESCHERICHIA FREUNDII)

The organisms in this group are gram-negative motile rods that are generally lactose fermenting. The colonies on Mac-Conkey agar may be colorless to pale pink, produce H_2S, grow on Simmons citrate, and are indole negative, methyl red positive, and Voges-Proskauer negative. They may have to be distinguished from *Arizona, Salmonella,* and possibly *Proteus.* The **negative lysine decarboxylase reaction** and **growth in KCN broth** distinguish these organisms from *Arizona* and *Salmonella.* The negative urease test distinguishes them from *Proteus.*

BETHESDA-BALLERUP GROUP

The organisms in this group are related to the *Citrobacter* group and are gram-negative rods that are nonmotile and form colorless colonies on MacConkey agar. On TSI agar they produce a *Salmonella*-like pattern (alkaline slant, acid butt, H_2S). Clinically, they are harmless and therefore must be differentiated from *Salmonella.* The Bethesda-Ballerup group has most of the characteristics of the *Citrobacter* group. **The organisms grow in KCN medium and are lysine decarboxylase negative,** while salmonellae give converse reactions. A polyvalent antiserum* is available for serologic identification. There may be serologic cross-reactions with *Salmonella* typing sera (O and Vi).

---

*Difco Laboratories, Detroit, Mich.

*Difco Laboratories, Detroit, Mich.

Table 11-11. *Salmonella-Arizona-Citrobacter* division*

Substrate or test	Salmonella group	Arizona group	Citrobacter group
Lactose	–	+ or ×	+ or ×
Dulcitol	+	–	d
Gelatin	–	(+)	–
KCN	–	–	+
Lysine decarboxylase	+	+	–
Arginine dihydrolase	– or (+)	– or (+)	(+)
Ornithine decarboxylase	+	+	– or +
Malonate	–	+	–

*From Ewing and Edwards: The principal divisions and groups of Enterobacteriaceae and their differentiation, Atlanta, 1962, U. S. Department of Health, Education, and Welfare, Public Health Service, Communicable Disease Center.

Note: The majority of salmonellae ferment dulcitol promptly, but S. *typhi*, S. *pullorum*, S. *paratyphi* A, S. *cholerae-suis*, and a few others do not do so. Members of the *Arizona* group are uniformly negative on this substrate. S. *paratyphi* A is lysine negative. S. *typhi* is ornithine negative.

+ = positive in 1 or 2 days; – = negative; (+) = delayed positive; × = late and irregularly positive; d = different biochemical types; – or + = majority of strains negative but positive varieties occur.

ALKALESCENS-DISPAR GROUP

These organisms are nonmotile gram-negative anaerogenic bacteria related to *E. coli*. On MacConkey, SS, and TSI agars they are similar to *Shigella* but can be differentiated by the use of antisera.*

PROTEUS-PROVIDENCE GROUP
Proteus

Proteus vulgaris is part of the normal intestinal flora. *Proteus morganii* may cause summer diarrhea in children (food infection). Outside the intestinal tract, both are pathogens and are often resistant to treatment.

LABORATORY DIAGNOSIS
Morphology

Proteus organisms are motile, gram-negative rods that vary somewhat in size and thickness (hence the name). On blood agar the colonies often swarm, forming a thin transparent veil with an undulating periphery. They produce an ammoniacal odor and at times hemolysis. Strains lacking the H antigen do not swarm (are not motile). The swarming of the motile forms can be inhibited by increasing the agar concentration to 5-8% or by incorporating chloral hydrate or phenylethyl alcohol. McConkey agar and the more inhibitory enteric selective

*Difco Laboratories, Detroit, Mich.

media such as SS and bismuth sulfite agar also suppress swarming.

Biochemical reactions

Some *Proteus* organisms liquefy gelatin and are nonlactose fermenters, but they usually ferment glucose and may or may not produce H_2S. They are variably aerogenic and anaerogenic and hence on TSI may be confused with *Salmonella* and *Shigella*. They produce an enzyme called urease, which hydrolyses urea. *Salmonella* and *Shigella* are urease negative (Table 11-12).

Urease test:

Principle: Urea hydrolysis produces ammonium carbonate which shifts the neutral pH of the Christensen urea agar to the alkaline side, as evidenced by the red color of the phenol red indicator.

$$H_2NC = NH_2 + 2H_2O \xrightarrow{\text{Urease}} 2NH_3 + CO_2$$
$$\underset{\text{Urea}}{\overset{\|}{O}}$$

Technique: Streak slant. *Proteus* produces hydrolysis within 3 hr., as evidenced by a pink-red color. The *Klebsiella-Enterobacter* group gives a delayed (18 hr.) reaction. PathoTec* test papers may also be used to prove the presence of urease.

*Warner-Chilcott Laboratories Division, Warner-Lambert Pharmaceutical Co., Morris Plains, N. J.

Table 11-12. *Proteus-Providence* division*

Substrate or test	Proteus group				Providence group	
	vulgaris	*mirabilis*	*morganii*	*rettgeri*	Subgroup A	Subgroup B
Indole	+	–	+	+	+	+
Voges-Proskauer						
37° C.	–	–	–	–	–	–
22° C.	– or +	+ or –	–	–	–	–
Simmons citrate	d	d	–	+	+	+
Hydrogen sulfide (TSI)	+	+	–	–	–	–
Urease	+	+	+	+	–	–
Gelatin—22° C.	+	+	–	–	–	–
Lysine decarboxylase	–	–	–	–	–	–
Arginine dihydrolase	–	–	–	–	–	–
Ornithine decarboxylase	–	+	+	–	–	–
Gas from glucose	+	+	+	– or +	+	–
Mannitol	–	–	–	+	–	d
Adonitol	–	–	–	+	+	–
Inositol	–	–	–	+	–	+
Maltose	+	–	–	–	–	– or +

*From Ewing and Edwards: The principal divisions and groups of Enterobacteriaceae and their differentiation, Atlanta, 1962, U. S. Department of Health, Education, and Welfare, Public Health Service, Communicable Disease Center.

Note: Gas volumes formed from glucose are relatively small (a bubble to about 15%).

+ = positive in 1 or 2 days; – = negative, no reaction; d = different biochemical types; – or + = majority of strains negative but positive varieties occur; + or – = majority of cultures positive but negative varieties occur.

Phenylalanine deaminase test:

Principle: The *Proteus-Providence* group produces the enzyme phenylalanine deaminase which, in the presence of oxygen, removes alanine groups from L-phenylalanine, resulting in the formation of phenylpyruvic acid, which with ferric iron produces a gray-brown compound. PathoTec test papers give results in 5-10 min. A micromethod is available.

Micromethod: Transfer a single colony (enter only the dome of the colony) to 0.3 ml. 0.2% aqueous L-phenylalanine. Incubate at 35° C. for 10 min. and add 2 drops 8% FeCl₃ solution. Immediate development of a green color indicates a positive test (conversion of substrate to phenylpyruvic acid).

As *Proteus mirabilis* responds to penicillin, *Proteus* groups should either be identified or penicillin disks should be included in the sensitivity test.

Serology

Proteus OX-19, OXK, and OX-2 are agglutinated by sera from patients with rickettsial diseases (**Weil-Felix reaction**), probably due to a common antigen.

Providence

These organisms are gram-negative motile rods that do not ferment lactose. On TSI they may ferment glucose, but fail to produce H₂S; if they do not produce gas, they resemble *Shigella*. They are urease negative and differ from *Shigella* by growing on Simmons citrate and by being motile and phenylalanine deaminase positive.

PSEUDOMONAS

Pseudomonas aeruginosa may be found in small numbers in the normal intestinal flora, but it may assume pathogenic proportions if patients are on antibiotic therapy. It may be cultured from wounds (blue-green pus), ears, bile, diarrheic stool in children, and urine. It is important because of its resistance to treatment and its tendency to attack debilitated patients.

Pseudomonas species are gram-negative rods that move by means of polar flagellae (they do not belong to the Enterobacteriaceae) and may have some tendency to swarm. They are catalase and oxidase positive. They do not ferment sugar (glucose) but produce carbohydrate breakdown by **oxidation,** thus producing gluconic acid, but no gas. Oxidation is utilization, not fermentation.[56] To determine whether the carbohydrate is broken down by oxidation (O) or fermentation (F), an OF medium is used.

LABORATORY DIAGNOSIS
Morphology

Culture: On blood agar two types of colonies may be found. Usually they are moist, flat, gray, and shiny, but they may also be dry with scalloped edges. They produce a sweetish aromatic odor and a greenish fluorescence that extends into the surrounding agar. Beta hemolysis is also seen. The water-soluble greenish fluorescent color develops better at room temperature and on exposure to sunlight. The pigment formation depends on the medium (see differential diagnosis). The tendency to swarm, which interferes with colony counts of urinary specimens, can be suppressed by media deficient in sodium chloride and other salts.[57]

They produce diffuse turbidity in broth.

On TSI agar they produce a neutral or alkaline reaction and flat shiny colonies. They have to be separated from the similarly biochemically inactive Achromobacteraceae, which includes the genera *Alcaligenes, Achromobacter,* and *Flavobacterium* (see discussion of differential diagnosis).

Biochemical identification

Oxidase tests:

Kovacs test: Place a 6 cm.[2] piece of Whatman No. 1 filter paper in a petri dish and then place 2 or 3 drops 1% liquid solution tetramethyl-*p*-phenylenediamine dihydrochloride on the center of the paper. The test colony is removed with a platinum loop and streaked onto the reagent-impregnated paper. The colony turns dark purple in 5-10 sec. if the reaction is positive, i.e., if *Pseudomonas* is present.

Cytochrome oxidase test (p-aminodimethylaniline oxalate test):
Reagent:
1. Alpha-naphthol (1%) in ethyl alcohol (96%)
2. Aqueous solution of *p*-aminodimethylaniline oxalate (1%)

Mix by gently tapping.

Technique: Ewing and Johnson suggest the following procedure: Spread 2-3 drops of reagent over an 18 hr. culture. Within 30 sec. (time is critical) *Pseudomonas* colonies take on a blue color.

One drop of reagent may also be applied to filter paper. One colony is rubbed into the reagent spot, and if the organism is *Pseudomonas,* an immediate blue color develops.

PathoTec test papers: An oxidase test paper is available.*

Urease test: Most *Pseudomonas* species contain slowly acting urease (see discussion of *Proteus*).

Nitrate reduction test: *Pseudomonas* rapidly reduce nitrates to nitrites and to gaseous nitrogen.

Principle: The reduction of nitrates (NO_3) leads to the formation of nitrites (NO_2) and may progress to liberation of nitrogen (N).

In test 1 the medium is examined for the presence of nitrites. If none are present, test 2 is performed to discover residual nitrates. If none are found, it can be assumed that the reduction of the nitrates has proceeded beyond the nitrite stage.

Reagents:
1. Sulfanilic acid:
    Sulfanilic acid, 8 gm.
    Acetic acid (5N),† 1000 ml.
2. Alpha-naphthylamine:
    Alpha-naphthylamine, 5 gm.
    Acetic acid (5N),† 1000 ml.

Indole nitrite medium (contains nitrate), nitrate agar, and the reagents listed are commercially available.‡

Test 1: Inoculate nitrate broth (must be free of nitrites) with pure culture and incubate at 35° C. for 12-24 hr. To 10 ml. culture broth add 0.2 ml. sulfanilic acid and 0.2-0.3 ml. alpha-naphthylamine in drops. A red color indicates nitrites. The pH of the medium must be acid. A control test must be performed on the uninoculated broth.

Test 2: Reduce residual nitrate to ni-

---

*Warner-Chilcott Laboratories Division, Warner-Lambert Pharmaceutical Co., Morris Plains, N. J.
†Glacial acetic acid, 290 ml.; distilled water to 1000 ml.
‡Baltimore Biological Laboratory, Baltimore, Md.

trite with a reducing agent such as zinc dust and repeat the nitrite test. The presence of nitrate can also be proved by the addition of 1 drop diphenylamine H_2SO_4 reagent (1 crystal of diphenylamine in 1 drop of H_2SO_4). Blue color development indicates nitrates. Pure nitrogen can sometimes be seen as gas bubbles.

Interpretation: Test 1 detects nitrate-positive organisms that reduce nitrate to nitrite but do not go any further; therefore no gas appears. Nitrate-negative organisms fail to reduce nitrate and therefore no red color or gas appears. Test 2 will confirm the presence of unreduced nitrate.

Nitrite-positive organisms reduce nitrate to nitrite and then progress to break down nitrite to liberate ammonia or nitrogen; thus gas bubbles may be seen. If the utilization of nitrate and nitrite is complete, tests 1 and 2 will be negative except for gas formation.

DIFFERENTIAL DIAGNOSIS OF PSEUDOMONAS

Nonpigmented *Pseudomonas* must be differentiated from *Alcaligenes, Mimeae, Herellea, Achromobacter, Flavobacterium,* and *Aeromonas.*

The following criteria may be used (Table 11-13): pigment production, OF medium and motility, Sellers agar, phenol red agar with 10% lactose, phenol red agar with 10% glucose, nitrate reduction, and citrate utilization.

Pigment production

The pigment production of *Pseudomonas,* which is often absent on routine media, can be stimulated by "Tech"* medium to enhance pyocyanin production and by "Flo"* medium to enhance fluorescein production.[58] The addition of Cetrimide[59] (cetyl trimethyl ammonium chloride) to "Tech" medium (Pseudogel agar*) renders this medium selective for *P. aeruginosa* by inhibition of other organisms.

Mimeae and Herellea[60]

These organisms are found in the intestinal tract but may also be cultured from the vagina, skin, or respiratory system.

They are small, blunt-ended gram-negative coccobacilli and rods that form low, gray, smooth, nonhemolytic, foul-smelling colonies resembling enteric colonies on blood agar. TSI reaction shows a neutral or alkaline slant and a neutral butt. They are relatively inert fermentatively and oxidatively and are catalase positive. *Mimeae* and *Herellea* grow on EMB and MacConkey agar and can thus be distinguished from *Neisseria,* which does not grow on these media. The gram stain reveals gram-negative diplococci, diplobacilli, and occasional small rods and filaments; the diplococcic forms resemble *Neisseria.*

Lack of motility and fluorescence and the absence of nitrate reduction differentiate both organisms from *Pseudomonas.*

Some strains of *Mimeae* are oxidase positive and, because of the appearance of the gram stain, may suggest *Neisseria.* They do not utilize carbohydrates, either fermentatively or oxidatively.

---

*Baltimore Biological Laboratory, Baltimore, Md.

Table 11-13. Differentiation of cultures giving group V TSI reactions

	Pseudomonas	*Flavobacterium*	*Alcaligenes*	*Achromobacter*	*Mimeae*	*Herellea*
Pigment	Blue-green	Tan	–	–	–	–
Motility	+	Variable	Variable	Variable	–	–
10% glucose oxidation	±	–	–	–	–	+ (Acid)
10% lactose oxidation	–	–	–	–	–	+ (Acid)
Nitrate reduction	+	–	Variable	–	–	–
Oxidase	+	+	Delayed	–	Variable	–
Citrate utilization	+	–	+	+	0	+

Herellea is oxidase negative and utilizes carbohydrates by oxidation, not by fermentation.

OF medium with glucose and Sellers medium are helpful in identifying *Pseudomonas, Mimeae,* and *Herellea.*

OF basal medium*: *P. aeruginosa* can be differentiated from the other genera mentioned by the production of an oxidative reaction in OF basal medium (oxidation-fermentation medium) of Hugh and Leifson (Table 11-14).

Technique: Inoculate two tubes of each medium from a young agar slant culture to be tested. Stab the media once with a straight needle, penetrating almost to the bottom of the agar. Cover one tube of each pair with a 4-5 mm. layer of sterile mineral oil or melted petrolatum. Incubate the tubes for 48 hr. or longer. Record "acid," "acid and gas production," or "no change in color" (and pH). Also record whether or not the organism is

*Baltimore Biological Laboratory, Baltimore, Md.

motile, i.e., whether the organism has grown only along the line of inoculation or whether it has grown out away from the line of inoculation. Comparisons with uninoculated control tubes should be made (Table 11-14).

Changes in covered agar are considered due to true fermentation, while changes in the open tubes are due to oxidative utilization of the carbohydrates present. If the carbohydrate is not utilized by either method, there is no acid production in either tube.

Controls:
Oxidation: *Pseudomonas* (oxidizer, nonfermenter)
Fermentation: *E. coli* (fermenter, aerogenic)
Inactive: *Alcaligenes faecalis* (nonoxidizer, nonfermenter)

Sellers agar* [61]: It is a differential medium for identification of nonfermentative gram-negative bacilli that do not acidify TSI agar.

Technique: Just before inoculation add 0.15 ml. or 2 drops of a sterile 50% aqueous solution of dextrose by letting it run down the glass opposite the slant. Inoculate Sellers agar slants by stabbing into the butt and streaking the slant. Incubate for 24 hr. at 35° C. and examine. Typical reactions are listed in Table 11-15. Some *Pseudomonas* cultures may require incubation for 2 days to produce a typically alkaline reaction in the butt. The yellow band reaction, due to oxidation of the added dextrose, may disappear after 24 hr.

Under ultraviolet light only the *Pseudo-*

*Baltimore Biological Laboratory, Baltimore, Md.

Table 11-14. Reactions in OF basal medium

	Open	Covered	Motility
Pseudomonas	Acid*	–	+
Alcaligenes	–	–	+
Mimeae	–	–	–
Herellea	Acid	–	–
Shigella	Acid	Acid	–
Salmonella	Acid + Gas	Acid + Gas	+

*Yellow.

Table 11-15. Reactions on Sellers agar

	Pseudomonas aeruginosa	Mima polymorpha	Herellea	Alcaligenes
Slant				
Fluorescence	+	–	–	–
Blue color	–	+	+	+
Yellow band				
Dextrose oxidized	–	–	+	–
Butt				
Alkaline (blue)	+	–	–	±
Anaerobic growth	+	–	–	+
Nitrogen				
Gas produced	+	–	–	+

Table 11-16. *Klebsiella-Aerobacter-Serratia* division*

Substrate or test	Klebsiella group	Aerobacter group Sub-group A	Sub-group B	Hafnia group 37° C.	Hafnia group 22° C.	Aerobacter group Subgroup C 37° C.	22° C.	Serratia group
Gas from glucose	+	+	+	+	+	+	+	d
Gas from inositol	+	–	+	–	–	+	+	–
Gas from glycerol	+	–	+	+	+	d	(+)	–
Gas from cellobiose	+	+	+	+	+	d	(+)	–
Sorbitol	+	+	+	–	–	+	+	+
Raffinose	+	+	+	–	–	+	+	+
Lysine decarboxylase	+	–	+	+	+	d	+	+
Arginine dihydrolase	–	+	–	–	–	–	–	–
Ornithine decarboxylase	–	+	+	+	+	+	+	+
Gelatin—22° C.	–	(+)	×		–		+	+
Motility	–	+	+	d	+	+	+	+

*From Ewing and Edwards: The principal divisions and groups of Enterobacteriaceae and their differentiation, Atlanta, 1962, U. S. Department of Health, Education, and Welfare, Public Health Service, Communicable Disease Center.

Note: When gas is formed from glucose by *Serratia*, the volumes are small (10% or less). *Aerobacter* subgroup A corresponds to *Aerobacter cloacae*; subgroup B corresponds to *Aerobacter aerogenes*; subgroup C corresponds to *Aerobacter liquefaciens* (a psychrophilic bacterium).

+ = positive in 1 or 2 days; – = negative; (+) = delayed positive; × = late and irregular positive; d = different biochemical types.

---

monas fluoresces, the fluorescein production being stimulated by the magnesium sulfate and mannitol present.

Achromobacter species[62]

These species are gram-negative rods that are sometimes motile, are nonchromogenic, and are saprophytes of soil and water.

Alcaligenes faecalis

This organism, though found in stool, does not belong to the Enterobacteriaceae, but rather to the Achromobacteraceae.

It is a sometimes motile gram-negative rod that is chemically inactive on routine media. On MacConkey agar it produces small colorless colonies that may be mistaken for those of a pathogen. On TSI agar it gives an alkaline reaction throughout the medium.

Chromobacter species

These are saprophytic, motile gram-negative rods that produce a nondiffusable violet pigment. They may be confused with *Serratia* or with *Pseudomonas*.

Table 11-17. *Klebsiella-Aerobacter-Serratia* division*

Substrate or test	Klebsiella and Aerobacter groups	Hafnia group 37° C.	22° C.	Serratia group
Gas from glucose	+	+	+	d
Gas from cellobiose	+	+	+	–
Gas from glycerol	d	+	+	–
Sorbitol	+	–	–	+
Raffinose	+	–	–	–
Arabinose	+	+	+	–
Methyl red	–	+	–	
Voges-Proskauer	+	d	+	+
Gelatin—22° C.	d		–	+

*From Ewing and Edwards: The principal divisions and groups of Enterobacteriaceae and their differentiation, Atlanta, 1962, U. S. Department of Health, Education, and Welfare, Public Health Service, Communicable Disease Center.

Note: When gas is formed from glucose by *Serratia*, the volumes are small (10% or less).

+ = positive in 1 or 2 days; – = negative; d = different biochemical types.

Table 11-17a. Differentiation of Enterobacteriaceae by biochemical tests[*]

Substrate or test	Escherichieae		Edwardsielleae	Salmonelleae			Klebsiella		
	Escherichia	Shigella	Edwardsiella	Salmonella	Arizona	Citrobacter	Klebsiella	cloacae	aerogenes
Indole	+	– or +	+	–	–	– or +	–	–	–
Methyl red	+	+	+	+	+	+	–	–	–
Voges-Proskauer	–	–	–	–	–	–	+	+	+
Simmons citrate	–	–	–	d	+	+	+	+	+
Hydrogen sulfide (TSI)	–	–	+	+	+	+	–	–	–
Urease	–	–	–	–	–	d^w	+	+ or –	–
KCN	–	–	–	–	–	+	+	+	+
Motility	+ or –	–	+	+	+	+	–	+	+
Gelatin—22° C.	–	–	–	–	(+)	–	–	(+) or –	– or (+)
Lysine decarboxylase	d	–	+	+	+	–	+	–	+
Arginine dihydrolase	d	– or (+)	–	+ or (+)	+ or (+)	d	–	+	–
Ornithine decarboxylase	d	d†	+	+	+	d	–	+	+
Phenylalanine deaminase	–	–	–	–	–	–	–	–	–
Malonate	–	–	–	–	+	d	+	+ or –	+ or –
Gas from glucose	+	–†	+	+	+	+	+	+	+
Lactose	+	–†	–	–	d	d	+	+	+
Sucrose	d	–†	–	–	–	d	+	+	+
Mannitol	+	+ or –	–	+	+	+	+	+	+
Dulcitol	d	d	–	d††	–	d	– or +	–	–
Salicin	d	–	–	–	–	d	+ or (+)	+ or (+)	+
Adonitol	–	–	–	–	–	–	+	– or +	+
Inositol	–	–	–	d	–	–	+	d	+
Sorbitol	+	d	–	+	+	+	+	+	+
Arabinose	+	d	–	+††	+	+	+	+	+
Raffinose	d	d	–	–	–	d	+	+	+
Rhamnose	d	d	–	+	+	+	+	+	+

[*]Courtesy Dr. P. R. Edwards and Dr. W. H. Ewing, Communicable Disease Center, Atlanta, Ga.

†Certain biotypes of *S. flexneri* produce gas; *S. sonnei* cultures ferment lactose and sucrose slowly and

‡*S. typhi, S. cholerasuis, S. enteritidis* bioser. *paratyphi* A and *pullorum,* and a few others ordinarily do

§Gas volumes produced by cultures of *Serratia, Proteus,* and *Providence* are small.

+ = 90% or more positive in 1 or 2 days; – = 90% or more negative; d = different biochemical types

w = weakly positive reaction.

Aeromonas species[63]

These are saprophytic gram-negative motile rods that are oxidase positive and may have to be distinguished from *Pseudomonas.*

KLEBSIELLA-ENTEROBACTER (AEROBACTER)[64]

Edwards and Ewing differentiate the nonmotile *Klebsiella* and the motile *Aerobacter,* for which they suggest the name *Enterobacter.*

Klebsiella

These organisms are nonmotile, encapsulated, gram-negative, short rods.

Morphology: On MacConkey agar they produce pink mucoid colonies that may "string" when touched with the inoculating loop.

Biochemistry: They are active fermenters of lactose and of other sugars with production of acid and gas. They are ornithine decarboxylase[62] negative and grow on synthetic alginate medium. *Klebsiella* are Voges-Proskauer, urease, and lysine decarboxylase positive.

Enterobacter (Aerobacter)

Enterobacter species are motile, gram-negative, short rods that are morphologically similar to *Klebsiella.*

Biochemically, they are ornithine decarboxylase positive and grow on synthetic

Klebsielleae					Pecto-bacterium	Proteeae					
Aerobacter							Proteus			Providence	
hafnia		liquefaciens		Serratia		vulgaris	mirabilis	morganii	rettgeri	alcali-faciens	stuartii
37° C.	22° C.	37° C.	22° C.		25° C.						
-	-	-	-	-	- or +	+	-	+	+	+	+
+ or -	-	+ or -	- or +	-	+ or -	+	+	+	+	+	+
+ or -	+	- or +	+ or -	+	- or +	-	- or +	-	-	-	-
(+) or -	d	+	+	+	d	d	+ or (+)	-	+	+	+
-	-	-	-	-	-	+	+	-	-	-	-
-	-	d	-	d^w	d^w	+	+	+	+	-	-
+	+	+	+	+	+ or -	+	+	+	+	+	+
+	+	d	-	+	+ or -	+	+	+	+	+	+
-			+	+	+ or (+)	+ or (+)	+	-	-	-	⌣
+	+	+ or -	+	+	-	-	-	-	-	-	-
-	-	-	-	-	-	-	-	-	-	-	-
+	+	+	+	+	-	-	+	+	-	-	-
-	-	-	-	-	-	+	+	+	+	+	+
+ or -	+ or -	-	-	-	- or +	-	-	-	-	-	-
+	+	+	+	+ or -§	- or +	+ or -	+	d	- or +	+ or -	-
- or (+)	- or (+)	d	(+)	- or (+)	d	-	-	-	-	-	-
d	d	+	+	+	+	+	d	-	d	d	d
+	+	+	+	+	+	-	-	-	+ or -	-	d
-	-	-	-	-	-	-	-	-	-	-	-
d	d	+	+	+	+	d	d	-	d	-	-
-	-	d	d	d	-	-	-	-	d	+	-
-	-	+	+	d	- or (+)	-	-	-	+	-	+
-	-	+	+	+	-	-	-	-	-	-	d
+	+	+	+	-	+	-	-	-	-	-	-
-	-	+	+	-	+ or (+)	-	-	-	-	-	-
+	+	-	-	-	d	+	-	-	+ or -	-	-

decarboxylate ornithine.
not ferment dulcitol promptly. S. *cholerasuis* does not ferment arabinose.

[+, (+), -]; (+) = delayed positive; + or - = majority of cultures positive; - or + = majority negative;

alginate medium.* They ferment lactose and most sugars with production of acid and gas. The urease reaction is variable, but most are negative.

Serratia-Hafnia

According to Ewing and Edwards, the genera *Serratia* and *Hafnia* belong to the tribe *Klebsiella*, though they ferment lactose late or not at all.

SERRATIA

These organisms are gram-negative, motile (peritrichous flagellae), long rods

*Bacto-decarboxylase medium base plus Bacto-1-ornithine HCl (0293), Difco Laboratories, Detroit, Mich.

that ferment lactose late or not at all. Some form a red pigment, which is more pronounced when the organism is grown at 22° C. and in the dark. Nonpigmented *Serratia* must be differentiated from late lactose-fermenting *E. coli*, *Shigella*, *Proteus-Providence*, and possibly *S. typhi*. *Serratia* can be differentiated from *Proteus* by the absence of the prompt urease reaction and from *Providence* by the absence of the prompt phenylalanine deaminase test. It can be differentiated from *Shigella* and *E. coli* by growth in KCN broth, a positive Voges-Proskauer reaction, and a negative methyl red test. It can be differentiated from *S. typhi* by citrate utilization of Simmons citrate (*S.*

typhi and S. *paratyphi* A are Simmons citrate negative, in contradistinction to the other salmonellae).

HAFNIA

According to Edwards and Ewing, *Hafnia* belongs in the same division as *Serratia,* which can be differentiated from *Hafnia* by liquefaction of gelatin at 22° C. and utilization of sorbitol. The colonies are colorless to slightly pink on Mac-Conkey agar; lactose is either not fermented or ferments late.

DIFFERENTIAL DIAGNOSIS: The *Hafnia-Serratia* group may give TSI reactions that can be confused with the reactions of the *Proteus-Providence* group, with late lactose-fermenting *E. coli,* and rarely with no H₂S-producing *Salmonella. Hafnia* and *Serratia* give a negative methyl red test at 22° C. and a positive Voges-Proskauer reaction and fail to hydrolyze urea promptly. *E. coli* and *Proteus-Providence* are methyl red positive and Voges-Proskauer positive.

SALMONELLA[65]

These organisms are pathogens that can be isolated from feces, urine, and blood. They may also be found in bile and bone marrow or in sputum in cases of pneumonia. They are gram-negative motile bacilli that fail to ferment lactose so that they produce colorless colonies on Mac-Conkey and SS agar.

LABORATORY DIAGNOSIS

Specimen: In the early stages of the infection inoculate 10 ml. of the patient's blood into 10 times its volume of broth. Clotted blood may also be used. Feces are suitable for isolation at any time during the disease and convalescence. It must be noted that there may be very few pathogens in relation to the abundance of nonpathogenic organisms. Rectal swabs and fecal specimens after cathartics are useful. See discussion of handling fecal specimens (p. 533) and of mailing these specimens (p. 535).

Cultural and biochemical tests

The cultural steps leading to inoculation of TSI have been described (p. 561). On TSI most *Salmonella* cultures give an acid butt with gas and H₂S and alkaline slants. S. *typhi* is anaerogenic on TSI and produces a small amount of sulfide salt and no gas. Gas-forming (aerogenic) strains that fail to produce H₂S are infrequent (S. *paratyphi* A and S. *typhisuis*) and must be differentiated from late lactose-fermenting *E. coli.* Salmonellae are motile, fail to grow in KCN medium, and are urease and indole negative and lysine decarboxylase positive (Table 11-11).

Blood cultures: Bile as a medium is superior to trypticase soy broth.

Serologic identification

This is based on the fact that flagellate bacteria possess not only a **thermostable somatic O antigen** but also a **thermolabile flagellar H antigen.** Nonflagellate bacteria contain only the O antigen. A third antigen is the **Vi antigen,** which is a peripheral body antigen and is thermolabile in contradistinction to the thermostable O antigen. The Vi antigen may interfere with the agglutination of freshly isolated bacteria by anti-O antigen sera. Three antisera are thus available: anti-O, anti-H, and anti-Vi.*

Salmonella contains the somatic, heatstable O antigen and can be grouped by the use of polyvalent O antisera. Subgroups of the O antigen are identified by the use of O grouping sera, e.g., sera for subgroups A, B, C, etc. Type identification is established by the use of H typing sera for heat-labile flagellar antigens such as antigens a, b, c, etc. Most salmonellae are diphasic, and each phase may contain one H antigen or more.

The polyvalent O antisera are used in the slide agglutination test. If positive agglutination occurs, proceed further to identify the group to which the organism belongs by using the individual *Salmonella* O antisera groups A through E, including Vi. The Vi antigen is present in some *Salmonella* strains and may block the activity of the O antigens. If agglutination is observed with polyvalent serum and with one of the group sera and if the biochemical tests are consistent with *Salmo-*

---

*Difco Laboratories, Detroit, Mich.

nella, the culture is reported as containing *Salmonella.*

Macroscopic slide test: Prepare a dense suspension (about 1 ml.) of the organism taken from a solid medium. Divide a microscope slide into two sections by marking with a wax pencil. Place 1 drop *Salmonella* O polyvalent antiserum* onto one section of the slide and 1 drop normal saline solution onto the other. This will serve as a negative control. Transfer 1 loopful of the bacterial suspension to the saline solution and 1 loopful to the antiserum. Rock the slide for 1-2 min. Positive agglutination will be rapid and complete.

If the culture reacts with *Salmonella* polyvalent O antiserum but does not react with the specific *Salmonella* O antisera groups, it should be checked with *Salmonella* Vi antiserum. If there is no agglutination with the *Salmonella* Vi antiserum at this point, the culture may be regarded as not of the *Salmonella* genus. If the culture reacts with the *Salmonella* Vi antiserum, the culture suspension in saline solution should be heated to 100° C. in a boiling water bath for 30 min. and cooled. After cooling, the heated culture should be retested with the individual *Salmonella* O antisera groups A, B, C₁, etc., the *Salmonella* Vi antiserum, and with polyvalent Bethesda-Ballerup antiserum. If the organism does not react with the Vi antiserum after heating, but, for instance, does react with *Salmonella* O antiserum group D, it is most likely *Salmonella typhosa* and the diagnosis should be confirmed by testing an unheated saline suspension of the culture with *Salmonella* H antiserum group d. If the heated culture continues to react with Vi antiserum and does not react with any of the *Salmonella* O antisera, the organism may be *Citrobacter* and should be tested in KCN broth.

Serologic agglutination test (Widal reaction):

Principle: By means of a slide test, the patient's serum is examined (and titered) for the presence of antibodies to *Salmonella* by the use of a suspension of specially prepared corresponding bacterial

*Difco Laboratories, Detroit, Mich.

antigens. If the antibody is present, it will agglutinate the antigen. Sera must be tested for agglutinating properties for somatic (O), flagellar (H), and Vi antigens.

Technique: Add the patient's serum in varying dilutions to a constant amount of antigen in a slide test.

1. With a 0.2 ml. pipette, deliver 0.08, 0.04, 0.02, 0.01, and 0.005 ml. quantities of the patient's serum to the rings or squares of a glass slide from left to right.
2. Mix the contents of the antigen vial, and by means of the dropper provided, place 1 drop antigen on each quantity of serum in one row.
3. Mix the serum-antigen mixture in the row with a wooden applicator stick, moving from right to left.
4. Rotate the slide for 3 min.
5. The highest dilution producing agglutination represents the serum titer. Dilutions: 1:20, 1:40, 1:80, 1:160, and 1:320.
6. If the titer is greater than 1:320, dilute the serum 1:10 with saline solution, and repeat test. The dilutions will then be 1:200, 1:400, 1:800, etc.

Interpretation:

1. High-titer O (1-160 or more) and low-titer H: active infection
2. High-titer H (1-160 or more) and low titer O: postvaccination and postinfection
3. High-titer Vi: suggests carrier state

Salmonella typhosa infection

If typhoid fever is suspected on clinical grounds, bismuth sulfite agar should be added to the list of primary media. *S. typhosa* produces black colonies with a metallic sheen on this medium, while other *Salmonella* are usually dark green with black centers.

In typhoid fever the blood culture may be positive in the first week of the disease, before the stool culture is positive.

Arizona group

These organisms are gram-negative, short motile rods that are closely related to salmonellae. On MacConkey agar they produce colorless colonies. On TSI agar they produce a *Salmonella*-like pattern (alkaline slant, acid butt, H₂S). *Arizona* differs from *Salmonella* by liquefying gelatin slowly in 7-20 days and by slowly utilizing malonate and lactose. If *Arizona* does not form H₂S, it has to be distinguished from *E. coli* and *Citrobacter*. *Arizona* will grow on Simmons citrate; *E. coli* will not. *Arizona* is lysine decarboxylase positive and KCN negative, while *Citrobacter* gives opposite reactions.

The **Bethesda-Ballerup group** may also give *Salmonella*-like reactions on MacConkey and TSI agars (see p. 561).

SHIGELLA

This group consists of gram-negative nonmotile rods that are nonlactose fermenters. Some ferment mannitol, while others do not. Except for *S. dysenteriae*, most are catalase positive.

Dysentery bacilli are difficult to isolate, especially after the first few days. A specimen of feces without pus and blood-streaked mucus is usually negative. Specimens obtained from the rectum on a swab and plated immediately give best results.

LABORATORY DIAGNOSIS

Culture: Stool is planted on differential and selective media, and as in *Salmonella* infections, colorless (lactose negative) or almost colorless colonies are transferred to urea agar and triple sugar iron agar. Organisms that produce acid but no gas in butt, alkaline slant, and no hydrogen sulfide on TSI and that are nonmotile are treated with polyvalent *Shigella* group antisera* (Table 11-8). Cultures which show the characteristics of *Shigella* but fail to react with antisera should be suspended in saline solution and heated at 100° C. for ½ hr. and then retested since heat-labile K antigen may inhibit O agglutination.

Serologic identification

Macroscopic slide test: Divide a microscope slide into two sections by marking with a wax pencil. Place 1 drop *Shigella* antiserum onto one section and 1 drop 0.5% saline solution onto the other section. This will serve as negative control. Transfer 1 loopful of the culture taken from a solid medium to the saline solution and 1 loopful to the antiserum. Mix well to emulsify the mixtures. Tilt the slide back and forth for 1-2 min. to enhance agglutination. Positive agglutination will be rapid and complete. Perform this procedure with polyvalent group A antiserum; if no reaction occurs, proceed to polyvalent groups B, C, and D and to the *Alkalescens-Dispar* group.

A positive reaction with a polyvalent group antiserum identifies the organism as a member of that *Shigella* group. Final identification of the specific type within a group is accomplished by using individual type-specific sera.*

Members of the *E. coli* related *Alkalescens-Dispar* group give cultural reactions very similar to *Shigella* and can be serologically differentiated (see p. 568).

Biochemical identification

Shigella fails to grow on Simmons citrate and does not hydrolyze urea, but grows on KCN medium and does not contain phenylalanine deaminase or lysine decarboxylase (Table 11-10).

PASTEURELLA

Four species of *Pasteurella* are human pathogens: *P. pestis*, *P. pseudotuberculosis*, *P. multocida*, and *P. tularensis*. They are short, at times elliptical, gram-negative rods that show bipolar staining, are nonmotile (with the exception of *P. pseudotuberculosis*, which shows some motility at 20° C.), grow aerobically on most media, and do not produce hemolysis.

Pasteurella pestis

Plague is caused by *P. pestis*, a short, thick, straight, gram-negative bacillus with rounded ends that sometimes occurs in pairs or in very short chains. Bipolar staining and the presence of many swollen vacuolated forms (involution forms) on 3% sodium chloride agar are characteristic.

---

*Difco Laboratories, Detroit, Mich.

*Difco Laboratories, Detroit, Mich.

Plague, one of the most devastating of all human infectious diseases, is primarily a disease of rats and is transmitted by the rat flea to other rats; man is only incidentally involved. The organism produces an endotoxin that is utilized for the production of a toxoid for immunization.

LABORATORY DIAGNOSIS

Smear: Make smears from pus (bubo, sputum) and fix with methyl alcohol 3-5 min. instead of with heat, which interferes with the bipolar staining. Stain one smear with gram stain and another with Loeffler methylene blue. Bipolar staining is characteristic and is best seen with Wayson stain.

Wayson stain for bipolar staining:
Solution A:
  Basic fuchsin, 0.2 gm.
  Methylene blue, 0.75 gm.
  Absolute ethyl alcohol, 20.9 ml.
Solution B:
  5% phenol in water, 200 ml.
Add solution A to solution B. Stain for a few seconds, wash, and dry.

Culture: Material from patients consists of fluid aspirated from skin lesions, lymph nodes, or flea bites. Blood may also be used. At autopsy the spleen should be cultured.

Culture media: Use brain-heart infusion broth. After 24 hr. of cultivation at 35° C., clouding of the medium can be observed. Bacterial clumps appear after 3-4 days.

After 2 days of incubation at 35° C. on blood agar, there appear delicate, transparent, minute, colorless 0.1-0.2 mm. colonies that may become mucoid and darken centrally. The slow growth is characteristic. The organisms grow well on Loeffler medium.

Biochemically the organism does not utilize sucrose, but is able to grow in the presence of bile (MacConkey agar). It is nonmotile and indole negative. Chemical reactions are used mainly to differentiate *P. pestis* from other *Pasteurella* (Table 11-18).

Serology: Bacteria are agglutinated by immune serum (patient's serum). Use an avirulent strain or formalin-killed organisms as antigen.

Table 11-18. Differentiation of *Pasteurella* group

	Pasteurella multocida	*Pasteurella pseudotuberculosis*	*Pasteurella pestis*
Optimal temperature	37° C.	30° C.	28° C.
Motility at 20° C.	−	+	−
Sucrose utilization (acid, no gas)	+	Variable	−
Indole production	+	−	−
Pathogenicity for mice	+	−	+
Growth in the presence of bile (MacConkey)	−	+	+
Methyl red test	−	+	+
Methylene blue reductase	+	+	−
H₂S production	+	+	−

Bacteriophage typing: Lysis of colonies by specific bacteriophage is a rapid method of identification. Filter paper strips containing lyophilized virus are available from certain centers, e.g., U. S. Public Health Service, Department of Health, Education, and Welfare, San Francisco, Calif.

Virulence: The organisms are pathogenic to mice and to guinea pigs (danger to laboratory personnel). Inoculate a white mouse or guinea pig subcutaneously or intraperitoneally with 24 hr. broth culture. Death occurs in 2-4 days. Autopsy will reveal multiple abscesses.

Fluorescent microscopy: Staining with fluorescent antibodies can be utilized.

Pasteurella pseudotuberculosis[66]

Pasteurella pseudotuberculosis produces tuberculosis-like lesions in many wild animals and in animals kept as pets, e.g., cats, canaries, etc. Human infections produce a picture of gastroenteritis or acute appendicitis.

ISOLATION

Material: Obtain material from bile, feces, macerated lymph nodes, etc.

Morphology: The organism is a pleomorphic, gram-negative rod that may exhibit coccoid and ovoid forms.

Culture: The organism will grow on all routine media at 22°-30° C. and after 24 hr. will form minute 1-2 mm. colonies.

Biochemical reactions are shown in Table 11-18.

This species can be biochemically differentiated from other *Pasteurella* on the basis of motility (motile at 20° C.), on the basis of phage typing, agglutination, and fluorescent antibody technique.

Pasteurella multocida

Pasteurella multocida produces severe gastroenteritis in fowl, birds, domestic animals, and man.

Isolation

Material: Clinical specimens include sputum, saliva, pus, macerated tissue, etc.

Morphology: The organism is a gram-negative, oval to coccoid short structure measuring 0.3-1.25μ. The individual cell shows polar staining, the middle remaining almost unstained (safety-pin appearance).

Culture: In broth the organism forms wooly masses. It grows readily on blood agar in the form of transparent droplike colonies. It does not thrive on media containing bile. For biochemical activity, see Table 11-18. It utilizes sucrose to form acid without gas. The organism characteristically is very sensitive to penicillin.

Pasteurella tularensis

Tularemia is caused by *P. tularensis*, a small nonmotile gram-negative, pleomorphic coccoid, and strictly aerobic organism that produces a fatal septicemia (tularemia) in rodents, especially rabbits. It is transmitted to man by handling infected animals or material and by the bite of insects such as ticks, lice, fleas, etc. The wood tick *(Dermacentor andersonii)* is an intermediate host in which the organism is transmitted through the egg stage.

Morphology: The organism occurs as a gram-negative rod or as small cocci. It varies from 0.3-0.7μ in length, the smallest organisms being slightly larger than rickettsiae. The organism is dangerous to handle in the laboratory.

Laboratory diagnosis

Two laboratory methods are available for the diagnosis of tularemia: (1) culture and (2) agglutination tests.

The agglutination tests are specific and, as serum is easily obtainable, are most frequently used. A skin test is also available.

Culture: It is seldom possible to successfully culture human material directly. The human material may consist of sputum, lymph nodes, blood, or exudate from a wound. Inoculation of a guinea pig is the best procedure. The organism does not grow on plain agar. Blood glucose cystine agar is the preferred medium. Addition of sterile guinea pig spleen segments to the water of condensation improves the medium. Small, viscid, transparent to milky colonies appear slowly in 2-7 days. Embryonated egg is an excellent culture medium.

Guinea pig inoculation: The material should be ground in a mortar and suspended in saline solution. Inoculate material from patient's ulcer, regional lymph gland, or effusion subcutaneously into the abdomen of a guinea pig. The animal dies within 1 wk., presenting gray, granular caseation of enlarged lymph glands of the groin and a great number of white areas of necrosis over the enlarged spleen and liver. Cultures are obtained from blood, spleen, heart, or liver of the guinea pig. Direct smears should be stained with **Wayson stain.**

Caution: Laboratory infection is common. Animal inoculation should not be made unless the workers are immune.

Agglutination tests:

Identification of the organism: A commercially available *P. tularensis* antiserum* can be used for direct serologic identification. This serum can also serve as a positive control for the slide agglutination test.

Identification of the antibody in the patient's serum: By slide or tube technique the patient's serum will agglutinate *P. tularensis*. Because of the danger involved in handling the organisms from the patient, strain No. 38, distributed by the National Institutes of Health, should be used

---

*Difco Laboratories, Detroit, Mich.

as antigen and tested with the patient's serum. It is avirulent, smooth, easily cultured, and highly agglutinable. A *P. tularensis* slide test antigen is also commercially available.*

Test tube agglutination test: Because of frequent cross-agglutination between *P. tularensis* and *Brucella melitensis* and *abortus,* sera from suspected persons should be set up with both *P. tularensis* and *B. melitensis* (or *abortus*) organisms in dilutions from 1:10-1:2560.

Technique: Mark tubes from 1-10. Add 0.8 ml. saline solution to the first tube and 0.5 ml. to the others. Pipette 0.2 ml. test serum into first tube, mix (dilution 1:5), and transfer 0.5 ml. of mixture of first tube to second tube, mix, and repeat. Discard 0.5 ml. from ninth tube. Add 0.5 ml. antigen to each tube and shake. The tenth tube is the antigen control. The final serum dilutions are 1:10, 1:20, 1:40, 1:80, 1:160, 1:320, 1:640, 1:1280, and 1:2560.

Incubate test tubes in a water bath at 35° C. for 2 hr. and then place in a refrigerator overnight. Record the result after 2 hr. in the water bath. The highest titer indicates the specific reaction. If the serum is from a patient with tularemia, the *P. tularensis* antigen will be agglutinated in higher dilution and earlier than the *Brucella* antigen. If the serum is from a patient with undulant fever, the reverse will be true. Should the serum agglutinate tularemia and undulant fever organisms to the same titer, agglutination absorption tests will have to be performed. Cross-reaction with *Proteus* OX-19 has also been reported. The antigen is commercially available.

Repeated agglutination tests are necessary to appreciate the fall or rise of a given titer. After the first week, agglutination of the organism with the patient's serum is usually positive. Positive reactions persist for many years or life.

Skin test: The intracutaneous test[67] with bacterial protein (detoxified) is highly specific and will be positive as early as the third day of symptoms.

---

*Difco Laboratories, Detroit, Mich.

BORDETELLA

The genus *Bordetella* consists of three species that have an absolute requirement for nicotinic acid and are associated with respiratory infections. They are gram-negative coccobacilli and include *B. pertussis, B. parapertussis,* and *B. bronchiseptica.*

Bordetella pertussis

Bordetella pertussis is the causative organism of whooping cough.

LABORATORY DIAGNOSIS

Laboratory diagnosis includes lymphocyte count and isolation of pertussis bacillus by cough plate and/or nasopharyngeal swab.

Blood: The leukocyte count in the paroxysmal phase is usually 15,000-40,000, with about 60-80% lymphocytes.

Culture[68]:

Cough plate: Hold an uncovered plate of Bordet-Gengou medium 4-6 in. in front of the patient's mouth during several expulsive coughs.

Nasopharyngeal swab: Pass a sterile swab of Dacron on a soft wire through the nose and into the nasopharynx, leave it in place for about 30 sec., and then remove and streak plate with swab. This method is superior to the cough plate method.[69]

• • •

For primary culture the organism requires blood agar containing potato infusion and 20% sheep blood (**Bordet-Gengou medium**). The growth is slow, requiring 2-4 days to become visible. As penicillin suppresses the growth of gram-positive organisms, the use of two plates is suggested, one without penicillin and one containing 1 unit penicillin/ml. medium.

Incubate at 35° C. under increased CO_2 tension in a candle jar. Examine several times during the first 48 hr. and with a sterile scalpel cut out any molds or spreading contaminants. Then examine twice daily for *B. pertussis,* using a hand lens and placing the plates (uncovered) over a substage lamp. Do not discard as negative for 1 wk. The colonies are smooth, raised, glistening, pearly, and nearly transparent. They are surrounded by a small zone of hemolysis which is not sharply defined.

Cultures are positive for about 1 mo. after onset of whooping cough if untreated. During the first 2 wk. of the disease the culture is positive in over 90% of cases.

Morphology: The organism is a coccoid bacillus and is gram-negative, nonmotile, and often shows polar staining. It does not occur in chains and does not show pleomorphic threads. The cells stain faintly, decolorize readily, and measure less than 1μ in length.

Biochemical reaction: These organisms are inert (Table 11-19).

Differential diagnosis: B. pertussis should be differentiated from *Haemophilus influenzae*, which is also a gram-negative rod found in sputum and morphologically similar to B. pertussis. B. pertussis must also be distinguished from B. parapertussis and B. bronchiseptica. These organisms are morphologically indistinguishable but can be separated biochemically and serologically (Table 11-9).

Agglutination tests: B. pertussis and B. parapertussis antisera are available for rapid identification of culture by the slide test method.

Bordetella bronchiseptica

Bordetella bronchiseptica shows all the characteristics of the species except that it is motile. It reduces nitrates to nitrites. It grows more rapidly than B. pertussis on Bordet-Gengou medium (2-3 days), and the colonies are larger.

HAEMOPHILUS

Haemophilus species can be differentiated on the basis of (1) cultural characteristics such as the requirement of **growth factor X,** which is considered to be hemin, a thermostable substance present in blood, and/or of **factor V,** which is considered to be coenzyme I, di- or triphosphopyridine nucleotide, which is thermolabile and supplied by blood, bacteria, and yeast (blood also contains an enzyme that counteracts factor V); and (2) the presence or absence of hemolysis on blood agar.

Classification of Haemophilus on basis of growth factors and hemolysis:

Factors X and V: *H. influenzae* (nonhemolytic), *H. haemolyticus* (hemolytic)

Factor X only: *H. ducreyi, H. vaginalis,* etc.

Factor V only: *H. parainfluenzae* (nonhemolytic), *H. parahaemolyticus* (hemolytic)

Haemophilus influenzae

This organism is a gram-negative small rod that may or may not be encapsulated. Six types of *H. influenzae* (A to F) are distinguished serologically. The most important one is type B, which causes most of the serious infections in infants and children such as septicemia, endocarditis, and meningitis. The nonencapsulated forms are not type specific and are part of the normal laryngeal flora.

LABORATORY DIAGNOSIS

Gram stain: The organism is a small, nonmotile, gram-negative, pleomorphic coccobacillus that sometimes appears as

Table 11-19. Differential characteristics of *Bordetella* and *Haemophilus*

	B. pertussis	B. bronchiseptica	B. parapertussis	H. influenzae
Motility	–	+	–	–
Growth on Bordet-Gengou medium	+	+	+	–
Reduction of nitrates	–	+	+	–
Hemolysis on 20% blood agar	+	+	+	– or +
Factors X and V needed	–	–	–	+
Indole production	–	–	–	+ (80%)
Urease production	–	4 hr.	+	–

long filaments. The average length is 1-1.5μ and the average thickness is 0.3μ. The form of the organism is dependent on the age of the culture.

Culture: For culture the organism requires both X and V growth factors and is best isolated on chocolate agar under increased tension in a CO_2 jar. The organism grows best around colonies of other bacteria, particularly staphylococci, a behavior pattern that is called the **satellite phenomenon.** The staphylococci provide coenzyme I. Instead of streaking the plate with *S. aureus,* the plate may be painted with a swab dipped in a mixture of 1 mg. beta-diphosphopyridine nucleotide added to 2 ml. 0.01% sodium thioglycollate in sterile water. The plate is allowed to dry and is then inoculated. Strips impregnated with factors V and X are commercially available.*

Use a second plate containing 0.2 units penicillin/ml. agar and streak with a few lines of staphylococci. Incubate both plates at 35° C. in a CO_2 jar. The colonies are small, clear, colorless, and non-hemolytic, with a dewdrop appearance and a mousy odor. The capsule of pathogens is best developed in an 8 hr. culture; older colonies may lose it.

Chocolate agar is superior to blood agar, which may contain substances that are bactericidal and depress factor V.

Serologic identification: Agglutination slide tests and quellung slide tests are available for serologic identification. If positive results are obtained with polyvalent serum, typing with A and B antisera follows.

Haemophilus vaginalis[70]

Haemophilus vaginalis requires only factor X for growth (not factor V, and therefore the satellite phenomenon is not needed). It is a short, gram-negative rod that does not grow on EMB. It grows best in the CO_2 jar on sheep blood (not human blood) and in thioglycollate medium without methylene blue, the indicator of oxidation-reduction.

This organism has been isolated from

*Case Laboratories, Chicago, Ill.

the human genitourinary tract (prostate, vagina, urine), and may not actually belong to the *Haemophilus* genus. It shares this uncertainty of classification with *H. aprophilus,* which has been identified in cases of endocarditis.

Haemophilus ducreyi

Haemophilus ducreyi is the causative organism of an ulcerative venereal disease—chancroid or "soft chancre" (Plate 12).

LABORATORY DIAGNOSIS

Direct smear: The ulcer base is cleaned and material from the growing edge is smeared on a slide. The organism is a gram-negative, ovoid to cylindric bacillus occurring singly, in clumps, or in chains of two to four. It varies in length from 1.1-1.5μ and has an average diameter of 0.6μ. It may be intra- or extracellular and is accompanied by polymorphonuclear cells. It may be plentiful or very scarce, and the smear may only help to exclude granuloma inguinale. Smears of aspirated material from abscessed inguinal lymph nodes may also show only a very few organisms.

Culture: The organism requires blood (growth factor X, but not V). On 30% rabbit blood agar at 35° C., very small (0.5-1 mm. in diameter), smooth, glistening colonies appear after 24 hr. Defibrinated rabbit blood that has been stored in the refrigerator for 3-4 days prior to use is an excellent medium if, after inoculation, it is incubated in a CO_2 jar at 35° C.

Haemophilus aegyptius (Koch-Weeks bacillus)

Haemophilus aegyptius is one of the agents of infectious conjunctivitis. For growth it requires both factors X and V. Morphologically and culturally it is indistinguishable from *H. influenzae.*

Haemophilus haemolyticus and Haemophilus parahaemolyticus

These two hemolytic species require both factors V and X. They may be mistaken for hemolytic streptococci on blood agar.

Haemophilus parainfluenzae

Haemophilus parainfluenzae is a non-hemolytic species and requires only factor V. It is normally found in the upper respiratory tract.

GRANULOMA INGUINALE

Granuloma inguinale is a venereal disease which, in the United States, is almost confined to Negroes. It is characterized by granulomatous lesions involving the external genitalia, the anal area, and at times the face.

The cause of the disease is not clearly understood, but it is probably due to a bacterial organism called *Donovania granulomatis*. It can be cultured in the yolk sac of the chick embryo and is seen in direct smears of the lesions (Plate 13).

Laboratory diagnosis

Donovan bodies:

Smears: Scrape the lesions and squash the material between two slides. Dry the resulting two smears and stain with Wright stain. Large mononuclear cells are seen which contain many Donovan bodies. These are straight to slightly

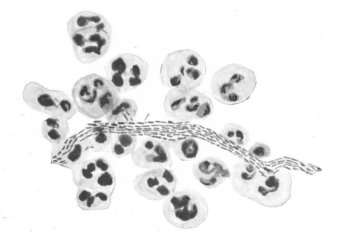

Plate 12. *Haemophilus ducreyi* from a chancroid. (Gram stain; oil-immersion lens.)

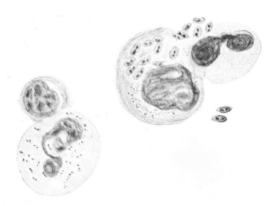

Plate 13. Donovan bodies of granuloma inguinale. Oil-immersion field showing encapsulated forms in a ruptured endothelial leukocyte and diplococcus forms in a polymorphonuclear leukocyte. (Giemsa stain.)

curved rods that stain purple and are surrounded by a pink-staining ovoid capsule.

Tissue sections: Biopsies of the lesion stained with hematoxylin and eosin show the previously mentioned mononuclear cells containing Donovan bodies.

OTHER GROUPS OF AEROBIC GRAM-NEGATIVE RODS

Moraxella lacunata may be the cause of a form of conjunctivitis in man (**Morax-Axenfeld conjunctivitis**).

It is a gram-negative, plump, short bacillus measuring about $2\text{-}3\mu$ in length and up to 1.5μ in diameter. It is frequently paired. It grows slowly on blood agar and after 5-6 days the colonies measure 2-3 mm. in diameter. It grows well on Loeffler medium.

Actinobacillus is a gram-negative organism that forms moist to mucoid colonies. There are several species that are serologically related. They produce ulcerating, granulomatous to purulent lesions in the subcutaneous and deep tissues of cattle and horses. The superficial lesions contaminate the drinking water which, when consumed by man, allows bacteria to cause human infection.

Actinobacillus mallei (Malleomyces mallei)

This is the causative organism of **glanders,** an infectious disease of horses.

LABORATORY DIAGNOSIS

This organism is dangerous to handle in the laboratory.

Specimen: Examine pus from one of the discharging lesions or material from an incised nodule.

Morphology:

Smear: The organism is a gram-negative, slender, long, often beaded rod, which at times is slightly curved and varies from $0.4\text{-}0.8\mu$ in length. In older cultures long filaments are found. The ends are clubbed. It stains poorly with gram stain and stains best with methylene blue.

Culture: For primary isolation the medium must contain glycerol. On Loeffler agar, small, opaque, slimy colonies appear slowly, while on blood agar, methemoglobin formation produces brownish-colored colonies. As the culture ages the colonies have a tendency to flow together so that a heavy, shiny, brownish mass is produced. On glycerin agar slants the colonies appear slowly; they are yellowish at first, and then become brownish. In broth the organism grows slowly, producing diffuse clouding, which in older cultures settles to the bottom of the tube as a mucoid viscid ring.

Serology: An antigen is available that is precipitated by immune serum that contains complement-fixing antibodies before cutaneous ulcerating lesions appear, thus eliminating dangerous bacteriologic procedures. An extract, **mallein,** is available for diagnostic cutaneous and conjunctival tests.

Animal inoculation: The organism is pathogenic to guinea pigs. Exudate or pure culture material is injected subcutaneously and in 4-5 days an abscess forms. The **Straus reaction** involves the appearance of caseating testicular necrosis 1-2 wk. after intraperitoneal injection of the *Actinobacillus* into guinea pigs. *Brucella* may produce a similar reaction.

Pseudomonas pseudomallei (Malleomyces pseudomallei)

Although *P. pseudomallei* is motile, this organism resembles *A. mallei* morphologically and in its cultural appearance. It is the causative agent of **melioidosis** (pseudoglanders), a disease that is characterized by multiple soft tissue sinuses and abscesses in its chronic form.

P. pseudomallei grows on routine media, is catalase positive, reduces methylene blue, and is not pigmented.

GRAM-NEGATIVE MICROAEROPHILIC NONSPORE-FORMING BACILLI

BRUCELLA[71, 72]

The species are *Br. abortus* (var. *bovis*), *Br. melitensis,* and *Br. suis.*

Brucellosis, or undulant fever,[73-76] is caused by a small gram-negative bacillus, *Br. abortus* or *Br. suis.* The former is the bovine strain from cattle, and the latter is the porcine strain from swine.

Brucellosis is a disease of animals that is transmitted to man. Infection may occur through the skin from contact with infected animals or by mouth from the ingestion of infectious dairy products. A similar disease, Malta or Mediterranean fever, is due to the caprine strain, *Br. melitensis,* from goats.

During the first week of the disease, and often during the febrile stage of recurrence, the organism may be found in blood culture. Culture of the urine and feces is usually not successful. After the second week, specific agglutinins may be demonstrated in the blood serum. Agglutinins may remain in the blood for several months or for many years, but sometimes they disappear a few months after recovery.

LABORATORY DIAGNOSIS

SMEAR: The organism varies in length from $0.3-2.3\mu$ and has an average diameter of 0.4μ. It is a gram-negative coccobacillus. It is found intracellularly on smears of blood cultures and is seen to fill the cytoplasm of polymorphs.

CULTURE: Best results are obtained with blood cultures. However, specimens of urine, pus, bone marrow, and lymph node are also used.

Medium: Trypticase soy broth or agar in an atmosphere of 2-10% CO_2 (candle jar) is used. Place 5-10 ml. blood into 50 ml. trypticase soy broth with 10% CO_2 and incubate at 35° C. for 4-7 days. After 7 days of incubation, mix the culture and transfer 1 loopful of blood culture to a trypticase soy agar plate and incubate for 4 days at 35° C. in a CO_2 jar. Reincubate blood culture for another 7 days, replenishing the CO_2 if necessary. After 7 days, streak the blood culture again; this process may have to be repeated a third time before the culture can be reported as negative. After 4 days, examine the agar plate for small (2-3 mm.), transparent, smooth, well-defined, soft, spheroidal colonies that later become opalescent due to a brownish tinge. **Smooth colonies** can be differentiated from rough ones by tilting the plate 45 degrees and examining it under transmitted light with the low-power objective of the microscope. The rough colonies appear darker than the smooth ones. Make a gram stain of suspicious colonies and perform a **slide agglutination test** with polyvalent antiserum, using smooth colonies only. If the test with polyvalent antiserum is positive, use the dye plate method for species differentiation.

Dye plate method (dye sensitivity): Species differentiation is made according to their characteristic sensitivity to dyes. Prepare filter paper strips impregnated with Thionine, 1:20,000; basic fuchsin, 1:25,000; and methyl violet, 1:100,000. Inoculate trypticase soy agar and place filter paper strips on surface. After incubation under increased CO_2 tension, clear zones will appear close to the strips (Table 11-20).

Brucella differentiation kits are available commercially.*

AGGLUTINATION TESTS: The test tube

---

*Difco Laboratories, Detroit, Mich.

Table 11-20

Species	CO_2 requirements on initial isolation	Growth in presence of			H_2S production
		Thionine (1:20,000)	Basic fuchsin (1:25,000)	Methyl violet (1:100,000)	
Brucella abortus	+	–	+	+	+ for first 2 days only
Brucella suis	–	+	–	–	+ throughout 4 days
Brucella melitensis	–	+	+	+	0 to ± throughout 4 days

method is recommended, with antigen prepared with avirulent National Institutes of Health *Br. abortus* strain No. 256. One antigen is used for the diagnosis of all three forms of brucellosis. Cross-reaction with *Pasteurella tularensis* may occur.

Tube dilution method:

Technique: Use fresh (not inactivated) serum, free from hemolysis.

Set up 11 small tubes and add 0.9 ml. saline solution to the first tube and 0.5 ml. to the others. To the first tube add 0.1 ml. serum, mix by drawing it in and out of the pipette 7 or 8 times, and transfer 0.5 ml. to the second tube. Continue in like manner through the tenth tube, discarding 0.5 ml. and leaving tube 11 for a negative control.

To all tubes add 0.5 ml. diluted antigen (National Institutes of Health strain No. 256) and mix. The dilutions of the serum are from 1:20-1:10,240.

Incubate for 48 hr. in a water bath at 37.5° C. before making the final reading. The titer is the highest dilution showing complete (4+) agglutination. Do not use serum when hemolysis is present. Hemolysis causes nonspecific clumping.

Slide test methods: Commercially available *Brucella* antigens* as well as polyvalent and type-specific antisera* allow rapid slide agglutination techniques.

Rapid slide method:

Technique: Use slides that contain six rows of rings painted with alkyd resin paint, five or six to the row. Serum and antigen must be at room temperature.

Shake the antigen thoroughly. Place 0.08, 0.04, 0.02, 0.01, and 0.005 ml. amounts of serum in a row of circles. Place 1 drop antigen on each quantity of serum. Mix the serum and antigen in each circle in the row with a wooden applicator, working from the smallest quantity of serum to the largest. Lift the plate and tilt it back and forth for no more than 3 min. Read in indirect light against a dark background and determine the highest serum dilution that still gives agglutination of the antigen.

ANIMAL INOCULATION: Guinea pigs (300-600 gm.), which must be tested for

---

*Difco Laboratories, Detroit, Mich.

the absence of *Brucella* agglutinins, are injected subcutaneously (if culture is mixed) or intraperitoneally (if culture is pure) with 2 ml. material. After 8 wk., test for *Brucella* agglutinins. If present, kill animal and look for granulomatous lesions in the spleen, liver, and testes.

GRAM-NEGATIVE ANAEROBIC NONSPORE-FORMING BACILLI

BACTEROIDES

These organisms are gram-negative, generally nonmotile, nonencapsulated, and nonspore-forming rods. They are **obligate anaerobes,** and all pathogens within the group more or less produce gas.

They are commonly found in the mouth and in the intestinal and urogenital tracts. Pathologically, they may be responsible for lung and brain abscesses, peritonitis, and appendicitis.

LABORATORY DIAGNOSIS

Smear: Gram-negative, slender, pleomorphic rods with rounded ends are seen. Some species produce filamentous forms and have round, swollen bodies.

Culture: The organism grows slowly in thioglycollate broth and may require 2 wk. before it can be recovered. The organism may be transferred from thioglycollate broth to blood agar in an anaerobic jar, where it slowly develops to form small, clear, colorless colonies.

The organisms are often "lost" on routine culture since they are obligate anaerobes. No growth appears on the plates; and the thioglycollate, which may show growth of gram-negative rods, is routinely plated on aerobic culture plates. Thus another day elapses and by this time the organisms in thioglycollate may have died.

The organism is difficult to culture even under complete anaerobiasis. Subculture should be made on several tubes of media to assure survival of the organism. Most species require blood. Hemolysis is rarely seen. The various species can be differentiated on the basis of biochemical reactions, but they are difficult to perform because of the requirement of strict anaerobiasis. Some strains produce pigment.

FUSOBACTERIUM FUSIFORME

Fusobacterium fusiforme is a gram-negative, nonmotile rod with pointed ends; it is part of the normal flora of the mouth and is associated with fusospirochetal disease (**Vincent's angina**), an ulcerative infection of the mouth and larynx.

LABORATORY DIAGNOSIS

Smear: Smears are stained with crystal violet. The organism is a somewhat pleomorphic gram-negative rod with pointed to rounded ends. It is slightly bent at times and often occurs in pairs, the blunt ends touching. It is nonmotile and varies from 8-16μ in length and from 0.5-1μ in diameter.

Culture: The organism is an anaerobe that grows on blood agar with a narrow zone of hemolysis and produces a foul odor (H_2S). Ascitic fluid agar is a good medium for isolation.

GRAM-POSITIVE NONSPORE-FORMING BACILLI

LACTOBACILLUS

Lactobacillus acidophilus occurs in the stool of newborn infants and in adults in the mouth, gastrointestinal tract, and vagina (**Döderlein's bacillus**) as well as in the stomach (**Boas-Oppler bacillus**) during pyloric obstruction. It may be found along with yeast in sputum specimens. There is some relationship between *Lactobacillus* counts in saliva and dental caries.

LABORATORY DIAGNOSIS

Smear: It is a gram-positive, nonspore-forming, nonmotile rod that varies in length and thickness.

Culture: It is a microaerophilic to anaerobic organism that ferments glucose. It grows on thioglycollate broth at 35° C., requiring several days and a pH of 6.1-6.8 for growth. The organism grows better when CO_2 is added.

Lactobacilli are the test organisms in the turbidimetric assay methods for folic acid and vitamin B_{12}. Cultures of lacto-

Table 11-21. Characteristic properties of *Listeria* and corynebacteria

	Listeria monocytogenes	*Coryne-bacteria*
Catalase	+	+
Motility	+ at 20° C. ± at 37° C.	–
Glucose (acid only)	+	+
Hemolysis	+ (beta)	–
Indole	–	–
Salicin (acid only)	+	–
Nitrate reduction	–	+
Methyl red	+	–

bacilli are used clinically to normalize the intestinal and vaginal flora.

CORYNEBACTERIACEAE

The family Corynebacteriaceae includes the genera *Listeria*, *Corynebacterium*, and *Erysipelothrix* (Table 11-21).

Listeria

Listeria monocytogenes[77-79] is a short, gram-positive, nonspore-forming, motile rod. It is a facultative anaerobe that is catalase positive and produces hemolysis on blood agar. Because of these characteristics, plus the fact that the rods may be very short and tend to occur in pairs, *Listeria* may be mistaken for streptococci. Spontaneous infections of animals (rabbits, chickens, etc.) are transmitted to other animals or to man. Pregnant women may transfer the infection transplacentally to the fetus (abortion) or to newborn infants via the genital tract. The most important clinical infections are meningitis, pneumonia, and septicemia.

LABORATORY DIAGNOSIS

Smear: Gram-positive rods are characteristic. They are small, measuring 0.5-2μ in length and 0.4μ in diameter. They may be single, parallel, or at angles to each other. They may be somewhat pleomorphic, with coccoid forms appearing in smears of cultures. They stain uniformly, lacking the granularity of corynebacteria, but are motile, while corynebacteria are nonmotile (Table 11-21). At times long filamentous forms appear.

Culture: Blood agar plate and thioglycollate broth are used. Good motility occurs at 20° C. in broth. Tissue must be left in the refrigerator for at least 24 hr. before it is ground and cultured. Round, soft, transparent colonies that produce beta hemolysis are seen on blood agar at 35° C. after 24 hr. **Smooth** and **rough forms** occur together. The smooth forms appear as previously described and have a smooth surface. Under the oblique light of the microscope they have a bluish opalescence. The rough forms have irregular edges and folds on the surface that radiate from a central elevation. Hemolysis is only poorly developed. Many transitions between smooth and rough forms can be found. The organisms characteristically survive 8 wk. when placed in 20% sodium chloride and stored in the refrigerator; this is helpful in culturing *Listeria* from contaminated autopsy and surgical material because other organisms fail to survive.

Motility: Use motility agar incubated at 20° C. *Listeria* are motile.

Biochemical reactions: The biochemical reactions of *Listeria* are as follows:

Glucose, maltose, fructose: acid

Sucrose, sorbitol, xylose: acid, delayed, longer than 3 days

Manitol, insulin, starch: no utilization or fermentation

Indole, H_2S, urease, oxidase: negative

Nitrates: not reduced

Methyl red, catalase: positive

Animal inoculation: Inject 1 loopful of saline-suspended culture into the conjunctival sac of a rabbit or guinea pig. Purulent conjunctivitis will sometimes result after about 8 hr., but usually a period of 2-5 days should be allowed. The conjunctivitis will heal spontaneously.

Listeriosis is a common disease of animals and therefore the usual inoculation routes cannot be used.

Corynebacterium diphtheriae

Corynebacterium diphtheriae is a small, slender, nonmotile, gram-positive rod that is at times curved and is characterized by irregular staining. It produces a powerful exotoxin that gives rise to a pseudomembranous inflammation and may involve the tonsils, pharynx, nose, vagina, conjunctiva, and wounds. *C. ulcerans* has a similar action.

Classification: Three types of *C. diphtheriae* are distinguishable on the basis of their gross cultural characteristics on blood tellurite medium. This classification has little value since all types produce the same toxin.

1. Gravis: The colonies are dry, rough, and grayish blue. They have a matt surface and show a raised center with radiating sulci. The edges are irregular. Hemolysis is often seen after 48 hr. or more.
2. Mitis: The colonies are round, convex, smooth, and greenish blue to black (after 24 hr.). The edges are smooth. Hemolysis occurs after 28 hr.
3. Intermedius: The colonies are grayish black and have a matt surface and raised center. No sulci are present, and the edges are irregularly outlined.

LABORATORY DIAGNOSIS

PRESUMPTIVE DIAGNOSIS:

Material: Obtain material from the tonsils in the acute phase and from the nasopharynx in the chronic or carrier stage. Smears and cultures must be obtained prior to therapy.

Smear: The organism is a gram-positive, straight, or slightly bent rod that may vary in length from 0.8-4 or 5μ. The ends are usually rounded, but at times may be nodular or pointed. The organisms form V- and L-shaped patterns as well as packages of parallel forms and "Chinese-letter" arrangements. Older cultures may be pleomorphic. The smears may be stained with methylene blue or gram stain. Albert stain reveals metachromatic granules. The direct smear is not an adequate tool for the diagnosis of diphtheria because diphtheroids and actinomycetes resemble *C. diphtheriae*.

Culture: Culture swab on blood agar and on Loeffler medium. Examine both, especially the **Loeffler slant,** after 18 hr., when grayish-white, soft, 1 mm. colonies that can be easily emulsified in water may be seen on the slant. These colonies are smeared and stained. If suspicious on the basis of the gram stain, the colonies are transferred from Loeffler slant to serum-cystine-thiosulfate-tellurite agar (Tinsdale medium) plate for the production of characteristic colonies. This medium is stabbed as well as streaked because the brown to black halo is first noted around the stabs.

Tinsdale medium: On serum-cystine-thiosulfate-tellurite agar, *C. diphtheriae* forms smooth, shiny, black to grayish colonies with (very important) black halos. H_2S is produced by the action on cystine and it then reacts with the tellurite in the medium. The halo is best seen after 48 hr., but may appear after 24 hr. *C. ulcerans* gives a similar picture. It may be isolated from skin ulcers or throat lesions. Most bacteria form black colonies on Tinsdale medium, but they are devoid of the brown to black halo. Included in this list of bacteria that produce black colonies are the following: diphtheroids (nonpathogenic corynebacteria), streptococci, staphylococci, *Neisseria*, pneumococci, *Klebsiella, Haemophilus,* and *E. coli.* Included in the group of **nonpathogenic diphtheroids** are the following: *C. acnes,* which is anaerobic and may be found on the skin, in the vagina, and in the spinal fluid, and *C. xerosis, hofmanni,* and *ulcerans.*

If black colonies with black halos appear on the Tinsdale medium, the organism is transferred again to Loeffler medium or to **Pai egg medium** to confirm the characteristic morphology. Smears should not be made directly from Tinsdale medium. If the smears from Loeffler medium again suggest *C. diphtheriae,* send a report to the physician and to the hospital ward stating that the organisms morphologically resemble *C. diphtheriae.*

Chemical reactions: Chemical reactions are not reliable, though characteristically *C. diphtheriae* ferments dextrose without gas and fails to ferment sucrose.

DEFINITIVE DIAGNOSIS:

Demonstration of toxicity—virulence tests: These tests include animal inoculations or the agar diffusion test. One of these tests must be performed on all suspicious cultures.

Animal inoculation (in vivo method): Rabbits or guinea pigs are used. The hair of the animal is shaven with an electric clipper so that the skin of the back and flanks is exposed. Inject 0.1 ml. of 2-3 ml. broth suspension of an 18 hr. growth of bacteria on Loeffler slant intracutaneously into the nonimmune animal. Five hours later 500 units of diphtheria antitoxin are given intravenously and at the same time 0.1 ml. bacterial suspension is injected intracutaneously into a different site. A virulent toxigenic strain may be used as a control. If the test is positive, 48 hr. after the injection into a guinea pig a necrotic area will appear on the skin. This necrotic response is not found in the area injected after the administration of diphtheria antitoxin.

Agar diffusion test: Prepare petri plates using a special agar media, which is prepared as follows:
1. Proteose-peptone agar,* 20 gm.
2. Lactic acid, 0.7 ml. in 500 ml. distilled water
3. Sodium hydroxide (4%), 1.5 ml.

Bring to boil, filter, adjust to pH 7.8 with 1N hydrochloric acid, and refilter through fluted filter paper.

Prepare filter paper strips saturated with 50 units diphtheria toxin and place on top of freshly prepared and just-gelled agar plate. Allow to dry completely in incubator (3 hr.). Streak saline emulsion of unknown *C. diphtheriae* and of known positive and negative diphtheria control bacteria at right angles to the centrally placed impregnated filter strip. Incubate plate at 35° C. If the diphtheria bacilli are toxin producing, a precipitation line will form between the impregnated filter paper and the bacterial streak.

NOTE: After 48 hr., secondary lines may form which are not related to toxin production.

Erysipelothrix

This organism is widely distributed in animals and is important as a cause of an infectious disease in swine. It causes skin

---

*Difco Laboratories, Detroit, Mich.

lesions in man, but very seldom produces a generalized disease.

It is a gram-positive, nonmotile rod that is slender, straight, and often paired. It may be curved (S shaped) and may give rise to long, slender, tangled filaments.

The organism is catalase negative (*Listeria* and *Corynebacterium* are catalase positive) and reduces nitrates. It is weakly saccharolytic and may produce H_2S.

The organism grows well at 35° C. on blood agar. Cystine-glucose-blood agar (see discussion of *Pasteurella*) is a good medium for primary plating.

Animal inoculation: Intraperitoneal injection of 0.25 ml. bacterial suspension will kill mice in 2-4 days.

MYCOBACTERIA[80]

The genus *Mycobacterium* includes the following:

1. Pathogens: *M. tuberculosis* (var. *hominis*), *M. bovis* (var. *bovis*), *M. avium* (birds and pigs), *M. ulcerans* (skin in man), *M. leprae* (human leprosy), *M. paratuberculosis* (cattle), *M. lepraemurium* (rat leprosy)
2. Saprophytes (including potential pathogens): *M. phlei* (soil), *M. smegmatis* (soil), *M. fortuitum* (soil, cattle, cold-blooded animals, man), *M. marinum* (salt-water fish, man), etc.
3. Unclassified atypical acid-fast organisms (including potential pathogens): (a) photochromogens (*M. kansasii*, the yellow bacillus, Runyon group I), (b) scotochromogens (Runyon group II), (c) nonchromogenic strains (Battey type, Runyon group III), and (d) rapid growers (Runyon group IV)

LABORATORY DIAGNOSIS OF TUBERCULOSIS

Laboratory diagnosis and differentiation of mycobacteria includes special methods of collection and concentration, acid-fast smears, culture of acid-fast organisms, pigment studies, biochemical reactions and other differentiating tests, drug-susceptibility patterns, animal pathogenicity, and immunologic methods for detecting antibodies to *M. tuberculosis*.

Special methods of collection and concentration

TYPES AND HANDLING OF SPECIMENS: CONTAMINATED SPECIMENS:

Sputum: If the specimen is not processed immediately, store it in the refrigerator. Sputum of children may have to be obtained by gastric lavage, which in general should be avoided. Special, plastic, sterile, wide-mouth, screw-capped centrifuge tubes for the collection of sputum are available* in which the concentration procedure can be carried out, thus minimizing the handling of infectious material.

The first morning expectoration provides the best specimen; it is superior to a large pooled specimen, which may be heavily contaminated and/or toxic to tubercle bacilli and may also dilute a single positive contribution.

Methods employing heated aerosols are successful in stimulating sputum production if expectoration is difficult. They are preferable to gastric lavage.

Gastric contents: Gastric contents should be collected directly into 5 ml. 15% trisodium phosphate or into 1 ml. 10% sodium bicarbonate (to reach pH 7). The normal acidity and enzymatic activity of the gastric juice are detrimental to tubercle bacilli. Since saprophytic tubercle bacilli on smears are indistinguishable from pathogenic forms, the gastric material should only be cultured, not smeared. Digest with sodium hydroxide or with NAC. Positive cultures must be carefully identified before reporting as *M. tuberculosis*. The use of gastric aspiration should be avoided.

Urine: Allow 24 hr. specimen to stand overnight in the refrigerator. If specimen is received in a gallon jug, transfer it to a clean Ehrlenmeyer flask; it is difficult to decant from jugs without disturbing the sediment. Cover mouth of flask. Discard upper portion, saving the lower 300-400 ml. Centrifuge the saved portion in multiple centrifuge tubes and combine the sediments. Digest with sodium hydroxide as for sputum.

*Falcon Plastics Division, Becton, Dickinson & Co., Rutherford, N. J.

A first morning specimen is preferred since it is less contaminated than a 24 hr. specimen. Cleaning of the genitalia will prevent contamination with smegma bacilli. Positive smears must be interpreted with caution, and positive cultures must be carefully identified before reporting as *M. tuberculosis*.

Feces[81]: The first morning specimen is collected in a clean, wide-mouth glass jar. Add 3 vol. water, mix well, and filter through several thicknesses of gauze. The filtrate is saturated with sodium chloride and left undisturbed for 30 min. to allow the bacteria to rise to the surface. Collect this floating material with a large spoon, place in a wide-mouth bottle, and add an equal volume of 1N NaOH solution. Shake in a paint shaker and incubate at 35° C. for 3 hr., shaking every 30 min. Add 1N hydrochloric acid to neutralize the mixture to sterile litmus paper, centrifuge, and use sediment as inoculum.

Tissues: Tissues from surgical or autopsy specimens should be homogenized using a mortar and pestle or glass tissue homogenizers (see Chapter 16).

Skin: Acid-fast organisms of skin lesions should be cultured at 30° C. since *M. ulcerans* and *M. balnei* fail to grow at 35° C.

NONCONTAMINATED SPECIMENS: Noncontaminated specimens include catheterized urine specimens, clear body fluids such as pleural, pericardial, and peritoneal fluids, and cerebrospinal fluid. Do not use a digestion method because it unavoidably leads to loss of vital bacteria. Centrifuge specimens at high speed and use sediment for smear, culture, and animal inoculation.

Cerebrospinal fluid: Spinal fluid examination should be done promptly. If there is a pellicle, it should be spread on a slide, fixed, and stained for acid-fast bacteria. If no pellicle is found, centrifuge the specimen, decant supernatant, and use sediment for smears, culture, and animal inoculation.

CONCENTRATION AND DECONTAMINATION METHODS:

1. *N*-Acetyl-L-cysteine (NAC) digestion method. This method is milder, but contaminating bacteria may survive.
2. NaOH digestion method (proteolytic).
3. Trisodium phosphate concentration method. May be used as holding medium.
4. Clorox digestion method. Can be used for smears only.

The purpose of these methods is to destroy contaminating organisms while allowing tubercle bacilli to survive so that they can be concentrated, cultured, stained, and injected into animals. Because the strong mineral acids and alkali that are conventionally used for concentration are harmful to the tubercle bacillus, the use of a milder proteolytic digestion method is suggested (NAC). Several methods are available.

***N*-Acetyl-L-cysteine (NAC) digestion method**[82-84]:

Reagents:

1. Phosphate buffer (M/15, pH 6.8):
   Solution A (stock standard):
   Na_2HPO_4 (M/15), 9.47 gm./L.
   KH_2PO_4 (M/15), 9.07 gm./L.
   Solution B (working standard, pH 6.8):
   Na_2HPO_4 (M/15), 50 ml.
   KH_2PO_4 (M/15), 50 ml.
   Check with pH meter or pH paper.
2. *N*-Acetyl-L-cysteine–sodium hydroxide digestant (50 ml.):
   NaOH (1N, 4%), 25 ml.
   Sodium citrate (0.1M, 2.9%), 25 ml.
   N-Acetyl-L-cysteine (20%) or *N*-acetyl-L-cysteine powder,* 0.25 gm.
   Sterilize the three solutions by autoclaving and store in the refrigerator. Use within 24 hr. after mixing solutions.
3. Bovine albumin (0.2%) in saline solution (0.85%). Adjust to pH 7.0 with 10% NaOH. Sterilize by Seitz filtration.

Procedure:

1. To 10 ml. sputum specimen collected in a 50 ml. sterile, disposable, plastic, screw-capped centrifuge tube add an equal volume of *N*-

---

*Sigma Chemical Co., St. Louis, Mo.

acetyl-L-cysteine–sodium hydroxide solution. (The volume of sputum should not exceed one fifth the volume of the tube.)

2. Mix in a Vortex mixer for 5-30 sec., or until digested.
3. Let stand at room temperature for 15 min. to decontaminate.
4. Fill tube to within ½-¾ in. of the top with sterile M/15 phosphate buffer, pH 6.8.
5. Centrifuge at (or near) 300 rpm for 15 min.
6. Carefully decant supernatant fluid. Retain sediment.
7. Prepare a smear from the sediment. (If direct drug-susceptibility tests are to be done, it is necessary to roughly quantitate the numbers of acid-fast organisms in the sediment. For this purpose use an inoculating loop 3 mm. in diameter and spread the material over an area approximately 1 × 2 cm.)
8. Stain by the acid-fast method.
9. Add 2 ml. 0.2% bovine albumin fraction V in 0.85% saline solution to the remaining sediment.
10. Using 1 ml. of this sediment, make a 1:10 dilution with sterile water.
11. Inoculate media as follows, using 0.1 ml. specimen for each tube or plate:
    (a) Lowenstein-Jensen slants: two tubes from undiluted sediment and two tubes from 1:10 dilution
    (b) 7H 10 base with OADC supplement: one plate from undiluted sediment and one plate from 1:10 dilution

The NAC digestion procedure lowers the viscosity of mucoid and purulent specimens and is not harmful to acid-fast bacteria. This method is "on trial" at this time. It leads to an increased number of contaminants even if the 1N NaOH concentration is increased to 7%.

NaOH digestion method: Transfer specimen into a heavy, round-bottomed, screw-capped tube and add an equal amount of autoclaved 4% sodium hydroxide. Mix and then shake forcefully for 15 min. in a paint shaker; centrifuge at 3000 rpm for 15 min. Decant supernatant, add 1 drop bromthymol blue to sediment, and neutralize it accurately with sterile 1N hydrochloric acid. Use sterile Pasteur pipettes to obtain specimen for smears, cultures, and animal inoculation. If the volume of the sediment is too small, use sterile phosphate buffer, pH 6.6, for dilution. (Bromthymol blue: acid—yellow; alkaline—blue.) Use sterile Pasteur pipettes to obtain specimen for smears, cultures, and animal inoculation. If the volume of the sediment is too small, use sterile buffer, pH 6.6, for dilution.

Trisodium phosphate concentration method: This method is suitable for mailing contaminated specimens since trisodium phosphate is relatively nontoxic to tubercle bacilli. An equal volume of 10% trisodium phosphate is added to the specimen. The mixture is shaken in a paint shaker for 15 min. and centrifuged at 300 rpm for 15 min. Decant supernatant and add 10 ml. sterile saline solution, mix, and recentrifuge. The supernatant is poured off and the sediment is ready for plating.

Clorox (5.25% sodium hypochlorite) digestion method: This concentration method can be used only for the preparation of smears because it kills the organisms.

Mix one half to equal parts of Clorox with specimen. Allow to stand for 15 min. Centrifuge at 3000 rpm for 30 min. Decant supernatant and prepare smear from sediment.

Acid-fast smear

The acid-fast smear reveals the following:

1. **Morphology:** size and shape, e.g., polymorphic (*M. avium*), long (Runyon group I); shape, e.g., long and thin (*M. tuberculosis*), straight, curved; and structure, e.g., beaded (*M. tuberculosis*), crossbanding (*M. kansasii*), solid (*M. leprae*), branched
2. Acid-fast property of the bacillus, e.g., weak, strong
3. A rough estimate of the number of organisms

Acid-fast bacilli found in the sputum smear nearly always represent tubercle bacilli and indicate that the patient is

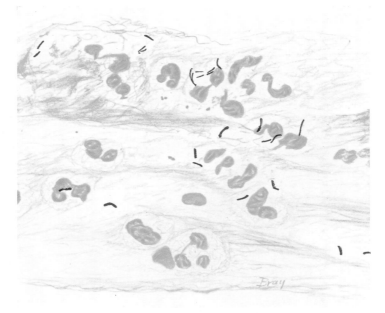

Plate 14. Tubercle bacilli in sputum. (Acid-fast stain.)

infectious. Sputum smears may be used to follow the **response to treatment.** Three sputum specimens should always be examined. Positive smears of urinary sediments or of gastric contents must be interpreted with great caution since they may contain acid-fast saprophytes. Smears are the basis of the direct drug-susceptibility testing method.

Direct smears and smears of concentrated material or of cultures are stained for acid-fast bacteria by the Kinyoun, Ziehl-Neelsen, or fluorescent dye methods.

Morphology: In the case of *M. tuberculosis* the positive smear shows straight, slightly curved, thin rods that require special staining because of their lipid content. Once stained, they are not readily decolorized (acid fast). In cultures the bacteria are often coccoid, filamentous, and branching (hence mycobacteria). Staining is not uniform; it is accentuated by granules and interrupted by poorly stained segments. Acid-fast bacteria are difficult to stain with gram stain, but they are gram positive. The average number of bacilli per slide or field is sometimes reported as the Gaffky number, though the number of bacilli in the direct smear is not a good index of the severity of the disease.

Method of reporting: If fewer than three organisms per slide are found, request another specimen. Report 3-9 organisms as rare, 10 as few, and over 10 as numerous.

STAINS FOR ACID-FAST BACILLI:

Kinyoun method: See routinely employed stains, p. 538.

Ziehl-Neelsen staining method:

Reagents:
1. Carbolfuchsin (mordant and dye):
   Saturated solution of basic fuchsin (10 gm. basic fuchsin in 100 ml. 95% ethyl alcohol), 10 ml.
   Aqueous solution of crystalline phenol (5%), 90 ml.
2. Acid-alcohol (decolorizing agent):
   HCl (concentrated), 3 ml.
   Ethyl alcohol (95%), 97 ml.
3. Counterstain:
   Methylene blue, 0.3 gm.
   Distilled water, 100 ml.

Procedure:
1. Fix the smear by heating on a slide warmer for 2 hr. at 65° C. or overnight.
2. Place a piece of filter paper (cut

slightly smaller than the slide) over the smear.

3. Cover smear with carbolfuchsin.
4. Steam for 5 min. **Do not boil and do not allow slide to dry.** (If an electric staining rack is used, allow up to 15 min. time.)
5. Wash with distilled water.
6. Decolorize with acid alcohol for 2 min.
7. Wash with distilled water.
8. Counterstain with methylene blue for 30-60 sec.
9. Wash in distilled water, dry, and examine.

Fluorescent dye method:
Truant fluorescent dye[85]**:**
Reagents:

1. Stain:
   Auramine, 1.5 gm.
   Rhodamine, 0.75 gm.
   Glycerol, 75 ml.
   Phenol, 10 ml.
   Distilled water, 50 ml.

Filter through glass wool to clarify. Solutions keep several months at 4° C. or at room temperature. Store in dark bottle.

2. Decolorant solution (acid-alcohol): HCl (0.5%) in ethanol (70%)
3. Counterstain (potassium permanganate): 0.5 gm. potassium permanganate in 100 ml. distilled water. Store in dark bottle.

Procedure:

1. Prepare smear using new slides.
2. Fix smears by heating on slide warmer for 2 hr. at 65° C. or overnight.
3. Cover smear with auramine-rhodamine dye.
4. Stain for 15 min. at room temperature, 37° C., or 60° C.
5. Rinse off stain with distilled water.
6. Decolorize for 2-3 min. with acid-alcohol.
7. Wash with distilled water.
8. Flood smear for 2-4 min. with 0.5% potassium permanganate.
9. Rinse, dry, and examine.
10. Confirm all positive smears by restaining of the original smear by the acid-fast method.

The reagent is a fluorescent dye that stains mycobacteria selectively. No antigen-antibody reaction is involved in this procedure.

The fluorescent dye method allows rapid scanning of smears with 100× total magnification. Positive smears can be confirmed by overstaining with acid-fast stain. Patients on drug therapy may discharge organisms that stain by fluorescent methods but not by the conventional acid-fast stains.

Culture of acid-fast organisms

Culture allows observation of the following:

1. **Rate of growth:** slow grower, over 7 days, or rapid grower, less than 7 days, dysgony, e.g., saprophytes
2. **Temperature of growth,** e.g., no growth at 22° C. (*M. tuberculosis,* etc.), growth at 22° C. (*M. kansasii*)
3. **Color and effect of exposure to light,** e.g., photochromogens and nonphotochromogens
4. **Shape and texture of colony** (microcolonial characteristics): rough (*M. tuberculosis*), smooth (*M. kansasii*), variable (Runyon groups II and IV), flat or heaped up colonies, large (*M. smegmatis*), small (*M. tuberculosis*)

There are three basic types of **media.**

Liquid media[86]**:** Liquid media are not suitable for primary isolation because clouding is produced by *M. tuberculosis* and by atypical tubercle bacilli.

Dubos Tween-albumin broth (TAB): Use dehydrated Dubos broth base to prepare 1 L. Autoclave at 121° C. for 15 min. and cool to 50°-56° C. Add 100 ml. 5% saline bovine albumin fraction V*, pH 7, adjusted by the addition of 2-4 drops 10% NaOH. Sterilize by filtration. Add 10 ml. 50% sterile glucose in water and place 5 ml. into sterile 20 × 150 mm. screw-capped tubes. Incubate for 12 hr. at 35° C. to test for sterility.

Synthetic media: Middlebrook 7H 10 with OADC supplement is a synthetic medium which, because of its agar base, is transparent. It allows recognition of early (3 wk.) growth and of microcoloni-

---

*Armour Laboratories, Chicago, Ill.

al characteristics of various types of mycobacteria. With this clear medium it is possible to "read through" the contamination. The medium permits more accurate drug-susceptibility testing because drugs are not subject to potential inactivation by inspissation since they can be added after sterilization.

Egg media: Lowenstein-Jensen and Petragnani media are the most commonly used egg media. They are opaque; therefore early colonies may be missed. Drug-resistant organisms frequently fail to grow on these media. Drugs incorporated into egg media may lose some of their potency during the process of inspissation.

Lowenstein-Jensen medium: The tubes should be allowed to lie almost horizontally and with the caps loosened until the inoculum dries on the slant. Incubate at 35° C. 6-8 wk. in the dark. Do not allow cultures to dry out. Cultures of patients under treatment and cultures of bovine organisms may grow very late. Examine and aerate tubes once a week. Before discarding, examine smears of culture surface microscopically. Expose tubes to light and examine for pigment production after growth appears.

Middlebrook 7H 10 medium: Incubate Middlebrook 7H 10 plates with OADC supplement in upright position under CO_2 in permeable polyethylene bags[87] at 35° C. for 3 wk. in the dark or in **Mylar CO_2-impermeable bags** containing heavily seeded plates of growing *M. phlei.* Examine plates only once at 3 wk., both macroscopically and microscopically with a dissecting microscope.

Middlebrook plates are reported as follows:

4+	Over 500 colonies (confluent growth)
3+	Between 200-500 colonies (almost confluent growth)
2+	100-200 colonies
1+	50-100 colonies
Actual count	Below 50 colonies

Culture differentiation of mycobacteria

Culture differentiation is based on (1) microcolonial characteristics on Lowenstein-Jensen and Middlebrook 7H 10 agar; (2) pigment production in the dark, following exposure to light for 1 hr., or fol-

lowing exposure for 2 wk.; and (3) rate of growth at 22°, 37°, and 45° C.

Microcolonial characteristics of mycobacteria on Lowenstein-Jensen medium: Fregnan and Smith[88] describe the following types.

Human type: Small, wrinkled, dry, and umbilicated at times, with beige to pale-yellow color. They are friable, easily detached from the surface, and have a "cabbage appearance." They appear in about 6 wk. and emulsify with difficulty.

Bovine type: Moist, pale, somewhat nipplelike, and small, with color similar to human type. They grow slowly, appearing in about 8 wk. They are tiny, adhere to the surface, and emulsify rapidly.

Avian type: Colonies appear in about 3 wk. and are smooth, hemispherical, and faintly yellow to gray.

Atypical types: Yellow to orange and pink, usually moist, soft, creamy, and usually smooth. Proliferative growth appears in a few days. The atypical types are able to grow at room temperature.

Microcolonial characteristics of mycobacteria on Middlebrook 7H 10 agar with OADC enrichment: Vestal and Kubica[89] describe the following forms.

Rough (R): Dry, white, or buff colonies which microscopically are composed of filaments or pseudocords that often produce a dark central spot. This type of colony suggests *M. tuberculosis* but is also found in other mycobacteria, i.e., *M. bovis, M. kansasii,* and some rapid-growing mycobacteria. It is important to remember that tuberculosis organisms always grow in the rough form on 7H 10 medium with supplement.

Smooth (S): Colonies are circular, with raised central areas sloping to an irregular or undulated periphery. This type of colony is seen in *M. avium,* in group III nonphotochromogens, and in group II scotochromogens.

Several other smooth types of colonies such as smooth D, T, K, etc. are described.

Pigment studies[90]

Mycobacteria can be classified according to whether pigment appears during growth when light is present or excluded or whether it does not appear at all, irregardless of light exposure. Exclusion of air interferes with pigment production, which is best seen in young cultures.

Exposure to light for one hour:

Light source: Use a 30- to 60-watt lamp. The culture tubes should be 8-10 in. from the light source.

Procedure:

1. Select cultures with well-isolated colonies (grown in dark).
2. Loosen cap on culture tube.
3. Remove whole shield from culture and cover half of slant with one half of the shield.
4. Expose to light for 1 hr. as directed.
5. Replace whole shield and incubate at 35° C. in the dark for 6-12 hr. or overnight.
6. Check for pigmentation by comparing pigment of colonies on both exposed and shielded portions of the tube.

If results are not clear cut, compare with other tube of same specimen which has remained in the dark.

NOTE: Tests must be made with actively growing cultures. (Up to 5 or 6 days **after** colonies have appeared is usually satisfactory. Older cultures should not be used.)

Interpretation: M. kansasii and *M. marinum* will develop yellow pigment within 1 hr.

Exposure to continuous light for two weeks[91]:

Light source: Use a 36 in., cool white, 30-watt light bulb (General Electric fluorescent bulb). Place cultures approximately 8 in. from the light source. The light intensity should be 150 candles/sq. ft. Measure with a Weston Master No. 3 light meter.

Procedure:

1. Prepare two Lowenstein-Jensen slants so as to have well-isolated colonies.
2. Treat tubes as follows:
   (a) Light tube (1 tube):
       (1) Shield from light.
       (2) Incubate for 2 wk. in dark.
       (3) Remove shield and expose to light for 2 wk.

(b) Dark tube (1 tube):
    (1) Incubate for 4 wk. and shield from light.
3. Compare pigmentation of colonies on both sets of cultures at the end of 4 wk.

Interpretation: All colonies of photochromogens may require 2 wk. of exposure before developing pigment.

Biochemical reactions and other differentiating tests

Semiquantitative catalase test[92]:

Principle: Acid-fast bacteria contain catalase, an enzyme that liberates O_2 from hydrogen peroxide.

Reagent:

Tween 80–hydrogen peroxide mixture (1:1):

1. Tween 80 (10% in distilled water)
2. Hydrogen peroxide (Superoxol*) (30%)

Inoculation of media: Add 0.1 ml. of a 7-day-old TAB culture to a Lowenstein-Jensen butt tube.† Incubate at 35° C. for 1-2 wk.

Technique:

1. Remove cultures from incubator and add 1 ml. Tween 80–hydrogen peroxide mixture to Lowenstein-Jensen culture.
2. Allow cultures to remain stationary for 5 min.
3. Measure column of bubbling in mm.
4. Record as follows: < 40 mm. or > 50 mm.

Interpretation: Isoniazid-resistant *M. tuberculosis* are catalase negative. All mycobacteria contain catalase; some "atypical" mycobacteria contain an increased amount (> 50 mm.), while *M. tuberculosis* contains < 40 mm.

Niacin test[93]:

Principle: Niacin produced by the organism forms a color compound with cyanogen bromide and aniline. Cyanogen

---

*Merck & Co., Rahway, N. J.
†Lowenstein-Jensen butt tubes: Dispense 5 ml. Lowenstein-Jensen medium in 20 × 150 mm. screw-capped test tubes. Inspissate tubes in upright position in a water bath at 85° C. for 60 min. Remove tubes and incubate at 35° C. overnight to check for sterility of medium.

bromide is tear gas and must be used under a well-ventilated fume hood.

Reagents:
1. Sterile water or saline solution
2. Aniline (4% in ethyl alcohol)
3. Cyanogen bromide (10% aqueous)

Procedure:
1. Add 1 ml. sterile water or saline solution to the culture slant of the test organism. Colonies should be present at least 3 wk. before the test is performed and may require 8-9 wk. after colonies have appeared before yielding a positive test.
2. Slant the culture so that the fluid covers the colonies and let it remain in this position for 15 min.
3. Remove 0.5 ml. of this aqueous extract* and transfer to a 16 × 125 mm. screw-capped test tube.
4. Add 0.5 ml. aniline and 0.5 ml. cyanogen bromide to the extract.
5. Mix and observe for the formation of a yellow color. If niacin is present, the color appears almost immediately throughout the solution.

Controls:
1. Niacin-positive culture (known *M. tuberculosis*)
2. Niacin-negative culture (e.g., known group III nonphotochromogen)
3. Saline control on uninoculated tube of medium

Results: The test is positive when the development of a yellow color indicates the presence of niacin. No color change indicates absence of niacin, therefore the test is negative.

Interpretation: M. tuberculosis is the only niacin-positive mycobacterium.

NOTE: Stock solutions of aniline and cyanogen bromide may be prepared and stored in brown bottles in the refrigerator. If either solution changes color or precipitates, it should be discarded and a fresh solution prepared. The 10% cyanogen bromide solution is close to saturation and therefore storage in the refrigerator may cause precipitation. However,

warming to room temperature will bring about solution of most of the compound.

Neutral red test:

Principle: Virulent strains of *M. tuberculosis* are able to bind neutral red in an alkaline aqueous solution. Nonvirulent strains and saprophytes will not take up the dye.

Procedure:
1. Place 5 ml. 50% v/v methanol into each of a series of small screw-capped centrifuge tubes and inoculate with two large colonies from each of the cultures.
2. Incubate the tubes for 1 hr. at 35° C. and then centrifuge to pack the organisms. Decant the alcohol.
3. Add 5 ml. alcohol to each tube, resuspend the organisms by shaking the tubes, and repeat step 2.
4. Add 5 ml. alkaline barbiturate buffer (sodium barbital, 1 gm.; sodium chloride, 5 gm.; and distilled water, 100 ml.) and 1 ml. 20% aqueous solution of neutral red to each tube. Shake the contents and incubate the tubes for 30 min. at room temperature.

Interpretation: After incubation, neutral red–positive strains exhibit varying degrees of pink or red staining. Negative strains remain unchanged. Virulent strains are neutral red positive; saprophytes and atypical mycobacteria are neutral red negative.

Cord formation:

Principle: Virulent strains form cords that consist of bacteria aligned parallel, side to side, and end to end.

Procedure:
1. Grow the test strains on egg media slants.
2. Incubate the cultures for 3-7 days at 35° C. without disturbing.
3. By means of serologic or Pasteur pipettes and with as little agitation as possible, transfer 1 drop of water from condensation to a slide. Do not smear or streak.
4. Dry, fix, and stain the smears using the acid-fast technique.
5. Examine the smears under high-power, dry, and oil-immersion objectives.

---

*Rotate tube so that the slant faces downward, insert pipette along glass side, and remove extract without touching slant. Tube may be used again since the colonies have not been disturbed.

Interpretation: Virulent tubercle bacilli grow in long strands or serpentine cords, whereas avirulent types form no particular arrangement. Sometimes positive cording may be seen by viewing the side of the culture under a scanning lens.

Drug-susceptibility patterns

Untreated *M. tuberculosis* is usually susceptible to isoniazid, *p*-aminosalicylic acid (PAS), and streptomycin. Runyon groups III and IV are resistant.

DRUG-SUSCEPTIBILITY TESTING[94]: There are many variables in these tests such as (1) type of test done (direct or indirect), (2) choice of drugs and their concentrations, and (3) choice of medium.

TYPES OF TESTS:
1. Direct tests: Undiluted or diluted sputum is used as inoculum of drug-containing media. Results may be reported in 3 wk.
2. Indirect tests: Growth from primary cultures is used as inoculum of drug-containing media, and the results are therefore delayed for 6 wk.

Direct tests: Direct tests should be performed on all specimens with positive smears.

Choice of drugs and their concentrations: Streptomycin (2 μg), isoniazid (0.2 μg), and PAS (2 μg) are the drugs that are used.

Choice of medium: Use Middlebrook 7H 10 agar with OADC enrichment.

Preparation of medium for drug-susceptibility testing: A **Felsen plate** is used. The first quadrant contains dyed medium without any drug. The second quadrant contains isoniazid, the third contains streptomycin, and the fourth contains PAS.

The amount of drug or dye stock solution to be added to 200 ml. Middlebrook 7H 10 agar with OADC enrichment is as follows:
1. 1 ml. 5 μg/ml. Congo red as control
2. 0.4 ml. 100 μg/ml. isoniazid
3. 0.4 ml. 1000 μg/ml. streptomycin
4. 0.4 ml. 1000 μg/ml. PAS (add enough dilute NaOH to dissolve)

Solutions 1, 2, and 4 are sterilized by autoclaving; solution 3 is prepared from sterile vials.

Direct drug-susceptibility testing[95]: Two inocula are recommended in setting up the sensitivity plates. One is inoculated with the undiluted concentrate, while the other is inoculated with the diluted concentrate. Standardization of the inocula is necessary for reliable test results since overinoculation may exaggerate the incidence of primary resistance due to spontaneous drug-resistant mutants.

Procedure:
1. Stain and read smears of digested sputa.
2. Dilute the concentrates of positive specimens with sterile distilled water on the basis of smear results as follows:

No. of AFB per oil-immersion field	Dilutions of concentrate for use as inocula
Less than 1	Undiluted and 10^{-1}
1-10	10^{-1} and 10^{-2}
More than 10	10^{-2} and 10^{-3}

3. Inoculate drug media in Felsen quadrant plates with each of the two dilutions selected. Use 3 drops from a Pasteur capillary pipette for each quadrant.
4. Incubate at 35° C. for 3 wk. in Mylar bags with *M. phlei.*
5. Examine plates for growth, both macroscopically and microscopically with a dissecting microscope fitted with a 10× ocular lens.
6. Record bacterial growth **per quadrant** as follows:

Confluent	++++
Almost confluent	+++
Approximately 100 colonies	++
50-100 colonies	+
Below 50	Actual count

7. Report results obtained with both dilutions of inocula.

NOTE: Since spontaneous drug-resistant mutants may appear in heavily inoculated media, readings on specimens giving 4+ growth in the control quadrants may not be valid.

Animal pathogenicity

Not all laboratory animals are equally susceptible to various types of tubercle bacilli. The guinea pig is most sensitive to the human and bovine types, the rabbit to the bovine and avian species, and the mouse to some of the atypical forms.

Guinea pig inoculation: Use two guinea pigs that are negative to intracutaneous injections of 0.1 ml. 5% old tuberculin. The concentrated neutralized specimen (see p. 593) is injected subcutaneously into the groin and at 6 wk. the animals are killed. At autopsy examine for tubercles in the inguinal lymph nodes, liver, and spleen. Smears of these tubercles must contain acid-fast organisms and tissue sections should confirm the diagnosis of tuberculosis. Involvement of the lymph nodes alone is not enough; the spleen and liver must be involved to prove invasion by the organism. Involvement of the lung only indicates spontaneous tuberculosis and nullifies the test. If the guinea pig dies within 21 days, the test should be repeated.

Isoniazid-resistant tubercle bacilli may fail to produce disease in guinea pigs.

Rabbits are injected intravenously with cultures of bovine or avian tuberculosis.

Immunologic methods for detecting antibodies to Mycobacterium tuberculosis[96-98]

The suggested test is the gel double-diffusion technique, which is based on the Ouchterlony precipitin reaction in gels. This test may lend itself to rapid screening of large groups of individuals for active cases of tuberculosis.

Unclassified (atypical) mycobacteria

A scheme for the separation of medically significant strains of unclassified acid-fast bacilli has been developed by Runyon.[90]

Group I: photochromogenic mycobacteria (yellow bacillus, *M. kansasii*)
Group II: scotochromogenic mycobacteria (orange bacillus)
Group III: nonphotochromogenic mycobacteria (Battey-avium-swine complex)
Group IV: rapid-growing mycobacteria

PHOTOCHROMOGENS (M. KANSASII)[91]

To establish the diagnosis of group I mycobacteria, all cultures for tubercle bacilli are incubated in the dark except for short weekly examinations. When colonies appear, they should be exposed to light for 1 hr. (see p. 597). If the cultures are old, 2 wk. of exposure may be needed (see p. 597). The photochromogenic *M. kansasii* develops yellow pigment after 1 hr. of exposure. Photochromogenic mycobacteria produce severe pulmonary disease in man and are most common in the northern, midwestern, and southwestern regions of the United States. The organisms are long and the smear, fixed in formalin and stained with Ziehl-Neelsen stain, shows **crossbanding** of the rods.

SCOTOCHROMOGENS

Scotochromogens develop yellow to orange pigmentation while incubating in the dark. Aside from a few isolated cases of pulmonary disease and occasional lymphadenitis, most strains are thought not to be disease producing.

NONPHOTOCHROMOGENS (BATTEY AND OTHER GROUPS)[99]

Nonphotochromogens form smooth colonies that usually do not form pigment in the dark or after exposure to light for 1 hr. or 2 wk. Some strains acquire a faint yellow tinge. Identification of this group is important because these strains are **drug resistant** and produce pulmonary disease which is difficult to treat. Other strains within this group are called J & V and Radish strains. They fail to hydrolyze Tween 80 within 21 days.[100]

RAPID-GROWING MYCOBACTERIA

Colonies form in less than 7 days. These strains have been isolated from superficial and deep lesions. *M. fortuitum,*[101, 102] *M. smegmatis,*[102] and *M. phlei*[103] should be identified by name rather than being reported as rapid growers. The **arylsulfatase test**[104] will distinguish *M. fortuitum* from *M. phlei* and *M. smegmatis*. *M. fortuitum* during 3 days of incubation will release phenolphthalein from tripotassium phenolphthalein disulfate so that its presence can be detected with sodium carbonate. *M. phlei* and *M. smegmatis* fail to break the compound even after 1 wk. of incubation. *M. fortuitum* is pathogenic to albino mice. A rapidly growing subculture of *M. tuberculosis* must not be mistaken for *M. fortuitum*.

Mycobacterium leprae (Hansen's bacillus)[105, 106]

The causative organism of leprosy is *M. leprae*. The organism is a straight or slightly curved rod that is 1-8μ long and 0.3-0.5μ in diameter. It is strongly acid fast and stains evenly.

LABORATORY DIAGNOSIS

The only procedure available is the acid-fast smear.

Acid-fast smear: Obtain smears from nasal secretion, skin nodules, or ulcers on nasal septum and stain by acid-fast or fluorescent (auramine) methods.

Observe for large numbers of acid-fast bacilli in the lepra cells (endothelial cells); a rounded mass or globus is the characteristic arrangement.

Scrapings from the entire thickness of the skin by the **Wayson technique** is recommended.[107] Pinch an area of the skin between the thumb and forefinger, using sufficient pressure to blanch the skin. Make an incision about 5 mm. in length, going through the full thickness of the skin but not into the fatty tissue. Scrape the cut surfaces and make smears for staining.

Inoculate guinea pigs with material showing acid-fast bacilli in order to eliminate tuberculosis bacilli. Leprosy bacilli are not pathogenic for guinea pigs. *M. leprae* is difficult to culture and requires minced chick embryo.

ACTINOMYCETACEAE

The genus *Nocardia*, an obligate aerobe, and the genus *Actinomyces*, an obligate anaerobe, are members of the family Actinomycetaceae and are transition forms between bacteria and fungi, showing some similarity to tubercle bacilli, to *Corynebacterium diphtheriae*, and to fungi.

Nocardia asteroides and brasiliensis

Nocardia causes localized granulomatous lesions but is also able to cause generalized systemic infections resembling tuberculosis (**nocardiosis**).

LABORATORY DIAGNOSIS

Material: Examination of pus or sputum may show sulfurlike granules which may be white, cream colored, yellow, or red.

Smear: Make direct smear or make smear after concentration; use gram stain and modified Kinyoun stain. *Nocardia* is gram positive and weakly acid fast.

Wet preparation: Use 10% potassium hydroxide.

Concentration method (Ajello): Mix equal portions 10% trisodium phosphate and sputum in a centrifuge tube and allow to digest at room temperature until the sputum becomes clear (about 4 hr.). Centrifuge the cleared sputum for 15 min. at 2000 rpm and neutralize the sediment with 2N hydrochloric acid before inoculating media.

Acid-fast stain: Use Kinyoun stain and decolorize with 1% sulfuric acid in water, which has a light decolorizing action.

Culture: Use blood agar, thioglycollate broth, and Sabouraud dextrose agar. Surface growth occurs in broth, with a pellicle often growing upward on the wall of the tube. Slide or cover slip cultures show slowly branching mycelia.

Slide culture technique: Fill the concavities of culture slides with heated chlamydospore agar, using a quantity sufficient to bring the surface of the medium to a level just higher than the surrounding surface of the slide. Inoculate the surface of the medium. Place cover slip over inoculum so that it is in contact with the medium and the surrounding slide. Place slide culture in sterile petri dish, which is lowered into a jar containing a moist paper towel. Incubate at 35° C.

Growth is relatively rapid on blood agar, appearing in as little as 2 days. The colonies are similar to those on Sabouraud agar.

On Sabouraud dextrose agar, 5-10 mm. colonies develop slowly in 4-5 days. They are folded, elevated, tan to yellow, and produce aerial hyphae. The latter distinguish them from the otherwise similar colonies of some species of mycobacteria.

This distinction is important since *Nocardia* survives concentration methods, grows on acid-fast culture media in 1-2 wk., and is acid fast. Substrate hyphae, which are not observed in mycobacteria, may also be seen. Smears of cultures show short branching filaments and bacillary and coccoid forms that are partially acid fast.

BIOCHEMICAL REACTIONS: The following tests can be used to distinguish *N. asteroides* from *N. brasilienses,* and to distinguish both from *Streptomyces* species.

Casein hydrolysis test: Suspend 5 gm. skimmed milk powder* in 15 ml. distilled water. Dissolve 1 gm. agar in 50 ml. water. Autoclave separately and cool to 47° C. Mix milk and agar and pour into five sterile petri dishes. Each culture is heavily streaked once across, incubated at 28° C., and observed for 7-14 days for clearing of the opaque casein underneath and around the colonies.

N. asteroides is incapable of hydrolyzing casein, whereas *Streptomyces* species and other *Nocardia* can hydrolyze this protein.

Growth in gelatin:
Medium:
1. Gelatin, 4 gm.
2. Distilled water, 1000 ml.

Adjust to pH 7. Dispense 5 ml. into tubes and autoclave at 121° C. for 5 min. Inoculate with organism from Sabouraud dextrose agar. It may take over 3 wk. of incubation at room temperature before growth appears.

Interpretation: **N. asteroides** will not grow, *Streptomyces* species will grow poorly, and *N. brasilienses* shows good growth.

Decomposition of L-tyrosine and xanthine: Suspend 0.5 gm. L-tyrosine (or 0.4 gm. xanthine)—both are insoluble—in 100 ml. nutrient agar, autoclave, mix, and pour into petri dishes. Each plate is heavily streaked once across, incubated at 28° C., and examined at 14 and 21 days for the disappearance of the crystals underneath and around the growth.

N. asteroides does not decompose tyrosine or xanthine. *N. brasiliensis* decomposes tyrosine only, and *Streptomyces* decomposes both.

Animal toxicity: *N. asteroides* is the

only species pathogenic to man and laboratory animals, e.g., guinea pigs and mice. Mix the growth of several slants with 5% hog gastric mucin and inject 1 ml. of this mixture intraperitoneally into at least two guinea pigs. At autopsy after spontaneous death or after killing one guinea pig after 2 wk. and the other after 4 wk., examine for lesions containing mycelia.

Actinomyces israelii and bovis

These species are the causative organisms of actinomycosis. *A. israelii* is usually isolated from human sources and *A. bovis* from cattle.

LABORATORY DIAGNOSIS

Material: Pus, sputum, or scrapings from sinus tracts are used.

Examination for and of sulfur granules: Pour the material into a petri dish, spread thinly, and examine for the so-called sulfur granules, which are colonies of the fungus and are often pearly gray and translucent instead of yellow. When placed on a slide, they are not easily mashed (distinguishing them from caseous particles). The sulfur granules appear typically in serosanguineous pus, often containing mucoid material. Study a granule in 10-20% potassium or sodium hydroxide. Make an impression preparation of a granule by mashing between two slides; lift the slides apart, stain by the Gram method, and make a culture.

In the pus the unstained granule (Fig. 11-8) is a tangled mass of small, branching septate filaments that tend to be arranged radially at the periphery of the granule (the ray fungus). In granules from tissue the tips of the filaments are sometimes surrounded by hyaline or gelatinous material, giving the appearance of clubbed ends.

Gram stain: The fungus is gram positive, and the tips of the filaments tend to break up into bacillary and coccoid forms. The gelatinous material forming the clubbed end is gram negative. If granules are not found, smear the pus or sputum and examine for gram-positive, fine, short rods and filaments which break up into bacillary and coccoid forms. True branching is rarely seen.

---

*Difco Laboratories, Detroit, Mich.

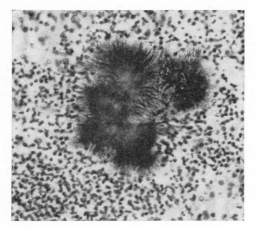

Fig. 11-8. Sulfur granules in pus. (Hematoxylin-eosin stain.)

Culture: The material is aerobically and anaerobically cultured. If granules are found, they should be washed in sterile saline solution, ground against the wall of the container with a sterile glass rod, and then used as inoculum.

Culture media: Brain-heart infusion agar (BHI) with 0.2% dextrose is the medium of choice. One plate is incubated in an anaerobic jar containing 5% CO_2 at 35° C. Duplicate BHI plates are incubated aerobically at 35° C. and in a CO_2 jar at 35° C. Suspicious colonies are subcultured to thioglycollate broth. Most strains of *A. israelii*, which are usually isolated from human sources, produce rough (R) colonies on BHI agar. After 7-10 days these rough colonies are a dull white and have irregular surfaces and edges. They feel dry and crumbly and do not adhere to the agar surface. In thioglycollate broth they produce large lobulated "bread-crumb" type colonies as well as discrete granules. Gram stains of the cultures show gram-positive branched elements.

A. bovis produces smooth (S) colonies which, after 7-10 days on BHI agar, are large, convex, round, dull white, glistening, and smooth. They vary in consistency from soft to firm. In thioglycollate broth they vary from "bread-crumb" type growth to diffuse growth at the bottom of the tube and mucoid ropes. Gram stain shows gram-positive diphtheroid forms.

DIFFERENTIAL DIAGNOSIS: *A. israelii* and *A. bovis* must be differentiated from (1) *A. naeslundii*, a common, nonpathogenic, catalase-negative inhabitant of the mouth, which grows aerobically and tolerates 10% bile salts, and from (2) anaerobic diphtheroids (*Corynebacterium acne*), which are catalase positive (Table 11-22).

Biochemical reactions: *Actinomyces* are catalase and indole negative and fail to liquefy gelatin. *A. israelii* differs from *A. bovis* in that it does not reduce nitrate and does not hydrolyze starch. *A. bovis* reacts oppositely.

STREPTOMYCES

These organisms are saprophytic earth, dust, and field bacteria, some of which are used for the production of antibiotics. They cause mycetomas and usually form sulfur granules (grains), which in most strains are large and vary in color from pink to red, depending on the species. For differentiation from *Nocardia,* see p. 602.

GRAM-POSITIVE SPORE-FORMING BACILLI

All bacilli in this group are able to form spores under unfavorable circumstances. Their normal habitat is soil and the intestine of man and animals. Outside the bowel some species are disease producing. Spores are resistant to the usual disinfectants and to some extent to heat. These bacilli can therefore be used in sterilization control (**bacterial spore strips**).

BACILLACEAE

Classification:
Bacillus: Aerobic; no distention or only slight distention of bacilli during sporulation
    I. Pathogenic
        A. *Bacillus anthracis*
    II. Nonpathogenic
        A. *Bacillus subtilis*
Clostridium: Anaerobic; exotoxin production
    I. Spores—central; eccentric; subterminal
        A. Distention of bacilli during sporulation
            1. Motile
                (a) *Clostridium septicum*
                (b) *Clostridium botulinum*
                (c) *Clostridium sporogenes*

Table 11-22. Differentiation of *Actinomyces bovis* and anaerobic diphtheroids*

Tests	Actinomyces bovis	Anaerobic diphtheroids
Catalase test	Catalase negative (after 1-2 wk. of growth on brain-heart infusion agar, place 1 drop fresh 3% H_2O_2 directly on a colony; bubbling will not appear)	Catalase positive (after 1-2 wk. of incubation, place 1 drop fresh 3% H_2O_2 directly on growth; bubbles of gas will form)
Litmus milk	No reaction	Clots and digests milk; reaction may require 2-3 wk.
Gelatin with dextrose	No change	Liquefies gelatin; reaction may require 2-3 wk.
Reaction to dextrose	Growth not stimulated by dextrose; some strains may be inhibited by dextrose	All stains greatly stimulated by dextrose; some strains grow very slowly without dextrose
Animal injection	Pathogenic to mice	Not pathogenic to mice

*From Newer concepts and techniques in clinical diagnostic bacteriology, St. Louis, 1959, The Catholic Hospital Association of the United States and Canada.

B. No distention of bacilli during sporulation
   1. Motile
     (a) *Clostridium bifermentans*
   2. Nonmotile
     (a) *Clostridium perfringens*
II. Spores—terminal
  A. Spores round
   1. Motile
     (a) *Clostridium tetani*
  B. Spores oval
   1. Motile
     (a) *Clostridium tertium*

GRAM-POSITIVE AEROBIC SPORE-FORMING BACILLI
Anthrax bacillus

Anthrax bacillus is a large, gram-positive, nonmotile organism with square ends; it often occurs in chains (bamboo-rod appearance) and is encapsulated. It produces the carbuncle-like lesion of anthrax (malignant pustule). The pulmonary form is called **woolsorter's disease.**

LABORATORY DIAGNOSIS

Gram stain: A gram-positive, spore-forming, rectangular, large rod (4-8μ in length and 1-2μ in diameter) occurring in chains of two or more is seen. The **capsule** appears only as a faint halo with gram stain, while in Wright-stained preparations it stands out as a pink rim surrounding the dark-blue bacillus. Refractile, small, oval spores may be found free, in groups, or centrally within the bacillus

in cultured material, but not in tissue.

Culture: The organism grows well on blood agar and forms (if there is not too much contamination) rough, flat, granular colonies with irregular margins. The colonies are opaque when viewed by transmitted light and are tough and stringy. When examined with the microscope, the colonies appear to be composed of filaments resembling wavy hair, **caput medusae.** This picture is characteristic for pathogenic forms of *B. anthracis.* The nonpathogenic forms often produce smooth colonies.

Apart from the differences in microcolonial appearance, features that distinguish virulent forms from **nonpathogenic anthrax-like organisms** are as follows: *B. anthracis* lacks motility, fails to reduce methylene blue broth in 48 hr., is pathogenic for guinea pigs, and is sensitive to penicillin; 10 units of penicillin/1 ml. agar will suppress the growth of anthrax bacilli. Almost all nonpathogenic anthrax-like organisms are motile, reduce methylene blue broth in 48 hr., and are not pathogenic to laboratory animals.

In thioglycollate broth the organism concentrates close to the surface.

In stab cultures of gelatin it shows the characteristic **fir-tree** appearance after 3 days of incubation at room temperature.

Toxicity testing: For animal inoculation 0.25 ml. of broth culture should be injected subcutaneously into the dorsal region of two guinea pigs. Death will occur after a short terminal illness in from 48 hr. to 3-5 days. At autopsy anthrax bacilli can be demonstrated in the tissues.

Serologic tests: In the **Ascoli thermo-precipitin test** the anthrax antigen in a saline tissue extract is precipitated by the addition of serum containing anthrax-precipitating antibodies.

Bacillus subtilis (Hay bacillus)

Bacillus subtilis may be found as a contaminant of wounds. It is motile, catalase and H_2S positive, and able to curdle milk and to reduce nitrates. Gram stain shows a slender gram-positive rod. Ovoid spores are seen which do not distend the bacillary body. Rough, wrinkled colonies are formed on blood agar. The organism is insensitive to penicillin.

GRAM-POSITIVE ANAEROBIC SPORE-FORMING BACILLI
Clostridia

These organisms are anaerobic gram-positive (at least when young) rods that form spores. Older organisms are easily decolorized and may appear to be gram negative. The natural habitat is soil and the intestinal tract of animals and man. Most are saprophytic soil bacteria that decompose proteins. The pathogens produce powerful exotoxins. With the exception of *Cl. botulinum,* all clostridia are associated with wound infections. The most important ones are *Cl. tetani,* the causative organism of tetanus; *Cl. perfringens, Cl. edematiens, Cl. septicum, Cl. sporogenes,* and *Cl. histolyticum,* the causative organisms of gas gangrene; and *Cl. botulinum,* the causative organism of botulism.

Characteristics that aid in the identification of clostridia include spore formation (shape and location), motility, microcolonial features on blood agar, liquefaction of gelatin, fermentation of glucose, lactose, and sucrose, indole formation, and nitrate reduction (Table 11-23).

Laboratory diagnosis

Material: Use debrided wound tissue or aspirated fluid from wounds and swabs.

The latter is least satisfactory. The tissue should be cultured immediately, preferably in the operating room. Use cooked meat medium or thioglycollate broth.

Smears: Clostridia are large, cylindric, straight rods, though curved and irregular forms appear in old cultures. *Cl. perfringens* is encapsulated, although most species are not. Young cultures are strongly gram positive.

Motility: All species, with the exception of *Cl. perfringens,* are slowly motile (peritrichal flagella).

Spores: Location may vary even in a given species, and several days of growth in an alkaline medium may be required to produce spores. The medium should be sugar-free so that acid production does not lower the pH.

Culture: For anaerobic culture techniques, see p. 541. The basic media of choice are cooked meat medium, thioglycollate broth, and blood agar. Most species are strict anaerobes.

Special selective media: The use of selective inhibitory media is indicated because many of the organisms infecting wounds are falcultative anaerobes capable of overgrowing clostridia colonies. The most frequently used inhibitory media are **chloral hydrate–sodium azide blood agar** and **sorbic acid–polymyxin broth.** As all inhibitory media may also restrict the organisms that they are designed to select, parallel cultures on routine media must not be omitted.

Chloral hydrate–sodium azide blood agar: To liquid and cooled blood agar add 1 ml. 1% solution of chloral hydrate and 2 ml. 1% solution sodium azide. Both solutions should be sterilized by Seitz filtration.

Sorbic acid–polymyxin broth: To 100 ml. thioglycollate broth add 0.12 gm. sorbic acid. After autoclaving, add 1.5 mg. polymyxin. The inhibitory media will tend to prevent spreading of contaminating organisms (*Proteus* and *Pseudomonas*). As a further step to prevent spreading, keep the agar surface dry by including calcium chloride in the anaerobic jar.

Biochemical reactions:

Gelatin liquefaction: Add 10% gelatin to infusion broth, adjust to pH 7.4, distribute in tubes, and autoclave. Clostridia liquefy gelatin.

Indole test: Culture the organism for 3 days in thioglycollate medium without glucose. The medium is then tested with Ehrlich reagent (see p. 566). Clostridia are indole negative.

Nitrate reduction: To thioglycollate medium without glucose add 0.1% sodium nitrate and 0.1% glucose. This medium is inoculated with pure culture and incubated from 12-24 hr. at 35° C. It is then tested with sulfanilic acid and alpha-naphthylamine reagents (see p. 570 and Table 11-23).

Toxicity testing: Two guinea pigs are injected intramuscularly with 0.2 ml. thioglycollate broth. One is protected by antitoxin; the other will succumb in 1-2 days. To initiate necrosis, 2.5% calcium chloride in the inoculum may be necessary.

Stormy fermentation of milk: Boil deep milk tubes containing 0.1% peptone and a pinch of iron filing and then cool to 49° C. Inoculate with specimen and keep in water bath at 49° C. If pure culture, stormy fermentation will occur after 2 hr. of incubation. If mixed culture, make transfer on anaerobic plate and repeat test after 12 hr.

Differential carbohydrate fermentation media (Table 11-23): Add 10% solution of sugar (5% salicin) sterilized by Seitz filtration to thioglycollate medium without glucose to form a final concentration of 1%. Acid production as an index of carbohydrate fermentation is detected by adding 0.05% aqueous solution of bromthymol blue (acid—yellow) to a small portion of medium removed with a sterile pipette.

On the basis of fermentation reaction, three main groups can be established:

Glucose negative: *Cl. tetani*

Glucose positive and lactose negative: *Cl. sporogenes, Cl. botulinum, Cl. edematiens*

Glucose and lactose positive: *Cl. perfringens, Cl. septicum*

CLOSTRIDIUM PERFRINGENS (CLOSTRIDIUM WELCHII)

Clostridium perfringens is commonly found in the intestinal tract of man and animals. It is the most important contributor to the production of **gas gangrene**. Serologically, types A to S can be distinguished.

Laboratory diagnosis

Gram stain: *Cl. welchii* is a short, thick, gram-positive rod, 0.8-1.2μ in diameter and 4μ in length. The parallel sides are straight and the ends are rounded. Spores are seldom seen but, if present (in alkaline pH), they are ovoid, central, or terminal. The organism is nonmotile and is encapsulated.

Culture: In 24 hr. under anaerobic

Table 11-23. Clostridia

	Digestion of cooked meat medium	Spores	Glucose	Lactose	Sucrose	Gelatin liquefaction	Motility	Milk	Nitrate reduction
Cl. perfringens (Cl. welchii)	G -	Rare, eccentric	+	+	+	+	-	A, G, C	+
Cl. septicum	G -	Ovoid, eccentric	+	+	-	+	+	A	+
Cl. edematiens (Cl. novyi)	G -	Ovoid, eccentric	+	-	-	+	+	G, C	-
Cl. botulinum	G	Ovoid, eccentric	+	-	-	+	+	D	-
Cl. tetani	—	Terminal, round	-	-	-	+	+	—	-
Cl. sporogenes	G	Ovoid, eccentric	+	-	-	+	+	D	+

A = acid; G = gas; C = clot; D = digestion.

conditions, opaque, smooth 2-4 mm. colonies with translucent edges appear on blood agar. At times the periphery of the colony is striated and the medium beneath and around the colonies shows beta hemolysis. Growth in cooked meat broth is seen in a few hours and is evidenced by gas production and the pink color of meat. Stormy fermentation is rapidly produced in milk. The organisms ferment glucose, maltose, lactose, and sucrose and liquefy gelatin (Table 11-23).

Nagler reaction: In media containing human sera, *Cl. welchii* produces opalescence (Nagler reaction), which is inhibited by *Cl. welchii* antitoxin and which is due to lecithinases produced by the organism. A **lactose-egg yolk-milk** agar with one half of the plate covered with antitoxin and then dried is superior to Nagler medium. Both halves are streaked with the organism to be tested.

CLOSTRIDIUM EDEMATIENS

Clostridium edematiens is primarily a soil organism.

Laboratory diagnosis

Gram stain: Gram stain reveals gram-positive rods measuring 2-5μ in length and up to 1.2μ in diameter. The organism is motile and nonencapsulated. It readily forms ovoid, central, or preterminal spores that have a wider diameter than the bacillus. They may be found free.

Culture: The organism is a strict anaerobe and is very sensitive to free oxygen. Cooked meat medium produces moderate growth only, even if all oxygen is carefully removed by heating of the medium prior to inoculation. Rounded, 2-3 mm., shiny, uneven, hemolytic colonies appear on blood agar in 48 hr., provided contact with oxygen is prevented. They have irregular edges and may have some tendency to spread.

Biochemical reactions: All types liquefy gelatin and are indole negative. Most types ferment glucose (Table 11-23).

CLOSTRIDIUM SEPTICUM

Clostridium septicum is a gram-positive, motile rod that is 2-6μ long, and up to 0.6μ in diameter. The rods have parallel sides and rounded ends. Filamentous forms are common. Young colonies are gram positive, while older ones are frequently gram negative. The ovoid spores are subterminal and distend the organism. Under strict anaerobiasis at 35° C. there appear on blood agar rounded hemolytic (alpha to beta), transparent, somewhat spreading colonies with irregular edges. For biochemical reactions, see Table 11-23.

CLOSTRIDIUM SPOROGENES

Clostridium sporogenes is a thin, gram-positive rod with rounded edges. It is not encapsulated and forms subterminal ovoid spores that are frequently found free. It is aerobic and naturally nonpathogenic, but enhances the pathogenicity of other clostridia. Glistening to yellow-gray-white, rounded, hemolytic colonies with rhizoid projections are formed on blood agar. The colonies are soft and have a tendency to flow. For biochemical reactions, see Table 11-23.

CLOSTRIDIUM TETANI

Tetanus is a disease characterized by severe toxemia and absence of bacteremia. Cultivated soil is rich in *Cl. tetani,* which is also found in the intestinal tract of man and animals.

Laboratory diagnosis

Material: Use excised wound tissue.

Smear: The organism is a slender rod that frequently gives rise to filamentous forms. The cells are not encapsulated; they are motile, and are strongly gram-positive when young. They have terminal globoid spores that distend the organisms and do not stain with gram stain (**drumstick appearance**).

Culture: The organism is a strict anaerobe. It grows well on blood agar, where it forms shiny, granular, 2-5 mm., hemolytic, transparent colonies that give rise to spreading pseudopods and to swarming. There are, however, nonmotile (nonspreading) forms of *Cl. tetani.* The colonies have a burnt-flesh odor.

Biochemical reactions: *Cl. tetani* does not ferment sugars or liquefy gelatin.

Animal inoculation and protection: Inject 0.25 ml. supernatant of cooked meat broth culture or emulsified fresh wound material intramuscularly into the thigh muscles of two mice, one of which has been protected by subcutaneous injection of 0.5 ml. (1500 units) of tetanus antitoxin 1 hr. prior to the inoculation. If the material is solid, a pocket has to be formed which must be closed airtight with collodion. Calcium chloride (2.5%) in the inoculum may be necessary to initiate necrosis. If the test is positive, after a few hours the hind leg of the unprotected mouse will be first to show the characteristic rigid spasms of tetanus which later, at the slightest provocation, involves the whole animal.

Determination of toxin production: To prove the presence of toxin in the patient's serum, inject mice subcutaneously as follows:

Mouse 1: 0.5 ml. serum
Mouse 2: 0.5 ml. serum + 0.5 ml. tetanus antitoxin (1:10)
Mouse 3: 0.5 ml. serum + 0.5 ml. diphtheria antitoxin (1:10)
Mouse 4: 0.5 ml. serum previously heated to 100° C. for 30 min.

If toxins are present in the serum, mouse 2 and 4 will live, and mouse 1 and 3 will die.

CLOSTRIDIUM BOTULINUM[108]

This organism does not multiply in the living body of human beings but grows in inadequately preserved meat, vegetables, and fruit. It is widely distributed in soil and causes **botulism** by the ingestion of preformed toxins formed under anaerobic conditions. The toxins are extremely dangerous, and any suspected material must be handled with great care so that not even the smallest amounts come in contact with the skin or mucous membrane. The toxins are rapidly destroyed by boiling. Five types of the organism (A to E), each with its specific toxin, have been described, but only two types of toxin, A and B, are important as the cause of botulism in the United States. Chickens are susceptible to A, but not to B. Toxin of A causes weakness of the neck (**limber neck**) in chickens, with death in 24 hr.

Laboratory diagnosis

Smear: The organism is a gram-positive rod that is 4-8μ long and 1μ in diameter. It is often paired, at times in chains. The spores are ovoid, short, terminal, or subterminal. The organism is motile, strictly anaerobic, and nonencapsulated.

Culture:
Material: Use ground food.
Media: The organism is cultured on blood agar and cooked meat medium. At 35° C. under strict anaerobiasis, 2-3 mm. slightly hemolytic colonies appear on blood agar. These colonies appear slightly brown under transmitted light.

Determination of toxin production: The test is made on suspected food. Filter 10 ml. fluid or extract, boil one portion 30 min. to destroy the toxin, and inoculate mice intraperitoneally with 0.5 ml., one with the unheated and another with the heated portion (negative control). If positive, the mouse inoculated with the unheated portion will show dyspnea and decrease of respiration from 120-160 to 20-30/min. with costal breathing and will die in 3 or 4 hr. The control mouse will not be affected. Protection tests with mice immunized with specific antitoxins may be used to determine the type.

VIBRIOS AND SPIRILLA (SPIRILLACEAE)
Vibrio comma[109]

Vibrio comma causes **cholera,** recent outbreaks of which have been reported in India, Indonesia, and the Philippines.

The organism is a curved, motile, nonspore-forming, gram-negative, aerobic rod with a single polar flagellum.

LABORATORY DIAGNOSIS

Smear: The organisms vary in length from 2-4μ and measure about 0.5μ in diameter. They appear singly or are arranged end to end, producing S curves. Straight forms may appear in cultures.

Stain particle of mucous stool by the Gram method, using 1:10 carbolfuchsin as counterstain. Observe for typical comma-shaped vibrios.

Culture: The organism is able to grow in a strongly alkaline medium of pH 8.4-9.5, but is very sensitive to acidity. It fails to grow on SS or EMB media but will grow on blood agar. At 35° C. under aerobic conditions, moist, glistening, soft, whitish colonies appear on blood agar. These colonies produce greenish discoloration and clearing of the surrounding agar (hemodigestion) but no true hemolysis (**El Tor vibrio** produces hemolysis). Beef extract agar containing 0.5% NaCl and 0.5% medium taurocholate (pH 8) is a good plating medium.

In broth a pellicle usually forms in 24 hr.

The identity of the colony is established by smear morphology and by biochemical and serologic reactions.

Biochemical reactions: Gelatin is liquefied, nitrate is reduced, lactose is not at all or only slowly fermented, and indole is formed. The latter two reactions are responsible for the **cholera red reaction.** Note that this reaction is also given by nonpathogenic vibrios and is therefore of somewhat limited value.

Cholera red test: Culture organism in peptone solution. After 3-8 days examine for surface growth in hanging drop preparation and in stained smear.

Test the peptone tube after 18-24 hr. for cholera red reaction by adding 5 drops concentrated sulfuric acid and observe for red color.

Fermentation reaction: Acid (no gas) is produced by fermentation of glucose and fructose, but lactose fermentation is delayed.

Serology: The H antigen is nonspecific. Vibrios are divided into six groups (I to VI) by means of the O antigen. All known pathogens belong to group I. In addition, each comma bacillus contains A, B, and C antigens which form the basis for two specific antisera: anti-AB (Ogawa) and anti-AC (Inoba) antisera, or a mixture of both. Rough (R) forms are agglutinated by saline solution, which therefore must be used as a control.

Vibrio fetus[110-112]

Vibrio fetus is a common cause of abortion in sheep and cattle, but has also been cultured from human beings, primarily in relation to pregnancy and to the neonatal period.

LABORATORY DIAGNOSIS

Material: The material most commonly used consists of body cavity fluids of stillborn fetuses, segments of necrotic placentas, and cervical or vaginal mucus; rarely semen or smegma is used.

Smear: The organism is a gram-negative, curved cell resembling *V. comma.* Spiral, S-shaped, coccoid, and filamentous forms are common in older cultures. The organism is motile (having one polar flagellum).

Dark-field examination of a fresh preparation may be helpful in identification of the organism.

Culture: The organism is a microaerophilic bacillus that requires incubation in a candle jar in the presence of 10% CO_2. Semisolid media containing 0.75-0.1% agar such as **thiol medium**[*] and thioglycollate medium without indicator but with 0.07% agar[†] are suggested. These media are distributed in 5 ml. tubes and are inoculated by stabbing. On rabbit blood agar the colonies are smooth (S) or rough (R), buff, translucent, and nonhemolytic, but at times they may be mucoid or even crumbly.

It grows in the upper one third of thioglycollate medium. It does not grow on SS, EMB, or MacConkey agar.

Biochemical reactions: Most strains are catalase positive. Nitrates are reduced, but carbohydrates are not oxidized or fermented. Indole and H_2S are not produced. The organism will grow in 0.1% agar broth containing 2.5% sodium chloride, but it will fail to grow when the concentration of sodium chloride reaches 3.5%.

Animal inoculation: Pregnant guinea pigs abort after intraperitoneal inoculation.

Serology: Agglutinins appear in the serum and in the cervical-vaginal mucus.

Spirillum minus

Spirillum minus is a rigid, corkscrew-like organism that usually displays two or three (sometimes up to six) undulations and bipolar flagella. It measures 3-5μ in

---

[*]Difco Laboratories, Detroit, Mich.

[†]Baltimore Biological Laboratory, Baltimore, Md.

length, and in the process of moving it rotates around its long axis. It is gram-negative, but Giemsa stain is preferred for smears and tissue imprints.

The organism causes **sodoku,** or **rat-bite fever,** which may follow the bite of a rat, mouse, or other rodent.

LABORATORY DIAGNOSIS

Laboratory diagnosis is based on demonstration of the organism in the exudate of the primary or secondary skin lesion, in blood, and in smears of regional lymph nodes. The blood smears and tissue imprints are stained with Giemsa stain.

The **dark-field technique** is excellent for the examination of wet preparations.

Animal inoculation: As the direct examination of human material is usually unsatisfactory and as the organism cannot be cultured, the clinical material should be injected subcutaneously or intraperitoneally into guinea pigs or white mice. Blood smears or heart imprints are examined by the dark-field technique or by the Giemsa staining method 14-17 days after inoculation. White mice must be examined for *S. minus* prior to inoculation since they may normally harbor these organisms.

MISCELLANEOUS ORGANISMS
STREPTOBACILLUS
Streptobacillus moniliformis[113]

Nonspirillar rat-bite fever is due to an organism that laboratory and wild rats harbor in the nasopharynx—*Streptobacillus moniliformis.*

It is a pleomorphic gram-negative rod that is nonmotile and measures 2-3μ in length. In culture, the organism gives rise to long, branching filaments, often exhibiting spindle-shaped swellings.

LABORATORY DIAGNOSIS

Material: Pus, joint fluid, and blood are the most suitable specimens.

Smear: Direct smears of clinical material contain pleomorphic gram-negative rods. The routine media (thioglycollate broth, blood agar, and trypticase soy broth with CO_2) should be employed, provided they are enriched with ascitic fluid (20%) or serum (10-30%).

Culture: After 48 hr. on blood agar, small, round, colorless, hemolytic colonies appear. Under the dissecting microscope the colonies reveal peripheral filaments. After 4 days, accompanying L_1 or **pleuro-pneumonia-like** colonies between or in the center of the original colonies may be found by microscopic examination (100×).

Serologic tests: Patients develop agglutinating antibodies in the course of rat-bite fever.

SPIROCHETES (TREPONEMATACEAE)

Treponemas are elongated, motile, flexible, corkscrew-like organisms that divide transversely. They vary in length from 4-16μ and most forms cannot be stained by the usual dyes. They can be detected by dark-field microscopy and **silver impregnation** methods. Most are difficult to culture or cannot be propagated on artificial media at all.

Included in the family of Treponemataceae are the genera *Treponema, Leptospira,* and *Borrelia.*

Treponema
TREPONEMA PALLIDUM

Treponema pallidum is a delicate spirochete 6-14μ long and 0.2μ thick; it is the causative organism of **syphilis.**

Laboratory diagnosis

Laboratory diagnosis includes dark-field examination and serologic tests for syphilis (**STS**) (see Chapter 14). The usual methods of smear and culture are not satisfactory.

Dark-field examination: Clinically, syphilis is divided into three stages. *T. pallidum* may be demonstrated by dark-field microscopy in the ulcer of the **primary chancre** or in the aspirate of enlarged inguinal lymph nodes of the primary disease. It may also be found in the cutaneous and mucosal lesions of **secondary syphilis.**

Method: Squeeze or scrape ulcer base to stimulate the release of serum. Press slide against moist ulcer base and cover immediately with cover slip. Examine with dark-field illumination (Fig. 11-9).

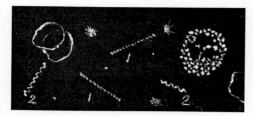

Fig. 11-9. Dark-field microscopy showing, **1,** *Treponema pallidum* and, **2,** other spirals (contaminating organisms).

T. pallidum is a slender spiral with close regular curves like a corkscrew. It is motile, moving forward and backward and rotating on its long axis but still retaining its rigid curves. In ulcerated lesions and on mucous membranes it is often found with other spiral forms, especially *T. macrodentium, T. microdentium,* and *B. vincentii.*

Serologic tests for syphilis: Two types of antibodies are formed in response to the invasion of the human body by *T. pallidum.* One group of antibodies is directed against the treponema and its components and are therefore classified as **treponemal antibodies.** They are tested for with treponemal antigens such as the **Reiter treponema strain** or its protein. The other group of antibodies forms in response to the tissue damaged by the action of the spirochetes, and they are classified as **nontreponemal antibodies** or **reagins.** They are measured by the use of **nontreponemal antigens,** e.g., cardiolipin-lecithin-cholesterol antigens.

Nontreponemal tests: **VDRL** and its various modifications such as Rapid Plasma Reagin, Plasmacrit, Rapid Plasma Reagin Card, etc. are nontreponemal tests.

Interpretation: The nontreponemal tests are not specific, but rather indicate the presence of a chronic disease that may be syphilis. This lack of specificity is offset by the fact that they are well standardized, reproducible, and easily performed with a small amount of equipment and skill. When determined quantitatively, they can be used to follow treatment and cure.

Treponemal tests: In recent years many treponemal tests such as the *Treponema*

pallidum immobilization test (TPI) and the *Treponema pallidum* complement-fixation test (TPCF) have been described; both use the Nichols treponema strain or the **fluorescent treponema antibody test** (FTA), the Reiter protein complement-fixation test (RPCF), and the Kolmer-Reiter protein test (KRP) with the Reiter treponema strain or its protein.

Indications: The main indications are (1) to distinguish biologic false positive reactions, which usually consist of reactive reagin tests, from the truly specific reactions, and (2) to establish the diagnosis of **late syphilis** in which nontreponemal tests are usually nonreactive.

Details of these tests are given in the section dealing with serology.

• • •

Other treponemas indistinguishable morphologically from *T. pallidum* are found in **yaws** (*T. pertenue*) and in **pinta** (*T. herrejoni*). Pinta occurs chiefly in Central and South America and is nonvenereal. The comparative morphology of the spiral organisms of chief interest in medical diagnosis may be seen in Fig. 11-10.

Leptospira

These organisms are tightly coiled, thin spirochetes, the ends of which may be turned at a sharp angle to form a hook. The organisms measure $5\text{-}15\mu$ in length and about 1μ in diameter.

LABORATORY DIAGNOSIS[114]

Smears: The Giemsa stain will demonstrate leptospirae in smears of body fluids, while silver impregnation methods (Levaditi and Fontana) are useful for tissue sections.

Dark-field examination: It is useful for the examination of urine, but positive findings must be confirmed by culture and animal inoculation.

Culture: Fletcher medium* is the medium of choice for isolation of leptospirae from blood, urine, and various tissues such as kidneys. Inoculate four tubes with 1 or 2 drops of specimen or tissue emulsion and incubate at 26° C. up to 5 wk.

---

*Difco Laboratories, Detroit, Mich.

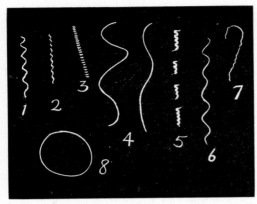

Fig. 11-10. Dark-field microscopy showing spiral organisms. Diagram showing comparative morphology of the following: **1,** *Treponema macrodentium;* **2,** *Treponema microdentium;* **3,** *Treponema pallidum;* **4,** *Borrelia vincentii;* **5,** *Spirillum minus;* **6,** *Borrelia recurrentis;* **7,** *Leptospira icterohaemorrhagiae;* **8,** erythrocyte (7.5μ) for comparison.

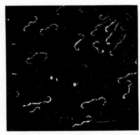

Fig. 11-11. *Leptospira icterohaemorrhagiae.* (×950.) (From Handbuch der path. Mikro-organismen. Band VII.)

When the top layer turns turbid, remove 1 drop with a sterile pipette and examine under dark-field microscopy.

Animal inoculation: As cultures are frequently contaminated, animal inoculation is a necessary diagnostic step. Four young guinea pigs (less than 150 gm.) or young hamsters are injected intraperitoneally with 0.5 ml. of specimen such as urine, milk, tissue emulsion, etc. Heart blood and intraperitoneal fluid of the test animals should be cultured every sixth day unless death occurs, at which time the autopsy will reveal hemorrhagic spots in the lungs and other organs.

Serologic tests: These include complement-fixation, agglutination, and agglutination-lysis tests. The antigens and control antisera are commercially available. As in all serologic tests, positive findings in a single specimen are of limited value, but a fourfold rise in titer is significant.

FTA Leptospira: Fluorescent-labeled antileptospiral globulins are available for identification of the more commonly encountered leptospirae.

LEPTOSPIRA ICTEROHAEMORRHAGIAE

This organism is the cause of **Weil's disease** (infectious jaundice), which is characterized by sudden onset, fever, prostration with generalized aching and muscular pains, and later jaundice. Kidney damage and jaundice are the rule, but either or both may be absent. The wild rat is the reservoir of infection, and the causative organism is found in the urine of the rats and in stagnant water or sewage contaminated by rats.

In the United States *L. icterohaemorrhagiae* is the most common cause of infectious jaundice in man (Weil's disease), but it is also pathogenic for dogs (Fig. 11-11). *L. canicola* is the common cause of leptospirosis in the dog (Stuttgart's disease) and occasionally infects man (**canicola disease**).

Other strains reported in the United States include *L. pomona,* found in swine, cattle, and horses (the cause of pomona fever or swineherd's disease in man), *L. autumnalis* (Fort Bragg or pretibial fever), *L. grippotyphosa* (water or mud fever), and *L. bataviae* (Indonesian Weil's disease).[115]

Borrelia

These spirochetes are 8-10μ long with flat spirals of various sizes and thin, tapered ends. They are easily stained with aniline dyes.

BORRELIA VINCENTII

Borrelia vincentii is a 3-10μ long microaerophilic or anaerobic spirochete with flat, irregular loops. It occurs in symbiosis with **fusiform bacilli,** mainly in neglected oral mucosa.

Laboratory diagnosis

The gram-stained smear is used for the laboratory diagnosis of *B. vincentii.*

BORRELIA RECURRENTIS

This organism is one of the causative agents of **relapsing fever** in man.

The disease is characterized by a febrile stage of 3-10 days' duration, ending by crisis and recurring at intervals of about a week. There are several types of the disease, varying in different localities and transmitted by different vectors, but the organisms are practically alike. The European type and the Central African type are chiefly louse-borne, whereas the types in northern Africa, in Central and South America, in Spain,[116] and in the United States (Texas, California, Colorado, and Kansas) are transmitted by a tick (some species of *Ornithodorus*). Infection is caused by contamination of the bite lesion with the body fluids of the crushed louse or with the excretory wastes of the tick.

Laboratory diagnosis

During the febrile stage, examine a fresh drop of blood microscopically, with the usual direct lighting or by dark-field illumination and stain smears with Wright or Giemsa stain (Fig. 11-12). In the afebrile stage between paroxysms, when the organisms have agglutinated and mostly disappeared from the bloodstream, inoculate a mouse with about 0.2-0.5 ml. of blood and examine the mouse's blood (obtained from the tail) in 2 days and daily thereafter for 5-10 days.

Morphology: The spirochete is a motile spiral with a flexible body and 3-12 loose, irregular coils and measures about 15-30μ in length.

RICKETTSIAE

Rickettsiae are obligate, intracellular, gram-negative organisms which, like most bacteria, can be stained with aniline dyes and appear as small pleomorphic rods or cocci that measure 0.3-1μ in length and can therefore just be seen under the light microscope. The organisms contain RNA and DNA, and the electron microscope reveals an electron-dense nucleus and a cell membrane. They differ from viruses by maintaining their own, though limited, enzyme systems. They cannot be Seitz filtered. They stain best with Giemsa stain.

Rickettsiae can only be propagated in laboratory animals, tissue cultures, and yolk sacs of fertile eggs. For a more detailed discussion, see the following section on viruses, as the laboratory investigation of both infectious agents is similar.

Insects (lice, flies, ticks, and mites) are the natural reservoir of these organisms. Rickettsiae do not produce disease in the arthropods that transmit the organisms to man, but in man they cause diseases characterized by fever and rash.

Numerous diseases are caused by rickettsiae (Table 11-24). The following are immunologically distinct groups:

> Typhus group
>   Epidemic typhus
>   Endemic typhus
>   Tsutsugamushi (scrub typhus)
> Spotted fever group
>   Rocky Mountain spotted fever
>   Rickettsialpox
>   Q fever
>   Boutonneuse fever (Mediterranean fever)
>   South African tick-bite fever
>   Queensland tick typhus
> Trench fever

Epidemic typhus (Old World) is transmitted from man to man by the louse (*Pediculus humanus*) and is caused by *R. prowazekii*.

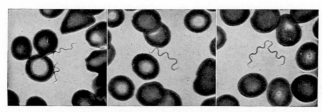

Fig. 11-12. *Borrelia recurrentis* in blood. (From Todd and Sanford: Clinical diagnosis, Philadelphia, 1939, W. B. Saunders Co.)

Table 11-24. Important rickettsial diseases of man

Disease	Rickettsia	Vector
Typhus		
Epidemic	*R. prowazekii*	Louse
Endemic	*R. mooseri*	Flea
Spotted fevers		
Rocky Mountain		
spotted fever	*R. rickettsii*	Tick
Mediterranean		
fever	*R. conorii*	Tick
South African		
tick-bite fever	*R. pijperi*	Tick
Rickettsialpox	*R. akari*	Mite
Tsutsugamushi	*R. tsutsugamushi*	Mite
Q fever	*R. burneti*	Tick
Trench fever	*R. wolhynica*	Louse

Brill's disease is a mild or modified form of epidemic typhus.

Endemic typhus in this country is transmitted by the rat flea (*Xenopsylla cheopis*) from rat to man and to rats. It is caused by *R. typhi* or *R. mooseri*. Endemic typhus is called murine typhus.

Tsutsugamushi fever (**scrub typhus**) is transmitted by mites (*Trombicula akamushi* and *Trombicula deliensis*) and is caused by *R. tsutsugamushi* or *orientalis*.

Rocky Mountain spotted fever, western type, is transmitted by the wood tick (*Dermacentor andersoni*). The eastern type of spotted fever is transmitted from animals to man by the dog tick (*Dermacentor variabilis*), and both types of spotted fever are caused by *R. rickettsii*. Spotted fever is usually called Rocky Mountain spotted fever.

Rickettsialpox is caused by *R. akari* and is transmitted by mites (*Allodermanyssus sanguineous*) which are found on mice.

Q fever is caused by *R. burneti* or *diaporica*. The vector is not known, but it is probably a tick.

Bullis fever is a rickettsial disease that is synonymous with Rocky Mountain spotted fever. The vector is probably the Lone Star tick, *Amblyomma americanum*.

Boutonneuse fever (**Mediterranean fever**) is caused by *R. conorii* and is transmitted by a tick (*Rhipicephalis sanguineous*).

South African tick-bite fever is caused by *R. rickettsii* (var. *pijperi*) and others and is transmitted by the dog ticks *Haemaphysalis leachi* and *Rhipicephalus sanguineous*.

Queensland tick typhus is thought to be transmitted by the tick *Ixodes holocyclus* and belongs to the spotted fever group.

Trench fever, common during World War I, is transmitted by the body louse (*Pediculus humanus*). It is presumably caused by *R. wolhynica* or *R. quintana*.

LABORATORY DIAGNOSIS

For a more detailed discussion, see the following section on viruses; the viral methods of investigation also apply to rickettsiae.

Smear: Not helpful unless it is of vector, tissue, or egg culture.

Culture: Routine culture methods are not suitable.

Fertile egg cultures: Rickettsiae grow readily in the yolk sac of the developing chick embryo (chickens must not have been on antibiotics).

Tissue culture: Intracellular localization of rickettsiae is a diagnostic feature.

Animal inoculation: Susceptible laboratory animals are the guinea pig, mouse, and rabbit. Inject 3 ml. ground clotted blood intraperitoneally in several guinea pigs for the diagnosis of typhus and spotted fever.

Serologic tests: Perform the following tests: agglutination reaction of **Weil-Felix,** complement-fixation test with specific antigens, agglutination of specific rickettsiae, hemagglutination inhibition, and fluorescent antibody test.

The serologic tests become positive rather late in the course of the disease. A rise in the titer, proved on subsequent tests, is of greater importance than a single measurement.

Fluorescent antibody technique: Up to the present time the technique has been used for the identification of endemic and epidemic typhus.

Weil-Felix reaction (Table 11-25): Set up agglutinations with *Proteus* OX-19 and OX-2 and Kingsbury strain OXK. A positive reaction usually occurs after the

Table 11-25. Weil-Felix reaction

Disease	Serologic reactions			Complement-fixation test
	OX-19	OX-2	OXK	
Epidemic typhus	++	−	−	+
Endemic typhus	++	−	−	+
Tsutsugamushi fever	−	−	++	+
Mediterranean fever	+	+	+	+
South African tick fever	+	−	−	+
Rickettsialpox	−	−	−	+
Q fever	−	−	−	+

fourth day and is definite by the eighth day. The reaction is positive in typhus (epidemic and endemic) and in spotted fever, but typhus usually gives a strongly positive test with only OX-19, whereas spotted fever may be positive with only one of the other strains or with more than one strain. Agglutination in dilution 1:160 is positive; dilution 1:80 is suspicious. A positive reaction may occur in typhoid fever, in relapsing fever, and in undulant fever but without a progressive rise in titer. Tsutsugamushi fever gives a strongly positive reaction with OXK, but negative reactions with other strains. Rickettsialpox, Bullis fever, trench fever, and Q fever give negative reactions with all strains. Cross-agglutination between *P. tularensis* and *Proteus* OX-19 may occur.

Antibiotics do not interfere with the Weil-Felix reaction.

Rickettsiae in tissue sections: Wolf et al.[117] described a 12 min. Wright buffer sequence suitable for staining rickettsiae in formalin-fixed tissue (see Chapter 16).

METHODS IN VIROLOGY[118]

Viruses are the smallest microorganisms known. They can only be visualized by the electron microscope. They are characterized by their ultramicroscopic size and by the fact that they can only propagate within cells. As a result of virus infection and replication, the involved cell may develop intracytoplasmic or intranuclear inclusion bodies.

Definition: The **intracellular virus** is a strictly intracellular infectious organism that possesses only one type of nucleic acid, either RNA or DNA, is reproduced from its own genetic material, is unable to grow or to divide by binary fission, and is devoid of a Lipmann system of enzymes. The virus, when it leaves the cell (**extracellular virus**), acquires a protein coat.

Viruses occupy a position between living and nonliving matter. They can be crystallized like an inanimate chemical substance but are capable of limitless multiplication.

Viruses have a **chemical composition** similar to the composition of **genes** of tissue cells. Like the nucleic acid of the genes, virus nucleic acid is able to store information and to transmit it to other nucleic acid molecules and to reproduce itself. While gene reproduction is controlled, virus reproduction is devoid of any control system and spreads from cell to cell.

CLASSIFICATION OF VIRUSES

Viruses are divided into two groups, depending on whether they contain RNA or DNA.

RNA viruses: RNA viruses include enterovirus, myxovirus, influenza virus, respiratory syncytial virus, rabies virus, measles virus, reovirus, and arbovirus.

DNA viruses: DNA viruses include adenovirus and herpesvirus.

Virus diseases can be classified according to the **tropism** of the virus, e.g., its affinity for a particular kind of cell. This classification is not entirely satisfactory because a virus may have more than one tropism and different groups of viruses may have the same tropism.

The classification according to tropism is as follows:

    Generalized diseases
      Smallpox
      Vaccinia
      Measles
      Rubella
      Varicella
      Yellow fever
    Diseases of nervous system
      Poliomyelitis
      Rabies
      Encephalitis

Diseases of respiratory tract
Influenza
Common cold
Atypical pneumonia
Diseases of skin and mucous membranes
Herpes simplex and zoster
Diseases of eye
Trachoma
Inclusion conjunctivitis
Diseases of liver
Infectious hepatitis
Yellow fever
Infectious mononucleosis

According to **various characteristics** such as RNA contents, size of virus particles, mode of spread, and result of treatment with diethylether, viruses are collected into several groups: arboviruses, reoviruses, herpesviruses, RS viruses (respiratory syncytial virus), enteroviruses (poliovirus, Coxsackie viruses A and B, ECHO viruses), and adenoviruses (myxoviruses, parainfluenza viruses).

LABORATORY DIAGNOSIS[119]

Laboratory diagnosis includes (1) virus isolation, i.e., isolation of the causative agent; (2) serologic tests, i.e., demonstration of a rise in the specific antibody titer in the course of the disease; and (3) examination of tissue for characteristic pathologic changes.

Collection and handling of clinical material

Label and identify each specimen separately. Do not use water-soluble ink.

Types of specimen: Use stool (walnut size), rectal swabs, throat washings (15 ml. sterile nutrient broth) or throat swabs, cerebrospinal fluid, clotted blood (15-20 ml.), and tissue specimens. Other specimens may consist of pleural fluid, contents of vesicles, urine, scrapings of skin lesions, etc. The material should be obtained fresh when the patient is admitted, and a similar specimen should then be collected about 2 wk. after the onset of symptoms. All material—even if contaminated—should be collected in sterile containers using sterile technique, frozen, and kept frozen. Freeze-drying techniques may also be used. To prevent drying out, swabs should be placed in 1 ml. nutrient broth or in **Hanks balanced salt solution.**[*]

If shipping is required, the material should be packed and shipped on dry ice. If facilities for freezing are not available, the material may be placed in 50% buffered glycerin.

Collection of specimens for serologic tests: Two or three specimens of blood (15-20 ml.) are drawn at suitable intervals with sterile syringes and discharged into sterile screw-capped test tubes. The blood is allowed to clot and the serum separated under sterile technique. The serum is then stored in the deep freeze, but it must be prevented from absorbing CO_2, which renders it anticomplementary. All sera are examined at the same time with identical antigen and reagents.

Handling of autopsy specimens: Specimens should be collected under sterile conditions and immediately deposited in the deep freeze.

Methods of virus isolation

Before isolation is attempted it is necessary to remove bacteria and particles from the material. This is accomplished by the use of bacterial filters of progressively decreasing porosity such as Berkfeld filters, Seitz filters, etc.

Further preparation of the specimen includes the addition of antibiotics that will not harm the virus such as penicillin and streptomycin and, finally, differential centrifugation.

Tissue culture: The virus can be cultivated in growing tissue suspended in nutrient medium. Not all viruses grow on all cells; **monolayer cell cultures** as well as **permanent cell strain cultures** of various tissues are commercially available. They include tissue cultures sensitive to a wide range of viruses, such as **human amnion** and **HeLa cells.** These cultures are inoculated, and as viral growth develops, **cytopathogenic changes** of individual cells may be produced (Fig. 11-13). These are visualized when fragments of the culture are removed, stained on a cover slip, and examined microscopically. The affected cells become granular, round up, shrivel,

---

[*]Becton, Dickinson & Co., Rutherford, N. J.

Table 11-26. Practical diagnostic tests for viral diseases of man*

Virus	Clinical presentation	Specimens for isolation	Available tests
Respiratory			
Influenza	Acute respiratory disease	Throat washings or swabs, nasal excretions	CF, EE, FA, HI
Parainfluenza	Pharyngitis, croup, bronchiolitis	Sputum, throat washings	CF, CPE, HI
Adenovirus	Acute respiratory illness, pneumonia, pharyngitis, coryza, conjunctivitis	Throat swab, rectal swab, stool, CSF, conjunctival secretion	CF, CPE, HI, N
RS	Bronchiolitis, pneumonia, coryza	Throat swab, nasal swab	CF, CPE, HI, N
Psittacosis	Pneumonia	Throat washings, sputum, blood	CF, EE, FA, I, IA, N
Central nervous system			
Poliovirus	Paralysis, aseptic meningitis, undifferentiated respiratory illness	Throat washings and swabs, rectal swabs, CSF, blood, urine	CF, CPE, FA, IA, N
ECHO	Aseptic meningitis, paralysis, exanthem, respiratory disease, diarrhea	Throat washings and swabs, rectal swabs, CSF, blood, urine	CF, CPE, FA, HI, N
Insect-borne encephalitis	Acute febrile disease, encephalitis, aseptic meningitis	Blood, throat washings, CSF, urine, brain and other tissues (if fatal)	CF, CPE, HI, IA, N
Herpes	Encephalitis, aseptic meningitis	Blood, CSF, brain tissue (if fatal)	CF, CPE, EE, FA, I, IA, N
Mumps	Encephalitis	Saliva, blood, urine, milk, brain tissue (if fatal)	CF, CPE, EE, HI, IA, N, skin test
Lymphocytic choriomeningitis	Aseptic meningitis	Blood, CSF, brain tissue (if fatal)	CF, CPE, HI, IA, N
Rabies	Fatal systemic disease	Saliva, throat and eye swabs, CSF	CF, FA, IA, N, NB
Aseptic meningitis	Meningitis	CSF	CF, CPE, N
Exanthems			
Variola-vaccinia	Smallpox, eczema vaccinatum	Vesicle, pustular or scab material	CF, CPE, EE, FA, HI, I, N, precipitin test
Varicella-herpes zoster	Chickenpox, herpes zoster	Vesicle, pustular or scab material	CF, CPE, FA, I, N, Ouchterlony gel reaction
Rubeola	Measles, pneumonitis, encephalomyelitis	Blood, urine, throat swabs, conjunctival secretion	CF, CPE, HI, N
Rubella	Rubella, neonatal defects	Blood, urine, throat washings and swabs	CF, EE, FA, IA, N interference test
Miscellaneous			
Lymphogranuloma venereum	Genital, inguinal, pelvic, anorectal, extragenital	Buboes, lymph nodes	CF, I, Frei test
Colorado tick fever	Acute febrile disease	Blood, throat washings, stool	CF, CPE, EE, HI, IA, N
Obscure febrile diseases	Acute fever	Throat washings, stool, CSF	CF, N

*From Schaeffer: Hosp. Prac. 1:3, 1966.

CF = complement fixation; CPE = cytopathogenic effect in tissue culture; EE = embryonated eggs; FA = fluorescent antibodies; HI = hemagglutinoinhibition; I = inclusion bodies; IA = inoculation into animals; N = neutralization; NB = Negri bodies.

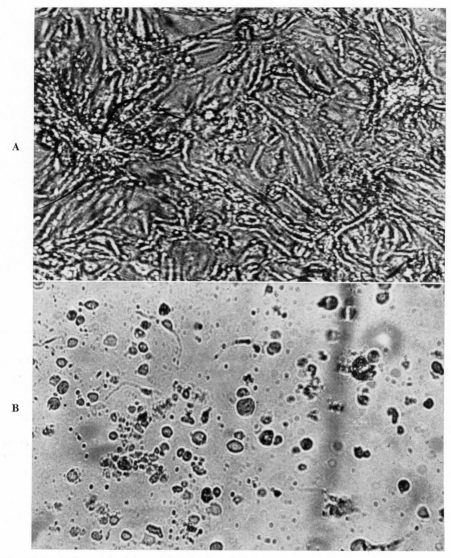

Fig. 11-13. Effect of poliovirus on monkey kidney tissue culture. **A,** Before infection there is a continuous layer of polygonal cells. **B,** After inoculation the cells degenerate, demonstrating viral cytopathogenic effect. Two days after infection most cells have died; survivors are swollen or shrunken and show pyknotic nuclei. (From Schaeffer: Hosp. Pract. **1:**51, 1966.)

and finally disappear. The following viruses produce **cytopathogenic changes:** Coxsackie, ECHO, herpesvirus, adenovirus, vaccinia, influenza, etc. The disappearing cells form areas of necrosis within the sheets of cultured cells called **plaques.** The morphology of these plaques is characteristic for certain viruses and can be brought out as areas of decolorization by staining the living cells with vital dyes. Specific immune sera will inhibit the cytopathogenic effect.

Cultivation of virus in the chick embryo: In most cases the fertile eggs are incubated for 10-12 days at 37°-38° C. before they are inoculated. Several different locations may be chosen for the inoculation, depending on the nature of the virus:

Egg inoculation (Fig. 11-14): **Chorio-**

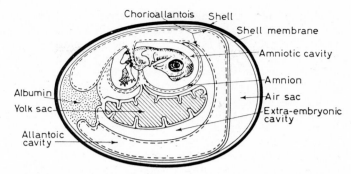

Fig. 11-14. Diagram of developing chick embryo. (From Baker: Handbook of bacteriological technique, London, 1962, Butterworth & Co.)

allantoic inoculation of vaccinia, variola, and herpes simplex viruses produces characteristic pocks.

Allantoic inoculation is used for influenza, Newcastle disease, and mumps viruses.

Amniotic sac inoculation is used for the isolation of influenza virus from throat washings.

Yolk sac inoculation is adopted for primary isolation of members of the psittacosis–lymphogranuloma venereum group and for neurotropic viruses.

Inoculation of laboratory animals: The tissue culture and the embryonated egg inoculation have largely replaced the laboratory animal in the virus laboratory. Nevertheless, intracerebral inoculation of the suckling mouse is necessary for the cultivation of Coxsackie and arboviruses and the virus of lymphocytic choriomeningitis.

Serologic tests

Serologic tests are retrospective methods employing acute and convalescent sera which contain antibodies, the nature of which can be elicited by in vitro antigen-antibody reactions. In response to the infection, various antibodies such as neutralizing, complement fixing, etc. appear, all at the same time or at various times, and of varying titers. Two specimens must be obtained, one on admission and one at a later date, the time interval varying from a few days to 2 wk. A fourfold increase in antibody titer is considered diagnostic. The serologic tests include

neutralization, hemagglutination inhibition, complement fixation, precipitation, agglutination, and immunofluorescence.

Neutralization: When a specific immune serum is added to the corresponding virus, the virus is rendered noninfective or is neutralized. Any one of the methods of virus propagation discussed lends itself to neutralization. The immune serum and the virus are mixed and kept in contact for a short period of time and then the virus is inoculated into the original system. Under the influence of the immune serum the expected virus effect must be prevented. This expected effect will vary according to the system used; e.g., in cell cultures the cytopathogenic effect will be absent, plaques will fail to form, or hemadsorption will not take place.

Hemagglutination and hemagglutination inhibition tests: These tests are based on the principle that the suspensions of certain viruses will cause agglutination of red blood cells. If specific immune serum is introduced into this system, it will inhibit the agglutination of the red cells in proportion to the amount of antibody present in the serum.

These tests are useful for the identification of myxoviruses, poxviruses, and some groups of arboviruses and adenoviruses.

Complement-fixation test: In viral and rickettsial diseases, complement-fixing specific immune antibodies appear at various times, some in 2 wk., others in the third or fourth week. They are usually not found in the wake of vaccinations with virus. The test follows the principle of all complement-fixation tests and is of value only if performed as a quantitative procedure. Phase one combines the antigen with the inactivated immune serum and complement, and in phase two the hemolytic system of sheep cells and hemolysin is added as indicator of complement fixation. The binding of the complement to the antigen-antibody complex is evidenced by the absence of hemolysis. Many of the virus antigens are commercially available.

Agglutination, precipitation, and flocculation tests: All these names describe similar phenomena of clumping of antigen by the action of antibodies. If the antigen is large, the term **agglutination** is used; if it is small, it is **precipitated** out of suspension; and if both phenomena occur, the process is called **flocculation.** The agar diffusion method of Oudin-Ouchterlony can also be used as a **precipitation** method.

Fluorescent antibody technique: This technique is used primarily for the diagnosis of rabies and influenza.

Direct method: The fluorescein-labeled antiserum is directly applied to the smear (the antigen).

Indirect method: The antigen is first treated with unlabeled specific immune serum, which may be the patient's serum. The homologous antigen in a smear or tissue slide will fix the antibodies or the antibody molecules of the immune serum in situ. The excess immune serum is washed off. The fixed gamma globulin is detected by fluorescent anti-gamma globulin of the same species as produced the unlabeled immune globulin.

Tissue examination

The diagnosis of some viral diseases can be made on the basis of pathologic anatomic tissue patterns and/or the presence of **inclusion bodies** which may be found in the nucleus, the cytoplasm, or both. Inclusion bodies are either pure virus particles, as is the case in adenoviruses, or they are virus-directed cell proteins or virus by-products. They are acido-philic solid structures surrounded by a clear zone. The involved cells or nuclei are usually enlarged. They are helpful in the diagnosis of cytomegalic inclusion disease, molluscum contagiosum, verruca vulgaris, herpes infections, inclusion encephalitis, and rabies.

Electron microscopic examination of some viruses reveals the presence of two structures that probably represent developmental stages of the virus. One is called the **elementary body** and measures 300 mμ. It consists of an electron-dense nucleus surrounded by a capsule. Contrary to "true" viruses, it contains both RNA and DNA. The other structure is much larger (1500 mμ) and resembles microsomes of normal cells. Both structures, when suitably stained, can just be seen by the light microscope.

SELECTED VIRUS GROUPS
Adenoviruses

Clinically, adenoviruses produce upper respiratory infections and forms of atypical pneumonia.

Laboratory diagnosis

Cytologic examination of sputum: The ciliated cells show abnormalities known as **ciliocytophthoria,** which is not specific for adenovirus infections, for it is also seen in influenza.

Fluorescent microscopy: Fluorescent microscopy is a sensitive test for detecting adenovirus in infected cells.

Serology: The complement-fixation test is the most useful procedure for diagnosis.

Cat-scratch disease virus

Cat-scratch disease is probably caused by a virus related to the lymphogranuloma venereum group.

Laboratory diagnosis

The intradermal skin test is used for diagnosis of cat-scratch disease.

Enteroviruses

Polioviruses, Coxsackie viruses, or ECHO viruses may produce no symptoms or may lead to an upper respiratory infection, myocarditis, meningitis, pleurodynia, and herpangina.

Laboratory diagnosis

Laboratory diagnosis includes isolation of the virus from pharyngeal washings and stool in tissue culture, detection and titer of neutralizing antibodies in the patient's serum, and detection and titer of complement-fixing antibodies in the patient's serum.

Reoviruses

Reoviruses are related to the enteroviruses and ECHO viruses. They are responsible for upper respiratory infections and diarrhea in newborn infants and small children.

Laboratory diagnosis

Diagnosis involves virus isolation by means of the cytopathogenic effect in tissue cultures or by the plaque method and demonstration of complement-fixing antibodies.

Arboviruses

Arboviruses have an arthropod-vertebrate cycle, the arthropod being the vector while the vertebrate is the reservoir. Man is an incidental host. The vector is frequently a mosquito *(Culex, Anopheles,* or *Aedes)* or a tick, and the disease in man may be a form of encephalitis, fever, or dengue.

Laboratory diagnosis

Serology: The neutralization test is used. The virus grows readily in the cerebrum of baby mice. This growth can be inhibited (neutralized) by immune serum. After adaptation, arboviruses grow well in tissue cultures of HeLa cells, chicken embryonic cells, and hamster kidney cells.

Herpes virus group

Depending on its localization, this virus produces a variety of clinical pictures, most of them harmless diseases or infections, though some may lead to death. If localized in the skin, the virus produces herpes simplex; in the mouth or vagina it leads to stomatitis and vaginitis; in the eye, to conjunctivitis; and in the central nervous system, to meningoencephalitis.

Laboratory diagnosis

Tissue examination: Intranuclear inclusions are found in giant cells. Herpes elementary bodies can be seen by electron microscopy in the fluid of vesicles. The fluorescent antibody technique offers a rapid method of diagnosis.

Culture: Herpes virus grows best in the chick embryo, but it also grows in HeLa cells, monkey kidney, and human amniotic cell cultures, where it produces a cytopathogenic effect.

Animal inoculation: Intracerebral or intraperitoneal injection into suckling mice provides a rapid method (3 days) of identification.

Serology: Rising titers of neutralizing and complement-fixing antibodies should be demonstrated.

Rabies virus

Rabies virus infects the central nervous system, but it also multiplies in the salivary glands, lacrimal glands, and lungs and therefore may be secreted in saliva, tears, and upper respiratory excretions. If it is present in the saliva, the virus is transmitted by the bite of an affected animal. It multiplies in the wound and is propagated along the neural pathways to the central nervous system. In the brain it produces a viral type of encephalitis characterized by the appearance of **Negri bodies.** They are round to oval eosinophilic bodies that vary in size from 2-10 μ. They are found in the cytoplasm of ganglion cells. They are most commonly found in Ammon's horn, in Purkinje cells, and in pyramidal cells of the cerebral cortex.

The disease produced by the virus is called **rabies** (often referred to as **hydrophobia**) and is a fatal infectious disease of the central nervous system. It is transmitted by bite from animal to animal and from animal to man. Dogs usually succumb to the disease in 5 days, while the human incubation period usually varies from 4-6 wk., although it may be much shorter or longer. There are two types of virus—the dog type and the wildlife type.

Laboratory diagnosis

Laboratory diagnosis is based on staining of impressions and of smears for Negri bodies using Sellers stain, examination of stained tissue sections, rabies fluorescent antibody test, and complement-fixation test.

Material: Use the salivary gland and brain of the animal. The head should be shipped in dry ice. Small animals such as bats may be fixed in 10% formalin. Ship spinal fluid, saliva, and throat swabs in dry ice in sealed ampules.

Animal inoculation: Inoculate infant white mice intracerebrally.

Sellers staining method: This method[120] was first published in 1927.

Without previous fixation, and while the impression preparation or smear is still moist, dip it into the stain and remove it at once. Rinse in tap water and dry without blotting. When properly stained, the smear by transmitted light appears reddish violet in thin areas and purplish in thicker areas.

Sellers stain: Make a saturated solution of basic fuchsin and also a saturated solution of methylene blue in absolute methyl alcohol (acetone-free). Prepare the stain as follows, using first only 2 ml. of the basic fuchsin solution.

1. Basic fuchsin solution, 2-4 ml.
2. Methylene blue solution, 15 ml.
3. Methyl alcohol, absolute (acetone-free), 25 ml.

Mix and make a trial stain. If too bluish, add 0.5 ml. more fuchsin solution and make another trial stain. Repeat until satisfactory. Usually not more than 3 ml. fuchsin solution will be necessary.

The stain improves after standing 24 hr. and keeps indefinitely if evaporation is prevented. It may be made in larger quantities and stored.

Under the low-power objective locate thin areas containing large nerve cells and examine with the oil-immersion lens.

The **Negri bodies,** located in the cytoplasm of the large nerve cells and often extracellularly, are round or oval, stain cherry red, and contain blue-staining granules or masses that are usually clearly visible. The cytoplasm of the nerve cells stains somewhat purplish blue and the nucleus more deeply blue. The background (stroma) is rose pink. Nerve fibers are deeper pink, bacteria are deep blue, and erythrocytes are copper colored.

Procedure for rabies fluorescent antibody test:

Materials:
1. Normal mouse brain suspension stored in 1 ml. amounts in freezer
2. Rabid mouse brain suspension stored in 1 ml. amounts in freezer
3. Antirabies conjugate stored in 0.2 ml. amounts in freezer
4. Positive control slides that are already fixed in acetone and stored in freezer

Preparation of smears:
1. Remove a 1 mm. thick cross section of Ammon's horn with scissors or scalpel and place on wooden tongue depressor. Touch a special double-ringed slide very lightly to the brain cross section. Make duplicate impression smears on the same microscope slide. Make at least two slides per animal.
2. Allow slides to air dry for about 30 min.
3. Drop slide into Coplin jar containing acetone at freezer temperature. Store the Coplin jar and a supply of acetone permanently in the freezer; a temperature of 20° C. is sufficient.
4. Allow at least 4 hr. for fixation (overnight preferable).
5. Remove slide from acetone and allow to drain dry while still in the freezer.

Staining:
1. Remove slide from freezer and allow to warm to room temperature.
2. Prepare two portions of antirabies conjugate and dilute each with an equal volume of mouse brain suspension or follow directions enclosed with the conjugate.
3. Use normal brain suspension for dilution 1 and infected brain suspension for dilution 2. CAUTION! The

infected brain suspension contains live rabies virus!

4. Cover one smear with a small drop of dilution 1 and cover the other smear with a drop of dilution 2.
5. Place at 35° C. in humid chamber for 30 min. Use large petri dishes with wet toweling in top.
6. Rinse slides with buffered saline solution and place in staining rack. Then immerse staining rack in buffered saline solution for 10 min.
7. Rinse slide in distilled water to prevent formation of salt crystals.
8. Blot dry with bibulous paper. (When the slides are drained dry, the fluorescence seems to fade.)
9. Mount in glycerin medium (90% glycerol and 10% buffer at pH 7.0).
10. Carefully apply cover slip to omit air bubbles.

Interpretation: First examine the control smear stained with dilution 1. Since only normal mouse brain was contained in the suspension, the labeled antirabies antibody should stain any rabies antigen that was present in the smear. The stained particles will appear as Negri bodies, as fine, dustlike, green material, or usually as both. If no green material is evident, the smear is negative. Color varies with the filter combinaton used.

If any positive slides are found, the smear stained with dilution 2 must be examined. Since rabies antigen was present in this suspension, the labeled antirabies antibody should have been absorbed; hence it is not available for staining. Therefore no stained particles should be seen in this smear. If any green staining material is seen, the test is not conclusive.

A positive interpretation can be made only when staining **is** seen in the smear treated with dilution 1 but **not** seen in the smear treated with dilution 2.

Myxoviruses

Myxoviruses include influenza viruses (types A and B), mumps virus (myxovirus parotidis), parainfluenza virus, Newcastle disease virus (myxovirus multiforme), and RS virus (respiratory syncytial virus).

Laboratory diagnosis

Hemagglutination: Myxoviruses agglutinate the red cells of guinea pigs, chickens, sheep, and human group O cells. The agglutination is produced by adsorption of the virus onto the red cells, from where it can be eluted again.

Hemadsorption: Infected tissue culture cells adsorb red cells added to the culture. This hemadsorption can be prevented by immune serum.

Sensitivity to ether: Ether inactivates myxoviruses.

Measles virus

Laboratory diagnosis

Material: Obtain from blood and pharyngeal washings.

Cytologic examination of nasal and pharyngeal smears: Multinucleated giant cells with eosinophilic intranuclear and intracytoplasmic inclusions can be seen.

Tissue examination: Sections reveal multinucleated giant cells in lymphatic tissue (**Warthin-Finkeldey type giant cell**).

Tissue culture: Human amniotic cells form a suitable medium. The virus produces two changes: syncytial or giant cell formation and transformation of the polygonal cells into spindle and stellate forms.

Serologic tests: Complement-fixation and neutralization tests are used. Rubella studies are particularly important in pregnancy because of the risk of damage to the fetus by rubella virus.

Cytomegaloviruses[121, 122]

This term includes the virus formerly called **salivary gland virus,** which only locally involves the parotid gland, and **cytomegalic inclusion disease virus,** which produces generalized **cytomegalic inclusion disease.** An increasing number of infections with this virus has been reported in adults with neoplastic diseases, leukemia, or tissue transplants.

Laboratory diagnosis

Histopathology: It must be noted that the characteristic inclusions may be very few and may be missed when only a single section is examined. The involved cell is enlarged, at times to four times its normal size. The nucleus, which is also enlarged, is pushed to the cell base and contains an acidophilic inclusion that is surrounded by a clear ring, giving rise to the characteristic owl-eye appearance.

Exfoliative cytology: Cells bearing inclusions have been found in urine, saliva, and gastric washings.

Virus isolation: Cultures of human embryonic skin and muscle cells support the virus. The cultured virus is suitable for neutralization and complement-fixation tests.

Psittacosis-lymphogranuloma venereum group
(Bedsonia infections)

In this group are the psittacosis-ornithosis virus and the lymphogranuloma venereum virus.

PSITTACOSIS

Psittacosis is a respiratory disease of man acquired from contact with birds. The clinical picture varies from an upper respiratory infection to pneumonia.

Laboratory diagnosis

Material: Use sputum and blood.

Virus isolation: The virus can be isolated by inoculation of the yolk sac or by intracerebral, intranasal, or intraperitoneal injection into mice.

Serology: Use complement-fixation and agglutination tests.

ORNITHOSIS

Bedsonia isolated from parrots, parrakeets, canaries, and lovebirds, produce a disease in man called **psittacosis.** Bedsonia isolated from chickens, ducks, turkeys, pheasants, and pigeons produce **ornithosis.**

LYMPHOGRANULOMA VENEREUM

Lymphogranuloma venereum is a venereal disease characterized by enlargement of the regional lymph nodes which become adherent, break down, and tend to form sinuses. This glandular enlargement may follow a primary skin lesion (papule, pustule, or vesicle), usually unobserved, or urethritis and is accompanied by systemic symptoms of an infection.

Laboratory diagnosis

Smears: Make a smear of pus from infected lymph nodes and stain with Giemsa stain for elementary bodies.

Tissue sections: The lymph nodes have a characteristic, though not diagnostic, appearance.

Frei skin test: It is a delayed skin sensitivity reaction to an inactivated antigen (**Lygranum**).

Complement-fixation test: A commercial antigen, Lygranum, may be used.

Trachoma virus

Trachoma is a virus disease of the conjunctiva and cornea.

Laboratory diagnosis

Conjunctival epithelial scrapings: Allow scraped material to dry on a microscope slide, fix with absolute methyl alcohol (acetone-free) for 5 min., and stain with dilute Giemsa stain.

The viruses may appear as small coccoid bodies, called **elementary bodies,** grouped in clusters or pairs; may appear singly; or may appear as intracellular inclusions. The latter are masses of elementary bodies. This inclusion body cannot be differentiated from the inclusion conjunctivitis virus. The trachoma inclusion is rich in carbohydrates and stains with iodine.

Cytology of expressed follicular material: It contains masses of macrophages, necrotic mononuclear cells, and cell debris.

Inoculation of yolk sac: See p. 619.

Hepatitis virus

Viral hepatitis occurs in two forms: infectious hepatitis due to hepatitis virus A and serum hepatitis due to hepatitis virus B. These two viruses are closely related.

HEPATITIS VIRUS A

Infectious hepatitis occurs sporadically or in epidemics and has an incubation period of 10-15 days. The disease is characterized by jaundice, nausea, abdominal pain, anorexia, and fever.

Laboratory diagnosis

Laboratory diagnosis includes the urinary, hematologic, serum enzymatic, and biochemical findings of hepatitis.

In the course of the disease the virus can be found in the stool, the blood, and the duodenal juice. The virus has been cultured in chick embryo and tissue cultures.[123] No specific laboratory test exists at this time for hepatitis virus A or B. Various hemagglutination tests have been described, but they are also positive in other diseases.

HEPATITIS VIRUS B[124]

Serum hepatitis is due to hepatitis virus B, which is transmitted by parenteral inoculation of infected blood or blood derivatives and by unsterilized needles and syringes. The incubation period lasts 8-26 wk., after which time a disease is produced that is similar to infectious hepatitis.

The virus is restricted to man and is found in the blood only. It is not present in the stool, urine, or nasopharyngeal washings.

The most common sources of serum hepatitis are transfusions, the risk increasing with their number, and pooled plasma. The incidence varies from 3-20%. The virus cannot be detected in plasma or blood by any method, though many tests such as transaminase determination and thymol turbidity measurement have been suggested. Careful screening of donors and rejection of donors with a history of jaundice or of drug addiction together with the elimination of all unnecessary transfusions, help to reduce the incidence of posttransfusion hepatitis. It has been suggested that 20 ml. of gamma globulin, which has some protective action against hepatitis, be administered to all recipients of blood transfusions.

The virus can be inactivated by heating plasma protein fraction to 60° C. for 10 hr., by storage of pooled plasma at 32° C. for 6 mo., and by the use of a combination of ultraviolet irradiation and 0.3% beta-propiolactone. Careful washing of the red cells also reduces the incidence of hepatitis.

Variola and vaccinia viruses

The variola and vaccinia viruses are poxvirus variolae (**smallpox**), poxvirus officinalis (**vaccinia virus**), poxvirus bovis (**cowpox**), and poxvirus mollusci (**molluscum contagiosum virus**).

Laboratory diagnosis

Laboratory diagnosis involves **microscopic examination** of the contents of the pustule and of scrapings obtained from its floor and sides. The material can be stained for elementary bodies by the method of Gutstein or examined unstained with the electron microscope.

Gutstein method[125]:
Stain:
1. Methyl violet (1% aqueous), equal parts
2. Sodium bicarbonate (2% aqueous), equal parts

Technique: Allow smear to air dry. Fix in methyl alcohol for 30 min. and filter stain onto slide. Cover slide and incubate at 37° C. for 20-30 min. Rinse in distilled water, air dry, and examine under oil-immersion lens.

Interpretation: Elementary bodies stain light violet.

Virus isolation: Use blood in the pre-eruption stage and saliva and pustular material in the later stages. The virus may be isolated by inoculation of the chorioallantoic membrane of the embryonated egg and tissue culture.

Serology: Antibodies in the patient's serum may be detected by the hemagglutination inhibition test, neutralization test, and complement-fixation test.

Varicella–herpes zoster virus

Chickenpox is a very contagious, generalized exanthematous disease, while herpes zoster is a localized skin disease of very low infectivity that occurs in individuals with limited immunity.

Laboratory diagnosis

Smears of the scrapings of the base of the vesicles reveal intranuclear inclusions and multinucleated giant cells. (Poxviruses also show intracytoplasmic inclusions.)

Smears of the contents of the vesicle may show elementary bodies (see Gutstein method) that can be differentiated from the elementary bodies of smallpox by **electron microscopy.**

The virus is isolated in tissue culture using blood, spinal fluid, vesicular contents, and pharyngeal and nasal washings.

The complement-fixation test is used for detection of antibodies.

Mycoplasma species (Eaton pleuropneumonia-like organisms, PPLO)[126-130]

Mycoplasma species are independent organisms and are not L forms of bacteria, which they resemble. *Mycoplasma* strains have been recovered from the upper respiratory tract, urogenital tract, brain, and blood in human beings. There are four antigenically distinct species, the most important being *M. pneumoniae.*

Laboratory diagnosis

Material: Use sputum, throat washings (normal saline solution), and oral-pharyngeal swabs. Specimens are immediately transferred, at the bedside, to 5 ml. trypticase soy broth containing 0.5% horse serum or bovine albumin. To suppress bacterial contamination, penicillin, polymyxin B, or thallium acetate should be added since mycoplasma are resistant to these agents. Specimens should be cultured at once or frozen at −65° C.

Culture:

Media:

1. PPLO medium* to which 200 ml./L. pooled horse serum and 100 ml./L. 25% extract of fresh bakers' yeast has been added
2. Diphasic agar, an agar plate overlayered by broth and enriched like the PPLO medium

Colonies are observed by oblique transillumination with the dissecting microscope (30-60×). *M. pneumoniae* colonies appear slowly within 5-10 days, are small (measuring 30-100μ in diameter), granu-

lar, and half submerged in agar. They are beta hemolytic in 24-48 hr., and the appearance of some organisms can be likened to fried eggs.

Small spheres are formed in broth.

Serologic tests:

Complement-fixation test: The cultured organisms provide a satisfactory antigen.

Fluorescent antibody technique: Sections of the thorax of a chick embryo infected with PPLO are treated with fluorescein-tagged antibody (direct method) or fluorescein-tagged antiglobulin if the indirect method is used.

Convalescent sera usually show a variety of immunologic reactions such as false positive serologic tests for syphilis, cold hemagglutinins, and agglutinins for *Streptococcus MG.*

REFERENCES

1. Cowan, S. T., and Steel, K. J.: Manual for the identification of medical bacteria, London, 1965, Cambridge University Press.
2. Harris, A. H., and Coleman, M. B.: Diagnostic procedures and reagents, ed. 4, New York, 1963, American Public Health Association, Inc.
3. Bailey, W. R., and Scott, E. G.: Diagnostic microbiology, ed. 2, St. Louis, 1966, The C. V. Mosby Co.
4. Spaulding, E. H., and Emmons, E. K.: Amer. J. Nurs. **58:**1238, 1958.
5. Freeman, M. A., and Barwell, C. F.: J. Hyg. **58:**337, 1960.
6. Hart, D.: J.A.M.A. **172:**1019, 1960.
7. Smith, R. E., Pease, N. M., Reiquam, C. W., and Beatty, E. C.: Amer. J. Clin. Path. **44:**698, 1965.
8. Castaneda, M. R.: Proc. Soc. Exp. Biol. Med. **64:**114, 1947.
9. Darkfield microscopy, Atlanta, 1962, U. S. Department of Health, Education, and Welfare, Public Health Service, Communicable Disease Center.
10. Thayer, J. D., and Martin, J. E.: Public Health Rep. **79:**49, 1964.
11. Brumfitt, W., and Percival, A.: J. Clin. Path. **17:**482, 1964.
12. Smith, L. G., Thayer, W. R., Malta, E. M., and Utz, J. P.: Ann. Intern. Med. **54:**66, 1961.
13. Leigh, D. A., and Williams, J. D.: J. Clin. Path. **17:**498, 1964.
13a. Kass, E. H.: Arch. Intern. Med. (Chicago) **105:**194, 1960.
14. Trainer, T. D.: Amer. J. Clin. Path. **41:**101, 1964.
15. Leading article: Brit. Med. J. **1:**1325, 1965.
16. Bacteriology Committee, Association of Clinical Pathologists: J. Clin. Path. **18:**1, 1965.

---

*Difco Laboratories, Detroit, Mich.

17. Gill, F. A., and Hook, E. W.: Amer. J. Med. **39**:780, 1965.
18. Petersdorf, R. G., and Sherris, J. C.: Amer. J. Med. **39**:766, 1965.
19. Jawetz, E.: Arch. Intern. Med. (Chicago) **110**:141, 1962.
20. Expert committee on antibiotics: Bull. WHO **210**:3, 1961.
21. Petersdorf, R. G., and Plorde, J. J.: Ann. Rev. Med. **14**:41, 1963.
22. Hallman, L.: Bakteriologie und Serologie, ed. 3, Stuttgart, 1961, Georg Thieme Verlag.
23. Estela, L. A., and Shuey, H. E.: Amer. J. Clin. Path. **40**:591, 1963.
24. Williams, R. E. O.: Bull. WHO **19**:153, 1958.
25. Ayoub, E. M., and Wannamaker, L. W.: J.A.M.A. **187**:908, 1964.
26. Montgomerie, J. Z., Kalmanson, G. M., and Guze, L. B.: Amer. J. Med. Sci. **251**:184, 1966.
27. Petran, E. I.: Amer. J. Clin. Path. **41**:224, 1964.
28. Roy, S. B., Sturgis, G. P., and Massell, B. F.: New Eng. J. Med. **254**:95, 1956.
29. Todd, E. W.: J. Exp. Med. **55**:267, 1932.
30. Tillett, W. S., and Francis, T., Jr.: J. Exp. Med. **52**:561, 1930.
31. MacLeod, C. M., and Avery, O. T.: J. Exp. Med. **73**:183, 1941.
32. Wood, H. F., and McCarty, M.: Amer. J. Med. **17**:768, 1954.
33. Anderson, H. C., and McCarty, M.: Amer. J. Med. **8**:445, 1950.
34. Stollerman, G. H., et al.: Amer. J. Med. **15**:645, 1953.
35. Wood, H. F., and McCarty, M.: J. Clin. Invest. **30**:616, 1951.
36. Ivler, D., Chairman: Ann. N. Y. Acad. Sci. **128**:1, 1965.
37. Rogers, D. E., Chairman: Ann. N. Y. Acad. Sci. **65**:57, 1956.
38. Van Prohaska, J., Mock, F., Bake, W., and Collins, R.: Surg. Gynec. Obstet. **112**:1, 1961.
39. Elston, H. R., and Fitch, D. M.: Amer. J. Clin. Path. **42**:346, 1964.
40. White, A.: J. Lab. Clin. Med. **58**:334, 1961.
41. Wilson, E., Foter, M., and Lewis, K.: Appl. Microbiol. **7**:22, 1959.
42. Nahmias, A. J., and Eichkoff, T. C.: New Eng. J. Med. **265**:177, 1961.
43. Editorial: Brit. Med. J. **2**:361, 1961.
44. Schaub, I. G., and Merritt, C. D.: Bull. Hopkins Hosp. **106**:25, 1960.
45. Litsky, B. Y.: Hosp. Manage. **100**:34, 1965.
46. Litsky, B. Y.: Hosp. Manage. **101**:82, 1966.
47. Army Medical School: J. Bact. **38**:119, 1939.
48. Graber, C. D., Scott, R. C., Dunkelberg, W. E., and Dirks, K. R.: Amer. J. Clin. Path. **39**:360, 1963.
49. Danielsson, D.: Acta Dermatovener. **74**:80, 1965.
50. Hess, E. V., Hunter, D. K., and Ziff, M.: J.A.M.A. **191**:91, 1965.
51. Spink, W. W.: Arch. Intern. Med. (Chicago) **106**:433, 1960.
52. Rosen, F. S.: New Eng. J. Med. **264**:919, 1961.
53. Smith, H. H., and Anderson-Langmuir, C.: Amer. J. Clin. Path. **45**:218, 1966.
54. Rogers, K. B., and Taylor, J.: Bull. WHO **24**:59, 1961.
55. Batshon, B. A.: Amer. J. Clin. Path. **45**:125, 1966.
56. Hugh, R., and Leifson, E.: J. Bact. **66**:24, 1953.
57. Schneierson, S. S.: J. Bact. **82**:621, 1962.
58. King, E. O., Ward, M. K., and Raney, D. E.: J. Lab. Clin. Med. **44**:301, 1954.
59. Brown, V. I., and Lowbury, E. J.: J. Clin. Path. **18**:752, 1965.
60. Green, G. S., Johnson, R. H., and Shively, J. A.: J.A.M.A. **194**:1065, 1965.
61. Sellers, W.: J. Bact. **87**:46, 1964.
62. Ashby, D. J. B., and Kwantes, W.: J. Clin. Path. **14**:670, 1961.
63. Ewing, W. H., Hugh, R., and Johnson, J. G.: Studies on the Aeromonas group, Atlanta, 1961, U. S. Department of Health, Education, and Welfare, Public Health Service, Communicable Disease Center.
64. Fife, M. A., Ewing, W. H., and Davis, B. R.: The biochemical reactions of the tribe Klebsielleae, Atlanta, 1965, U. S. Department of Health, Education, and Welfare, Public Health Service, Communicable Disease Center.
65. Edwards, P. R., and Ewing, W. H.: Manual for enteric bacteriology, Atlanta, 1951, U. S. Department of Health, Education, and Welfare, Public Health Service, Communicable Disease Center.
66. Mair, N. S., Mair, H. J., Stirk, E. M., and Carson, J. G.: J. Clin. Path. **13**:432, 1960.
67. Forshay, L.: J. Infect. Dis. **51**:286, 1932.
68. Kendrick, P., Miller, J. J., and Lawson, G. M.: American Public Health Association year book, New York, 1935-1936, American Public Health Association, Inc.
69. Brooks, A. M., Bradford, W. L., and Berry, G. P.: J.A.M.A. **120**:883, 1942.
70. Gardner, H. L., and Dukes, C. D.: Amer. J. Obstet. Gynec. **69**:962, 1955.
71. Castaneda, M. R.: Bull. WHO **24**:73, 1961.
72. Martin, W. J., Schirgen, A., Kelly, P. J., and Beahess, O. H.: Proc. Staff Meet. Mayo Clin. **24**:717, 1960.
73. Huddleson, I. F.: Brucellosis in man and animals, New York, 1943, The Commonwealth Fund.
74. Gould, S. E., and Huddleson, I. F.: J.A.M.A. **109**:1971, 1937.
75. Keller, A. E., Pharris, C., and Gaub, W. H.: J.A.M.A. **107**:1369, 1936.
76. Simpson, W. M.: Ann. Intern. Med. **15**:408, 1941.

77. Barber, M., and Okubadejo, O. A.: Brit. Med. J. 2:735, 1965.
78. Gray, M. L., Seeliger, H. P. R., and Potel, J.: Clin. Pediat. 2:614, 1963.
79. Gray, M. L.: Ann. N. Y. Acad. Sci. 98: 686, 1962.
80. Kubica, G. P.: Current concepts in the isolation and identification of clinically significant mycobacteria, Atlanta, 1965, U. S. Department of Health, Education, and Welfare, Public Health Service, Communicable Disease Center.
81. Petroff, S. A.: Bull. Hopkins Hosp. 26: 276, 1915.
82. Kubica, G. P., Kaufman, A. J., and Dye, W. E.: Amer. Rev. Resp. Dis. 89:284, 1964.
83. Mulcahy, J. D., Moffitt, G. W., and Cameron, G. M.: J. Conf. State & Prov. Public Health Lab. Directors 23:159, 1965.
84. Kubica, G. P., Dye, W. E., Cohn, M. L., and Middlebrook, G.: Amer. Rev. Resp. Dis. 87:775, 1963.
85. Truant, J. P., Brett, W. A., and Thomas, W.: Henry Ford Hosp. Med. Bull. 10:287, 1962.
86. Karlson, A. G., Martin, J. K., and Harrington, R.: Mayo Clin. Proc. 39:410, 1964.
87. Kubica, G. P., Kaufmann, A. J., and Beam, R. E.: Amer. J. Clin. Path. 41:452, 1964.
88. Fregnan, G. D., and Smith, D. W.: J. Bact. 83:819, 1962.
89. Vestal, A. L., and Kubica, G. P.: Amer. Rev. Resp. Dis. 94:247, 1966.
90. Runyon, E. H.: Med. Clin. N. Amer. 43: 273, 1959.
91. Wayne, L. G., and Doubek, J. R.: Amer. J. Clin. Path. 42:431, 1964.
92. Wayne, L. G.: Amer. Rev. Resp. Dis. 86: 651, 1962.
93. Konno, K.: Science 124:985, 1956.
94. Weyer, E. M.: Ann. N. Y. Acad. Sci. 130: 681, 1966.
95. Cannetti, G., et al.: Bull. WHO 29:565, 1963.
96. Froman, S., et al.: Amer. J. Clin. Path. 42: 340, 1964.
97. DeGroat, A., Anastassiadis-Aries, U. E., and White, M. F.: Amer. J. Clin. Path. 41:441, 1964.
98. Parlett, R. C.: Ann. N. Y. Acad. Sci. 98: 637, 1962.
99. Volini, F., Colton, R., and Lester, W.: Amer. J. Clin. Path. 43:39, 1965.
100. Wayne, L. G., Doubek, J. R., and Russell, R. L.: Amer. Rev. Resp. Dis. 90:588, 1964.
101. Gordon, R. E., and Smith, M. E.: J. Bact. 69:502, 1955.
102. Jones, W. D., and Kubica, G. P.: Amer. J. Med. Techn. 30:187, 1964.
103. Gordon, R. E., and Smith, M. E.: J. Bact. 66:41, 1953.
104. Wayne, L. G.: Amer. J. Clin. Path. 36: 185, 1961.
105. Soule, M. H.: Ann. N. Y. Acad. Sci. 54: 34, 1951.
106. Soule, M. H.: Int. J. Leprosy 32:195, 1964.
107. Maddock, R. K.: J.A.M.A. 148:44, 1952.
108. Eadie, G. A., Molner, J. G., Solomon, R. J., and Aach, R. D.: J.A.M.A. 187:134, 1964.
109. Mukerjee, S.: Brit. Med. J. 2:546, 1964.
110. King, E. O.: Ann. N. Y. Acad. Sci. 98: 700, 1962.
111. Kilo, C., Hagemann, P. O., and Marzi, J.: Amer. J. Med. 38:962, 1965.
112. Eden, A. N.: J. Pediat. 68:297, 1966.
113. McGill, R. C., Martin, A. M., and Edmunds, P. N.: Brit. Med. J. 1:1213, 1966.
114. Galton, M. M.: Ann. N. Y. Acad. Sci. 98: 675, 1962.
115. Jeghers, H.: Bull. New Eng. Med. Center 15:61, 1953.
116. Ferron, E. D.: Rev. Clin. Esp. 20:283, 1946.
117. Wolf, G. L., Cole, C. R., Sasloaw, S., and Carlisle, H. N.: Stain. Techn. 41:3, 1966.
118. Horstman, D. M.: Amer. J. Med. 38:738, 1965.
119. Lennette, E. H., and Schmidt, N. J.: Diagnostic procedures for virus and rickettsial diseases, ed. 3, New York, 1964, American Public Health Association, Inc.
120. Sellers, T. F.: Amer. J. Public Health 17: 1080, 1927.
121. Carlstrom, G.: Acta Paediat. Scand. 54: 17, 1965.
122. Duvall, C. P., et al.: Ann. Intern. Med. 64:531, 1966.
123. Editorial: Brit. Med. J. 1:534, 1962.
124. Senior, J. R.: Gastroenterology 49:3, 1965.
125. Gutstein, M.: J. Path. Bact. 45:313, 1937.
126. Morton, H. E.: Ann. N. Y. Acad. Sci. 98: 670, 1962.
127. Hayflick, L.: Trans. N. Y. Acad. Sci. 27: 817, 1965.
128. Grayston, J. T., et al.: J.A.M.A. 191:97, 1965.
129. Forsyth, B. R., Bloom, H. H., Johnson, K. M., and Chanock, R. M.: J.A.M.A. 191: 92, 1965.
130. Griffin, J. P., and Crawford, Y. E.: J.A.M.A. 193:1011, 1965.

Chapter 12

Methods in mycology

FUNGI

Fungi are nonphotosynthetic microorganisms (lacking chlorophyll) that differ from bacteria by the size of their individual components and by a more complex morphology. Fungi possess a cell wall, cytoplasm, and nuclei. Each fungus (**thallus**) consists of a vegetative portion, the **mycelium,** and a reproductive portion, the reproductive mycelium (**spores**).

STRUCTURE

Fungi are roughly divided into yeast-like and moldlike varieties (see classification). Moldlike fungi produce long branching filaments called **hyphae** that may be divided by septa into segments so that so-called **septate hyphae** are produced, in contradistinction to nonseptate hyphae. The mass of hyphae is called mycelium. The part of the fungus that projects above the surface of the medium is called **aerial mycelium,** and the part that penetrates into the medium is called **vegetative mycelium.** The reproductive mycelium produces spores, which are called asexual **spores** when they are formed without previous fusion of the nuclei. If nuclear fusion occurs, the resulting spores are called sexual. The fungi of medical importance belong to a collective group called **Fungi Imperfecti,** in which the sexual form of reproduction is either imperfectly known or not observable at all.

CLASSIFICATION OF PATHOGENIC FUNGI

For the purpose of rapid clinical grouping, fungi can be classified as follows:

Fungi with bacterial characteristics
  Actinomyces (see Chapter 11)—anaerobic

Nocardia—aerobic; somewhat acid fast
  Streptomyces—aerobic
Fungi that form hyphae (mycelial fungi)
  Dermatophytes—*Microsporum, Trichophyton,* and *Epidermophyton*
  Maduromycosis—*Madurella* and *Allescheria*
  Chromoblastomycosis—*Hormodendron* and *Phialophora*
  Miscellaneous group, usually nonpathogenic—*Aspergillus, Mucor, Penicillium, Rhizopus,* and *Hemispora*
Fungi with the characteristics of yeast, i.e., reproduce by budding (blastosporulation)
  Cryptococcus
  Candida
  Geotrichum
  Diphasic fungi that produce both mycelial (at room temperature) and yeast (at 37° C.) forms in vivo and in vitro
  Histoplasma
  Blastomyces
  Sporotrichum
  Coccidioides

Fungi may also be classified according to the specific location and depth to which they may affect the host.

Superficial mycoses (dermatophytes) that affect the outermost layer of skin and hair
  Microsporum—affects skin and hair of scalp and face; body only occasionally; nails not involved
  Trichophyton—attacks skin, nails, and hair
  Epidermophyton—attacks nails and skin; hair not involved
  Malassezia furfur—found in skin scrapings
Cutaneous and subcutaneous mycoses (mycetomas)
  Chromoblastomycosis organisms
  Rhinosporidium
  Sporotrichum
  Candida
Systemic mycoses
  Actinomyces
  Nocardia
  Blastomyces
  Cryptococcus
  Coccidioides
  Candida
  Geotrichum

DIAGNOSIS OF FUNGUS INFECTIONS

Diagnosis is based on direct examination of wet material, examination of stained material, culture, animal inoculation, serologic methods such as complement-fixation tests, agar precipitation techniques, etc.

COLLECTION OF SPECIMENS

Effort should be made to collect specimens for fungus examinations as free from bacterial contamination as possible. Place specimens of hair, skin, and nails in sterile petri dishes.

Hair: Pluck out some of the infected hairs so that the roots may also be examined. Other hairs selected for examination should be cut off about ¼ in. from the scalp. The remaining portion, including the root, should be used for culture.

In scalp ringworm infections caused by *Microsporum audouinii* and *canis,* the infected hair fluoresces when exposed to **ultraviolet light** in a dark room. Epilate the fluorescing hairs.

Skin: Cleanse the skin thoroughly with 70% alcohol and with a sterile scalpel shave off thin layers of the epidermis, avoiding the drawing of blood. Obtain shavings from several sites of the lesion, including the margin and the apparently normal skin just beyond the margin.

Nails: Obtain specimens of nails after cleaning them thoroughly with soap, water, and 70% alcohol by scraping the surface of the nails almost down to the nail bed.

Pus: When abscesses are present, using aseptic technique collect pus with needle and syringe before incision. From draining sinuses, collect as much pus as possible by aspirating with a sterile pipette after thorough cleansing (soap, water, and alcohol) of the site of the sinus opening. Gentle pressure or massage over the sinus tract (when not contraindicated) may be helpful. When only a small amount of pus can be obtained, leave it in the pipette and deliver it to the laboratory promptly. More material is needed than for a bacteriologic examination. The use of cotton swabs for specimens is seldom satisfactory.

Sputum: Collect fresh specimens of sputum after the patient has brushed his teeth and rinsed his mouth thoroughly. Collect the specimen directly in a sterile petri dish. In cases of suspected *Candida* infections, material should be smeared directly onto slides.

It requires less time to collect a specimen properly than to identify contaminants.

CONCENTRATION OF SPUTUM
FOR FUNGUS CULTURE

The method suggested by Sanford[1] is as follows. Mix a fresh early morning specimen with equal parts of a 1% pancreatin solution in phosphate buffer, pH 7.5. Shake well and incubate at 35° C. for 1-1½ hr. or until liquefied, shaking occasionally. Centrifuge the liquefied specimen at 3000 rpm for 20 min. and decant the supernatant. Mix the small amount of sediment (0.1-0.2 ml.) well and use for inoculation of culture plates and for direct microscopy.

METHODS OF EXAMINATION[2, 3]
DIRECT EXAMINATION—WET PREPARATION USING SODIUM HYDROXIDE

Hair: Place segments of hair in a few drops of 10% sodium hydroxide on a microscope slide. Place a cover slip on the preparation and heat gently over a Bunsen burner. Clearing may require several heatings of short duration. Examine the cleared specimen under low and high power for spores and mycelial elements.

In *Trichophyton* infections the spores tend to be arranged in chains within the substance of the hair (Fig. 12-1).

In *Microsporum* infections the spores are arranged in a mosaic pattern in the peripheral layers of the hair (Fig. 12-2).

In *Piedria* infections, white or black nodules are located along the hair shaft.

Skin: Clean the area thoroughly with tincture of green soap, water, and 70% alcohol. With a sterile blade shave off a layer of the epidermis at the margin of the lesion. Just scraping the dry superficial scales is not sufficient. Mount a portion directly in 10% potassium or sodium hydroxide under a cover glass. Warm gently (Fig. 12-3).

The specimen should be examined

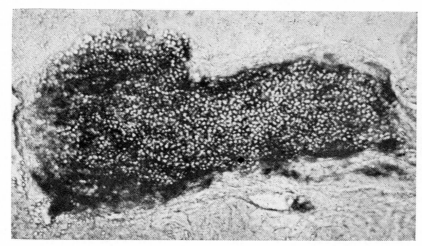

Fig. 12-1. Hair stump infected with *Trichophyton tonsurans*. Arthrospores are within the substance of the hair (endothrix pattern). (Courtesy McNeil Laboratories, Fort Washington, Pa.)

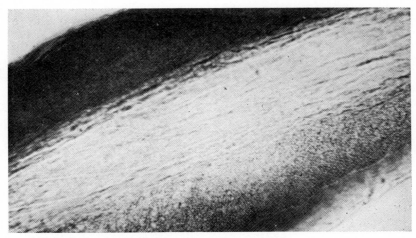

Fig. 12-2. Hair infected with *Microsporum audouinii*. Arthrospores are in the outer portion of the hair along both sides (ectothrix pattern). (Courtesy McNeil Laboratories, Fort Washington, Pa.)

without too much delay since some of the fungi tend to disintegrate in the hydroxide after about 24 hr. The other portion is used for culture.

Examine for mycelial elements and spores. Most hyphae are septate, change little in diameter, and form straight or wavy lines (Figs. 12-4 and 12-5).

Artefacts: Cotton fibers, cellulose fibers, cholesterol deposits, and debris may be mistaken for hyphae (Fig. 12-6).

Nails: Examine nail scrapings by the same procedure used for skin specimens.

Pus, sputum, and other material: Mount some of the material, selecting any suspicious colonies or granules, in 10% potassium or sodium hydroxide under a cover glass. The general class may often be recognized in the fresh material, but the species is determined from cultures. In the direct examination of a wet preparation using sodium hydroxide, care

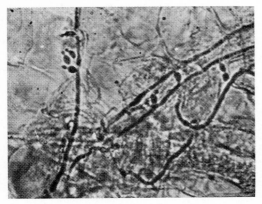

Fig. 12-3. Hyphae and budding cells of *Candida albicans* in epidermal scale. (Courtesy McNeil Laboratories, Fort Washington, Pa.)

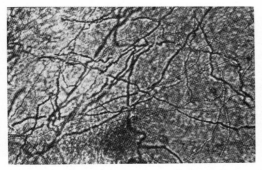

Fig. 12-4. Young hyphae of *Trichophyton* in epidermal scale. They appear as dark or light lines, depending on whether they are sharply in focus. (Courtesy McNeil Laboratories, Fort Washington, Pa.)

must be taken to recognize elastic tissue fibers, which are not segmented, and cotton fibers, which are irregular and flat (Fig. 12-7).

CULTURE

Methods are explained in the discussions of the various fungi.

The purpose of culture media is to support the growth of fungi and to suppress the accompanying bacterial flora as well as to prevent secondary contamination of the medium that may occur with long periods of incubation.

Occasionally what are thought to be contaminants may be the etiologic or coetiologic agent or agents.

Choice of media: Several media should be inoculated with clinical material, e.g., Sabouraud agar with and without antibiotics, blood agar, and the media mentioned in the following discussion. They are commercially available. Most fungi are aerobic. Thioglycollate broth is indicated for the culture of *Actinomyces*. The type of medium used will somewhat depend on the specimen and on the degree of bacterial contamination.

Usually the specimen is inoculated into Sabouraud dextrose agar with and without cycloheximide and chloramphenicol and incubated at 35° and 25° C. The use

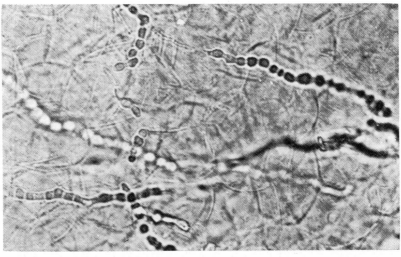

Fig. 12-5. Old hyphae of *Trichophyton* in epidermal scale, broken up into chains of arthrospores. (Courtesy McNeil Laboratories, Fort Washington, Pa.)

of both media and both temperatures will decide whether a fungus is diphasic, i.e., whether it has a yeast and a mycelial phase.

The culture plates may be lightly sealed with Parafilm to prevent drying, for they should be kept for 4-8 wk. before being discarded as negative. Contaminants and saprophytes usually grow quickly, while most pathogens grow at a slower rate.

Once growth has been obtained the

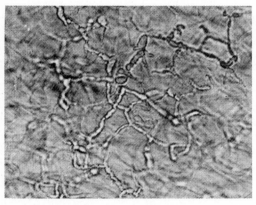

Fig. 12-6. Mosaic artefact showing deposits of cholesterol and debris among epithelial cells. It is differentiated from fungal hyphae by (1) arrangement in spaces between cells, (2) abrupt changes in diameter, (3) tapering and indefinite terminations, and (4) characteristic reentrant angles at points of abrupt change in width.

organism may be transplanted to special media such as chlamydospore agar to stimulate spore production.

It is advisable to use only a few media because the morphology of the fungi varies on different media.

Colonial characteristics: The colony should be examined for **pigment** formation, **texture** (glabrous, cottony, or woolly), **rate of growth**, and **morphology** (folded, flat, heaped, etc.).

Media for isolation and identification of fungi

Routine media:

Sabouraud dextrose agar: Sabouraud medium without antibiotics is used routinely for the isolation of fungi. Its low pH supresses bacterial growth. The addition of **antibiotics** makes the medium even more selective for the isolation of pathogenic fungi (with certain exceptions) since saprophytic fungi and bacteria are supressed. It is therefore used for contaminated specimens such as skin, sputum, etc. The following fungi are sensitive to **cycloheximide:** *Cryptococcus neoformans, Candida krusei* and *tropicalis* (not *C. albicans*), *Trichosporum cutaneum, Mucor, Rhizopus, Allescheria boydii, Aspergillus fumigatus.*

Nocardia asteroides and *Actinomyces* are sensitive to **chloramphenicol.**

Media with added antibiotics are **inactivated** at 35° C. and, if antibiotic

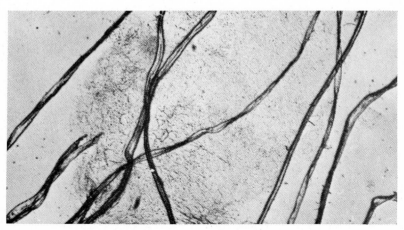

Fig. 12-7. Cotton fibers in KOH. (Courtesy McNeil Laboratories, Fort Washington, Pa.)

activity is desired, are effective only at room temperature.

Brain-heart infusion agar (BHI) with cycloheximide and chloramphenicol: This is a good medium for systemic fungi. Incubate at room temperature if antibiotic activity is desired.

BHI blood agar contains 6% blood.

Littman oxgall agar: The addition of streptomycin makes this medium, which contains bile and crystal violet, more selective than Sabouraud agar. It is suggested for the cultivation of dermatophytes.

SPECIAL MEDIA:

Media for stimulation of sporulation: The media used are **potato-dextrose agar, neutral wort agar, chlamydospore agar,** and **cornmeal agar.** The addition of 1% Tween 80 stimulates the production of chlamydospores of *C. albicans.* Neutral wort agar is useful for the differentiation of *Trichophyton* species, and rice grain medium is helpful in the differentiation of *Microsporum* species. These media are inoculated by cutting into the surface.

Slide culture

Purpose: The culture of fungi on glass slides in a moist chamber allows observation of the undisturbed relationship between the reproductive and vegetative mycelia.

Procedure:
1. Place a slide on a bent glass rod in the bottom of a petri dish. Cover and sterilize.
2. Prepare Sabouraud dextrose agar plates with about 15 ml. agar per plate. Permit to solidify. Use agar blocks about 1 cm. square and 2-3 mm. deep.
3. Using sterile technique, place block of agar on slide in petri dish.
4. Inoculate centers of four sides of agar block with fungus to be studied.
5. Cover inoculated block with sterile cover slip.
6. With sterile technique, add 8 ml. sterile water to bottom of petri dish.
7. Incubate at 25° C. until sporulation occurs.

8. When spores appear, carefully lift off cover slip and lay aside, with fungus growth upward.
9. Lift agar square from slide and discard.
10. Place 1 drop lactophenol cotton blue on this slide and cover with a clean cover slip. Obtain clean slide, place 1 drop lactophenol cotton blue near one end, and cover with original cover slip, placing mycelial surface down.
11. Blot away excess mounting fluid from cover slips of the two preparations. When dry, seal edges with nail polish or preferably with asphalt tar varnish.

ANIMAL INOCULATION[4]

Purpose: This is done to evaluate pathogenicity and to study the tissue phase. The skin of guinea pigs, white mice, and rabbits can be infected with dermatophytes. *Histoplasma, Cryptococcus,* and *Coccidioides* are pathogenic to mice. Guinea pigs and mice can be infected with *Nocardia* and *Blastomyces.*

Gastric mucin for enhancing pathogenicity of fungi: Gastric mucin accelerates the action of pathogenic fungi when a mixture of organisms and mucin is inoculated intraperitoneally into experimental animals.

Material: Gastric mucin of the granular type is used.*

Preparation:
1. Emulsify 5 gm. gastric mucin in 95 ml. distilled water in a Waring blendor for 5 min.
2. Autoclave for 15 min. at 120° C.
3. Cool to room temperature.
4. Adjust to pH 7.3 with 10% sodium hydroxide.
5. Check sterility by culturing.
6. Store in refrigerator.

Use: Mix equal parts of the 5% gastric mucin suspension and the fungus spore suspension and inject the mixture (1 ml.) intraperitoneally into the experimental animal.

---

*Wilson Laboratories Division, Wilson & Co., Inc., Chicago, Ill.

FLUORESCENT ANTIBODY TECHNIQUE

The fluorescent antibody method has many advantages over conventional methods. The technique is more rapid, the organisms do not need to be viable and are easily spotted even if there are only a few, and the morphology of the fluorescent cell can be appreciated.

Fluorescent methods have been used for the diagnosis of *Cryptococcus neoformans, Candida albicans, Sporotrichum schenkii, Histoplasma capsulatum,* and *Blastomyces dermatitidis.*

MOUNTING FLUIDS AND STAINS

Lactophenol cotton blue:
1. Phenol crystals (melted in water bath and then weighed), 20 gm.
2. Lactic acid, 20 gm.
3. Glycerin, 40 gm.
4. Cotton blue, 0.05 gm.
5. Distilled water, 20 ml.

Sodium or potassium hydroxide: Use 10% sodium or potassium hydroxide in water.

Parker's superchrome blue-black ink: Mix equal parts of blue-black ink and 20% aqueous sodium hydroxide.

India ink (Littman):
1. India ink, 15 ml.
2. Merthiolate (aqueous, 1:1000), 30 ml.
3. Tween 80 (aqueous, 1:100), 0.1 ml.

Filter before use.

Methylene blue: Mix 2.5% methylene blue in 95% alcohol.

WET PREPARATION USING LACTOPHENOL COTTON BLUE

Technique: Clean microscope slide with silicone-coated paper and add a few drops of lactophenol cotton blue; add a small drop of 95% alcohol separately. With a rigid, sterile inoculating needle remove a segment of aerial mycelium, dip it quickly into the alcohol drop, and transfer to the mounting fluid. Tease the segment apart using two needles, apply cover slip, and examine under the low- and high-power objectives of the microscope.

Stains: The following stains should be available: Wright, gram, Giemsa, and modified acid-fast (decolorizing agent, 0.5% aqueous sulfuric acid).

TISSUE PREPARATIONS

Tissue slides made from surgical and autopsy specimens as well as from experimentally injected animals are stained with hematoxylin-eosin stain, MacCallum-Goodpasture stain (which stains all gram-positive fungi), PAS stain (periodic acid–Schiff stain), mucicarmine stain, Gomori methenamine silver nitrate stain, and Gridley stain. (For details of tissue examination, see Chapter 16.)

SEROLOGIC TESTS[5]

The following tests are employed in the diagnosis of coccidioidomycosis, histoplasmosis, and blastomycosis: complement-fixation tests, precipitin tests, and collodion agglutination. Cross-reactions and many other factors make these tests difficult to interpret. Two serum samples should be obtained, one early in the course of the disease and one 2 or 3 wk. later. A sharp rise in the titer followed by a fall may be significant.

SKIN TESTS

Intradermal tests are outside the scope of the general laboratory.

YEASTLIKE FUNGI
Candida

Species of *Candida* are often found on mucous membranes (mouth, vagina, intestines, etc.), on moist portions of the skin (between toes and fingers and in axillary, inguinal, and intergluteal regions), and less frequently around and in the nails (paronychia, onychia) and in the respiratory tract.

LABORATORY DIAGNOSIS

Material: Scrapings from skin or nails (KOH preparations) and sputum, stool, body fluids, urine, and vaginal smears are used.

Specimens should be examined when fresh and should not be allowed to stand at room temperature because the organism multiplies on standing.

Smear and wet preparation: Hyphae and oval budding yeastlike cells can be seen in skin and nails. In stool, urine, etc. the oval budding cells predominate. The hyphae are characteristically constricted at the level of the septa (Fig. 12-3).

The approximate number of organisms per field should be included in the report since the finding of only a few organisms may lack clinical significance. On the basis of the wet preparation the organisms should be reported as *Candida* species.

Culture: The organisms grow well on most media at room temperature and at 35° C. Most grow in the presence of chloramphenicol and cycloheximide, a characteristic that can be used effectively for isolation of the yeast from contaminated specimens.

Media: Use Sabouraud agar with and without antibiotics at room temperature and at 35° C. It must be noted that **some** *Candida* species are sensitive to cycloheximide; therefore 50 units penicillin and streptomycin/ml. media may be added instead. Soft white to tan smooth colonies will appear on both plates (Fig. 12-8), and microscopic examination reveals thin-walled budding cells accompanied by mycelia and pseudomycelia in the deeper and peripheral portions of the colony. The term **"pseudomycelium"** is applied to a tubular cell originating from a blastospore that elongates and remains in contact with the mother cell. The term "**blas-**

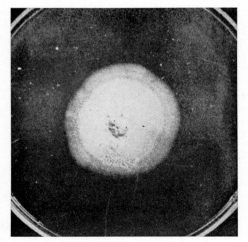

Fig. 12-8. *Candida albicans.* Colony 5 wk. old showing pasty appearance with honeycombed edge. (From Dobes: Southern Med. J. 36:614, 1943.)

tospore" connotes a spore produced by a budding process along the mycelium (*b* part of Fig. 12-9, *A*).

Differential diagnosis

The finding of yeast cells in cultures incubated at room temperature and at 35° C. is suggestive of any one of the following species of fungi: *Candida, Cryptococcus, Geotrichum,* and *Trichosporon.*

If the culture is pure, the differential diagnosis is made on the basis of a wet preparation.

Candida species give rise to budding cells, with pseudomycelia and mycelia penetrating the deeper portions of the agar. If *Candida* is suggested by the morphology, transfer a segment of culture to **cornmeal** or **chlamydospore agar** (see discussion of identification of *C. albicans*).

Cryptococcus fails to produce a mycelium and can be differentiated from *Candida* species and from true yeast by the single-budding cells surrounded by a wide capsule (India ink preparation).

If a mycelium is present, the yeast may be either *Geotrichum* or *Trichosporon.*

Geotrichum species give rise to septate hyphae and rectangular arthrospores.

Trichosporon produces arthrospores as well as blastospores.

If the organism is a member of the *Candida* species, it must be determined whether it is *C. albicans,* the only member of *Candida* that is definitely pathogenic.

IDENTIFICATION OF CANDIDA ALBICANS: The usual criteria are production of chlamydospores and of characteristic blastospore patterns, fermentation tests, reduction of dyes such as tetrazolium or gentian violet, and production of germ tubes in serum.

Production of chlamydospores: Use cornmeal or chlamydospore agar (cut-streak plate). With a straight, heavy inoculating wire make a cut into the agar at a 45-degree angle, extending across and down through to the bottom of the plate. Use control streak with known *C. albicans* culture. Incubate at room temperature up to 5 days and examine daily. When control streak shows chla-

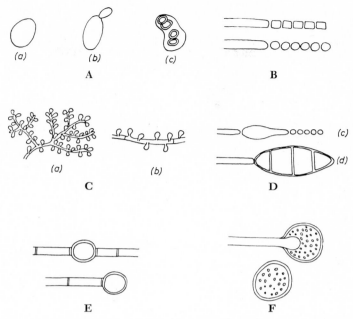

Fig. 12-9. A, Yeast cells: a, yeast cell, b, blastospore, and c, ascospore. B, Arthrospores. C, Conidiophores. D, Type of microconidia, c, and type of macroconidia, d. E, Chlamydospores. F, Sporangiospores. (From Baker: Handbook of bacteriological technique, London, 1962, Butterworth & Co.)

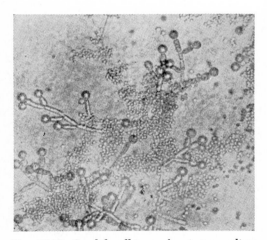

Fig. 12-10. *Candida albicans* showing mycelium and characteristic masses of spores and terminal chlamydospores. (From Dobes: Southern Med. J. **36:**614, 1943.)

walled, macroconidic, and 8-12μ in diameter (Fig. 12-10).

Blastospore pattern on cornmeal cut-streak plate: All *Candida* species have mycelia with blastospores, the name given to budding spores. *C. albicans* blastospores occur in large ball-like groups at the junction of the mycelial segments, distinguishing it from other species except *C. stellatoidea*, which is distinguished by star-shaped colonies on blood agar. The blastospores of *C. tropicalis* are irregularly distributed, occurring both between and at the joints, whereas those of *C. parakrusei* and *C. krusei* appear chiefly at the joints. The blastospores of *C. krusei* are arranged in characteristic whorls. *C. albicans*, in addition to mycelia and blastospores, also shows chlamydospores.

Fermentation test: Transplant the culture three times every 24 hr. to a tube of beef extract agar and incubate at 35° C.

Inoculate the third-generation culture into sugar tubes for fermentation. Inoculate 2% solutions of glucose, maltose,

mydospores, examine test streak. If chlamydospores are present, diagnose as *C. albicans*.

Chlamydospores are formed terminally on enlarged hyphae and are thick

Table 12-1. *Candida* fermentation

	Dextrose	*Lactose*	*Maltose*	*Sucrose*
C. albicans	Acid and gas	–	Acid and gas	Acid
C. krusei	Acid and gas	–	–	–
C. tropicalis	Acid and gas	–	Acid and gas	Acid and gas
C. pseudotropicalis	Acid and gas	Acid and gas	–	Acid and gas
C. stellatoidea	Acid and gas	–	Acid and gas	–
C. parapsilosis (parakrusei)	Gas	–	–	–

– = no reaction.

sucrose, and lactose in 8 ml. peptone water containing Andrade indicator with a saline suspension of the organisms. The latter is prepared by adding 2 ml. sterile saline solution to the third-generation beef extract broth. The tubes are equipped with Durham tubes and cotton plugs. Note the production of gas and acid or of gas alone after 48 hr. of incubation at 35° C. (Table 12-1).

Andrade indicator: Dissolve 0.5 gm. acid fuchsin in 100 ml. distilled water. Add 16 ml. 0.1N NaOH and allow to stand overnight. The color should change from pink to brown and then to yellow. If necessary, add small amounts of 0.1N NaOH. (Acid = pink.)

Tetrazolium reduction: Various species of *Candida* have different capacities to reduce monotetrazolium compounds (**Pagano medium**), producing different color intensities of the colonies.

C. albicans	Cream to light pink
C. krusei	White (spreading)
C. tropicalis	Deep red
C. stellatoidea	Light red

Four of the tests can be combined on a four-quadrant Felsen plate containing a chlamydospore agar in one quadrant and a sucrose medium, a lactose medium, and a tetrazolium medium in the other quadrants.[6]

Production of germ tubes in serum[7]: Inoculate 0.5 ml. human serum with the organism and incubate at 35° C. Examine the specimen microscopically 1½ hr. later and again in another 1½ hr. *C. albicans* is unique in its ability to form germ tubes under these conditions.

Serologic tests: Serologic tests have no value in the diagnosis of *Candida* infections.

Animal inoculation: Only *C. albicans* is lethal to rabbits; death occurs within 1 wk. following intravenous inoculation of 1 ml. of a 1% suspension of the organisms in sterile saline solution.

Histopathology: In tissue preparations, *Candida* produces mainly mycelia, which are difficult to see in sections stained with hematoxylin-eosin but can be visualized well with PAS stain.

Cryptococcus neoformans (Torula)

Infection due to the yeastlike organism *Cryptococcus neoformans* (Plate 15) is known as cryptococcosis. Although it is sometimes called European blastomycosis, it is not an infection due to *Blastomyces*. Since the organism has a tendency to invade the central nervous system, one of the common clinical manifestations is torula meningitis.

LABORATORY DIAGNOSIS

Material: Sputum, spinal fluid, urine, and serous exudates are used.

Smear and wet preparation: In 10% KOH, unicellular, large budding yeast cells are seen and no mycelia are formed. India ink preparations show a well-developed capsule. The addition of 0.1% toluidine blue to the spinal fluid differentiates pink-staining cryptococcal cells from deep blue-staining leukocytes. Red blood cells remain unstained. The yeast cells are large, round, thick walled, and 5-15μ in diameter. The buds are attached to the parent cell by a narrow neck. A wide polysaccharide capsule surrounds both cells.

Stained smears are not of much value because the nucleus is gram positive and

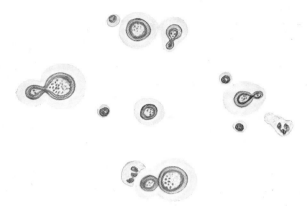

Plate 15. *Torula* in spinal fluid. (Greenthal stain; high-power magnification.)

the capsule is not stained. Wright stain colors the organism deep blue so that it resembles lymphocytes. (This should be remembered when examining spinal fluid sediments.)

Culture: Large amounts of the original specimen (5 ml. spinal fluid, 20 ml. pleural fluid, etc.) may have to be concentrated to yield positive findings in early cases of cryptococcosis.

Blood agar: In 2-10 days, mucoid, yeastlike, white to cream colonies grow at 35° C. and at room temperature (3-4 days' delay). The ability to grow at 35° C. differentiates pathogenic from nonpathogenic forms of *Cryptococcus* because saprophytic strains usually grow at room temperature only.

BHI agar: The organism may require an enriched medium and therefore BHI agar should be included among the media used. *C. neoformans* is sensitive to **cycloheximide;** isolation should not be attempted on media containing this antibiotic.

Differential diagnosis

C. neoformans must be differentiated from other yeastlike fungi that grow at 35° C. and at room temperature. *C. neoformans* does not produce mycelia on cornmeal agar, while *Candida* species do (see section on identification of *C. albicans*). Septate hyphae and barrel-shaped spores differentiate *Geotrichum*.

Special tests:

Urease test: *Cryptococcus* is the only yeastlike fungus that hydrolyzes urea.

Animal inoculation: *C. neoformans* is pathogenic to mice.

Histopathology[8, 9]**:** *Cryptococcus* is the only yeastlike fungus in which the capsule contains acidic polysaccharides. The capsule may be overlooked in sections stained with hematoxylin-eosin and may stain poorly with PAS. The capsules of cryptococci stain metachromatically with toluidine blue and are colored by mucicarmine, colloidal iron, and Alcian blue. The latter two are the more sensitive methods.

Geotrichum candidum

Geotrichum candidum is a yeastlike fungus that reproduces by **arthrospores.** It is saprophytic but may cause infections of the skin and of the respiratory and gastrointestinal tracts that closely resemble candidiasis.

LABORATORY DIAGNOSIS

Smear and wet preparation: Yeastlike cells are seen on smears and wet preparations.

Culture: The organism grows readily on Sabouraud agar with and without antibiotics. At first yeastlike colonies form and rapidly develop central mycelia that may be aerial or buried within the agar. They are made up of rectangular microscopic arthrospores that readily break off.

They are typically rectangular with square or round ends and show little tendency to round up (Fig. 12-9, *B*).

Trichosporon

Trichosporon produces white, soft mycelial masses on hair shafts. It grows readily on Sabouraud agar, producing cream-colored yeastlike colonies that are smooth at first, but soon become wrinkled. Arthrospores, mycelium, and blastospores are seen microscopically.

SYSTEMIC MYCOSES

By definition, systemic mycotic infections involve all organs of the body, but they may involve only a few or, at one stage, may be restricted to a single organ, e.g., the skin.

DIPHASIC FUNGI
Histoplasma capsulatum[10-13]

Histoplasmosis is a fungus disease caused by *Histoplasma capsulatum* (Plate 16). It is a soil saprophyte, the spores of which are inhaled by man and animals.

The organism appears in two phases: a **tissue phase,** the form in which it exists in tissues, and a **mycelial phase,** the form in which it exists when cultured at room temperature. The **yeast phase** is similar to the tissue phase and occurs when the fungus is cultured at 35° C.

LABORATORY DIAGNOSIS

Material: It may consist of imprints of lymph nodes, liver, spleen, and bone marrow and of blood smears. In disseminated histoplasmosis, examine the buffy coat of blood and bone marrow. In pulmonary infections the sputum should be cultured.

Imprints and smears: Imprints and smears are best stained with Giemsa or Wright stain. The organism is found in the tissue or **yeast phase. Macrophages** (reticulum cells) contain intracytoplasmic organisms that are small, round to oval, and measure 1-4μ in diameter. They have a distinct wall, within which is a wide achromatic zone and a crescentic nucleus-like structure. They are somewhat similar in appearance to *Leishmania,* but have no kinetoplast. The organism is gram positive.

Culture: Most **clinical material** contains the yeast phase of the organism, which in sputum survives from 1-2 wk. at refrigerator temperature but fails to do so at room temperature. The media should be inoculated immediately.

Media: Use BHI blood agar without antibiotics or plain blood agar, BHI agar with antibiotics, and Sabouraud dextrose agar with and without antibiotics.

Immediately inoculate two plates of BHI blood agar, two plates of Sabouraud agar without antibiotics, and two plates of Sabouraud agar with antibiotics. Incubate one set of plates at 35° C. and one set at room temperature.

The organism forms the mycelial phase at room temperature, while it grows in the yeast phase at 35° C. The antibiotics at 35° C. prevent the growth of the yeast phase of *H. capsulatum,* as they do of all diphasic fungi.

Mycelial phase: After 10-14 days of incubation at 25° C. (room temperature) on Sabouraud dextrose agar or on BHI agar, white, fluffy colonies with fine aerial mycelia form. As the culture ages it acquires a tan color. The first spores that appear and can be seen on wet preparations are **microconidia,** which are round to pyriform sessile or stalked structures measuring 2-3μ in diameter. They are borne on lateral **conidiophores** arising from **septate hyphae.** Large **macroconidia** called **chlamydospores,** which are **tuberculated** and measure 8-25μ in diameter, develop later (Fig. 12-11).

In order to obtain the characteristic chlamydospores it may be necessary to transplant the culture to sporulation media such as **chlamydospore** or **cornmeal agars.**

Yeast phase: The mycelial phase can be converted to the yeast phase by subculturing a colony to BHI agar and incubating at 35° C. To avoid drying of the medium, the petri dishes should be surrounded with Parafilm. After 2-3 days, small, white to cream-colored, moist, convex colonies will appear at the periphery of the original inoculum. Wet preparations will show small, oval, thin-walled cells that exhibit budding and measure 2-4μ.

Tissue phase, animal inoculation, and

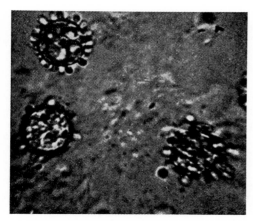

Fig. 12-11. *Histoplasma capsulatum.* Culture showing characteristic tuberculated spores. (From Reid et al.: J. Lab. Clin. Med. **27**:419, 1942.)

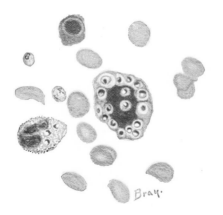

Plate 16. *Histoplasma capsulatum* in bone marrow smear.

histopathology: The tissue phase is similar to the yeast phase.

Technique: The original clinical material or the culture may be injected intraperitoneally into mice. Mix sputum, gastric washings, or ground tissue with equal parts of sterile saline solution until liquefied. Add 10,000 units penicillin and 1000 units streptomycin/ml. specimen. (If the specimen is not contaminated, this procedure is not necessary.) Inject 1 ml. of the mixtures **intraperitoneally** into two or three **mice.** Kill the mice after 4 wk. and examine the spleen and liver, which

contain the yeast phase. On slides stained with hematoxylin-eosin it is difficult to discover the unstained outlines of the organisms within the cytoplasm of macrophages. The PAS stain is not reliable for the detection of histoplasmosis. Other carbohydrate reactions give better results, e.g., **Gomori methenamine silver stain** and **Gridley stain.**

Serologic tests: A skin test and a **complement-fixation test** with yeast phase and tissue phase antigens are available. To be diagnostic the titer of the complement-fixation test must be over 1:32 and should rise within a period of about 6 wk. The titer may persist for several weeks or months and then fall rapidly, or it may remain elevated for as long as 1 yr., even in the event of clinical recovery. Pulmonary cavitation is usually accompanied by a rise in titer, while in the case of single pulmonary nodules the serologic methods are of no value.

Newer serologic methods include the fluorescent antibody technique[14] and agar gel precipitin reaction[15] and are used in addition to such serologic tests as histoplasmin-latex agglutination[16] and histoplasmin-collodion agglutination.[17]

Blastomyces dermatitidis

North American blastomycosis, or **Gilchrist's disease,** is caused by *Blastomyces dermatitidis.*

LABORATORY DIAGNOSIS

Material: Pus, sputum, tissue biopsies, body fluids, or scrapings from the border of cutaneous lesions may be utilized.

Smears and wet preparation: Make preparation in 10% potassium or sodium hydroxide and search for doubly contoured (thick-walled) spherical bodies, some of which will be seen budding (Fig. 12-12), distinguishing them from *Coccidioides immitis*, which reproduces by endosporulation. The inner portion of the blastomyces shows marked granulation which may be seen best in a smear stained with **Wright stain.** The organisms measure 7-15μ in diameter and are devoid of a capsule. A wide neck connects the single bud to the parent cell.

Unstained wet preparations may be

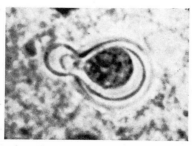

Fig. 12-12. Blastospore of *Blastomyces dermatitidis.* (Oil-immersion lens; ×1200.)

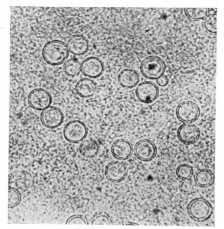

Fig. 12-13. *Blastomyces dermatitidis.* Budding forms in exudate. (×500.) (Courtesy Dr. Francis D. Smith.)

ringed with nail polish; after a few hours, examine for **single germ tubes** (mycelial filaments) originating from the spheroidal bodies.

Culture: The fungus is **biphasic;** there is a **yeast phase** at 35° C., which is similar to the **tissue phase,** and a **mycelial phase** at room temperature.

Media: BHI blood agar and Sabouraud agar should be inoculated in duplicate; incubate one set at room temperature and one at 35° C. The cultures should be held for 4 wk. before considered negative and must therefore be sealed with Parafilm to prevent drying.

On Sabouraud agar at room temperature the mycelial phase produces woolly colonies with white aerial hyphae and a central small elevation that later turns buff and brown. On microscopic examination the colonies reveal septate hyphae and round to pyriform **microconidia,** 3-8μ in size, on **lateral conidiophores.**

On BHI blood agar at 35° C. the yeast phase leads to wrinkled, waxy, gray to tan colonies, which on microscopic examination are seen to be composed of cells 7-15μ in diameter that show single budding (Fig. 12-13).

Skin tests: A skin test antigen is available.

Serologic tests. The **complement-fixation test** is valuable in following the disease since the titer usually rises gradually as the disease progresses and disappears upon recovery. The test has no value in diagnosis of the disease.

Tissue phase and histopathology: Using PAS, Gomori methenamine silver, or Gridley stains, the yeastlike, thick-walled, single-budding organisms will be seen in **giant cells** or macrophages.

Paracoccidioides brasiliensis (Blastomyces brasiliensis)

In **South American blastomycosis,** the cutaneous lesions of which are similar to those of coccidioidal granuloma, the organisms *(P. brasiliensis)* found in the tissues appear as doubly contoured spherical bodies like those of *Blastomyces dermatitidis* in North American blastomycosis, but some of the bodies of *P. brasiliensis* will show **multiple budding** (small spherical, oval, or elongated buds).

LABORATORY DIAGNOSIS

Material: Pus, blood, sputum, and tissue are used.

Smear and wet preparation: Unstained preparations reveal cells with refractile walls that give rise to several buds which may vary in size or be uniform and appear to be "pinched off" at the site of attachment.

Culture: The organism is **biphasic.** Inoculate two sets of BHI blood agar and Sabouraud agar. Incubate one set at room temperature and the other set at 35° C.

Mycelial phase: On Sabouraud agar at room temperature irregularly folded colonies with aerial mycelia slowly appear.

Wet preparations reveal septate hyphae and a few pyriform microconidia, sessile or on short stalks. As the mycelial phase is not diagnostic, it is necessary to convert it to the yeast phase by subculturing it to BHI blood agar and incubating at 35° C.

Yeast or tissue phase: On BHI blood agar at 35° C. the colonies are yeastlike, wrinkled, waxy, and white to gray and grow slowly. Wet preparations reveal thick-walled round spheres 6-30μ in diameter with multiple budding.

Histopathology: The yeast or tissue phase can also be produced by injection of the mycelial phase into the **testes of guinea pigs** which, after several weeks, develop an orchitis accompanied by draining sinuses. The thick-walled structures can be demonstrated by PAS, Gomori methenamine silver, and Gridley stains.

Coccidioides immitis

Coccidioidomycosis (coccidioidal granuloma, San Joaquin fever, or valley fever) can be either a relatively mild granulomatous lung disease that is usually self-limiting or a progressive and frequently fatal disease.

The fungus occurs in the soil of only a few areas in America. The spores, which are carried by wind and air, enter the human body through the respiratory tract.

LABORATORY DIAGNOSIS

Material: Sputum, tissue, pus, and pleural fluid are used.

Smear and wet preparation: Large, thick-walled, spherical bodies called **spherules** that vary from 10-80μ in diameter are seen. They contain small spherical or irregular **endospores** varying from 2-5μ in diameter. Some spherules are tightly filled with spores, while others show spores that are peripherally arranged. Other spherules are empty and broken and the spores are free (Fig. 12-14).

The slide may be sealed with fingernail polish. **Multiple** germ tubes (mycelial filaments) will be seen projecting from the spherules within 3-4 hr.

Culture: The organism is **biphasic** and grows readily on Sabouraud agar. Since it is resistant to the action of cyclohexi-

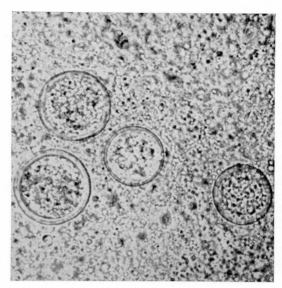

Fig. 12-14. *Coccidioides immitis* in pus from lymph node. (×600.) (From Stiles and Davis: J.A.M.A. **119**:765, 1942.)

mide and chloramphenicol, Sabouraud agar containing these antibiotics can be used as primary selective medium.

Mycelial phase: Inoculate Sabouraud agar, two plates with antibiotics and two plates without antibiotics. Incubate one plate of each set at room temperature and one plate of each set at 35° C. The fungus produces filamentous structures at room temperature as well as at 35° C.

A white aerial mycelium develops in a few days and imparts a white, cottony look to the originally smooth, gray, flat, moist colony. The growth may develop a brownish pigment on the reverse side so that the entire colony appears tan. Sporulation occurs in 7-14 days.

Microscopically the aerial mycelium shows hyphae segmented into cylindric or barrel-shaped spores measuring about 3-4μ; these are called **arthrospores** (Fig. 12-15). They are separated by empty cells. When the hyphae rupture, many of these spores are freed, thus making handling of cultures dangerous. Before wet preparations are prepared, the culture should be flooded with sterile normal saline solution that is injected into the culture tube through the unopened top.

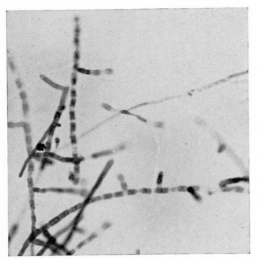

Fig. 12-15. *Coccidioides immitis.* Hyphae showing segmentation into arthrospores with characteristic light areas. (Lactophenol cotton blue stain.)

The differential diagnosis of fungi that are filamentous on culture at room temperature and at 35° C. includes *Coccidioides immitis* and species of *Allescheria* and of *Phialophora.*

Yeast phase: The conversion of the mycelial phase to the yeast phase should not be attempted because of the danger involved and also because it is seldom successful.

Animal inoculation: The material used may be a culture or clinical material without the benefit of prior culture.

The mycelial phase can be converted to the tissue phase by injecting 0.1 ml. saline suspension of spores and mycelium into the **testes of a guinea pig.** Within 1 wk. the animal will develop orchitis.

For direct animal inoculation with clinical material, cover the material with 10,000 units penicillin/ml. and 1000 μg streptomycin/ml. Shake for 1 hr., and centrifuge at 2500 rpm for 15 min. The sediment is suspended in sterile saline solution. Use the inoculation technique just given.

Histopathology: The spherules are visible in hematoxylin-eosin preparations, but they and their endospores are better visualized by the use of Gridley or PAS

stains. Immature spherules are devoid of endospores.

Skin tests: Skin tests are of little diagnostic value.

Serologic tests: Precipitins appear early in the disease (1-4 wk.) and then disappear. The immunodiffusion test[18] can be used as a screening test for precipitating antibodies. Complement-fixing antibodies do not appear at all in some cases, while in others they remain low, appear late, persist longer.

SUBCUTANEOUS MYCOSES

This group of fungi usually involves skin and subcutaneous tissue, but may spread to internal organs.

SPOROTRICHOSIS
Sporotrichum schenkii

This fungus produces a subacute and chronic disease called **sporotrichosis.**

LABORATORY DIAGNOSIS

Material: Obtain pus from an ulcerated lesion or aspirate from a nodule.

Smear and wet preparation: The tissue yeast phase consists of thin-walled, small, spherical to oval structures that are infrequently seen in human material. They can best be demonstrated on smears stained with PAS or Gomori methenamine silver stains. The fluorescent antibody technique may be used to discover scarce organisms.

Culture: The organism is **biphasic,** demonstrating a mycelial phase in cultures at room temperature and a yeast phase in tissues and cultures at 35° C. Use Sabouraud agar with antibiotics and BHI blood agar.

Mycelial phase: After 3-7 days on Sabouraud agar at room temperature, moist, white, smooth, leathery colonies appear that soon develop wrinkled or folded areas. They lack cottony aerial mycelia and after 1 wk. or so they turn brown and finally black.

Wet preparations reveal delicate septate hyphae 1-1.5μ in diameter and small pyriform conidia arranged in clusters on the ends of lateral conidiophores. In older cultures a second set of conidiophores appears on the sides of conidiophores and hyphae.

Tissue phase: The mycelial phase can be converted to the tissue phase by transfer to BHI blood agar and incubation at 35° C. The colonies are moist, cream-colored, soft, and yeastlike.

Wet preparations show small fusiform or oval budding cells.

Animal inoculation: The yeast phase may also be demonstrated by injecting a saline suspension of the mycelial form intratesticularly into several mice.

Histopathology: The organisms are difficult to find on sections stained with hematoxylin-eosin. PAS and Gomori methenamine silver stains are required to bring out the cells.

Serologic tests: Antibodies can be demonstrated in sporotrichosis.

MADUROMYCOSIS

Maduromycosis is a chronic granulomatous infection (**mycetoma**) usually involving the soft tissues and bones of the feet (**Madura foot**), rarely other parts of the body.

There are two types of mycetomas: (1) **actinomycetic mycetoma** resulting from infection by *Actinomyces* and (2) **maduromycotic mycetoma** caused by a variety of true fungi, i.e., *Allescheria boydii, Madurella mycetomi, Madurella grisea, Phialophora jeanselmei, Cephalosporium,* and *Aspergillus.*

True mycetomas must be distinguished from pseudomycetomas produced by bacteria.

Allescheria boydii

A. boydii is the most common causative agent of maduromycosis in the United States.

LABORATORY DIAGNOSIS

Material: Pus and curettings should be examined grossly for **grains** or **granules** that are small, irregularly shaped masses of fungus.

Smear and wet preparation: Examine granules in KOH and flattened under a cover slip. The granules are light colored and are composed of wide septate hyphae 2-3μ in diameter that contain numerous chlamydospores. The granules of *A. boydii* must be distinguished from those of

Actinomyces, which have a delicate mycelium (1μ wide or less), peripheral clubs that break up into diphtheroids, short branching segments, and do not form chlamydospores.

Culture: Use Sabouraud agar with penicillin and streptomycin and incubate at 35° C. Wash the granules overnight in normal saline solution containing penicillin and streptomycin (50,000 units penicillin and 100,000μ streptomycin/10 ml. saline solution) and then culture.

The colonies are filamentous and cottony, at first white but later becoming a dark brownish gray. The reverse side is gray to black.

Wet preparations reveal septate hyphae and brownish ovoid to clavate conidia that are borne singly but are aggregated into clusters. Most strains produce **ascospores.**

Histopathology: The grains are well-stained with hematoxylin-eosin and PAS stains.

RHINOSPORIDIUM[19, 20]

The causative organism of **rhinosporidiosis,** *Rhinosporidium seeberi,* has been found in nasal secretions and in nasal and other polypoid growths. Little is known about its source, the mode of transmission, or the portal of entry. It is found in the tissues as a thick-walled spherule, varying greatly in size (up to 250μ). The small forms are similar to those of *Blastomyces,* but budding is not present. Reproduction is by endosporulation. It has not been cultured, and it has not been possible to infect laboratory animals.

CHROMOBLASTOMYCOSIS[21, 22]

Chromoblastomycosis is a skin disease that may follow contamination of a wound with soil. It is caused by several fungi that produce dark colonies with black reverse sides and short gray aerial mycelia. The different species are distinguished by the types of conidiophores they form. There are three types of sporulation:

1. *Cladosporium (Hormodendrum)*-type sporulation: Ovoid spores in branching chains arise from the terminal cells of conidiophores that vary in length.

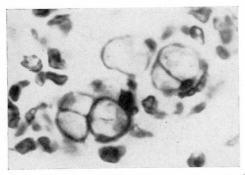

Fig. 12-16. Chromoblastomycosis organisms. Dark brown septate cells in tissue section of granuloma. (Hematoxylin-eosin stain.)

2. *Phialophora*-type sporulation: Spores escape from the bottom of cup-shaped openings of flask-shaped structures (phialides).

3. *Acrotheca*-type sporulation: Spores arise from the sides of conidiophores.

The fungi involved are species of *Cladosporium (Hormodendrum)* and *Phialophora.*

LABORATORY DIAGNOSIS

Material: Scrapings and biopsy tissue are used.

Culture: Use Sabouraud agar with cycloheximide and chloramphenicol and incubate at room temperature.

On Sabouraud agar, brown to black, flat to dome-shaped colonies that have a short aerial mycelium are formed. The fungi are identified, as previously mentioned, by the type of sporulation seen in wet preparations.

Histopathology: The brown septate bodies can readily be seen in sections stained with hematoxylin-eosin (Fig. 12-16).

CUTANEOUS MYCOSES
DERMATOMYCOSIS (FUNGI OF SKIN, NAILS, AND HAIR)

The dermatomycoses are known as **athlete's foot (tinea pedis), ringworm of the body (tinea corporis)** or **of the scalp (tinea capitis),** and **jock itch (tinea cruris).** Fungus infection of the nails is called **onychomycosis.**

The three most important causal agents of dermatomycosis are *Trichophyton* (10 or 12 species), *Epidermophyton* (1 species), and *Microsporum* (3 species).

LABORATORY DIAGNOSIS

Material: Using filtered ultraviolet light, select infected hairs. Hairs infected by *Microsporum audouinii* and *canis* show green **fluorescence.** *Trichophyton*-infected hairs do not or only slightly fluoresce. If hairs do not fluoresce, look for hairs with nodules or for stumps of hairs. Allow the hair to dry before culturing.

Obtain thin fragments or shavings from skin and nails after cleaning the area with 70% alcohol to remove surface bacteria. Place material in sterile petri dish.

Wet preparation: Examine hair or skin and nail shavings in KOH. In **tinea versicolor** this is the only method of examination available since the fungus *(Malassezia furfur)* does not grow on culture media. It shows septate hyphae mixed with thick-walled spherical cells. The other dermatophytes show branching septate hyphae and must be distinguished by culture.

Culture: If necessary, cut the specimen into small fragments with a sterile scalpel and transfer onto two plates of Sabouraud agar with cycloheximide and chloramphenicol. Incubate one set at room temperature and one set at 35° C. The specimen should be pressed into the agar. Examine the cultures every week.

Trichophyton

Trichophyton species invade hair (*T. rubrum* rarely), skin, and nails.

TRICHOPHYTON MENTAGROPHYTES (TRICHOPHYTON GYPSEUM)

Wet preparation: Wet preparations of hair usually show an ectothrix type of involvement (Figs. 12-2, 12-4, and 12-5) (the hair does not fluoresce).

Culture: On Sabouraud dextrose agar the colonies grow rapidly and are cottony or granular to powdery. The surface mycelium is white to beige. The reverse side is yellow at first, then brownish to red. Wet preparations of culture show nu-

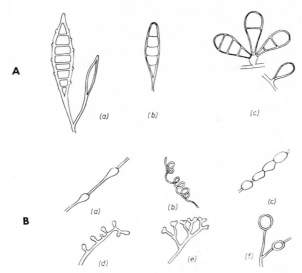

Fig. 12-17. A, Three types of macroconidia found in dermatophytes: **a,** fusiform macroconidia of *Microsporum*, with thick walls, 5-15 cells, and from 40-150μ in length; **b,** cylindric macroconidia of *Trichophyton*, with thin walls, 2-6 cells, and 10-15μ in length; and **c,** pear-shaped macroconidia of *Epidermophyton*, with moderately thick walls, 2-4 cells, 30-40μ in length, and often appearing in clusters. **B,** Other structures found in dermatophytes: **a,** racquet hypha; **b,** spiral hypha; **c,** hyphal swellings; **d,** pectinate hypha; **e,** antlerlike hypha; and **f,** chlamydospores. (From Baker: Handbook of bacteriological technique, London, 1962, Butterworth & Co.)

merous microconidia that are small and slender or somewhat spherical. They develop on lateral, terminal, simple, or branched conidiophores or along hyphae. Macroconidia are rarely seen; they are thin walled, septate (2-5 cells), and spindle or club shaped (*b* part of Fig. 12-17, *A*). In some strains numerous coiled hyphae, nodular bodies, and racquet hyphae are seen.

TRICHOPHYTON RUBRUM

T. rubrum rarely involves hair.

Culture: On Sabouraud dextrose agar the colony usually grows slowly and develops a white aerial mycelium. The margins may be glabrous. Some strains are velvety and change in color from white to cream to red. The reverse sides of most strains are deep red.

Wet preparations may reveal only a few or many microconidia arising from the sides of hyphae on short conidiophores. Macroconidia are rare; they are thin walled, elongated with blunt ends, and contain 3-8 cells.

T. rubrum may be differentiated from *T. mentagrophytes* by the use of 1% dextrose cornmeal agar; *T. rubrum* develops a red reverse side, while *T. mentagrophytes* fails to do so.

TRICHOPHYTON VIOLACEUM

Infected hair reveals an endothrix pattern (Fig. 12-1).

Culture: On Sabouraud dextrose agar the colony grows slowly and is waxy, slightly folded, and deep violet in color. Sometimes white aerial hyphae develop in subcultures. Chlamydospores are present and microconidia are absent in wet preparations.

TRICHOPHYTON TONSURANS

Wet preparations of hair reveal an endothrix growth pattern (Fig. 12-1).

Culture: On Sabouraud dextrose agar the colony develops slowly into a flat structure that later becomes heaped, folded, and even cerebriform with a depressed center. The aerial mycelium is fine and powdery and is yellow to reddish brown,

The reverse side is yellowish to mahogany red.

Wet preparations of the culture show numerous microconidia on short lateral conidiophores. They are elongated and delicate, but later become large and irregular. Macroconidia are rare.

TRICHOPHYTON SCHOENLEINII

Wet preparations of hair reveal an endothrix pattern (Fig. 12-1).

Culture: On Sabouraud dextrose agar the fungus grows slowly, producing folded, heaped, glabrous, waxy, leathery colonies that grow into and split the agar. The surface is white to tan and may be powdery.

Wet preparations of culture show irregular hyphae with clubbed ends (favic chandeliers) and numerous chlamydospores. Microconidia are very rare and macroconidia are absent.

Epidermophyton

Epidermophyton invades the skin and nails, but not hair. It usually has broad filaments with rectangular segments that tend to disintegrate in hydroxide. In culture it is characterized by numerous clavate macroconidia and the absence of microconidia. *Epidermophyton* does not fluoresce.

EPIDERMOPHYTON FLOCCOSUM

Culture: The colony is first powdery and greenish yellow and later becomes white and cottony. No microconidia are formed. **Macroconidia** are clavate and their appearance suggest snowshoes. They are numerous, contain 2-4 cells, and occur in groups of two or three (*c* part of Fig. 12-17, *A*). Chlamydospores are numerous.

Microsporum

Members of *Microsporum* invade hair and skin, but not nails.

LABORATORY DIAGNOSIS

Material: Hairs infected by *M. audouini* and *M. canis* show greenish fluorescence under **Wood's light** (filtered ultraviolet light). Shavings of involved skin should also be examined.

Wet preparation: Examine skin shavings and broken hairs, which reveal a sheath of spores surrounding the hair shaft. The spores are small, 2-3μ in diameter, and form a mosaic pattern. The hyphae grow down the hair but stop short of the bulb (Fig. 12-2).

Culture: Use Sabouraud agar containing cycloheximide and chloramphenicol and incubate at room temperature.

MICROSPORUM AUDOUINII

Culture: On Sabouraud agar the flat, velvety colonies appear slowly and are covered by dense compressed mycelia. Old cultures sometimes show grooves. The reverse side is usually reddish brown.

Microscopic examination usually reveals many chlamydospores. Microconidia and

Table 12-2. Laboratory diagnosis of epidemic ringworm in the United States

	Microsporum audouinii	*Trichophyton tonsurans*
Wood's lamp	Fluorescence; select hair for further study	No fluorescence; epilate hair stubs embedded in scalp
Examination of hair in 10% KOH	Small spores in mosaic on surface of hair (ectothrix)	Chains of large spores inside hair (endothrix)
Culture growth	Slow-growing, flat, velvety colony with pink- to salmon-colored reverse side	Rapid-growing, flat, or convex colony that later shows folded surface; reverse side tan to red color
Microscopic examination	Sterile mycelia and chlamydospores (*M. canis* and *M. gypseum* have characteristic spores)	Microconidia present; macroconidia rare
Special cultures	Does not grow on rice grain medium (*M. canis* and *M. gypseum* grow on rice grain medium)	Stimulated by thiamine (*T. mentagrophytes* and *T. rubrum* not stimulated)

macroconidia are rare. The latter, when present, are large, thick walled, and spindle shaped, with few or no septa. Commonly they are imperfectly formed. Knobby racquet hyphae are seen (*a* part of Fig. 12-17, *B*).

MICROSPORUM CANIS

Culture: On Sabouraud agar the colonies grow rapidly with woolly aerial mycelia and yellow-brown pigmentation in the periphery and in the agar. After 2-4 wk., concentric rings appear and the yellow reverse side becomes brown.

Microscopically, numerous spindle-shaped macroconidia are seen which have 8-15 cells, thick walls, and roughened ends (*a* part of Fig. 12-17, *A*). A few sessile microconidia can be detected.

MICROSPORUM GYPSEUM

Culture: On Sabouraud agar the organism grows rapidly and forms flat, coarse, powdery colonies with irregular borders and a dull orange to light brown pigmentation. The reverse side of the colony is dull yellow to tan.

Microscopically, numerous spindle-shaped, multicelled (3-9), slightly thick-walled macroconidia are seen. They are shorter and broader than those of *M. canis*. Microconidia are rare; when present, they are sessile.

SUPERFICIAL MYCOSES

Superficial mycotic infections involve the outermost layers of the skin and hair.

Malassezia furfur[23]

Malassezia furfur is the cause of **tinea versicolor** and is easily demonstrated in potassium or sodium hydroxide preparations of skin scales. Abundant mycelia and many groups or clusters of spherical or ovoid conidia are present.

Scotch tape may be used in the same way it is used in the diagnosis of oxyuriasis. Apply the tape to the affected skin area, then remove and examine for skin scales containing the fungus. Affected skin areas fluoresce under ultraviolet light, varying in color from yellow to brown.

Culture: The organism is very difficult to culture.

Trichosporon cutaneum

Trichosporon cutaneum produces soft nodules on the shafts of the hairs of the beard.

SAPROPHYTIC FUNGI

These fungi, which are not usually disease producing, are widely disseminated in nature and can be found as molds on decaying food articles. They are also responsible for focal human infections (otomycosis) and for generalized infections, mainly in debilitated patients.

Saprophytic fungi are important because (1) they exceed in number the fungi pathogenic to man, (2) they are common laboratory contaminants and must therefore be identified, and (3) they are **opportunist invaders** that attack individuals whose resistance is lowered by disease or forms of treatment.

Aspergillus fumigatus[24]

Aspergilli are frequently found in cultures and may represent the causative organisms of a disease process or they may be contaminants.

LABORATORY DIAGNOSIS

Material: Sputum, bronchial washings, and scrapings of cornea or external ear canal are used.

Smear and wet preparation: The wide septate hyphae of aspergilli can be seen in KOH preparations.

Culture: Most aspergilli are sensitive to cycloheximide.

The medium of choice is Sabouraud agar incubated at room temperature. The flat colony grows rapidly; it is white at first and then becomes bluish green and powdery.

Microscopically, septate hyphae are seen that give rise to conidiophores which have a stalk and a bulbous end called the **vesicle.** The vesicle is partially hidden by rows of **sterigmata,** which in turn give rise to chains of globose green conidia.

PHYCOMYCOSIS (MUCORMYCOSIS)[25]

Phycomycosis includes infections by *Mucor, Rhizopus, Absidia,* and similar Phycomycetes.

Mucor

The organism grows rapidly on Sabouraud agar, producing an aerial mycelium that is soft and white at first, but later becomes gray to brown.

Microscopically, nonseptate hyphae are seen that lack **rhizoids** (roots) and give rise to tall, single, erect sporangiophores with terminal **sporangia.**

Rhizopus

The organism grows rapidly on Sabouraud agar, producing a rich woolly mycelium that is white at first and later becomes gray with black and brown dots.

Microscopically the hyphae are **nonseptate** and give rise to long sporangiophores capped by spherical **sporangia** that contain spherical spores and a **columella.** The sporangiophores arise from nodes opposite rhizoids (rootlike structures).

Penicillium[26]

The fungus is a frequent contaminant of cultures and of food articles. On agar the colonies are rapidly growing and change from white to bluish green. The aerial mycelium produces numerous spores. Microscopically the spore-bearing hyphae form a characteristic **brush** (penicillus), an appearance produced by unbranched chains of conidia arising from branches of conidiophores.

GLOSSARY OF MYCOLOGIC TERMS

arthrospore Asexual spore formed by disarticulation of mycelium.

ascus Specialized saclike structure characteristic of Ascomycetes in which ascospores are produced.

blastospore Spore produced by a budding process along the mycelium or by a single spore.

budding Asexual reproductive process characteristic of unicellular fungi or spores involving formation of lateral outgrowth from parent cell that is pinched off to form a new cell.

chlamydospore Thick-walled resistant spore formed by direct differentiation of mycelium in which there is a concentration of protoplasm and nutrient material.

clavate Club shaped.

columella Persistent dome-shaped apex of the sporangiophore in some Phycomycetes.

conidiophore Specialized stalklike branch of mycelium on which conidia are developed either singly or in groups.

conidium Asexual spore that may have one or many cells and may be of any size and shape.

ectothrix Outside hair shaft.

endothrix Within hair shaft.

favic chandeliers Specialized hyphae that are curved, freely branching, and antlerlike in appearance. They are found in certain dermatophytes, especially *Trichophyton schoenleinii.*

fungus Chlorophyll-lacking saprophytic or parasitic member of the plant kingdom whose plant body is not differentiated into roots, stems, or leaves. In most species the fundamental structural unit is the mycelium.

fusiform Spindle shaped.

germ tube Tubelike process produced by a germinating spore that develops into the mycelium.

glabrous Smooth.

hyaline Glassy or transparent.

hyphae Filaments that make up the thallus, or body, of a fungus.

intercalary Refers to spores produced between two hyphal segments.

lateral Refers to spores produced on the side of the hypha thread.

macroconidium Large, often multicellular spore.

microoconidium Small single-celled spore.

micron One thousandth of a millimeter. It is represented by the Greek letter μ (pronounced mew), e.g., 10μ.

mycelium Mat of intertwined and branching threadlike hyphae.

nodes Those points on the stolon where the rhizoids are subtended.

perithecium Special round, oval, or beaked structure in which asci are formed.

phaeo Prefix meaning dark.

pleomorphism Degenerative change in a fungus that converts the colony into one that is completely sterile. Characteristic and diagnostic spores required for identification are lost and cannot be restored because pleomorphism is irreversible.

pyriform Pear shaped.

racquet mycelium Vegetative hyphae showing terminal swelling of segments, suggesting a tennis racquet in shape.

rhizoid Branched and rootlike radiating hyphae extending into the substrate.

ringworm Superficial fungus infection. The word was derived from the ancient belief that these infections were caused by wormlike organisms and from the fact that the lesions are often circinate or circular in form.

spirals Specialized tightly coiled branches of mycelia found in many fungi. Their function is unknown.

sporangiophore Specialized mycelial branch bearing a sporangium.

sporangium Closed structure within which asexual spores are produced by cleavage.

sporophore Specialized mycelial branch upon which spores are produced.

sterigmata Short or elongate specialized projections from sporophores on which spores are developed.

stolon A runner. A horizontal hypha that sprouts where it touches the substrate and forms rhizoids in the substrate.

stroma Cushionlike mat of fungus cells.

thallus Term used for the fungus plant.

tinea (ringworm) Term used to designate various types of superficial fungus infections, e.g., tinea capitis, ringworm of the scalp; tinea pedis, ringworm of the foot.

zygospore Thick-walled sexual spore found in Phycomycetes that is produced through fusion of two similar gametangia.

REFERENCES

1. Sanford, L. V., Mason, K. N., and Hathaway, B. M.: Amer. J. Clin. Path. **44**:172, 1965.
2. Ajello, L., Georg, L. K., Kaplan, W., and Kaufman, L.: CDC manual for medical mycology, Atlanta, 1963, U. S. Public Health Service Publication No. 994, Department of Health, Education, and Welfare, Communicable Disease Center.
3. Riddell, R. W.: Mycological techniques, Broadsheet No. 43, J. Clin. Path., 1962.
4. Strauss, R., and Klingman, A.: J. Infect. Dis. **88**:151, 1951.
5. Campbell, C. C.: Ann. N. Y. Acad. Sci. **89**:163, 1960.
6. Hayes, A., and Thompson, J. R.: Amer. J. Clin. Path. **41**:553, 1963.
7. MacKenzie, D. W. R.: J. Clin. Path. **15**:563, 1962.
8. Mowry, R. W., and Winkler, C. H.: Amer. J. Clin. Path. **32**:628, 1956.
9. Mowry, R. W.: Amer. J. Clin. Path. **34**:595, 1958.
10. Meleney, H. E.: Amer. J. Trop. Med. **20**:603, 1940.
11. Henderson, R. G., Pinkerton, H., and Moore, L. T.: J.A.M.A. **118**:885, 1942.
12. Reid, J. D., Scherer, J. H., Herbut, P. A., and Irving, H.: J. Lab. Clin. Med. **27**:419, 1942
13. Key, J. A., and Large, A. M.: J. Bone Joint Surg. **24**:281, 1942.
14. Shamiyeh, B., and Shipe, E. L.: Public Health Lab. **22**:198, 1964.
15. Klite, P. D.: J. Lab. Clin. Med. **66**:770, 1965.
16. Carlisle, H. N., and Saslaw, S.: J. Lab. Clin. Med. **51**:793, 1958.
17. Saslaw, S., and Campbell, C. C.: J. Lab. Clin. Med. **35**:780, 1950.
18. Huppert, M., and Bailey, J. W.: Amer. J. Clin. Path. **44**:369, 1965.
19. Caldwell, G. T., and Roberts, J. D.: J.A.M.A. **110**:1641, 1938.
20. Elles, N. B.: Arch. Ophthal. (Chicago) **25**:969, 1941.
21. Moore, M., Cooper, Z. K., and Weiss, R. S.: J.A.M.A. **122**:1237, 1943.
22. Silva, M.: Ann N. Y. Acad. Sci. **89**:17, 1960.
23. Keddie, F., Shadomy, J., and Barfatani, M.: J. Invest. Derm. **87**:641, 1963.
24. Seabury, J. H., and Samuels, M.: Amer. J. Clin. Path. **40**:21, 1963.
25. Lie Kian Joe and Njo Injo Tjoei Eng: Ann. N. Y. Acad. Sci. **89**:4, 1960.
26. Huang, S., and Harris, L. S.: Amer. J. Clin. Path. **39**:167, 1963.

Chapter 13

Water and milk examinations

STANDARD METHODS OF WATER ANALYSIS[1]

Apparatus:

Sample bottles: Use 4 oz. glass-stoppered bottles with stoppers and necks covered with tinfoil. In practice, when the examination can be made promptly, cork stoppers covered with thick paper or cloth may be used.

Pipettes: They should be accurate to within 2%. Plug the mouth end with cotton. Wrap in paper and sterilize.

Dilution bottles: Dilution tubes should have good stoppers and should hold twice the volume of water actually used.

Fermentation tubes: They should contain at least twice as much medium as the amount of water to be used.

Media: Use formulas given in *Standard Methods.*[1] Formulas for all media are also given in *Manual of Dehydrated Culture Media.*[*]

EXAMINATION

Examine samples promptly, impure water within 6 hr., and pure water within 12 hr. Keep at 6°-10° C. until examined. Record any variations from these limits.

The following routine procedures are most commonly used: (1) official count and (2) test for coli-aerogenes group.

Official count: Make such dilutions as will give from 30-300 colonies per plate. Shake samples and dilutions 25 times and plate at once, placing 1 ml. in the petri dish and adding 10 ml. agar at 40° C. Mix by tilting and rotating dish. Incubate 24 hr. at 37° C. Count with ×2½ lens.

Test for coli-aerogenes group: Plant in

six fermentation tubes (special rack) of lactose broth one 1 ml. and five 10 ml. amounts. If relatively impure, use smaller amounts. Record gas formation at 24 and 48 hr.: 0 = no gas; + or − = less than 10% gas; + = 10% or more. Ten percent gas in a tube at 24 hr. is strong evidence (positive presumptive test) of the presence of the coli-aerogenes group, but plate the tube showing gas formation in the smallest amount of water tested at the end of 48 hr. on eosin–methylene blue (EMB) medium. All of the tubes showing gas may be plated if desired. Mix the lactose broth in the fermentation tube and transfer the small amount which sticks to a 4 mm. wire loop to a test tube containing about 5 ml. sterile water. Mix with the loop and transfer a drop to one half of an EMB plate, spreading with a bent glass rod. Incubate 24 hr. Lactose-fermenting colonies on EMB practically confirm the presumptive test (partially confirmed test). If no typical colonies (*Escherichia coli* or *Aerobacter aerogenes*) appear, incubate another 24 hr. To complete the demonstration of the presence of this group, discard the plates showing no growth (anaerobic organisms) and from the other plates transfer two colonies most likely to be *E. coli* to agar slant and lactose broth fermentation tubes. Incubate 48 hr. and record gas formation at 24 and 48 hr. Make gram stains on those showing gas formation. Nonspore-forming gram-negative bacilli (agar slant) that ferment lactose with gas formation within 48 hr. (lactose broth fermentation tubes) are considered positive for *E. coli* (completed test). This is required when the partially confirmed test is doubtful and

---

[*]Difco Laboratories, Detroit, Mich.

in the case of the smallest gas-forming portion of each sample when fitness for drinking is considered.

For private supplies, three tubes of lactose broth may be sufficient: 0.1 ml., 1 ml., and 10 ml. Specimens are not examined unless collected properly in bottles sterilized at the laboratory. Specimens from open wells are not examined.

Test for free chlorine: Mix 1 ml. toluidine reagent with 100 ml. sample in a 100 ml. Nessler tube with graduation 300 mm. from the bottom. Let stand at least 5 min. until the maximum color has developed and compare with standards in similar tubes. Record in parts per million.

NOTE: Nitrites, ferric compounds, manganic compounds, chlorates, and organic coloring matter interfere. If the test is set in a dark cabinet 10 min., nitrites do not interfere. Do not let the test be exposed to direct sunlight.

Toluidine reagent: Dissolve 1 gm. orthotoluidine, melting point 129° C., in 1 L. of dilute hydrochloric acid (100 ml. concentrated acid diluted to 1 L.).

In preparation of permanent standards, two solutions are required. Mix as outlined in Table 13-1 and dilute to 100 ml. in Nessler tube.

Copper sulfate solution: Dissolve 1.5 gm. copper sulfate and 1 ml. concentrated sulfuric acid in distilled water and make up to 100 ml.

Potassium dichromate solution: Dissolve 0.025 gm. potassium dichromate and 0.1 ml. concentrated sulfuric acid in distilled water and make up to 100 ml.

Standards of potability: Not more than 10% of all 10 ml. portions will show presence of *E. coli* group.

Table 13-1. Preparation of permanent standards for content of chlorine

Chlorine (parts/million)	Copper sulfate solution (ml.)	Potassium dichromate solution (ml.)
0.05	0.4	5.5
0.10	1.8	10.0
0.20	1.9	20.0
0.50	2.0	45.0

Three or more of the five 10 ml. tubes show *E. coli* occasionally; this must not occur in more than (1) 5% of the samples when 20 or more samples have been examined or (2) 1 standard sample when less than 20 samples have been examined.

STANDARD METHODS OF MILK ANALYSIS[2]

Bacteriologic examination: Obtain samples of 10 ml. or more from well-mixed specimens, using sterile sampling pipette. Place into sterile bottles with stoppers and place in cracked ice if examination cannot be made at once.

Plate milk promptly. If more than 4 hr. after collection, state so in the report by giving time of collection and of plating.

Use the new standard beef extract agar.

Plate three dilutions: 1:100, 1:1000, and 1:10,000. If the character of the milk is known, other dilutions may be used, or one of the above dilutions may be omitted, but not less than two plates should be made for each sample of milk. In making dilutions, mix by shaking specimen rapidly 25 times (excursions of about 1 foot) in less than about 7 sec. Pour agar between 40°-45° C. Pour agar not later than 15-20 min. after portions of milk have been placed in the petri dish. Incubate 48 hr. at 37° C. Count and average all plates with 30-300 colonies. If there are none with this number, count the one nearest to 300. Count all colonies on each plate unless the number exceeds 300, in which case a part may be counted and the number estimated, but such counts are not as accurate. Count with a ×2½ lens. Report in round numbers with two significant left-hand digits. Express as colonies per milliliter or standard plate count per milliliter.

Sediment (dirt) test: Strain 1 pint sample of well-mixed milk through a cotton disk placed over a 1 in. opening. Filtering is hastened if milk is warmed. Special filtering apparatus and standard disks are obtainable. Spray disk with 10% formalin, attach to card for filing, and let dry. Compare with standards made by filtering pints of milk containing 1.25, 2.50, 3.75, and 5 mg. dirt/pint. Read as follows: 0 = clean; 1.25 = fairly clean; 2.5 =

slightly dirty; 3.75 = dirty; 5.0 = very dirty.

Determination of pus and long-chain streptococci: Centrifuge well-mixed portion of milk, smear sediment, and let dry. Fix with methyl alcohol 3-5 min. Blot dry. Wash with xylol, drain, and dry. Stain with Loeffler methylene blue. If overstained, decolorize carefully with alcohol. Confirm by culture (pp. 546 and 553).

Fat (Babcock method): Glassware, reagents, and apparatus should be standard. Heat centrifuge or tester to 55°-60° C. during test.

Speeds for centrifuge are as follows:

Diameter (in.): 10 12 14 16 18 20 22 24

Rate (rpm): 1074 980 909 848 800 759 724 693

Warm sample to 15°-20° C. and mix by pouring back and forth in clean vessels. Transfer 18 gm. (17.5 ml. pipette, blowing out last drop) to milk bottle and add 17.5 ml. concentrated sulfuric acid (specific gravity 1.82) at temperature of 15°-20° C. Mix until no curds remain. Centrifuge 5 min. at proper speed. Add hot water, over 60° C., to fill bulb of bottle. Centrifuge 2 min. Add hot water to top of graduated scale. Centrifuge 1 min. Set bottle in water bath (55°-60° C.) with water as high as top of fat column and leave it until the specimen (fat column) is the same as the temperature of the water bath. Remove the bottle and measure fat column with calipers, measuring from the lowest surface to the highest point of the upper meniscus. Reject all tests in which the fat column is not clear.

REFERENCES

1. Standard methods for the examination of water and waste water, ed. 11, New York, 1960, American Public Health Association, Inc.
2. Standard methods for the examination of dairy products, ed. 11, New York, 1960, American Public Health Association, Inc.

Chapter 14

Serology

Two principal kinds of serologic tests for syphilis are in general use today—the nontreponemal antigen tests and the treponemal antigen tests. A number of tests not described in this chapter will serve adequately as an aid in diagnosis; however, those included represent the most widely used of the older procedures and the newer tests of current interest.

Nontreponemal tests listed include the widely performed VDRL slide flocculation tests with serum and the VDRL slide flocculation tests with spinal fluid. These tests are quite practical and may be relied on for the diagnosis of most cases of syphilis.

From the treponemal antigen tests, a Reiter protein test (Kolmer) is included. This test is relatively easy to perform and serves as an important aid in problem cases.

Although the *Treponema pallidum* immobilization test (TPI) is the best known of the treponemal antigen tests, few laboratories have the equipment, time, and funds necessary for performing this test; therefore it is excluded from this section. It is available on special request from state health department laboratories. The fluorescent treponemal antibody test (FTA), which has proved to be at least as sensitive and specific as the TPI test,

Grateful acknowledgement is made to William J. Brown, M.D., Chief, Venereal Disease Branch, Communicable Disease Center, Atlanta, Georgia, United States Department of Health, Education, and Welfare, for permission to use material from the 1964 manual Serologic Tests for Syphilis.

has been included since this test may be performed in most laboratories.

In presenting these procedures for modern syphilis serology, the following general rules are offered for their use. In the presence of either clinical signs and symptoms or reactive spinal fluid findings and in the absence of a recent history of adequate syphilotherapy, a reactive VDRL test performed by an approved laboratory probably will justify treatment.

If serious doubt remains in patients with no history, signs, or symptoms of syphilis, a Reiter antigen test should be performed. If the Reiter test is reactive, treatment is indicated. If the Reiter test is nonreactive and there is still doubt, either the FTA or the TPI test may be utilized.

GENERAL INFORMATION

A test technique is composed of equipment, reagents, volumes, time periods, temperatures, and orders of procedure. Each of these factors may be of equal importance, and none can be disregarded with impunity. Technicians who make arbitrary changes in recommended techniques must assume full responsibility for the test results.

Although serologic tests for syphilis are not absolutely specific and some sera and spinal fluids are reactive in one test and nonreactive in another, analyses of conflicting serologic results in terms of diagnosis or prognosis should not be made by the technician. These decisions lie only within the province of the physician. Valid serologic test findings are, however, obtained when (1) standardized reagents and adequate controls are used, (2) technique recommendations are strictly adhered to, and (3) results are reported as specified for each procedure.

Each technician should test every new lot of reagent in parallel with one that is being used and that has acceptable reactivity before the new lot of reagent is placed in routine use. This procedure is recommended regardless of the source from which the new reagent is obtained. Other factors to be considered in the control of serologic tests are discussed in the following paragraphs.

Reporting serologic test results: In accordance with the recommendations in the 1953 report of the National Advisory Serology Council to the Surgeon General of the United States Public Health Service, the terms "reactive," "weakly reactive," and "nonreactive" have been substituted for the terms "positive," "weakly positive" or "doubtful," and "negative" in reporting test results.

In reporting results of quantitative reactions it is recommended that the end point titer be reported in terms of the greatest dilution in which the tested specimen produces a reactive (positive) result, and that the term "dils," a contraction of the word dilution, be used to identify these dilution reactivity end points. By this means, reactions of identical intensity will receive the same report in terms of dils when different testing methods are employed.

VDRL TESTS[1-4]

VDRL slide flocculation tests with serum:

Equipment:
1. Rotating machine adjustable to 180 rpm, circumscribing a circle ¾ in. diam. on a horizontal place.
2. Ring maker to make paraffin rings approximately 14 mm. diam.
3. Slide holder* for 2 × 3 in. microscope slides.
4. Hypodermic needles of appropriate sizes, with or without points.

Glassware:
1. Slides,* 2 × 3 in., with paraffin rings approximately 14 mm. diam.
2. Bottles,† 30 ml., round, screw capped (Vinylite or tinfoil lined) or glass stoppered, and narrow mouth.
3. Syringe, Luer type, 1 or 2 ml.

NOTE: Some of the 30 ml. glass-stoppered bottles now available are unsatisfactory for preparing a single volume of antigen emulsion for these tests due to an inward bulging of the bottom that causes the 0.4 ml. saline solution to be distributed only at the periphery. A satisfactory emulsion may be obtained if the 0.8 ml. saline solution covers the bottom surface of this type of bottle when double quantities of antigen emulsion are prepared. Round bottles of approximately 35 mm. diam. with flat or concave inner-bottom surfaces are satisfactory for preparing single volumes of antigen emulsion.

The low cost of plastic caps makes it unnecessary to clean them for reuse. The use of an unclean stopper or cap can be the cause of unsatisfactory emulsions.

Reagents:
1. Antigen:
   (a) Antigen for this test is an alcoholic solution containing 0.03% cardiolipin, 0.9% cholesterol, and sufficient purified lecithin to produce standard reactivity. During recent years this amount of lecithin has been 0.21 ± 0.01 %.
   (b) Each lot of antigen must be serologically standardized by proper comparison with an antigen of known reactivity.
   (c) Antigen is dispensed in screw-

---

*Glass slides with ceramic rings may also be used for the VDRL slide test with the following precautions. The rings must be high enough to prevent spillage when slides are rotated at prescribed speeds. Slides must be cleaned after each use so that serum will spread to the inner surface of the ceramic rings. This type of slide should be discarded if or when the ceramic ring begins to flake off since these particles may be mistaken for antigen particle clumps in the test sera, thereby causing a false reactive report.
†Catalog No. LG-1, MW-90525 (plain bottles); No. LG-1, MW-90530 (glass-stoppered bottles), Corning Glass Works, Corning, N. Y.

---

*May be obtained from Scientific Products Co., American Hospital Supply Corp., Evanston, Ill.

capped (Vinylite liners) brown bottles or hermetically sealed glass ampules and is stored at room temperature (73°-85° F.).

(d) The components of this antigen remain in solution at normal temperature so that any precipitate noted will indicate changes due to factors such as evaporation or additive materials contributed by pipettes. Antigen containing precipitate should be discarded.

2. Saline solutions:

(a) Buffered saline solution containing 1% sodium chloride. Formaldehyde (neutral, reagent grade), 0.5 ml. Secondary sodium phosphate (Na_2HPO_4 + $12H_2O$), 0.093 gm. Primary potassium phosphate (KH_2PO_4), 0.17 gm. Sodium chloride (ACS), 10 gm. Distilled water to make 1000 ml. This solution yields potentiometer readings of pH 6.0 ± 0.1 and is stored in screw-capped or glass-stoppered bottles.

(b) Saline solution (0.9%).

Add 900 mg. dry sodium chloride to each 100 ml. distilled water.

Preparation of sera:

1. Heat clear serum obtained from centrifuged clotted blood in a 56° C. water bath for 30 min. before being tested.

2. Examine all sera when removed from the water bath and recentrifuge those found to contain particulate debris.

3. Sera to be tested more than 4 hr. after the original heating period should be reheated at 56° C. for 10 min.

Preparation of slides:

1. Clean 2 × 3 in. glass slides with Bon Ami. Polish with soft cloth after drying. Slides are used once and discarded.

2. Paraffin rings are made by transferring heated paraffin to the slides by means of a hand-operated or an electrically heated ring-making machine. Care should be exercised to produce rings of the prescribed diameter.

NOTE: Glass slides with concavities or glass rings are not recommended for this test.

Preparation of antigen emulsion:

1. Pipette 0.4 ml. buffered saline solution to the bottom of a 30 ml. round, glass-stoppered or screw-capped bottle.

2. Add 0.5 ml. antigen (from the lower half of a 1 ml. pipette graduated to the tip) directly onto the saline solution while continuously but gently rotating the bottle on a flat surface. Temperature of buffered saline solution and antigen should be in the range of 23°-29° C. at time antigen emulsion is prepared.

NOTE: Antigen is added drop by drop, but rapidly, so that approximately 6 sec. are allowed for each 0.5 ml. antigen. Pipette tip should remain in upper third of bottle and rotation should not be vigorous enough to splash saline solution onto pipette. Proper speed of rotation is obtained when the outer edge of the bottle circumscribes a 2 in. diam. circle approximately three times per second.

3. Blow last drop of antigen from pipette without touching pipette to saline solution.

4. Continue rotation of bottle for 10 sec. more.

5. Add 4.1 ml. buffered saline solution from 5 ml. pipette.

6. Place top on bottle and shake from bottom to top and back approximately 30 times in 10 sec.

7. Antigen emulsion is then ready for use and may be used during 1 day.

Double this amount of antigen emulsion may be prepared at one time by using doubled quantities of antigen and saline solution. A 10 ml. pipette should then be used for delivering the 8.2 ml. vol. saline solution. If larger quantities of antigen emulsion are required, more than one mixture should be prepared. These aliquots may then be tested and pooled.

Stabilized antigen emulsion: If desired, VDRL antigen emulsion for use in all of the VDRL tests may be stabilized by the addition of benzoic acid. The use of this stabilized emulsion makes it unnecessary to prepare fresh emulsions each day tests are performed.

Reagents:
1. Benzoic acid (1% alcohol solution). Dissolve 1 gm. reagent grade benzoic acid in 100 ml. absolute ethyl alcohol. Store in a tightly sealed allglass container in the refrigerator at 6°-10° C. May be used as long as the solution remains clear.
2. VDRL antigen emulsion may be prepared in either single (5 ml.) or double (10 ml.) volumes.

Preparation of stabilized antigen emulsion:
1. Immediately after preparation of the emulsion, add 0.05 ml. 1% benzoic acid to each single volume (5 ml.) or 0.1 ml. to each double volume (10 ml.). Shake gently from bottom to stopper for 10 sec. Pipette benzoic acid solution with a 0.1 or 0.2 ml. capacity pipette graduated in hundredths.
2. Test each stabilized aliquot with control sera and pool all those of standard reactivity. Mix by swirling bottle gently.

Storage of stabilized antigen emulsion:
1. Store stock bottle of stabilized emulsion in a tightly stoppered bottle at 6°-10° C.
2. For use, remove the stock bottle from the refrigerator, swirl gently to mix, and remove an aliquot sufficient for one day's testing with a pipette. Return the stock bottle to the refrigerator immediately to avoid warming.
3. Allow the aliquot for each day's testing to stand at room temperature at least 30 min. before use. Check with control sera for standard reactivity each day before testing individual sera.
4. Use a new aliquot from the refrigerator each day.
5. The stock stabilized emulsion stored in the refrigerator may be used as long as it retains a standard level of reactivity as determined by testing control serum or sera.

Testing antigen-emulsion delivery needles:
1. It is of primary importance that the proper amount of antigen emulsion be used, and for this reason the needle used each day should be checked. Practice will allow rapid delivery of antigen emulsion, but care should be exercised to obtain drops of constant size.
2. For use in the slide qualitative test and slide quantitative test A, antigen emulsion is dispensed from a syringe fitted with an 18-gauge needle without a point that will deliver 60 drops antigen emulsion/ml. when syringe and needle are held vertically.
3. For use in slide quantitative test B, antigen emulsion is dispensed from a syringe fitted with a 19-gauge needle without a point which will deliver 75 drops antigen emulsion/ml. when syringe and needle are held vertically.
4. When allowed to stand, antigen emulsion should be gently mixed before use by rotating the bottle.

Preliminary testing of antigen emulsion:
1. Each preparation of antigen emulsion should first be examined by testing sera of known reactivity in the reactive, weakly reactive, and nonreactive zones. This is accomplished by the method described in the discussion of the VDRL slide qualitative test with serum. These tests should present typical results, and the size and number of antigen particles in the nonreactive serum should be optimum.
2. Only those antigen emulsions that have produced the designated reactions in tests performed with control sera (reactive, weakly reactive, and nonreactive) should be used. If antigen particles in the nonreactive serum tests are too large, the fault may be in the manner of preparing antigen emulsion, al-

though other factors are sometimes responsible.

3. An unsatisfactory antigen emulsion should not be used.

VDRL slide qualitative test with serum:

1. Pipette 0.05 ml. heated serum into one ring of a paraffin-ringed glass slide.
2. Add 1 drop (1/60 ml.) antigen emulsion onto serum.
3. Rotate slides for 4 min. (Mechanical rotators that circumscribe a ¾ in. diam. circle should be set at 180 rpm. Rotation by hand should circumscribe a 2 in. diam. circle 120 times/min.)
4. Read tests immediately after rotation.

NOTE: Serum controls of graded reactivity (reactive, weakly reactive, and nonreactive) are always included during a testing period to ensure proper reactivity of antigen emulsion at the time the tests are run.

Reading and reporting slide qualitative test results:

1. Read tests microscopically with low-power objective at 100× magnification. The antigen particles appear as short rod forms at this magnification. Aggregation of these particles into large or small clumps is interpreted as degrees of reactivity (Table 14-1).
2. **Zonal reactions** due to an excess of reactive serum component are recognized by irregular clumping and the loosely bound characteristics of the clumps. The usual reactive finding is characterized by large or small clumps of fairly uniform size. Experience will allow differentiation to be made between this type of reaction and the zonal picture wherein large and/or small clumps may be intermingled with free antigen particles. A zonal reaction is reported as reactive. In some instances this zoning effect may be so pronounced that a weakly reactive result is produced by a very strongly reactive serum. It is therefore recommended that all sera producing weakly reactive results in the qualitative test be retested using the quantitative procedure before a report of the VDRL slide test is submitted. When a reactive result is obtained on some dilution of a serum that produced only a weakly reactive result as undiluted serum, the report is reactive (see explanation of reading and reporting slide quantitative test results in the discussion of VDRL slide quantitative tests with serum).

VDRL slide quantitative test with serum: All sera that produce reactive or weakly reactive results in the qualitative VDRL slide test should be quantitatively retested by one of the two methods referred to as quantitative test A or B. Since both of these procedures in most instances provide for direct measurements of serum and saline solution, either method is efficient in regard to the technician's time and amount of glassware employed. Since quantitative test A uses serum dilutions of 1:2.5, 1:5, 1:10, etc., the alternate quantitative test B has been added for those laboratories that desire the doubling serum-dilution scheme of 1:2, 1:4, 1:8, 1:16, etc.

VDRL slide quantitative test A:

1. Place four 2 × 3 in. glass slides containing twelve 14 mm. paraffin rings in a five-place slide holder.
2. Place a glass slide with two parallel strips of masking or adhesive tape in the center space of the slide holder. Numbers identifying the sera to be tested (four on the two slides above the numbered slide and four on the two lower slides) are written on the adhesive strips.
3. Prepare 1:10 dilution of each serum to be tested quantitatively by adding 0.1 ml. heated serum to 0.9 ml. 0.9%

Table 14-1

Reading	Report
No clumping or very slight roughness	Nonreactive (N)
Small clumps	Weakly reactive (WR)
Medium and large clumps	Reactive (R)

saline solution, using a 0.2 ml. pipette graduated in 0.01 ml.

4. Mix the serum and saline solution thoroughly and then allow the pipette to stand in the test tube.

5. Using this 0.2 ml. pipette, transfer 0.05, 0.02, and 0.01 ml. quantities of the 1:10 dilution of the first serum into the fourth, fifth, and sixth rings, respectively.

6. With the same pipette, transfer 0.05, 0.02, and 0.01 ml. quantities of the first serum, undiluted, into the first, second, and third ringed areas, respectively.

7. Repeat this procedure with each serum and the accompanying 1:10 serum delution until each of the eight sera are pipetted onto the slides.

8. Add 1 drop (0.03 ml.) 0.9% saline solution to the second and fifth rings of each serum by vertical delivery from a 15-gauge hypodermic needle[*] fitted to a glass syringe.

9. Add 1 drop (0.04 ml.) 0.9% saline solution to the third and sixth rings of all eight sera by vertical delivery from the syringe fitted with the 13-gauge needle.[*] The six mixtures of each serum are then equivalent to dilutions of 1:1 (undiluted), 1:2.5, 1:5, 1:10, 1:25, and 1:50.

10. Rotate slides gently by hand for about 15 sec. to mix the serum and saline solution.

11. Add 1 drop (1/60 ml.) antigen emulsion to each ring using a syringe and needle as described in the technique for the slide qualitative serum test.

12. Complete tests by rotation of the slides in the manner prescribed for the VDRL slide qualitative test with serum.

13. Read results microscopically immediately after rotation. The highest serum dilution giving a reactive result (not weakly reactive) is reported as the reactivity end point

of the serum, e.g., reactive—1:25 dilution, or reactive—25 dils.

14. If all serum dilutions tested give reactive results, prepare a 1:100 dilution of that serum by diluting 0.1 ml. of the 1:10 serum dilution with 0.9 ml. 0.9% saline solution.

15. Pipette 0.05, 0.02, and 0.01 ml. amounts of this 1:100 serum dilution onto each ring and add enough saline solution to bring the volumes to 0.05 ml. Serum dilutions of 1:100, 1:250, and 1:500 are thus prepared. Test these dilutions of serum exactly as the lower dilutions are tested.

VDRL slide quantitative test B:

1. Place four 2 × 3 in. glass slides with 12 paraffin rings in a five-place slide holder, with a numbered slide in the center space exactly as described for slide quantitative test A.

2. Prepare a 1:8 dilution of each serum by adding 0.1 ml. heated serum to 0.7 ml. 0.9% saline solution, using a 0.2 ml. pipette graduated in 0.01 ml.

3. Mix the serum and saline solution thoroughly and then allow the pipette to stand in the test tube.

4. Using this pipette, transfer 0.04, 0.02, and 0.01 ml. quantities of the 1:8 serum dilution into the fourth, fifth, and sixth paraffin rings, respectively.

5. With the same pipette, transfer 0.04, 0.02, and 0.01 ml. undiluted serum into the first, second, and third paraffin rings, respectively.

6. Repeat this procedure with each serum and the accompanying 1:8 serum dilution until each of the eight sera are pipetted into their respectively numbered places on the slides.

7. Add 2 drops (0.01 ml. in each drop) 0.9% saline solution to the second and fifth rings of each serum by vertical delivery from a 23-gauge hypodermic needle[*] fitted to a glass syringe.

---

[*]Needles should be checked for proper drop size.

[*]Needles should be checked for proper drop size. Saline solutions may be delivered from a 19-gauge needle (0.02 ml./drop) and a 15-gauge needle (0.03 ml./drop).

8. Add 3 drops 0.9% saline solution (delivered in the same manner) of the same size to the third and sixth rings of each serum.

9. Rotate slides gently by hand for about 15 sec. to mix the serum and saline solution.

10. Add 1 drop (1/75 ml.) antigen emulsion to each ring, using a syringe and needle of appropriate size. CAUTION! Note that the amount of antigen emulsion used in this method has been reduced to 1/75 ml. to correspond with the reduced serum volume of 0.04 ml.

11. Complete tests in the manner described for the VDRL slide qualitative test with serum and read results microscopically immediately after rotation. By this method, the dilutions of each serum are 1:1 (undiluted), 1:2, 1:4, 1:8, 1:16, and 1:32.

12. If all serum dilutions tested produce reactive results, prepare a 1:64 dilution of that serum in saline solution. Add 7 parts saline solution to 1 part of the 1:8 serum dilution and test in three amounts as was done with the 1:8 serum dilutions. Dilutions prepared from the 1:64 dilution will be equivalent to 1:64, 1:128, and 1:256.

Reading and reporting slide quantitative test results:

1. Read tests microscopically at 100× magnification as described for the qualitative procedure.

2. Report results in terms of the greatest serum dilution that produces a reactive (not weakly reactive) result, in accordance with the examples given in Table 14-2.

NOTE: Under conditions of high temperature and low humidity which are sometimes present during the summer months in certain areas, antigen emulsion may be stored in the refrigerator but should be restored to room temperature before use. To avoid surface drying under these conditions, tests should be completed and read as rapidly as possible. Slide covers containing a moistened blotter may be employed.

VDRL tube flocculation tests with serum:

Equipment:

1. Kahn shaking machine (must be operated at 275-285 oscillations/min.).

2. Reading lamp, fluorescent or gooseneck type.

Reagents:

1. Antigen (VDRL slide flocculation test antigen).

Table 14-2

Test A					
Undiluted serum 1:1	Serum dilutions				Report
	1:2.5	1:5	1:10	1:25	
R	WR	N	N	N	Reactive, undiluted only, or 1 dil
R	R	WR	N	N	Reactive, 1:2.5 dilution, or 2.5 dils
R	R	R	WR	N	Reactive, 1:5 dilution, or 5 dils
WR	N	N	N	N	Weakly reactive, undiluted only, or 0 dils
WR	R	R	WR	N	Reactive, 1:5 dilution, or 5 dils

Test B					
Undiluted serum 1:1	Serum dilutions				Report
	1:2	1:4	1:8	1:16	
R	WR	N	N	N	Reactive, undiluted only, or 1 dil
R	R	WR	N	N	Reactive, 1:2 dilution, or 2 dils
R	R	R	WR	N	Reactive, 1:4 dilution, or 4 dils

R = reactive; WR = weakly reactive; N = nonreactive.

2. Saline solutions:
   (a) Buffered saline solution (1%). (Prepare as for the VDRL slide flocculation tests.)
   (b) Unbuffered sodium chloride solution (1%). Add 1 gm. dry sodium chloride (ACS) to each 100 ml. distilled water.

Preparation of sera:

1. Heat clear serum that has been removed from centrifuged whole clotted blood in a 56° C. water bath for 30 min. before being tested.
2. Examine all sera when removed from the water bath and recentrifuge those found to contain particulate debris.
3. Sera to be tested more than 4 hr. after being heated should be reheated at 56° C. for 10 min.

Preparation of antigen emulsion:

1. Prepare antigen emulsion as described for the VDRL slide flocculation tests.
2. Add 4 parts 1% sodium chloride solution to 1 part VDRL slide test emulsion. Mix well and allow to stand 5 min. or more (not more than 2 hr.) before use. This solution will be referred to as diluted antigen emulsion. Resuspend diluted antigen emulsion before use.

VDRL tube qualitative test with serum:

1. Pipette 0.5 ml. heated serum into a 12 × 75 mm. (outside dimensions) test tube.
2. Add 0.5 ml. diluted antigen emulsion to each serum.
3. Shake tubes on Kahn shaker for 5 min.
4. Centrifuge all tubes for 10 min. at force equivalent to 2000 rpm in a No. 1 I.E.C. centrifuge or equivalent to 1700 rpm in a No. 2 I.E.C. centrifuge* with horizontal heads.
5. Return tubes to the Kahn shaking machine and shake for exactly 1 min.

NOTE: Include reactive and nonreactive control sera in each test run.

---

*International Equipment Co., Boston, Mass.

Reading and reporting tube qualitative test results:

1. Read test results **as soon as secondary shaking period is completed** by holding tubes close to the shade of a reading lamp with a black background at approximately eye level. A shaded fluorescent desk lamp or a gooseneck-type lamp with a blue bulb is a satisfactory reading light source.
2. Record results as follows:
   Reactive: Visible aggregates in a clear or slightly turbid medium. All borderline reactions for which the observer has doubt regarding visible clumping should be reported as nonreactive.
   Nonreactive: No visible clumping or aggregation of antigen particles. Appearance is slightly turbid or granular. Definite silken swirl on gentle shaking occurs.

NOTE: Turbid or hemolyzed sera may cause completed tests to be too turbid for macroscopic reading and are therefore unsatisfactory specimens for this test. Zonal reactions due to excess of reactive serum component may appear to be very weak or, in rare instances, nonreactive. Whenever a zonal reaction is suspected, another test should be performed using 0.1 ml. heated serum and 0.4 ml. saline solution in place of the original 0.5 ml. serum. If a reactive finding is obtained with the smaller amount of serum, a reactive report should be issued.

VDRL tube quantitative test with serum:

1. Pipette 0.5 ml. freshly prepared 0.9% saline solution into each of five or more test tubes (12 × 75 mm.), omitting the first tube.
2. Add 0.5 ml. heated serum to the first and second tubes. (The first tube may be omitted if the VDRL tube qualitative test has been performed and if sufficient serum is not available.)
3. Mix and transfer 0.5 ml. from second to third tube.
4. Continue mixing and transferring

0.5 ml. from each tube to the next until the last tube is reached.

5. Mix and discard 0.5 ml. from last tube.

6. Add 0.5 ml. diluted antigen emulsion to each tube and proceed as described under VDRL tube qualitative test with serum.

Reading and reporting tube quantitative test results: The greatest serum dilution producing a definitely reactive result is reported as the reactivity end point, as shown in the examples given in Table 14-3.

VDRL tests with spinal fluid:
Equipment:

1. Kahn shaking machine (must be operated at 275-285 oscillations/min.).

Reagents:

1. Antigen (VDRL slide flocculation test antigen).

2. Saline solutions:
   (a) Buffered saline solution (1%). (Prepare as for the VDRL slide flocculation tests.)
   (b) Sodium chloride solution (10%). Dissolve 10 gm. dry sodium chloride (ACS) in 100 ml. distilled water.

Preparation of spinal fluid:

1. Centrifuge and decant each spinal fluid sample. Spinal fluid samples that are visibly contaminated or contain gross blood are unsatisfactory for testing.

2. Heat spinal fluid at 56° C. for 15 min. Cool to room temperature before testing.

Preparation of sensitized antigen emulsion:

1. Prepare antigen emulsion as described for the VDRL slide flocculation tests (see discussion of preparation of antigen emulsion).

2. Add 1 part of 10% sodium chloride solution to 1 part VDRL slide test emulsion.

3. Mix well and allow to stand at least 5 min. (but not more than 2 hr.) before use.

VDRL qualitative test with spinal fluid:

1. Pipette 1 ml. heated spinal fluid into a 13 × 100 mm. test tube. Include reactive and nonreactive spinal fluid controls in each test run.

2. Add 0.2 ml. sensitized antigen emulsion to each spinal fluid sample. Resuspend sensitized antigen emulsion immediately before use by inverting container several times.

3. Shake racks of tubes on Kahn shaking machine for 15 min.

4. Centrifuge all tubes for 5 min. at force equivalent to 1800 rpm in a No. 1 I.E.C. centrifuge or equivalent to 1600 rpm in a No. 2 I.E.C. centrifuge* with horizontal heads.

5. Return tubes to Kahn shaking machine and shake exactly 2 min.

Reading and reporting qualitative test results:

1. Read test results as soon as possible after the secondary shaking period by holding tubes close to the shade of a desk lamp having a black background.

   NOTE: Each tube may be held motionless or shaken gently during the reading. Excessive agitation should be avoided.

2. Report results as follows:
   Reactive: Definitely visible aggregates suspended in a water-clear or turbid medium. All borderline reactions for which the observer has doubt regarding visible clumping should be reported as nonreactive.
   Nonreactive: No aggregation; com-

Table 14-3

Un-diluted serum 1:1	Serum dilutions				Report
	1:2	1:4	1:8	1:16	
R	N	N	N	N	Reactive, undiluted only, or 1 dil
R	R	R	N	N	Reactive, 1:4 dilution, or 4 dils
R	R	R	R	N	Reactive, 1:8 dilution, or 8 dils

R = reactive; N = nonreactive.

*International Equipment Co., Boston, Mass.

plete dispersion of particles. Appearance is turbid or slightly granular. Definite silken swirl on gentle shaking occurs.

VDRL quantitative test with spinal fluid: Quantitative tests are performed on all spinal fluid samples found to be reactive in the qualitative test.

1. Prepare spinal fluid dilutions as follows:
   (a) Pipette 1 ml. 0.9% sodium chloride solution into each of five or more tubes.
   (b) Add 1 ml. heated spinal fluid to tube 1, mix well, and transfer 1 ml. to tube 2.
   (c) Continue mixing and transferring from one tube to the next until the last tube contains 2 ml. Discard 1 ml. from the last tube. The respective dilution ratios are 1:2, 1:4, 1:8, 1:16, 1:32, etc.
2. Test each spinal fluid dilution as described in the discussion of the VDRL qualitative test with spinal fluid.

Reading and reporting quantitative test results:

1. Read each tube as described in the discussion of VDRL qualitative test with spinal fluid.
2. Report test results in terms of the highest dilution of spinal fluid producing a reactive result. The term "dils," which expresses the same dilution reactivity end point, may be applied. Examples are given in Table 14-4.

KOLMER TEST

Equipment:

1. Racks, test tubes, and galvanized wire for 72 tubes.

Glassware:

1. Test tubes, Pyrex, 15 × 85 mm. outside dimensions.
2. Tubes, centrifuge, graduated, 15 ml. capacity, Pyrex.
3. Tubes, centrifuge, round-bottomed, 50 ml. capacity.

Reagents:

1. Antigen. Cardiolipin antigen for the Kolmer tests is an alcoholic solution

Table 14-4

Spinal fluid dilutions					
1:2	1:4	1:8	1:16	1:32	Report
N	N	N	N	N	Reactive,* undiluted only, or 1 dil
R	R	R	N	N	Reactive, 1:8 dilution, or 8 dils
R	R	R	R	N	Reactive, 1:16 dilution, or 16 dils

*Reactive finding with undiluted spinal fluid in the qualitative test.
R = reactive; N = nonreactive.

containing 0.03% cardiolipin, 0.05% lecithin, and 0.3% cholesterol. Each new lot of this antigen should be tested in parallel with a standard antigen in both qualitative and quantitative tests on reactive, weakly reactive, and nonreactive sera before being placed into routine use.

2. Saline solution:
   (a) Weigh 8.5 gm. dried sodium chloride (ACS) and 0.1 gm. magnesium sulfate or chloride crystals for each liter of saline solution.
   (b) Dissolve salts in distilled water. Freshly prepared saline solution should be used for each test run.
   (c) Place portion of saline solution sufficient for diluting complement to be used for completing the tests into refrigerator, allowing remainder to stand at room temperature (73°-85° F.).
3. Sheep red cells. Freshly collected sheep blood should be refrigerated for 48 hr. before being used.
4. Hemolysin.*
5. Complement serum:
   (a) Cell-free guinea pig serum can be obtained by centrifuging the tubes of blood and decanting serum from the clots when the laboratory practice is to bleed guinea pigs the day before the complement-fixation tests are performed. The serum from

*Available commercially from Baltimore Biological Laboratory, Baltimore, Md.

three or more guinea pigs should be pooled and returned to the refrigerator.

(b) Dehydrated complement serum should be restored to **original serum volume** by dissolving in the proper amount of buffered diluent or distilled water and storing in the refrigerator.

(c) Complement serum stored in the frozen state should be returned to the liquid state by allowing it to stand at room temperature or at 37° C. only long enough to melt. As protein content of these sera will tend to collect at the bottom of the tube during thawing, these tubes of serum should be adequately mixed by inversion and returned to the refrigerator (6°-10° C.).

Preparation of sera:

1. Centrifuge blood specimens and separate serum from the clot by pipetting or decanting.
2. Heat serum at 56° C. for 30 min. Previously heated sera should be reheated for 10 min. at 56° C. on day of testing.
3. Recentrifuge any serum in which visible particles have formed during heating.

NOTE: If complement-fixation reactions of maximum sensitivity are desired in the Kolmer quantitative test, it is necessary to remove the natural anti-sheep hemolysins from sera. This may be accomplished in the following manner:

(a) Pipette 1 ml. each serum into a small (12 × 75 mm.) tube and place in the refrigerator for 15 min. or more.

(b) Add 1 drop washed, packed sheep red cells to each serum and mix well.

(c) Return all tubes to the refrigerator for 15 min.

(d) Centrifuge all tubes, and separate the sera by decanting. Avoid carrying over cell residue from side walls or bottom of tubes.

(e) These sera are then heated at 56° C. for 30 min. Previously heated, absorbed sera should be reheated for 10 min.

Preparation of spinal fluid:

1. Centrifuge and decant all spinal fluid samples to remove cellular and particulate debris. Spinal fluid samples that are visibly contaminated or contain gross blood should not be tested.
2. Heat all spinal fluid samples at 56° C. for 15 min. to destroy thermolabile anticomplementary substances.

Preparation of sheep red cell suspension:

1. Filter an adequate quantity of preserved sheep blood through gauze into a 50 ml. round-bottomed centrifuge tube.
2. Add 2 or 3 vol. saline solution to each tube.
3. Centrifuge tubes at a force sufficient to pack the corpuscles in 5 min. (No. 1 I.E.C.* centrifuge at 2000 rpm or No. 2 I.E.C. centrifuge at 1700 rpm).
4. Remove supernatant fluid by suction through a capillary pipette, taking off upper white cell layer.
5. Fill tube with saline solution and resuspend cells by inverting and gently shaking tube.
6. Recentrifuge tube and repeat the process for a total of three washings. if supernatant fluid is not colorless on third washing, cells are too fragile and should not be used.
7. After supernatant fluid is removed from third washing, cells are poured or washed into a 15 ml. graduated centrifuge tube and centrifuged at previously used speed for 10 min. in order to pack cells firmly and evenly.
8. Read the volume of packed cells in the centrifuge tube and carefully remove supernatant fluid.
9. Prepare a 2% suspension of sheep cells by washing the corpuscles into a flask with 49 vol. saline solution.

*International Equipment Co., Boston, Mass.

Shake flask to ensure even suspension of cells.

EXAMPLE:

2.1 ml. (packed cells) × 49 = 102.9 ml. (saline solution required)

10. Pipette 15 ml. 2% cell suspension into a graduated centrifuge tube and centrifuge at previously used speed for 10 min. A 15 ml. aliquot of a properly prepared cell suspension will produce 0.3 ± 0.01 ml. of packed cells. CAUTION! Use only centrifuge tubes that have been tested for proper calibration in 15 ml. and cell-pack volume zones.

NOTE: When the packed cell volume is beyond the tolerable limits just stated, the cell suspension concentration should be adjusted. The quantity of saline solution which must be removed or added to the cell suspension to accomplish adjustment is determined according to the following formula:

$$\frac{\text{Actual reading of centrifuge tube}}{\text{Correct reading of centrifuge tube}} \times \text{Vol. cell}$$
suspension = Corrected vol. cell suspension

EXAMPLE 1:

Vol. cell suspension, 100 ml.
Centrifuge tube (15 ml.) reading, 0.27 ml.

$$\frac{0.27 \text{ ml.}}{0.3 \text{ ml.}} \times 100 \text{ ml.} = 90 \text{ ml.}$$

Therefore 10 ml. saline solution should be removed from each 100 ml. cell suspension. Saline solution may be removed by centrifuging an aliquot of the cell suspension and pipetting off the desired volume of saline solution for discard.

EXAMPLE 2:

Vol. cell suspension, 100 ml.
Centrifuge tube (15 ml.) reading, 0.33 ml.

$$\frac{0.33 \text{ ml.}}{0.3 \text{ ml.}} \times 100 \text{ ml.} = 110 \text{ ml.}$$

Therefore 10 ml. saline solution should be added to each 100 ml. hang cell suspension. An adjusted cell suspension should be rechecked by centrifuging a 15 ml. portion.

11. Place flask of cell suspension in refrigerator when not in use. Always shake before using to secure an even suspension because the corpuscles settle to the bottom of the flask when allowed to stand.

Preparation of antigen dilution:

1. Place the required amount of saline solution in a flask and add antigen drop by drop while continuously shaking the flask. Rinse the pipette. The amount needed may be calculated from the number of tubes containing antigen in the test and titrations. The test dose constitutes 0.5 ml. antigen dilution indicated on the label of the bottle, which is usually 1:150.
2. The antigen dilution is kept at room temperature in a stoppered flask.
3. The diluted antigen should stand at room temperature for at least 1 hr. before it is used.

Preparation of stock hemolysin dilution:

1. Prepare 1:100 stock hemolysin dilution as follows:

   Saline solution, 94 ml.
   Phenol solution (5% in saline solution), 4 ml.
   Glycerinized hemolysin (50%), 2 ml.

   Phenol solution should be mixed well with the saline solution before glycerinized hemolysin is added. This solution keeps well at refrigerator temperature but should be discarded when found to contain precipitate.
2. Each new lot of stock hemolysin dilution (1:100) should be checked by parallel titration with the previous stock hemolysin dilution before it is placed into routine use.
3. Dilutions of hemolysin of 1:1000 or greater are prepared by further diluting aliquots of the 1:100 dilution.

After these reagents are prepared, the complement and hemolysin titrations may be assembled.

Complement and hemolysin titrations:

1. Perform these two titrations simultaneously in the same rack.

2. Place 10 tubes (numbered 1-10) in one side of the rack for the hemolysin titration and eight tubes (numbered 1-8) in the other side for the complement titration. Add two other tubes to the rack, one for 1:1000 hemolysin solution and one for 1:30 complement dilution.

3. Prepare a 1:1000 dilution of hemolysin by placing 4.5 ml. saline solution in a test tube and adding 0.5 ml. 1:100 stock hemolysin solution by measuring from point to point in a 1 ml. pipette. Allow the solution to run into the tube a little above the level of the saline solution. Discard pipette. Mix thoroughly with a clean pipette, being sure to wash down all hemolysin solution adhering to the wall of the tube.

4. Pipette 0.5 ml. 1:1000 hemolysin solution into the first five tubes of the hemolysin titration.

5. Add the amounts of saline solution to the hemolysin titration tubes as shown in Table 14-5.

6. Proceed as shown in Table 14-6.

7. Prepare a 1:30 dilution of complement by adding 0.2 ml. guinea pig serum to 5.8 ml. saline solution, measuring from point to point in a 1 ml. pipette. Discard pipette. Mix thoroughly with a clean pipette, being sure to wash down all of the serum adhering to the wall of the tube.

8. Pipette 0.3 ml. of 1:30 complement into each of 10 tubes of the hemolysin titration.

9. Add the amounts of 1:30 comple-

Table 14-5*

	Tube No.									
	1	*2*	*3*	*4*	*5*	*6*	*7*	*8*	*9*	*10*
Saline solution (ml.)	None	0.5	1.0	1.5	2.0	0.5	0.5	0.5	0.5	0.5

*From Laboratory procedures for modern syphilis serology, U. S. Public Health Service, 1961.

Table 14-6*

Tube No.	Process	Final hemolysin dilution
1	None	1:1000
2	Mix; discard 0.5 ml.	1:2000
3	Mix; transfer 0.5 ml. to tube 6; discard 0.5 ml.	1:3000
4	Mix; transfer 0.5 ml. to tube 7; discard 1.0 ml.	1:4000
5	Mix; transfer 0.5 ml. to tube 8; discard 1.5 ml.	1:5000
6	Mix; transfer 0.5 ml. to tube 9	1:6000
7	Mix; transfer 0.5 ml. to tube 10	1:8000
8	Mix; discard 0.5 ml.	1:10,000
9	Mix; discard 0.5 ml.	1:12,000
10	Mix; discard 0.5 ml.	1:16,000

*From Laboratory procedures for modern syphilis serology, U. S. Public Health Service, 1961.

Table 14-7*

	Tube No.							
	1	*2*	*3*	*4*	*5*	*6*	*7*	*8*
Complement 1:30 (ml.)	0.2	0.25	0.3	0.35	0.4	0.45	0.5	0

*From Laboratory procedures for modern syphilis serology, U. S. Public Health Service, 1961.

Table 14-8*

	Tube No.							
	1	*2*	*3*	*4*	*5*	*6*	*7*	*8*
Saline solution (ml.)	1.3	1.3	1.2	1.2	1.1	1.1	1.0	2.5

*From Laboratory procedures for modern syphilis serology, U. S. Public Health Service, 1961.

Table 14-9. Complement titration (first stage)

Tube No.	Complement 1:30 (ml.)	Antigen dilution (ml.)	Saline solution (ml.)
1	0.2	0.5	1.3
2	0.25	0.5	1.3
3	0.3	0.5	1.2
4	0.35	0.5	1.2
5	0.4	0.5	1.1
6	0.45	0.5	1.1
7	0.5	0.5	1.0
8	0	0	2.5

Table 14-10. Hemolysin titration (complete)

Tube No.	Hemolysin dilution (0.5 ml.)	Complement 1:30 (ml.)	Saline solution (ml.)	Sheep cell suspension, 2% (ml.)
1	1:1000	0.3	1.7	0.5
2	1:2000	0.3	1.7	0.5
3	1:3000	0.3	1.7	0.5
4	1:4000	0.3	1.7	0.5
5	1:5000	0.3	1.7	0.5
6	1:6000	0.3	1.7	0.5
7	1:8000	0.3	1.7	0.5
8	1:10,000	0.3	1.7	0.5
9	1:12,000	0.3	1.7	0.5
10	1:16,000	0.3	1.7	0.5

ment to the complement titration tubes as shown in Table 14-7.

10. Add 0.5 ml. antigen dilution to each of the first seven tubes of the complement titration.

11. Add 1.7 ml. saline solution to each of the 10 tubes of the hemolysin titration.

12. Add the amounts of saline solution to the complement titration tubes as shown in Table 14-8.

13. Add 0.5 ml. 2% sheep red cell suspension to each tube of the hemolysin titration.

14. Shake each tube of the hemolysin titration to ensure even distribution of cells and place rack containing the two titrations in the 37° C. water bath for 1 hr.

At this point the complement titration and the completed hemolysin titration stand as shown in Tables 14-9 and 14-10.

15. Remove rack from water bath and read hemolysin titration.

The unit of hemolysin is the highest dilution that gives complete hemolysis. The use of dilutions lower than 1:4000 is not recommended.

Table 14-11*

Dilution containing 1 unit/ 0.5 ml.	Dilution containing 2 units/ 0.5 ml.	To prepare 2-unit hemolysin dilution, mix	
		1:100 hemolysin solution (ml.)	Saline solution (ml.)
1:4000	1:2000	0.3	5.7
1:5000	1:2500	0.2	4.8
1:6000	1:3000	0.2	5.8
1:8000	1:4000	0.15	5.85
1:10,000	1:5000	0.1	4.9
1:12,000	1:6000	0.1	5.9
1:16,000	1:8000	0.1	7.9

*From Laboratory procedures for modern syphilis serology, U. S. Public Health Service, 1961.

Hemolysin for the complement titration and test proper is diluted so that 2 units are contained in 0.5 ml.

16. Prepare a quantity of diluted hemolysin (containing 2 units/0.5 ml.) sufficient for the complement titration in accordance with Table 14-11.

Table 14-12. Complement titration (complete)*

Tube No.	Complement 1:30 (ml.)	Antigen dilution (ml.)	Saline solution (ml.)		Hemolysin (ml.)	Sheep cell suspension, 2% (ml.)	
1	0.20	0.5	1.3		0.5	0.5	
2	0.25	0.5	1.3		0.5	0.5	
3	0.30	0.5	1.2	37° C. water bath for 1 hr.	0.5	0.5	37° C. water bath for ½ hr.
4	0.35	0.5	1.2		0.5	0.5	
5	0.40	0.5	1.1		0.5	0.5	
6	0.45	0.5	1.1		0.5	0.5	
7	0.50	0.5	1.0		0.5	0.5	
8	None	None	2.5		None	0.5	

*From Laboratory procedures for modern syphilis serology, U. S. Public Health Service, 1961.

Table 14-13

Exact unit (ml.)	Full unit (ml.)	Two full units (ml.)	Dilution to use	Preparation		
				Complement serum (ml.)		Saline solution (ml.)
0.3	0.35	0.7	1:43	1	+	42
0.35	0.4	0.8	1:37	1	+	36
0.4	0.45	0.9	1:33	1	+	32
0.45	0.50	1.0	1:30	1	+	29

17. Add 0.5 ml. diluted hemolysin (containing 2 units hemolysin) to each of the first seven tubes of the complement titration.
18. Add 0.5 ml. 2% sheep red cell suspension to all eight tubes of the complement titration. The addition of hemolysin and cells to the complement titration should be completed without delay, preferably within 5 min. after rack is removed from the water bath.
19. Shake each tube of the complement titration to ensure even distribution of cells and return to the 37° C. water bath for 30 min. The completed complement titration is shown in Table 14-12.
20. Remove rack from water bath and read complement titration.

The smallest amount of complement giving complete hemolysis is the exact unit. The full unit is 0.05 ml. more than the exact unit.

For the complement-fixation tests, complement is diluted so that 2 full units are contained in 1 ml.

EXAMPLE:

Exact unit, 0.3 ml.
Full unit, 0.35 ml.
Dose (2 full units), 0.7 ml.

Dilution of complement to be employed in the test proper may be calculated by dividing 30 by the dose, i.e.,
$\dfrac{30}{0.7} = 43$ or 1:43 dilution of guinea pig serum.

Table 14-13 gives additional examples.

Occasionally hyperactive complement sera are encountered that yield titrations indicating 2 full units/ml. in dilutions greater than 1:43. These complements should be used at 1:43 dilution to accomplish satisfactory testing.

NOTE: Tubes of the complement or hemolysin titrations showing complete hemolysis may be removed and placed in refrigerator for later use as hemoglobin solutions for the reading standards (p. 672).

Kolmer qualitative tests with serum and spinal fluid:
1. Arrange test tubes in wire racks so that there are two tubes for each

serum and spinal fluid to be tested. Control sera of graded reactivity should be included. Number the first row of tubes to correspond to the serum and spinal fluid being tested. Three additional test tubes are included for reagent controls.

2. Pipette 0.5 ml. saline solution into each tube of the second row.
3. Add the following amounts of saline solution to the three control tubes:

   Antigen control, 0.5 ml.
   Hemolytic system control, 1 ml.
   Corpuscle control, 2.5 ml.

4. Pipette 0.2 ml. each serum to be tested into tubes 1 and 2.
5. Pipette 0.5 ml. each spinal fluid to be tested into tubes 1 and 2.
6. Pipette 0.2 ml. each control serum to be tested into tubes 1 and 2.
7. Add 0.5 ml. antigen dilution to the first tube of each test, either serum, control serum, or spinal fluid, and to the antigen control tube.
8. Allow test racks to stand for 10-30 min. at room temperature.
9. Prepare diluted complement during this interval. The amount needed is equivalent to 1 ml. for each tube of the test plus a slight excess.

   NOTE: The volume of complement serum to be diluted is determined by the amount of diluted complement necessary for the test proper. Dividing the number of ml. of diluted complement needed by the titration dilution factor (2 full units) will give the ml. of complement serum needed. Calculations may be made in accordance with Table 14-14.

10. Add 1 ml. of diluted complement (containing 2 full units) to all tubes of the serum, control serum, and spinal fluid tests, including the antigen control tube and the hemolytic system control tube.
11. Mix the contents of the tubes by shaking the racks well and place in the refrigerator at 6°-10° C. for 15-18 hr.
12. Prepare the volume of diluted hemolysin needed for the test proper,

Table 14-14*

Complement titration (2 full units)	Diluted complement needed (ml.)	Complement serum required (ml.)	Cold saline solution required (ml.)
1:43	43	1	42
1:43	215	5	210
1:37	37	1	36
1:30	210	7	203

*From Laboratory procedures for modern syphilis serology, U. S. Public Health Service, 1961.

Table 14-15

Hemolysin titer (2 units in 0.5 ml.)	Diluted hemolysin needed (ml.)	1:100 hemolysin required (ml.)	Saline solution required (ml.)
1:3000	30	1	29
1:4000	120	3	117
1:2500	25	1	24
1:2500	250	10	240

allowing 0.5 ml. (containing 2 units) for each tube. Prepare a slight excess. The following formula may be used for calculating the amounts of 1:100 hemolysin solution and diluent required to prepare the needed volume of diluted hemolysin.

$$\frac{100}{\text{Hemolysin titration dil factor (2 units)}} \times \text{Vol.}$$

diluted hemolysin needed (ml.) = Ml. 1:100 hemolysin required

Additional examples are given in Table 14-15.

13. Remove racks of tubes from the refrigerator at regular intervals and place immediately in the 37° C. water bath for 10 min. The interval will be determined by the length of time necessary to add hemolysin and sheep cell suspension to each rack.
14. Remove each rack from the water bath and add 0.5 ml. diluted hemolysin to all tubes of the test except the corpuscle control tube.
15. Add 0.5 ml. 2% sheep red cell suspension (prepared the previous day)

to all tubes. The 2% cell suspension should be agitated occasionally to ensure even suspension of cells during the period when this reagent is being added to the complement-fixation tests.

16. Mix the contents of the tubes thoroughly by shaking each rack before returning it to the 37° C. water bath for the secondary incubation. Examine the controls at 5 min. intervals. The period of secondary incubation will be determined by the length of time necessary to reproduce the predetermined reactivity pattern of the control serums. In all instances, however, the reading time should be at least 10 min. more than is required to hemolyze the antigen and hemolytic system controls but should not exceed a total of 60 min. incubation. When control sera are not available, the secondary incubation period will be terminated 10 min. after the hemolytic system control and the antigen control hemolyze. In no instance should this period extend beyond 1 hr.

17. Remove each rack of tubes from the water bath at the end of the secondary incubation period. Record observed hemolysis as described in the discussions of preparation of

reading standards (p. 673) and of reading and reporting test results (p. 673) except in those instances in which inhibition of hemolysis is noted in the control tube.

All sera and spinal fluids showing inhibition of hemolysis in the control tube should be returned to the 37° C. water bath for a period sufficient to complete 1 hr. of secondary incubation. At the end of this period these tests are removed from the water bath, and tube readings (including control tubes) are recorded.

Kolmer quantitative tests with serum and spinal fluid:

1. Place test tubes in wire racks, allowing eight tubes for each serum and six tubes for each spinal fluid to be tested. Include reagent controls and control sera of graded reactivity.

2. For each serum, pipette 0.9 ml. saline solution into tube 1 and 0.5 ml. saline solution into tubes 2, 3, 4, 5, 6, 7, and 8.

3. For each spinal fluid, pipette 0.5 ml. saline solution into tubes 2, 3, 4, 5, and 6.

4. Pipette the indicated amount of saline solution into each of the following reagent control tubes:
   Antigen control, 0.5 ml. saline sol.
   Hemolytic control, 1 ml. saline sol.
   Corpuscle control, 2.5 ml. saline sol.

Table 14-16. Outline of Kolmer qualitative test with serum and spinal fluid*

Tube No.	Serum (ml.)	Saline solution (ml.)	Antigen (ml.)	Shake rack well; allow to stand at room temperature for 10-30 min.	Complement, 2 full units (ml.)	Shake rack well; primary incubation 15-18 hr. at 6°-10° C. followed by 10 min. in 37° C. water bath	Hemolysin, 2 units (ml.)	Sheep cell suspension, 2% (ml.)	Shake rack well; secondary incubation in 37° C. water bath
1	0.2	None	0.5		1		0.5	0.5	
2	0.2	0.5	None		1		0.5	0.5	
Tube No.	Spinal fluid (ml.)								
1	0.5	None	0.5		1		0.5	0.5	
2	0.5	0.5	None		1		0.5	0.5	
Controls									
Antigen		0.5	0.5		1		0.5	0.5	
Hemolytic system		1.0	None		1		0.5	0.5	
Corpuscle		2.5	None		None		None	0.5	

*From Laboratory procedures for modern syphilis serology, U. S. Public Health Service, 1961.

Table 14-17*

Tube No.	Process	Serum dilution
1	Add 0.6 ml. of inactivated serum; mix and transfer 0.5 ml. to tube 8 (control) and to tube 2	Undiluted
2	Mix; transfer 0.5 ml. to tube 3	1:2
3	Mix; transfer 0.5 ml. to tube 4	1:4
4	Mix; transfer 0.5 ml. to tube 5	1:8
5	Mix; transfer 0.5 ml. to tube 6	1:16
6	Mix; transfer 0.5 ml. to tube 7	1:32
7	Mix: discard 0.5 ml.	1:64
8		Undiluted (control)

*From Laboratory procedures for modern syphilis serology, U. S. Public Health Service, 1961.

5. For each serum proceed as shown in Table 14-17.
6. For each spinal fluid proceed as shown in Table 14-18.
7. Add 0.5 ml. diluted antigen to the first seven tubes of each serum test, to the first five tubes of each spinal fluid test, and to the antigen control tube. Shake the racks to mix thoroughly.
8. Allow racks to stand at room temperature for 10-30 min.
9. Complete the tests as indicated in steps 9-17 of the technique for the performance of the Kolmer qualitative tests with serum and spinal fluid (pp. 670 and 671).

Preparation of reading standards:
1. Heat tubes of hemoglobin solution (saved from the titration or obtained from control tubes of current day's

Table 14-19. Outline of Kolmer quantitative tests with serum and spinal fluid*

		Antigen (ml.)		Complement, 2 full units (ml.)		Hemolysin, 2 units (ml.)	Sheep cell suspension, 2% (ml.)	
Tube No.	Serum (in 0.5 ml.)							
1	0.2 (undiluted)	0.5		1		0.5	0.5	
2	0.1 (1:2)	0.5		1		0.5	0.5	
3	0.05 (1:4)	0.5		1		0.5	0.5	
4	0.025 (1:8)	0.5		1		0.5	0.5	
5	0.012 (1:16)	0.5		1		0.5	0.5	
6	0.006 (1:32)	0.5		1		0.5	0.5	
7	0.003 (1:64)	0.5		1		0.5	0.5	
8	0.2 (undiluted, control)	None		1		0.5	0.5	
Tube No.	Spinal fluid (in 0.5 ml.)							
1	0.5 (undiluted)	0.5		1		0.5	0.5	
2	0.25 (1:2)	0.5		1		0.5	0.5	
3	0.125 (1:4)	0.5		1		0.5	0.5	
4	0.062 (1:8)	0.5		1		0.5	0.5	
5	0.031 (1:16)	0.5		1		0.5	0.5	
6	0.5 (undiluted, control)	None		1		0.5	0.5	
Reagent controls								
Antigen, 0.5 ml. saline solution		0.5		1		0.5	0.5	
Hemolytic system, 1.0 ml. saline solution		None		1		0.5	0.5	
Corpuscle, 2.5 ml. saline solution		None		None		None	0.5	

Column annotations: Shake rack well; allow to stand at room temperature 10-30 min. | Primary incubation 15-18 hr. at 6°-10° C. followed by 10 min. in 37° C. water bath | Shake rack well; secondary incubation in 37° C. water bath

*From Laboratory procedures for modern syphilis serology, U. S. Public Health Service, 1961.

tests) in the 56° C. water bath for 5 min.

2. Prepare a 1:6 dilution of 2% corpuscle suspension by adding 5 ml. saline solution to 1 ml. 2% suspension.

3. Prepare reading standards by mixing hemoglobin solution and cell suspension in the proportions given in Table 14-20.

4. Reading standards are prepared with one-half volumes of cell suspension and hemoglobin solution when performing the one-half volume tests.

Reading and reporting test results:

1. All serum and spinal fluid controls should show complete hemolysis.

2. Estimate the individual tube readings by comparison with the reading standards at the end of the secondary incubation period, and record degree of complement fixation noted, except for those specimens showing inhibition of hemolysis in the control tube.

3. Read the tubes that have been returned to the 37° C. water bath for a full hour's secondary incubation, estimating and recording the degree of complement fixation of each tube and control tube by comparison with the reading standards.

4. Report the results of the qualitative tests in accordance with Table 14-21.

5. Quantitative tests are reported in terms of the highest dilution giving a reactive result (1+, 2+, 3+, or 4+), as illustrated in Table 14-22.

NOTE: If a reactive result is obtained with the highest dilution of the regular quantitative test (1:64), higher dilutions may be prepared and tested.

Table 14-18

Tube No.	Process	Spinal fluid dilution
1	Add 0.5 ml. spinal fluid	Undiluted
2	Add 0.5 ml. spinal fluid; mix; transfer 0.5 ml. to tube 3	1:2
3	Mix; transfer 0.5 ml. to tube 4	1:4
4	Mix; transfer 0.5 ml. to tube 5	1:8
5	Mix; discard 0.5 ml.	1:16
6	Add 0.5 ml. spinal fluid	Undiluted (control)

Table 14-20

1:6 corpuscle suspension (ml.)	Hemoglobin solution (ml.)	Equivalent complement fixation	
		%	Record
3.0	0.0	100	4+
1.5	1.5	50	3+
0.75	2.25	25	2+
0.3	2.7	10	1+
0.15	2.85	5	±
—	3.0	0	–

Table 14-21. Kolmer qualitative test reporting*

Test tube reading	Control tube reading	Report	Test tube reading	Control tube reading	Report
4+	–	Reactive	3+	3+	Anticomplementary
3+	–	Reactive	3+	2+	Anticomplementary
2+	–	Reactive	3+	1+	Weakly reactive
1+	–	Reactive	3+	±	Reactive
±	–	Weakly reactive	2+	2+	Nonreactive
–	–	Nonreactive	2+	1+	Nonreactive
4+	4+	Anticomplementary	2+	±	Weakly reactive
4+	3+	Anticomplementary	1+	1+	Nonreactive
4+	2+	Weakly reactive	±	±	Nonreactive
4+	1+	Reactive			

*From Laboratory procedures for modern syphilis serology, U. S. Public Health Service, 1961.

Table 14-22*

Sera or spinal fluids							
	Dilutions						
Un-diluted	1:2	1:4	1:8	1:16	1:32	1:64	Report
4	3	1	–	–	–	–	Reactive, 1:4 dilution, or 4 dils
4	–	–	–	–	–	–	Reactive (4+), undiluted, or 1 dil
4	4	3	2	–	–	–	Reactive, 1:8 dilution, or 8 dils
4	4	4	4	4	1	–	Reactive, 1:32 dilution, or 32 dils
3	1	–	–	–	–	–	Reactive, 1:2 dilution, or 2 dils
1	–	–	–	–	–	–	Reactive (1+), undiluted, or 1 dil
2	1	±	–	–	–	–	Reactive, 1:2 dilution, or 2 dils
±	–	–	–	–	–	–	Weakly reactive
–	–	–	–	–	–	–	Nonreactive
4	4	4	4	4	4	4	See Note below

*From Laboratory procedures for modern syphilis serology, U. S. Public Health Service, 1961.

6. Report the results of the quantitative tests in accordance with Table 14-23 when the full hour's incubation at 37° C. is required.

Retesting anticomplementary sera* (modified Sachs method):

1. Heat 0.5 ml. serum in the 56° C. water bath for 15 min. If the serum has been previously inactivated, reheat for 5 min.
2. Add 4.1 ml. accurately titrated N/300 hydrochloric acid to the serum and invert several times. Allow to stand for 30 min. at room temperature.
3. Centrifuge for 10 min., save supernatant fluid, and discard sediment.
4. Add 0.4 ml. 10% sodium chloride solution to the supernatant fluid. Neutralization is not necessary.
5. Arrange two rows of five test tubes each and number 1-5. The second row contains the serum controls.
6. Pipette 0.5 ml. saline solution into tubes 3, 4, and 5 of both rows.
7. To both rows:
   (a) Add 1 ml. treated serum to tube 1.
   (b) Add 0.5 ml. treated serum to tubes 2 and 3.
   (c) Mix tube 3 and transfer 0.5 ml. to tube 4.
   (d) Mix tube 4 and transfer 0.5 ml. to tube 5.
   (e) Mix tube 5 and discard 0.5 ml. The five tubes of each row contain 0.1, 0.05, 0.025, 0.012, and 0.006 ml. of serum, respectively.
8. Add 0.5 ml. antigen dilution to each tube of the first row.

*Anticomplementary sera may also be retested by preparing serial twofold dilutions in saline solution, beginning with 1:2 and ending with 1:64. Each dilution of serum in 0.5 ml. amounts is tested in two tubes as test and control. Interpret test results in the same manner as described in the discussion of retesting anticomplementary spinal fluids (p. 675).

Table 14-23. Quantitative test reporting (after 1 hr. secondary incubation at 37° C.)*

Test tube reading	Control tube reading	Report†
4 4 4 4 4 2 –	4+	Anticomplementary
4 4 3 – – – –	2+	Reactive
4 4 1 – – – –	1+	Reactive
4 4 1 – – – –	±	Reactive
3 2 – – – – –	±	Reactive
4 4 1 – – – –	3+	Weakly reactive
3 2 – – – – –	1+	Weakly reactive
2 1 – – – – –	±	Weakly reactive
3 – – – – – –	±	Reactive
1 – – – – – –	±	Nonreactive
1 – – – – – –	1+	Nonreactive
2 – – – – – –	1+	Nonreactive
2 – – – – – –	2+	Nonreactive

*From Laboratory procedures for modern syphilis serology, U. S. Public Health Service, 1961.
†Quantitative designations of dilution end point or dils are omitted.

9. Add 0.5 ml. saline solution to each tube of the second row.
10. Shake rack of tubes to mix and allow to stand at room temperature for 10-30 min.
11. Add 1 ml. diluted complement to all tubes of both rows.
12. Shake rack to mix and place in refrigerator for 15-18 hr. at 6°-10° C.
13. Complete the test as described in the discussion of Kolmer qualitative tests with serum and spinal fluid (p. 669).
14. Record degree of hemolysis in both the test and control tubes.
15. All tubes of the second row may show complete hemolysis. However, the first and second tubes of the second row may show slight inhibition of hemolysis.

With nonreactive sera, the corresponding front tubes show the same degree of inhibition of hemolysis, and if the degree is slight, a nonreactive report may be rendered. With reactive sera, inhibition of hemolysis is much more marked in tubes of the front row. Report the results as reactive, weakly reactive, or nonreactive.

Retesting anticomplementary spinal fluids:
1. Heat the spinal fluid for 15 min. at 56° C.
2. Arrange two rows of five test tubes each and number 1-5.
3. Pipette 0.5 ml. saline solution into tubes 2, 3, 4, and 5 of both rows.
4. To both rows:
   (a) Add 0.5 ml. spinal fluid to tubes 1 and 2.
   (b) Mix tube 2 and transfer 0.5 ml. to tube 3.
   (c) Mix tube 3 and transfer 0.5 ml. to tube 4.
   (d) Mix tube 4 and transfer 0.5 ml. to tube 5.
   (e) Mix tube 5 and discard 0.5 ml.
5. Add 0.5 ml. antigen dilution to each tube of the first row.
6. Add 0.5 ml. saline solution to each tube of the second row.
7. Shake rack of tubes to mix and allow to stand at room temperature for 10-30 min.

8. Add 1 ml. diluted complement to all tubes of both rows, shake rack to mix, place in the refrigerator for 15-18 hr. at 6°-10° C., and complete test as described in the discussion of Kolmer qualitative tests with serum and spinal fluid (p. 669).
9. Interpret the results according to the following examples:

First row: 4 4 4 1 – ⎫
Second row: 4 1 – – – ⎬ Reactive

First row: 4 3 2 – – ⎫
Second row: 4 1 – – – ⎬ Reactive

First row: 4 1 – – – ⎫
Second row: 1 – – – – ⎬ Reactive

First row: 4 4 2 – – ⎫
Second row: 4 2 1 – – ⎬ Nonreactive

First row: 3 2 – – – ⎫
Second row: 3 1 – – – ⎬ Nonreactive

REITER PROTEIN ANTIGEN TEST[7-10] (ONE-FIFTH VOLUME KOLMER TEST)

Equipment:
1. Racks, test tubes, and galvanized wire for 72 tubes.

Glassware:
1. Test tubes, Pyrex, 12 × 75 mm. outside dimensions.
2. Tubes, centrifuge, graduated, 15 ml. capacity, Pyrex.
3. Tubes, centrifuge, round-bottomed 50 ml. capacity.
4. Pipette, 0.2, 0.25, or 0.5 ml. capacity.

Reagents:
1. Reiter protein antigen. This antigen is prepared from a culture of Reiter treponemes by cryolysis and ammonium sulfate precipitation. New lots of antigen should be tested in parallel with a standard antigen in both qualitative and quantitative tests on reactive, weakly reactive, and nonreactive sera before being placed into routine use.
2. Saline solution, sheep red cells, hemolysin, and complement serum are the same as for the Kolmer qualitative test.

Preparation of sera: Same as for the Kolmer test (p. 665).

Preparation of spinal fluid: Same as for the Kolmer test (p. 665).

Table 14-24

	Tube No.								
	2	3	4	5	6	7	8	9	10
Saline solution (ml.)	0.5	1.0	1.5	2.0	0.5	0.5	0.5	0.5	0.5

Table 14-25*

Tube No.	Process	Final hemolysin dilution
1	None	1:1000
2	Mix	1:2000
3	Mix; transfer 0.5 ml. to tube 6	1:3000
4	Mix; transfer 0.5 ml. to tube 7	1:4000
5	Mix; transfer 0.5 ml. to tube 8	1:5000
6	Mix; transfer 0.5 ml. to tube 9	1:6000
7	Mix; transfer 0.5 ml. to tube 10	1:8000
8	Mix	1:10,000
9	Mix	1:12,000
10	Mix	1:16,000

*From Laboratory procedures for modern syphilis serology, U. S. Public Health Service, 1961.

Preparation of sheep red cell suspension: Same as for the Kolmer test (p. 665).

Preparation of antigen dilution: Reiter protein antigen dilution is to be prepared just prior to its use in the test.

1. Place the required amount of saline solution in a flask or tube.
2. Draw up 0.05 ml. or more of Reiter protein antigen in the bottom half of a 0.1 ml. pipette, graduated to the tip, and add to the saline solution. (The test dose is 0.1 ml. antigen dilution, indicated on the bottle label, as determined by titration. The amount needed may be calculated from the number of tubes containing antigen in the test.)
3. Mix well by filling and emptying the pipette a few times in the diluted antigen solution.

Preparation of stock hemolysin dilution: Same as for the Kolmer qualitative test (p. 666).

Hemolysin and complement titrations:
1. Place 10 tubes (numbered 1-10) in a rack.
2. Prepare a 1:1000 dilution of hemolysin in tube 1 by adding 0.5 ml. 1:100 stock hemolysin to 4.5 ml. saline solution, measuring from point to point in a 1 ml. pipette. Discard pipette and with a clean one mix thoroughly, being sure to wash down all hemolysin solution adhering to the wall of the tube.
3. Pipette 0.5 ml. 1:1000 hemolysin solution into tubes 2-5.
4. Add the amounts of saline solution to tubes 2-10 as shown in Table 14-24.
5. Proceed as shown in Table 14-25.
6. Perform the hemolysin and complement titrations simultaneously in the same rack.
7. Use 12 × 75 mm. tubes. Place 10 tubes (numbered 1-10) in one side of the rack for the hemolysin titration and six tubes (numbered 1-6) in the other side for the complement titration.
8. Pipette 0.1 ml. of each of the hemolysin dilutions (1:1000-1:16,000) into each of the corresponding 10 tubes of the hemolysin titration.
9. Prepare a 1:50 dilution of complement by adding 0.1 ml. guinea pig serum to 4.9 ml. saline solution, measuring from point to point in a 0.2 ml. pipette. Discard pipette. Mix thoroughly with a clean 1 ml. pipette, being sure to wash down all serum adhering to the wall of the tube.
10. Pipette 0.1 ml. of 1:50 complement into each of the 10 tubes of the hemolysin titration.
11. Add the amounts of 1:50 complement and saline solution to the complement titration tubes as shown in Table 14-26.
12. Complete the hemolysin titration by the addition of 2% sheep cell suspension and saline solution in the

Table 14-26*

	Tube No.					
	1	*2*	*3*	*4*	*5*	*6*
Complement 1:50 (ml.)†	0.25	0.20	0.15	0.12	0.10	0
Saline solution (ml.)	0.25	0.30	0.35	0.38	0.40	0.60

*From Laboratory procedures for modern syphilis serology, U. S. Public Health Service, 1961.
†The complement dilution should be delivered to the bottom of the tubes. The quantity of 1:50 complement in the first two tubes may be measured with a 0.5 or 0.25 ml. pipette and in the last three tubes with a 0.2 ml. pipette.

Table 14-27*

Tube No.	Hemolysin (0.1 ml.)	Complement 1:50 (ml.)	Sheep red cell suspension, 2% (ml.)	Saline solution (ml.)
1	1:1000	0.1	0.1	0.4
2	1:2000	0.1	0.1	0.4
3	1:3000	0.1	0.1	0.4
4	1:4000	0.1	0.1	0.4
5	1:5000	0.1	0.1	0.4
6	1:6000	0.1	0.1	0.4
7	1:8000	0.1	0.1	0.4
8	1:10,000	0.1	0.1	0.4
9	1:12,000	0.1	0.1	0.4
10	1:16,000	0.1	0.1	0.4

*From Laboratory procedures for modern syphilis serology, U. S. Public Health Service, 1961.

Table 14-28*

Dilution containing 1 unit/ 0.1 ml.	Dilution containing 2 units/ 0.1 ml.	To prepare 2-unit hemolysin dilution, mix	
		1:100 hemolysin solution (ml.)	Saline solution (ml.)
1:4000	1:2000	0.1	1.9
1:5000	1:2500	0.1	2.4
1:6000	1:3000	0.1	2.9
1:8000	1:4000	0.1	3.9
1:10,000	1:5000	0.1	4.9
1:12,000	1:6000	0.1	5.9
1:16,000	1:8000	0.1	7.9

*From Laboratory procedures for modern syphilis serology, U. S. Public Health Service, 1961.

Table 14-29*

Exact unit (ml.)	Two exact units (ml.)	Test dose
0.25	0.5	0.2 ml. of 1:20 dilution
0.2	0.4	0.2 ml. of 1:25 dilution
0.15	0.3	0.2 ml. of 1:33 dilution
0.12	0.24	0.2 ml. of 1:42 dilution
0.10	0.2	0.2 ml. of 1:50 dilution

*From Laboratory procedures for modern syphilis serology, U. S. Public Health Service, 1961.

amounts and in the order indicated in Table 14-27.

13. Shake each tube of the hemolysin titration to ensure even distribution of cells and place rack containing the two titrations in the 37° C. water bath for 1 hr.

14. Remove rack from the water bath and read hemolysin titration. The unit of hemolysin is the highest dilution that gives complete hemolysis.

15. Prepare a quantity of diluted hemolysin, containing 2 units/0.1 ml., sufficient for the complement titration, as shown in Table 14-28.

16. Add 0.1 ml. diluted hemolysin (containing 2 units hemolysin) to each of the first five tubes of the complement titration.

17. Add 0.1 ml. 2% sheep red cell suspension to each tube of the complement titration.

18. Shake each tube of the complement titration to ensure even distribution of the cells and return the rack to the 37° C. water bath for ½ hr.

The smallest amount of 1:50 complement giving complete hemolysis is the exact unit. For use in the test, complement is diluted so that 2 exact units are contained in 0.2 ml.

EXAMPLE:

Exact unit, 0.15 ml.
Two exact units (dose), 0.30 ml.
Complement dilution used in titration, 1:50 ml.

Dilution of complement to be employed in the test proper may be calculated by dividing 50 by the dose and multiplying by the volume in which the dilution is to be contained, i.e.: $\dfrac{50}{0.3} \times 0.2 = 33$ or a 1:33 dilution of guinea pig serum.

Other examples are given in Table 14-29.

Qualitative tests with serum and spinal fluid:

1. Arrange 12 × 75 mm. test tubes in wire racks so that there are two tubes for each serum or spinal fluid to be tested. Control sera of predetermined reactivity must be included. Number the first row of tubes to correspond to the serum or spinal fluid being tested. Three additional test tubes are included for reagent controls (antigen, hemolytic system, and corpuscle).
2. Prepare a 1:5 dilution of each serum by adding 0.2 ml. serum to 0.8 ml. Kolmer saline solution. Mix well. Spinal fluid is tested undiluted.
3. Complete the tests as outlined in Table 14-30.
4. Mix contents of tubes thoroughly and return to 37° C. water bath. The period of secondary incubation will be determined by the length of time necessary to reproduce the predetermined reactivity pattern of the control serum. In all instances the reading time should be at least 10 min. more than the time necessary to hemolyze the antigen and hemolytic system controls and should

not exceed a total of 60 min. incubation.

5. Remove each rack of tubes from the water bath at the end of the secondary incubation period. Record observed hemolysis as described in the discussion of preparation of reading standards and of reading and reporting test results, except in those instances in which inhibition of hemolysis is noted in the control tube.

All serums and spinal fluids showing inhibition of hemolysis in the control tube should be returned to the 37° C. water bath. Read control tubes at 5 min. intervals and record test results when complete hemolysis is observed in the control tube (not longer than 1 hr. secondary incubation). Record test results in accordance with Table 14-32.

Quantitative tests with serum and spinal fluid:

1. Place 12 × 75 mm. test tubes in racks, allowing eight tubes for each serum and six tubes for each spinal fluid to be tested. Reagent control tubes are the same as for the qualitative tests.
2. For each serum, pipette 0.2 ml. saline solution into tubes 2-7 and 0.1 ml. into tube 8.

Table 14-30. Performance of one-fifth volume Kolmer test*

Tube No.	Serum (1:5) ml.	Saline solution (ml.)	Antigen (ml.)	Shake rack well; allow to stand at room temperature for 10-15 min.	Complement, 2 exact units (ml.)	Incubate 15-18 hr. at 6°-10° C. followed by 10 min. in 37° C. water bath	Hemolysin, 2 units (ml.)	Sheep cell suspension, 2% (ml.)
1	0.2	None	0.1		0.2		0.1	0.1
2	0.2	0.1	None		0.2		0.1	0.1
Tube No.	Spinal fluid (ml.)							
1	0.1	0.1	0.1		0.2		0.1	0.1
2	0.1	0.2	None		0.2		0.1	0.1
Controls								
Antigen		0.2	0.1		0.2		0.1	0.1
Hemolytic system		0.3	None		0.2		0.1	0.1
Corpuscle		0.6	None		None		None	0.1

*From Laboratory procedures for modern syphilis serology, U. S. Public Health Service, 1961.

3. Pipette 0.2 ml. serum (diluted 1:5) into tubes 1, 2, and 8.
4. Mix the contents of tube 2, transfer 0.2 ml. to tube 3, and so on to tube 7. Mix contents of tube 7 and discard 0.2 ml.
5. For each spinal fluid, pipette 0.3 ml. saline solution into tube 1, 0.2 ml. into tubes 2-5, and 0.1 ml. into tube 6.
6. Pipette 0.3 ml. spinal fluid into tube 1, mix well, and transfer 0.2 ml. to tubes 2 and 6. Mix tube 2, transfer 0.2 ml. to tube 3, and so on to tube 5. Mix tubes and discard 0.2 ml.
7. Add 0.1 ml. diluted antigen to the first seven tubes of each serum test and to the first five tubes of each spinal fluid test.
8. Add 0.2 ml. diluted complement to all tubes.
9. Shake the racks to mix thoroughly and place in the refrigerator at 6°-10° C. for 15-18 hr.
10. Complete the tests the following morning as indicated for the qualitative tests.
11. The end point titer is the highest dilution giving a reactive result. With both sera and spinal fluids, the first tube is considered to be undiluted, or 1 dil. Additional dilutions may be prepared and tested if no end point is obtained.

Retesting of anticomplementary sera:
Anticomplementary sera may be retested by preparing serial twofold dilutions in saline solution as described for the quantitative test, beginning with the 1:5 dilution and ending with 1:80. Each dilution of serum in 0.2 ml. amounts is tested in two tubes, as test and control, as described for the qualitative test. Results of these tests may be interpreted as reactive, without reference to titer, if the first serum dilution showing complete hemolysis in the control tube has a 3+ or 4+ reaction in the tube containing antigen. All other reactions would be reported as anticomplementary.

Preparation of reading standards:
1. Heat tubes of hemoglobin solution (saved from the titration) in the 56° C. water bath for 5 min.

2. Prepare a 1:7 dilution of 2% sheep cell suspension by adding 0.5 ml. 2% suspension to 3 ml. saline solution.
3. Prepare reading standards by mixing hemoglobin solution and cell suspension in the proportions given in Table 14-31.

Reading and reporting test results:
1. All serum and spinal fluid controls should show complete hemolysis.
2. Estimate the individual tube readings by comparison with the reading standards at the end of the secondary incubation period and record degree of complement fixation noted, except for those specimens showing inhibition of hemolysis in the control tube.
3. Read the tubes that have been returned to the 37° C. water bath for a full hour's secondary incubation, estimating and recording the degree of complement fixation of each tube and control tube by comparison with the reading standards.
4. Report the results of the qualitative tests in accordance with Table 14-32.

FLUORESCENT TREPONEMAL ANTIBODY TEST[11, 12]

Equipment:
1. Rotating machine, adjustable to 100 rpm, circumscribing a circle 3/4 in. diam. on a horizontal plane.
2. Incubator, adjustable to 37° C.
3. Dark-field fluorescent microscope assembly.
4. Blotting paper or filter paper sheets.
5. Diamond point stylus.

Table 14-31*

1:7 corpuscle suspension (ml.)	Hemoglobin solution (ml.)	Equivalent complement fixation	
		%	Record
0.7	None	100	4+
0.35	0.35	50	3+
0.175	0.525	25	2+
0.07	0.63	10	1+
0.035	0.665	5	±
None	0.7	0	−

*From Laboratory procedures for modern syphilis serology, U. S. Public Health Service, 1961.

Table 14-32. Kolmer qualitative test reporting*

Test tube reading	Control tube reading	Report	Test tube reading	Control tube reading	Report
4+	–	Reactive	3+	3+	Anticomplementary
3+	–	Reactive	3+	2+	Anticomplementary
2+	–	Reactive	3+	1+	Weakly reactive
1+	–	Reactive	3+	±	Reactive
±	–	Weakly reactive	2+	2+	Nonreactive
–	–	Nonreactive	2+	1+	Nonreactive
4+	4+	Anticomplementary	2+	±	Weakly reactive
4+	3+	Anticomplementary	1+	1+	Nonreactive
4+	2+	Weakly reactive	±	±	Nonreactive
4+	1+	Reactive			

*From Laboratory procedures for modern syphilis serology, U. S. Public Health Service, 1961.

Glassware:
1. Microscope slides 1 × 3 in. frosted end, and approximately 1 mm. thick.
2. Cover glasses, No. 1, 22 mm. sq.
3. Disposable capillary pipettes, 5¾ in. in length.*
4. Staining dish with removable glass tray. Inside dimensions—3⅝ × 2¾ × 2½ in. in height. Coplin staining jars may be used when few slides are involved.
5. Petri dishes, 150 mm. diam. and 15 mm. depth, or other appropriate cover.
6. Glass rods, approximately 100 × 4 mm., both ends fire polished.

Reagents:
1. Antigen:
   (a) *Treponema pallidum,* Nichols strain, extracted from rabbit testicular tissue in basal medium as recommended for the TPI test. This suspension should contain approximately 50 organisms per microscopic field, using a 450× dry objective. This is the antigen for the FTA test and may be stored in a refrigerator without added preservative.
   (b) Same as above but preserved by freeze drying, reconstituted with sterile distilled water to the original volume, and stored

in a refrigerator.* Careful attention should be given to mixing so as to break up clumps and to obtain an even distribution of treponemes. This may be accomplished with a disposable pipette equipped with a rubber bulb. Pull antigen into the pipette and expel five to six times.
2. Fluorescein-labeled antihuman globulin of proved quality. This may be obtained from commercial sources† or may be prepared locally using fluorescein isothiocyanate.
3. Diluted fluorescein conjugate. This may be prepared by diluting fluorescein-labeled antihuman globulin in phosphate buffered saline solution containing 2% Tween 80.‡ Optimum dilutions have been found in the range of 1:5-1:320. The dilution selected for a particular lot of fluorescein-labeled antihuman globulin is optimum when maximal fluorescence is obtained with strongly reactive sera and a large excess of antihuman globulin is not used.
4. Phosphate buffered saline (pH 7.2)

*Scientific Products Division, American Hospital Supply Corp., Evanston, Ill.; Harshaw Scientific Co., Cincinnati, Ohio.

*Baltimore Biological Laboratory, Baltimore, Md.; Difco Laboratories, Detroit, Mich.
†Sylvana Chemical Co., Orange, N. J.; Baltimore Biological Laboratory, Baltimore, Md.
‡Distributed by Hill Top Laboratories, Inc., Cincinnati, Ohio; Laboratory Center, Wilmington, Del.

(Bacto-Hemagglutination buffer No. 0512*).

5. Mounting medium consists of 1 part buffered saline solution plus 9 parts glycerin (reagent grade).

Preparation of sera:

1. Heat clear sera or diluted sera in a 56° C. water bath for 30 min. Allow to cool to room temperature before testing.
2. If sera have been heated on a previous day, reheat for 10 min. at 56° C.
3. Prepare a 1:10 serum dilution by adding 0.1 ml. serum to 0.9 ml. buffered saline solution. Discard pipette. Prepare a 1:200 serum dilution by adding 0.1 ml. of the 1:10 serum dilution to 1.9 ml. buffered saline solution. Discard pipette.

Preliminary test of antigen:

1. A new lot of antigen or in other respects an antigen of unknown quality should be compared with an antigen of known reactivity before being incorporated into the regular test procedure.
2. A satisfactory antigen preparation should not stain directly or nonspecifically with a diluted fluorescein conjugate of known quality.
3. Reaction patterns which have been established for control sera showing reactive, minimally reactive, and nonreactive results with an accepted antigen should be reproduced by the antigen of unknown quality.

Procedure:

1. On grease-free slides cut two circles approximately 1 cm. diam. with a diamond stylus.
2. With a capillary pipette smear approximately 0.01 ml. antigen within each circle and allow to air dry.
3. Immerse slides in acetone for 10 min., remove, and air dry.
4. Cover each antigen smear with approximately 0.03 ml. of a 1:200 dilution of the test serum. Each serum is to be tested in duplicate on a single slide.
5. Prevent evaporation of serum dilutions on smears by covering slides

with petri dish tops or bottoms which contain moistened filter paper.

6. Rotate slides at 100 rpm for 30 min. in an incubator at 37° C.
7. Rinse slides with buffered saline solution and soak in two changes of buffered saline solution for a total of 10 min. This may be followed with a distilled water rinse to remove salt crystals if desired.
8. Blot slides gently with filter paper.
9. Place approximately 0.03 ml. diluted fluorescein conjugate (previously diluted to the appropriate titer) on each smear. Spread conjugate with a glass rod in a circular pattern so that smears are completely covered.
10. Prevent evaporation with petri dish cover as in step 5.
11. Repeat steps 6, 7, and 8.
12. Place a very small drop of mounting medium on each smear and apply a cover glass.
13. Slides may be examined immediately or may be preserved for a more convenient time by placing them in a refrigerator at 6°-10° C.

NOTE: Output of the ultraviolet light source should be checked periodically. This may be acomplished by using a Weston Master No. 3 photoelectric exposure meter to determine the ultraviolet density at or immediately below the microscope stage level. Readings of 400 or more on this exposure meter when ultraviolet filters are employed indicate satisfactory ultraviolet light for fluorescent reading.

Controls: The following must be included in each test run and should be performed in duplicate.

1. A dilution of serum demonstrating moderate to strong reactivity (R).
2. A dilution of reactive serum that will produce a minimally reactive (2+) result.
3. A 1:200 dilution of serum demonstrating no reaction (N).
4. Antigen smear treated only with fluorescein-labeled antihuman globulin (nonspecific staining control).

Reading and reporting test results (Table 14-33):

---

*Difco Laboratories, Detroit, Mich.

Table 14-33

	Reading	Report
4+	Very strongly fluorescent	Reactive (R)
3+	Strongly fluorescent	Reactive (R)
2+	Minimally fluorescent	Reactive (R)
1+	Weakly fluorescent	Nonreactive (N)
− to ±	Vaguely visible	Nonreactive (N)

1. Smears are studied microscopically, using ultraviolet light and a high-power dry objective. The total magnification should approximate 450×.
2. Nonreactive smears should be checked with visible illumination in order to verify the presence of treponemes.

DISCUSSION[13-23]

The standard tests for syphilis (STS) seem to become positive after the first to the third week following the appearance of the primary lesion and to remain positive until treated, occasionally after prolonged treatment (Kolmer-fast blood in about 30% of persons with latent syphilis). Many persons with Kolmer-fast blood have positive spinal fluids. Less than 10% of persons show a positive reaction by the fifth day. The reagin titer increases rapidly for the first 4 wk. and then remains approximately stationary for about 6 mo.

A negative reaction implies absence of infection but never rules it out completely. In suspicious cases, repeat weekly for 8 wk. Repeatedly negative reactions indicate that there is no active syphilis. A positive reaction should be checked if there are no confirmatory clinical signs and symptoms. However, seropositive latent syphilis is a large part of all syphilis. Repeatedly positive reactions indicate syphilis, except in yaws, pinta, rat-bite fever (due to *Spirillum minus*), relapsing fever, trypanosomiasis, leprosy, disseminated lupus erythematosus, and possibly malaria and pellagra. Biologically false positive reactions may persist for years (or for life) and often indicate a collagen disease. A transient positive reaction may occur in infectious mononu-

cleosis, glandular tuberculosis, virus pneumonia, hyperproteinemia, after recent smallpox vaccination, and following influenzal infection and other infections with febrile reactions. These transient false positive reactions usually become negative within 6 mo.

Following vaccination, a small percentage of persons who had a primary reaction (vaccinia) gave a positive VDRL test and/or Kolmer test. Positive reactions occur during the second week and may occur for as long as 5 mo. During this time the false positive reaction will decrease without treatment. It also tends to decrease when the serum is allowed to stand over, becoming negative within a month or two.

In persons with treated and asymptomatic syphilis the serology often fluctuates from positive to negative to positive.

With spinal fluid, the tests are negative until there is involvement of the central nervous system. The percentage of positive reactions in paresis is approximately 100% and in tabes and meningovascular syphilis 60-80%.

A negative cord VDRL test and/or Kolmer test does not exclude syphilis in the child. A strongly positive reaction usually means that the baby has congenital syphilis, according to McCord. This is particularly true if the titer increases; if it decreases and soon disappears, this indicates passive transfer of reagin through the placenta (Fildes' law).

A study of the various serodiagnostic tests for syphilis in the United States seemed to indicate that the most widely used complement-fixation tests and flocculation tests are of relatively equal value. In untreated primary syphilis the percentage of positive reactions found was about 55-80%; in untreated secondary syphilis, approximately 100%; in variously treated tertiary syphilis, about 60-85%. There was in all about 1% false positive tests in normal presumably nonsyphilitic individuals, about 59.5% in leprosy, and about 14.5% in malaria. The percentage of false positive tests in the other groups (jaundice, pregnancy, malignant disease, and febrile diseases) was not significantly greater than in the normal individuals. Menstruation did not seem to affect the tests.

BIOLOGIC FALSE POSITIVE REACTIONS

The need for specific tests with which to identify the biologic false positive reaction sometimes obtained with a standard test for syphilis is being partially met by the use of antigens prepared from killed *Treponema pallidum,* as in the Reiter protein complement–fixation test (RPCF), *Treponema pallidum* immune adherence test (TPIA), and *Treponema pallidum* complement-fixation test (TPCF), and also by the use of live treponemes as in the fluorescent treponemal antibody test (FTA).

REFERENCES

1. Harris, A., Rosenberg, A. A., and Riedel, L. M.: J. Ven. Dis. Inform. **27**:169, 1946.
2. Harris, A., Rosenberg, A. A., and Del Veccio, E. R.: J. Ven. Dis. Inform. **29**:72, 1948.
3. Rosenberg, A. A., Harris, A., and Harding, V. L.: J. Ven. Dis. Inform. **29**:359, 1948.
4. Bossak, H. N., and Duncan, W. P.: Public Health Rep. **73**:836, 1958.
5. Kolmer, J. A.: Amer. J. Clin. Path. **12**:109, 1942.
6. Kolmer, J. A., Spaulding, E. H., and Robinson, H. W.: Approved laboratory technic, ed. 5, New York, 1951, Appleton-Century-Crofts, Inc.
7. Cannefax, G. R., and Garson, W.: Public Health Rep. **72**:335, 1957.
8. Bossak, H. N., Falcone, Virginia H., Duncan, W. P., and Harris, A.: Public Health Lab. **16**:39, 1958.
9. D'Alessandro, G., and Dardanoni, L.: Amer. J. Syph. **37**:137, 1953.
10. Wallace, A. L., and Harris, A.: Public Health Lab. **16**:27, 1958.
11. Deacon, W. E., Falcone, V. H., and Harris, A.: Proc. Soc. Exp. Biol. Med. **96**:477, 1957.
12. Deacon, W. E., Freeman, Elizabeth M., and Harris, A.: Proc. Soc. Exp. Biol. Med. **103**:827, 1960.
13. Smith, D. C.: South. Med. J. **39**:234, 1946.
14. Kline, B. S.: Amer. J. Clin. Path. **16**:68, 1946.
15. Barksdale, E. E.: Southern Med. J. **39**:229, 1946.
16. Hatz, B.: Amer. J. Clin. Path. **8**:39, 1938.
17. Cardon, L., and Atlas, D. H.: Arch. Dermat. & Syph. **46**:713, 1942.
18. Favorite, G. O.: Proc. Soc. Exp. Biol. Med. **52**:297, 1943.
19. Barnard, R. D.: Illinois Med. J. **77**:78, 1940.
20. McCord, J. R.: J.A.M.A. **105**:89, 1935.
21. Ven. Dis. Inform. **16**:189, 1935.
22. J.A.M.A. **104**:2083, 1935.
23. Ven. Dis. Inform. **18**:4, 1937.

Chapter 15

Toxicology– poisons and drugs

In recent years the multiplication of the number of potent drugs, newer insecticides and pesticides, and industrial compounds of a toxic nature has considerably increased the number of potential poisons. Acute or chronic poisoning with many of these agents may mimic a number of disease states or alter the symptoms of preexisting disease. In order to arrive at a correct diagnosis the determination of the presence or absence of toxic compounds in body fluids may be necessary. Even if there is a history of possible exposure to the toxic agent, for accurate diagnosis and therapy the actual demonstration of the presence of the toxic agent in the body may be necessary.

Toxic agents are rarely distributed evenly throughout the body, ethyl alcohol being an exception. Most toxic agents tend to accumulate in particular tissues of the body in accordance with their chemical nature and metabolic pathways. Thus lead is deposited in the bones, and arsenic tends to accumulate in keratin-rich tissues such as skin, hair, and nails. In general, the substances whose determinations are discussed in this chapter may be found in the body as the result of accidental or other exposure to toxic agents not normally found in the body (at least not in high concentrations), or they may be due to an overdose of drugs prescribed by the physician. Also the therapeutic levels of some drugs in the blood or other body fluids may be helpful in proper therapy.

Particularly in testing for inorganic elements such as arsenic, lead, and mercury, usually present in small amounts, contamination from reagents or other sources in the laboratory must be considered, and great care should be taken in scrupulous cleaning of glassware and testing of all reagents.

ETHYL ALCOHOL[1-4]

The determination of ethyl alcohol is probably the most frequently requested test in the forensic or clinical toxicology laboratory. The widespread use of alcoholic beverages renders this substance the most important single toxic agent that confronts us. Certain pathologic conditions or cerebral trauma may cause many symptoms indistinguishable from those of alcohol intoxication. Also an alcoholic odor on the breath that can result from the ingestion of only a small amount of alcohol can, together with the other symptoms, lead to an erroneous diagnosis of alcohol intoxication. Only by an accurate chemical analysis of a suitable body fluid (blood or urine) can a reliable diagnosis be assured.

Alcohol is readily absorbed and in a short time fairly evenly distributed in all body fluids. Some is excreted in the expired air; 2 L. of alveolar air is considered to contain about the same amount of alcohol as 1 ml. of blood or urine. The breath as ordinarily collected usually contains about 50% alveolar air.

Normally there are small amounts of

684

Table 15.1. Common poisons and their antidotes

Type of poison	Antidotes and treatment	Type of poison	Antidotes and treatment
Acids (acetic, vinegar, nitric, sulfuric, hydrochloric, and muriatic)	AVOID VOMITING! Give 1 cup milk of magnesia, later white of raw egg or cup of olive oil; apply heat if necessary	Food poisoning (ptomaines and botulism)	Cause vomiting with strong soapsuds or 1 tbs. mustard in glass of warm water, then give castor oil or Epsom salts; apply heat
Boric acid and borax	Give lots of water containing baking soda, 2 tsp. in each glass of water; follow with lemon juice; keep patient warm	Aspirin (Anacin, B.C. tablets, Stanback, A.P.C. tablets, and Empirin compound)	Give EMETICS* to cause vomiting; then universal antidote†; give aromatic spirits of ammonia, tsp. in ½ glass of water
Carbolic acid, phenol, sheep-dip, and cresol solution	Give 1 qt. water containing 2 tbs. pure alcohol or whiskey diluted half with water; continue with lots of warm water, then white of egg or olive oil	Phosphorus (rat and roach paste and matches)	Give large amount of peroxide mixed half with water; later give ½ cup liquid petrolatum or mineral oil; DO NOT GIVE OTHER FATS OR OTHER OILS! 0.5% copper sulfate solution
Alcohol (whiskey, paregoric, and morphine)	Give EMETICS* to cause vomiting; strong coffee as stimulant; aromatic spirits of ammonia	Tincture of iodine and Lugol solution	Give starch paste, tbs. salt in glass warm water to cause vomiting, then milk or white of egg
Alkalies (Drano, Saniflush, lye, and ammonia water)	Give large volumes of vinegar, lemon juice, or grapefruit juice; boric acid for use in eye; give milk, white of egg, flour in water, or olive oil. DO NOT GIVE EMETICS!	Mercury (bichloride, corrosive sublimate, etc.)	Give 2 raw egg whites in milk for every tablet of bichloride of mercury taken; if doctor not present yet, cause vomiting with strong soapsuds or EMETICS* and repeat egg white dose
Arsenic and Paris green (Rough on Rats)	Give large quantities of warm water and milk of magnesia freely, follow with castor oil; antidote from pharmacist; iron hydroxide with magnesium oxide	Barbiturates (Nembutal, Seconal, Amytal, Butisol, etc., and belladonna group)	Cause vomiting with strong soapsuds or EMETICS,* then give strong coffee, followed by Epsom salts; keep patient warm
Laxatives (phenolphthalein, Exlax, Phenolax, Feenamints, etc.)	Give EMETICS*	Mushrooms, strychnine, gasoline, and kerosene	Give UNIVERSAL ANTIDOTE† until doctor arrives; give EMETICS* to cause vomiting
Dexedrine and Benzedrine	Give EMETICS*	Cleaning fluids	Give EMETICS*
Insecticides (D.D.T., etc.)	Give EMETICS*	Nail polish remover and acetone	Give EMETICS* and UNIVERSAL ANTIDOTE†

*Emetics: 1 tbs. mustard
or
1 tbs. salt to glass warm water

†Universal antidote: Burnt toast, 2 parts; Milk of magnesia, 1 part; Strong tea, 1 part

alcohol in the blood, usually from 20-30 mg./100 ml. (0.02-0.03%). If the alcohol level in the blood is under 0.05%, this is usually considered presumptive evidence that the person is not under the influence of alcohol; levels of over 0.15% are usually considered evidence of definite intoxication.

Alcohol is best determined by distillation, followed by a colorimetric estimation in the distillate by the use of dichromate. The reaction is based on the reduction of the dichromate by alcohol, with the formation of the green chromous ion. Certain other volatile compounds, particularly methyl alcohol, formaldehyde, and paraldehyde, will also give the reaction; if an abnormal concentration of alcohol is found, these other substances must be tested for.

Reagents:
1. Picric acid solution (1%). Dissolve 10 gm. picric acid in distilled water and dilute to 1 L. The concentration of this reagent is not critical.
2. Standard dichromate reagent. Dissolve 3.333 gm. reagent grade potassium dichromate in 500 ml. distilled water. Add in small quantities, cooling after each addition, a total of 321 ml. concentrated sulfuric acid. Dilute to 1 L. with distilled water. Allow to stand overnight and then add additional distilled water if necessary to bring to 1 L. Store in a glass-stoppered bottle. Avoid contact with organic matter. Under these conditions the reagent is stable for 6 mo.
3. Anti-foam A emulsion.*
4. Standard alcohol solution. Dilute 2 ml. absolute ethyl alcohol to 1 L. with distilled water. This solution contains 0.16 gm. ethyl alcohol/100 ml. (the density of absolute alcohol being taken as 0.80 at room temperature).

Apparatus: An all-glass distilling apparatus is desirable. This is available commercially† or can be made from component parts, as described by Duboski and Shupe.[1]

---

*Dow Corning Corp., Midland, Mich.
†Scientific Glass Apparatus Co., Bloomfield, N. J.

Also required are 10 ml. glass-stoppered graduated cylinders.

Collection of specimen: Do not contaminate the specimens by using alcohol as an antiseptic; any of the available aqueous germicidal solutions may be used. Obtain about 8 ml. blood in a tube containing an anticoagulant (potassium oxalate, 20 mg., is satisfactory). Stopper and store in the refrigerator until examined. Random urine samples are not satisfactory as they may not be in equilibrium with venous blood. For best results, have the patient empty the bladder, discard the sample, then have him empty the bladder 30 min. later, and use this sample.

Procedure: Pipette 5 ml. blood or urine into the distilling flask. Rinse the pipette with 10-20 ml. water into the flask. Add 10-15 ml. picric acid solution and 5-10 drops of Anti-foam A. Attach the connecting tube and condenser and distill gently so that 10 ml. distillate is obtained in 10-12 min. in a graduated cylinder. Mix the distillate well. In one test tube place a 2 ml. aliquot of the distillate. In another tube place 2 ml. water as a blank. To each tube add 6 ml. dichromate solution (accurately measured). Heat in a boiling water bath for 15 min., cool to room temperature, and read in photometer at 600 nm., setting to zero with the blank solution. Obtain milligrams of alcohol in aliquot from previously prepared calibration curve.

$$\% \text{Alcohol} = \frac{\text{Vol. distillate}}{\text{Aliquot taken}} \times \frac{100}{\text{Ml. serum}} \times \frac{\text{Mg. in aliquot}}{1000}$$

Calibration curve: Add to 5 ml. alcohol-free blood (outdated bank blood is suitable) in the distilling flask 10 ml. standard alcohol solution (0.16 gm./100 ml. or 16 mg. in aliquot), add several drops Anti-foam A and 10-15 ml. picric acid, and distill as in the preparation of the sample. Collect exactly 10 ml. distillate and treat 2 ml. distillate (containing 3.2 mg. alcohol) with 6 ml. chromic acid solution as in the sample procedure. Repeat the procedure using 7.5, 5, and 2.5 ml. standard alcohol solution and 5 ml. blood. Two-milliliter aliquots of these distillates will contain 2.4, 1.6, and 0.8 mg. alcohol, respectively. Plot the amount of alcohol in the aliquot against the OD for the calibration curve. This curve is valid for the duration of the batch of dichromate solution used. If the sample aliquot reading corresponds to more than 4 mg., the determination must be repeated, using a smaller aliquot of the distillate.

It is customary to express the concentration of alcohol in percent (gm./100 ml.) and not in mg./100 ml., as is done with many clinical tests. All medicolegal specifications are stated in terms of gm./100 ml., and to avoid confusion all concentrations of alcohol should be expressed in these terms.

Determination of blood alcohol by microdiffusion[5, 6]: This method uses the Conway microdiffusion chamber and is simple and relatively rapid. It does not distinguish between ethyl alcohol and other volatile reducing substances but may be satisfactory for many routine purposes.

Reagents:
1. Acid dichromate. Dissolve 3.7 gm. reagent grade potassium dichromate in 150 ml. distilled water. Carefully add 280 ml. concentrated sulfuric acid and dilute to 650 ml.
2. Saturated potassium carbonate.
3. Standard alcohol solution. Dilute 2 ml. absolute ethanol to 1 L. with water. Since the density of absolute ethanol is 0.80, 2 ml. will weigh 1.60 gm.; hence the standard contains 0.160 gm./100 ml., or 160 mg.%.

Procedure: Pipette 1 ml. acid dichromate into the center compartments of a number of Conway dishes. In the outer compartment place 1 ml. saturated potassium carbonate. Dilute a portion of the blood sample 1:2 with water (1 ml. blood plus 1 ml. water). Add 1 ml. of the diluted blood to the outer compartment, seal, and mix sample and carbonate by gently swirling. If the chamber is of the type requiring a liquid seal, use saturated potassium carbonate. Also obtain a sample of normal blood containing no alcohol; use 1 ml. of a 1:2 dilution with water in a second dish as a blood blank and 1

ml. of a 1:2 dilution with the standard solution as a standard in another dish. The addition of blood to the standard is necessary since alcohol may diffuse from blood at a different rate than from a simple aqueous solution. Allow all dishes to stand for 1 hr. At the end of the diffusion, using a capillary pipette, transfer the acid dichromate from each center well to a separate tube graduated at 10 ml. Rinse center well with water several times and add to acid dichromate. Dilute to exactly 10 ml. with water. Also prepare a reagent blank by diluting 1 ml. of the acid dichromate to 10 ml. with water. Read OD of the solutions at 600 nm. against reagent blank.

Calculation:

$$\left(\frac{\text{OD unknown}}{\text{OD standard} - \text{OD blood blank}} \right)$$
$$\times \text{ Conc. of standard (gm.\%)}$$
$$= \text{ Conc. of alcohol in sample (gm.\%)}$$

Blood containing about 0.300 gm.% alcohol will reduce all the dichromate present so that higher concentrations will not further increase the color. Hence, when values over about 0.250 gm.% are obtained, the test should be repeated on a further dilution of the blood, using 1 ml. of a 1:4 dilution and making the appropriate correction in the calculation. It will be noted that with high alcohol concentrations the dichromate solution turns green fairly rapidly; in this case one could stop the diffusion sooner, e.g., after 20 min. The exact diffusion time is not important as long as all the samples, standards, and blanks diffuse for exactly the same time.

QUALITATIVE TESTS FOR METHANOL, FORMALDEHYDE, AND PARALDEHYDE[7]

If a positive test is obtained for alcohol and there is a possibility that one of these interfering substances may be present, qualitative tests should be run.

Reagents:
1. Chromotropic acid. Dissolve 0.5 gm. chromotropic acid or its disodium salt (Eastman No. P230, 4,5-dihydroxy,2,7-naphthalene disulfonic

acid, disodium salt) in 100 ml. water.

2. Concentrated sulfuric acid.
3. Potassium permanganate (5%). Dissolve 5 gm. potassium permanganate in 100 ml. distilled water.
4. Sodium bisulfite (0.15M). Dissolve 1.5 gm. sodium bisulfite in 100 ml. distilled water.
5. Dilute sulfuric acid. Add 10 ml. concentrated sulfuric acid to 90 ml. distilled water.
6. *p*-Hydroxybiphenyl (1%) in 0.5N sodium hydroxide. Dissolve 1 gm. *p*-hydroxybiphenyl (Eastman No. 2174, phenylphenol) in 100 ml. distilled water containing 2 gm. sodium hydroxide.
7. Copper sulfate (4%). Dissolve 4 gm. copper sulfate crystals in 100 ml. distilled water.

Procedure: If a positive test for alcohol has been obtained, add 1 ml. distillate to each of three test tubes. To one tube add 1 ml. dilute sulfuric acid and 10 drops potassium permanganate. Allow to stand for 10 min. and add sodium bisulfite solution drop by drop until the purple color disappears. Place this tube and one of the tubes containing the unoxidized distillate in an ice bath. To both tubes add 0.2 ml. chromotropic acid and 4 ml. concentrated sulfuric acid. Mix and place the tubes in a boiling water bath for 15 min. The appearance of a purple color in the untreated distillate indicates the presence of formaldehyde, whereas the appearance of a purple color in the oxidized distillate indicates the presence of methanol and/or formaldehyde.

To the third aliquot of the original distillate add 1 drop copper sulfate solution and 6 ml. concentrated sulfuric acid. Mix and add 0.2 ml. *p*-hydroxybiphenyl solution, shaking constantly. Place in boiling water bath for 3 min. and cool to room temperature. In the absence of formaldehyde, a pink color indicates the presence of paraldehyde.

ARSENIC[8-11]

The use of arsenic compounds is still widespread, including those in rat poisons, insecticides, paints, and dyes. Arsenic compounds are also used as drugs, though not to the same extent as formerly (e.g., in the treatment of syphilis). In the past, arsenic was probably the most common poison used with homicidal intent, and its detection and quantitative estimation have been the responsibility of the analytic toxicologist for many years. The clinical chemist may encounter a similar task since arsenic is still a frequently encountered metallic poison. The amount of arsenic "normally" present in the human body has been the subject of some controversy, but it seems apparent that small amounts are usually present due to minute quantities ingested with foods. Of the common foods, seafoods contain the largest amounts (up to 0.3 mg./100 gm.), except for fruits and vegetables contaminated by insecticidal spray residues.

Two methods for arsenic are given. The first, the Reinsch test, is a qualitative method for arsenic (as well as for antimony and mercury), and the second, the Gutzeit method, can be adapted to quantitative detection. In the Reinsch test the arsenic is deposited on a copper wire to isolate the element. In the Gutzeit method the arsenic, after digestion with oxidizing agents to destroy organic matter, is volatilized as arsine and detected by its reaction with mercuric bromide paper.

Reinsch test:
Reagent:
1. Concentrated hydrochloric acid (arsenic free), reagent grade, and a 10% solution of the acid made by diluting 1 vol. acid with 9 vol. distilled water.

Equipment: Pure copper wire, 20 gauge.

Procedure: Place 20-30 ml. urine or stomach washings in a 50 ml. Erlenmeyer flask. (It has been recommended that, if possible, larger quantities be used.) Make the material slightly alkaline with sodium hydroxide, evaporate to a volume of about 25 ml., make acid with hydrochloric acid, and proceed as given below. To the mixture add one-seventh its volume of concentrated hydrochloric acid. Prepare a spiral of copper wire by winding a length of 20-gauge copper wire around a pencil, allowing a straight length of about 6 in. as a handle. Clean the spiral to a bright luster by alternately dipping it into concentrated nitric acid and water; then rinse well with distilled water. Immerse the copper spiral in the acidified mixture and place on a steam bath for 1 hr., with occasional swirling. Add more 10% hydrochloric acid from time to time to maintain a constant volume. The copper spiral is then removed, washed well with water, and dried with filter paper. A dark coloration may indicate arsenic, antimony, or mercury. If the wire is not comparable in brightness to its original state, further tests may be performed. The copper spiral may be used quantitatively by placing it in the chamber of a Gutzeit apparatus, or the following test can be performed. Cut off the handle from the spiral and place the latter in a small glass thimble prepared by drawing out the upper end of a clean glass test tube. Suspend this through an opening in an asbestos mat and cover the end of the tube with a clean cover glass in which is placed a drop of water. Heat the portion of the thimble below the asbestos until the copper begins to turn red. This will drive off antimony, arsenic, and mercury, which will condense on the cover glass as a film. Bismuth will not sublime. Pick up the cover glass by touching the drop of water with a glass slide, and examine the film under low-power and high-power dry lenses. Antimony condenses as amorphous granular material, arsenic in octahedral crystals, and mercury as globules.

Gutzeit test:

Reagents:

1. Concentrated nictric acid, reagent grade.
2. Concentrated sulfuric acid, reagent grade.
3. Perchloric acid (70%), reagent grade.
4. Sodium bisulfite, reagent grade, granular.
5. Stannous chloride solution. Dissolve 40 gm. stannous chloride in distilled water and make up to 100 ml.
6. Sulfuric acid (10%). Add 10 ml. concentrated sulfuric acid carefully to about 70 ml. distilled water, cool, and make up to 100 ml.
7. Dry glass wool impregnated with lead acetate. A plug of glass wool sufficient to fill lower two thirds of volume of Gutzeit apparatus is saturated by immersing it in a solution of lead acetate (approximately 50 gm. in water to 100 ml.). It is then removed and air or oven dried and inserted into the column.
8. Cupric sulfate solution. Dissolve 10 gm. crystalline cupric sulfate in distilled water to make 100 ml.
9. Zinc metal, granular, arsenic free, reagent grade.
10. Mercuric bromide–methanol solution. Dissolve 5 gm. mercuric bromide in absolute methanol and dilute to 100 ml.; protect from light.
11. Filter paper strips impregnated with mercuric bromide. Immerse Whatman No. 1 or No. 4 filter paper, 12.5 or 15 cm., in the mercuric bromide solution for 5 min. Then remove with tweezers, air dry, and cut strips from the center of sheet to fit the small tube of the Gutzeit apparatus, leaving a tail protruding at the top to facilitate removal. Avoid touching the strip with the hands except at the tail end.

Special apparatus: Gutzeit apparatus is shown in Fig. 15-1. This may be made from parts found in the laboratory. The lower bottle has a capacity of about 50 ml.; the column is about 6 in. long and ¾ in. diam., and the small tube is about 3 in. long and has an inside diameter of 4-6 mm.

Procedure: For the digestion, place either 100 ml. urine, 20 ml. blood, 50 gm. hair, 50 ml. vomitus, or 50-100 gm. finely ground suspected food in a 300-500 ml. Kjeldahl flask. Add 10 ml. nitric acid to the urine, 20 ml. to the blood, 50 ml. to the vomitus, or 50-100 ml. to the food. To each flask add 5 ml. sulfuric acid and heat over a low flame under a fume hood until the volume is reduced and the first signs of darkening appear. As the solution darkens, care must be taken to prevent charring. Remove from the flame and add drop by drop 1 ml. of a mixture of

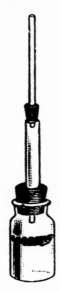

Fig. 15-1. Gutzeit apparatus.

1 part nitric acid to 2 parts perchloric acid. Resume heating gently. Repeat addition of acid until digest remains clear. Discontinue this treatment when a colorless to faintly yellow solution is obtained that does not darken further on heating. Continue boiling with stronger heating until dense white fumes cease evolving. Cool, cautiously add about 5 ml. water, and then transfer quantitatively to an Erlenmeyer flask with small portions of distilled water. Add 100 mg. sodium bisulfite and heat again until dense white fumes appear. Cool and transfer to a 50 ml. glass-stoppered cylinder with distilled water, add 3 drops stannous chloride solution, and dilute to 50 ml.

Prepare a standard blank by adding 200 mg. sodium bisulfite and 40 ml. 10% sulfuric acid to a flask, boil until white fumes appear, cool, add 6 drops stannous chloride solution, and dilute to 100 ml. with water. Prepare a number of the Gutzeit setups. Place glass wool impregnated with lead acetate in the column, as described earlier, and a strip of filter paper impregnated with mercuric bromide in each of the small tubes and connect to columns. Prepare a working standard by diluting 1 ml. stock standard to 200 with distilled water. This solution contains 5

μg arsenic/ml. In one Gutzeit bottle place 20 ml. digested sample; in three other bottles place 20 ml. standard blank, adding to one bottle 1 ml. working standard (5 μg arsenic) and to a second bottle 2 ml. standard (10 μg arsenic), the third bottle serving as a blank. To each bottle add 1 ml. copper sulfate solution and about 5 gm. arsenic-free zinc, stopper immediately, and set the column in a pan of water at 25° C. for 45 min. At the end of this time examine the filter paper strips. If arsenic is present, the lower end of the strip will be colored orange to brown, depending upon the concentration of the element. The amount in the sample aliquot may be estimated by comparison of the strip from the sample bottle with that from the standard bottles. It may be necessary to repeat the determinations using a smaller aliquot of the sample (adding 10% sulfuric acid to the bottle to bring the volume to 20 ml.) or with larger aliquots of sample.

Although antimony is not usually encountered, it will give a brown to black stain when present. It can be differentiated from arsenic by exposing the strip to fumes of concentrated hydrochloric acid; this will cause the antimony color to disappear, whereas a true arsenic stain will remain.

Calculation: The estimation of the amount of arsenic is made by comparison of the stains of sample and standards. For example, 100 ml. urine was digested and made up to 50 ml. A 20 ml. aliquot of this gave a stain that appeared to be roughly intermediate in size between those produced by 20 μg arsenic and 30 μg arsenic. Hence the aliquot would be estimated to contain about 25 μg arsenic. The total arsenic in the 100 ml. urine sample would then be:

$$25 \times \frac{50}{20} = 63 \ \mu g/100 \ ml. \ urine$$

This could be reported as 630 μg or 0.63 mg./L. urine.

Normal values and interpretation: The concentration of arsenic in blood is considered to be normal in the range of 6-20 μg/100 ml., and the urinary excretion is considered to be normal up to 0.1 mg./L.

In occupational exposure, excretion of more than 1 mg./L. is considered to indicate evidence of harmful exposure.

CARBON MONOXIDE IN BLOOD (CARBOXYHEMOGLOBIN)[12-14]

Carbon monoxide is toxic because its combination with hemoglobin (carboxyhemoglobin) is more stable than oxyhemoglobin; hence the hemoglobin combined with carbon monoxide is not available for the essential transport of oxygen to the tissues, and anoxia results. One part carbon monoxide/5000 parts air will produce about 20% saturation of the hemoglobin with some toxic symptoms when breathed for 1 hr. A hemoglobin saturation of over 60% is usually fatal.

Carbon monoxide is probably responsible for more deaths than any other poison. The main sources of carbon monoxide are illuminating gases and the incomplete combustion of fuels such as automobile exhaust fumes and improperly vented gas-fired heating appliances. Individuals with anemia or an increased metabolic rate are more susceptible to carbon monoxide intoxication.

Blood specimens for suspected carbon monoxide poisoning should be taken as soon as possible after exposure since the gas is gradually eliminated from the blood at a rate of about 15%/hr. when breathing pure air and much more rapidly under oxygen therapy. Heparinized blood is preferable for analysis; oxalate is said to cause low results. If analysis is not carried out as soon as the blood sample is secured, it may be preserved for a few hours in the refrigerator in a well-filled, tightly stoppered tube.

A spectrophotometric method for carbon monoxide is given in the chapter on hematology (p. 104). The following chemical method is based on the fact that carbon monoxide will reduce palladium chloride to metallic palladium. The method is quite specific in that there are few substances that will react under the conditions of the experiment.

Carbon monoxide is separated from the blood by diffusion in the Conway microdiffusion chamber.

Reagents:
1. Sulfuric acid (10%, w/v). Add 5.8 ml. concentrated sulfuric acid to about 80 ml. water, cool, and dilute to 100 ml.
2. Hydrochloric acid (0.1N). Dilute 8.5 ml. concentrated hydrochloric acid to 100 ml.
3. Potassium iodide (2%). Dissolve 1 gm. potassium iodide in 50 ml. water. Prepare just before use.
4. Palladium chloride solution (0.01N). Dissolve 88 mg. palladium chloride ($PdCl_2$) or 107 mg. $PdCl_2 \cdot 2H_2O$ in 100 ml. 0.1N hydrochloric acid. Store in brown bottle in refrigerator.

Procedure: Place 2 ml. palladium chloride solution in the inner chamber of a Conway diffusion dish. In the outer chamber place 1 ml. blood sample plus 2 ml. 10% sulfuric acid (sample) or 1 ml. water plus 2 ml. 10% sulfuric acid (blank). Place covers on dishes, mix by rotation, and allow to stand for 1 hr. If the dishes are of the type that require a liquid seal, use the 10% sulfuric acid.

Without disturbing the particles of metallic palladium that may be floating on the surface, carefully pipette 0.2 ml. of the liquid from the inner chamber of the sample dish and add to a cuvette. Also pipette 0.2 ml. of the palladium chloride solution from the inner chamber of the blank dish to another cuvette. To each cuvette add 10 ml. 2% potassium iodide, mix well, and read in photometer at 490 nm. within 5 min. against a blank of potassium iodide solution.

Calculations: Two milliliters of 0.01N palladium chloride will react with 0.01 mM. or 0.224 ml. carbon monoxide under standard conditions. Since 1 vol. carbon monoxide will combine with 1.36 gm. hemoglobin, reaction of all the palladium chloride would represent the formation of 0.224/1.36 or 0.165 gm. carboxyhemoglobin/ml. of blood, or 16.5 gm./100 ml. Hence:

$$\frac{\text{OD blank} - \text{OD sample}}{\text{OD blank}} \times \frac{16.5 \times 100}{\text{Hb}}$$

$$= \% \text{Saturation with carbon monoxide}$$

where Hb represents the grams of hemoglobin per 100 ml. in the blood sample.

If hemoglobin is not run, a normal value may be assumed.

For expected low results (under 20% saturation) the palladium chloride solution may be diluted 1:5 with 0.1N hydrochloric acid before addition of 2 ml. to the dishes. In this case the factor 16.5 in the equation is replaced by 3.3.

For somewhat more accurate results, after diluting the original blank palladium solution with 10 ml. potassium iodide, withdraw 3 ml. and further dilute 1:2 with potassium iodide solution. Then:

$$\frac{OD\ blank - OD\ sample}{OD\ blank - OD\ diluted\ (1:2)\ blank}$$
$$\times \frac{16.5 \times 50}{Hb} = \%\,Saturation$$

Theoretically this method does not require any further standardization if the palladium chloride solution is accurately made up. However, when first trying out the method, it may be well to run a few samples of known carbon monoxide content. The method for obtaining these is mentioned in the next section.

Simple qualitative test: Lake about 2-3 drops blood with about 2 ml. water (approximately 1:10 dilution). Add a small pinch (amount that can be piled on the flat end of a toothpick) of a mixture of equal parts of pyrogallic acid and tannic acid, mix by inverting, and allow to stand for 5-15 min. Run a negative control with normal blood and a positive control with blood treated with carbon monoxide (see below). Normal blood will assume a gray-brown color on addition of the reagent, while that containing carbon monoxide will have a pink tinge, depending upon the amount of the gas absorbed.

For a more quantitative procedure, dilute 0.1 ml. blood with 0.9 ml. water and add 1 ml. reagent composed of equal volumes of freshly prepared 2% aqueous solutions of pyrogallic acid and tannic acid. Mix the tubes by inversion and compare them with standards after 15 min.

To prepare standards, obtain at least 10 ml. pooled heparinized blood from a number of nonsmokers known to be free of any recent exposure to carbon monoxide. Place half the blood in each of two 250 ml. round reagent bottles. Displace the air in one bottle with 100% oxygen, stopper tightly, and rotate in a horizontal position around the long axis for 15-20 min. to saturate. Treat the other bottle similarly with carbon monoxide. The gas is conveniently obtained in small lecture cylinders from most laboratory supply houses. Rotate for about 20 min., flush with fresh carbon monoxide, and rotate an additional 20 min. CAUTION! Carbon monoxide must be used under a fume hood or out-of-doors in a strong breeze. Varying proportions of the two saturated blood samples may then be mixed to obtain standards varying from 100% oxygen to 100% carbon monoxide. When these standards are treated like the blood sample as described and placed in tubes that are well sealed with melted paraffin, they will remain satisfactory for several weeks. Permanent standards of oil colors may be obtained commercially.*

Normal values and interpretation: Normally there may be from 1-2.5% saturation of carbon monoxide in the blood. Individuals who smoke may have up to 5% saturation, and persons exposed to higher concentrations of carbon monoxide such as taxi drivers may have as much as 8% saturation. Symptoms may occur when the percent saturation reaches 20%; with over 30% saturation the symptoms may be severe. Death usually occurs with over 60% saturation, although occasionally only 40-50% may be fatal.

LEAD[15, 16]

Lead enters the body through the gastrointestinal and respiratory tracts and accumulates in the body (especially in bones). Intoxication is usually of a chronic nature because it is slowly absorbed and even more slowly excreted. As little as 2 mg. daily, ingested over a period of weeks, will lead to chronic lead poisoning. Early symptoms of lead poisoning include facial pallor, a mild grade of anemia with basophilic stippling of the erythrocytes, and a "lead line" on the gums. Symptoms of lead poisoning are due to the circulating lead and not to that in fixed deposits. However, often other

---

*Mine Safety Appliances Co., Pittsburgh, Pa.

conditions such as even mild acidosis may cause a release of the lead from the bone back into the blood, producing symptoms of poisoning.

Acute lead poisoning can be diagnosed only by chemical means or by history. Of importance is the presence of low-grade anemia, stippling of erythrocytes, and the presence of abnormal quantities of lead in the urine and blood.

In this method for the detection of lead the blood or urine is digested with acid to remove organic material; the lead is then extracted with dithizone in chloroform from a buffered solution. Cyanide is added to reduce the interference from other metals that also react with dithizone.

Reagents: Make up all reagents with water that has been distilled from an all-glass still.

1. Digestion reagent. Carefully mix 5 vol. nitric acid and 2 vol. sulfuric acid.
2. Buffer solution. Prepare in a glass-stoppered Pyrex bottle on which lines·have been marked, giving the volumes to which the solution is made. Dilute 118 gm. dibasic ammonium citrate and 75 ml. concentrated ammonium hydroxide to 250 ml. with distilled water. Add 5 gm. potassium cyanide (CAUTION!) and 2.5 gm. sodium sulfite. Extract with small volumes (2-3 ml.) of dithizone in chloroform (30 mg./L.) until the dithizone layer stays green. Add chloroform solution to bottle, stopper, and shake. Allow chloroform to settle and then remove by suction with the aid of a drawn-out glass tube extending to the bottom of the solution. After the extraction, add 500 ml. ammonium hydroxide solution.
3. Wash reagent. Dilute 5 gm. potassium cyanide and 250 ml. ammonium hydroxide with distilled water to 500 ml.
4. Phenol red. Dissolve 0.1 gm. phenol red in water to make 100 ml.
5. Perchloric acid (70%), reagent grade.
6. Dithizone solution. Dissolve 30 mg. dithizone (Eastman No. 3092, di-phenylthiocarbazone) in 1 L. of reagent grade chloroform.
7. Standards:
   A. Stock standard. Dissolve 366 mg. lead acetate (Pb($C_2H_3O_2$)$_2$ · $3H_2O$) in about 500 ml. distilled water; if necessary add glacial acetic acid drop by drop to obtain complete solution and then dilute to 1 L. Use only fresh crystals of the salt. This solution contains 0.2 mg. lead/ml.
   B. Working standard. Dilute 1 ml. stock standard to 100 ml. with distilled water. This solution contains 2 μg lead/ml.

Special apparatus: It is convenient to use special digestion tubes. Attach a 24/40 female standard taper joint giving an overall length of about 260 mm. to regular 25 × 200 mm. NPN digestion tubes. These tubes are fitted with standard glass stoppers to fit the joints. If these tubes are used, the digestion and extraction can be carried out in one tube, avoiding errors and the greater chance of contamination due to transfers of solutions. All glassware used for the digestion and extraction must be thoroughly cleaned and rinsed with dilute (1:3) nitric acid and then rinsed well with distilled water before use. The digestion can be carried out in 100 ml. Kjeldahl flasks and the extraction in 60 ml. separatory funnels, but there is a much greater chance of contamination.

Procedure: Add 2 ml. blood or 10 ml. urine to digestion tube. Add 5 ml. of the digestion reagent and a few glass beads. For a reagent blank, treat 5 ml. water exactly as the sample and carry it through all steps of the procedure. Digest over a microburner until thin white fumes fill the tube. Heat cautiously at first to avoid foaming. Allow to cool and add 20 drops 70% perchloric acid. Heat again through the following stages: yellow, colorless, yellow with frothing, colorless, and clear. Cool. (Keep digestion tube covered with a 50 ml. beaker whenever possible.)

Add 5 ml. water and mix by swirling. Add 4 ml. concentrated ammonium hydroxide and 1 drop phenol red solution. Cool and mix by swirling. If red color disappears, add more ammonia drop by drop with mixing until solution remains red. Add 10 ml. buffer solution (if digestion was carried out in Kjeldahl flasks, use the buffer solution to aid in quantitative transfer of digested solution to separatory funnel). Add 5 ml. dithizone solution, stopper, and shake hard. If dithizone layer is colored red at this point, add 5 ml. more of the dithizone reagent and shake again. In this case double the OD reading to obtain the correct value.

Draw off as much of the upper aqueous layer as possible with the aid of suction and wash by shaking with 10 ml. wash reagent. Remove as much of the aqueous layer as possible by suction. Pour into a colorimeter tube, stopper, and let stand until clear. Read in photometer at 510 nm., setting to zero with a chloroform blank. Subtract OD of reagent blank from that for samples.

Run standards by adding the following to digestion tubes: 4 ml. water to one tube, 2 ml. water and 2 ml. working standard (4 μg lead) to a second tube, and 4 ml. working standard (8 μg lead) to a third tube. To each tube add 10 ml. buffer and 5 ml. dithizone solution. Shake, remove aqueous layer, and wash as in sample procedure. Read in photometer at 510 nm., setting to zero with standard blank. Calculate K for standards.

$$\text{Mg. lead/100 ml.} = \frac{K \times OD \times 100}{\text{Ml. sample used}}$$

Normal values and interpretation: Most of the lead in blood is in the erythrocytes, and whole blood is more satisfactory for analysis than serum. The average value is 0.03 mg./100 ml. blood (0.0-0.05 mg.). In lead poisoning the values have ranged from 0.06 mg./100 ml. up to 0.24 mg. or over. The upper limit of normal lead excretion is 0.08 mg./24 hr., and 0.1 mg./24 hr. indicates mild exposure but not poisoning. Most patients with lead poisoning excrete more than 0.15 mg./24 hr.

MERCURY[17-19]

Mercury compounds are used primarily as antiseptics, insecticides, and diuretics. In general, mercurous compounds are less lethal than mercuric compounds. Poisoning with mercury can occur after in-gestion, cutaneous application, rectal application, vaginal insertion, and even accidental intravenous injection of any of its compounds. All patients with mercury poisoning excrete mercury in the urine, but patients with symptoms rarely excrete less than 300 μg/24 hr.

In the following method the organic material is destroyed by heating with permanganate, and the mercury is extracted as the dithizone complex. Mercury is estimated by measuring the color of the dithizone solution before and after treatment with a reagent that destroys the mercury complex (this eliminates interference due to copper).

Reagents:
1. Sulfuric acid solution. Carefully add 1 vol. concentrated sulfuric acid to 2 vol. water.
2. Hydroxylamine hydrochloride (10%). Dissolve 10 gm. hydroxylamine hydrochloride in distilled water to make 100 ml.
3. Potassium permanganate, AR crystals.
4. Dithizone solution. Dissolve 5 mg. dithizone (diphenylthiocarbazone, Eastman No. 3092) in 1 L. chloroform. This solution should be kept in the refrigerator and is not stable for more than about 10 days.
5. Reversion solution. Dissolve 10.2 gm. potassium acid phthalate and 30 gm. potassium iodide in distilled water to make 500 ml. If necessary, a few drops of 5% sodium thiosulfate solution may be added to remove any free iodine. Shake the solution with several 10 ml. portions of the chloroform solution of dithizone, and discard the chloroform layer.
6. Diluting solution. Dilute 100 ml. sulfuric acid solution and 20 ml. hydroxylamine solution to 1 L.
7. Standards:
   A. Stock standard. Dissolve 1.354 gm. mercuric chloride in distilled water and dilute to 1 L.
   B. Working standard. Dilute 2 ml. stock standard to 100 ml. with distilled water. This solution contains 2 μg mercury/ml.

Procedure: Place an aliquot of urine (usually 25 ml.) in a 250 ml. flask and dilute to 50 ml. with distilled water. Add 10 ml. sulfuric acid solution and 1 gm. potassium permanganate. Fit with a reflux condenser and boil gently for 30 min. If the solution becomes decolorized during boiling, cool slightly, add 0.5 gm. more potassium permanganate, and continue boiling. If necessary, add more permanganate so that the permanganate color persists during the entire 30 min. of boiling. Cool the solution somewhat and add hydroxylamine hydrochloride solution drop by drop until the permanganate color disappears. Add 2 ml. more hydroxylamine solution and boil the mixture under reflux for 1 min. Then cool the solution and dilute to 100 ml. with distilled water. Shake a 25 ml. portion of this solution in a separatory funnel with 10 ml. of the dithizone solution. If the color of the chloroform layer indicates a low mercury content (color still green with very little brownish tinge), add the balance (75 ml.) of the digest and shake again. If the chloroform layer is green but with considerable brownish tinge, add 75 ml. diluting solution to the aqueous layer to make 100 ml. If the chloroform layer is almost clear orange, dilute a smaller aliquot of the digest to 100 ml. with the diluting solution and extract.

Allow the chloroform layer to separate completely and then filter through a small plug of cotton (inserted into the stem of the separatory funnel) into a photometer cuvette. Stopper the cuvette to avoid loss of chloroform by evaporation and read in photometer at 620 nm., setting to zero with chloroform as the blank. Refer to this OD reading as D_1. Transfer the solution to a small separatory funnel and shake with 10 ml. of the reversion solution. Again allow the chloroform layer to separate completely and filter through a plug of cotton into a cuvette. Read OD in the photometer (this reading is D_2). Calculate $D_2 - D_1$ value. Also set up a series of standards by adding 1, 2, 3, and 4 ml. working standard (2, 4, 6, and 8 μg of mercury, respectively) to 100 ml. diluting solution and carry through the extraction procedure using the dithizone and reversion solutions. Plot the $D_2 - D_1$ value for the standards against the amount of mercury in the standard. De-termine the amount of mercury in the sample aliquot from the curve, using the $D_2 - D_1$ value found for the sample; from this, calculate the amount of mercury in the total sample.

Normal values and interpretation: In normal individuals up to 6 μg mercury/ 100 ml. urine may be excreted. In patients with mercury poisoning or industrial exposure, larger amounts may be excreted; amounts up to 100 μg/100 ml. have been reported. Mercury is a cumulative poison, and traces may be found in the urine several months after exposure.

BARBITURATES[20-24]

Barbiturates are widely used medicinally as sedatives, hypnotics, and anesthetics and are among the most frequently encountered drugs in the field of toxicology. There are some 40 different barbiturates in use, listed under more than 150 different trade and pharmaceutical names. Barbiturate intoxication usually occurs after ingestion of the drug. Barbiturates are readily absorbed from the gastrointestinal tract, although the rate varies with individual compounds. In man, peak concentrations occur in the blood 3-12 hr. after ingestion, depending upon the compound used. Some of the barbiturates are largely excreted in the urine, whereas others are largely metabolized in the liver; some are partially excreted and partially metabolized. In general, the short-acting barbiturates are chiefly metabolized by the liver and the long-acting ones are excreted in the urine. Barbiturates are rather slowly eliminated from the body, and this may result in cumulative toxicity from continued large doses. In patients with impaired liver or kidney function, elimination may be still slower and cumulative poisoning is more likely to occur.

Because patients with barbiturate intoxication are often unconscious, detection of barbiturates in the blood and possible identification of the type of compound is helpful in treatment. No completely satisfactory colorimetric determination of barbiturates has been developed. Barbiturates can be determined and identified by ultraviolet spectroscopy; this requires a spectrophotometer capable of measuring wavelengths of 230-270 nm. Because such an instrument is not available in many laboratories, the method will not be described here.

The method described is a very simple and rapid colorimetric procedure that can be performed in any clinical laboratory. It has certain limitations in that not all barbiturates are detected equally well, but it is satisfactory for all screening purposes. The method is applicable to whole blood, plasma or serum, urine, gastric washings, or other fluids.

Reagents:
1. Chloroform, reagent grade.
2. Mercuric nitrate in phosphate buffer.
   Solution A: Add 0.2 ml. concentrated nitric acid to 1 gm. mercuric nitrate. Add water to make 50 ml.
   Solution B: Prepare a 0.15M phosphate buffer, pH 8.0, by dissolving 4.48 gm. anhydrous disodium phosphate (Na_2HPO_4) and 5.25 gm. monopotassium phosphate (KH_2PO_4) in water to make 500 ml. Check pH and adjust to 8.0 if necessary.
   Solution C: Mix 2 ml. of solution A with 50 ml. of solution B. Filter if turbid. This solution is stable at room temperature.
3. Diphenylcarbazone reagent. Dissolve 100 mg. *sym.*-diphenylcarbazone in 100 ml. chloroform. Allow to stand for a few days in the light to age. Transfer to a brown bottle and store in the refrigerator. This reagent is stable for several months.
4. Sulfuric acid (2N). Dilute 56 ml. concentrated sulfuric acid to 1 L.
5. Standards:
   A. Stock standard. Dissolve 50 mg. secobarbital sodium in water and dilute to 100 ml. in a volumetric flask. This contains 50 mg.% barbiturate. Store in refrigerator.
   B. Working standard. Dilute stock standard 1:10 and 1:5 to obtain 5 and 10 mg.% standards as needed.

Procedure: Place 1 ml. of sample in a 15-20 ml. glass-stoppered tube. Add 1 ml. water to one tube as a blank and 1 ml. standards to additional tubes. To each tube add 2 drops 2N sulfuric acid and 10 ml. chloroform. Stopper tightly and shake vigorously for 15 sec. Allow to stand for a few minutes for separation of the two phases. Withdraw and discard most of the upper aqueous phase with a disposable capillary pipette, and filter the chloroform layer through a 9 cm. piece of Whatman No. 31 filter paper into a clean tube. Add 1 ml. buffered mercuric nitrate to the filtered chloroform. Stopper and shake vigorously for 15 sec. Allow layers to separate, and remove and discard upper aqueous phase. Filter chloroform through Whatman No. 31 filter paper into a third tube. Pipette 5 ml. filtered chloroform from the second extraction to a dry cuvette. Add 1 ml. diphenylcarbazone solution, mix, and allow to stand for a few minutes. Read sample and standards against blank at 550 nm.

Calculation:

$$\text{Mg.\% barbiturate (secobarbital)} = \frac{\text{OD sample}}{\text{OD standard}} \times \text{Conc. of standard}$$

The method is sensitive to 1 mg. or less of barbiturate/100 ml. It cannot be used to identify the barbiturate or classify it as long or short acting. It is quantitative only when the barbiturate being measured is known and is read against a similar standard. Interference occurs only from the hydantoins.

Different barbiturates produce different intensities of color. If the color formed by secobarbital is taken as 100%, the amounts of color produced by other commonly used barbiturates are amobarbital, about 87%; pentobarbital sodium, diallylbarbituric acid, butethal, and hexobarbital sodium, about 72%; cyclobarbital, aprobarbital, and phenobarbital, about 54%; and butabarbital sodium, vinbarbital, and mephobarbital, about 40%. Barbituric acid and probarbital give very little color.

BROMIDE[25, 26]

Bromide determinations in blood may be required in instances of bromide intoxication from an overdose of sedatives containing bromides. In this method the bromide in a protein-free filtrate is oxidized by hypochlorite to bromate. After removal of the excess hypochlorite with sodium formate, the bromate reacts with added potassium iodide to liberate iodine, which is determined colorimetrically.

Reagents:

1. Zinc sulfate and sodium hydroxide for preparing Somogyi filtrate (p. 298).
2. Hydrochloric acid. Dilute 189 ml. concentrated hydrochloric acid to 1 L. with distilled water.
3. Calcium hypochlorite solution. Dissolve 15 gm. calcium hypochlorite (purified, 70% available chlorine) as completely as possible in 100 ml. distilled water and filter. Dilute 1 vol. filtrate with 3 vol. distilled water.
4. Calcium carbonate, powdered, reagent grade.
5. Sodium formate (20%). Dissolve 20 gm. sodium formate in distilled water to make 100 ml.
6. Potassium iodide solution. Dissolve 10 gm. potassium iodide in distilled water to make 100 ml.
7. Stock bromide standard. Dissolve 1.288 gm. sodium bromide or 1.489 gm. potassium bromide that has been dried for several hours at 110° C. in distilled water and dilute to 1 L. This solution contains 1 mg. bromide/ml.

Procedure: Prepare a 1:10 Somogyi filtrate from 1 ml. blood (p. 298). Set up a number of test tubes graduated at 10 ml. In one tube place 5 ml. blood filtrate and in a second tube place 1 ml. filtrate and 4 ml. distilled water. (Since the normal concentration of bromide is low and that in bromide poisoning is high, it is well to set up two different concentrations of the sample to allow for these possibilities.) Prepare a working standard by diluting 5 ml. stock standard to 100 ml. Pipette 1, 2, and 3 ml. working standard to test tubes and add distilled water to make 5 ml. These standards contain 0.05, 0.10, and 0.15 mg. bromide. Also add 5 ml. distilled water to another tube as a blank. To each tube, blank, standards, and samples add 0.3 ml. 2N hydrochloric acid and a pinch of calcium carbonate. There should be a slight excess of carbonate, as shown by a slight precipitate remaining in the tube. To each tube add 1 ml. calcium hypochlorite solution, mix, and heat in a briskly boiling water bath for 8 min. Remove from the bath, cool somewhat, and add 0.5 ml. 20% sodium formate solution. Mix and heat again in a boiling water bath for 8 min. Cool, add 3 ml. 2N hydrochloric acid to each tube, dilute to 10 ml., and mix. Add 1 ml. potassium iodide to each tube and read after 10 min. in a photometer at 420 nm., setting to zero with the reagent blank and timing the readings so that each is taken exactly 10 min. after the iodide is added.

Calculation: Calculate the K for the standards (p. 288). Then:

$$\text{Mg.\% bromide} = \text{OD} \times \text{K} \times \frac{\text{Dilution of blood}}{\text{Ml. aliquot taken}} \times 100$$

Method of Wuth: In this method proteins are precipitated with trichloroacetic acid, and the bromide in the filtrate is estimated by the brown color formed with the addition of gold chloride.

Reagents:

1. Trichloroacetic acid (10%). Dissolve 100 gm. TCA in water and dilute to 1000 ml.
2. Gold chloride (0.5%). Dissolve 0.5 gm. gold chloride ($AuCl_3,HCl,3H_2O$) in water and dilute to 100 ml.
3. Bromide standards:
   A. Stock standard. The same as for previous method.
   B. Working standard (0.2 mg./ml.). Dilute 10 ml. stock standard to 50 ml. with 10% TCA.

Procedure: To 8 ml. TCA add slowly and with constant swirling 2 ml. serum or working standard. Mix thoroughly and allow to stand for 10 min. Centrifuge and filter supernatant. Pipette 5 ml. filtrates (unknowns and standard) and 5 ml. 10% TCA (blank). Add 1 ml. gold chloride, mix, and let stand 5 min. Read in photometer at 440 nm. against blank.

Calculation:

$$\frac{\text{OD unknown}}{\text{OD standard}} \times 40 = \text{Mg.\% bromide}$$

Normal values and interpretation: Normally the bromide concentration of the blood is very low (under 3 mg.%).

Symptoms of bromide intoxication begin to appear when the concentration reaches 80-150 mg.%, there being considerable individual variation. With increasing bromide concentration, the symptoms become increasingly severe, and with values over 250 mg.% the patient may be demented.

SULFONAMIDES[27]

Some of these drugs (sulfanilamide, sulfapyridine, sulfathiazole, sulfamerazine, and sulfadiazine) are absorbed rapidly and appear in the blood, urine, and body fluids both in the free forms and conjugated with the acetyl radical, the proportion varying with each drug. The conjugated portion has a close relationship to the occurrence of toxic symptoms. The concentration of sulfadiazine in cerebrospinal fluid is about 70% of that in blood. The optimum blood concentration of the free (active) form of sulfanilamide is 7-10 mg./100 ml.; of sulfapyridine or sulfathiazole, 4-6 mg./100 ml.; of sulfadiazine, 8-12 mg./100 ml. and of sulfamerazine, 10-15 mg./100 ml. The optimum concentration of sulfanilamide in the urine is 50-100 mg./100 ml.

The drugs are excreted almost entirely by the kidneys and are retained in renal impairment. The conjugated form is less soluble (except sulfadiazine and sulfamerazine) and tends to crystallize out in the urinary tract, forming calculi.

Other sulfonamides (phthalylsulfathiazole, sulfaguanidine, and succinylsulfathiazole) are absorbed to a much less extent and are used as bacteriostatic agents in the intestinal tract. The blood level rarely exceeds 4-5 mg. sulfaguanidine, 0.1-1.5 mg. phthalylsulfathiazole, or 1-2 mg. succinylsulfathiazole per 100 ml.

Method of determination of sulfonamides: The procedure is the same for all of the sulfonamides. The sulfonamides react with sodium nitrite in acid solution to form a diazotized compound that couples with a naphthylamine to produce a purple-red color.

Reagents:
1. Trichloroacetic acid solution. Dissolve 15 gm. trichloroacetic acid in distilled water and dilute to 100 ml.
2. Sodium nitrite. Dissolve 0.1 gm. sodium nitrite in 100 ml. distilled water. This should preferably be prepared fresh as needed, though it will keep for a few days in the refrigerator.
3. Coupling reagent. Dissolve 100 mg. N-(1-naphthyl)ethylenediamine dihydrochloride (Eastman No. 4835) in 100 ml. distilled water. Store in a dark bottle in the refrigerator.
4. Hydrochloric acid solution (4N). Dilute 40 ml. concentrated hydrochloric acid to 100 ml. with distilled water.
5. Ammonium sulfamate solution. Dissolve 0.5 gm. ammonium sulfamate in 100 ml. distilled water.
6. Standards: In theory a separate standard should be made up for each sulfonamide, using as standard the substance being determined, e.g., a sulfanilamide standard for sulfanilamide determinations, a sulfaguanidine standard for sulfaguanidine determinations, etc. Because of the large number of different sulfonamides in use, it is usually not worth while to do this. One sulfonamide standard can be used for all determinations, with the use of an appropriate factor. If most of the determinations are to be one particular sulfonamide, this one can be used as a standard. Since the molecular weights of sulfapyridine, sulfadiazine, and sulfamerazine are close together, it may be most convenient to use one of these as a standard.
   A. Stock standard. Dissolve 100 mg. sulfonamide in about 800 ml. water with the aid of gentle heating. Cool and dilute to 1000 ml. This solution contains 0.1 mg. sulfonamide/ml.
   B. Working standard. Dilute 50 ml. stock standard and 200 ml. 15% trichloroacetic acid to 1000 ml. with water. This solution contains 0.005 mg. sulfonamide/ml.

Procedure for blood (free form): Into a 50 ml. flask put 15 ml. distilled water and slowly add 1 ml. oxalated blood. Let stand 2-3 min. until laked. Add 4 ml. 15% trichloroacetic acid solution while shaking. Let stand 15 min. and filter. Transfer 10 ml. filtrate to a 50 ml. Erlenmeyer flask or test tube. Also make up a blank from 10 ml. distilled water and two standards, one with 5 ml. stock standard and 5 ml. distilled water (0.025 mg. sulfonamide) and one with 10 ml. stock standard (0.050 mg.) To each tube or flask add 1 ml. sodium nitrite solution, mix, and let stand 3 min. Add 1 ml. sulfamate solution, mix, and let stand 2 min. Add 1 ml. coupling reagent, mix, and let stand 10 min. Read in photometer at 540 nm., setting to zero with blank tube.

Calculations: Calculate the K for the standards (p. 288). Then:

$$\text{Mg.\% sulfonamide} = K \times OD \times \frac{\text{Dilution of blood}}{\text{Aliquot filtrate}} \times 100 \times F$$

or for the proportions used above:

$$\text{Mg.\% sulfonamide} = K \times OD \times 200 \times F$$

where F is the factor for the sulfonamide if the standard and the sample are not the same drug. The values for F are given in Table 15-2. The factors for other compounds can be determined from their molecular weight as follows:

$$F = \frac{\text{Mol. wt. drug}}{\text{Mol. wt. standard}}$$

For example, if sulfadiazine is used as

the standard and Gantrisin is being determined, $F = \frac{267.3}{250.2}$. When the same compound is being determined as is used in the standard, the factor is 1. Some of the sulfonamide exists in the blood in conjugated form. Since the free form is the active compound, estimations of the conjugated form are of little clinical significance.

Procedure for cerebrospinal fluid: This procedure is the same as that for blood. When the concentration of sulfonamide is low, it is best to use 14 ml. water and 2 ml. cerebrospinal fluid (giving a 1:10 dilution).

Procedure for urine: Make accurate and appropriate dilutions of the urine. For sulfanilamide, sulfapyridine, sulfathiazole, sulfamerazine, and sulfadiazine it is usually 1:100; for sulfaguanidine and succinylsulfathiazole, 1:5. Make a trichloroacetic acid filtrate of the diluted urine and proceed as for blood. The calculations are the same as for blood except that the results must be multiplied by the original dilution of the urine.

NOTE: Procaine (Novocain) gives the same color reaction as the sulfonamides and should not be used as an anesthetic. Use piperocaine (Metycaine) or dibucaine (Nupercaine), which do not give the reaction.

Phenobarbital gives a positive reaction. In amounts usually present in urine the reaction is delayed.

Table 15-2. Conversion factors* (theoretical)

	Sulfa-nilamide	Sulfa-pyridine	Sulfa-thiazole	Sulfa-diazine	Sulfa-merazine	Succinyl-sulfa-thiazole
Molecular weight	172.14	249.17	255.22	250.17	264.30	355.00
Standards						
Sulfanilamide		1.45	1.48	1.45	1.54	2.06
Sulfapyridine	0.69		1.02	1.00	1.06	1.42
Sulfathiazole	0.68	0.98		0.98	1.04	1.39
Sulfadiazine	0.69	1.00	1.02		1.06	1.42
Sulfamerazine	0.65	0.94	0.97	0.95		1.34
Succinylsulfathiazole	0.48	0.70	0.72	0.70	0.74	

*When one sulfonamide is used as a standard in determining another one, multiply by the factor given. The factors for sulfaguanidine may be determined from its anhydrous molecular weight of 214.24. For phthalylsulfathiazole, the molecular weight is 403.42, for Gantrisin, 267.30, and for sulfacetimide, 214.

Indole also gives the reaction.

Carinamide does not give the reaction directly but will do so after being broken down, as in the test for conjugated sulfonamides.

Other substances that give a positive test are aniline, benzidine, hydrazine, naphthylamine, orthotoluidine, *p*-dimethylaminobenzaldehyde, *p*-aminobenzoic acid, sulfanilic acid, benzocaine, Larocaine, and tetracaine (Pontocaine).

Cocaine and Halocaine give negative reactions.

A false positive reaction is obtained if the nitrous acid formed is not neutralized by sufficient ammonium sulfamate solution. Care should be taken to measure accurately the nitrite and sulfamate solutions.

MORPHINE[28]

Morphine is used primarily as an analgesic and sedative. Like the other opium alkaloids, it is readily absorbed from the gastrointestinal tract; however, it is two to four times as toxic when given parenterally. Morphine disappears from the blood fairly rapidly and is excreted in the urine and feces. The quantitative determination of morphine in biologic materials offers considerable difficulties. The following method for the qualitative detection of morphine in urine may be of value in instances of suspected morphine intoxication.

Reagents:

1. Concentrated hydrochloric acid, reagent grade.
2. Sodium hydroxide (50%). Dissolve 10 gm. sodium hydroxide in 10 ml. distilled water.
3. Extraction solvent. Mix together 8 vol. reagent grade chloroform and 2 vol. reagent grade isobutanol.
4. Sodium carbonate, reagent grade, anhydrous powder.
5. Sodium phosphate solution. Dissolve 9.47 gm. anhydrous dibasic sodium phosphate (Na_2HPO_4) in distilled water to make 1 L.
6. Sodium hydroxide (0.5N). Dissolve 10 gm. sodium hydroxide in distilled water to make 1 L.
7. Concentrated phosphoric acid (85%), reagent grade.
8. Ammoniacal silver nitrate. Dissolve 10 gm. silver nitrate in 100 ml. distilled water. Add concentrated ammonium hydroxide drop by drop until the precipitate first formed just redissolves. Then add concentrated phosphoric acid drop by drop to a pH of about 8.5 (test paper). Again add concentrated ammonium hydroxide drop by drop until the precipitate just dissolves.

Procedure: Add 5 ml. concentrated hydrochloric acid to 50 ml. urine and autoclave at 15 lb. pressure for 30 min. Cool and add 2 ml. 50% sodium hydroxide solution and an excess of sodium carbonate anhydrous powder until the pH is approximately 8.5. Extract in a separatory funnel with 250 ml. extraction solvent. Discard the aqueous layer and wash the solvent layer by shaking with 50 ml. sodium phosphate solution; discard the aqueous layer. Extract the solvent layer with 25 ml. 0.5N sodium hydroxide solution and discard the solvent layer. Add 1 ml. concentrated phosphoric acid to the alkaline solution and then add sodium carbonate anhydrous powder until the pH is about 8.5. Add 2 ml. ammoniacal silver nitrate solution. Extract with 125 ml. extraction solvent and discard the aqueous layer. Wash the solvent layer with 25 ml. sodium phosphate solution. Filter the solvent layer through double-fast filter paper and evaporate to dryness on a steam bath.

Transfer small portions of the residue to a spot plate and apply the color reagents given below. Add 1 drop reagent to the residue, mix with a small stirring rod, and note the colors formed. Compare the colors with those from a small amount of actual morphine.

Froehde reagent: Dissolve by gently heating 50 ml. sodium molybdate in 10 ml. concentrated sulfuric acid. Make up fresh as needed. This reagent gives a violet color, changing to green to brown-red to blue.

Marquis reagent: Add 2 or 3 drops 40% formaldehyde solution to 3 ml. concentrated sulfuric acid. Prepare fresh as needed. This reagent gives a peach-red color, changing to violet to blue-violet.

PARA-AMINOBENZOIC ACID[29]

Para-aminobenzoic acid has been used in the treatment of rickettsial diseases in which a blood level of 30-60 mg.% is desirable. It may be determined in blood by the method used for the sulfonamides. Prepare a 1:20 dilution of the blood as for sulfonamides. Because of the higher blood levels found, use an aliquot of 3 ml. filtrate plus 7 ml. distilled water. The procedure is the same as for blood. The sulfonamide standard can be used. Since the molecular weight of *p*-aminobenzoic acid is 137.1, the factor for a sulfanilamide standard is 0.80, and for a sulfapyridine or sulfathiazole standard the factor is 0.55.

Calculation:

$$Mg.\%\ PAB = K \times OD \times \frac{20}{3} \times 100 \times F$$

PARA-AMINOSALICYLIC ACID (PAS)[29]

This drug is used in the treatment of tuberculosis. It may be determined by the formation of an orange color with Ehrlich reagent.

Reagents:

1. Trichloroacetic acid solution (7.5%). Dissolve 75 gm. trichloroacetic acid in distilled water to make 1000 ml.
2. Sodium hydroxide (1N).
3. Hydrochloric acid (1N).
4. Ehrlich reagent. Dissolve 3 gm. *p*-dimethylaminobenzaldehyde (Eastman No. 95) in 7 ml. sulfuric acid and dilute to 1 L. with distilled water.
5. Standards:
   A. Stock standard. Dissolve 100 mg. *p*-aminosalicyclic acid in 7.5% trichloroacetic acid to make 100 ml.
   B. Working standard. Dilute 1 ml. stock standard to 200 ml. with 7.5% trichloroacetic acid. This solution contains 0.005 mg./ml. *p*-aminosalicylic acid.

Procedure for blood: Add 0.5 ml. blood to 9.5 ml. 7.5% trichloroacetic acid in a centrifuge tube. Mix, allow to stand for a few minutes, and centrifuge. To 2 ml. clear supernatant add 0.5 ml. 1N sodium hydroxide, 1 ml. water, and 1 ml. Ehrlich reagent and mix. Set up a blank using 2 ml. 7.5% trichloroacetic acid instead of the sample and two standards, one with 1 ml. working standard plus 1 ml. 7.5% trichloroacetic acid (0.005 mg.) and one with 2 ml. working standard (0.010 mg.). Treat exactly the same as sample aliquots. If the photometer requires larger volumes of solution, one may use double quantities of all solutions (filtrates, standards, and reagents). Read in photometer at 470 nm., setting to zero with blank.

Calculations: Calculate the K for the standards. Then:

$$Mg.\%\ PAS = K \times OD \times \frac{Dilution\ of\ filtrate}{Aliquot\ taken} \times 100$$

or for the aliquots just given:

$$Mg.\%\ PAS = K \times OD \times \frac{20}{2} \times 100 = K \times OD \times 1000$$

Normal values: Therapeutic blood levels are in the range of from 4-8 mg.%.

Procedure for urine: Dilute the urine 1:500 with distilled water. In a graduated tube place 1 ml. diluted urine and 3 ml. 1N hydrochloric acid. Prepare a working standard by diluting 1 ml. stock standard to 100 ml. with 7.5% trichloroacetic acid. To one standard tube add 1 ml. standard (0.01 mg.) and 1 ml. trichloroacetic acid solution; to the other standard tube add 2 ml. standard (0.02 mg.). Also prepare a blank from 2 ml. 7.5% trichloroacetic acid. To each standard tube and blank add 2 ml. 1N hydrochloric acid. Heat standards and samples in a boiling water bath for 30 min. Cool and make up to 4 ml. with water. To the sample tubes add 3 ml. 1N sodium hydroxide, 1 ml. distilled water, and 2 ml. Ehrlich reagent. To the standard and blank tubes add 4 ml. 1N sodium hydroxide and 1 ml. Ehrlich reagent. Read in photometer, setting to zero with the blank tube.

Calculations: Calculate to the K for the standards. Then:

Gm. PAS/100 ml. urine $= K \times OD \times$

$$\frac{\text{Dilution of urine}}{\text{Aliquot taken}} \times \frac{100}{1000}$$

Since the standards are expressed in milligrams, for the dilution and aliquots used:

Gm. PAS/100 ml. urine $= K \times OD \times$

$$\frac{500}{1} \times \frac{1}{10} = K \times OD \times 50$$

Normal values: The amount excreted in the urine is usually between 70 and 80% of the ingested dose.

ISONIAZID[30]

Isoniazid (isonicotinic acid hydrazide) is used in the treatment of tuberculosis. The drug is readily absorbed by the digestive tract and is rather rapidly excreted by the kidneys. If it is desirable to determine the concentration of the drug in serum, the following method can be used. In this method the isoniazid reacts with a special reagent to give an orange color that is determined photometrically. The reaction is rather specific; the only common drug that interferes is nicotinamide.

Reagents:
1. Metaphosphoric acid (20%). Dissolve 20 gm. metaphosphoric acid in distilled water to make 100 ml.
2. Diammonium phosphate (16.5%). Dissolve 16.5 gm. diammonium phosphate $(NH_4)_2HPO_4$) in distilled water to make 100 ml.
3. Sodium pentacyanoamineferroate (0.2%). Since this material is not available commercially, prepare as follows. In a flask place 10 gm. finely powdered sodium nitroprusside and 32 ml. concentrated ammonium hydroxide. Mix to dissolve and allow to stand overnight in the refrigerator. Then add 100 ml. ethyl alcohol and mix. Filter off the yellow crystals using a Buechner funnel, wash with small portions of absolute methanol and ether, and then draw air through crystals until dry. Store crystals in desiccator. Dissolve 200 mg. crystals in distilled water containing 1.5 ml. concentrated ammonium hydroxide and dilute to 100 ml.

4. Standards:
   A. Stock standard. Dissolve 100 mg. isoniazid in 100 ml. water and store in the refrigerator. This solution contains 1 mg./ml. and is stable for about 1 wk.
   B. Working standard. Dilute 1 ml. stock standard to 100 ml. with distilled water. Prepare fresh as needed. The standard contains 0.01 mg./ml.

Procedure for serum: Mix 2 ml. serum with 4 ml. water in a centrifuge tube and add 2 ml. 20% metaphosphoric acid. Mix and allow to stand for 10 min. and centrifuge strongly. Pipette 4 ml. clear supernatant to another tube, add 1 ml. diammonium phosphate solution and 1 ml. pentacyanoaminoferroate solution, and mix. Also set up a blank containing 4 ml. water and two standards, one containing 2 ml. water and 2 ml. working standard (0.02 mg. isoniazid) and one containing 4 ml. working standard (0.04 mg. isoniazid), and treat the same as unknowns. Let stand 10 min. and read in photometer at 420 nm., setting to zero with blank.

Calculations: Calculate the K for the standards. Then:

$$\text{Mg.\% isoniazid} = K \times OD \times \frac{\text{Vol. of filtrate}}{\text{Aliquot used}}$$

$$\times \frac{100}{\text{Ml. serum used}}$$

For the aliquots used, this reduces to:

$$\text{Mg.\% isoniazid} = K \times OD \times \frac{8}{4} \times \frac{100}{2}$$

$$= K \times OD \times 100$$

Procedure for cerebrospinal fluid: For cerebrospinal fluid use 4 ml. fluid plus 2 ml. water and 2 ml. metaphosphoric acid to make filtrate. The procedure is the same as for blood. The calculations are the same, allowing for the larger volume of cerebrospinal fluid used.

SALICYLATES[31]

In the treatment of rheumatic fever with salicylates it has been suggested that a level of approximately 35 mg.% or more is necessary for adequate therapeutic effect. A daily dose of about 10 gm. sodium salicylate is required to maintain the optimum level. The peak blood level occurs 24-48 hr. after beginning of therapy. The drug is rapidly excreted by the kidneys, and usually very little remains in the plasma longer than 48 hr. after the drug is discontinued. The concentration of salicylates in the red cells is negligible; hence plasma or serum is used for analysis.

In the following method of analysis the salicylates are extracted from the plasma as salicylic acid with ethylene dichloride and are estimated by means of the purple color formed with ferric nitrate. The method is not suitable for quantitative estimation in urine because of interfering substances but could be used for a qualitative test.

Reagents:
1. Ethylene dichloride, reagent grade.
2. Hydrochloric acid (approximately 6N). Dilute 70 ml. concentrated hydrochloric acid to 1 L. with distilled water.
3. Ferric nitrate solution. Dissolve 1 gm. ferric nitrate and 0.5 ml. concentrated nitric acid in distilled water to make 100 ml.
4. Standards:
   A. Stock standard. Dissolve 0.580 gm. sodium salicylate in distilled water to make 250 ml. This solution contains 2 mg. salicylic acid/ ml. Store in refrigerator.
   B. Working standard. Dilute 20 ml. stock standard to 100 ml. with distilled water. This solution contains 0.4 mg./ml. salicylic acid.

Procedure: Place 2 ml. plasma or serum, 0.5 ml. 6N hydrochloric acid, and 30 ml. ethylene dichloride in a glass-stoppered bottle or flask of approximately 60 ml. capacity. Also prepare other bottles containing 1 ml. working standard (0.4 mg. salicylic acid) and 2 ml. working standard (0.8 mg.), adding the acid and ethylene dichloride to each. Stopper and shake vigorously for 5 min. by hand or preferably in a shaking machine. Transfer to centrifuge tubes and centrifuge for 5 min. for complete separation of the layers. Carefully pipette 20 ml. lower ethylene dichloride layer to dry glass-stoppered flask or bottle and add 10 ml.

water and 0.25 ml. ferric nitrate solution. Shake 5 min. Allow the layers to separate completely, centrifuge if necessary, and transfer the colored upper layer to a photometer cuvette. Read sample and standards at 540 nm., setting to zero with a blank consisting of 10 ml. water and 0.25 ml. ferric nitrate solution.

Calculation: Calculate the K for the standards.

$$\text{Mg.\% salicylic acid} = K \times OD \times \frac{100}{2}$$
$$= K \times OD \times 50$$

Method of Trinder[32]**:** This method is more rapid and requires a smaller amount of serum. It is very useful for quick and accurate determination of salicylate poisoning in children. A combined reagent containing mercuric chloride to precipitate the protein and ferric nitrate is used to form the color that is read directly in the supernatant after centrifugation.

Reagents:
1. Dissolve 40 gm. mercuric chloride in about 900 ml. water and add 10 ml. concentrated hydrochloric acid and 40 gm. ferric nitrate. Dissolve the salt and dilute to 1 L. Filter if turbid.
2. Standards:
   A. Stock standard. Use the same stock standard as in the previous procedure.
   B. Working standard. Dilute stock standard 1:10 to make a 20 mg.% working standard.

Procedure for serum or plasma: Add 1.8 ml. water to 0.2 ml. serum or plasma. Also prepare a blank with 2 ml. water and a standard with 0.2 ml. of the standard plus 1.8 ml. water. To each tube add 2 ml. of the reagent. Mix well and then centrifuge strongly. Decant clear supernatant and read samples and standard against blank at 540 nm.

Calculation: Since sample and standard have been treated similarly:

$$\frac{OD \text{ sample}}{OD \text{ standard}} \times 20 = \text{Mg.\% salicylate}$$

Procedure for urine: Treat the urine similar to serum, making a preliminary dilution of 1:5 with water. Another dilution may be required, depending upon the concentration of salicylate in the urine. Also prepare a blank by adding 0.2 ml. diluted urine to 2 ml. of the reagent; then add 1.6 ml. water and 0.2 ml. of 85% phosphoric acid. If centrifugation is necessary, centrifuge both the unknown and the blank. Read blank against water and subtract OD obtained from that of the urine sample. The calculations are the same as before, multiplied by any factor for the dilution of the urine.

PHENOTHIAZINE

Many of the tranquilizer drugs used are derivatives of phenothiazine (chlorpromazine, promazine, prochlorperazine, etc.), as are antihistaminics. The physician may wish to determine whether the patient has been taking one of these drugs. The following test is very simple to perform and indicates the presence or absence of the drug in the urine, together with a rough estimate of the amount being ingested. It is based on a color reaction with ferric chloride in the presence of acid and an oxidizing agent.

Reagent:
1. Dissolve 1 gm. ferric chloride in 250 ml. water. Add 100 ml. concentrated nitric acid and 50 ml. 70% perchloric acid.

Procedure: To 1 ml. urine add 1 ml. reagent, mix, and note the color that develops within 20 sec. A positive reaction is the development of a pink to violet color. A rough estimate of the amount of the drug ingested may be made. A 1+ color reaction gives a light yellowish pink and indicates an intake of approximately 5-20 mg./day; a 2+ reaction, a salmon pink, 20-70 mg./day; a 3+ reaction, light lavender, 70-120 mg./day; a 4+ reaction, a darker violet, over 120 mg./day. A color chart for this reaction is available in an article by Forrest and Forrest.[33]

REFERENCES

1. Dubowski, K. M., and Shupe, L. M.: Amer. J. Clin. Path. **22:**709, 1952.
2. Harger, R. H.: J. Lab. Clin. Med. **20:**746, 1935.
3. Shupe, L. M., and Dubowski, K. M.: Amer. J. Clin. Path. **22:**109, 1952.
4. Lundquist, F.: In Glick, D., editor: Methods of biochemical analysis, New York, 1959, Interscience Publishers, Inc., vol. 7, p. 217.
5. Winnick, T.: Industr. Engin. Chem. (anal. ed.) **14:**523, 1942.
6. MacLeod, L. D.: J. Biol. Chem. **181:**323, 1949.
7. Feldstein, M., and Klendshoj, N. C.: J. Forensic Sci. **2:**39, 1957.
8. Gettler, A. O.: Amer. J. Clin. Path. **2:**76, 1939.
9. Helwig, C. A.: Amer. J. Clin. Path. **13:**96, 1943.
10. Gettler, A. O., and Kaye, S.: J. Lab. Clin. Med. **35:**146, 1950.
11. Kaye, S., and Goldbaum, L. R.: In Gradwohl, R. H. B.: Legal medicine, St. Louis, 1954, The C. V. Mosby Co.
12. Gettler, A. O., and Freimuth, H. C.: Amer. J. Clin. Path. **7:**79, 1942.
13. Harper, P. V.: J. Lab. Clin. Med. **40:**634, 1952.
14. Berniger, H., and Smith, R.: Clin. Chem. **5:**127, 1959.
15. Bessman, S. P., and Layne, E. C., Jr.: J. Lab. Clin. Med. **45:**159, 1955.
16. Kehoe, R. A., Homann, F. T., and Cholak, J.: J. Industr. Hyg. **15:**257, 1933.
17. Locket, S.: Clinical toxicology, St. Louis, 1957, The C. V. Mosby Co.
18. Hubbard, D. M.: Industr. Engin. Chem. (anal. ed.) **12:**768, 1946.
19. Gray, D. J. S.: Analyst **77:**436, 1952.
20. Goldbaum, R. L.: Ann. Chem. **24:**1604, 1952.
21. Broughton, P. G. M.: Biochem. J. **63:**207, 1956.
22. Walker, J. T., Fisher, R. S., and MacHugh, J.: Amer. J. Clin. Path. **18:**451, 1948.
23. Wallenius, G., Zaar, B., and Lausing, E.: Scand. J. Clin. Lab. Invest. **15:**252, 1963.
24. Baer, D. M.: Amer. J. Clin. Path. **44:**114, 1965.
25. Greenberg, R.: J. Lab. Clin. Med. **28:**779, 1943.
26. Frankel, S.: Lab. Dig. **22:**12, 1959.
27. Bratton, A. C., and Marshall, E. K.: J. Biol. Chem. **128:**537, 1939.
28. Kaye, S.: Handbook of emergency toxicology, ed. 2, Springfield, Ill., 1961, Charles C Thomas, Publisher.
29. Smalley, A. E.: Bull. Inst. M. Lab. Technol. **14:**109, 1949.
30. Scardi, V., and Bonavita, V.: Clin. Chem. **3:**728, 1957.
31. Brodie, B. B., Udenfriend, S., and Coburn, A. F.: J. Pharmacol. **80:**114, 1944.
32. Trinder, P.: Biochem. J. **57:**301, 1954.
33. Forrest, I. S., and Forrest, F. M.: Clin. Chem. **6:**11, 1960.

Chapter 16

Methods of tissue examination

All specimens delivered to the tissue laboratory from surgery must be adequately identified, e.g., patient, origin, date, surgeon, and clinical diagnosis. On arrival to the laboratory, each specimen is numbered and entered in an acquisition book. The assigned number identifies the specimen throughout all procedures. Identification and numbering of autopsy specimens is usually taken care of by the morgue attendant.

Work area: The handling of a large number of surgical specimens is aided by a specially designed stainless steel table situated close to a sink, microphone, light, and disposal unit (Fig. 16-1). It is equipped with two rubber belts that can be moved manually in either direction. The specimens to be described and examined are lined up on the belt closest to the pathologist. As he completes the description, examination, and sectioning of each specimen, he places it on the rear belt to move it away from the work area.

Bacteriologic workup: It is important that specimens which may require bacteriologic examination be sent to the laboratory in sterile containers without formalin. Using sterile technique, the surgeon should obtain specimens from lymph nodes or lungs, and material from abscesses, ulcers, sinus tract, and joints. Failure to do so may prevent a definitive diagnosis in some cases.

See Chapter 11 for handling of tissue specimens.

TECHNIQUE FOR PROCESSING TISSUES

There are several methods of processing tissue that can be used to assess variations in tissue patterns, e.g., frozen section technique, paraffin section technique, celloidin technique, electron microscopy, and, more recently, the application of electron microscopy techniques to light microscopy.

CRYOSTAT FROZEN SECTION TECHNIQUE

The open-top type of cold chamber microtome cryostat* allows preparation of thin frozen sections, which reach paraffin section quality with frozen section speed. The cryostat frozen section technique is useful in histochemistry, biochemistry, and immunochemistry because cellular structures and chemical substances are well preserved. The details of the technique are well described in the manual published by the American Society of Clinical Pathologists.[1]

Prefreezing with carbon dioxide or ethyl chloride[2] by using a special attachment to the cylinder (Quick-Freezing Device*) greatly speeds up the procedure.

PARAFFIN SECTION TECHNIQUE

This technique necessitates the following steps: fixation, dehydration, clearing, impregnation, blocking, embedding, section cutting, staining, and mounting. Calcified or ossified specimens have to be decalcified after adequate fixation.

Fixation

Adequate fixation is the most important step in tissue preparation. It is a step that cannot be retraced after the processing of the tissue is completed.

---

*International Equipment Co., Boston, Mass.

705

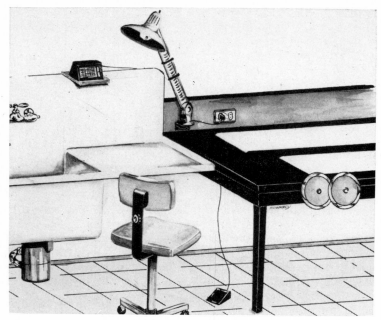

Fig. 16-1. Table for surgical pathology.

Specimens should be cut into thin (3 mm.) blocks and fixed as soon as possible after removal. The purpose of fixation is to prevent autolysis and putrefaction, to preserve the tissue details, to harden the tissues, to alter the refractive index of the various cell components so that they can be differentiated from each other, and to induce a mordant action with some stains. The agents employed as fixatives are formaldehyde (formalin), mercuric chloride, potassium dichromate, ethyl alcohol, etc., as well as various combinations of these (compound fixatives).

Fixatives:

Formaldehyde (formalin): Formaldehyde is a gas that is water soluble, about 40% by weight. It is used as a 10% solution.

Formalin:
1. Formaldehyde (40%), 10 ml.
2. Water, 90 ml.

Formalin is usually acid due to the formic acid content. It should be neutralized by covering the bottom of the container with calcium carbonate.

Zenker fluid:
1. Potassium dichromate, 2.5 gm.
2. Mercuric chloride, 5 gm.

3. Distilled water, 100 ml.

Just before using, add glacial acetic acid to each 20 ml. of solution.

Before staining the fixed tissue with alum hematoxylin, remove mercuric chloride by the following method.

Method for removing mercury:
1. Deparaffinize sections (see p. 709).
2. Place in alcoholic iodine (1 gm. iodine and 100 ml. 80% alcohol).
3. Rinse in tap water.
4. Place in 5% aqueous sodium thiosulfate solution ("hypo") for 5 min.
5. Wash in running tap water 10-20 min. and rinse in distilled water.

Decalcification

Bone specimens must be fixed before they are decalcified. There are several methods of decalcification: 5% nitric acid in distilled water, 5% formic acid in 5% formalin in distilled water, chelating agents, ion exchange resins, and electrolytic action.

Decal* is a commercial solution that, after fixation in formalin, provides rapid

---

*Scientific Products Co., American Hospital Supply Corp., Evanston, Ill.

(12 hr.) decalcification of most bone specimens.

Dehydration, clearing, impregnation, blocking, and embedding

The purpose of embedding media is to permit the cutting of thin sections. The media used are paraffin, celloidin, Carbowax (a water-soluble wax preparation), and plastics (e.g., epoxy resin).

Epoxy embedding: This method represents the application of electron microscopy techniques to light microscopy. Epoxy-embedded specimens can be examined by either light or electron microscopy. This form of embedding has the following advantages: (1) ultrathin sections ($1-8\mu$ thick) can be cut with mechanically driven heavy-duty instruments using hard-grade steel knives and (2) the sections allow superior resolution and are almost free of artefacts.

Resumé of technique[3]: The tissue blocks are fixed in phosphate-buffered 5% gluteraldehyde, cut to $2 \times 2 \times 0.1$ cm. size, and placed in 0.1N phosphate buffer for 12 hr. They are postfixed in 1% osmium tetroxide. The slices are dehydrated in a series of solutions of ethyl alcohol, infiltrated with Araldite, and embedded. The cut sections are floated on warm 1% gelatin on a glass slide, to which they become attached by drying and baking at 60° C. As some biologic stains do not react with epoxy-embedded tissue, the commercial polychromatic stain Paragon-1301* may be used as a rapid and satisfactory method of staining.[4]

Automatic tissue processor: This machine mechanically transfers the tissues from reagent to reagent by day and by night. It reduces the time required in each reagent by continuous agitation and by warming some of the reagents.

Paraffin wax embedding: Prior to embedding in wax, which is immiscible with water, the tissues have to be dehydrated by immersion in increasing strengths of ethyl alcohol. They are carried from 50 to 70, 90, and 100% alcohol. Following dehydration the sections have to be cleared in so-called clearing agents such as chloroform, benzine, xylene, etc. After clearing, the tissues are impregnated with paraffin wax heated to 45°-60° C. Following this step, the tissues are transferred from the final wax bath to a mold filled with liquid wax, which is then quickly cooled. This process is called blocking.

Embedding molds and embedding boxes, each consisting of two L-shaped pieces of cast lead and a baseplate, are available commercially.*

For embedding, the tissues must be thoroughly dehydrated and cleared. Some tissues are hardened considerably by alcohol and xylene. Another dehydrating agent, **dioxane** (diethylene dioxide), has been recommended as causing less hardening than the usual reagents. It is miscible in all proportions with water and alcohol and dissolves paraffin readily when heated but only slightly when cold. While it may be used directly from water, it is probably best to put the tissues through a mixture of dioxane and alcohol, equal parts, then in dioxane, and then in dioxane containing paraffin in the oven at about 40° C. before placing them in the paraffin bath.

Celloidin embedding:
1. Alcohol (95%), 24 hr. or longer.
2. Absolute alcohol, two changes, 24 hr. or longer.
3. Absolute alcohol and ether, equal parts, 24 hr. or longer.
4. Thin celloidin, 24 hr.-1 wk.
5. Thick celloidin, 24 hr.-1 wk.
6. Mount on blocks of vulcanized fiber, harden in chloroform for 1-2 hr., and place in 80% alcohol for 1 hr. or longer. The blocks may be kept permanently in 80% alcohol. Cut and stain.

Thick celloidin:
1. Dry celloidin, 30 gm.
2. Ether and absolute alcohol, mixture of equal parts, 450 ml.

Thin celloidin:
1. Thick celloidin, 100 ml.
2. Ether and absolute alcohol mixture, 100 ml.

Very thin celloidin: This is used for

---

*Paragon Co., New York, N. Y.

*Lipshaw Manufacturing Co., Detroit, Mich.

fixing sections on slide. Dissolve 0.75 gm. celloidin in 100 ml. alcohol-ether (equal parts).

Section cutting

Sections are cut by machines called microtomes. During the process of cutting the sections become somewhat compressed and have to be flattened out prior to their attachment to slides. The quality of the section depends to a great extent on the condition of the knife (Table 16-1). The knife should be 120 mm. long and have a 14-degree plane wedge cutting edge. The knife must be kept in good shape by honing (yellow Belgian water stone) and by stropping on a leather strap. Knife-sharpening machines are available commercially.

Trim the paraffin block containing the tissue so that the surface to be cut forms a rectangle. Set the paraffin microtome to cut sections 6-8μ. As sections are cut, they form a ribbon. Using a camel's hair brush and forceps, transfer the sections to a pan of warm water (40°-45° C., not hot enough to melt the paraffin). The sections should become flat and smooth on the surface of the water.

Separate sections with a heated scalpel (or tissue lifter), mount on slide with albumin fixative, drain, and place in a slide box in drying oven.

Preparation of microscopic sections on 35 mm. film[5, 6]

Paraffin sections of good quality are transferred onto 35 mm. plastic film and covered with a plastic spray. This method, which is excellent for serial sections, allows incorporation of the sections with the autopsy protocol and projection with a 35 mm. projector.

Staining

The various theories of staining are not uniformly accepted. The physical theory explains staining on the basis of adsorption, absorption, and solubility, whereas the chemical theory explains it on the basis of chemical union. Acid-reacting components of a cell combine with alkaline dyes, and alkaline areas react with acid

Table 16-1. Defects encountered in section cutting*

Defect	Cause
Block does not ribbon	Paraffin too hard; dull knife; knife angle wrong
Ribbon is curved	Knife edge not uniformly sharp; edges of block not parallel; knife not parallel to block
Sections compressed	Dull knife; soft paraffin; knife tilt to vertical; paraffin on knife edge; sections too thin
Ribbon tears and splits	Nicked knife edge; dirt or grit on knife edge or in block
Crumbling of sections	Incomplete fixation; dull knife; incomplete dehydration; paraffin too soft
Sections roll up	Dull knife; knife tilt too vertical
Sections adhere to knife	Paraffin on upper edge of block or on edge of knife; dull knife
Sections are alternately thick and thin	Knife loose; blocks too large; tilt of knife not sufficient to clear bevel; paraffin block too warm

*Modified from Manual of histologic and special staining technics, ed. 2, New York, 1960, McGraw-Hill Book Co.

dyes. Most fat stains are examples of staining based on the relatively greater solubility of the dye in fat than in the dye solvent.

DIAGNOSTIC STAINING PROCEDURES: Hematoxylin-eosin is the most commonly used stain. In recent years an attempt has been made to develop staining methods that are specific for certain substances of diagnostic importance. These staining procedures must be reliable, easily controlled, and applicable in the general laboratory. Such stains are available for lipids, organic substances such as iron and calcium, pigments such as melanin and hemoglobin, some amino acids such as tyrosine, nucleic acids, carbohydrates, and some enzymes.

Hematoxylin-eosin stain:
Solutions:
Harris hematoxylin solution:
1. Hematoxylin crystals, 5 gm.
2. Alcohol (95%), 50 ml.
3. Ammonium or potassium alum, 100 gm.
4. Distilled water, 1000 ml.
5. Mercuric oxide, 2.5 gm.

Dissolve the hematoxylin in the alcohol and the alum in the water by heating. Mix the two solutions. Bring the mixture to a boil as rapidly as possible; then remove from heat and add the mercuric oxide. Reheat the solution about 1 min. until it becomes dark purple, and promptly remove the container from the flame and plunge it into a basin of cold water. The solution is ready to use when cool.

The addition of 2-4 ml. glacial acetic acid/100 ml. stain improves the nuclear details. With van Gieson stain, omit the acid.

Ammonia water: Use 3 drops ammonia/1000 ml. water.

Staining procedure:
1. Xylene, 2 min.
2. Xylene, 2 min.
3. Absolute alcohol, 1 min.
4. Absolute alcohol, 1 min.
5. Alcohol (95%), 1 min.
6. Alcohol (95%), 1 min.
7. Alcohol (70%), 1 min.
8. Wash in tap water, 10 min.
9. Harris hematoxylin, 15 min.
10. Tap water, 4 dips.
11. Acid alcohol (1%), 4 dips.
12. Tap water, 4 dips.
13. Ammonia water, 4 dips (or until blue).
14. Distilled water, 15 min.
15. Eosin, 2 min.
16. Alcohol (95%), 1 min.
17. Alcohol (95%), 1 min.
18. Absolute alcohol, 1 min.
19. Absolute alcohol, 1 min.
20. Xylene, 2 min.
21. Xylene, 2 min.
22. Xylene, 2 min.
23. Drain on filter paper and mount in Permount* before drying.

---

*Fisher Scientific Co., St. Louis, Mo.

The **first 8 steps** of the procedure are listed in all other staining methods under one step—"deparaffinize."

The **last 8 steps** are referred to in all staining methods as "dehydrate, clear, and mount."

Results:
Nuclei—blue
Cytoplasm—pink

Defects in completed sections

Some defects will carry over from the cutting and floating processes, e.g., wrinkles, tears, etc. (Table 16-2).

Mounting

The purpose of mounting media is to preserve the specimen, to cement the cover slip to the slide, and to render the specimen transparent (high refractive index). Some media are water soluble (gum media), and others are not miscible with water (resinous media). One of the best artificial media is Permount.

STAINS FOR CONNECTIVE TISSUE

Connective tissue consists of mesenchymal cells (fibrocytes and fibroblasts) that are embedded in a ground substance which they enrich by the production of extracellular substances—collagen, elastin, and reticulin. The interfibrillar ground substance contains acid mucopolysaccharides in association with proteins. The tis-

Table 16-2

Defect	Cause
Sections have tendency to fall off slide	Albumin layer dissolved (usually by alkaline stain); paraffin lost in floating process
Sections are wavy	Sections of uneven thickness
Sections appear opaque	Insufficient clearing
Sections stain irregularly	Paraffin not completely removed; uneven thickness; inadequate fixation
Sections contain foreign pigment	Acid formalin; mercuric fixatives; not treated with iodine

sue mucopolysaccharides are hyaluronic acid, mucoitin-sulfuric acid, and chondroitin sulfuric acid. These polysaccharides can be oxidized with periodic acid to yield an aldehyde that gives a purple color with basic fuchsin (Hotchkiss, McManus, Schiff).

Connective tissue stains include Mallory phosphotungstic acid–hematoxylin stain, van Gieson stain, Masson trichrome stain, Wilder reticulum stain, periodic acid–Schiff stain, and Verhoeff elastic stain.

Mallory phosphotungstic acid–hematoxylin stain (PTAH)

Fixation: Fix tissue in Zenker fluid. If formalin-fixed tissue is used, mordant tissue in Zenker fluid for 1-12 hr. before embedding.

Solution:
1. Hematoxylin, 1 gm.
2. Phosphotungstic acid, 20 gm.
3. Distilled water, 1000 ml.

Dissolve the hematoxylin and the phosphotungstic acid separately in distilled water by gently heating. When cool, combine the solutions and make up to 1 L.

Add 5 ml. 1% potassium permanganate to ripen.

Staining procedure:
1. Deparaffinize sections. If fixed in Zenker fluid, remove mercuric chloride.
2. Stain with PTAH for 12-24 hr.
3. Differentiate in 95% alcohol and check under the microscope.
4. Absolute alcohol, 2 days.
5. Xylene, 2 days.
6. Mount in Permount.

Results:
Nuclei, fibroglia, myoglia, neuroglia, fibrin, and cross-striation of muscle fibers—blue
Collagen, reticulin, and ground substance of bone—yellow to brick red
Elastic fiber—purple

Van Gieson stain for collagen

Fixation: Fix tissue in 10% formalin.
Solutions:
Weigert iron hematoxylin solution: See procedure for Masson trichrome stain.

Van Gieson solution:
1. Acid fuchsin (1% aqueous solution), 2.5 ml.
2. Picric acid (saturated aqueous solution), 97.5 ml.

Staining procedure:
1. Deparaffinize sections.
2. Weigert iron hematoxylin solution, 10 min.
3. Wash in distilled water.
4. Counterstain with van Gieson stain, 1-3 min.
5. Alcohol (95%).
6. Absolute alcohol, two changes.
7. Xylene, two changes.
8. Mount in Permount. Add 3 drops saturated alcoholic picric acid for each 50 ml. of xylene used in clearing. Mount from acidified xylene.

Results:
Collagen—red
Muscle and cornified epithelium—yellow
Nuclei—blue to black

Masson trichrome stain[7, 8*]

Fixation: Fix tissue in Bouin solution or 10% formalin. Mordant sections of formalin-fixed material in Bouin solution for 1 hr. at 56° C. or overnight at room temperature.

Technique: Paraffin; cut sections at 6μ.
Solutions:
Bouin solution:
1. Picric acid (saturated aqueous solution), 75 ml.
2. Formaldehyde (37-40%), 25 ml.
3. Glacial acetic acid, 5 ml.

Weigert iron hematoxylin solution:
Solution A:
1. Hematoxylin, 1 gm.
2. Alcohol (95%), 100 ml.
Solution B:
1. Ferric chloride (aqueous, 29%), 4 ml.
2. Distilled water, 95 ml.
3. Concentrated hydrochloric acid, 1 ml.

Working solution: Mix equal parts of solution A and solution B.

---

*From Manual of histologic and special staining technics, ed. 2, New York, 1960, McGraw-Hill Book Co.

Biebrich scarlet-acid fuchsin solution:
1. Biebrich scarlet (aqueous, 1%), 90 ml.
2. Acid fuchsin (aqueous, 1%), 10 ml.
3. Glacial acetic acid, 1 ml.

Phosphomolybdic-phosphotungstic acid solution:
1. Phosphomolybdic acid, 5 gm.
2. Phosphotungstic acid, 5 gm.
3. Distilled water, 200 ml.

Aniline blue solution:
1. Aniline blue, 2.5 gm.
2. Acetic acid, 2 ml.
3. Distilled water, 100 ml.

Light green solution:
1. Light green, 5 gm.
2. Distilled water, 250 ml.
3. Glacial acetic acid, 2 ml.

Heat water, dissolve light green, cool, filter, and add acid.

Acetic water solution (1%):
1. Glacial acetic acid, 1 ml.
2. Distilled water, 100 ml.

Staining procedure:
1. Deparaffinize sections.
2. Mordant in Bouin fixative for 1 hr. at 56° C. or overnight at room temperature.
3. Cool and wash in running water until yellow color disappears.
4. Rinse in distilled water.
5. Weigert iron hematoxylin solution for 10 min. Wash in running water 10 min.
6. Rinse in distilled water.
7. Biebrich scarlet-acid fuchsin solution for 15 min. Save solution.
8. Rinse in distilled water.
9. Phosphomolybdic acid–phosphotungstic acid solution for 10-15 min. before aniline blue solution. Aqueous phosphotungstic acid (5%) for 15 min. before light green counterstain. Discard solution.
10. Aniline blue solution for 5-10 min. or light green solution for 1 min. Save solution.
11. Rinse in distilled water.
12. Acetic water 1% for 3-5 min. Discard solution.
13. Alcohol (95%).
14. Absolute alcohol, two changes.
15. Xylene, two changes.
16. Mount in Permount or balsam.

Results:
Nuclei—black
Cytoplasm, keratin, muscle fibers, and intercellular fibers—red
Collagen and mucus—blue

NOTE: For central nervous system (CNS) sections, change timing schedule as indicated in steps listed.
7. Biebrich scarlet-acid fuchsin solution for 1-2 min.
9. Phosphomolybdic acid–phosphotungstic acid solution for 10-30 min.
10. Aniline blue solution for 15-20 min.

Wilder reticulum stain[9]*

Fixation: Fix tissue in formalin, Zenker fluid, or Helly fluid.

Technique: Paraffin, celloidin, or frozen sections; cut sections at 6-10μ.

Solutions:
Phosphomolybdic acid solution:
1. Phosphomolybdic acid, 10 gm.
2. Distilled water, 100 ml.

Uranium nitrate solution:
1. Uranium nitrate, 1 gm.
2. Distilled water, 100 ml.

Ammoniacal silver solution: To 5 ml. 10.2% aqueous solution of silver nitrate add 28% ammonia water drop by drop until the precipitate that forms is almost dissolved. Add 5 ml. 3.1% sodium hydroxide and barely dissolve the resulting precipitate with a few drops of ammonia water. Make the solution up to 50 ml. with distilled water. Use at once. Glassware must be acid-clean.

Reducing solution:
1. Distilled water, 50 ml.
2. Neutral formaldehyde (40%), 0.5 ml.
3. Uranium nitrate (1% aqueous solution), 1.5 ml.

Make fresh just before use.

Gold chloride solution:
1. Gold chloride solution (1%), 10 ml. Break glass vial (15 gr.) in graduated cylinder with 100 ml. distilled water for 1% solution.

*From Manual of histologic and special staining technics, ed. 2, New York, 1960, McGraw-Hill Book Co.

2. Distilled water, 40 ml.
Sodium thiosulfate ("hypo") solution:
1. Sodium thiosulfate, 5 gm.
2. Distilled water, 100 ml.
Nuclear fast red (Kernechtrot) stain:
Dissolve 0.1 gm. nuclear fast red in 100 ml. 5% solution aluminum sulfate with aid of heat. Cool, filter, and add grain of thymol as a preservative.
Staining procedure:
1. Deparaffinize.
2. Remove mercury precipitates if fixed in Zenker fluid.
3. Wash well in distilled water.
4. Phosphomolybdic acid solution for 1 min. (oxidizer).
5. Rinse well in running water or cells will hold the yellow.
6. Dip in 1% aqueous uranium nitrate for 5 sec. or less (sensitizer).
7. Wash in distilled water for 10-20 sec.
8. Place in ammoniacal silver solution for 1 min.
9. Dip very quickly in 95% alcohol and place immediately into:
10. Reducing solution for 1 min.
11. Rinse well in distilled water.
12. Tone in gold chloride solution for 1 min. or until sections lose their yellow color and turn lavender. Too much toning will make sections red. Check individually under microscope.
13. Rinse in distilled water.
14. Place in 5% sodium thiosulfate solution for 1-5 min.
15. Wash well in tap water.
16. Counterstain, if necessary, with alum hematoxylin-eosin or nuclear fast red. Rinse well in distilled water.
17. Alcohol (95%).
18. Absolute alcohol, two changes.
19. Xylene, two changes.
20. Mount in Permount or balsam.
Results:
Reticulum fibers—black
Collagen—rose color
Other tissue elements—depends on counterstain used

Periodic acid–Schiff stain (PAS)

The Schiff reaction is based on the oxidation of glycol groups to aldehydes, which are replaced by organic radicals that in turn combine with acid to form the red color. Hematoxylin eosin–stained slides can be restained directly with periodic acid–Schiff stain.

Control: Diastase treatment of the slides removes glycogen.

Fixation: Fix tissue in 10% formalin or Zenker fluid.

Solutions:

Schiff leucofuchsin solution: Dissolve 1 gm. basic fuchsin in 200 ml. distilled water and bring to boiling point. Cool to 50° C. and filter. Add 20 ml. normal hydrochloric acid. Cool and add 1 gm. anhydrous sodium bisulfite. Allow to stand in dark for 48 hr. until solution becomes straw colored. Keep in brown bottle in refrigerator. A few drops of the reagent should rapidly turn 10 ml. 40% formaldehyde purple.

Periodic acid solution (0.5%):
1. Periodic acid crystals, 0.5 gm.
2. Distilled water, 100 ml.
Normal hydrochloric acid solution:
1. Concentrated hydrochloric acid, 83.5 ml.
2. Distilled water, 916.5 ml.
Light green counterstain stock solution (0.2%):
1. Light green crystals, 0.2 gm.
2. Distilled water, 100 ml.
3. Glacial acetic acid, 0.2 ml.
Light green working solution:
1. Light green stock solution, 10 ml.
2. Distilled water, 50 ml.
Staining procedure:
1. Deparaffinize.
2. Remove mercury if fixed in Zenker fluid.
3. Rinse in distilled water.
4. Periodic acid solution, 5 min.
5. Rinse in distilled water.
6. Schiff reagent, 15 min.
7. Wash with running water for 10 min. until pink.
8. Light green for 5 sec.
9. Alcohol (95%).
10. Absolute alcohol, two changes.
11. Xylene, two changes.
12. Mount in Permount.
Results:
Polysaccharides, mucopolysaccharides, glycoproteins, and glycolipids—pink
Mucin, hyaline, colloid, basement mem-

brane, amyloid, fungi, glycogen, Gaucher cells, megakaryocytes, and blast cells—Schiff positive
Nuclei—blue
Background—pale green

Verhoeff elastic tissue stain

Fixation: Fix tissue in 10% formalin.
Solutions:
Elastic tissue stain: Dissolve 1 gm. hematoxylin in 22 ml. absolute alcohol in a test tube with the aid of heat. Filter and add 8 ml. 10% aqueous solution of ferric chloride and 8 ml. iodine solution (2 gm. iodine and 4 gm. potassium iodide dissolved in 100 ml. distilled water).
Ferric chloride solution:
1. Ferric chloride, 2 gm.
2. Distilled water, 100 ml.
Van Gieson stain:
1. Acid fuchsin (1% aqueous solution), 5 ml.
2. Picric acid (saturated aqueous solution), 100 ml.
Sodium thiosulfate ("hypo") solution:
1. Sodium thiosulfate (5% aqueous solution).
Staining procedure:
1. Deparaffinize sections.
2. Verhoeff elastic tissue stain, 15 min.
3. Wash in distilled water.
4. Differentiate in 2% ferric chloride solution for a few seconds; examine under low-power lens for proper differentiation.
5. Sodium thiosulfate (5%), 1 min.
6. Wash in tap water for 5 min.
7. Counterstain in van Gieson stain, 1 min.
8. Differentiate in 95% alcohol.
9. Absolute alcohol, two changes.
10. Xylene, two changes.
11. Mount in Permount.
Results:
Elastic fibers—blue-black
Nuclei—blue-black
Collagen—red
Other tissues—yellow

STAINS FOR CELLULAR PRODUCTS

The most common intracellular products are fat, glycogen, mucin, and amyloid.

STAINS FOR FAT

Almost all lipids can be stained with the Sudan stains and oil red O stain, in which they are selectively soluble. Nile blue sulfate stain allows differentiation of neutral fats (which stain pink) from fatty acids (which stain blue to violet). Osmic acid identifies unsaturated fats.

Scarlet red (Sudan IV)—Herxheimer

Fixation: Fix tissue in 10% formalin.
Solutions:
Glycerin jelly:
1. Gelatin, 40 gm.
2. Water, 210 ml.
3. Glycerin, 250 ml.
4. Phenol crystals, 5 gm.
Soak gelatin in water, add glycerin and phenol, and warm until dissolved.
Scarlet red (Sudan IV) stain:
1. Alcohol (70%), 50 ml.
2. Acetone, 50 ml.
3. Scarlet red in excess.
Filter.
Staining procedure:
1. Wash thoroughly in water.
2. Freeze, cut, and place in water.
3. Dip in 50% alcohol and stain in scarlet red, 5-15 min.
4. Dip in 50% alcohol and transfer to water.
5. Stain in acid hematoxylin, 3-5 min.
6. Wash in water.
7. Dip in ammonia water (2 drops ammonia to 50 ml. water) until blue.
8. Wash in water.
9. Mount in glycerin jelly or Abopon,* a water-miscible mounting medium.
Results:
Fat—orange to red
Nuclei—blue

Nile blue sulfate stain

Fixation: Fix tissue in 10% formalin.
Solution:
1. Nile blue sulfate, 1.5 gm.
2. Distilled water, 100 ml.
Staining procedure:
1. Cut frozen sections and float in water.
2. Nile blue sulfate solution, 20 min.
3. Wash in tap water.

---

*Valnor Corp., Brooklyn, N. Y.

4. Differentiate in 1% acetic acid water until pink color is clear. Check under the microscope.
5. Wash well in distilled water.
6. Mount in Abopon or glycerin jelly.

Results:

Neutral fats—pink

Fatty acids—blue to violet

Nuclei and elastic tissue—dark blue

Osmium tetroxide stain for fat

Fixation: Fix tissue in 10% formalin.

Solution:

Osmic acid solution:

1. Osmium tetroxide, 1 gm.
2. Distilled water, 100 ml.

Staining procedure:

1. Cut frozen section and float in water.
2. Osmium tetroxide, 24 hr.
3. Water, several changes, 6-12 hr.
4. Absolute alcohol, 6 hr.
5. Wash in distilled water.
6. Mount in glycerin jelly or Abopon.

Results:

Fat—black

Background—yellow to brown

STAINS FOR CARBOHYDRATES AND MUCOPROTEINS (MUCIN)

In some phases of surgical pathology the demonstration of mucus within cells is of considerable importance in the classification of tumors. Most mucins contain several glycoproteins and can therefore be detected by stains for carbohydrates. Best carmine stain is specifically for glycogens. Other carbohydrate stains depend on (1) the oxidation of glycols to aldehydes, which are demonstrated with the Schiff stain; (2) the metachromasia of certain dyes such as toluidine blue; and (3) the carboxyl groups in carbohydrates, which can be stained with the PAS stain, colloidal iron stain,[10] Alcian blue stain, and Alcian green stain.[11] Solutions of ferric salts are selectively taken up by mucin and can be demonstrated by the ferrocyanide reaction. Mucicarmine is an empirical stain for mucin.

Mucin is usually divided into **connective tissue** and **epithelial mucins**. The connective tissue mucins should be stained with dyes reacting with the acidic groups of the carbohydrates, e.g., colloidal iron stain or Alcian blue. Toluidine blue metachromasia can also be used. The epithelial mucins are PAS positive, and as most of them also contain acidic groups, they can also be stained with Alcian blue or the colloidal iron stains. The PAS stain may be combined with Alcian blue to give superior results in the staining of epithelial mucin.[12]

Best carmine stain for glycogen[13]*

Fixation: Tissue must be fixed in absolute alcohol. Since glycogen is soluble in water, take the tissue directly from the fixative to the clearing agent and then to paraffin.

Technique: Paraffin; cut sections of 6μ.

Solutions:

Carmine stock solution:

1. Carmine, 2 gm.
2. Potassium carbonate, 1 gm.
3. Potassium chloride, 5 gm.
4. Distilled water, 60 ml.

Boil gently and cautiously for several minutes. Cook in open dish (evaporating dish). When cool, add 20 ml. strong ammonia water. Keep in refrigerator.

Carmine working solution:

1. Stock carmine solution, 10 ml.
2. Ammonia water (28%), 15 ml.
3. Methyl alcohol, 15 ml.

Differentiating solution:

1. Absolute alcohol, 20 ml.
2. Methyl alcohol, 10 ml.
3. Distilled water, 25 ml.

Staining procedure:

1. Deparaffinize sections.
2. Dip slides in very thin solution of celloidin and dry for a few seconds.
3. Place in water to harden for a few seconds.
4. Stain in Harris hematoxylin solution for 15 min.
5. Differentiate in acid alcohol. Allow the nuclei to remain slightly dark because ammonia slightly decolorizes them.
6. Place in working solution of carmine for 20-30 min. Carry a control slide for checking.

---

*From Manual of histologic and special staining technics, ed. 2, New York, 1960, McGraw-Hill Book Co.

7. Place in the differentiating solution for a few seconds.
8. Wash quickly in 80% alcohol.
9. Alcohol (95%).
10. Absolute alcohol, two changes.
11. Xylene, two changes.
12. Mount in Permount.

Results:
Glycogen—pink to red
Nuclei—blue

Mayer mucicarmine stain[13]*

Fixation: Any well-fixed tissue.
Technique: Paraffin; cut sections at 6μ.
Solutions:
Weigert iron hematoxylin solution:
Solution A:
1. Hematoxylin, 1 gm.
2. Alcohol (95%), 100 ml.
Solution B:
1. Ferric chloride (29% aqueous solution), 4 ml.
2. Distilled water, 95 ml.
3. Concentrated hydrochloric acid, 1 ml.

Working solution: Mix equal parts of solutions A and B. Prepare fresh.
Metanil yellow solution:
1. Metanil yellow, 0.25 gm.
2. Distilled water, 100 ml.
3. Glacial acetic acid, 0.25 ml.
Mucicarmine stain:
1. Carmine, 1 gm.
2. Aluminum chloride (anhydrous), 0.5 gm.
3. Distilled water, 2 ml.

Mix stain in small test tube. Heat over small flame for 2 min. Liquid becomes almost black and syrupy. Dilute 1:4 with tap water for use.
Staining procedure:
1. Deparaffinize sections. Remove mercury precipitates through iodine and "hypo" solutions if necessary.

NOTE: Use control slides.
2. Stain for 7 min. in working solution of Weigert iron hematoxylin.
3. Wash in tap water for 5-10 min.
4. Place in diluted mucicarmine solution for 30-60 min. or longer. Check

control slide with microscope after 30 min.
5. Rinse quickly in distilled water.
6. Stain in metanil yellow solution for 1 min.
7. Rinse quickly in distilled water.
8. Rinse quickly in 95% alcohol.
9. Dehydrate in two changes of absolute alcohol, clear with two or three changes of xylene, and mount in Permount.

Results:
Mucin—deep rose to red
Nuclei—black
Other tissue elements—yellow

Crystal violet amyloid stain[14]*

Fixation: Fix in formalin (10%) or alcohols.
Technique: Paraffin; cut sections at 6μ.
Solutions:
Crystal violet stock solution:
1. Crystal violet, to saturate, approximately 14 gm.
2. Alcohol (95%), 100 ml.
Crystal violet working solution:
1. Crystal violet stock solution, 10 ml.
2. Distilled water, 300 ml.
3. Concentrated hydrochloric acid, 1 ml.
Staining procedure:
1. Deparaffinize sections.
2. Stain in crystal violet working solution for 1-2 min. Use control slide. Check with microscope.
3. Rinse well in tap water.
4. Mount in Abopon.
5. Seal edges of cover slip with fingernail polish.

Results:
Amyloid—purple-violet
Other tissue elements—blue

STAINS FOR BACTERIA
Kinyoun acid-fast stain

Fixation: Fix tissue in 10% formalin.
Solutions:
Kinyoun carbolfuchsin solution:
1. Basic fuchsin, 4 gm.
2. Phenol crystals, melted, 8 ml.

---

*From Manual of histologic and special staining technics, ed. 2, New York, 1960, McGraw-Hill Book Co.

*From Manual of histologic and special staining technics, ed. 2, New York, 1960, McGraw-Hill Book Co.

3. Alcohol (95%), 20 ml.
4. Distilled water, 100 ml.
Acid-alcohol (1%):
1. Concentrated hydrochloric acid, 1 ml.
2. Alcohol (70%), 99 ml.
Methylene blue stock solution:
1. Methylene blue, 1.4 gm.
2. Alcohol (95%), 100 ml.
Methylene blue working solution:
1. Methylene blue stock solution, 10 ml.
2. Tap water, 90 ml.
Staining procedure:
1. Deparaffinize sections. Remove mercury precipitates through iodine and "hypo" solutions if necessary.
2. Kinyoun carbolfuchsin, 1 hr.
3. Wash well in tap water.
4. Differentiate in two changes of 1% acid-alcohol until tissue is pale pink.
5. Wash well in tap water.
6. Counterstain in methylene blue working solution for a few seconds.
7. Dehydrate, clear, and mount in Permount.
Results:
Acid-fast bacteria—bright red
Background—light blue

Levaditi method for staining spirochetes in blocks

Fixation: Fix blocks 1 mm. thick in 10% formalin.
Technique: Embed tissue in paraffin after staining is complete.
Solutions:
Silver nitrate solution:
1. Silver nitrate, 1.5-3 gm.
2. Distilled water, 100 ml.
The stronger solution of silver nitrate is preferable for biopsy specimens.
Reducing solution:
1. Pyrogallic acid, 4 gm.
2. Formalin, 5 ml.
3. Distilled water, 100 ml.
Staining procedure:
1. Rinse block of tissue in tap water.
2. Place in 95% alcohol for 24 hr.
3. Transfer to distilled water and leave until the tissue sinks to the bottom of the container.
4. Place in freshly prepared aqueous silver nitrate solution and keep at

35° C. in the dark for 3-5 days, changing the solution three times.
5. Wash in distilled water.
6. Place in reducing solution for 24-72 hr. at room temperature in the dark.
7. Wash in distilled water.
8. Dehydrate in 80%, 95%, and absolute alcohol.
9. Clear in oil of cedarwood.
10. Embed in paraffin in the usual manner.
11. Cut sections at 5μ and mount on slides.
12. When dry, remove the paraffin with xylene.
13. Mount in Permount.
Results:
Spirochetes—black
Background—yellow

MacCallum-Goodpasture stain for bacteria in tissue*

Fixation: Fix tissue in 10% formalin.
Technique: Paraffin; cut thin sections.
Solutions:
Goodpasture stain:
1. Basic fuchsin, 0.59 gm.
2. Aniline, 1 ml.
3. Phenol crystals (melted), 1 ml.
4. Alcohol (30%), 100 ml.
Gram iodine solution:
1. Iodine, 1 gm.
2. Potassium iodine, 2 gm.
3. Distilled water, 300 ml.
Stirling gentian violet stain:
1. Gentian violet (crystal violet), 5 gm.
2. Absolute alcohol, 10 ml.
3. Aniline, 2 ml.
4. Distilled water, 88 ml.
Saturated picric acid solution:
1. Picric acid, 1.18 gm.
2. Distilled water, 100 ml.
Staining procedure:
1. Deparaffinize sections.
2. Place in Goodpasture stain, 10 min.
3. Wash in distilled water.
4. Differentiate in full-strength formalin for a few minutes to fix the Goodpasture stain.
5. Wash in distilled water.

---

*From Manual of histologic and special staining technics, ed. 2, New York, 1960, McGraw-Hill Book Co.

6. Counterstain in saturated aqueous picric acid, 3-5 min.
7. Wash in water.
8. Differentiate in 95% alcohol.
9. Wash in water.
10. Stain in Stirling gentian violet solution, 3 min.
11. Wash in water.
12. Place in gram iodine solution, 1 min.
13. Rinse in water. Blot, but leave moist.
14. Place in a solution of equal parts aniline and xylene, several changes.
15. Xylene, two changes.
16. Mount in Permount.

Results:
Gram-positive organisms—blue
Gram-negative organisms—red
Other elements—various shades of red to purple

NEUROHISTOLOGY

The nervous tissue consists of two components: nerve cells (neurons) and neuroglia, the specialized connective tissue surrounding them. The nerve cells contain neurofibrils, Nissl substance, pigment, and other structures. They give rise to nerve fibers (axons) which are classified according to their coverings: (1) some fibers are without any covering, (2) some fibers are surrounded by a layer of flattened cells, and (3) some fibers are surrounded by a myelin (lipid) sheath and flattened cells.

The handling of nerve tissue (fixative, processing, and cutting) follows the outline given for routine tissues. The routine staining methods such as hematoxylin-eosin, Mallory PTAH, and the stains for fat are employed for other tissues.

Cresylecht violet solution for Nissl substance*

Fixation: Fix tissue in 10% formalin.
Technique: Use paraffin sections.
Solution:
Cresylecht violet solution (0.1%):
1. Cresylecht violet, 1 gm.
2. Distilled water, 1000 ml.

---

*From Manual of histologic and special staining technics, ed. 2, New York, 1960, McGraw-Hill Book Co.

3. Glacial acetic acid, 3 ml.
4. Sodium acetate, 0.205 gm.
Adjust pH to 3.5 before use.
Staining procedure:
1. Deparaffinize sections through two changes of xylene and absolute alcohol.
2. Leave slides in second change of absolute alcohol overnight at 30° C.
3. Stain with 0.1% cresylecht violet solution, 1-2 hr.
4. Differentiate rapidly in 95% alcohol in a flat dish until background is clear. Differentiation may be hastened by adding a few drops of glacial acetic acid to the alcohol.
5. Dehydrate in two changes of absolute alcohol, clear in xylene, and mount in Permount.

Results:
Nissl substance—intense purple
Nuclei—purple
Background—clear

Luxol fast blue–periodic acid Schiff–hematoxylin stain

Fixation: Fix tissue in 10% formalin.
Technique: Use paraffin or frozen sections.
Solutions:
Luxol fast blue solution (0.1%):
1. Luxol fast blue MBS,* 0.1 gm.
2. Alcohol, (95%), 100 ml.
Dissolve dye in alcohol. Add 5 ml. 10% acetic acid to each 1000 ml. solution. This solution is stable.
Lithium carbonate solution (0.05%):
1. Lithium carbonate, 0.05 gm.
2. Distilled water, 100 ml.
Schiff leucofuchsin solution: Bring 200 ml. distilled water to a boil, remove from flame, and when bubbling ceases add 1 gm. basic fuchsin and stir until dissolved. Cool to 50° C. and filter. Add 20 ml. 1N hydrochloric acid solution. Cool to 25° C. Add 1 gm. anhydrous sodium bisulfite. Keep in dark for 2 days at room temperature. Store in brown bottle in refrigerator. Stable for several months or until it turns pink.

---

*E. I. DuPont de Nemours & Co., Inc., Wilmington, Del.

Sulfurous acid solution:
1. Sodium metabisulfite (10% aqueous solution), 6 ml.
2. Hydrochloric acid (1N aqueous solution), 5 ml.
3. Distilled water, 100 ml.

Periodic acid solution (0.5%):
1. Periodic acid, 0.5 gm.
2. Distilled water, 100 ml.

Staining procedure:
1. Deparaffinize sections.
2. Place overnight in 0.1% Luxol fast blue solution in oven at 60° C.
3. Rinse off excess stain in 95% alcohol.
4. Rinse in distilled water.
5. Place in 0.05% lithium carbonate solution for a few seconds.
6. Differentiate in 70% alcohol, 20-30 sec.
7. Place in second solution of 0.05% lithium carbonate, 20-30 sec.
8. Differentiate in 70% alcohol.
9. Rinse in distilled water. If differentiation is incomplete, repeat steps 7 and 8.
10. Place in 0.5% periodic acid solution for 5 min.
11. Rinse in two changes of distilled water.
12. Place in Schiff solution, 15-30 min.
13. Place in three changes of sulfurous acid solution, 2 min. each.
14. Wash in tap water for 5 min.
15. Stain in Harris hematoxylin, 1 min.
16. Wash in tap water, 5 min. Differentiate briefly in acid alcohol; "blue" in tap water.
17. Dehydrate with two changes of 95% alcohol and absolute alcohol; clear with two to three changes of xylene, and mount in Permount.

Results:
Myelin—blue-green
Fungi and PAS-positive elements—rose to red
Nuclei—dark blue
Cytoplasmic nucleoproteins—bluish purple
Capillaries—red

STAINING OF FUNGI

Fungi contain various polysaccharides that can effectively be stained by the following methods: periodic acid-Schiff stain, Alcian blue stain, and toluidine blue O stain, which stains fungal elements metachromatically. The imperfect fungi, which contain a large amount of mucin, stain selectively with mucicarmine. Gomori methenamine silver stain is an excellent silver impregnation method for the demonstration of fungi in formalin-fixed tissue, irrespective of whether they are dead or active. Gridley stain, which gives good results, is a modified PAS procedure in which 4% chromic acid is used as an oxidizing agent in conjunction with Coleman's modification of the Schiff reagent. In Chapter 12 the most suitable stains for the visualization of a particular fungus in tissues are mentioned under the heading of histopathology.

Gomori methenamine silver nitrate stain*

Fixation: Fix tissue in 10% formalin.
Technique: Use paraffin sections.
Solutions:
Chromic acid (5%):
1. Chromic acid, 5 gm.
2. Distilled water, 100 ml.
Silver nitrate solution (5%):
1. Silver nitrate, 5 gm.
2. Distilled water, 100 ml.
Methenamine solution (3%):
1. Hexamethylenetetramine (USP),† 3 gm.
2. Distilled water, 100 ml.
Borax solution (5%):
1. Borax (photographic grade),‡ 5 gm.
2. Distilled water, 100 ml.
Methenamine silver nitrate stock solution:
1. Silver nitrate (5% solution), 5 ml.
2. Methenamine (3% solution), 100 ml.

A white precipitate forms, but immediately dissolves when the solution is shaken. Clear solution remains usable for months when stored in the refrigerator.
Methenamine silver nitrate working solution:
1. Borax (5% solution), 2 ml.
2. Distilled water, 25 ml.

Mix and add 25 ml. methenamine silver nitrate stock solution.

---

*From Manual of histologic and special staining technics, ed. 2, New York, 1960, McGraw-Hill Book Co.
†Fisher Scientific Co., St. Louis, Mo.
‡Eastman Kodak Co., Rochester, N. Y.

Sodium bisulfite solution (1%):
1. Sodium bisulfite, 1 gm.
2. Distilled water, 100 ml.

Gold chloride (0.1%):
1. Gold chloride (1% solution), 10 ml.
2. Distilled water, 90 ml.

This solution may be used repeatedly.

Sodium thiosulfate ("hypo") solution (2%):
1. Sodium thiosulfate, 2 gm.
2. Distilled water, 100 ml.

Light green stock solution:
1. Light green SF yellowish, 0.2 gm.
2. Distilled water, 100 ml.
3. Glacial acetic acid, 0.2 ml.

Light green working solution:
1. Light green stock solution, 10 ml.
2. Distilled water, 50 ml.

Staining procedure:
1. Deparaffinize sections. Slides previously stained with most other stains may be used by removing cover glasses in xylene and running through alcohols to water. Subsequent chromic acid treatment will remove any remaining stain.

NOTE: Run a control slide.
2. Oxidize in 5% chromic acid solution for 1 hr.
3. Wash in running tap water for a few seconds.
4. Rinse in 1% sodium bisulfite for 1 min. to remove any residual chromic acid.
5. Wash in tap water for 5-10 min.
6. Wash with three or four changes of distilled water.
7. Place in methanamine silver nitrate working solution in oven at 58°-60° C. for 30-60 min. until section turns yellowish brown. Use paraffin-coated forceps to remove slide from this solution and dip in distilled water. Check for adequate silver impregnation with microscope. Fungi should be dark brown at this stage.
8. Rinse with six changes of distilled water.
9. Tone in 0.1% gold chloride solution for 2-5 min.
10. Rinse in distilled water.
11. Remove unreduced silver with 2% sodium thiosulfate ("hypo") solution for 2-5 min.
12. Wash thoroughly in tap water.
13. Counterstain with light green working solution for 30-45 sec.
14. Dehydrate with two changes of 95% alcohol plus absolute alcohol, clear with two to three changes of xylene, and mount in Permount.

Results:
Fungi—sharply delineated in black
Mucin—taupe to dark gray
Inner parts of mycelia and hyphae—old rose
Background—pale green

Alcian blue stain (with or without orange G)[15]

Fixation: Fix tissue in 10% formalin.
Technique: Use paraffin sections.
Solution:
1. Alcian blue 8GX, 1 gm.
2. Distilled water, 97 ml.
3. Glacial acetic acid, 3 ml.

Staining procedure:
1. Deparaffinize sections.
2. Acetic acid (3%), 2 min.
3. Alcian blue solution, 15 min.
4. Distilled water.
5. Ethyl alcohol series through 95%.
6. Orange G (1%) in 80% alcohol, 3-5 sec.*
7. Dehydrate, clear, and mount in Permount.

Results:
Without orange G:
    Fungal gel—turquoise blue
    Hyphal walls—light blue
    Hyphal cytoplasm—colorless
With orange G:
    Fungal gel—turquoise
    Hyphal walls—green-orange
    Hyphal cytoplasm—orange

Toluidine blue O stain[15]

Semipermanent preparation (several days):
Fixation: Fix tissue in 10% formalin.
Technique: Use paraffin sections.
Solution:
1. Ammonium molybdate (5%), equal parts.
2. Potassium ferrocyanide (1%), equal parts.

---

*Overstaining can be corrected with 0.5% NH_4OH in absolute alcohol.

Staining procedure:
1. Deparaffinize sections.
2. Aqueous solution of toluidine blue O (0.5%), 1 min.
3. Distilled water.
4. Dehydrate, clear, and mount in Permount.

Results:
Hyphae—purple or blue-green

STAIN FOR RICKETTSIAE IN SECTIONS OF FORMALIN-FIXED TISSUE

Wright buffer stain[16]

Fixation: Fix tissue in 10% formalin.
Technique: Use paraffin sections.
Staining procedure:
1. Deparaffinize sections.
2. Wright stain, 6 min.
3. Wright buffer stock solution, 6 min.

Results:
Rickettsial wall—pink
Chromatin body—blue

CYTOLOGY

MALIGNANT CELLS

Malignant cells are characterized in general by relatively large (and abnormal) nuclei and small amounts of cytoplasm, by the presence of prominent nucleoli, by marked variation in size, shape, and staining property, being usually hyperchromatic, and by exhibiting atypical or irregular mitoses. Cancer cells may be found by the smear technique in puncture biopsy material, in vaginal secretion,[17, 18] in prostatic secretion,[19] in urine, in gastric contents, in bronchial aspirations, in cavity fluids, and in sputum. A diagnosis of malignancy made from stained smears should be considered tentative and should be checked by tissue sections.

Papanicolaou method of staining

Fixation: Fix smears before drying in equal parts of ether and 95% alcohol for 5-15 min. The smears may be left in the fixative for 3 days if necessary, but prolonged fixation affects the staining reaction.

Solutions:
EA$_{36}$ *stain:* First prepare a 10% aqueous solution of each of the three dry stains to be used, and from each of these prepare a 0.5% solutions of the stain in 95% alcohol by adding 5 parts of the aqueous solution to 95 parts of **absolute** alcohol. Use the alcoholic solutions, filtering just before using.
1. Light green SF yellowish, 45 ml.
2. Bismark brown, 10 ml.
3. Eosin yellowish, 45 ml.
4. Phosphotungstic acid, 0.2 gm.
5. Lithium carbonate (saturated aqueous solution), 1 drop.

Orange G-6 solution: Prepare a 10% aqueous solution of orange G-6 (OG$_6$[*]) by heating. To 5 parts of this solution add 95 parts absolute alcohol. Use this alcoholic solution.
1. Orange G-6 solution, 100 ml.
2. Phosphotungstic acid, 0.015 gm.

The amount of phosphotungstic acid used varies from 0.010-0.025 gm., the larger amount giving a sharper contrast.

Staining procedure:
1. Rinse in 70% alcohol, 50% alcohol, and distilled water.
2. Stain in Harris hematoxylin (without acetic acid) for 5-10 min.
3. Rinse in distilled water.
4. Rinse three or four times in 0.5% aqueous solution of hydrochloric acid.
5. Rinse thoroughly in water.
6. Leave for 1 min. in a weak solution of lithium carbonate (3 drops saturated aqueous solution/100 ml. water). Rinse thoroughly in water.
7. Rinse in distilled water, 50% alcohol, 70% alcohol, 80% alcohol, and 95% alcohol.
8. Stain for 1 min. in the orange G-6 solution.
9. Rinse five to ten times in each of two jars containing 95% alcohol.
10. Stain in EA$_{36}$ (or EA$_{50}$) for 2 min.
11. Rinse five to ten times in each of three jars containing 95% alcohol (not the same alcohol which was used after orange G-6 solution).
12. Rinse in **absolute** alcohol, then in a mixture of equal parts of absolute alcohol and xylene, and then in xylene.

[*]National Aniline Division, Allied Chemical Corp., New York, N. Y.

13. Mount in Clarite, Canada balsam, or gum damar.

NOTE: A shorter method of staining may be used for immediate examination.

1. Without previous fixation, apply stain EA_{36} (or EA_{50}) for about 5 min. Wash off excess stain with 95% alcohol.
2. Rinse in **absolute** alcohol and then xylene, and mount (or study after smearing with immersion cedarwood oil).

The nuclei will be faintly stained, but when desired the smears can be restained by the longer method.

MUSEUM SPECIMENS

Tissue received for museum specimens should be placed immediately into Kaiserling I solution and left for 1-5 days. Wash tissue briefly and place into Kaiserling II solution for 1-6 hr. Change tissue to Kaiserling III solution for 1-2 hr. or until natural color is restored, wash free from all traces of alcohol and fixing fluid (running water overnight), and then transfer to Kaiserling IV solution, in which specimens are kept permanently.

To prepare tissue for exhibition, cut fresh surface if necessary, place in alcohol 1-2 hr. to freshen color, and then place in a museum jar of suitable size and shape and in such a position as to show up the important areas. Cover tissue well with Kaiserling IV solution. Seal the jar with melted asphalt cement, being careful to see that there are no air holes along the margin of the top.

Before sealing, insert a label along the side of the jar in such a way as not to obstruct the picture of the tissue. This label should give the accession number, the diagnosis, the name of the patient, and the date and should be written in pencil on white card paper and dipped in paraffin. A similar label on a gummed label should be stuck on the outside of the jar and covered with paraffin.

Kaiserling solutions:
Kaiserling I:
1. Formalin (40%), 200 ml.
2. Water, 1000 ml.
3. Potassium nitrate, 15 gm.
4. Potassium acetate, 30 gm.
Kaiserling II:
1. Alcohol (80%).
Kaiserling III:
1. Alcohol (95%).
Kaiserling IV:
1. Potassium acetate, 200 gm.
2. Glycerin, 400 ml.
3. Water, 2000 ml.
4. Phenol, 3 or 4 ml., may be added to prevent molds.

REFERENCES

1. Commission of Continuing Education: Manual for workshop on cryostat frozen section and freeze substitution techniques, Chicago, 1961, American Society of Clinical Pathologists.
2. Wiedmann, F. E.: Stain Techn. **40:**1, 1965.
3. Grimley, P. M., Albrecht, J. M., and Michelitch, H. J.: Stain Techn. **40:**357, 1966.
4. Spurlock, B. O., Skinner, M. S., and Kattine, A. A.: Amer. J. Clin. Path. **46:**252, 1966.
5. Pickett, J. P., and Sommer, J. R.: Arch. Path. **69:**239, 1960.
6. Sommer, J. R., and Pickett, J. P.: Arch. Path. **71:**6, 669, 1961.
7. Masson, P. J.: J. Tech. Methods **12:**75, 1929.
8. Lillie, R. D.: Histopathological technic and practical histochemistry, New York, 1948, McGraw-Hill Book Co., p. 196 (A.F.I.P. Modification).
9. Wilder, H. C.: Amer. J. Path. **11:**817, 1935.
10. McManus, J. F. A., and Mowry, R. W.: Staining methods: histological and histochemical, New York, 1960, Paul B. Hoeber, Inc., pp. 133-139.
11. Putt, F. A., and Hukill, P. B.: Arch. Path. **74:**169, 1962.
12. Mowry, R. W., and Winkler, C. H.: Amer. J. Path. **32:**628, 1956.
13. Mallory, F. B.: Pathological technique, Philadelphia, 1942, W. B. Saunders Co., pp. 127, 130.
14. Lieb, D.: Amer. J. Clin. Path. **17:**413, 1947.
15. Moore, E. J.: Stain Techn. **40:**23, 1965.
16. Wolf, G. L., Cole, C. R., Saslow, S., and Carlisle, H. N.: Stain Techn. **41:**185, 1966.
17. Papanicolaou, G. N.: Science **95:**438, 1942.
18. Papanicolaou, G. N., and Trout, H. F.: Diagnosis of uterine cancer by the vaginal smear, New York, 1943, The Commonwealth Fund.
19. Herbut, P. A., and Lubin, E. N.: J. Urol. **57:**542, 1947.

Appendix

Table of normal values

	Clinical chemistry	
Test	*Sample*	*Values*
A/G ratio	Serum	1.5-2.5
Albumin	Serum	4-5.5 gm.%
Aldolase	Serum	6.1-21.3 dihydroxyacetone units
Amino acid nitrogen	Plasma	3.5-7 mg.%
	Urine	50-200 mg./24 hr.
Ammonia	Urine	0.5-1 gm./24 hr.
Ammonia nitrogen	Whole blood	35-100 μg%
Amylase (diastase)	Serum	60-200 Somogyi units
	Urine	35-260 units/hr.
Atherogenic index (AI)	Serum	Below 50 units
BEI	Serum	3.2-6.4 μg%
Bilirubin (all methods)		
Direct	Serum	0.1-0.4 mg.%
Total	Serum	0.3-1.3 mg.%
Indirect	Serum	0.2-0.8 mg.%
BMR		±10% of Dubois standards
Bromsulphalein (BSP)		
2 mg./kg. body weight	Serum	Not more than 15% after 30 min.
5 mg./kg. body weight	Serum	0-5% after 45 min.
Calcium	Serum	8.5-10.5 mg.%
	Urine	50-400 mg./24 hr.
Cephalin-cholesterol		
flocculation	Serum	No flocculation
Ceruloplasmin (copper		
oxidase)	Serum	35-65 I.U. (15-35 mg.%)
Chloride	Serum	98-110 mEq./L. (575-645 mg.% as NaCl)
	Whole blood	77-88 mEq./L. (450-515 mg.% as NaCl)
	Urine	10-15 gm./24 hr. as NaCl
Cholesterol, total	Serum	150-270 mg.%
Cholesterol esters	Serum	68-74% of total cholesterol
Cholinesterase	Serum	40-80 units
Copper	Serum	70-150 μg%
	Urine	Up to 40 μg/day
CO_2-combining power	Plasma	24-34 mM./L. (53-76 vol.%)
CO_2 content	Plasma	20-25 mM./L. (45-55 vol.%)
Creatine	Serum	0.5-0.9 mg.%
Creatine phosphokinase		
(CPK)	Serum	0-5 μg/hr./ml.
Creatinine	Serum	0.6-1.2 mg.%
	Urine	1-1.5 gm./24 hr.

Table of normal values—cont'd

Clinical chemistry—cont'd		
Test	*Sample*	*Values*
ET$_3$	Serum	11-17% after 2 hr. of incubation
Fat tolerance	Serum or plasma	Increase to 17.5 mEq./L. fatty acids
Fatty acids		
Esterified	Serum	7-14 mEq./L.
Free	Serum or plasma	0.35-1.2 mEq./L.
Fibrinogen	Plasma	200-400 mg.%
Galactose tolerance	Whole blood	Index up to 160 mg.%
Globulin	Serum	1.5-3 gm.%
Glucose		
Folin-Wu method	Whole blood	80-125 mg.%
Somogyi method	Whole blood	65-95 mg.%
	Serum or plasma	80-115 mg.%
Glutamic oxalacetic transaminase (GOT)	Serum	8-30 Reitman-Frankel units
Using diazonium salt	Serum	8-30 units (same as Reitman-Frankel method)
Glutamic pyruvic transaminase (GPT)	Serum	5-25 Reitman-Frankel units
Using diazonium salt	Serum	5-25 units (same as Reitman-Frankel method)
Hippuric acid synthesis		
Intravenous	Urine	0.7-1.6 gm./hr.
Oral	Urine	3-3.5 gm./4 hr.
Hydroxybutyrate dehydrogenase (HBD)	Serum	56-125 I.U./L.
Icterus index	Serum	2-6 units
Iron	Serum	70-150 μg%
Iron-binding capacity, total	Serum	200-400 μg%
Isocitric dehydrogenase (ICD)	Serum	238-686 KGA units/ml.
Lactic dehydrogenase (LDH)	Serum	41-98 units
	Urine	550-2050 units in 8 hr. specimen
Using tetrazolium salt	Serum	27-77 I.U.
Leucine aminopeptidase (LAP)		
Adults	Serum	5-20 units
Infants	Serum	5-24 units
Adults	Urine	2-18 units/24 hr.
Levulose tolerance	Whole blood	Not more than 26-30 mg.% above fasting level
Lipase	Serum	0-1 unit
Magnesium	Serum	1.6-2.1 mEq./L.
	Urine	0.1-0.2 gm./24 hr.
Nonprotein nitrogen (NPN)	Whole blood	25-45 mg.%
Oxygen capacity		
Men	Whole blood	20.7 vol.% (15.4 gm. Hb)
Women	Whole blood	19 vol.% (14.2 gm. Hb)
Oxygen saturation	Arterial blood	95-97%
	Venous blood	60-85%
pH	Venous blood	7.32-7.42
	Arterial blood	7.35-7.45
	Urine	4.8-7.6 (average 6)

Table of normal values—cont'd

Test	Sample	Values
Clinical chemistry—cont'd		
Phosphatase, acid		
Bessey-Lowry		
Men	Serum	0.13-0.63 B-L unit
Women	Serum	0.01-0.56 B-L unit
Using alpha-naphthylphos-		
phate	Serum	1-1.9 I.U./L.
Phosphatase, alkaline		
Bessey-Lowry		
Adults	Serum	0.8-2.3 B-L units
Children	Serum	2.8-6.7 B-L units
Using phenolphthalein mono-		
phosphate	Serum	9-35 I.U.
Phospholipids	Serum	150-350 mg.% (average 230 mg.%); 6-14 mg.% lipid phosphorus
Phosphorus, inorganic		
Adults	Serum	2.5-5 mg.%
Children	Serum	3.5-6 mg.%
Adults	Urine	0.78-1.1 gm. (1.8-2.5 P_2O_5)
Potassium	Serum	4-5.6 mEq./L. (16-22 mg.%)
Prostatic acid phosphatase	Serum	Up to 0.15 units
Protein, total	Serum	6-8 gm.%
Protein-bound iodine (PBI)	Serum	4-8 μg%
Prothrombin time	Serum	70-100% (11-15 sec.)
Sodium	Serum	135-145 mEq./L. (310-335 mg.%)
TBI		
Euthyroid	Serum	0.9-1.1
Hyperthyroid	Serum	Less than 0.9
Hypothyroid	Serum	Greater than 1.1
T_4 by column chromatography	Serum	3.0-6.4 μg%
Thymol turbidity	Serum	0-5 units
Thyroxine-binding globulin		
capacity	Serum	12-20 μg thyroxine-binding capacity/100 ml.
Total lipids	Serum	400-1000 mg.%
Total nitrogen	Urine	10-16 gm./24 hr.
Triglycerides	Serum	40-145 mg.% (1.4-4.9 mEq./L.)
Urea	Serum or whole blood	22-40 mg.%
	Urine	10-40 gm./24 hr.
Urea nitrogen	Serum or whole blood	10-18 mg.%
Uric acid	Serum	2.5-8 mg.%
	Urine	0.4-0.8 gm./24 hr.
Urobilinogen	Urine	0.4-1 mg./day
	Feces	30-220 mg./100 mg. of stool or 40-280 mg./day
Zinc sulfate turbidity	Serum	2-8 units

Hematology			
Bleeding time (Ivy)		Bone marrow differential count	
Average	4 min.	Reticuloendothelial cells	0-1%
Range	1-7 min.	Myeloblasts	0-2%
		Promyelocytes	1-5%
Blood volume		Myelocytes	
Males	52-70 ml./kg.	Neutrophilic	5-25%
Females	53-62 ml./kg.	Eosinophilic	0-3%
		Basophilic	0-0.5%

Table of normal values—cont'd

Hematology—cont'd

Bone marrow differential count—cont'd

Metamyelocytes	10-20%
Band granulocytes	15-30%
Neutrophilic granulocytes	10-25%
Eosinophils	0-5%
Basophils	0-0.5%
Lymphocytes	5-20%
Monocytes	0-3%
Plasma cells	0-5%
Nucleated RBC	
Rubriblasts	1-5/100 WBC
Prorubricytes	1-6/100 WBC
Rubricytes	5-25/100 WBC
Metarubricytes	2-20/100 WBC
Myeloid:erythroid ratio	3-8:1
Megakaryocytes	1-2 or more/high-power dry field

Clot retraction

Begin	1 hr.
Complete	24 hr.

Coagulation time (Lee-White) 10-12 min.
(8.5-15.5 min.)

Differential count

Adults

Neutrophils	56-65%
Band granulocytes	1-5%
Lymphocytes	25-34%
Monocytes	4-5%
Eosinophils	0.5-4%
Basophils	0-1.5%

Children

	Birth (%)	2 mo.-2 yr. (%)	2-8 yr. (%)	8-16 yr. (%)
Polymorphs (neutrophils)	45-65	30	30-50	50-60
Band granulocytes	6-12	3	3	2-5
Eosinophils	2	2.5	2.5	2.5
Basophils	0.5	0.5	0.5	0.5
Lymphocytes	26-35	59-63	60-39	30-40
Monocytes	5	5	4	5

Eosinophilic count 150-300/mm.^{3}

Erythrocytic count

Males

Average	4.8 million/mm.^{3}
Range	4.4-5.4 million

Females

Average	4.3 million/mm.^{3}
Range	3.8-5 million

Hematocrit

Males	40-52 vol.%/100 ml.
Females	38-47 vol.%/100 ml.

Children

Birth	45-65 vol.%
2 yr.	30-40 vol.%
8 yr.	32-42 vol.%

Hemoglobin

Males	14.9 gm.% (15.4 ± 1.5)
Females	13.7 gm.% (14.2 ± 1.5)

Children

Birth	21.5 gm.% (23.9 ± 3.0)
4 wk.	16 gm.% (15.3 ± 3.0)
2 mo.	13.5 gm.% (13.1 ± 2.2)
1 yr.	12 gm.% (11.6 ± 1.5)
4 yr.	13 gm.% (12.2 ± 1.5)

Leukocyte count

Birth	9000-30,000 WBC/mm.^{3}
2 mo.-2 yr.	6000-17,000 WBC/mm.^{3}
2-8 yr.	6000-13,000 WBC/mm.^{3}
8-16 yr.	5000-13,000 WBC/mm.^{3}
16-21 yr.	4500-11,000 WBC/mm.^{3}

Mean corpuscular hemoglobin (MCH)
29 ± 2$\mu\mu$g

Mean corpuscular hemoglobin concentration (MCHC) 34 ± 2%

Mean corpuscular volume (MCV) 87 ± 5μ^3

Methemoglobin 0-3% total hemoglobin
(0.03-0.13 gm./100 ml.)

Osmotic fragility

0.30% saline solution	100% hemolysis
0.40% saline solution	50-95% hemolysis
0.55% saline solution	0% hemolysis

Partial thromboplastin time (kaolin-activated) 30-45 sec.

Platelet count

Average	260,000/mm.^{3}
Range	145,000-350,000/mm.^{3}

Prothrombin consumption time Longer than
21 sec.

Prothrombin time 11-12.8 sec.

Red cell count See erythrocyte count
Reticulocyte count 0-2%

Sedimentation rate (Wintrobe)

Men	0-9 mm.
Women	0-15 mm.
Children	0-13 mm.

White cell count See leukocyte count

Table of normal values—cont'd

Urinary hormones	
Catecholamines	20-180 μg/day
Hydroxyindolacetic acid (HIAA)	2-9 mg./day
Hydroxysteroids	10-15 mg./day
17-Ketosteroids	
Males	10-18 mg./day
Females	6-15 mg./day
Vanillyl mandelic acid (VMA)	2-14 mg./day

Kidney function tests	
Creatinine clearance (endogenous)	100-120 ml./min.
Concentration test (sp. gr.)	1.030 or more
Dilution test (sp. gr.)	1.002-1.001
Inulin clearance (average)	123 ml./min./1.73 m.²
PAH clearance (average)	634 ml./min./1.73 m.²
Phenolsulfonphthalein test (PSP)	26% excretion after 15 min.
	40% excretion after 30 min.
Urea clearance	
Maximal	70-110% of normal (75 ml./min.)
Standard	70-110% of normal (54 ml./min.)

Cerebrospinal fluid	
Cells	1-5/mm.³
Chlorides	113-127 mEq./L.
Glucose	45-100 mg./100 ml.
Protein	20-45 mg./100 ml.
Urea	8-28 mg./100 ml.

Index

A

ABH substance, secretion of, and Lewis system, 252
ABO
  blood groups
    and ABO typing, 236-241
    exclusion of paternity by, 255
  erythroblastosis, 183
    laboratory diagnosis, 278-279
  hemolytic disease of newborn; see ABO erythroblastosis
Absorption
  of antibodies, 271
  chromatography, 291
  of cold agglutinins, 274
  spectra of hemoglobin and derivatives, 102, 103
Abt-Downey test for fetal hemoglobin, 170
Acanthocheilonema perstans, 489
Acanthocytes, 135
Accuracy and precision in laboratory, 3
Acetate buffer, 433, 434
Acetest, 35
Acetic acid and heat test of urine, 18
Acetic water solution, 711
Acetoin reaction, 566
Acetylcholine, effect of cholinesterase on, 390
Acetylsulfadiazine crystals, 54
Acetylsulfaguanidine crystals, 53
Acetylsulfapyridine crystals, 54
Acetylsulfathiazone crystals, 53, 54
Achilles tendon reflex time as test of thyroid function, 427
Achromobacter species, 573
Acid
  alcohol, 538
  gastric, measurement, 443-444
  hematin technique in hemoglobinometry, 98
  phosphatase, determination of, 402, 404, 405
Acid-base
  balance in blood, 349-350
  metabolism, kidney in, 16
Acid-ether concentration for trematodes, 492
Acid-fast
  routine, 531
  smear
    Mycobacterium leprae, 601
    tubercle bacilli, 593

Acid-fast—cont'd
  stain
    Kinyoun, 715-716
    for mycobacteria, 538
    for pus, 525
Acidity, gastric, concentration of, 444-445
Acidosis and alkalosis, changes in blood pH and CO_2 content, table, 350
Acids, standard, preparation, 432
Acid-serum test (Ham) for nocturnal hemoglobinuria, 175
Ackerman-Meyers rapid screening method of iodine separation, 417
Acquired hemorrhagic disorders, 224
ACTH
  Thorn test of circulating eosinophils, 122
  in urine, determination of, 72
Actinobacillus mallei, 585
Actinomyces bovis and anaerobic diphtheroids, differentiation, table, 604
Actinomyces israeli and *bovis*, 602-603
Actinomycetaceae, 601-603
Actinomycosis, 602
Aculute pellets in hemoglobinometry, 99
Adaptations, bacterial, 529
Addis count, 56-57
Addison's disease
  Robinson-Power-Kepler test, 342-343
  serum potassium in, 340
Adenoviruses, 620
Adrenal
  function tests, 78, 79
  medulla, 79
Adrenocortical hormones, 73
Aerobacter aerogenes in water, test for, 652
Aerobacter species, 574
Aerobes, obligate, growth of, 529
Aerobic bacilli
  gram-negative, 560-588
  gram-positive spore-forming, 604-605
Aeromonas species, 574
Afibrinogenemia, 224
Agammaglobulinemia, 201
Ag antigen, 240
Agar
  blood; see Blood agar
  chlamydospore, 634, 636
  chocolate, 542, 557
  cornmeal, 634, 636

Agar—cont'd
 diffusion test for *Corynebacterium diphtheriae,* 590
 gel electrophoresis for hemoglobin separation, 170, 172, 173
Agars for Enterobacteriaceae, 561
Agglutination test(s)
 Bordetella pertussis, 582
 Brucella, 585-587
 Pasteurella tularensis, 580-581
 serologic, *Salmonella,* 577
 viruses, 620
Agglutination-inhibition tests for pregnancy, 92
Agglutinins
 cold, 273, 274
  nonspecific, of anti-A₁, anti-H, and anti-I, 239
  specificity and hemolytic activity, 181
 for *Streptococcus MG,* 552
Agglutinogens, Rh-Hr, 243
Agranulocytosis, 187-188
Ahaptoglobinemia, 166
Ajello concentration method for *Nocardia,* 601
Albers-Schönberg disease, 187
Albert stain, 538
Albumin
 globulin, and protein, total, determination of, 320-329
 test, blood group antibodies, 266
 titration of antibodies, 272
 in urine, tests for, 18, 19
Albuminuria
 false or accidental, 19
 functional, 20
Albu-Stix, 19
Albutest, 19
Alcaligenes faecalis, 573
Alcian blue stain, 719
Alcohol
 determination methods, 686, 687
 intoxication, possible erroneous diagnosis, 684
Alder's anomaly, 144
Aldolase, determination of, 384-385
Aldosterone, 78-79
Aldosteronism, 78, 79
Alkalescens-Dispar group, 568
Alkali denaturation method for fetal hemoglobin, 170
Alkaline
 hematin technique in hemoglobinometry, 98
 incineration method of Barker for iodine separation, 415-417
 phosphatase
  in clinical diagnosis, 402
  determination of, 403, 404
  heat-stable, as index of placental function, 94
  leukocytic (APGL), in pregnancy, 89
  stain, 127, 128
  test of liver function, 369
 pyrogallol method for anaerobic cultures, 541
Alkalosis and acidosis, changes in blood pH and CO₂ content, table, 350
Alkaptonuria and alkapton bodies, 26
Alleles, multiple, Wiener's nomenclature and theory, 242
Allergic reactions from transfusion, 263

Allescheria boydii, 645
Alpha hemolysis, 529
Alpha hemolytic streptococci, 547
Alpha-hydroxybutyrate dehydrogenase (HBD), 385-387
Alpha-naphthylphosphate, acid phosphatase using, 405-406
Alsever solution, 190
Amato bodies, 144
Amebas
 free-living, in soil, 468
 intestinal, human, differential diagnosis, table, 466
 species, characteristics, 465-468
Amebiasis, serologic diagnosis, 465
Amebic gel diffusion precipitation test, 465
Amino acid nitrogen, 317-319
 test for, 22
Amino acids
 in plasma, liver function and, 362
 in urine, tests for, 21-23
Aminoaciduria, 21-23
 Dent's classification (modified after Holt), 29
 overflow, 24
 renal, 23-24
Ammonia, blood, determination of, 316-317
Ammoniacal silver solution, 711
Ammoniomagnesium phosphate crystals, 56
Ammonium biurate crystals, 52, 56
Ammonium sulfate test for myoglobin in urine, 40
Amniotic fluid, 520-521
 examination in erythroblastosis fetalis, 276-277
Amorphous
 phosphates, 56
 sediment in urine, 50, 52
Amount of urine, 13
Amylase
 methods of determination, 387-389
 tests, duodenal contents, 447
 urinary, 447
Amyloid
 disease, Congo red test for, 430
 in multiple myeloma, 201
Anaerobes
 obligate, growth of, 529
 sensitivity determination of, 545
Anaerobiasis, indicator of, 542
Anaerobic
 cultures, 541-542
  handling, 531
 diphtheroids and *Actinomyces bovis,* differentiation, table, 604
 gram-negative nonspore-forming bacilli, 587-588
 gram-positive spore-forming bacilli, 605-608
 streptococci, 550-551
Anaero-jar, 541
Analysis, gastric, 443-446
Ancylostoma braziliense, 482
Ancylostoma caninum, 482
Ancylostoma duodenale, 482
Andrade indicator for identification of *Candida albicans,* 638
Androgens, 73
Anemia(s)
 aplastic, 184-185

Anemia(s)—cont'd
 blood cells in diagnosis, 138-139
 classification, 115, 154
 Cooley's or Mediterranean, 167
 erythrokinetic evaluation, 155
 Heinz body, congenital, 179
 hemolytic
  acquired, 179
  autoimmune, 180-182
  common features and methods of investigation, 167-169
  congenital nonspherocytic, 176
   erythrocyte enzyme deficiencies in, 409
  crises, 166
  diagnosis, 160
  enzyme-deficient, 176
  due to extracorpuscular defects, 179
  due to intracorpuscular defects, 167-179
  due to isoantibodies, 182-184
  toxic, 184
 of infection, 159
 iron-deficiency, 158-159
 in lupus erythematososus, 192
 macrocytic, 155-158
 megaloblastic, 155
 microcytic, and microcytic hypochromic, 158-
  160
 myelophthisic, 186-187
 nonmegaloblastic, 155
 normocytic, 160-185
  normochromic, 161
 pernicious, 155, 157
 pyridoxine (vitamin B_6)-deficiency, 159
 red blood count in, 114
 severe, variations in red cell counting in, 112
 sickle cell, 174
 sideroachrestic hypochromic, 159
Aniline
 blue solution, 711
 test for pentose in urine, 32
Animal
 inoculation; *see* Inoculation, animal
 pathogenicity, tubercle bacilli, 599-600
 toxicity, *Nocardia*, 602
Anion exchange resin method for iodine separation, 414
Anisocytosis, 134, 161
Anopheles mosquito, 495, 496
Anthrax bacillus, 604-605
Anti-A₁ lectin, 238
Anti-A serum, 238
Antibiotic(s)
 bacterical and bacteriostatic, 544
 in combination, test tube testing of, 545
 fungi media with, 633
 neutralizing agents, 530
 sensitivity of bacteria, 543-546
 solutions in sensitivity determination of, 545
Antibodies
 of ABO system, 239
 absorption of, 271
 and antigens, 232-236
 anti-Rh, production of, 183
 atypical, screening of blood donor and recipient for, 259
 blood group, detection and identification, 265-
  271

Antibodies—cont'd
 characteristics, summary, table, 233
 cold, 273, 274
  atypical, in A₁ and A₂ subgroups, 238-239
  elution of, 274-275
 in crossmatching, table, 268-270
 definition, 232
 of Duffy system, 252
 elution of, 271-272
 in erythroblastosis fetalis, 275, 276
 fluorescein-labeled, 539
 heterophil, in mononucleosis, 188, 190, 191
 of Ii system, 255
 of Kell system, 251
 Lewis, tests for, 253
 of Lu system, 255
 of MNSU system, 251
 names and actions, 232
 of P and Jay system, 251
 platelet, 273
 saline-acting, and albumin-acting, thermal
  amplitude of, 181
 titration of, 272-273
 treponemal and nontreponemal, 611
 white cell, 273
Antibody reactions, of streptococci, 551-552
Anti-C agglutinin, 238
Anticoagulant(s)
 in blood specimens, 284-285
 choice of, in obtaining blood, 98
 circulating
  hemorrhagic diseases due to, 225-226
  or plasma factor defect, tests to distinguish,
   213
  test for, 214-215
 in coagulation procedures, 208
 therapy, 219
Antidotes to common poisons, table, 685
Antigen
 dilution, preparation
  in Kolmer test, 666
  in Reiter test, 676
 emulsion
  preparation in VDRL slide flocculation tests
   with serum, 657
  stabilized, VDRL, 658
Antigen-antibody reaction, 234
Antigenic structure of pneumococci, 556
Antigens
 of ABO system, 239
 altered, 240
 and antibodies, 232-236
 in coliform bacteria, 566
 definition, 232
 of Duffy system, 251-252
 of Ii system, 255
 of Kell system, 251
 of Kidd system, 254
 Lewis, in infants, 253
 low-incidence and high-incidence, 255
 of Lu system, 255
 of MNSU system, 251
 of P and Jay system, 251
 serologic identification of *Salmonella*, 576
 variations with age, 240
Antiglobulin
 crossmatch, 260

Antiglobulin—cont'd
   test, 234-236
      blood group antibodies, 266-267
      nongamma globulin, 236
      of red cells of newborn infant in erythro-
         blastosis fetalis, 278
      two-stage, for Lewis antibodies, 253
Anti-H lectin, 238
Antihemophilic factor in coagulation, 207
Antiplatelet factor, 227
Anti-Rh
   antibodies, 246
   testing sera, 245-246
Antistreptolysin O titer, 551
Antithrombin, plasma, test, 215
Anulocytes, 134
Anuria, 13
Aplastic anemias, 184-185
Apoferritin, 158
Apparatus for water analysis, 652
Appendix, 722-726
Aqueous dissolution technique for concentration
      of cells in sputum, 523-524
Arboviruses, 621
Arizona group, differentiation of, from *Salmo-
      nella*, 577
Arsenic
   methods of determination, 688-691
   uses of, 688
Artefacts, fungal hyphae and, 631, 633
Arteriosclerotic kidney disease, classification and
      manifestations, table, 70
Arthritis
   synovial fluid analysis in, 517
   synovianalysis in, table, 520
Arthrospores
   Coccidioides immitis, 643
   Geotrichum candidum reproduced by, 639
Asbestos bodies in sputum, 524
Ascaris lumbricoides, 482, 483, 484
Ascoli thermoprecipitin test for anthrax bacilli,
      605
Ascorbic acid
   determination, 429-430
   method of Cr^{51} blood volume determination,
      110
Ashby technique for red blood cell survival
      time, 166
Aspergillus fumigatus, 649
Asthma, Curschmann's spirals in, 521, 524
Atherogenic index (AI), 381
Atherosclerosis
   lipoproteins in pathogenesis of, 380, 381, 382
   polyunsaturated fatty acids in studies on, 380
   role of cholesterol in, 375
Athlete's foot, 646
Atomic
   absorption
      analysis, examination of hair by, 451
      spectrophotometry, 290-291
   weights, table, 435
Auer body, 140
Autoagglutinins, cold, test for, 274
AutoAnalyzer, 297, 298
Autoantibodies, 179-180
Autoclaving, sterilization by, 530

Autohemolysis
   quantitative test, 164
   screening test, 163
Autoimmune
   hemolytic anemias, 180-182
   reactions in lupus erythematosus, 193
Automatic tissue processor, 707
Automation
   in clinical laboratory, 294-298
   in laboratory, 2
   protein-bound iodine by, 420
Autopsy tissue, examination, 534

B

Babcock method for fat in milk, 654
Bacillaceae, classification, 603-604
Bacilli
   Boas-Oppler, 446
   dysentery, 578
   gram-negative, 560-588
   gram-positive, 588-608
   morphologic structure, 528
Bacillus subtilis, 605
Bacitracin, sensitivity of streptococci to, 549
Bacteremia, 532
Bacteria
   chemical composition and growth, 529
   collection and handling of specimens, 530
   definition and morphologic classification, 526
   division, 526
   enteric gram-negative, 560-564
   gram stain reaction, 528
   morphology, 526-528
   oxygen requirements, 541-542
   sensitivity to antibiotics, 543-546
   staining methods, 538-540
   stains for, 715-717
   in urine
      estimating number of, methods, 535
      significance, 48
Bacterial
   cultures and smears, handling, 531
   enzymes and toxins, 528-529
   infections, hemolytic anemia with, 184
   spore strips, 530
   vaccine, 546
Bactericidal antibiotics, 544
   area, surgical specimens, 705
   method of milk analysis, 653
   specimens, collection, handling, and shipment,
      535
   survey, staphylococcal infections in hospitals,
      554-555
Bacteriology
   clinical, introduction, 526
   indicators in, 543
   methods of examination, 537-543
   quality control, 7-9
Bacteriophage typing of *Pasteurella pestis*, 579
Bacteriostatic antibiotics, 544
Bacteroides, 587
Bagassosis, sputum in, 524
Balantidium coli, characteristics, 469
Bandrowski base, 389
Barbiturates
   effect on basal metabolic rate, 426

Barbiturates—cont'd
  intoxication, determination of, 696
  wide use of, 695
Barfoed reagent, 33
Barker alkaline incineration method of iodine
      separation, 415-417
Bartonellosis, hemolytic anemia with, 184
Basal metabolism, 424-427
Bases, standard, preparation, 432
Basic nutrient media, 542
Basket cells, 144
Basophil(s)
  count, absolute, 122
  maturation, 147
  tissue, or mast cell, 148
Basophilic
  megaloblast, 133
  normoblast, 131
  stippling, 136, 137
Battey nonphotochromogens, 600
Bedsonia infections, 624
Beef tapeworm, 471-473
Beer's law, 285, 287, 288, 289
Bence Jones protein, 20-21
  in multiple myeloma, 197, 198, 199
Benedict-Talbot basal metabolism standards for
      children, 426
Benedict test
  modified qualitative, for fructose and pentose
      in urine, 31
  for sugar reducing substances in urine
    qualitative, 27
    quantitative, 29-30
Benzidine
  dihydrochloride, myeloperoxidase stain with,
      128, 129
  test
    for blood in stool, 453
    modification for urine, 39
Berthelot reaction, 311
Best carmine stain for glycogen, 714-715
Beta hemolysis, 529
Beta hemolytic streptococci, 547, 548
Beta-hydroxybutyric acid in urine, Hart test for,
      35
Bethesda-Ballerup group, 567
  Salmonella-like reactions, 578
Beutler screening tests for glucose-6-phosphate
      dehydrogenase, pyruvate kinase, and
      glutathione reductase deficiencies, 178
Bg antigen, 240
Bial orcin test for pentose in urine, 32
Bicarbonate, titration of, in duodenal aspirate,
      448
Biebrich scarlet-acid fuchsin solution, 711
Bile
  pigments
    and derivatives in stool, tests for, 453-454
    liver function tests based on, 355-362
    removal of, 36
    tests for, 35-38
  solubility test for pneumococci, 555-556
  specimen, 532
Biliary calculi, analysis, 431
Bilirubin
  cord blood, 183
  direct-reacting, 357

Bilirubin—cont'd
  Jendrassik-Grof method, 357-358
  Malloy-Evelyn method, 358-359
  metabolism, 355
  principle, 356
  serum, test in hemolytic anemia, 164
  standardization, 359
  in stool, occurrence, 454
  tests for, 35-36
Biochemical
  identification of *Shigella*, 578
  reactions
    Actinomyces, 603
    clostridia, 605-606, 607
    Listeria, 589
    mycobacteria, 597
    Nocardia, 602
    Proteus, 568
    Salmonella, 576
    Vibrio comma and *fetus*, 609
  tests
    Enterobacteriaceae differentiated by, table,
        574-575
    in group differentiation of Enterobacteria-
        ceae, 562, 564
    synovial fluid, 519
Biochemistry of amniotic fluid, 520
Biologic
  false positive reactions, syphilis, 683
  fluids, examination, 507-525
  methods, oxygen exhaustion, 541
  pregnancy tests, 90-92
Bismuth sulfide agar, 561
Blastocystis brasiliensis, 642-643
Blastocystis dermatitidis, 641-642
Blastocystis hominis, characteristics, 469, 470
Blastomycosis
  North American, 641
  South American, 642
Blastospore, 636
  pattern on cornmeal cutstreak plate, 637
Bleeding
  patient, investigation of, 209-223
  time, methods for measuring, 209
Blocking, paraffin section technique, 707
Blood; *see also* Hematologic
  acid-base balance, 349-350
  agar
    Cryptococcus neoformans, 639
    Enterobacteriaceae, 561
    staphylococci, 553
    streptococci, 547
  alcohol in, 686, 687
  ammonia, determination of, 316-317
  bank blood transfusions, 265
  banking
    quality control in, 2
    terms, glossary, 279-281
  and blood components in clinical use, 265
  bromide in, determination, 697
  cells
    color plate, 126
    grouping, methods, 237
    nomenclature, 96
    origin, 95
    origin and maturation, 130
    packed, in transfusions, 265

Blood—cont'd
  cells—cont'd
    red; *see* Erythrocytes *and* Red blood cells
    white; *see* Leukocytes *and* White blood cells
  in cerebrospinal fluid, 510
  chimeras, 241
  clot; *see also* Clot
    method for L.E. cells, 192
  clotting; *see* Coagulation
  coagulation; *see* Coagulation
  collection
    for coagulation tests, 208
    for donor selection, 258
  composition, 95
  constants, 114-115
  constituents
    changes on standing, 285
    determination of, importance, 283
  count
    in acute leukemias, 194
    in chronic leukemias, 195
    in pertussis, 581
  crossmatching, 259-260
  cultures, 532
    organisms isolated from, 536
  defibrination with glass beads, 98
  deproteinization methods, 298-299
  derivatives
    in coagulation procedures, 208
    transfusions of, 265
  in disease, clinical composition factors, 283
  donor selection, 257-258
  examination, methods, 96-97
  factors, certain, approximate frequencies, table,
    267
  flagellates, 500-504
  flukes, 494
  formation, 95
  fresh
    examination, 96
    use in transfusions, 265
  galactose determination, 365
  in gastric juice, determination of, 445
  glucose determination, 299-307
  group
    antibodies, detection and identification, 265-
      271
    systems, 236-257
  grouping in disputed paternity, tests, 255-256
  groups; *see also* Groups *and* Subgroups
    A and AB, subgroups, 238-240
    ABO, 236-241
    and blood typing, 232-258
    Diego system, 255
    Duffy system, 251-252
    Ii system, 225
    Kell system, 251
    Kidd system, 254
    Lewis system, 252-254
    Lutheran system, 255
    MNSU, 259-260
    P and Jay system, 251
    specific substances A and B, 262
  hemoglobinuria and hematuria, 38-40
  hydrogen ion concentration in, 348-350
  indices, 114-115
  intestinal parasites in, examination, 462

Blood—cont'd
  lead in, method of determination, 693-694
  lipids, 371-382
  lipoproteins in, 380
  microanalysis, 293-294
  nonprotein nitrogen in, 310-313
  para-aminobenzoic acid in, determination of,
    701
  para-aminosalicylic acid in, determination of,
    701
  pregnancy tests, 89
  salicylates in, determination of, 703
  samples, preservation of, 285
  serum; *see* Serum
  smear, 124-130
    in acute leukemias, 194
    examination for malarial parasites, 496-500
    peripheral, nonhematologic cells in, 154
  specimens
    collection, 284-285
    obtaining, 97
  in stool, tests for, 452-453
  storage and "storage lesion," 262
  sugar
    effects of epinephrine and of insulin on, 306
    normal values and pathologic interpreta-
      tion, 301
  sulfonamides in, 698-699
  transfusions; *see* Transfusions
  for transfusions, choice of, 261
  urea clearance, 64-65, 66
  urea nitrogen (BUN) determination, 308-310
  uric acid in, 313-314
  in urine, causes, 47
  values, average normal, at different age levels,
    113
  volume determination, 109-110
Bloor method, modified, cholesterol determina-
    tion, 373
Blue diaper syndrome, 38
Boas-Oppler bacilli, 446, 588
Bone
  disease, alkaline phosphatase in, 403, 404
  marrow
    in acute leukemias, 194
    in agranulocytosis, 188
    in aplastic anemias, 185
    aspiration, choice of site, 202
    biopsy, surgical method, 203
    blood formation in, 95
    cells peculiar to, 204-205
    culture, 532
    in disease, 205
    examination, 202-205
    in hemolytic anemia, 166
    in lupus erythematosus, 192
    macroglobulinemia, 200
    in mononucleosis, 188
    in multiple myeloma, 197
    in myelophthisic anemia, 187
    in polycythemia vera, 185
    smears, examination, 203-204
    specimen, methods of obtaining, 202-203
    staining of smears and of touch prepara-
      tions, 203
    in thrombocytopenic purpura, 227
  specimens, decalcification, 706

Boothby and Sandiford, modification of DuBois normal standards, basal metabolism, 424
Bordetella species, 581, 582
Bordet-Gengou medium, 581
Borrelia recurrentis, 613
Borrelia vincentii, 612
Bottles, sample, for water analysis, 652
Botulism, 608
Bouin solution, 710
Boutonneuse (Mediterranean) fever, 614
Brain-heart infusion agar (BHI)
   Cryptococcus neoformans, 639
   with cycloheximide and chloramphenicol for fungi, 634
Brecker-Cronkite phase microscopy method of counting platelets, 123-124
Brewer jar for anaerobic cultures, 541
Brewer methemoglobin reduction test, 177
Brill's disease, 614
Brine flotation method for intestinal parasites in feces, 460
Bromelin method of Pirofsky-Mangum for titration of antibodies, 273
Bromide intoxication, methods of determination, 696-698
Bromine water test for melanin in urine, 45
Bromsulphalein test (BSP), 367-369
Bronchial
   casts in sputum, 521
   secretion in fibrocystic disease of pancreas, 449
Brucella species, 585-587
Brucellosis, 585-587
Buffer solutions, 433-434
Buffy coat smears, 125
Bullis fever, 614
Burr cells, 134, 135, 161
Butanol extractable iodine (BEI), 420-421

C

Cabot rings, 133, 136, 137
Calcium
   carbonate crystals, 52, 55
   in coagulation, 206
   determination, 329-331
   oxalate crystals in urine, 51, 52
   in urine, Sulkowitch test for, 57
Calculations
   formulas for, 434, 435, 436
   with photometric readings, 288-289
Calculi
   biliary, analysis, 431
   urinary, 66-71
Candida albicans, identification of, 636-638
Candida species, 635-638
Candle jar method for carbon dioxide production, 541
Canicola disease, 612
Capillary
   blood, obtaining specimens, 97
   fragility test, 209-210
Capsular swelling
   pneumococcus typing, 556
   with *Streptococcus MG* antiserum, 552

Carbohydrate
   fermentation
      differential media for clostridia, 606
      gonococcus, 558
      meningococcus, 559
   metabolism
      glucose tolerance tests in studies of, 301
      liver function tests based on, 365-366
Carbohydrates, stains for, 714-715
Carbolfuchsin-Kinyoun stain for mycobacteria, 538
Carbon dioxide
   content of blood, measurement, 343
   content and combining power, 346-348
   production, candle jar method, 541
   volume percent calculation, table, 347
Carbon monoxide
   in blood, 691-692
   saturation, hemoglobinometry, 99
Carboxyhemoglobin, 691
   absorption spectra, 102, 103
   physical characteristics, 101, 103
Carmine stain for glycogen, 714-715
Carotene and vitamin A determination, 427-429
Casein hydrolysis test for *Nocardia,* 602
Casts
   in sputum, 521
   in urine, 47, 48
Catalase test
   semiquantitative, for mycobacteria, 597
   for streptococci, 549
Catecholamines in urine, 79-83
Cat-scratch disease virus, 620
Cell
   count
      leukocyte, 130
      reticulocyte, 139, 140
   grouping, 237, 238, 239, 240
Celloidin embedding, 707
Cells
   blood; *see* Blood cells
   hematopoietic, morphology, 130-154
   with inclusion bodies, in urine, 50
   L.E., 192, 193
   nonhematologic, in peripheral blood smear, 154
   tumor, in peripheral blood, 154
Cellular products, stains for, 713-715
Cellulose acetate electrophoresis
   hemoglobin separation by, 172
   protein separation by, 326
Centrifugation in coagulation procedure, 5
Cephalin-cholesterol flocculation test, 362-363
Cerebrospinal fluid
   chemical examination, 511-512
   chloride in, 342
   collection of specimens, 510
   cultures, organisms isolated from, 536
   deproteinization, 298
   in disease, 515-517
   enzymes, 512
   handling of specimens, 532
   microscopic examination, 512-514
   normal values, table, 726
   physical examination, 510-511
   protein in, determination of, 323
   secretion, 507
   serologic examination, 514-515

Cerebrospinal fluid—cont'd
  sulfonamides in, determination of, 699
  tubercle bacilli in, 592
Ceruplasmin
  determination, 389-390
  in serum copper determination, 336
Cestodes (tapeworms), 470-478
Chagas' disease, 502
Chancre, dark-field examination, 610
Chancroid
  culture, 533
  Haemophilus ducreyi from, plate, 584
Charcot-Leyden crystals in sputum, 522, 524
Chediak-Higashi syndrome, 144
Chemical
  disinfection, 531
  examination
    cerebrospinal fluid, 511-512
    gastric juice, 445-446
    serous fluids, 508
    stool, 452-457
    urine, 18-46
  method of oxygen exhaustion, 541
  preservation of urine, 12
  test for cystine, 55
Chemistry, clinical, 283-437
  quality control in, 2-5
  table of normal values, 722-724
Chick embryo, cultivation of virus in, 618, 619
Chickenpox, 625
Children, leukocytes in, 118, 119
Chilomastix mesnili, characteristics, 468-469
Chimeras, blood, 241
Chlamydospore agar
  Candida, 636
  fungi, 634
Chlamydospores
  Histoplasma capsulatum, 640
  production of, 636-637
Chloral hydrate and phenylethyl alcohol media
    for staphylococci, 553
Chloral hydrate–sodium azide blood agar media
    for clostridia, 605
Chloramphenicol, fungi sensitive to, 633
Chloric acid oxidation method for butanol ex-
    tractable iodine, 421
Chloride determination, 340-343
Chlorides
  in cerebrospinal fluid, 512
  in sweat, screening tests for, 449-451
  in urine, Fantus test for, 57
Chloridometer, sweat tests with, 450
Chlorine in water, 653
Chloroform, preservation of urine by, 12
Chocolate agar, 542
  gonococcus culture on, 557
Cholera, 608
  red test, 609
Cholesterol
  crystals in sputum, 522
  determination, 372-375
  levels in various diseases, 374, 375
  in liver disease, 369
Cholinesterase
  activity of, measurement, 390-391
  serum level determination in liver disease, 370

Choriomeningitis, lymphocytic, cerebrospinal
    changes, 515
Chorionic gonadotropin, human, 89, 90
Christmas disease, 225
Chromatography
  absorption, 291
  amino acids in urine determined by, 21, 22
  column, thyroxine by, 421-424
  explanation, 291
  gas-liquid, 293
  paper, 292
  partition, 292
  protein in cerebrospinal fluid determined by,
    512
  sugar in urine determined by, 28-29
  thin-layer, 293
Chromatotube, ring-supported, for paper chro-
    matography, 29
Chromobacter species, 573
Chromoblastomycosis, 645
Chromosomes, sex, 141, 142, 143
Circulating
  anticoagulants
    hemorrhagic diseases due to, 225-226
    tests for, 213, 214, 215
  eosinophil count, 121-122
Citrate utilization, 566
Citrobacter group (*Escherichia freudii*), 567
Clearance tests of kidney function, 60-66
Clearing, paraffin section technique, 707
Clinical
  bacteriology, introduction to, 526
  chemistry; *see* Chemistry, clinical
  laboratory, automation in, 294-298
  material, organisms most likely to be isolated
    from, 535-537
Clinitest tablets, 28
Clonorchis sinensis, life cycle, 491
Clorox digestion method for tubercle bacilli de-
    contamination, 593
Clostridia species, 605-608
Clot
  formation
    cerebrospinal fluid, 511
    and fibrinolysis, schema, 213
    serous fluids, 508
  lysis, 211, 213, 214
  retraction, 211-212
  timers, 210
Clotting; *see also* Coagulation
  visualization of, method, 5
Clumping factor of staphylococci, slide test for,
    554
Co^{60}-B_{12}, urinary excretion of, 157
Coagulase test for staphylococci, 553
Coagulation
  aim, 205
  defects, transfusion therapy, 228
  factor defects, hemorrhagic diseases due to,
    224-225
  factors, 205, 206, 207
    in pregnancy, 89
  mechanism, scheme of, 205-207
  phase I, tests for, 220-223
  phase II, tests for, 215-219
  phase III, tests for, 211
  phases of, 205, 206

Coagulation—cont'd
  procedures, blood derivatives and reagents used in, 208
  quality control in, 5
  test(s)
    collection of blood for, 208
    requirements, table, 211
  time
    mixtures, table, 215
    of recalcified plasma, 210-211
    tests for, 210-211
Cocci
  gram-negative, 556-560
  gram-positive, 546-556
Coccidioidal granuloma, 643
Coccidioides immitis, 643-644
Coccidioidomycosis, 643
Coenzymes, 384
Cold
  agglutinins; *see* Agglutinins, cold
  antibodies, 273-274
Cole test, 32, 33
Coli-aerogenes group, test for, in water examination, 652-653
Collagen, Van Gieson stain for, 710
Collection of specimens; *see* Specimens, collection
Colloidal gold curves and tests, 514
Colonies of bacteria, 529
  in urine, counting, 535
Color
  index and mean corpuscular hemoglobin, 115
  sputum, 521
  stool, 452
  urine, 14-15
Colorimeter, 285-289
Colorimetric
  methods of hemoglobinometry, 98
  tablets and strips, tests for urine, 19
Column chromatography, thyroxine by, 421-424
Combustion methods of oxygen exhaustion, 541
Complement, 233
  antiglobulin test, 236
  -fixation test
    amebiasis, 465
    histoplasmosis, 641
    toxoplasmosis, 505
    viruses, 619
  and hemolysin titrations
    Kolmer test, 666-669
    Reiter test, 676-677
Computers in laboratory, 2
Concentration
  of cells in sputum, aqueous dissolution technique, 523-524
  method, Ajello, *Nocardia,* 601
  methods
    of feces examination for intestinal parasites, 459, 460
    for trematodes, 492-493
    for tubercle bacilli and handling of specimens, 591-593
  test of kidney function, Fishberg, 59
Concretions
  in sputum, 521
  in stool, 452
Congenital hemorrhagic disorders, 223-224

Congo red test for amyloid disease, 430
Conjunctiva, flora normally present in, 529
Connective tissue
  description, 709
  stains, 709-713
Consistency
  of sputum, 521
  of stool, 452
Conversion table, percent transmittance-optical density, 287
Cooked meat medium for anaerobic cultures, 541
Cooley's anemia, 167
Coombs test, 234-236
Copper
  oxidase determination, 389-390
  in serum, determination of, 336-337
  sulfate solution in preparation of permanent standards for content of chlorine in water, 653
  in urine, determination of, 337-338
Coproporphyrins, 40, 41, 42, 43, 44
Cord
  blood bilirubin, 183
  formation of tubercle bacilli, 598-599
Cornmeal agar
  Candida, 636
  fungi, 634
Coronary heart disease, lipoproteins in, 381, 382
Corpuscular constants, 114-115
Corticosteroids, 73
Corynebacteriaceae, 588-591
Corynebacterium diphtheriae, 589-590
Cough plate, pertussis, 581
Coulometric titration, chloride determination by, 343
Coulter counter
  erythrocyte and leukocyte counting with, 120
  platelet count by, 124
  for red blood cells, 113
Coumarin drugs, effect on prothrombin time, 217, 218
Count
  leukocyte, differential and absolute, 130
  official, water examination, 652
  reticulocyte, 139, 140
Counting chamber, red blood cell, 110, 111
Cover glass method for blood smear preparation, 125
Cr^{51} blood volume determination, 109-110
C-reactive protein, 551-552
Creatine
  conversion to creatinine, 314
  phosphokinase (CPK) determination, 391-393
  procedures for, 315, 316
Creatinine
  in blood, determination of, 314-316
  clearance (endogenous), 63
  level of specimen, 11
Creeping eruption, 482
Cresylecht violet solution for Nissl substance, 717
Crithidial form of hemoflagellates, 501
Crosby thrombin test for paroxysmal nocturnal hemoglobinuria, 175-176
Crossmatching, 258-263
  antibodies encountered in, table, 268-270
  emergency procedures, 260-261

Crossmatching—cont'd
  methods, 259
  technique, 259-260
Cryoglobulinemia, 200
Cryoglobulins, tests for, 327-328
Cryostat frozen section technique, 705
Cryptococcosis, 638
Cryptococcus neoformans, 638-639
Crystalline sediment in urine, 52
Crystals
  in alkaline urine, 56
  in sputum, 522, 524
  sulfonamide, in urine, 51, 53, 54, 55
  in urine, 51-56
  in wet preparation of synovial fluid, 518, 519
Culture
  media
    for antibiotic sensitivity determination, 544
    for blood, 532
  methods, 540-542
    Staphylococcus aureus, 553-554
Culture(s); *see also* Laboratory diagnosis
  Actinobacillus mallei, 585
  Actinomyces, 603
  anaerobic, 541-542
  anthrax bacillus, 604
  bacterial, 530, 531, 532, 534
  bacterioides, 587
  Blastomyces dermatitidis, 641
  blood, 532
  bone marrow, 532
  Brucella, 586
  Candida, 636
  cerebrospinal fluid, 515
  clostridia, 605, 606, 607, 608
  Corynebacterium diphtheriae, 589
  Cryptococcus neoformans, 639
  Enterobacteriaceae, 561, 562, 563, 564
  fungi, 632-633
    handling, 531
  Fusobacterium fusiforme, 588
  Geotrichum candidum, 639
  giving group V TSI reactions, differentiation, table, 571
  gonococcus, 557
  Haemophilus, 583, 584
  Histoplasma capsulatum, 640
  Lactobacillus, 588
  Leptospira, 611
  Listeria, 589
  lymphocyte, 149
  meningococcus, 559
  mixed, direct sensitivity testing of, 544
  mycobacteria, 595, 596
  Nocardia, 601-602
  organisms most likely to be isolated from, 535-537
  Pasteurella, 579, 580
  pertussis, 581, 582
  pneumococci, 555
  protozoa, 465
  Pseudomonas, 570
  pus, 525
  rickettsiae, 614
  Salmonella, 576
  Shigella, 578
  Staphylococcus, 553

Culture(s)—cont'd
  stock, 7, 8
  Streptobacillus moniliformis, 610
  streptococci, appearance of, 547
  of synovial fluid, 519
  Trichophyton, 646, 647, 648
  Vibrio, 608, 609
Curschmann's spirals in sputum, 521, 524
Cutaneous mycoses, 646-649
Cutting sections, 708
Cyanide nitroprusside test for cystine, 23
Cyanmethemoglobin method, hemoglobinometry, 99
Cycloheximide, fungi sensitive to, 633
Cylindroids in urine, 48
Cystine
  chemical test for, 55
  crystals, 55
  cyanide nitroprusside test for, 23
Cystinuria, 23
Cytochrome oxidase test for *Pseudomonas*, 570
Cytochromes, 40
Cytology, 720-721
  cerebrospinal fluid, 513
Cytomegaloviruses, 623

D

Dacie method for osmotic fragility of erythrocytes, 162
Dangers of transfusions, 264-265
Dark-field examination
  bacteria, 537
  in syphilis, 533
  Treponema pallidum, 610-611
Davidsohn test for infectious mononucleosis, 190
Decalcification, paraffin section technique, 706
Decontamination methods for tubercle bacilli, 592-593
Defects
  in complete tissue sections, 709
  in section cutting, table, 708
Defibrination
  with glass beads, 98, 208
  syndrome, 225
Dehydration, paraffin section technique, 707
Dent's classification of aminoaciduria (modified after Holt), 23
Dermatomycosis, 646-649
Detergents, sterilization by, 392
Detoxicating function, liver function tests based on, 366-367
Diabetes mellitus
  glucose tolerance test in diagnosis, 301
  tolbutamide diagnostic test for, 306
Diacetylmonoxime, reaction of urea with, 308
Diagnex test, 443
Diagnostic staining procedures, 708-709
Dialysis, concentration of urine protein for electrophoresis by, 21
Diameter, mean, of red blood cells, 116
Diaphorase deficiency in inborn metabolic errors, 410-411
Diastase
  methods of determination, 387-389
  in pancreatic juice, tests for, 447

Diazonium salt, glutamic oxalacetic transaminase, 407-408
2,6-Dichlorophenol-indophenol sodium solution, 429
Dicumarol in anticoagulant therapy, 209
Diego (Di) blood group system, 255
Dientamoeba fragilis, characteristics, 465, 467
Differential
  blood count
    bone marrow, 203
    cerebrospinal fluid, 513
    in polycythemia vera, 185
    serous fluids, 509
    synovial fluid, 517
  leukocyte count, 118, 130
  media
    bacteria, 542, 543
    Staphylococcus, 553
  partial thromboplastin time (PTT), 221
  test for infectious mononucleosis, 190, 191
Digestion methods for concentration and decontamination of tubercle bacilli, 592-593
di Guglielmo's disease, 194-195
Dilution
  bottles for water analysis, 652
  curve for prothrombin concentration in plasma, 217
Dioxane, tissue dehydrator, 707
Diphasic fungi, 640-644
Diphenylcarbazone in chloride determination, 340
Diphtheria, tests for, 589, 590
Diphtheroids
  anaerobic, and *Actinomyces bovis,* differentiation, table, 604
  nonpathogenic, 590
Diphyllobothrium latum, 473, 474, 475
Diplococcus pneumoniae (pneumococcus), 555
Dipylidium caninum, 478
Dirt test, milk, 653
Disease
  affecting basal metabolic rate, 426
  cerebrospinal fluid changes in, 515-517
  and disk-thioglycollate methods of sensitivity determination with anaerobes, 545
  hemorrhagic, 223-228
  sensitivity test of antibiotics, 543-544
  sputum in, 524
Disseminated lupus erythematosus, 191-193
Dittrich's plugs in sputum, 521
DNA viruses, 615
DNAse test agar, 554
Döderlein's bacillus, 588
Dog tapeworm, 478
Döhle bodies, 144, 145
Donath-Landsteiner hemolysin, biphasic type, detection, 182
Donor, universal, 261-262
Donors, blood, selection of, 257-258
Donovan bodies of granuloma inguinale, 584
Downey cells, 148
Dracunculus medinensis, 489
Drugs
  effect on basal metabolic rate, 426
  and poisons, toxicology, 684-704
  in urine, qualitative estimation of, 57

Drug-susceptibility patterns, *Mycobacterium tuberculosis,* 599
Dry-ash method
  of Barker, protein-bound iodine separation, 415
  thyroxine by column chromatography, 423
Dry heat sterilization, 530
Dualists, theory of blood cell origin, 95
DuBois normal standards, basal metabolism, 424
Dubos Tween-albumin broth (TAB), 595
Duffy (Fy) blood group system, 251-252
Duke method of measuring bleeding time, 209
Duodenal
  aspirate, titration of bicarbonate in, 448
  aspiration of rhabditiform larvae, 486
  contents
    enzyme tests, 447
    intestinal parasites in, examination, 462
  fluid changes in fibrocystic disease, 449
  secretion, 446
Dwarf tapeworm, 476, 477, 478
Dye-dilution principle, blood volume measurement, 109
Dye plate method and dye sensitivity test, *Brucella,* 586
Dysentery bacilli, 578

E

EA$_{36}$ stain, 720
Ears
  bacterial infectious, handling of specimens, 534
  cultures, organisms isolated from, 536
Eaton pleuropneumonia-like organisms (PPLO), 626
Echinococcus granulosus, 474-476, 477
Eclampsia, 89
Edema of lung, sputum in, 524
EDTA in obtaining blood for specimens, 98
Education, continued, in laboratory medicine, 1
Egg
  inoculation, viruses, 618-619
  media for *Mycobacterium tuberculosis,* 596
Ehrlich
  benzaldehyde test for urobilinogen in urine, 37
  dimethylaminobenzaldehyde reagent, 37
  reagent for urobilinogen tests, 360
El Tor vibrio, 609
Elastic tissue
  fibers in sputum, 522, 523
  stain, Verhoeff, 713
Electrolytes in urine, qualitative estimation of, 57
Electron microscopy
  blood examination, 96
  virus examination, 620
Electronic counters for red blood cells, 113
Electrophoresis
  cellulose acetate, protein separation by, 326
  fractionation of serum proteins by, 324-328
  hemoglobin, 171
  of lactic dehydrogenase isozymes, 398
  of lipoproteins, 380, 381
  in macroglobulinemia, 201
  paper, for Bence Jones protein, 21

Electrophoresis—cont'd
  of paraproteins, 197, 198, 199
  protein in cerebrospinal fluid, 512
  serum, in lupus erythematosus, 193
  starch gel, starch block, or agar gel, for separation of fetal hemoglobin, 170
  thin-layer, in aminoaciduria, 22
Electrophoretic protein fractions, changes with disease, table, 327
Elliptocytes, 135
Elliptocytosis, hereditary, 167
Elution
  of antibodies, 271-272
  of cold antibodies, 274-275
Embedding, 707
Encephalitis, St. Louis, cerebrospinal changes, 515
Endo agar, 561
Endolimax nana, characteristics, 467
Endothelial cell, 151
Endotoxins, bacterial, 529
Enriched media, 542
Entamoeba
  characteristics, 465
  medium of Cleveland and Collier, 465
Entamoeba histolytica, high-power field, color plate, 467
Enteric gram-negative bacteria, 560-564
Enterobacter species, 574
Enterobacteriaceae
  differentiation by biochemical tests, table, 574-575
  group differentiation by biochemical tests, 562, 564
  laboratory diagnosis, 560-564
  lactose-fermenting, differentiation, 565
  principal groups, chart, 559
Enterobius vermicularis, 479-480
Enterococcus group of streptococci, 550
Enteropathogenic *Escherichia coli* (EPEC), 566-567
Enteroviruses, 620-621
Enzymatic methods for staphylococci, 553-554
Enzyme
  test, specific, for glucose in urine, 30
  titration of antibodies, 272-273
Enzyme-deficient hemolytic anemias, 176
Enzymes, 382-411
  action and reaction, 382
  aldolase, 384
  alpha-hydroxybutyrate dehydrogenase, 385
  amylase (diastase), 387
  bacterial, 528
  in cerebrospinal fluid, 512
  ceruloplasmin (copper oxidase), 389
  cholinesterase, 390
  creatine phosphokinase, 391
  in erythrocytes, deficiencies in inborn metabolic errors, 408-411
  isocitric dehydrogenase, 393
  lactic dehydrogenase, 395
  leucine aminopeptidase, 399
  lipase, 401-402
  in liver disease diagnosis, 370
  pancreatic, 447
  phosphatases, 402

Enzymes—cont'd
  transaminases, 406
  units, 382, 383
Enzyme-treated cells, Coombs technique with, 236
Eosinopenia, 147
  classification, 120
Eosinophil count, circulating, 121-122
Eosinophilia, 147
Eosinophils
  maturation, 146
  variation in number, 147
Epidermophyton infections of skin and nails, 648
Epinephrine tolerance test, 306
Epithelial cells in urine, 50
Epoxy embedding, tissue, 707
Equipment for coagulation procedures, 5-6
Equivalents, table, 436
Errors
  in blood counts with Coulter counter, sources of, 121
  in circulating eosinophil count method, 121
  in clinical chemistry, sources of, 2
  in Coombs technique, sources of, 235-236
  in disk sensitivity testing, 544
  in hematocrit determination, 107
  in hematology, detection of, 6
  in hemoglobin methods, sources of, 100
  in red cell
    counting, 112
    and reverse typing, 240-241
  in Rh_o testing, 245
  in white cell counting, 120
Erysipelothrix, 590-591
Erythremia, 113, 185
Erythroblastosis
  ABO, 183
    laboratory diagnosis, 278-279
  fetalis, 182-183, 275-278
    amniotic fluid examination, 276-277
    paternal testing and fetal testing, 276
    postnatal studies, 277-278
    prenatal studies and maternal testing, 275
Erythroblasts, 161
Erythrocyte
  enzyme deficiencies in inborn metabolic errors, 408-411
  mean, cross section and measurements in different clinical conditions, 115
  uptake of I^{131}-labeled triiodothyronine (ET_3), 413
Erythrocytes; *see also* Red blood cells
  in blood smear examination, 129
  in stained smear, variation, 134-140
  in urine, 47
Erythrocytic inclusions, 137
Erythrocytosis, 113
  anoxic, 186
  physiologic, 114
Erythroid marrow hyperplasia, 166
Erythrokinetic evaluation of anemia, 155
Erythroleukemia, 194-195
Erythropoiesis, 131-140
Esbach quantitative method of testing urine for protein, 19
Escherichia coli
  description, 564

Escherichia coli—cont'd
enteropathogenic, 566
in water, standards, 652, 653
Escherichia freundii, 567
Estriol assay, placental, 94
Estrogens, 72
Ethyl alcohol determination, 684
Ethylenediaminetetraacetic acid (EDTA)
calcium titration with, 329, 330, 331
disodium salt of, as anticoagulant, 284
Ethylhydrocupreine hydrochloride, 556
Euglobulin
clot lysis, 214
screening test in macroglobulinemia, 200
Examination
in bacteriology, methods, 537-543
biologic fluid, 507-525
cerebrospinal fluid, 510-515
fungi, methods, 630-635
milk, standard methods, 653-654
pus, 525
sputum, 521-524
stool, 452-457
tissue, methods, 705-721
urine
chemical, 18-46
microscopic, 46-56
physical, 13-18
water, standard methods, 652-653
Exchange transfusions
choice of blood for, 261
in erythroblastosis fetalis, 278
Exocrine secretions, changes in fibrocystic disease, 449
Extracorpuscular defects, hemolytic anemias due to, 179
Extramedullary hematopoiesis, 131
Exudates
tests, 509
total protein in, 508
Eye cultures, organisms isolated from, 536

F

Factors X and V, *Haemophilus,* 582, 583, 584
Fairbanks and Beutler spot test for G-6-PD, 176
Falling drop method of measuring specific gravity of urine, 17
False positive reactions, biologic, syphilis, 683
Fanconi syndrome, 23
Fantus test for chlorides in urine, 57
Fat
in feces
examination for, 452
in steatorrhea, 455, 456
in milk, Babcock method of analysis, 654
stain for, 713-714
tolerance test, 381
in urine, significance, 49
Fatty
acid
crystals in sputum, 522
esters, determination, 376-377
acids
free (unesterified), determination, 377-378
polyunsaturated, 380
Febrile reactions, transfusion, 263

Fecal
fat and enzymes, estimation in pancreatic fibrosis, 451
porphyrins, screening test for, 42
Feces
collection of specimen, 533
examination, 452-457
Gram staining method for, 539
intestinal parasites in, examination, 459-462
preservation of specimens, 461
in parasitology, 504
tubercle bacilli in, 592
urobilinogen in, procedure, 361-362
worm eggs in, Stoll counting technique, 484-485
Femoral vein, obtaining infant's blood from, 97
Fenwal plasmaphoresis set, 265
Ferata cell, 151
Fermentation reaction
test
Candida, 637-638
for glucose in urine, 31
tubes for water analysis, 652
Vibrio comma, 609
Ferments, media identifying, 542
Ferric chloride test
for melanin in urine, 45
for phenylpyruvic acid in urine, 24
of urine, 34-35
Ferritin, 158
Ferro and Ham, direct method of total cholesterol determination, 374
Ferrohemoglobin solubility test, 173
Fetal hemoglobin, 168, 169, 170, 171
Fibrindex, 212
Fibrinogen
blood content, liver function and, 362
in coagulation, 206
deficiency tests, 212-213
determination, 328-329
increased, in cerebrospinal fluid, test, 511
titer, 212-213
Fibrinolysis
clot formation and, 213
excessive, screening tests for, 213
Fibrinolytic activity
in clot retraction, 212
fluorometric assay of, 214
Fibrin-stabilizing factor in coagulation, 207
Fibrocystic disease of pancreas, 449-451
Fibrometer, 219
Ficin titration of antibodies, 273
Filariae, 487, 488, 489
Filariform larvae of worms, 480, 485, 486
Film, 35 mm., preparation of microscopic sections on, 708
Filtrates, protein-free, 298-299
Filtration of bacteria, 531
Fish tapeworm, 473, 474, 475
Fishberg concentration tests, 59
Fisher-Race linked gene theory, 244
Fisher's
modification of Ehrlich reagent, 44
nomenclature, Rh factor, 243-244
Fi-Test, 212
Fixation of tissue, paraffin section technique, 705
Fixatives, paraffin section technique, 706

Flagellates
 blood and tissue, 500-501
 intestinal, morphologic differentiation, 468
 species, characteristics, 468, 469
Flame photometry, 290
 in potassium determination, 339
 in sodium determination, 338
Fletcher medium, leptospirae, 611
Flocculation tests
 in liver disease, 362-365
 in lupus erythematosus, 193
 slide, VDRL, 656-659
 tube, VDRL, 661-662
Flora, normal, in human beings, 529-530
Flotation methods, intestinal parasites in feces, 459, 460
Fluids
 amniotic, 520-521
 biologic examination, 507-525
 cerebrospinal, 510-517
 serous, 507-510
 from serous cavities, handling of specimens, 533
 synovial, 517-520
Flukes, 492-493
 blood, 494
 of man, table, 491
Fluorescence spot tests for glucose-6-phosphate dehydrogenase, pyruvate kinase, and glutathione reductase deficiencies, 178, 179
Fluorescent
 antibody test
  bacteria, 539
  enteropathogenic *E. coli,* 567
  fungi, 635
  group A streptococci, 549-550
  indirect, in amebiasis, 465
  lupus erythematosus, 193
  Mycoplasma, 626
  Neisseria gonorrhoeae, 557-558
  rabies, 622-623
  treponemal, 655, 679-682
  typhus, 614
  viruses, 620
 dye method, tubercle bacilli, 595
 microscopy
  blood examination by, 96
  for identification of amebas, 465
Fluorescytes, 97
Fluoride as blood preservative, 285
Fluorometric assay of fibrinolytic activity, 214
Fluorometry, 291
Foam test for bilirubin, 36
Folic acid deficiency, 157-158
Folin-Wu
 filtrate, 298, 299
 method, blood glucose determination, 300
Foreign bodies in sputum, 521, 522
Formaldehyde
 qualitative test for, 687-688
 tablets, preservation of urine by, 12
 tissue fixative, 706
Formalin
 preservation of urine by, 12
 in tissue fixation, 706

Formalin-ether sedimentation for stool examination, intestinal parasites, 460
Formalin-fixed tissue, stain for rickettsiae in sections of, 720
Formiminoglutamic acid (FIGLU) in urine, determination of, 158
Formol-gel test, macroglobulinemia, 200
Formulas for calculations, 434, 435, 436
Fouchet reagent, 36
Fragility of erythrocytes
 mechanical, 164
 osmotic, 161-163
Franklin method, bilirubin test, 36
Freezing point determination of urine, 17-18
Friedman test for pregnancy, 90
 quantitative, 93
Froehde reagent, morphine determination, 700
Frog tests for pregnancy, 91, 92
Frogs, care of, for pregnancy tests, 92
Frozen section technique, 705
Fructose
 conversion, 365
 tolerance test, 366
 in urine
  Benedict qualitative test for, 27, 31
  Selivanoff test for, 31
FSH in urine, determination, 71
FTA Leptospira, 612
Fuchs-Rosenthal counting chamber, 121, 122
Fungi
 collection of specimens, 630
 cultures, 632, 633, 634
  and smears, handling, 531
 description, 629
 diphasic, 640-644
 direct examination, 630-632
 Imperfecti, 629
 methods of examination, 630-635
 mounting and staining, 635
 pathogenic, classification, 629
 pathogenicity of, gastric mucin for enhancing, 634
 saprophytic, 649-650
 of skin, nails, and hair, 646-649
 in sputum, 523
 staining, 718-720
 structure, 629
 yeastlike, 635-640
Fusobacterium fusiforme, 588

G

Gaffkya tetragena, 555
Galactose
 conversion, 365
 determination, 308
 tolerance test, 365-366
 in urine
  Benedict qualitative test for, 27
  mucic acid test for, 32
Galactose-1-phosphate uridyl transferase, erythrocyte deficiency of, 409
Galactosemia, 24
 spot-screening test for, 32-33
Galactosuria, 32
Gametocytes, 496
γ-A antibodies, 233

γ-G antibodies, 232
Gamma globulin neutralization test, 236
Gamma globulins
  antibodies, 232
  immune, 180
  and immunoglobulins, 197-199
  increased, zinc sulfate turbidity test, 364, 365
Gamma hemolysis, 529
Gamma hemolytic streptococci, 547
γ-M antibodies, 232
Gas gangrene production, 606
Gaseous sterilization, 531
Gas-liquid chromatography, 293
Gasometric
  analysis, 343-346
  methods in hemoglobinometry, 98
Gaspak, 541
Gastric
  acid measurement, 443-444
  acidity, concentration of, 444-445
  analysis, 443-446
  contents, tubercle bacilli in, 591
  juice, gross examination, 445
  mucin for enhancing pathogenicity of fungi,
    634
  secretion, measurement, 444
Gastrointestinal tract cultures, organisms, iso-
    lated from, 536
Gaucher's disease, 201
Gelatin liquefaction, clostridia, 605
Genital tract
  cultures, organisms isolated from, 536
  infections, investigation of, 533
Genotypes
  Duffy, 252
  of Lu system, 255
  Rh, determination of, 247
  Rh-Hr, 248, 249
Geotrichum candidum, 639
Gerhardt ferric chloride test, 34-35
Germ tubes in serum, production by *Candida
    albicans*, 638
Giardia lamblia, characteristics, 469
Giemsa stain, blood cells, 125, 127
Gilchrist's disease, 641
Glanders, 585
Glandular fever, 188
Glanzmann, thrombasthenia, 226
Glass beads, defibrination with, 98, 208
Glassware
  for coagulation procedures, 5
  siliconizing, 208
Glitter cells in urine, 47
Globulin
  albumin, and protein, total, determination of,
    320-329
  in cerebrospinal fluid, tests, 511
  in serous fluids (Rivalta test), 508
Globulins, antibodies, 232
Glomerular
  filtration rate, 62
  nephritis, classification and manifestations,
    table, 68, 69
Glossary
  of blood banking terms, 279-281
  of mycologic terms, 650-651

Glucose
  in cerebrospinal fluid, 512
  concentration, postprandial, 305
  determination, 299-307
  specific enzyme test for, 30
  tolerance
    curves, 304
    tests, 301-307
      effects of preceding 48 hr. diets on, chart,
        302
      intravenous, 305
      normal response, 303
      one-dose test, 303-304
      one-hour two-dose test, 304-305
    pancreatic function, 448
  in urine
    Benedict qualitative test for, 27
    fermentation test for, 31
    Somogyi quantitative test for, 30-31
  in whole blood, changes on standing, 285
Glucose-6-phosphate dehydrogenase
  deficiency, screening tests for, 176-179
  low erythrocyte levels in inborn metabolic er-
    rors, 409
Glucuronates in urine, 33
Glutamic oxalacetic transaminase (GOT)
  in cerebrospinal fluid, 512
  and glutamic pyruvic transaminase (GPT),
    298, 406, 407
Glutathione
  reductase
    deficiency, tests for, 178
    in erythrocytes, inborn metabolic errors and,
      409
  stability test, 179
Glycerin jelly, formula, 713
Glycogen
  best carmine stain for, 714-715
  formation, 365
Glycosuria, 26
Gm groups and rheumatoid factor, 519
Gmelin test
  for bile
    in stool, 453
    in urine, 35
  Harrison's modification, 36
GN broth (Hajna), 560
Gold chloride solution, 711-712
Gomori methenamine
  silver nitrate stain, 718
  silver stain, histoplasmosis, 641
Gonadotropin, chorionic, human (HCG), 89
Gonococci in cervical smear, color plate, 557
Gonococcus, laboratory diagnosis, 556-558
Gonorrhea, collection of specimen and culture,
    533
Goodpasture stain, bacteria in tissue, 716
Gordiacea, 487
Gout, synovial fluid in, 518
Gowers diluting fluid, 110
Gram stain
  Actinomyces, 602
  anthrax bacillus, 604
  bacteria reaction, 528
  Cl. edematiens, 607
  Cl. welchii, 606
  Haemophilus influenzae, 582

Gram stain—cont'd
   iodine stain, 716
   pus examination, 525
Gram staining method, 539
Gram-negative
   aerobic, nonspore-forming bacilli, 560-585
   anaerobic nonspore-forming bacilli, 587-588
   cocci, 556-560
   microaerophilic nonspore-forming rods, 585-587
Gram-positive
   cocci, 546-556
   nonspore-forming bacilli, 588-603
   spore-forming bacilli, 603-608
Granular casts in urine, significance, 48
Granulation, toxic, 145, 146
Granulocytes, band and segmented, 141
Granulocytic
   leukemia, acute, 194
   series, white blood cells, 140-148
Granuloma
   coccidioidal, 643
   inguinale, 584-585
      diagnosis, 533
Grape cell, 197
Gravimetric method of Pernokis, Freeland, and
      Kraus, total lipid determination, 372
Gravindex test for pregnancy, 92, 93
Gridley stain, histoplasmosis, 641
Griess nitrite test of urine, 535
Ground itch, 481
Group A streptococci, 547, 549
Group O
   serum and anti-C, 238
   universal donor, tests, 261-262
Groups B, C, and D streptococci, 550
Groups, blood; *see* Blood groups
Guaiac test for blood in stool, 452
Guanase
   deficiency in inborn metabolic errors, 410
   in diagnosis of liver disease, 370
Guillaim-Barré syndrome, cerebrospinal fluid in,
      517
Guinea pig inoculation
   Pasteurella tularensis, 580
   tubercle bacilli, 600
Guinea worm, 489
Guthrie test, 24
Gutstein method, variola and vaccinia viruses,
      625
Gutzeit
   apparatus, 690
   test for arsenic, 689-691

H

H disease, 24
Haden modification of Folin-Wu method of
      filtration, 298
Haemophilus species, 582-584
Haff disease, 40
Hafnia, 576
Hageman factor in coagulation, 207
Hair
   examination by atomic absorption analysis, 451
   fungi of, 646, 647, 648
   in fungus infections, collection of specimens
      and direct examination, 630, 631

Hajna broth, 560
Ham's acid-serum test for nocturnal hemoglo-
      binuria, 175
Hand sweat test in fibrocystic disease, 449
Hand-Schüller-Christian disease, 201
Hanging-drop method, examination of bacteria,
      537
Hansen's bacillus, 601
Haptoglobins, 39, 160
   serum, tests in hemolytic anemia, 165-166
"Harleco" Dripak bilirubin standard, 359
Harris hematoxylin solution, 709
Harrison's modification of Gmelin test, 36
Hart test for beta-hydroxybutyric acid in urine,
      35
Hartrup disease, 24
Hart's syndrome, 24
Hay bacillus, 605
Heat
   and acetic acid test of urine, 18
   precipitation test for Bence Jones protein, 20
   production in body, measurement, 424
Heated aluminum silver electrode sweat test, 451
Heat-resistance test for *Streptococus faecalis,*
      550
Heat-stable alkaline phosphatase as index of
      placental function, 94
Heavy-chain disease, 197
Heinz
   bodies, 137
      in toxic hemolytic anemias, 179
   body anemia, congenital, 179
Heller
   ring test, 18
   table, modified, analysis of urinary calculi, 67
Helminths, 470-494
   scientific and common names and habitat,
      table, 463
Hemagglutination
   and hemagglutination-inhibition tests, viruses,
      619
   technique, in amebiasis, 465
   test in toxoplasmosis, 505
Hemagglutination-inhibition tests
   for pregnancy, 92
   for viruses, 619
Hemangiomas, thrombocytopenia with, 227
Hemastix reagent strips, 39
Hematest reagent tablets, 164, 165
Hematin, acid and alkaline, hemoglobinometry,
      98
Hematocrit
   determination, purpose and errors, 107
   in polycythemia vera, 185
   volume of packed red cells, 106-107
Hematoidin crystals in sputum, 522
Hematologic findings
   agranulocytosis, 187-188
   aplastic anemia, 185
   erythroblastosis fetalis, 183
   hemolytic
      anemias, 180, 184
      transfusion reactions, 184
   hereditary spherocytosis, 167
   leukemias, chronic, 195, 196
   lupus erythematosus, 192
   mononucleosis, 188

Hematologic findings—cont'd
  multiple myeloma, 197
  myelophthisic anemia, 187
  polycythemia vera, 185
Hematology
  methods in, 95-228
  quality control in, 6
  table of normal values, 724-725
Hematopoietic
  cells, morphology of, 130-154
  principle, 155
Hematoxylin phosphotungstic acid stain, Mallory,
    710
Hematoxylin-eosin stain, 709
Hematuria, 40
  causes, 47
Hemoconcentration, 186
Hemocytoblast, 131
Hemocytometer, improved Neubauer ruling on,
    110
Hemoflagellates, 500-504
Hemoglobin
  A, 168, 170, 171
  A_2, 168, 172, 174
  abnormal
    further identification, 173-175
    laboratory investigation, 169-173
    with thalassemia, 168
  absorption spectra, 102, 103
  breakdown, 160
  C, 175
  composition, 98
  D, 173, 174, 175
  E, 174
  electrophoresis, 171
  F, 168, 169, 170, 171
  H, 174, 175
  M, 175
  mean corpuscular, 114, 115
  normal values at different age levels, 114
  physical measurements as methods of deter-
    mination, 101
  S, 173, 174, 175
  serum, test in hemolytic anemia, 164-165
  spectroscopic examination, 39
  in urine, free, 38
  values, normal, 100
Hemoglobinemia, 160
  test with Hematest reagent tablets, 164-165
Hemoglobinometry, 98-106
Hemoglobinopathies, 168-175
Hemoglobinuria, 38-40, 160
  paroxysmal nocturnal, 175-176
Hemohistioblast, 131
Hemolysin
  and complement titrations
    Kolmer test, 666-669
    Reiter test, 676-677
  dilution, stock, preparation of, in Kolmer test,
    666
  test, soluble, for *Streptococcus faecalis,* 550
Hemolysins
  cold, monothermal, screening test, 181-182
  Donath-Landsteiner, biphasic type, detection,
    182
Hemolysis, 542
  alpha, beta, and gamma, 529

Hemolysis—cont'd
  methods, 160
  of streptococci, 547
Hemolytic
  anemias; *see* Anemias, hemolytic
  disease of newborn (HDN), 182-183, 275-
    279; *see also* Erythroblastosis
    comparison of ABO and Rh, table, 279
  jaundice, cause, 356
  reactions, transfusion, 263, 264
  streptococci, 547
  transfusion reactions, 184
Hemophilia, 225
Hemorrhage, subarachnoid, cerebrospinal
    changes, 515
Hemorrhagic diseases, 223-228
Hemosiderin, 158
  in urine, 39
Heparin
  in anticoagulant therapy, 219
  in blood ammonia determination, 316
  laboratory use, 284
  in obtaining blood for specimens, 98
  therapy, blood clotting time test for control
    of, 210
Hepatitis, 624, 625
Hereditary
  elliptocytosis, 167
  hemorrhagic disorders, 223-224
  spherocytosis, 167
Herellea, 571, 572
Hermaphroditic trematodes, 492
Hermaphroditism, chromosomal sex pattern in,
    142
Herpes
  virus group, 621
  zoster, 625
Herxheimer scarlet red (Sudan IV) stain, 713
Heterophil antibodies in mononucleosis, 188,
    190, 191
Heterozygotes, detection of G-6-PD deficiency
    in, 178
Hicks-Pitney modification of thromboplastin
    generation test, 222
Hippuric acid synthesis tests, oral and intrave-
    nous, 366-367
Histiocytosis X, 201
Histopathology of fungi, 638, 639, 642, 643,
    645, 646
Histoplasma capsulatum, 640-641
Histoplasmosis, 640
Hogben test for pregnancy, 91
Holt modification of Dent's classification of
    aminoaciduria, 23
Homocystinuria, 26
Hookworm larvae, differential diagnosis, 486
Hookworms, 480, 482
Hormone test for pregnancy, 91
Hormones
  definition, 71
  pituitary, in urine, determination, 71
  steroid, 72
  thyroid, 411, 412, 413
  urinary, and their metabolites, 71-84
Hospitals, staphylococcal infections in, bacterio-
    logic survey, 554-555
Howell-Jolly bodies, 133, 136, 137

Hr factors, 242, 243, 244
Human chorionic gonadotropin (HCG), 89, 90
Hyaline casts in urine, significance, 48
Hydatid or echinococcus cyst, 474, 475, 476, 477
Hydrochloric acid
  in determination of gastric contents, 445
  standard solution, 432
Hydrogen ion concentration (pH)
  in blood, 348-350
  of urine, 15-16
  values, 433
Hydrophobia, 621
Hydroxysteroids in urine, determination, 73, 76
17-Hydroxysteroids, urinary, modified Porter-
          Silber method, 77-78
Hymenolepis, 476, 477, 478
Hypercholesterolemia and atherosclerosis, 375
Hyperchromasia, 134
Hypercupremia, 338
Hyperglycemia, conditions with, 301
Hyperheparinemia, 226
Hyperplasia, marrow, erythroid, 166
Hyphae
  Candida, 635
  fungi, 629, 631, 632
Hypochromasia, 135
Hypocupremia, 338
Hypofibrinogenemia
  acquired, 25
  congenital, 224
Hypogammaglobulinemia, 201
Hypoglycemia
  conditions with, 301
  due to insulin, test of gastric contents, 446
  unresponsiveness, 306
Hypohaptoglobinemia, 166
Hypoprothrombinemia, 225

I

I[131]
  -labeled triiodothyronine, erythrocyte uptake
     of, 413
  triolein test, 448
  uptake by thyroid gland, 411
Icterus index, 356
Ictotest, 36
Idiopathic autoimmune hemolytic anemia, 180
Ii blood group system, 255
Immunocyte, 148
Immunoelectrophoresis of paraproteins, 198, 199,
     200
Immunoglobulins (Ig), 197-199
  groups, 232
Immunohematology, introduction to, 179
Immunologic
  pregnancy tests, 92-93
  slide test, quantitative, for pregnancy, 93
  thrombocytopenic purpura (ITP), 227
Immuno-plate test for pregnancy, 92
Impregnation, paraffin section technique, 707
IMViC reactions, *Escherichia,* 565-566
Incineration
  alkaline, Barker method of iodine separation,
     415-417
  butanol extractable iodine, 421
Inclusion bodies, viral diseases, 620

India ink for staining fungi, 635
Indican in urine, tests for, 38
Indicators in bacteriology, 543
Indole
  production, 565-566
  test, clostridia, 606
Infants
  blood specimens from, obtaining, 97
  leukocytes in, 118, 119
  newborn
    ABO hemolytic disease, 278-279
    collection of urine from, 12
    cultures from, organisms isolated from, 536
Infarction of lung, sputum in, 524
Infection(s)
  anemia of, 159
  intestinal parasitic, of man, table, 463
  in proliferative disorders, 201
  staphylococcal, in hospitals, 554-555
  wound, clostridia in, 605
Infectious mononucleosis, 188-191
  cells, 148
Infusora (ciliates), 469
Ink for staining fungi, 635
Inoculation
  animal
    Actinobacillus mallei, 585
    Brucella, 587
    Candida albicans, 638
    Clostridium tetani, 607-608
    Coccidioides immitis, 644
    Corynebacterium diphtheriae, 590
    Erysipelothrix, 591
    fungi, 634
    leptospirae, 612
    Listeria, 589
    rickettsiae, 614
    Spirillum minus, 610
    tubercle bacilli, 600
    Vibrio fetus, 609
    viruses, 619
  of media, liquid and solid, technique, 540
Inoculum concentration in antibiotic sensitivity
     determination, 544
Inorganic phosphorus, determination, 331-333
Insulin
  test, gastric secretion, 446
  tolerance test, 306
Intestinal
  flagellates, morphologic differentiation, table,
     468
  nematodes, 479-487
  parasites
    methods of examination, 459-462
    ova of, color plate, 471
  parasitic infections of man, table, 463
  sporozoa, 500
  tract, flora normally present in, 529
Intracellular products, stains for, 713-715
Intracorpuscular defects, hemolytic anemias due
     to, 167-179
Intrauterine transfusion in erythroblastosis fetalis,
     277
Intubation method, gastric analysis, 443-445
Inulin clearance, 62
Involution and L forms, bacterial, 529
Iodamoeba bütschlii, characteristics, 467-468

Iodine
  butanol extractable, 420-421
  inorganic, separation from protein-bound io-
    dine, 414-420
  protein-bound, 413-420
  radioactive; *see* I[131]
  staining of protozoa, 464
  test for bile in urine, 36
Iron
  content method of Wong, 100-101
  hematoxylin stain
    for intestinal parasites, 461-462
    for protozoa, 464
  influence on occult blood tests of stool, 453
  metabolism, 158
  requirements, 159
  serum, measurement, 334-336
  stain, blood smears, 138
Iron-binding capacity, serum, measurement, 334,
    335, 336
Iron-deficiency anemia, 158-159
  blood cells in diagnosis, 138, 139
Isoantibodies, hemolytic anemias due to, 182-184
Isocitric dehydrogenase (ICD)
  determination, 393-395
  in differential diagnosis of jaundice, 370
Isoniazid (isonicotinic acid hydrazide), concen-
    tration in serum, determination, 702
Isospora hominis, 500
Isotope technique, red blood cell survival time,
    166
Isozymes in lactic dehydrogenase, 397-398
Ivy method of measuring bleeding time, 209

J

Jaffe reaction, 314
Jaundice
  bilirubin values, 360
  causes and types, 356
  congenital hemolytic or acholuric, 167
  icterus index, 356
  infectious, 612
  laboratory findings, table, 355
  types, 36
Jendrassik-Grof method, serum bilirubin deter-
    mination, 357-358
Jock itch, 646
Joint fluid, 507
  handling of specimens, 533
Jordan's anomaly, 144
Jugular vein, obtaining infants blood from, 97

K

Kaiserling solutions, 721
Kala-azar, laboratory diagnosis, 502
Kaolin
  activated partial thromboplastin time (PTT),
    221
  modification of thromboplastin generation test,
    222
Kaplow simplified myeloxidase stain using benzi-
    dine dihydrochloride, 128
Karyotypes
  abnormal, in hematologic conditions, 143
  human, female, 142

Kell (K) blood group system, 251
Kernechtrot stain, 712
Ketone bodies in urine, tests for, 34-35
Ketosteroids in urine, determination, 73-76
Ketostix, 35
Kidd (Jk) blood group system, 254
Kidney
  in acid-base metabolism, 16
  clearance tests, 60-61
  diseases, classification and manifestations, ta-
    ble, 68-70
  function tests, 58-66
    choice of, table, 58
    table of normal values, 726
Kingsbury-Clark method of testing urine for pro-
    tein, 18-19
Kinyoun
  acid-fast stain, 715-716
  carbolfuchsin stain for mycobacteria, 538
Kjeldahl flask, 319, 320
Klebsiella, morphology and biochemistry, 574
Klebsiella-Aerobacter-Serratia division, tables,
    573
Kleihauer, acid dilution method of, demonstra-
    tion of fetal hemoglobin by, 170-171
Klinefelter's syndrome, 142
Knee with gout, synovial fluid from, 518
Koch-Weeks bacillus, 584
Kohn one-step rapid staining technique (modi-
    fied) for intestinal protozoa, 462
Kolmer
  one-fifth volume test (Reiter protein antigen
    test), 675-679
  qualitative tests with serum and spinal fluid,
    669-671
  quantitative tests with serum and spinal fluid,
    671-672
  test for syphilis
    complement and hemolysin titrations, 666-
      669
    equipment, glassware, and reagents, 664
    antigen and stock hemolysin dilutions, 666
    sera, spinal fluid, and sheep red cell sus-
      pension, 665-666
Kovac reagent, 566
Kovacs oxidase test, *Pseudomonas*, 570
Krystanin, appearance of elements stained with,
    46

L

L forms, bacterial, 529
Labile factor in coagulation, 207
Laboratory
  clinical, automation in, 294-298
  diagnosis
    ABO erythroblastosis, 278-279
    Actinobacillus mallei, 585
    Actinomyces israeli and *bovis*, 602-603
    Allescheria boydii, 645
    anthrax bacillus, 604
    Aspergillus fumigatus, 649
    Bacteroides, 587
    Blastomyces dermatitidis, 641-642
    Bordetella pertussis, 581
    Borrelia recurrentis, 613
    Brucella, 586-587

Laboratory—cont'd
  diagnosis—cont'd
    Candida, 635-636
    chromoblastomycosis, 646
    clostridia, 605-608
    Coccidioides immitis, 643
    Corynebacterium diphtheriae, 589-590
    Cryptococcus neoformans, 638-639
    cytomegaloviruses, 623-624
    dermatomycosis, 646
    Enterobacteriaceae, 560-564
    enteropathogenic *E. coli,* 567
    fibrocystic disease, 449-451
    Fusobacterium fusiforme, 588
    Geotrichum candidum, 639
    gonococcus, 556-558
    granuloma inguinale, 584-585
    Haemophilus, 582-584
    hepatitis, 625
    herpes virus, 621
    Histoplasma capsulatum, 640-641
    Lactobacillus, 588
    leishmaniasis, 502
    leprosy, 601
    Leptospira, 611-612
    Listeria, 588-589
    measles virus, 623
    meningococcus, 559-560
    Mycoplasma, 626
    myxoviruses, 623
    Nocardia, 601-602
    Paracoccidioides brasiliensis, 642-643
    Pasteurella, 579-581
    pneumococci, 555-556
    Proteus, 568-569
    protozoa, 462
    Pseudomonas, 570-571
    rabies virus, 622-623
    rickettsiae, 614-615
    ringworm, table, 648
    Salmonella, 576
    Shigella, 578
    Spirillum minus, 610
    Sporotrichum schenkii, 644-645
    Staphylococcus, 553
    Streptobacillus moniliformis, 610
    streptococci, 546-547
    Treponema pallidum, 610-611
    trypanosomiasis, 503-504
    tuberculosis, 591-600
    variola and vaccinia viruses, 625
    Vibrio, 608-609
    virus groups, selected, 620, 621, 622, 623, 624
    viruses, 616
  evidence of hemolytic transfusion reactions, 264
  findings
    jaundice, early, table, 355
    leukemias, 194, 195
    mononucleosis, 188, 190
    polycythemia vera, 185, 186
    in pregnancy, 89
  infection, tularemia, 580
  investigation
    of bleeding patient, 209-223
    cerebrospinal fluid, 510-515

Laboratory—cont'd
  investigation—cont'd
    of pus, 525
    serous fluids, 507
    sputum, 521-524
    steatorrhea, 455-457
    synovial fluid, 517-519
  methods for determination of
    blood constituents, availability of, 283
    Staphylococcus aureus, 553-554
  quality control in, 1-10
  results, recording and reporting, 8
  rules, 1
  tests
    thyroid function, 411
Labstix in measuring pH of urine, 16
Lactic acid
  dehydrogenase
    increased, in cerebrospinal fluid, 512
    in serous fluids, 508
  in gastric contents, determination, 445
Lactic dehydrogenase (LDH)
  determination, 395-399
  in diagnosis of liver disease, 370
Lactobacillus, 588
Lactophenol cotton blue, staining of fungi, 635
Lactose
  tolerance test in steatorrhea, 457
  in urine
    Benedict qualitative test for, 27
    mucic acid test for, 32
    Rubner test for, 33
Lactose-egg yolk-milk agar, *Clostridium welchii,* 607
Lactose-fermenting Enterobacteriaceae, differentiation, 565
Lancefield
  group A streptococci, 547
  groups A, C, and D streptococci, 550
Landsteiner's rule, 237
Lange nitroprusside test, 34
Larva migrans
  cutaneous, 482
  visceral, 484
    rhabditiform, differential diagnosis, 486
    unsheathed, 489
L.E. cells, 192, 193
Lead
  intoxication, 692-694
  poisoning, anemia in, 184
Lectin
  anti-A₁ and anti-H, 238
Lee-White method, coagulation time, 210
Leishman-Donovan (L.D.) bodies, 501
Leishmania, 501-502
Leishmanial form of hemoflagellates, 501
Leishmaniasis, visceral, laboratory diagnosis, 502
Leprosy, 601
Leptocytes, 135
Leptomonad form of hemoflagellates, 501
Leptospira, 611-612
Letterer-Siwe disease, 201
Leucine
  aminopeptidase (LAP)
    determination, 399-401
    test, 448

Leucine—cont'd
  crystals, 55
  test for, 56
Leukemia
  chronic granulocytic differentiation from mye-
      lophthisic anemia, 187
  chronic lymphatic, lymphocytosis in, 150
Leukemias, 194-196
Leukemoid reaction, 118
Leukoagglutinins, 273
Leukocyte
  in blood smear examination, 130
  concentration of, smears of buffy coat, 125
  count
    correction for nucleated red blood cells, 120
    with Coulter counter, 120
    diagrammatic respresentation, 117
    variations, 118
  culture technique, 143
  differential count, 130
  groups, 257
  in infants and children, 118, 119
  in urine, significance, 47
  values, relative and absolute, 131
Leukocytic alkaline phosphatase (APGL) in
      pregnancy, 89
Leukocytosis, 118
  causes, 145, 146
Leukopenia
  calculation of leukocyte count in, 117
  causes, 146
  classification, 120
  definition, 119
Levaditi method for staining spirochetes in
      blocks, 716
Levulose
  conversion, 365
  determination, 308
  tolerance test, 366
  in urine, Selivanoff test for, 31
Lewis (Le) blood group system, 252-254
Liebermann-Burchard reaction, cholesterol de-
      termination, 372
Light green solutions, 711, 712
Light-chain disease, 198
Lignin or lignocellulose test for sulfonamides in
      urine, 57
Lipase
  determination, 401-402
  test of duodenal contents, 447
Lipid
  phosphorus, determination, 375-376
  pneumonia, sputum in, 524
Lipids
  blood, 371-382
  doubly refractile, in urine, 49
  total, gravimetric method of Pernokis, Free-
      land, and Kraus, 372
Lipoproteins, methods of estimation, 380-382
Liquid media, inoculation of, technique, 540
Listeria, 588-589
Littman oxgall agar, 634
Liver
  disease
    effect on prothrombin time, 217
    thymol turbidity in, 363, 364
  flukes, ova of, 494

Liver—cont'd
  function tests
    based on
      bile pigments, 355-362
      carbohydrate metabolism, 365-366
      detoxicating function, 366-367
      plasma protein changes, 362
      Bromsulphalein test, 367-369
      classification, 355
      flocculation tests, 362-365
      miscellaneous, 369-371
      summary, 370-371
  involvement in infectious mononucleosis, 191
  role in body, 354
Lloyd reagent, 314, 316
Loa loa, 489
Loeffler
  methylene blue stain, 539
  slant, *C. diphtheriae,* 589
Longitudinal sinus, obtaining infant's blood from,
      97
Lowenstein-Jensen medium, *M. tuberculosis,* 596
Lugol solution, 37
Lung
  abscess, sputum in, 524
  infarction and edema, sputum in, 524
Lupus erythematosus, systemic, 191-193
Luteal hormones, 73
Lutheran (Lu) blood group system, 255
Luxol fast blue-periodic acid Schiff-hematoxylin
      stain, 717-718
Lymphatic leukemia, chronic, 196
Lymphoblasts, 148, 195
Lymphocytes
  in cerebrospinal fluid, increase of, 513
  culture, 149
  maturation, 148
  normal percentage, 119
  pathologic forms, 148, 149
  proliferative disorders, 196
  variation in number, 149, 150
Lymphocytic
  choriomeningitis, cerebrospinal changes in, 515
  leukemia, acute, 194
Lymphocytoid cell, 149
Lymphocytosis, 149-150
Lymphogranuloma venereum, 624
Lymphopenia, 120, 150
Lymphoproliferative disorders, 196
Lysis, clot, 211, 213, 214

M

M and N blood types, exclusion of paternity by,
      256
MacCallum-Goodpasture stain for bacteria in
      tissue, 716-717
MacConkey agar, 561
Machines for measuring basal metabolism, 424,
      425
Macroconidia, 640, 647
Macrocytes, 134, 136
Macrocytic anemias, 155-158
Macrogametocytes, 496
Macroglobulinemia, 200
Macroglobulins, test for, 327
Macrohematocrit, Wintrobe method, 106

Macrophages
  Histoplasma capsulatum, 640
  resembling intestinal protozoa, 470
Macroscopic
  examination, intestinal parasites in feces, 459
  mucus, blood, and pus in stool, 452
  slide test
    Salmonella, 577
    Shigella, 578
Madura foot, 645
Maduromycosis, 645
Magnesium determination, 333-334
Malabsorption
  and steatorrhea, 454-457
  tests, 448
Malaria
  differential diagnosis in Wright-stained blood
    smears, 498, 499
  laboratory findings, 500
  pigment, 137
  therapeutic or accidental, difference from na-
    tural malaria, 494
Malarial parasites, 494, 495, 496, 497, 500
Malassezia furfur, 649
Malignancy associated changes (MAC) in gran-
    ulocytes, 144
Malignant
  cells
    in serous fluids, tests, 509
    in sputum, 523
    staining, 720
  disease, sputum in, 524
Malleomyces mallei and *pseudomallei,* 585
Mallory phosphotungstic acid hematoxylin
    (PTAH) stain, 710
Malloy-Evelyn method, serum bilirubin determi-
    nation, 357, 358
Maltose in urine, Barfoed test for, 33
Mannitol salt agar, pathogenic staphylococci,
    553
Manometric apparatus, Van Slyke, 344
Maple sugar urine disease, 24
Marble bone disease, 187
Marquis reagent, morphine determination, 700
Marrow; *see* Bone marrow
Massive transfusions, 265
Masson trichrome stain, connective tissue, 710-
    711
Mast cells, 148
Mayer mucicarmine stain, 715
May-Hegglin
  anomaly, 145
  type of thrombocytopathia, thrombasthenia,
    and thrombocytopenia, 226
Mean corpuscular
  hemoglobin (MCH), 114
  hemoglobin concentration (MCHC), 115
  volume (MCV), 114
  diameter of red blood cells, 116
Measles virus, 623
Mechanical fragility of erythrocytes, 164
Meconium ileus, 449
Media; *see also* Laboratory diagnosis
  Actinomyces, 603
  Blastomyces dermatitidis, 642
  Brucella, 586
  Candida, 636

Media—cont'd
  clostridia, 605
  culture, selection of, 542-543
  Enterobacteriaceae, 561
  fungi isolation and identification, 633-634
  Histoplasma capsulatum, 640
  liquid and solid, inoculation of, 540
  M. tuberculosis, 595-596
Mediterranean
  anemia, 167
  fever, 614
Megakaryoblasts, 152
Megakaryocytes, 152-153
Megaloblastic
  anemias, 155
  erythropoiesis, 131, 133
Megaloblasts, 133
Megalocytes, 134
Melanin in urine, tests for, 45-46
Melioidosis, 585
Meningitis, colloidal gold curves, chart, 514
Meningococcus, 558-560
Mercuric nitrate in chloride determination, 340
Mercury
  removal from tissue specimens, 706
  poisoning, 694-695
Merozoites, 495
Merthiolate-iodine-formalin stain (MIF) for
    preservation of intestinal parasites,
    461
Metabolic errors, inborn, erythrocyte enzyme de-
    ficiencies in, 408-411
Metabolism
  basal; *see* Basal metabolism
  definition of, 424
  iron, 158
Metabolites and hormones, urinary, 71-84
Metamyelocytes, 141
Metanil yellow solution, 715
Metaplasia, myeloid, 186
Metarubricytes, 132, 133
Methanol, qualitative test for, 687-688
Methemalbumin, 160
  absorption spectra, 102
Methemalbuminemia, 166
Methemoglobin
  absorption spectra, 102, 103
  reduction test of Brewer, 177
  spectrophotometric method of determination,
    105
Methemoglobinemia, 175
Methenamine silver nitrate solutions, 718
Methyl red test, 566
Methylene blue stain for diphtheria bacilli, 539
Microaerophilic gram-negative nonspore-forming
    bacilli, 585-587
Microanalysis of blood constituents, 293-294
Microangiopathy, thrombotic, 227
Microbiology
  methods in, 526-626
  quality control in, 7-9
Micrococcus tetragenus, 555
Microcolonial characteristics of mycobacteria on
    Lowenstein-Jensen medium and Mid-
    dlebrook 7H 10 agar, 596
Microconidia, 640, 642
  in *Trichophyton* culture, 647, 648

Microcytes, 134

Microcytic anemias and microcytic hypochromic anemias, 158-160

Microdiffusion, blood alcohol determination by, 687

Microfiliariae, 487-488, 489

Microgametocytes, 496

Microhematocrit method, 107

Micro-Kjeldahl method for determination of total nitrogen, 319-320

Micromethod

blood glucose determination, 301

for detection of erythrocyte G-6-PD deficiency, 176-177

for nonprotein nitrogen, 311-312

for prothrombin time, 219

rapid, for recording red cell osmotic fragility, 163

for starch gel electrophoresis of hemoglobin, 172

Microorganisms; *see* Bacteria

Microscopic examination

cerebrospinal fluid, 512-514

feces

for free fat, 455

for intestinal parasites, 459

for protozoa, 464-465

gastric contents, 446

pancreatic juice, 449

pus, 525

serous fluids, 508

sputum, 522-523

urine, 46-56

Microscopic sections, preparation on 35 mm. film, 708

Microscopy, blood examination by, 96

Microsporum infections of hair, 630

and skin, 648-649

Microtome cryostat frozen section technique, 705

Microtomes, tissue section cutting, 708

Microzone method, hemoglobin separation, 173

Middlebrook 7H 10 medium, 596

Milk

analysis, standard methods, 653-654

stormy fermentation, test for clostridia, 606

Milliequivalents, 435, 436, 437

Millimicron and nanometer, 286

Millon test, 26

Mimeae, 571, 572

MNSU blood group system, 259-260

Mörner reagent, 56

Moist heat sterilization, 530

Monoblasts, 150, 195

Monocytes, 150, 151

Monocytic leukemia, acute, 194

Monocytosis, 151

Mononucleosis, infectious, 188-191

cells, 148

cerebrospinal fluid in, 515, 517

Monospot slide test for infectious mononucleosis, 191

Morax-Axenfeld conjunctivitis, 585

Moraxella lacunata, 585

Morphine intoxication, method of determination, 700

Morphology

Bordetella pertussis, 582

gonococcus, 556-558

hematopoietic cells, 130-154

meningococcus, 559-560

Mycobacterium tuberculosis, 594

Pasteurella, 580

Pneumococci, 555-556

Proteus, 568

Pseudomonas, 570

Staphylococcus, 553

streptococci, 546

Morula cell, 197

Mosquito, cycle of malarial parasites in, 495, 496

Motility test, 537, 538

Motivation of laboratory medicine, 1

Mott cell, 197

Mounting media for tissue sections, 709

and staining of fungi, 635

Mouse method, pneumococci, 556

Mouth, flora normally present in, 529

Mucic acid test for galactose or lactose in urine, 32

Mucicarmine stain, Mayer, 715

Mucin clot production (Ropes test), synovial fluid, 517-518

Mucins, stains for, 714

Mucoproteins, stains for, 714-715

Mucor, 650

Mucormycosis, 649

Mucous strands in urine, 48

Mucoviscidiosis, 449-451

Multiple myeloma, 196-200

cells, 152

Museum specimens, tissue preparation, 721

Mutations, bacterial, 529

Mycelial phase, *Histoplasma capsulatum,* 640

Mycelium, fungi, 629

Mycetoma, 645

Mycobacteria

biochemical reactions and other differentiating tests, 597-599

culture differentiation, 596

laboratory diagnosis, 591-600

pigment studies, 596-597

rapid-growing, 600

species, 591

stain for, 538

unclassified (atypical), 600

Mycobacterium

kansasii, 600

leprae, 601

tuberculosis; see also Tubercle bacilli

antibodies to, immunologic methods, 600

drug-susceptibility patterns, 599

laboratory diagnosis, 429-432

Mycologic terms, glossary, 650-651

Mycology, methods in, 629-651

Mycoplasma pneumoniae, 626

Mycoses

cutaneous, 646-649

subcutaneous, 644-646

superficial, 649-650

systemic, 640-644

Myelin globules in sputum, 522

Myeloblasts, 140, 195

Myelocytes, 141
Myelofibrosis or myelosclerosis with myeloid
    metaplasia, 186-187
Myelogenous leukemia, chronic, 195
Myeloid series, white blood cells, 140-148
Myeloma
    cells, 197
    multiple, 196-200
        plasma cells in, 152
    paraproteinemia, laboratory diagnosis, 199
Myeloperoxidase stain, 128, 129
Myelophthisic anemia, 186-187
Myeloproliferative disorders, 185-187
Myoglobin
    absorption spectra, 102
    in urine, tests for, 40
Myoglobinuria, causes, 40
Myxoviruses, 623

N

N-Acetyl-L-cysteine (NAC) digestion method,
    tubercle bacilli decontamination, 592-
    593
Naegeli type, acute monocytic leukemia, 194
Nagler reaction, *Cl. welchii,* 607
Nails
    fungi of, 646, 648
    specimens for fungus examination, 630
Nanometer, 286
Nasopharyngeal swab, pertussis, 581
Nasopharynx, bacterial infections, handling of
    specimens, 534
Natelson Microgasometer, 345, 346
    for determining carbon dioxide content and
        combining power, 347-348
    oxygen determination with, 352-353
Necator americanus, 480-482
Needles, antigen-emulsion delivery, testing, 658
Negri bodies in rabies, 621, 622, 623
Neisseria
    description, 556
    differentiation, table, 558
    gonorrhoeae, 556-558
    meningitidis, 558-560
Nematodes, 478-492
    female, cross sections, drawings, 479
Neoplastic cells in urine, 50
Nephritis, glomerular, classification and manifes-
    tations, table, 68, 69
Nephrosis, classification and manifestations, ta-
    ble, 69, 70
Nerve
    cells, components, 717
    fibers, classification, 717
    tissue, 717, 718
Nessler solution, 310
Neubauer ruling, improved, on hemocytometer,
    110, 111
Neurohistology, 717-718
Neutral red
    technique, basophil count, 122
    test, *M. tuberculosis,* 598
Neutralization test
    for immune anti-A and anti-B, 262
    viruses, 619
Neutropenia, classification, 120

Newborn
    babies; *see* Infants, newborn
    testing in erythroblastosis fetalis, 277, 278
Niacin test, mycobacteria, 597-598
Nicotinamide adenine dinucleotide (NAD), con-
    version, 383, 384
Niemann-Pick disease, 201
Nile blue sulfate stain, 713-714
Nissl substance, cresylecht violet solution for, 717
Nitrate reduction
    clostridia, 606
    test, *Pseudomonas,* 570-571
Nitrazine paper test for measuring pH of urine,
    16
Nitrogen
    amino acid, 317-319
        test for, 22
    blood urea, determination, 308-310
    nonprotein, 310-313
    still, 320
    total, by micro-Kjeldahl method, 319-320
Nitroprusside tests of urine, 34
Nocardia asteroides and *brasiliensis,* 601-602
Nongamma globulin-antiglobulin test, 236
Nonglucose sugars, determination of, 307-308
Nonne-Apelt test, cerebrospinal fluid, 511
Nonphotochromogens, mycobacteria, 600
Nonprotein nitrogen (NPN), determination of,
    310-313
Nontreponemal antigen tests for syphilis, 655
Normal
    solutions, 431, 432
    values, table of, 722-726
Normoblastic erythropoiesis, 131
Normoblasts
    basophilic, 131
    in hemolytic anemia, 161
    orthochromic, 132
    polychromatophilic, 132
    variations in, 133
Normocytic anemias, 160-185
North American blastomycosis, 641
Nose, bacterial infections, handling of specimens,
    534
Nuclear
    fast red (Kernechtrot) stain, 712
    sexing, methods of, 142
Nuclei of mature neutrophil and eosinophil, sex
    difference in, 141
Nucleus pulposus, ruptured, cerebrospinal fluid
    in, 515

O

Obermayer test for indican in urine, 38
Obligate anaerobes, *Bacteroides,* 587
Occultest tablets, 39
Odor
    of sputum, 521
    of stool, 452
    of urine, 14
OF basal medium, 572
Official count, water examination, 652
Oliguria, 13
Onchocerca volvulus, 489
Onychomycosis, 646

Optical density and transmittance percentage, conversion table, 287

Optochin
disk test, difference between pneumococci and alpha streptococci, 556
sensitivity of streptococci to, 549

Orange G-6 solution, 720

Orcein-acetic acid stain, blood smear, 142

Organisms most likely to be isolated from clinical material, 535-537

Orinase
diagnostic response curves in nondiabetic and diabetic subjects, chart, 307
test for diabetes mellitus, 306

Ornithine carbamyl transferase (OCT)
in diagnosis of liver disease, 370
inborn metabolic errors and, 410

Ornithosis, 624

Orthochromic
megaloblast, 133
normoblast, 132

Orthotoluidine test for blood in stool, 453

Osazone test of urine, 28

Osmium tetroxide stain for fat, 714

Osmolality
of serum and other biologic fluids, 354
of urine, 17

Osmometer, 18

Osmotic
fragility of erythrocytes, 161-163
pressure, 354

Osteoblasts in bone marrow, 204

Osteoclasts in bone marrow, 205

Osteofibrosis, 187

Osteopetrosis, 187

Osteosclerosis, diffuse, 187

Ova of intestinal parasites, color plate, 471

Overflow aminoaciduria, 24

Ox cell hemolysin test for infectious mononucleosis, 191

Oxalates in obtaining blood for specimens, 98

Oxidase test
gonococcus, 557
meningococcus, 559
Pseudomonas, 570

Oxime method of determining blood urea nitrogen, 308-309

Oxygen
absorption by thioglycollate medium, 542
capacity method, hemoglobinometry, 98
content
of blood, measurement, 343
and capacity, 350-353
exhaustion methods, 541
requirements of bacteria, 541-542
tension, reduced, production of, 541
volume percent calculation, table, 347

Oxyhemoglobin
absorption spectra, 102, 103
method, hemoglobinometry, 99

Oxyuris vermicularis, 479
ovum of, in urine, 51

P

P and Jay blood group system, 251
P and P method, prothrombin time, 219

Packed cells
in blood transfusions, 265
red, volume of, hematocrit, 106-107

PAH clearance test, 61-62

Pancreas, fibrocystic disease of, 449-451

Pancreatic
enzymes, 447
function
secretin and pancreozymin stimulation test of, 447-448
tolerance tests, 448
juice, analysis, 446-449

Pancreatitis, lipase determination in, 402

Pancreozymin and secretin stimulation test of pancreatic function, 447-448

Pandy test, cerebrospinal fluid, 511

Papain titration of antibodies, 273

Papain-treated sheep erythrocytes, tests with, for mononucleosis, 191

Papanicolaou
smear technique for serous fluids, 509
staining method, 720-721

Paper
chromatography
amino acids in urine determined by, 21
sugar in urine determined by, 28-29
technique, 292
electrophoresis
for hemoglobin separation, 172
of lipoproteins, 380
of paraproteins, 197, 198, 199
protein separation by, 324-326
of urine for Bence Jones protein, 21

Pappenheimer bodies, 137

Para-aminobenzoic acid, determination of blood levels, 701

Para-aminosalicylic acid (PAS), method of determination, 701-702

Paracoccidioides brasiliensis, 642-643

Paraffin
section technique, 705-709
wax embedding, tissue, 707

Paragonimus westermani, ovum of, 494

Paraldehyde, qualitative test for, 687-688

Paramyloid in multiple myeloma, 201

Paraproteins, 197, 198, 199

Parasites
intestinal
methods of examination, 459-462
ova of, color plate, 471
malarial, 494, 495, 496, 497, 500
preservation of specimens, 504
red blood cell, 494-504
in sputum, 522
in stool, 452
Toxoplasma, 504-505
in urine, 50

Parasitic infections, intestinal, of man, table, 463

Parasitology
methods in, 459-506
quality control, 9

Paroxysmal nocturnal hemoglobinuria (PNH), 175-176

Partial thromboplastin time (PTT), 220-221

Partition chromatography, 292

Pasteurella
description, 578

Pasteurella—cont'd
  group, differentiation, table, 579
  multocida, 580
  pestis, 578-579
  pseudotuberculosis, 579-580
  tularensis, 580-581
Paternity, disputed, blood grouping tests in, 255-256
Pathogenic staphylococci, 553
Pathology, surgical, table for, 706
PathoTec test papers, 570
Paul-Bunnell test for infectious mononucleosis, 190
Pelger-Huët anomaly, 145
Penicillium, 650
Pentose in urine
  Benedict qualitative test for, 27, 32
  occurrence, 31
  various tests for, 32
Pepsin test, gastric analysis, 445
Pepsinogen, pepsin and, 445
Peptostreptococcus, 550-551
Perchloric acid method, iodine separation, 415
Pericardium, fluid from, handling of specimens, 533
Periodic
  acid solution, 712
  acid–Schiff stain (PAS), connective tissue, 712-713
Peritoneum, fluid from, handling of specimens, 533
Pernicious anemia, 155, 157
Pernokis, Freeland, and Kraus, gravimetric method of total lipid determination, 372
Peroxidase stain, 128, 129
pH; *see also* Hydrogen ion concentration
  in blood, 348-350
  values, 433
Phage typing of staphylococci, 554
Phagocytic
  cells in sputum, 522, 524
  monocytes, 151
Phase microscopy
  blood examination by, 96
  method of Brecker-Cronkite, platelet count, 123-124
Phenistix, 24
Phenol
  derivatives in urine, 46
  preservation of urine by, 12
Phenolphthalein
  monophosphate, alkaline phosphate using, 404-405
  in titration of gastric acid, 444
Phenolsulfonphthalein test of kidney function, 59-60
Phenothiazine compounds in urine, test for, 704
Phenotypes
  Duffy, 252
  of Lu system, 255
  Rh, determination of, 246
  Rh-Hr, 248-249
Phenylalanine
  bioassay (Guthrie test), 24
  deaminase test, *Proteus,* 569
  determination in blood, quantitative fluorometric, 25

Phenylethyl alcohol and chloral hydrate media for staphylococci, 553
Phenylhydrazine reaction of urine, 28
Phenylketonuria, 24
Phenylpyruvic oligophrenia, 24
Pheochromocytomas, 79
Phloroglucinol test, 33
Phosphatase
  acid, determination, 402, 404, 405
  alkaline
    in clinical diagnosis, 402
    determination, 403
    test of liver function, 369
Phosphatases, determination, 402-406
Phosphate
  buffer, 434
  excretion index (PEI), 333
  inorganic, normal values and pathologic interpretation, 332
Phosphatides, determination, 375-376
6-Phosphogluconic dehydrogenase in erythrocytes, inborn metabolic errors and, 409
Phospholipids, determination, 375-376
Phosphomolybdic acid solution, 711
Phosphomolybdic-phosphotungstic acid solution, 711
Phosphorus, inorganic, determination, 331-333
Phosphotungstic acid hematoxylin stain (PTAH), Mallory, 710
Photochromogens, mycobacteria, 600
Photoelectric colorimeter, 286-289
Photometric
  method in hemoglobinometry, 99
  readings, calculations with, 288-289
Photometry, flame, 290
Phthalate buffer, 433
Phycomycosis, 649
Physical
  examination
    cerebrospinal fluid, 510-511
    serous fluids, 507-508
    of sputum, 521-522
    of stool, 452
    of urine, 13-18
  measurements as methods of hemoglobin determination, 101
Picrate solution, alkaline, with creatinine solution, reaction, 314
Pigment
  production
    by pathogenic staphylococci, 553
    Pseudomonas, 571
  studies, mycobacteria, 596-597
Pigments, bacterial, 528
Pileggi and Kessler, direct method of thyroxine iodine determination, 423
Pilocarpine iontophoresis technique, 450
Pinta, 611
Pinworms, 9, 479
Pipettes, 294, 295
  blood, cleaning of, 100
  cleaning of, 113
  for water analysis, 652
Pipetting machine, automatic, 295
Pirofsky-Mangum, bromelin method of, titration of antibodies, 273

Pituitary gland hormones, 71
Placental
   estriol assay, 94
   function in established pregnancy, evaluation
      of, 93-94
Plague, 578, 579
Plasma
   amino acid nitrogen in, 318, 319
   antithrombin test, 215
   ascorbic acid in, 429
   carbon dioxide content and combining power,
      346, 347, 348
   cells
      function, increase, and pathologic forms, 152
      origin and maturation, 151
      proliferative disorders, 196
   chloride in, 342
   clotting time, 210-211
   in coagulation procedures, 208
   creatinine in, 314
   diluted, clot lysis, 214
   electrophoretic pattern of, 324
   factor defect or circulating anticoagulants,
      screening tests to distinguish, 213
   fibrinogen in, 329
   flow, renal, 61-62
   proteins, changes in, liver function tests based
      on, 362
   prothrombin concentration in, dilution curve
      for, 217
   refractive index in hemoglobin determination,
      101
   salicylates in, determination, 703
   sodium in, 339
   thrombin time test, 214-215
   thromboplastin, 206
      antecedent (PTA), 207
      component in coagulation, 207
   transfusions, 265
   uric acid in, 313, 314
Plasmablast, 151
Plasmacyte, 151
Plasmacytoid cell, 149
Plasmaphoresis, 265
Plasmodia, 494, 495, 496, 497, 498, 499
Platelet
   adhesiveness, test for, 212
   antibodies, 273
      in serum, test for, 227
   count, 122-124
   defects, hemorrhagic diseases due to, 226-228
   groups, 257
   survival studies, 227
   transfusions, 265
   in blood smear examination, 130
Platelets
   in coagulation, 207
   estimation of, 6
   formation, 152, 153
   function and quantity, tests, 211-212
   functions, 226
   values and variation in number, 153, 154
Pleurae, fluid from, handling of specimens, 533
Pleuropneumonia-like organisms (PPLO), 626
Plumbism, anemia in, 184
Pneumococci, laboratory diagnosis, 555-556

Pneumococcus typing, capsular swelling (quel-
      lung), 556
Pneumoconiosis, sputum in, 525
Pneumocystis carinii, 505
Pneumonia
   acute lobar, toxic granules in, 146
   lipid, sputum in, 524
Poikilocytes, 135, 136
Poikilocytosis, 161
Poisons
   common, and their antidotes, table, 685
   and drugs, toxicology, 684-704
   potential, increase in, 684
Poliomyelitis, cerebrospinal fluid in, 517
Polyacrylamide gel electrophoresis, protein sepa-
      ration by, 326
Polychromasia, 135
Polychromatophilic
   megaloblast, 133
   normoblast, 132
Polycythemia, 185-186
   causes, 113
   variations in red cell counting in, 112
   vera, 114
Polykaryocyte, 153
Polymorphs
   normal percentage, 119
   segmented, pathologic forms, 144-145
   variation in number, 145, 146
Polyneuritis, cerebrospinal fluid in, 517
Polyunsaturated fatty acids, 380
Polyuria, 13
Pork tapeworm, 473, 474
Porphobilinogen, test for, 44-45
Porphyria, 44-45
Porphyrins, 40-44
   biosynthesis, 41
   tests for, 41-44
Porter-Silber method, modified, for extraction of
      urinary 17-hydroxysteroids, 77-78
Postprandial blood glucose test, 305
Potability, water, standards of, 653
Potassium
   chlorate, saturated aqueous, 38
   dichromate solution in preparation of perma-
      nent standards for content of chlorine
      in water, 653
   oxalate
      as anticoagulant in blood specimens, 284
      in blood ammonia determination, 316
      and sodium fluoride as blood preservative,
         285
   serum, determination, 339-340
Pour plate method, inoculation of solid media,
      540
Precipitin test
   group, for group A streptococci, 549
   Lancefield grouping of streptococci by, 547
Precision and accuracy in laboratory, 3
Preeclampsia and eclampsia, 89
Pregnancy, laboratory findings, 89
   tests, 89-94
   vomiting of, 89
Preservation
   of blood samples, 285
   of specimens of parasites, 504

Preservation—cont'd
  of urinary sediment, 47
  of urine specimens, 12
Pressure, cerebrospinal fluid, 510
Price-Jones method, mean diameter of red blood cells, 116
Proconvertin and prothrombin method, 219
Proliferative disorders of plasma cells and lymphocytes with protein abnormalities, 196-202
Prolymphocyte, 148
Promegakaryocyte, 152
Promegaloblast, 133
Promonocyte, 150
Promyelocytes, 140
Pronormoblast, 131
Proplasmacyte, 151
Prorubricyte, 131
  PA type, 133
Prostatic acid phosphatase, 404
Protein
  antigen test, Reiter, 655, 675-679
  Bence Jones, 20-21
  crossmatch, 259
  fractions, electrophoretic, changes with disease, table, 327
  plasma, changes in, liver function tests based on, 362
  removing from urine, 20
  serum, groups, 256-257
  total
    in arthritis, 519
    in cerebrospinal fluid, 511-512
    determination of, 320-329
    in exudates and transudates, 508
  in urine, tests, 18-21
Protein-bound iodine (PBI), 413-420
Protein-free filtrates, 298-299
Proteins, myeloma, in serum, 197
Proteinuria, 20
Proteus, laboratory diagnosis, 568-569
Proteus-Providence group, 568-569
Prothrombin
  in coagulation, 206
  consumption test, 220
  time
    in newborn infants, 218
    one-stage (Quick), 215-219
    other methods, 219
    serum, 220
    sodium oxalate solution in determination of, 285
    test for liver disease, 369
Protozoa, 9, 462-470
  class name, and incidence of infection, table, 463
  culture of, 465
  laboratory diagnosis, 462
  stained, drawings, 464
  stool examination, 462-465
Protozoan parasite, *Toxoplasma gondii,* 504
Providence organisms, 569
Prussian blue reaction of hemosiderin, 39
Pseudo-B antigen, 240
Pseudomonas
  description, 569
  differential diagnosis, 571

Pseudomonas—cont'd
  laboratory diagnosis, 570-571
  pseudomallei, 585
Pseudomycelium, 636
Psittacosis, 624
Purpura
  fulminans, 224
  immunologic thrombocytopenic, 227
  Schoenlein-Henoch, 224
  senilis, 224
  thrombotic thrombocytopenic, 227
Pus
  and blood in urine, three-glass test, 40
  collection for fungus examination, 630
  content, 525
  examination, 525
    in fungus infection, 631
  and long-chain streptococci determination, milk analysis, 654
  and purulent exudates, smears and cultures, 533-534
  sulfur granules in, in actinomycosis, 602, 603
Pyelonephritis, 70
Pyknocytes, 134
Pyknotic cell, 145
Pyridoxine-deficiency anemia, 159
Pyrogallol method, anaerobic cultures, 541
Pyroninophilic cell, 149
Pyruvate kinase (PK)
  deficiency, tests for, 178
  low erythrocyte levels in inborn metabolic errors, 409

Q

Q fever, 614
Qualitative estimation of drugs and electrolytes in urine, 57
Qualitative test(s)
  for carbon monoxide, 692
  for methanol, formaldehyde, and paraldehyde, 687-688
  with serum
    slide, VDRL, 659
    and spinal fluid, Kolmer, 669-671
    and spinal fluid, Reiter, 678
    tube, VDRL, 662
  with spinal fluid, VDRL, 663
Quality control
  in blood banking, 2
  chart, 4
  in clinical chemistry, 2-5
  in coagulation, 5
  in hematology, 6
  in microbiology, 7-9
  need for, 1
  in parasitology, 9
  in tissue laboratory, 9
Quantitative
  estimation of sugar in urine, Benedict method, 29-30
  fluorometric phenylalanine determination in blood, 25
  methods of diagnosing pregnancy, 93
  test(s)
    for glucose in urine, Somogyi, 30-31

Quantitative—cont'd
 test(s)—cont'd
  with serum
   slide, VDRL, 659-661
   and spinal fluid, Kolmer, 671-672
   and spinal fluid, Reiter, 678-679
   tube, VDRL, 662-663
   with spinal fluid, VDRL, 664
  for urine for bacteria, 535
 urinalysis, 58
Queensland tick typhus, 614
Quellung, capsular swelling test, 552, 556
Quick one-stage prothrombin time, 215-219

R

RA cell, 519
Rabies, 621
 virus, 621-623
Radioactive iodine; *see* I[131]
Rana pipiens, frog test for pregnancy, 91
Rapid slide test
 Brucella, 587
 for infectious mononucleosis, 191
 for lupus erythematosus, 193
Rat tapeworm, 477-478
Rat-bite fever, 610
RA-Test, 519
Reactions, transfusion, 263-279
Reagent blank, 288
Reagents for coagulation procedures, 5, 208
Red blood cells; *see also* Erythrocytes
 cerebrospinal fluid, 513
 color plate, 132
 count, 110-114
  with Coulter counter, 120
  diagrammatic representation, 112
 destruction
  evaluation, 155
  methods, 160
 erythropoiesis, 131-140
 exogenous and endogenous agents causing hemolytic anemia, 184
 inclusions, 161
 Lewis, typing for, 252-253
 mean diameter, 116
 mechanical fragility, 164
 of newborn infant, typing, grouping, and antiglobulin testing in erythroblastosis fetalis, 278
 normal values at different age levels, 114
 nucleated, correction of white cell count for, 120
 number of, variations, 113, 114
 osmotic fragility, 161-163
 packed, volume of, hematocrit, 106-107
 parasites in, 494-504
 pathology, 154, 155
 production, evaluation, 155
 sedimentation rate, 107-109
 in sputum, 522, 524
 survival time, 166, 167
Reducing substances
 in cerebrospinal fluid, 512
 in urine
  differentiation of, 27

Reducing substances—cont'd
 in urine—cont'd
  nonsugar, 33-34
  tests for, 26-33
Reed-Sternberg cell, 153
Rees-Ecker method of counting platelets, 124
Refractive index
 of plasma, hemoglobin determination by, 101
 of urine, 16
Refractometer, 17
Reilly bodies, 144
Reinsch test for arsenic, 688-689
Reiter
 protein antigen test (one-fifth volume Kolmer test), 655, 675-679
 qualitative tests with serum and spinal fluid, 678
 quantitative tests with serum and spinal fluid, 678-679
 treponema strain, 611
Relapsing fever, 613
Renal; *see also* Kidney
 aminoaciduria, 23-24
 plasma flow, 61-62
Reoviruses, 621
Replacement method, oxygen exhaustion, 541
Reporting Kolmer tests, 673, 674, 680
Respiratory metabolism, physiology and measurement, diagram, 425
Retesting anticomplementary
 sera, modified Sachs method, 674-675
 spinal fluids, 675
Reticulocytes, 138, 139, 140
Reticulocytosis, 161
Reticuloendothelial elements in bone marrow, 204
Reticulum
 cell, 131
 stain, Wilder, 711-712
Rh
 blood groups and blood grouping, 241-250
 erythroblastosis, 182
 factor
  discovery and incidence, 241
  variants, 247, 250
 genotypes, determination, 247
 phenotypes, determination, 246
 types, eight, tables, 242
 typing, 245-246
Rh₀ factor, 241, 242, 243
Rhabditiform larvae of worms, 480, 481, 485, 486
Rhabditis hominis larvae, differential diagnosis, 486
Rheumatic fever, salicylates in, determination of blood levels, 702
Rheumatoid factor, tests for, 519
Rh-Hr
 blood types, exclusion of paternity by, 256-257
 phenotypes and genotypes, 248-249
 relationships, 242, 243, 244
Rhinosporidium, 645
Rhizopus, 650
Rickettsiae
 description and diseases caused by, 613-614
 laboratory diagnosis, 614-615

Rickettsiae—cont'd
in sections of formalin-fixed tissue, stain for, 720
Rickettsial diseases, para-aminobenzoic acid in, determination of blood level, 701
Rickettsial pox, 614
Rieder cell, 149
Ringworm, 646
epidemic, laboratory diagnosis, table, 648
Risa for blood volume determination, 109
Rivalta test, globulin in serous fluids, 508
RNA viruses, 615
Robinson-Power-Kepler test for Addison's disease, 342-343
Rocky Mountain spotted fever, 614
Ropes test, synovial fluid, 517-518
Ross-Jones test, cerebrospinal fluid, 511
Rothera nitroprusside test, 34
Roundworms, 9, 478-492
Rubner test for lactose in urine, 33
Rubriblast, 131
PA type, 133
Rubricyte, 132
PA type, 133
Rules, safety, in bacteriology laboratory, 7
Rumpel-Leede test, 209-210
Ruptured nucleus pulposus, cerebrospinal fluid in, 515
Russell bodies, 151

S

Sabin and Feldman, dye test of, in toxoplasmosis, 505
Sabouraud dextrose agar, fungi media, 633
Sachs
buffered glycerol-sodium chloride solution, 560
method, modified, retesting anticomplementary sera, 674-675
St. Louis encephalitis, cerebrospinal changes, 515
Salicylates, blood levels, determination, 702-704
Saline
crossmatch, 259
titration of antibodies, 272
tube method, blood group antibodies, 266
Saline-agglutinating anti-Rh₀ (D), tube test with, 245
Saliva
blood group substances in, test for, 253-254
changes in fibrocystic disease, 449
Salkowski test for leucine, 56
Salmonella
laboratory diagnosis, 576-577
typhosa, infection, 577
Salmonella-Arizona-Citrobacter division, table, 568
Salzman method, platelet adhesiveness, 212
Sample bottles for water analysis, 652
San Joaquin fever, 643
Sanford method, osmotic fragility of erythrocytes, 161, 162
Saponin hemolysis technique, malarial parasites, 500
Saprophytic fungi, 649-650
Sarcina, 555
Sarcinae, 446

Satellite phenomenon, 583
Scalp veins, obtaining infant's blood from, 97
Scarlet red (Sudan IV), Herxheimer, stain for fat, 713
Schiff
leucofuchsin solution, 712, 717
stain, connective tissue, 712
Schilling
count, 130
method, urinary excretion of Co^{60}-B_{12}, 157
type, acute monocytic leukemia, 194
Schistocytes, 161
Schistosoma, life cycle, 493
Schistosomes, 493, 494
Schizogony, 495
Schizont, 495, 496
Schlesinger test for urobilin, 36-37
Schoenlein-Henoch purpura, 224
Scotochromogens, mycobacteria, 600
Screening
of donor and recipient for atypical antibodies, 259
tests for porphyrins, 41, 42
Scurvy, 224
Secretin and pancreozymin stimulation test of pancreatic function, 447-448
Sections
cutting, 708
tissue
staining methods, 708-709
techniques of preparation, 705
Sediment
of serous fluids, microscopic examination, 508, 509
test, milk analysis, 653
Sedimentation
rate of red blood cells, 107-109
of trematodes, 492-493
Selective media, 542, 543
Selivanoff test for levulose in urine, 31
Sellers
agar, 572
staining method, rabies virus, 622
Semen
collection and examination, 87-88
in urine, 50
Semiquantitative test, bacteria in urine, 535
Semisolid medium technique, bacteria examination, 537
Sensitivity
of bacteria to antibiotics, 543-546
determination with anaerobes, 545
testing
Mycobacterium tuberculosis, 545
staphylococci, 554
streptococci, 549
sulfonamide, 546
Serologic
diagnosis of gonococci, 558
examination of cerebrospinal fluid, 514-515
grouping of streptococci, 547, 548
identification
Haemophilus influenzae, 583
Salmonella, 576-577
Shigella, 578

Serologic—cont'd
  investigation
    of autoimmune hemolytic anemia, 180-181
    of enteropathogenic *E. coli,* 567
  tests
    amebiasis, 465
    anthrax bacillus, 605
    Coccidioides immitis, 644
    fungi, 635
    histoplasmosis, 641
    Leptospira, 612
    lupus erythematosus, 192-193
    meningococcus, 560
    mononucleosis, comparison of, 191
    rickettsiae, 614
    for syphilis (STS), 611
      nontreponemal and treponemal tests, 655
      positive and negative reactions, 682-683
      reporting results, terminology, 656
    viruses, 619-620
Serology, 655-683
  Actinobacillus mallei, 585
  in bacteriology, 8
  coliform bacteria, 566
  Proteus, 569
  Vibrio comma and *fetus,* 609
Serotonin 5-hydroxytryptamine, 83
Serous
  cavities, fluids from, handling of specimens, 533
  fluids, examination, 507-510
Serratia, 575
Serum
  acid phosphatase in, 402
  alkaline phosphatase
    determination, 402
    test of liver function, 369
  anticomplementary, retesting, modified Sachs method, 674-675
  bilirubin, methods of determination, 356-360
  calcium determination, 329, 330
  carbon dioxide content and combining power, 346
  chloride, determination, 341
  cholesterol levels, 374, 375
  in coagulation procedures, 208
  copper in, 336-337
  creatine and creatinine, procedures for, 315, 316
  deproteinization of, 298
  fatty acid esters in, 376-377
  glutamic oxalacetic transaminase (SGOT) and serum glutamic pyruvic transaminase (SGPT), 370, 406, 407
  grouping, 237-238, 239, 240
  hepatitis, 625
  iron and serum iron-binding capacity, 334-336
  isoniazid in, determination, 702
  magnesium in, 333
  in mononucleosis, findings, 188, 190, 191
  osmolality, 354
  paper electrophoretic pattern of, 325
  phospholipid in, 375, 376
  potassium determination, 339-340
  preparation
    in Kolmer test for syphilis, 665
    in VDRL slide flocculation tests, 657

Serum—cont'd
  protein groups, 256-257
  protein-bound iodine in, 413
  proteins, fractionation by electrophoresis, 325-328
  prothrombin time, 220
  salicylates in, determination, 703
  sodium in, determination, 338-339
  and spinal fluid
    Kolmer tests with, 669-672
    Reiter tests with, 678-679
  tests in hemolytic anemia, 164-166
  triglycerides, micromethod of Van Handel and Zilversmit, 378-380
  uric acid in, 313, 314
  VDRL tests with, 656-663
Sex chromosomes, 141-143
  difference in nuclei of mature neutrophil and eosinophil, 141
SF medium, 551
Sheep red cell suspension, preparation in Kolmer test for syphilis, 665-666
Shigella, 578
Shigella-Escherichia division, table, 565
Shreds in urine, 48
Sia test, macroglobulinemia, 200
Sickle
  cell anemia, disease, and trait, 174
  cells, 135-136
Sideroachrestic hypochromic anemias, 159
Sideroblasts, 138
Siderocytes, 137
Siderophilin, 158
Siliconization in coagulation procedures, 6
Siliconizing glassware, 208
Silver electrode, heated aluminum sweat test, 451
Silverman needle, bone marrow biopsy with, 203
Sinus tract cultures, organisms isolated from, 536
Sinuses, bacterial infections, handling of specimens, 534
Sinusoidal cell in bone marrow, 204
Skin
  flora normally present in, 529
  fungi of, 646, 648
  in fungus infections, collection of specimens and direct examination, 630
  test, *Pasteurella tularensis,* 581
  tests, 635
  tubercle bacilli on, 592
Slants, 541
Sleeping sickness, 502
Slide
  agglutination test for enteropathogenic *E. coli,* 567
  culture
    fungi, 634
    technique, *Nocardia,* 601-602
  method
    blood smear preparation, 124
    cell grouping, 237
  test
    clumping factor of staphylococci, 554
    Brucella, 587
    Rh factor, 245
  tests, VDRL, 656-661

Slides, preparation in VDRL flocculation tests, 657
SMA-12 AutoAnalyzer, 297
Smears; *see also* Laboratory diagnosis
  acid-fast tubercle bacilli, 593
  Actinobacillus mallei, 585
  bacterial and fungus, handling, 531
  Bacteroides, 587
  Blastomyces dermatitidis, 641
  blood, 124-130
  Brucella, 586
  Candida, 635
  clostridia, 605, 607, 608
  Corynebacterium diphtheriae, 589
  Cryptococcus neoformans, 638
  diplococci, 555
  Enterobacteriaceae, 560
  Fusobacterium fusiforme, 588
  gonococcus, 556, 557
  granuloma inguinale, 584
  Haemophilus ducreyi, 583
  Histoplasma capsulatum, 640
  Lactobacillus, 588
  leptospirae, 611
  Listeria, 588
  meningococcus, 559
  Mycobacterium leprae, 601
  Nocardia, 601
  Pasteurella pestis, 579
  rabies virus, 622, 623
  staphylococcus, 553
  Streptobacillus moniliformis, 610
  Vibrio, 608, 609
Smudge cell, 145
Snapper-Scheid bodies, 145
Sodium
  determination, 338-339
  hydroxide
    digestion method, tubercle bacilli decontamination, 593
    preparation for fungus examination, 630-632
    standard solution, 432
  metabisulfite method, diagnosis of sickle cell disease, 174
  oxalate solution as anticoagulant in blood specimens, 285
  p-aminohippurate (PAH) clearance, 61-62
  thiosulfate solution, 712
Solid media, inoculation of, technique, 540
Solutions
  buffer, 433-434
  standard, 431, 432
Somogyi
  filtrate, 298, 299
  method, blood glucose determination, 300
  quantitative test for glucose in urine, 30-31
Somogyi-Nelson method
  galactose or levulose determination, 308
  glucose determination, 302
Sorbic acid-polymyxin broth, clostridia media, 605
South African tick-bite fever, 614
South American blastomycosis, 642
Specific gravity
  copper sulfate method for hemoglobin determination, 101
  of urine, 16-17

Specimens
  collection
    in alcohol determination, 686
    bacteria, 530
    blood, 284-285
    cerebrospinal fluid, 510
    Enterobacteriaceae, 560
    feces, 533
    fungi, 630
    serous fluids, 507
    sputum, 521
    stool, for protozoa examination, 462-464
    tubercle bacilli, 591-595
    urine, 11-12
    viruses, for serologic tests, 616
  museum, tissue preparation, 721
  of parasites, preservation of, 504
  Salmonella, 576
  surgical, handling, 705
  types, for virus investigation, 616
Spectrophotometric
  analysis of amniotic fluid in erythroblastosis fetalis, 276-277
  methods for determination of hemoglobin derivatives, 103-106
Spectrophotometry, atomic absorption, 290-291
Spectroscopic
  examination of blood, hemoglobin determination by, 101, 103
  test
    for hemoglobinuria, 39
    for myoglobinuria, 40
Speegrav, 17
Spermatozoa
  count and morphology, 88
  in urine, 50
Spherocytes, 135, 136, 137, 161
Spherocytosis, hereditary, 167
Spinal fluid; *see also* Cerebrospinal fluid
  anticomplementary, retesting, 675
  preparation in Kolmer test for syphilis, 665
  and serum
    Kolmer tests with, 669-672
    Reiter tests with, 678-679
  VDRL tests with, 663-664
Spirillaceae, 608-610
Spirillum minus, 609-610
Spirochetes, 610-613
  in blocks, Levaditi method for staining, 716
Spirometer type closed circuit metabolism apparatus, 425
Spore strips, bacterial, 530
Spores
  bacterial, 528
  fungi, 629, 630
Sporogony, 495
Sporotrichosis, 644-645
Sporotrichum schenckii, 644-645
Sporozoa, intestinal, 500
Sporozoite, 495, 496
Spot-screening test for galactosemia, 32-33
Spotted fever, 614
Sputum, 521-524
  cultures, organisms isolated from, 537
  in disease, 524
  flora normally present in, 529
  in fungus infection, 630, 631

Sputum—cont'd
  handling of specimens, 534
  intestinal parasites in, examination, 462
  tubercle bacilli in, 591, 594
Squamous cells in urine, 50
SS agar, 561
Stabilized antigen emulsion, VDRL, 658
Stable factor in coagulation, 207
Stain(s)
  for acid-fast tubercle bacilli, 594-595
  for bacteria, 715-717
    routinely employed, 538, 539
  for carbohydrates and mucoproteins, 714-715
  for cellular products, 713-715
  for connective tissue, 709-713
  for fat, 713-714
  Gram, reaction of bacteria to, 528
  for Rickettsiae in sections of formalin-fixed
    tissue, 720
Stained preparations of sputum, 523
Staining
  in bacteriology, methods, 538-540
  blood smear, techniques, 125-129
  cellular products, 713, 714, 715
  connective tissue, 710, 711, 712, 713
  diagnostic, 708-709
  fungi, 635, 718-720
  Gram method, 539
  intestinal parasites, 461-462
  Papanicolaou method, 720-721
  protozoa, 464, 465
  rabies virus, 622, 623
  tissue sections, 708-709
  urinary sediment, 46
Standard
  deviation, calculation of, 3-5
  loop method, bacteria in urine, 535
  solutions, 431, 432
Staphylococcal infections in hospitals, bacterio-
    logic survey, 554-555
Staphylococci, 553, 554, 555
Starch
  gel electrophoresis
    hemoglobin separation by, 170, 172
    protein separation by, 326
  tolerance test, pancreatic function, 448
  zone method of electrophoresis, study of lipo-
    proteins, 381
Steam, sterilization by, 530
Steapsin test of duodenal contents, 447
Steatorrhea
  causes, 454, 455
  I[131] triolein test, 448
  laboratory investigation, 455-457
Stem cell, 131
Stercobilin in stool, 454
Sterilization in bacteriology, 530-531
Sternal puncture technique, 202
Steroid hormones, 72
Steroids, ketogenic, in urine, determinations, 73,
    76
Stimulation test for adrenal function, 78
Stirling gentian violet stain, 716
Stoll egg-counting technique, 484-485
Stomach; *see also* Gastric
  bacteria normally present in, 529

Stool; *see also* Feces
  analysis, 452-457
  examination for protozoa, 462-465
  specimens in parasitology, 9
Storage
  of blood, 262
  of culture media, 540
  diseases, 201
Stormy fermentation of milk, test for clostridia,
    606
Straus reaction, 585
Streak plate and streak-pour plate, inoculation
    of solid media, 540
Streptobacillus moniliformis, 610
Streptococcal extract, preparation of, 548-549
Streptococci
  anaerobic, 550-551
  catalase test for, 549
  description, 546
  laboratory diagnosis and morphology, 546-547
  long-chain, and pus, determination in milk
    analysis, 654
  sensitivity testing, 549
  serologic groups, 547
Streptococcus
  agalactiae, 550
  dysgalactiae, 550
  faecalis, 550
  MG, agglutinins for, 552
  pyogenes, 547
Streptolysin O, 551
Streptomyces, 603
Stromal cells in bone marrow, 204
Strongyloides stercoralis, 485-486
Stuart-Prower factor in coagulation, 207
Subarachnoid hemorrhage, cerebrospinal fluid
    changes, 515
Subcutaneous mycoses, 644-646
Subgroups of ABO blood groups, 238, 239, 240
Sudan IV, scarlet red, Herxheimer, 713
Sugar
  blood, normal values and pathologic interpre-
    tation, 301
  reducing substances, 26-33
  in serous fluids, 508
  in urine, paper chromatography in identifica-
    tion of, 28-29
Sugars, nonglucose, determination, 307-308
Sulfanilamide crystals, 54
Sulfhemoglobin
  absorption spectra, 102, 103
  spectrophotometric method of determination,
    105-106
Sulfisoxazole crystals, 53
Sulfonamide
  crystals in urine, 51, 53, 54, 55
  intoxication, 698
  sensitivity tests, 546
Sulfonamides
  absorption and excretion, 697-698
  conversion factors, table, 699
  method of determination, 698-700
  in urine, qualitative analysis, 57
Sulfosalicylic acid test of urine, 18-19
Sulfur granules in pus in actinomycosis, 602, 603
Sulfuric acid, standard solution, 432
Sulkowitch test for calcium in urine, 57

Suppression test for adrenal function, 78
Supravital stain, 129
Surgical
    pathology, table, 706
    tissue, examination, 534
Swabs and transport media for cultures and smears, handling, 531
Sweat tests in fibrocystic disease, 449-451
Symptomatic autoimmune hemolytic anemia, 180
Synovial fluid, 517-520
Synovianalysis in arthritis, table, 520
Syphilis
    biologic false positive reactions, 683
    causative organism, 610
    dark-field examination, 533
    serologic tests for (STS)
        discussion, 682-683
        nontreponemal and treponemal antigen tests, 655
    tests for, 611
    VDRL tests, 656-664
Syringe pipette, 295
Systemic
    lupus erythematosus (S.L.E.), 191-193
    mycoses, 640-644

T

Table for surgical pathology, 706
Taenia
    saginata, characteristics, 471-473
    solium, 473, 474
Tapeworms, 9
    beef, 471-473
    description, 470
    diagnosis, 470-471
    dog, common, 478
    dwarf, 476, 477, 478
    fish, 473, 474, 475
    in man, differential characteristics, table, 473
    mature segments, drawings, 471
    orders of medical importance, 345
    park, 473, 474
    rat, 477-478
    scolices, drawings, 470
Target cells, 134, 135
Tart cells, 151
    in lupus erythematosus, 193
Tauber test for pentose in urine, 32
Technologist, laboratory, 7
Telangiectasia, hereditary hemorrhagic, 224
Test tube
    agglutination test, *Pasteurella tularensis,* 581
    dilution method, sensitivity of bacteria to antibiotics, 544-545
    method of cell grouping, 237
Tests
    for ABO blood grouping, 237-238
    in ABO hemolytic disease of newborn, 278-279
    for amino acids in urine, 21-23
    antiglobulin or Coombs, 234-236
    for anti-Rh antibodies, 246
    basal metabolism, 424-427
    for bile
        pigments and derivatives in stool, 453-454
        in urine, 35-38
    for blood group antibodies, screening, 266-267

Tests—cont'd
    blood grouping, in disputed paternity, 255-256
    for blood in stool, 452-453
    for circulating anticoagulant, 214-215
    for clotting factor defects, 211
    of coagulation
        phase I, 220-223
        phase II, 215-219
        phase III, 211
    Congo red, for amyloid disease, 430
    glucose tolerance, 301-307
    for high isoagglutinin titer of group O blood, 261-262
    for immune anti-A and anti-B (neutralization test), 262
    kidney
        clearance, 60-61
        function, 58-66
            table of normal values, 726
    liver function, 354-371
    milk, 653-654
    miscellaneous, 427-431
    for mononucleosis, 190, 191
    for overall clotting ability, 210-211
    platelet function and quantity, 211-212
    pregnancy, 89-94
    for presence of urine, 12-13
    for protein in urine, 18-21
    for Rh factor, 245, 246
    for rheumatoid factor, 519
    screening for excessive fibrinolysis, 213
    for sugar reducing substances in urine, 26-33
    for syphilis, 611
    thyroid function, 411-427
    for tubular function, 65
    for vascular function, 209-210
    water, 652-653
Tetanus, 607
Tetrazolium
    reduction, *Candida,* 638
    salt, lactic dehydrogenase using, 398-399
Thalassemia, 167-168
Thayer-Martin medium, gonococcus smears on, 557
Thin-layer chromatography (TLC), 293
    and electrophoresis in aminoaciduria, 22
Thioglycollate medium, absorption of oxygen by, 542
Thiouracil, effect on basal metabolic rate, 426
Thomas-Seligson pipette, 295
Thormählen test for melanin in urine, 45
Thorn ACTH test, 122
Three-glass test for hematuria, 40
Throat
    cultures, organisms isolated from, 537
    infections, bacterial, handling of specimens, 534
Thrombin
    in coagulation procedures, 208
    test (Crosby) for nocturnal hemoglobinuria, 175
    time test, 214-215
Thromblasthenia, 226
Thrombocytes, 153
Thrombocythemia, 227, 228
Thrombocytopathia, 226

Thrombocytopenia
classification, 154
congenital, 226
with hemangiomas, 227
Thrombocytopenic purpura, immunologic, 227
Thrombocytosis, 227
Thromboplastin
generation test (TGT), 222-223
time, partial, 220-221
types and production, 206
Thrombotest method, prothrombin time, 219
Thrombotic microangiopathy, 227
Thymol
as blood preservative, 285
turbidity and flocculation test, 363-364
urine preservation by, 12
Thyroglobulin autoprecipitin test, 427
Thyroid
activity, basal metabolic rate as test of, 424
function tests, 411-427
gland
physiology, 411
radioactive iodine uptake by, 411
Thyroid-binding index (TBI), 412-413
Thyroid-stimulating hormone suppression test, 427
Thyrotropic hormone, function, 411
Thyroxine
by column chromatography, 421-424
effect on basal metabolic rate, 426
effect on thyroid secretion, 427
Thyroxine-binding globulins (TBG), 412, 413
Tick typhus, Queensland, 614
Tick-bite fever, South African, 614
Tinea
pedis, corporis, capitis, and cruris, 646
versicolor, 649
Tinsdale medium, *C. diphtheriae*, 590
Tissue
autopsy and surgical, examination, 534
basophil, 148
connective, stains for, 709-713
culture, viruses, 616, 618
examination
methods, 705-721
viruses, 620
flagellates, 500-504
laboratory, quality control in, 9
nerve, staining methods, 717-718
phase, *Histoplasma capsulatum,* 640, 641
preparations, fungi, 635
processing, technique, 705-709
processors, automatic, 707
sections
complete, defects in, 709
serous fluid sediment, 509
staining methods, 708-709
thromboplastin, 206
tubercle bacilli in, 592
Tissue-inhabiting nematodes, 487-489
Titan yellow dye in magnesium determination, 333
Titration
of antibodies, 272-273
of bicarbonate in duodenal aspirates, 448

Titrations, complement and hemolysin
Kolmer test for syphilis, 666-669
Reiter test, 676-677
Tj^a^ blood group system, 251
Töpfer reagent, 444
Tolbutamide diagnostic test for diabetes mellitus, 306
Tolerance tests of pancreatic function, 448
Tollens test, 33
Toluene sulfonic acid (TSA) test, 20
Toluidine
blue method, basophil count, 122
blue O stain, 719-720
reagent, test for free chlorine in water, 653
Toluol (toluene), preservation of urine by, 12
Torula, 638-639
Total
nitrogen determination, 319-320
protein, albumin, and globulin determinations, 320-329
Tourniquet test, 209-210
Toxic
agents, accumulation in body, 684
granulation, 145, 146
hemolytic anemias, 184
Toxicity testing
anthrax bacillus, 604
clostridia, 606
Toxicology, 684-704
Toxin production, *Cl. botulinum* and *tetani,* 608
Toxins, bacterial, 529
Toxocara canis and *cati,* 484
Toxoplasma gondii, 504-505
Toxoplasmosis, 504, 505
Trachoma virus, 624
Tranquilizer drugs, derivatives of phenothiazine, test for presence in urine, 704
Transaminase
determination, 406-408
in liver disease, 370
increased, in cerebrospinal fluid, 512
Transferrin, 158
Transfusion
method, red blood cell survival time, 166
reactions, 263-279
hemolytic, 184
therapy of coagulation defects, 228
Transfusions
blood-derivative, 265
choice of blood for, 261
dangers of, 264-265
exchange
choice of blood for, 261
in erythroblastosis fetalis, 278
intrauterine, in erythroblastosis fetalis, 277
massive, 265
plasma, 265
platelet, 265
Transmittance percentage and optical density, conversion table, 287
Transparency
cerebrospinal fluid, 511
and color, amniotic fluid, 520
synovial fluid, 517
and general appearance of serous fluids, 507
and turbidity of urine, 15

Transudates
  tests, 509
  total protein in, 508
Trematodes, 9, 492-493
Trench fever, 614
Trephine technique, bone marrow specimen, 202
Treponema pallidum
  description and laboratory diagnosis, 610-611
  immobilization test (TPI), 655
Treponemal
  antibody test, fluorescent, 655, 679-682
  antigen tests for syphilis, 655
  tests for syphilis, 611
Treponemataceae, 610-613
Trialists, theory of blood cell origin, 95
Trichinella spiralis, 490, 492
Trichloroacetic acid filtrate, 299
Trichomonas hominis, characteristics, 469
Trichomonas vaginalis in urine, 50
Trichophyton infections of skin, hair, and nails,
    646, 647, 648
Trichosporon, 640
  cutaneum, 649
Trichostrongylus, 486-487
Trichrome stain, Masson, 710-711
Trichuris trichiura, 479
Tricresol, preservation of urine by, 12
Triglycerides, serum, micromethod of Van Handel
    and Zilversmit, 378-380
Triiodothyronine, I131-labeled, erythrocyte up-
    take of, 413
Triphenyl tetrazolium chloride (TTC) test (Uro-
    screen), 535
Triple
  phosphate crystals, 52, 56
  sugar iron (TSI) agar, 561, 563, 564
Tris buffer, 434, 435
Trisodium phosphate concentration method,
    tubercle bacilli, 593
Tropism of virus, classification of disease accord-
    ing to, 615-616
Truant fluorescent dye, 595
Trypanosoma, forms of, 501
Trypanosomal form of hemoflagellates, 501
Trypanosomes, 502-504
Trypanosomiasis, laboratory diagnosis, 503-504
Trypsin
  in feces, test for, 454
  tests, duodenal contents, 447
  titration of antibodies, 273
Tryptophan test, cerebrospinal fluid, 512
Tsetse flies, sleeping sickness due to bite of, 502
TSH suppression test, 427
Tsutsugamushi fever, 614
Tube
  dilution method, *Brucella*, 587
  tests
    for Rh factor, 245
    VDRL, 661-663
Tubeless gastric analysis, 443
Tubercle bacilli
  acid-fast, staining, 594-595
  concentration methods and handling of speci-
    mens, 591-595
  decontamination methods, 592-593
  in sputum, 591, 594

Tuberculosis
  isoniazid in, 702
  laboratory diagnosis, 591-600
  para-aminosalicylic acid in, 701
  sputum in, 524
Tubular
  absorption, 65
  function, tests for, 65
  reabsorbed phosphate (TRP), 333
Türk
  cells, 148, 149
  diluting fluid, 116
Tularemia, 580
Tumor cells in peripheral blood, 154
Turbidity tests in liver disease, 363, 364
Turkel needle, bone marrow specimen, 202
Turner's syndrome, 142
Typhoid fever, culture, 577
Typhus, epidemic, 613
Typing, blood
  ABO, 236-241
  blood groups and, 232-258
Tyrosine
  crystals, 55
  test for, 56
L-Tyrosine and xanthine, decomposition of,
    Nocardia, 602
Tyrosinuria, 26

U

UCG titration test for pregnancy, 92, 93
Ultracentrifuge method of estimating lipopro-
    teins, 380
Ultraviolet radiation, sterilization by, 531
Undulant fever (brucellosis), 585-587
Universal donor, 261-262
Unstained bacteria, examination of, 537
Uranium nitrate solution, 711
Urea
  clearance, 64, 65, 66
  determination, 308-310
  tests for, 13
Urease
  method, blood urea nitrogen determination,
    309, 310
  test
    Cryptococcus, 639
    Proteus, 568
    Pseudomonas, 570
Uric acid
  in blood, determination of, 313-314
  crystals, 51
Uricase for uric acid determination, 313
Urinalysis, 11-84; *see also* Urine
  quantitative, 58
Urinary
  amylase, 447
  calculi, 66-71
  hormones
    and metabolites, 71-84
    table of normal values, 726
  reducing substances, differentiation, 27
  sediment, 46-58
  tract cultures, organisms isolated from, 537
Urine
  acetone bodies in, tests for, 34-35

Urine—cont'd
  Addis count, 56-57
  alcohol in, determination of, 686
  amino acid nitrogen in, 318, 319
  amino acids in, tests for, 21-23
  amount, 13
  ascorbic acid in, 429
  bile in, tests, 35-38
  blood in, tests, 38-40
  calcium in, determination, 330, 331
  casts in, 47, 48
  chemical examination, 18-46
  chloride in, determination, 341, 342
  clouding, 15
  collection and handling of specimen, 534
  color, 14-15
  copper in, 337-338
  creatine and creatinine in, 315, 316
  crystalline and amorphous sediment in, 51, 52
  crystals in, 51-56
  erythrocytes in, 47
  examination
    in hemolytic anemias, toxic, 184
    in lupus erythematosus, 193
  extraneous structures in, 56
  hippuric acid in, tests, 366-367
  hydrogen ion concentration, 15-16
  intestinal parasites in, examination, 462
  lead in, method of determination, 693-694
  leukocytes in, significance, 47
  magnesium in, 334
  mercury in, method of determination, 695
  microscopic examination, 46-56
  morphine in, method of determination, 700
  odor, 14
  osmolality, 354
    and freezing point determination, 17-18
  para-aminosalicylic acid in, determination, 701-702
  phenol derivatives in, 46
  phenothiazine compounds in, test for, 704
  phosphates in, determination, 332
  physical examination of, 13-18
  in pregnancy, 89
  pregnancy tests, 89-94
  presence of, tests for, 12-13
  protein in, determination, 323
  removing protein from, 20
  residual, 14
  salicylates in, determination, 703-704
  screening tests for bacteria, 535
  sodium in, 339
  specific gravity and refractive index, 16-17
  specimens
    collection, 11
    preservation, 12
  sugar in, paper chromatography in identification of, 28-29
  sugar reducing substances in, tests for, 26-33
  sulfonamide crystals in, 51, 53, 54, 55
  sulfonamides in
    determination, 699-700
    qualitative analysis, 57
  tests
    in hemolytic anemia, 166
    for protein, 18-21

Urine—cont'd
  three-glass test, 40
  total solids, 17
  transparency and turbidity, 15
  tubercle bacilli in, 591-592
  urea nitrogen in, determination, 309-310
  uric acid in, determination, 314
  urobilinogen in, procedure, 361
Urinometer, 17
Urobilin
  test for, 36-37
  and urobilinogen, fecal, test for, 453-454
Urobilinogen
  excretion, 356
  in stool, conditions causing increase and decrease, 454
  in urine
    and feces, tests, 360-362
    tests for, 37
Urolithiasis, 66
Uroporphyrin, 40, 41, 42, 43, 44

V

Vaccine, bacterial, 546
Vaccinia virus, 625
Vacutainers, 284
Vagina, flora normally present in, 529
Vaginal cytology in pregnancy, 89
Valley fever, 643
Van Gieson stain for collagen, 710
Van Handel and Zilversmit, micromethod of determination of serum triglycerides, 378-380
Van Slyke apparatus
  carbon dioxide content and combining power determination, 347
  gasometric analysis by, 344-346
  oxygen content and capacity determination, 350-352
Van Slyke-Neill pipette, 344, 345
Vanillyl mandelic acid (VMA), 81-83
Varicella-herpes zoster virus, 625-626
Variola virus, 625
Varney phosphorus jar, 541
Vascular
  defects, hemorrhagic diseases due to, 224
  fragility, increased, 224
  function, tests for, 209-210
VDRL
  slide
    flocculation tests with serum, 656-659
    qualitative test with serum, 659
    quantitative tests with serum, 659-661
  tests with spinal fluid, 663-664
  tube
    flocculation tests with serum, 661-662
    qualitative and quantitative tests with serum, 662
Venous blood, obtaining specimens, 97, 284
Verhoeff elastic tissue stain, 713
Veronal buffer, 434, 435
Vibrio, 608-609
Vincent's angina, 588
Virocytes, 148, 188
Virology methods, 615-620
  microbiology with reference to, 526-626

Virulence
  of *Pasteurella pestis,* 579
  tests, *Corynebacterium diphtheriae,* 590
Virus
  diseases
    classification, 615-616
    diagnostic tests, table, 617
    groups, selected, 620-626
Viruses
  characteristics, composition, and classification,
    615-616
  isolation methods, 616, 618, 619
  laboratory diagnosis, 616
Visual colorimeter, 286
Vitamin A and carotene determination, 427-429
Vitamin B$_6$-deficiency anemia, 159
Vitamin B$_{12}$
  deficiency, detection of, 157
  and pernicious anemia, 155, 157
Vitamin C deficiency, 224
Vitamin K
  in formation of clotting factors, 217, 218
  tolerance test in liver disease, 369
Voges-Proskauer reaction, 566
Volemetron method, blood volume determina-
    tion, 109
Vomiting of pregnancy, 89
von Willebrand's disease, 225, 226

W

Water bath in coagulation procedures, 5
Waterhouse-Friderichsen syndrome, 224
Watson, fecal urobilin and urobilinogen screen-
    ing procedures, 453-454
Watson-Schwartz test for porphobilinogen, 44-45
Wayson
  stain for bipolar staining, *Pasteurella pestis,*
    579
  technique of skin scraping, leprosy diagnosis,
    601
Weigert iron hematoxylin solutions, 710
Weights, atomic, 434, 435
Weil-Felix reaction, rickettsiae, 614-615
Weil's disease, 612
Wet preparation
  Blastomyces, 641
  Candida, 635
  Cryptococcus neoformans, 638
  examination of bacteria, 537
  fungi, 635
Wet-ash method
  thyroxine by column chromatography, 423
  of Zak, protein-bound iodine separation, 417
Whipworm, 479
White blood cells; *see also* Leukocytes
  absolute count, 130
  antibodies (leukoagglutinins), 273
  in cerebrospinal fluid, count, 512-513
  count, 116-121
    total, estimation from stained blood smear, 6
  morphology, 140-154
  pathology, 187-202

White blood cells—cont'd
  in serous fluids, count, 508-509
  in sputum, 522, 524
  synovial fluid, 517
Whooping cough, 581
Widal reaction, *Salmonella,* 577
Wiener's nomenclature and theory of multiple
    alleles, 242
Wilder reticulum stain for connective tissue, 711-
    712
Wilson's disease, 24
  serum copper levels in, 338
Wintrobe
  macrohematocrit method, 106
  sedimentation rate, 108
Witebsky substance, 262
Wöllner enzyme test II, modified, for mono-
    nucleosis, 191
Wong, iron content method of, 100-101
Wood fiber test for sulfonamides in urine, 57
Woolsorter's disease, 604
Work area, surgical specimens, 705
Worms, 470-494
Wort agar, neutral, for fungi, 634
Wound
  cultures, organisms isolated from, 537
  infections, clostridia in, 605
Wright
  buffer stain for rickettsiae, 720
  stain, 125
    for pus, 525
Wuchereria bancrofti, 488, 489

X

Xanthine and L-tyrosine, decomposition, *No-
    cardia,* 602
Xanthochromia, cerebrospinal fluid, 511
Xenopus laevis, frog test for pregnancy, 91
X-ray film method for feces, 454
D-Xylose excretion test of fecal fat, 456-457

Y

Yaws, 611
Yeast
  cells, 637
  phase, *Histoplasma capsulatum,* 640, 641
  in urine, 48
Yeastlike fungi, 635-640

Z

Zak method of iodine separation, 417-420
Zeiss-Winkel hand spectroscope, 101
Zenker fluid, tissue fixative, 706
Ziehl-Neelsen staining method, tubercle bacilli,
    594-595
Zinc sulfate
  centrifugal flotation, intestinal parasites in
    feces, 459-460
  turbidity test, 364